Standards of Psychiatric and Mental Health Nursing Practice

"Standards of Care" pertain to professional nursing activities that are demonstrated by the nurse through the nursing process. These involve assessment, diagnosis, outcome identification, planning, implementation, and evaluation. The nursing process is the foundation of clinical decision making and encompasses all significant action taken by nurses in providing developmentally and culturally relevant psychiatric mental health care to all patients.

STANDARD I. ASSESSMENT

The psychiatric-mental health nurse collects patient health data.

Rationale

The assessment interview, which requires linguistically and culturally effective communication skills, interviewing, behavioral observation, record review, and comprehensive assessment of the patient and relevant systems, enables the psychiatric-mental health nurse to make sound clinical judgments and plan appropriate interventions with the patient.

STANDARD II. DIAGNOSIS

The psychiatric-mental health nurse analyzes the assessment data in determining diagnoses.

Rationale

The basis for providing psychiatric mental health nursing care is the recognition and identification of patterns of response to actual or potential psychiatric illnesses, mental health problems, and potential comorbid physical illnesses.

STANDARD III. OUTCOME IDENTIFICATION

The psychiatric-mental health nurse identifies expected outcomes individualized to the patient.

Rationale

Within the context of providing nursing care, the ultimate goal is to influence mental health outcomes and improve the patient's health status.

STANDARD IV. PLANNING

The psychiatric-mental health nurse develops a plan of care that is negotiated among the patient, nurse, family, and health care team and prescribes evidence-based interventions to attain expected outcomes.

Rationale

A plan of care is used to guide therapeutic interventions systematically, document progress, and achieve the expected patient outcomes.

STANDARD V. IMPLEMENTATION

The psychiatric-mental health nurse implements the interventions identified in the plan of care.

Rationale

In implementing the plan of care, psychiatric-mental health nurses use a wide range of interventions designed to prevent mental and physical illness, and promote, maintain, and restore mental and physical health. Psychiatric-mental health nurses select interventions according to their level of practice. At the basic level, nurses may select counseling milieu therapy, promotion of self-care activities, intake screening and evaluation, psychobiological interventions, health teaching, case management, health promotion and health maintenance, crisis intervention, community-based care, psychiatric home health care, telehealth, and a variety of other approaches to meet the mental health needs of patients. In addition to the intervention options available to the basic-level psychiatric-mental health nurse, at the advanced level the APRN-PMH may provide consultation, engage in psychotherapy, and prescribe pharmacological agents in accordance with state statutes or regulations.

Standard Va. Counseling
Standard Vb. Milieu Therapy
Standard Vc. Promotion of Self-Care Activities
Standard Vd. Psychobiological Interventions
Standard Ve. Health Teaching
Standard Vf. Case Management
Standard Vg. Health Promotion and Health Maintenance
The following interventions (Vh–Vj) may be performed only by the APRN-PMH.
ADVANCED PRACTICE INTERVENTIONS Vh–Vj
Standard Vh. Psychotherapy
Standard Vi. Prescriptive Authority and Treatment
Standard Vj. Consultation

STANDARD VI. EVALUATION

The psychiatric-mental health nurse evaluates the patient's progress in attaining expected outcomes.

Rationale

Nursing care is a dynamic process involving change in the patient's health status over time, giving rise to the need for data, different diagnoses, and modifications in the plan of care. Therefore, evaluation is a continuous process of appraising the effect of nursing and the treatment regimen on the patient's health status and expected outcomes.

Reprinted with permission from American Nurses Association, Statement on the Scope and Standards of Psychiatric-Mental Health Nursing Practice, ©2000, American Nurses Publishing, Washington, D.C.

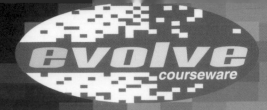

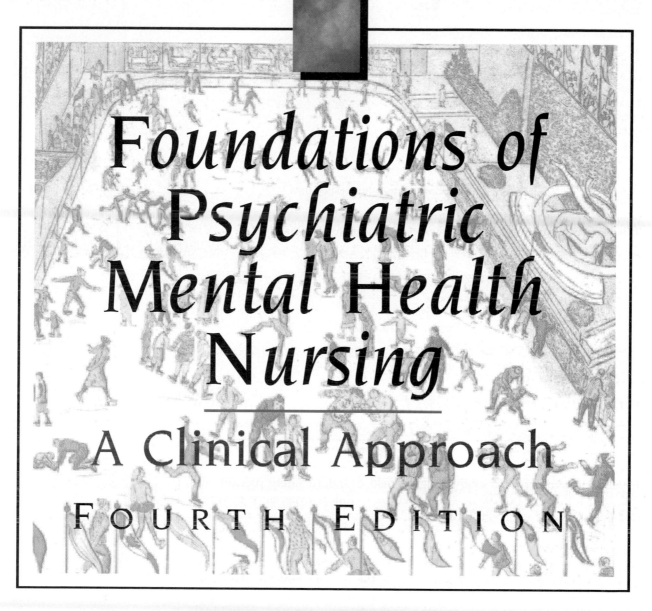

Foundations of Psychiatric Mental Health Nursing

A Clinical Approach

FOURTH EDITION

Elizabeth M. Varcarolis, RN, MA

Professor Emeritus
Formerly Deputy Chairperson, Department of Nursing
Borough of Manhattan Community College
New York, New York

Associate Fellow
Albert Ellis Institute for Rational
Emotive Behavioral Therapy (REBT)
New York, New York

Unit photographs by Steven Mark Leopold

SAUNDERS
An Imprint of Elsevier

SAUNDERS
An Imprint of Elsevier

The Curtis Center
Independence Square West
Philadelphia, Pennsylvania 19106

Vice President, Publishing Director: Sally Schrefer
Senior Editor: Terri Wood
Senior Developmental Editor: Robin Levin Richman
Project Manager: Frank Polizzano
Copy Editing Supervisor: Marian A. Bellus
Production Manager: Guy Barber
Illustration Specialist: Bob Quinn
Senior Book Designer: Ellen B. Zanolle

Library of Congress Cataloging-in-Publication Data

Varcarolis, Elizabeth M.
Foundations of psychiatric mental health nursing: a clinical approach / Elizabeth M.
Varcarolis.—4th ed.

p. ; cm.

Includes bibliographical references and index.

ISBN 0-7216-8896-9

1. Psychiatric nursing.   I. Title.
   [DNLM: 1. Mental Disorders—nursing.   2. Psychiatric Nursing.
   WY   160 V278f 2002]

RC440 .F58 2002 610.73'68—dc21   2001020320

NOTICE

Psychiatric nursing is an ever-changing field. Standard safety precautions must be followed, but as new research and clinical experience broaden our knowledge, changes in treatment and drug therapy become necessary or appropriate. Readers are advised to check the most current product information provided by the manufacturer of each drug to be administered to verify the recommended dose, the method and duration of administration, and contraindications. It is the responsibility of the treating licensed prescriber, relying on experience and knowledge of the patient, to determine dosages and the best treatment for each individual patient. Neither the publisher nor the editor assumes any responsibility for any injury and/or damage to persons or property arising from this publication.

THE PUBLISHER

To the memory of
Josiah and Ruth Merrill
to whom I owe so much and think of every day

Always to my husband
Paul
My partner, lover, best friend, and life companion;
your love and devotion mean everything to me

To the memory of important people in my life recently absent;
they will
always have a place in my heart:
Gary Greenwald—long time friend and "Dutch Uncle"
John Payne—supportive colleague and sharer of laughter
Shirley Wiley Denning   A lifelong cheerful and happy presence
Joannie Duell—A caring, spirited, and mischievous new friend in Arizona

Acknowledgments

I owe a great deal to many for their support and contributions to this text.

- Always first, I express my gratitude to the authors who have either written new chapters for this edition or have updated previous chapters, keeping the material current and relevant. I have been fortunate to work with professionals who brought their clinical expertise, knowledge, and clarity of thought to the readers of this text.
- My thanks to authors of the third edition, whose influence on the content and completeness of this text is still apparent: Thomas Wenzka, Susan Mejo, Jeannemarie Baker, Helene S. (Kay) Charron, Francesca Profiri, Peggy Miller, Anne Cowley Herzog, Michelle Conant Dan-El, and Carla E. Randall.
- Special thanks to Kay Charron for her creative work on the Instructors Electronic Resource, and her contribution of the multiple choice questions found both at the end of chapters and on the Evolve website.
- To my typist, Patty Romo, who has been with me through all four editions. She reads my mind and my handwriting (no mean feat), and rarely misses a beat. She is to be congratulated for her patience and expertise.
- To Steven Leopold, who worked hard and well to supply the unit opening photographs. I am so happy to have him with me for this edition . . . what an artful job.
- I am so proud and excited to have the work of Aida Whedon on this edition's cover. Aida was always a caring, enthusiastic supporter and teacher and later, friend, from first grade onward. She is part of my memory of very special people who greatly influenced my childhood and thus my whole life. I thank her son, Tony, for permission to use this picture.
- Many kudos go the staff at W.B. Saunders who helped to plan, develop, and make comprehensible reams of unending manuscript pages.

  To Terri Wood, Senior Editor, who shared in the vision for the fourth edition. Terri supplied vast amounts of reference material, worked hard to make this fourth edition an artistically appealing and unique text, and provided useful feedback from the "field." Thank you.

  To Robin Levin Richman, Senior Developmental Editor, who labored hand-in-glove with me through the minutia of galleys, pages, and manuscript dilemmas. Her influence is seen in the clarity, continuity, and smoothness evident throughout the text. Thank you.

  To Cathy Ott, Senior Editorial Assistant, whose responsive presence at the other end of the phone took care of many questions and concerns faster than immediately. Thank you.

  To the editorial staff, including senior copy editor Marian Bellus, who corrected and queried obsessively in order to make this text as error-free as possible. Thank you.

  To the designer, Ellen B. Zanolle, who did a magnificent job designing the book and the production staff who set the pages so they are appealing and inviting as well as easy to read. Thank you.

- A huge debt of gratitude goes to the educators and clinicians who reviewed the manuscript pages and offered valuable suggestions, ideas, opinions, criticisms, and contributions. All were welcomed and greatly helped refine and strengthen the individual chapters. I thank you all.

Sharon Y. Baron, MSN, RN, CS, CGP
Private Practice
The Wellness Community of Philadelphia
Havertown, Pennsylvania

Karen Ann Benson, PhD, ARNP
Seattle University
Seattle, Washington

L. Lee Boyles, MS, RN, LCDC
Neosho Community College
Ottawa, Kansas

Vicki Wecas Britt, MSN, RN, CS
Private Practice
Johnstown, Pennsylvania
University of Pittsburgh
Pittsburgh, Pennsylvania

Lydia Ann DeSantis, PhD, MNEd, MPh, MA, RN, CTN
University of Miami
Coral Gables, Florida

Lurelean B. Gaines, MSN, RN
East Los Angeles College
349th Gen Hospital USAR
Los Angeles, California

Benita W. Harris, PhD, MSN, RN
Delaware Technical and Community College
Georgetown, Delaware

Coleen Heckner, MS, RN, CS-P
Private Practice
Baltimore, Maryland

Kathleen Ibrahim, MA, RN, CS
New York State Psychiatric Institute
New York, New York

Susan L. Jones, PhD, RN
Kent State University
Kent, Ohio

Nancy Lisbeth Kostin, MSN, RN
Madonna University
Livonia, Michigan

Susan Jane Lewis, PhD, ARNP, CS
Department of Veterans Affairs Medical Center
Louisville, Kentucky

Charlotte Lorentson, MSN, RN, CS, BC
Eastern State Hospital
Williamsburg, Virginia

Yvonne Lovett, MSN, RN
Wayne County Community College
Detroit, Michigan

Marc S. Micozzi, PhD, MD
College of Physicians
University of Pennsylvania
Philadelphia, Pennsylvania

Pamela J. Nelson, MS, BSN, RN
Bethel College
St. Paul, Minnesota

Netha Burnaman O'Meara, MSN, BS, RN, CNS
Educational Consultant
Houston, Texas

Susan M. O'Toole, MSN, RN, CS
Allegheny General Hospital
Pittsburgh, Pennsylvania

Terri Pensabene, PhD, RN
University of Texas at Arlington
Arlington, Texas

Eris J. Perese, MS, RN
University of Buffalo
Buffalo, New York

Anne W. Ryan, MSN, RN, C, MPH
Chesapeake College
Wye Mills, Maryland

Jana C. Saunders, PhD, RN, CS
Medical College of Georgia
Athens, Georgia

Willa Y. Taite Sawyer, BSN, RN
Memphis Mental Health Institute
Memphis, Tennessee

Marie Smith, MA, RN, CS
Bronx Community College
Private Practice
New York, New York

Martha J. Thie, EdD, MSN, RN
University of Indianapolis
Indianapolis, Indiana

Dorothy A. Varchol, MSN, MA, RN, C
Cincinnati State Technical and Community College
Cincinnati, Ohio

Jeanne Venhaus Stein, MSN, RN
St. Louis Community College at Meramec
St. Louis, Missouri

Contributors

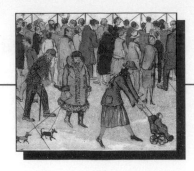

CARROL ALVAREZ, MS, BS, CS

Clinical Faculty, University of Washington, Seattle, Washington
Chapter 24: Anger and Aggression

PENNY S. BROOKE, MS, JD, APRN

Professor/Coordinator of Service-Learning, University of Utah College of Nursing, Salt Lake City, Utah
Chapter 8: Legal and Ethical Guidelines for Safe Practice

SUSAN CAVERLY, CS, ARNP

Clinical Instructor/Researcher, Department of Psychosocial and Community Health, School of Nursing, University of Washington, Seattle, Washington
Chapter 6: Mental Health Nursing in Community Settings

PATRICIA A. CLAYBROOK, MA

Clinical Instructor in Psychology, Mount St. Mary's College, Los Angeles, California
Unit VI: A Nurse Speaks

CHERRILL W. COLSON, MA, CS, EDD

Assistant Professor, Department of Nursing, Hostos Community College, City University of New York, Bronx; Clinical Specialist, Leake and Watts Children's Services, Yonkers, New York
Chapter 31: Disorders of Children and Adolescents

MARYANN FELDSTEIN, EDD, RN, CS

Former Director, Graduate Program in Psychiatric Mental Health Nursing, Columbia University School of Nursing; Private Practice, Individual and Family Therapy, New York, New York
Unit VIII: A Nurse Speaks

SALLY K. HOLZAPFEL, MSN, RN, CETN, CGNP

Clinical Assistant Professor, University of Medicine and Dentistry of New Jersey, Newark; Geriatric, Wound, Ostomy, and Continence Nurse Practitioner, Department of Veterans Affairs, New Jersey Health Care System, Lyons, New Jersey
Chapter 33: Psychosocial Needs of the Older Adult

KATHLEEN IBRAHIM, MA, CS

Assistant to Director of Nursing for Staff Development, New York State Psychiatric Institute, New York, New York
Chapter 17: People With Eating Disorders

KATHY A. KRAMER-HOWE, MA, MSW

Member NASW, Member National Council of Hospice Professionals, Paradise Valley, California
Chapter 30: Care for the Dying and for Those Who Grieve
Unit VII: A Social Worker Speaks

GLORIA KUHLMAN, DNSC, RN

Professor and Assistant Director of Nursing, Ohlone College, Fremont, California; Clinical Nurse Specialist, Veterans Administration Medical Center, Palo Alto, California
Chapter 32: Adults Requiring Specialized Interventions
Chapter 36: Alternative and Complementary Therapies and Practices

CATHERINE M. LALA, MSN, NP-P, RN, C

Adjunct Clinical Instructor, Psychiatric Nursing, New York University, New York; Nurse Practitioner in Psychiatry, Metropolitan Center for Mental Health, and Advanced Practice Nurse, St. Clare's Behavioral Health Center, Denville, New Jersey, and Mental Health Clinic of Passaic, Passaic, New Jersey
Chapter 34: Therapeutic Groups
Unit II: A Nurse Speaks

MARY LESNIAK, MS, RN, C

Director, Behavioral Health Services, Gnaden Huetten Memorial Hospital, Lehighton, Pennsylvania
Unit V: A Nurse Speaks

LOUISE MODIR, MA, RN, C

Adjunct Faculty, Regis University School for Professional Studies, Denver, Colorado; Clinical Psychiatric Nurse, Psychiatric Services, Rockford Memorial Hospital, Rockford, Illinois
Unit VII: A Nurse Speaks

ELORA AFICIONADO ORCAJADA, MSN, RN, CS, CASAC

Assistant Professor, Borough of Manhattan Community College, New York, New York
Unit III: A Nurse Speaks

JOHN A. PAYNE, MA, BS (Deceased)

Assistant Professor of Nursing, Borough of Manhattan Community College; Supervisor/Director of Nursing, Director of Nursing/Senior Management Consultant for Longterm Care and Psychiatry; Harlem Hospital Center, New York, New York
Unit I: A Nurse Speaks

JOHN RAYNOR, PHD

Professor, Borough of Manhattan Community College, City University of New York, New York, New York
Chapter 3: Biological Basis for Understanding Psychotropic Drugs

DENISE SAINT ARNAULT, PHD

Assistant Professor of Nursing, Adjunct Faculty in Anthropology, Core Faculty Asian Studies, Michigan State University, East Lansing, Michigan
Chapter 7: Culturally Relevant Mental Health Nursing

SHARON SHISLER, RN, CS

Clinical Nurse Specialist—Mental Health; Psychiatric Liaison, Greenwich Hospital; Group Therapist, Greenwich AIDS Alliance, White Plains Day Care Center, Greenwich, Connecticut
Unit IV: A Nurse Speaks

KATHLEEN SMITH-DiJULIO, MA, BSN

Lecturer, University of Washington, Seattle, Washington
Chapter 25: Family Violence
Chapter 26: Sexual Assault
Chapter 27: Care of the Chemically Impaired

MARGARET SWISHER, MSN, RN

Assistant Professor of Nursing, Montgomery County Community College, Blue Bell, Pennsylvania
Chapter 5: Mental Health Nursing in Acute Care Settings

JULIUS TRUBOWITZ, EDD

Assistant Professor, Queens College, City University of New York, Flushing, New York
Chapter 2: Relevant Theories and Therapies for Nursing Practice

ELIZABETH M. VARCAROLIS, MA, RN

Professor Emeritus, Formerly Deputy Chairperson, Department of Nursing, Borough of Manhattan Community College, New York, New York; Associate Fellow, Albert Ellis Institute for Rational Emotive Behavioral Therapy (REBT) New York, New York
Chapter 1: Mental Health and Mental Illness; Chapter 4: Psychiatric Mental Health Nursing and Managed Care Issues; Chapter 9: Assessment Strategies and the Nursing Process; Chapter 10: Developing Therapeutic Relationships; Chapter 11: The Clinical Interview and Communication Skills; Chapter 12: Understanding Stress and Holistic Approaches to Stress; Chapter 13: Understanding Anxiety and Anxiety Defenses; Chapter 14: Anxiety Disorders; Chapter 15: Somatoform and Dissociative Disorders; Chapter 16: Personality Disorders; Chapter 18: Mood Disorders: Depression; Chapter 19: Mood Disorders: Bipolar; Chapter 20: Schizophrenia and Other Psychotic Disorders; Chapter 21: Cognitive Disorders; Chapter 22: Crisis; Chapter 23: Suicide; Chapter 28: Severe Mental Illness: Crisis Stabilization and Rehabilitation; Chapter 29: Psychological Needs of the Medically Ill; Chapter 30: Care for the Dying and for Those Who Grieve; Chapter 35: Family Therapy

MARIKEN E. WOGSTAD-HANSEN, PHD, MA, LP, RN, CNS

Clinical Specialist, Adult Psychiatric and Mental Health Nursing; Licensed Psychologist; Independent Contractor, Chrysalis Mental Health Clinic, Chrysalis, A Center for Women, Minneapolis, Minnesota
Unit IX: A Nurse Speaks

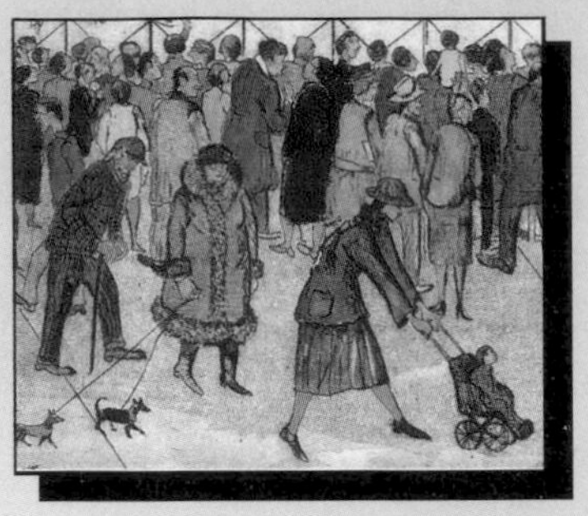

To the Student

Psychiatric nursing challenges us to understand human behavior. In the chapters that follow you will learn about people with psychiatric disorders and how to provide them with quality nursing care. As you read, keep in mind these special features.

A Nurse Speaks

provides personal stories of individual nurses in various practice settings

A Nurse Speaks

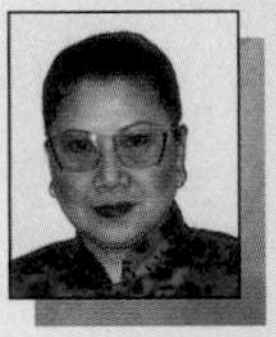

ELORA AFICIONADO ORCAJADA

I went to nursing school to become a nurse. It never dawned on me to become a teacher; nursing and teaching were two different things, I thought. Even a Master's degree at Columbia University did not fan the fires of teaching in me. I knew I was a nurse, a real dedicated nurse. I was, still am.

Right after nursing school, I was hired as a clinical instructor at the hospital I trained at. At that time a lot of medical doctors taught at the nursing school, and we worked, hand in hand with them. I believed I was equipped with the necessary skills and knowledge and I passed these to the next batch of Florence Nightingales, who not only equated nursing as a respectable profession but also primarily shared Florence's genuine concern for the infirm. Teaching and nursing grew simultaneously in me. They became synonymous in the practice of my profession when I started teaching at a community college, and I realized I had the passion and joy of teaching. Seeing our students metamorphose from being shy and passive to responsible and professional nurses became a source of pride and fulfillment. Years of working in different roles and different settings served as my solid groundwork for my vast knowledge and experience.

As teachers, how do we hone and whet the blunt blades of student nurses who come into our fold? How do we transform a tiny and ordinary pebble into a beautiful and expensive pearl but through constant and rigid friction?

Students enrolled in the Associate Degree Nursing Program never fail to amaze me. A small percentage of them are young but most of them are older, mature, working, and have families to take care of while they take the step to upgrade themselves.

Lena is a working mother with a teenage daughter and an 80-year-old father who although is still alert and independent is now showing signs of aging. Lena stated that being a nurse will allow her to take care of her loved ones and herself when illness affect the family. She claimed her knowledge will help her better understand those afflicted with diseases.

Mimi, a single mother of a 2-year-old son, stated that she is doing a payback to the nurses who took good care of her ill child in the hospital. She observed how these nurses were so committed in helping her son return to health.

Fe has chosen nursing as a profession because of the "ideal figure" she saw in the hospital and can never forget who was holding her grandmother's hand until she gasped her last breath on this earth.

Some go back to school with goal of nursing as a second profession or the fulfillment of a dream that was set aside for various reasons. A big percentage of the population are minorities, struggling to make a productive contribution while taking care of their own needs and their families' future in an increasingly productive multicultural society.

During the orientation program, student's handbooks or handouts are distributed. We make them aware of the college's expectations, requirements, rules and routine, etc.

Felnor, a working woman in her mid twenties and an A student in her preclinical courses, experienced a shocking revelation when she reached the clinical stage of nursing. She was astonished that she barely made a B in her first semester course. However, she had the desire to improve her grades; she came to me for advice. She was able to figure out that she has to improve her study habits and possibly request a change of shift and off days from her work. She learned to structure her time, set priorities in terms of short- and long-term goals. She graduated with honors.

Our practice of meeting each student individually on a one-to-one initial interview makes us aware of their problems and needs as well as their strengths, which we tap in several ways. We reiterate our expectations and ask them what they expect from us in return. Again, we internalize the value of self-discipline and perseverance. We also emphasize the importance of skill and safe practice in the care of clients.

Cultural diversity of our students can work to their

194

Vignettes

describe and individualize clients with specific psychiatric disorders

558 UNIT 5 ■ Psychobiological Disorders: Severe to Psychotic

Vignette

■ *Tom is a 37-year-old man who is currently an inpatient at the Veterans Administration Hospital. He has been separated from his wife and four children for 6 years. His medical records state that because of his illness (which Tom describes as "hearing voices a lot"), he has been in and out of hospitals for 17 years. Tom is an ex-Marine who first "heard voices" at the age of 19, while he was stationed in Okinawa; he subsequently received a medical discharge.*

The hospitalization was precipitated by an exacerbation of auditory hallucinations. "I thought people were following me. I hear voices, usually a woman's voice, and she's tormenting me. People say that it happens because I don't take my medications. The medications make me tired and I can't have sex." Tom also admits to using cocaine and marijuana. He is aware that marijuana and cocaine increase his paranoia and that taking drugs usually precedes hospitalization but says that "they make me feel good." Tom finished 11 years of school but did not graduate from high school. He says that he has no close friends. He was in prison for 5 years for manslaughter and told the nurse, "I was in prison because I did something bad." He was abusing alcohol and drugs at the time, and drug abuse has been related to each subsequent hospitalization.

Ms. Lally is Tom's primary nurse. When Tom meets the nurse, he is dressed in pajamas and bathrobe. His hygiene is good and he is well nourished. He tells the nurse that he does not sleep much because "the voices get worse at night." Ms. Lally notes in Tom's medical record that he has had two episodes of suicidal ideation. During those times, the voices were telling him to jump "off rooftops" and "in front of trains."

During the first interview, Tom only occasionally makes eye contact and speaks in a low monotone. At times, he glances about the room as if distracted, mumbles to himself, and appears upset.

Nurse: Tom, my name is Ms. Lally. I will be your nurse while you're in the hospital. We will meet every day for 30 minutes at 10 AM. During that time, we can discuss areas of concern to you.

Tom: Well . . . don't believe what they say about me. I want to start a new . . . Are you married?

Nurse: This time is for you to talk about *your* concerns.

Tom: Oh . . . *(Looks furtively around the room, then lowers his eyes.)* Someone is trying to kill me, I think . . .

Nurse: You appear to be focusing on something other than our conversation.

Tom: The voices tell me things . . . I can't say . . .

Nurse: I don't hear any voices except yours and mine. I am going to stay with you. Tell me what is happening and I will try to help you.

Tom: The voices tell me bad things.

Ms. Lally stays with Tom and encourages him to communicate with her. As Tom focuses more on the nurse, his anxiety appears to lessen. His thoughts become more connected, he is able to concentrate more on what the nurse is saying, and he mumbles less to himself.

The full nursing care plan for Tom is found at the end of this chapter.

Catatonia: Withdrawn Phase

The essential feature of catatonia is abnormal motor behavior. Two extreme motor behaviors are seen in clients with catatonia: extreme motor agitation and extreme psychomotor retardation (with mutism, even stupor). Other behaviors identified with catatonia include posturing, waxy flexibility, stereotyped behavior, extreme negativism or automatic obedience, echolalia, and echopraxia. The onset of catatonia is usually abrupt and the prognosis favorable. With chemotherapy and improved individual management, severe catatonic symptoms are rarely seen today. Useful nursing strategies are discussed in the following sections.

COMMUNICATION GUIDELINES

Clients in the withdrawn phase of catatonia can be so withdrawn that they appear comatose. They can be mute and may remain so for hours, days, or even weeks or months if they are not treated with antipsychotic medication. Although such clients may not appear to pay attention to events going on around them, the client is acutely aware of the environment and may remember events accurately at a later date. A withdrawn client has special needs, and the nurse can use the following guidelines. Developing skill and confidence in working with withdrawn clients takes practice. Refer to your communication card for guidelines on communicating with a withdrawn client.

SELF-CARE NEEDS

When a client is extremely withdrawn, physical needs take priority. A client may need to be hand fed or tube fed for adequate nutritional status to be maintained. Normal control over bladder and bowel functions can be interrupted. Assessment of urinary or bowel retention must be made and acted on when found. Incontinence of urine and feces may cause skin breakdown and infection. Because physical movements may be minimal or absent, range-of-motion exercises need to be carried out to prevent

Assessment Guidelines

at the end of each Assessment section in the nursing process part of clinical chapters provide summary points for client assessment

380 UNIT IV ■ Psychobiological Disorders: Moderate to Severe

Box 16–2 Nursing Assessment Guide for People with Personality Disorders

- What is the presenting problem according to the client? What is it according to others (e.g., family, employer, police)?
- Who has identified and defined the problem?
- What is the client's emotional state? Is the client:
  - Suspicious
  - Anxious
  - Experiencing helplessness
  - Expressing boredom
  - Unconcerned
  - Lacking in empathy
  - Lacking remorse for hurting others
  - Suffering from low self-esteem
- What particular circumstances or stress precipitated the behavior?
- How is the client handling the problem? How has the client handled problems in the past?
- Is the client suicidal? Self-mutilating?
- How would the client like to see the problem resolved?
- Does the client have any meaningful or lasting relationships? Friends, lovers, family?
- What is the client's developmental history?
- Is the client employed? What is the pattern of employment?
- How does the behavior affect the job or role functioning?
- What is the client's physical condition and status?
- What behaviors or defenses does the client exhibit?
  - Manipulation

Assessment Guidelines

PERSONALITY DISORDERS

1. Does client have a medical disorder or another psychiatric disorder that may be responsible for symptoms?
2. Assess for suicidal or homicidal thoughts—if yes, will need immediate attention.
3. Assessment about personality functioning needs to be viewed within the person's ethnic, cultural, and social background.
4. Personality disorders are often exacerbated following the loss of significant supporting people or in a disruptive social situation.
5. A change in personality in middle adulthood or later signals the need for a thorough medical work-up or assessment for unrecognized substance abuse disorder.

Cluster A Disorders (Odd, Eccentric)

Figure 16–2 shows the DSM-IV-TR criteria for cluster A disorders.

PARANOID PERSONALITY DISORDER

Individuals with paranoid PD greatly fear that others will exploit, harm, or deceive them, to the point of endangering their lives. Even when no evidence exists, clients with paranoid PD interpret all experience from the perspective that they have been done irreversible damage by others; therefore, people with paranoid PD are extremely reluctant to share information about themselves. Compliments or loyalty is misread as manipulation or attempts to disempower

Research Findings

boxes in abstract format in most clinical chapters introduce you to scientific methodology and present the latest results of psychiatric studies

CHAPTER 20 ■ Schizophrenia and Other Psychotic Disorders 543

RESEARCH FINDINGS

The Use of Cognitive Therapy for Treating Delusions

Objective

To assess the effectiveness of cognitive therapy in modifying delusions in clients seen in routine clinical practice.

Methods

Eighteen clients with chronic delusions were treated using cognitive therapy, after the method of Chadwick and Lowe. A single-case multiple-baseline experimental design was used, including a control treatment. Each subject was used as his or her own control.

Results

Six clients showed a reduction in the conviction of their delusions during cognitive therapy but not during the control treatment. Seven clients did not show any change in the conviction of their delusions. Five clients showed a variable response. There was no decrease to zero in the degree of conviction for any of the clients. All of them reported that the therapy had helped them, while six said, without being asked, that they had experienced changes in psychotic thinking.

Conclusions

One third of the clients with chronic delusions who were treated in this study responded to delusion modification with a reduction in the degree of conviction in their delusions. Change within cognitive therapy sessions predicted outcome, as did change in the conviction in delusion during baseline. Finally, the goal of cognitive therapy to treat delusions should be to reduce stress as well as the degree of conviction in the delusions.

Source: Jakes, S., Rhodes, J., and Turner, T. (1999). Effectiveness of cognitive therapy for delusions in routine clinical practice. *British Journal of Psychiatry*, 175:331–335.

These measures can help the client better focus

to solve problems related to environmental

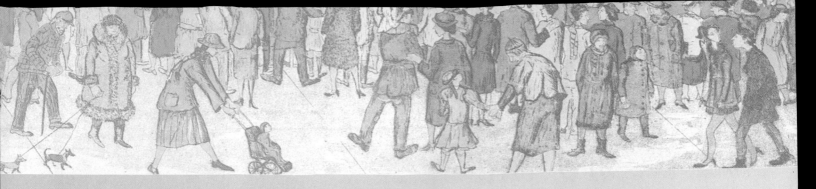

Case Studies

in clinical chapters present client histories in nursing process format

562   UNIT 5 ■ Psychobiological Disorders: Severe to Psychotic

Visit the **Evolve** website at
http://evolve.elsevier.com/Varcarolis
for more Case Studies.

CASE STUDY 20–1 *Working With a Person Who Is Paranoid*	
ASSESSMENT	This case study refers to Tom, the most frigüent in this chapter. After the initial interview, Ms. Lally divides the data into objective and subjective components.
OBJECTIVE DATA	■ Speaks in low monotone ■ Poor eye contact ■ Well nourished, adequate hygiene ■ States that he has auditory hallucinations ■ Has history of drug abuse cocaine and marijuana	■ Has no close friends ■ Was first hospitalized at age 19 and has not worked since that time ■ Has had suicidal impulses twice ■ Imprisoned 5 years for violent acting out (manslaughter) ■ Thoughts scattered when anxious
SUBJECTIVE DATA	■ "Someone is trying to kill me . . . I think." ■ "I don't take my medicine. It makes me tired and I can't have sex." ■ "The voices get worse at night, and I can't sleep." ■ Voices have told him to "jump off rooftops" and "in front of trains."	
SELF-ASSESSMENT	On the first day of admission, Tom assaults another male client, stating that the other client accused him of being a homosexual and touched him on the buttocks. After assessing the incident, the staff agrees that Tom's provocation came more from his own projections (Tom's sexual attraction to the other client) than from anything the other client did or said. Tom's difficulty with impulse control frightens Ms. Lally. She has concerns regarding Tom's impulse control and the possibility of Tom's striking out at her, especially when Tom is hallucinating and highly delusional. Ms. Lally mentions her concerns to the nursing coordinator, who suggests that Ms. Lally meet with Tom in the day room until he demonstrates more control and less suspicion of others. After 5 days, Tom is less excitable, and the sessions are held in a room set aside for client interviews. Ms. Lally also speaks with a senior staff nurse regarding her fear. By talking to the senior nurse and understanding more clearly her own fear, Ms. Lally is able to identify interventions to help Tom regain a better sense of control.	
NURSING DIAGNOSIS	Ms. Lally formulates two nursing diagnoses on the basis of her assessment data. 1. **Disturbed thought processes** related to alteration in biochemical compounds, as evidenced by persecutory hallucinations and intense suspiciousness. ■ Voices have told him to "jump off rooftops" and "in front of trains." ■ "Someone is trying to kill me, I think." ■ Abuses cocaine and marijuana, although these increase paranoia, because "it makes me feel good."	

Nursing Care Plans

in clinical chapters are often linked to the Case Studies and follow the nursing process

CHAPTER 20 ■ Schizophrenia and Other Psychotic Disorders   565

Visit the **Evolve** website at
http://evolve.elsevier.com/Varcarolis
for the other Nursing Care Plan diagnoses and for
more Nursing Care Plans.

NURSING CARE PLAN 20–1   *A Person With Paranoia: Tom*

NURSING DIAGNOSIS

Disturbed thought processes: related to alteration in biochemical compounds, as evidenced by persecutory hallucinations and intense suspiciousness.

Supporting Data

■ Voices have told him to "jump off rooftops" and "in front of trains."
■ "Someone is trying to kill me, I think."
■ Abuses cocaine and marijuana although paranoia increases: "It makes me feel good."

Outcome Criteria: Tom will state that he is able to function without interference from his "voices" by discharge.

SHORT-TERM GOAL	INTERVENTION	RATIONALE	EVALUATION
By (date), Tom will state that he feels comfortable with the nurse.	1a. Meet with Tom each day for 30 minutes. 1b. Use clear, unambiguous statements. 1c. Provide activities that need concentration and are noncompetitive.	1a. Short, consistent meetings help establish contact and decrease anxiety. 1b. Minimizes potential for misconstruing of messages. 1c. Increases time spent in reality-based activities and decreases preoccupation with delusional and hallucinatory ex-	*GOAL MET* By the end of the first week, Tom says he looks forward to meeting with "my nurse."

Visit the **Evolve** website
for pre-tests and post-tests,
more Case Studies and Nursing Care Plans,
Learning Activities, and MORE!

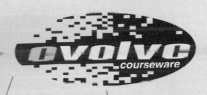

Critical Thinking and Chapter Review

at the end of each chapter provide scenario-based critical thinking problems and multiple-choice questions for study and review. Answers to the multiple-choice questions are in the IM part of the Instructor's Electronic Resource

CHAPTER 19 ■ Mood Disorders: Bipolar   519

Visit the **Evolve** website at
http://evolve.elsevier.com/Varcarolis
for additional self-study exercises.

Critical Thinking and Chapter Review

Critical Thinking

1. Donald has been taking lithium for 4 months. During his clinic visit, he tells you, his caseworker, that he does not think he will be taking his lithium anymore because he feels great and he is able to function well at his job and at home with his family. He tells you his wife agrees that "he has this thing licked."

   A. What are Donald's needs in terms of teaching?
   B. What are the needs of the family?
   C. Write out a teaching plan, or use an already constructed plan. Include these issues with sound rationales for the following teaching topics:

   ■ Use of alcohol, drugs, caffeine, over-the-counter medications
   ■ Need for sleep, hygiene
   ■ Types of community resources
   ■ Signs and symptoms of relapse

   D. Role play with a classmate how you could teach this family about bipolar illness and approach effective medication teaching, stressing the need for compliance and emphasizing those things that may threaten compliance.
   E. What referral information (websites, associations) could you give Donald and his family if they asked where they can access further information regarding this disease?

Chapter Review

Choose the **most appropriate answer.**

1. A major principle that should be observed when a nurse communicates with a client experiencing elated mood is

   1. use calm, firm approach
   2. give expanded explanations
   3. make use of abstract concepts
   4. encourage lightheartedness and joking

2. An outcome for a person in the continuation of treatment phase of bipolar disorder is

   1. client will avoid involvement in self-help groups
   2. client will adhere to medication regime
   3. client will demonstrate euphoric mood
   4. client will maintain normal weight

3. A medication teaching plan for a client receiving lithium should include

   1. rationale for lithium maintenance
   2. dietary teaching to restrict daily sodium intake
   3. importance of blood draws to monitor serum potassium level
   4. seeking medication change if side effects are troublesome

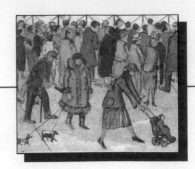

To the Instructor

AS WE SPEAK

Our lives and times are fast-paced. Medicine, neuropsychiatry, society, and our system of health care delivery continue to change with remarkable speed, taking twists and turns that are not always foreseeable. *Foundations of Psychiatric Mental Health Nursing, 4th edition,* moves forward to keep step with these changes through the addition of new information, while keeping the hallmarks of past editions.

Cultural aspects of the nurse's assessment are more critical as American society becomes even more culturally diverse, comprised of people with many different backgrounds and religious and spiritual beliefs (Chapters 7 and 9). It is now recognized through research and study that many of the alternative and complementary therapies in use by various cultures may prove beneficial for the greater population (Chapter 36). Since people often choose those practices with which they are more culturally comfortable, we are wise to include cultural health practices in our holistic assessment. Spiritual and religious beliefs and rituals may affect the body and mind in healthful ways and, when facilitated, may be a part of the healing process. Therefore, holistic approaches to client care need to include how our clients find comfort and peace in their religious or spiritual practices, so that we may support, when possible, these practices (Chapters 9 and 29).

The role of the psychiatric nurse practitioner/advanced practice nurse continues to expand. Nurses teach stress reduction techniques, work in prisons, work with clients with severe mental illness who are in crisis and in rehabilitation, care for the dying and their families, and provide and teach alternative and complementary approaches to promote health and prevent illness.

With the many changes in the health care system, including insurance companies dominating the care for many through Health Maintenance Organizations (HMOs) and Behavioral Health Maintenance Organizations (BHMOs), specific legal and ethical issues are raised. The shortage of nurses highlights the dilemma of nurses who are asked to work outside their expertise. Finally, consider a therapist who is only reimbursed by the insurance company for 15 to 20 therapy sessions for a client who has complex and long-term mental health needs. Difficult questions arise surrounding the constraints of health care and our current behavioral health care system. How do we remain advocates for those under our care? These and other issues are addressed in this new edition.

CONTENT NEW TO THIS EDITION

New content for the fourth edition includes the following:

- **Managed care issues** as they affect psychiatric nursing (Chapter 4)
- **Holistic approaches to stress** (Chapter 12)
- **Rehabilitation of the severely mentally ill in the community** (Chapter 28)
- **End-of-life care for the dying and their families** (Chapter 30)
- **Forensic nursing** and the psychiatric needs of the incarcerated client (Chapter 32)
- **Alternative and complementary therapies** (Chapter 36)

Updated information is provided for the following:

- **New DSM-IV-TR, 2000** taxonomy and criteria are used throughout
- **Psychotropic drug information,** both new and updated, is found in all clinical chapters, in Appendix D, and on the Evolve website for the book

- **New NANDA-approved nursing diagnoses** are used in all nursing process sections
- **NIC/NOC classifications for interventions and for outcomes** are introduced in Chapter 9 and used throughout when appropriate
- **New Scope and Standards of Psychiatric-Mental Health Nursing Practice, 2000,** of the American Nurse's Association and American Psychiatric Nurse's Association are incorporated throughout, and listed opposite the inside front cover for easy reference

NEW FEATURES

While many familiar features are retained and updated, we have added the following to inform, heighten understanding, and engage the reader:

- **Assessment Guidelines** are boxed summary points for client assessment, found at the end of each assessment step in the nursing process section of all clinical chapters
- **Research Findings,** located in most clinical chapters, are in abstract format and give students a basic awareness of the latest, most up-to-date results of scientific studies on psychiatric topics (e.g., new therapies), while introducing students to scientific methodology
- **Evolve Website** includes student pre- and post-tests, psychotropic drug information, web links, additional case studies and nursing care plans, multimedia resources, learning activities, and other self-study activities. Reminders referring the student to the Evolve website are placed throughout the text (1) at the beginning of the chapter, (2) just before the Case Study in clinical chapters, (3) just before the Nursing Care Plan in clinical chapters, (4) after the Summary in all chapters, and (5) just before the Critical Thinking and Chapter Review section in all chapters
- **New, vibrant, full-color design** gives the book an open, spacious feeling, while incorporating a wealth of information

- **Mental Health Continuum** is a visual representation of the way in which psychobiological mental disorders are placed on a range from moderate to severe (anxiety, somatoform/dissociative, personality, and eating disorders) and from severe to psychotic (mood-depression and mania, schizophrenia, and other psychotic disorders and cognitive disorders).
- **Case Studies** in clinical chapters present individualized histories of clients with specific psychiatric disorders and help the reader translate theory into practice. Each Case Study presents the first nursing diagnosis through all the steps of the nursing process. Additional nursing diagnoses in nursing process format are found on the Evolve website.
- **Nursing Care Plans,** in nursing process format, are derived from and follow the Case Studies. Additional nursing diagnoses for the care plans in the book as well as additional Nursing Care Plans are found on the Evolve website.
- **Vignettes** with a personal touch are brief, descriptive characterizations of clients with specific psychiatric disorders, to enhance the text discussion.
- **A Nurse Speaks** showcases nurses who speak from personal experience in their own practice to a variety of real issues that psychiatric nurses face in clinical practice. For example, a **nurse manager** discusses how nurses can deal with the legal and ethical issues in floating to units where they do not feel prepared to practice safely (Unit V). A **nurse in private practice** discusses her frustration with the managed care system when a client needs more than the insurance company is prepared to cover financially (Unit VIII). Nurses discuss their experiences in a variety of settings, e.g., **forensic setting** (Unit VI), **community mental health setting** (Units II and VII), and **group practice** (Unit IV). A nurse-psychologist addresses her practice of using **alternative and complementary therapies.** A psychiatric nurse clinician talks about her **dual role of clinician and teacher** in Unit III. One of my favorites is a personal account of the **growth of psychiatry and the role of the psychiatric nurse** since the Korean War (Unit I).

FAMILIAR FEATURES WITH A NEW PERSPECTIVE

The following features have been updated to reflect new knowledge and to introduce students to the clients they may encounter in psychiatric nursing and the nurses who care for them:

ORGANIZATION OF THE TEXT

Organized by units, chapters have been grouped to emphasize the clinical perspective and facilitate locating information. All clinical chapters are organized in a clear, logical, and consistent format with nursing process as the strong, visible framework. Prevalence of disorders and comorbidity have been added, since knowing that comorbid disorders are often part of the clinical picture of specific disorders helps students as well as clinicians understand how to better assess and treat their clients. The basic outline for clinical chapters is:

- Prevalence
- Comorbidity
- Theory
- Assessment
  - ♦**Overall Assessment:** appropriate assessment for a specific disorder, including assessment tools and rating scales. The rating scales included help to highlight important areas in the assessment of a variety of behaviors or mental conditions. Since many of the answers are subjective in nature, experienced clinicians use these tools as a guide when planning care, in addition to their knowledge of their clients.
  - ♦**Self-Assessment:** the nurse's own thoughts and feelings that may need to be addressed to give maximum care to the client and enhance self-growth in the nurse.
  - ♦**Assessment Guidelines:** the summary of specific areas to assess by disorder
- Nursing Diagnosis
- Outcome Criteria
- Planning
- Interventions
  - ♦Interventions follow the categories set by the *Scope and Standards of Psychiatric-Mental Health Care* (ANA, 2000). Various interventions for each of the clinical disorders are chosen based on which of them most fit specific client needs. There are **Basic Interventions**—counseling, self-care, milieu therapy, health teaching, case management, psychobiological interventions, health pro-

motion, and health maintenance and **Advanced Practice Interventions**—psychotherapy, prescriptive authority, and treatment and consultation.
  - ♦**Alternative and Complementary Therapies** are included for specific disorders.
- Evaluation

EXCITING NEW TEACHING AIDS

Instructor's Electronic Resource

In addition to the materials on the Evolve website, we offer a new Instructor's Electronic Resource (IER), which includes an Instructor's Manual, the PowerPoint image collection, and a Computerized Test Bank.

- **Instructor's Manual** includes annotated Chapter Outlines, Thoughts About Teaching the Topic, and Concept Maps.
- **PowerPoint** image collection of about 250 text and graphic slides includes cartoons that characterize client behaviors.
- **Computerized Test Bank** has over 930 NCLEX-style multiple-choice questions, complete with correct answers, rationales, cognitive levels, and stages of the nursing process.

I wish to thank all the educators who took the time to send in suggestions and feedback for the new edition of *Foundations of Psychiatric Mental Health Nursing*. I hope this edition helps facilitate your students' learning and appreciation for the practice of psychiatric mental health nursing.

BETSY VARCAROLIS

Contents

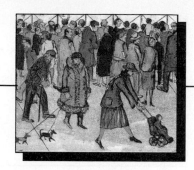

C h a p t e r 6

C h a p t e r 7

C h a p t e r 8

Unit III

C h a p t e r 9

C h a p t e r 10

C h a p t e r 11

Chapter 17

Chapter 18

Chapter 19

Chapter **20**

Schizophrenia and Other Psychotic Disorders   522
ELIZABETH M. VARCAROLIS

Chapter **21**

Cognitive Disorders   572
ELIZABETH M. VARCAROLIS

Unit **VI**

Psychiatric Emergencies   610

A Nurse Speaks   612
PATRICIA A. CLAYBROOK

Chapter **22**

Crisis   614
ELIZABETH M. VARCAROLIS

Chapter **23**

Suicide   638
ELIZABETH M. VARCAROLIS

Chapter 30

Care for the Dying and for Those Who Grieve 822
KATHY A. KRAMER-HOWE
ELIZABETH M. VARCAROLIS

Unit VIII

Lifespan Issues and Interventions 852

A Nurse Speaks 854
MARYANN FELDSTEIN

Chapter 31

Disorders of Children and Adolescents 856
CHERRILL COLSON

Chapter 32

Adults Requiring Specialized Interventions 886
GLORIA KUHLMAN

Foundations of Psychiatric Mental Health Nursing

FOURTH EDITION

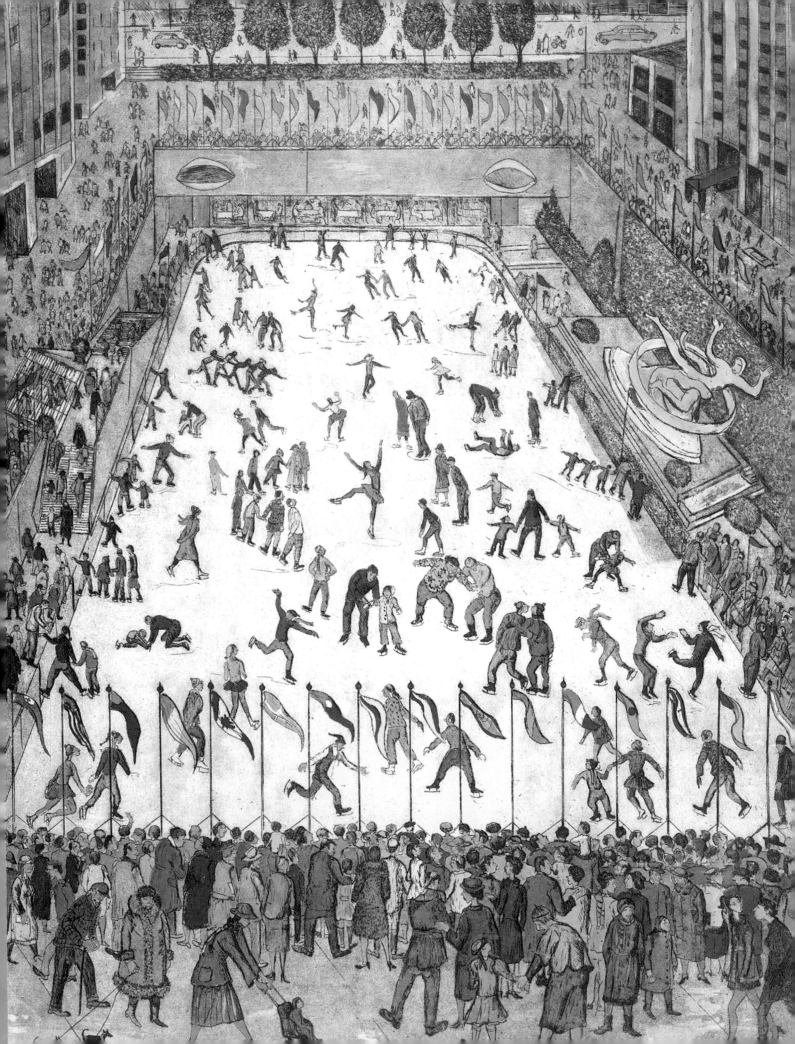

U n i t

I

Foundations in Theory

The most precious things in life
are not things.

ANONYMOUS

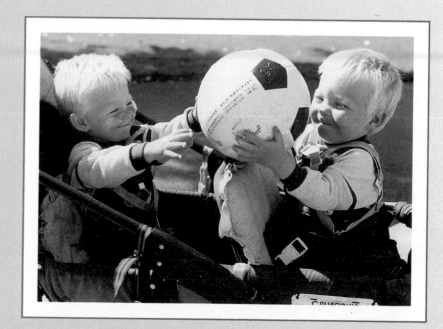

A Nurse Speaks

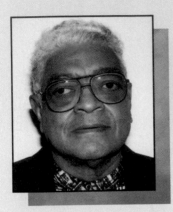

JOHN A. PAYNE*

Fifty years ago psychiatry was practiced in an environment vastly different from the one in which it is practiced today. Most clients were treated in large state hospitals, which were like small towns with their own store, restaurant, churches, farms, power plants, carpentry shop, and buildings housing thousands of clients and staff. There were buildings for admission and for treatment, infirmaries, chronic quiet units, and chronic disturbed units.

As nursing students, we were taught to care for clients who were receiving sedation, insulin shock, electric shock, malaria therapy, continuous hydrotherapy, wet packs, supraorbital lobotomies, physical restraints, and seclusion. All of these treatments were designed to make the clients more amenable to psychotherapy, to calm them, or for the safety of themselves or others. The disturbed wards were usually noisy and very active places in which clients acted out their psychoses both physically and vocally. Care for these clients was mostly custodial and involved keeping them clean, fed, safe, and calm.

I distinctly remember one client who was almost continuously kept in seclusion because of bizarre and aggressive behavior. He would not keep his clothes on, could not safely use eating utensils, and roared like a lion. Because of his behavior, he was frequently referred to as the Lion Man.

Keeping him clean and fed was a major project for the staff and always required several people. It was a frustrating experience because we all wanted to help him and see him behave in a more acceptable manner.

During the Korean War, I was away in the Air Force for four years. For three years I was a part of a system that treated young men for psychiatric problems by using many of the same modalities that were used in the state hospitals. The treatment there was somewhat more successful than that provided in the state hospitals because most of the men's visible signs of psychoses were of recent origin, having been caused by the stress of basic training or the stress of being in battle.

During my fourth year in the Air Force, psychotropic drugs were introduced. We began to use them very cautiously on our clients, with very limited success. As the doctors became more familiar with the drugs and increased the dosages, the results showed much improved behavior with most clients. Gradually no clients were being put into packs, and the hydrotherapy room was seldom used.

After being discharged from the Air Force, I returned to the hospital in which I had trained. As I went to the different buildings, I was surprised to see that here too there had been a decrease in the use of the old treatment modalities. Clients for the most part appeared much calmer; no clients were in seclusion all of the time, not even the Lion Man.

One day, while I was walking on the grounds with one of the charge attendants, he asked me if I knew who a client sitting on a bench talking with another client was. I said, "No. Who is he?" "That is the guy we used to call the Lion Man." What a change! The attendant told me that they had given him Thorazine and that within one week he was out of seclusion and keeping his clothes on. Gradually he began to socialize with staff and other clients. Within one month he was playing checkers, and within one year he was granted ground privileges.

---

*John Payne died in April, 2001, after a long illness.

Truly, the psychotropic drugs revolutionized the treatment of psychiatric clients.

Some psychotherapeutic modalities that had been used in smaller settings began to be used in the state hospitals. Group therapy, milieu therapy, and re-motivation therapy became the vogue, and with this the role of nursing became a more therapeutic one.

During President Kennedy's tenure in office, the Community Mental Health Bill was passed. This provided funds for moving the treatment of clients from the large state hospitals to the local hospital. Two things were significant about this legislation. First, all levels and modalities of treatment had to be provided to all residents within a specific "catch-ment area." Second, all disciplines (including nurs-ing) had to be represented on the treatment team.

States passed clients' bills of rights that released into the community thousands of clients who had spent many years in state hospitals. A part of the movement that was never adequate was the provision of group homes and follow-up supervision. This has led to our present situation of many actively psychotic ex-clients wandering our streets as homeless citizens. A change is going to come, and nursing is going to be an important part of that change. For now we have nurses in ever-increasing numbers who are becoming psychotherapists and psychiatric nurse practitioners. They will be leaders in providing care themselves and through mental health or psychiatric technicians—for nursing is still the only discipline that is proficient in providing 24-hour care to people in need.

Outline

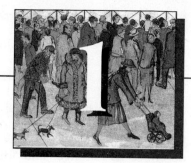

Mental Health and Mental Illness

ELIZABETH M. VARCAROLIS

Key Terms and Concepts

The key terms and concepts listed here also appear in color where they are defined or first discussed in this chapter.

attributes of mental illness

biologically based mental illness

clinical epidemiology

DSM-IV-TR—Diagnostic and Statistical Classification of Mental Disorders

epidemiology

mental disorders

mental health

myths and misconceptions (regarding mental illness)

prevalence rate

psychiatry's definition of normal mental health

psychobiological disorder

Objectives

After studying this chapter, the reader will be able to

1. Assess his or her own mental health using the five signs of mental health identified in this chapter (Table 1–1 and Figure 1–1).

2. Summarize factors that can affect the mental health of an individual and how these factors influence conducting a holistic nursing assessment.

3. Discuss some dynamic factors (including social climate, politics, myths, and biases) that contribute to making a clear-cut definition of mental health elusive.

4. Explain how epidemiological studies can improve medical and nursing care.

5. Demonstrate how the DSM-IV-TR multiaxial system can influence a clinician to consider a broad range of information before making a DSM diagnosis.

6. Compare and contrast the difference between a DSM-IV-TR diagnosis and a nursing diagnosis.

7. Give examples from your own culture of how consideration of norms and other cultural influences could affect making an accurate DSM-IV-TR diagnosis.

ental health professionals are faced with a multitude of problems in defining mental illness and mental health. Agreement on the definitions has been elusive throughout history. Early definitions were based on statistical measures. The term mental illness was applied to behaviors, described as "strange" and "different," that occurred infrequently and deviated from an established norm. Such criteria are inadequate because they suggest that mental health is based on conformity. If such definitions were used, nonconformists and independent thinkers such as Abraham Lincoln, Mahatma Gandhi, and Socrates would be judged mentally ill. There is a further problem in viewing those people whose behavior is statistically infrequent as mentally ill. Simply stated, the sacrifices of a Mother Teresa and the dedication of a Martin Luther King, Jr., are uncommon, but none of us would consider these much-admired behaviors to be signs of mental illness.

This chapter discusses concepts of mental health and mental illness. The reader is introduced to the concept of mental disorders as medical diseases that can be identified along a mental health continuum. You will see how mental disorders are categorized using the Diagnostic and Statistical Classification of Mental Disorders (DSM-IV-TR) and how nursing diagnoses can be utilized to ensure appropriate care. Mental health and managed care are discussed and the need to assess a person's cultural background and culture before a valid diagnosis can be made.

CONCEPTS OF MENTAL HEALTH AND ILLNESS

One approach to differentiating mental health from mental illness is based on what a particular culture regards as acceptable or unacceptable. In this view the mentally ill are those who violate social norms and thus threaten (or make anxious) those observing them. This definition seems partly true. The callous psychopathic person fits the definition, as does the sometimes wild manic person and the schizophrenic person who is displaying strange antics. However, this definition explicitly makes mental illness a relative concept. Many forms of unusual behavior can

be tolerated, depending on the prevailing cultural norms. People whose only problem is that they see things and hear things that no one else does may be put into a mental hospital, or they may be revered as visionaries, depending on the belief of their society (Leff 1981). The difficulty with defining mental illness through a particular behavior that is unacceptable to society is that it does not tell us what behavior a society should accept. Some totalitarian governments, to serve their own repressive goals, have classed all political dissidents as "mentally ill."

The field of mental illness is plagued by a host of myths and misconceptions. One myth is that to be mentally ill is to be different and odd. Another misconception is that to be healthy, a person must be logical and rational. All of us dream "irrational" dreams every night, and "irrational" emotions are not only universal human experiences but also essential to a fulfilling life. There are people who show extremely abnormal behavior and are characterized as mentally ill who are far more like the rest of us than different from us. There is no obvious and consistent line between mental illness and mental health. In fact, all human behavior lies somewhere along a continuum of mental health and mental illness.

Many psychiatrists still consider mental health, or normalcy, as the absence of psychopathology, but to many, mental health is far more than the absence of disease. Cambell's definition (1995) states that psychically normal (mentally healthy) persons are those who are in harmony with themselves and their environment. They conform to the cultural requirements or injunctions of their community. They may possess medical deviation or disease, but as long as this does not impair their reasoning, judgment, intellectual capacity, and the ability to make harmonious personal and social adaptation, they may be regarded as psychically sound or normal (Sadock 1999).

Psychiatry's definition of normal (mental health) changes over time and reflects changes in cultural norms, society's expectations and values, professional biases, individual differences, and the political climate of the time (Sadock 1999). For example, criticisms have come from various groups who believe that they were/are stereotyped (and unfairly) in the psychiatric community. Their concerns include the way in which the psychiatric community places an emphasis on the group's psychopathology rather than on health attributes. The psychology of women and the issues surrounding homosexuality are two very important examples but are by no means the only ones. This topic is discussed in more detail in the DSM-IV-TR axis system section in this chapter.

We are taught to evaluate our clients with mental health issues for their strengths and their areas of

The editor would like to thank Julius Trubowitz for his contribution to this chapter in the third edition of *Foundations of Psychiatric Mental Health Nursing*.

high functioning. You will find many attributes of mental health in some of your clients with mental health issues. It is these strengths that we build upon and encourage. By the same token, those who are "normal" or "mentally healthy" may have several areas of dysfunction at different times in their lives. We are all different, have different backgrounds (including siblings), and reflect different cultural influences even within the same subculture. We grow at different rates intellectually and emotionally, make different decisions at different times in our life, choose or choose not to evaluate our behaviors and grow within ourselves, have deep-seated spiritual beliefs or not, and so on. Understandably, then, there can be no one definition of mental health that fits all. However, there are some traits that mentally healthy people share and that contribute to a better quality of life. Some of these traits of "mentally healthy" people are depicted in Figure 1–1.

The following comments of a 40-year-old woman illustrate the continuum between illness and health as her condition changes from (1) deep depression to (2) mania to (3) health:

1. It was horror and hell. I was at the bottom of the deepest and darkest pit there ever was. I was worthless and unforgivable. I was as good as—no, worse than—dead.
2. I was incredibly alive. I could sense and feel everything. I was sure I could do anything, accomplish any task, create whatever I wanted, if only other people wouldn't get in my way.
3. Yes, I am sometimes sad and sometimes happy and excited, but nothing as extreme as before. I am much more calm. I realize now that, when I was manic, it was a pressure-cooker feeling. When I am happy now, or loving, it is more peaceful and real. I have to admit that I sometimes miss the intensity—the sense of power and creativity—of those manic times. I never miss anything about the depressed times, but of course the power and the creativity never bore fruit. Now I do get things done, some of the time, like

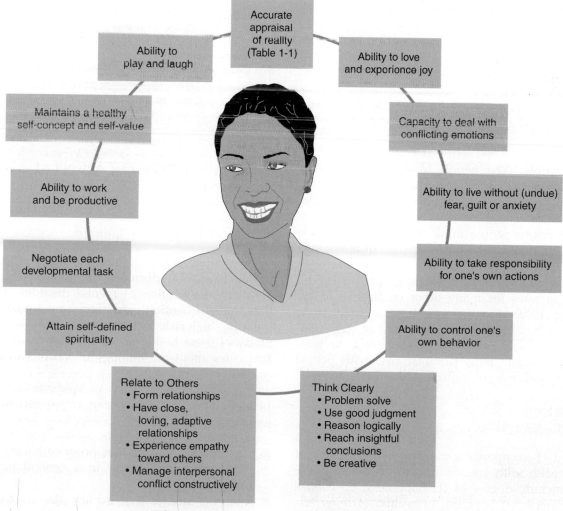

Figure 1–1 Some attributes of mental health.

TABLE 1–1   *Mental Health Versus Mental Illness*

SIGNS OF MENTAL HEALTH	SIGNS OF MENTAL ILLNESS
Happiness A. Finds life enjoyable B. Can see in objects, people, and activities their possibilities for meeting one's needs	**Major Depressive Episode** A. Loss of interest or pleasure in all or almost all usual activities and pastimes B. Mood as described by person is depressed, sad, hopeless, discouraged, "down in the dumps"
Control Over Behavior A. Can recognize and act on cues to existing limits B. Can respond to the rules, routines, and customs of any group to which one belongs	**Control Disorder, Under-socialized, Aggressive** A. A repetitive and persistent pattern of aggressive conduct in which the basic rights of others are violated
Appraisal of Reality A. Accurate picture of what is happening around one B. Good sense of the consequences, both good and bad, that will follow one's acts C. Can see the difference between the "as if" and "for real" in situations	**Schizophrenic Disorder** A. Bizarre delusions, such as delusions of being controlled B. Auditory hallucinations C. Delusions with persecutory or jealous content
Effectiveness in Work A. Within limits set by abilities, can do well in tasks attempted B. When meeting mild failure, persists until determines whether or not one can do the job	**Adjustment Disorder with Work (or Academic Inhibition)** A. Inhibition in work or academic functioning where previously there was adequate performance
A Healthy Self-concept A. Sees self as approaching one's ideals, as capable of meeting demands B. Reasonable degree of self-confidence helps in being resourceful under stress	**Dependent Personality Disorder** A. Passively allows others to assume responsibility for major areas of life because of inability to function independently B. Lacks self-confidence, e.g., sees self as helpless, stupid

Data from Redl, F., and Wattenberg, W. (1959). *Mental hygiene in teaching* (pp. 198–201). New York: Harcourt, Brace & World, and American Psychiatric Association (2000). *Diagnostic and statistical manual of disorders.* (4th ed., revised). Washington, DC: American Psychiatric Association.

most people. And people treat me much better now. I guess I must seem more real to them. I certainly seem more real to me. (Altrocchia 1980).

Finally, many people think that mental illness is incurable or that mental health treatment is not successful. However, the success rates for the treatment of many common mental disorders equal or exceed the success rates for many other medical disorders (Goldberg 1998). For example, people with panic disorder or bipolar disorder may have an 80% treatment success rate, major depression 60% to 80%, and schizophrenia 60%. Contrast that with people who have cardiovascular disease (Goldberg 1998):

■ Arthrectomy—52%
■ Angioplasty—41%

Table 1–1 compares some important aspects of mental health with specific mental disorders. These aspects include degree of (1) happiness, (2) control over behavior, (3) appraisal of reality, (4) effectiveness in work, and (5) healthy self-concept.

EPIDEMIOLOGY OF MENTAL DISORDERS

Applications of Epidemiology

Epidemiology is the quantitative study of the distribution of mental disorders in human populations. Once the distribution of mental disorders has been determined quantitatively, then epidemiologists can identify high-risk groups and high-risk factors. Study of these high-risk factors may lead to important clues about the etiology of various mental disorders.

The various applications of epidemiology are dependent upon three levels of investigation. (Regier and Burke 1999):

■ **Descriptive.** Studies that produce basic estimates of the rates of disorder in a general population and its subgroups.
■ **Analytic.** Studies that explore the rates of variation in illness among different groups, to identify

risk factors that may contribute to development of a disorder.

■ **Experimental.** Studies that test the presumed assumption between a risk factor and a disorder and seek to reduce the occurrence of the illness by controlling risk factors.

Each level of investigation supplies information that can be used to improve clinical practice and plan public health policies.

Clinical epidemiology represents a broad field that addresses what happens to people with illnesses who are seen by providers of clinical care. Studies use traditional epidemiological methods and are conducted in groups that are usually defined by illness or symptoms, or by diagnostic procedures or treatments given for the illness or symptoms. Clinical epidemiology includes studies of the

■ Natural history of an illness
■ Studies of diagnostic screening tests
■ Observational and experimental studies of interventions used to treat people with the illness or symptoms.

Results of epidemiologic studies are now routinely included in the DSM-IV-TR to describe the frequency of mental disorders. Analysis of epidemiological studies can assess the frequency with which symptoms appear together. For example, epidemiological studies demonstrated the significance of depression as a risk factor for death in people with cardiovascular disease and for premature death in people with breast cancer (Regier and Burke 1998).

Prevalence

The National Comorbidity Survey (NCS) (Kessler: NCS, 1990–1992) presents data from the first survey to have administered a structured psychiatric interview to a national probability sample in the United States. Data from this survey provide estimates of the lifetime and 12-month prevalence of psychiatric disorders in adults (18–55 years old) in the United States. The prevalence rate is the proportion of a population who has a mental disorder at a given time. About 28% of Americans over the age of 18 years (a group of more than 52 million) suffer from a mental or addictive disorder in a 1-year period (Goldberg 1998). See Table 1–2 for the prevalence of some psychiatric disorders in the United States.

MENTAL ILLNESS AND THE MENTAL HEALTH CONTINUUM

On April 14, 1999, legislation was proposed to help adults and children with the most severe mental illness obtain needed health insurance coverage. The legislation "recognizes and accepts severe mental illnesses as the real medical conditions they are" (NAMI 1999). This legislation would require full insurance parity for the most severe, biologically based mental illnesses, that is, mental disorders caused by neurotransmitter dysfunction, abnormal brain structure, inherited genetic factors, or other biological causes. Another term for this is psychobiological disorder. These biologically influenced illnesses include

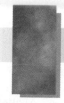

TABLE 1–2 *Prevalence of Psychiatric Disorders in the United States*

DISORDER	PREVALENCE IN A LIFETIME, %	PREVALENCE OVER 12 MONTHS, %
Any psychotic disorder	48.0	29.5
Any affective (mood) disorder	19.0	11.3
Major depression	17.1	10.3
Males	12.7	7.7
Females	21.3	12.9
Any anxiety disorder	24.9	17.2
Social phobia	13.3	7.9
Panic disorder	3.5	2.3
Any substance abuse	26.6	11.3
Alcohol dependence	14.1	7.2

From Goldberg, R. J. (1998). *Practical guide to the care of the psychiatric patient*, 2nd ed., p. 2. St. Louis: Mosby, based on Kessler, R. C., McGonagle, K. A., Zhao, S., et al: *Archives of general psychiatry* 1994; 51:18–19.

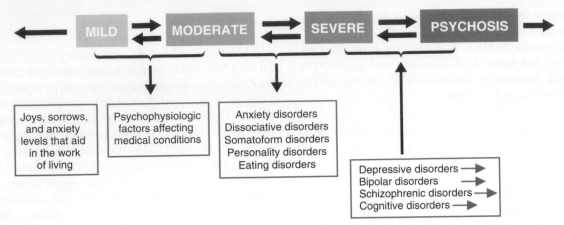

Figure 1–2 Mental health continuum of biologically based disorders.

- Schizophrenia
- Bipolar Disorder
- Major Depression
- Obsessive-Compulsive and Panic Disorders
- Posttraumatic Stress Disorder
- Autism

Other severe and disabling mental disorders include

- Anorexia Nervosa
- Attention-Deficit Hyperactivity Disorder

Therefore, many (not necessarily all) of the most prevalent and disabling mental disorders have been found to have strong biological influences. It is helpful to visualize these disorders along the Mental Health Continuum. This continuum will be used in each of the clinical chapters to identify the severity of the biologically influenced disorders. See Figure 1–2 for a conceptualization of biologically based disorders on the Mental Health Continuum.

The DSM-IV-TR (2000) cautions that the emphasis on the term mental disorder implies a distinction between "mental" disease and "physical" disorder, which is an out-of-date concept, and stresses mind-body dualism: ". . . there is much 'physical' in 'mental' disorders and much 'mental' in physical disorders." (APA 2000).

As nurses, we do not treat diseases; we care for people. If we believe that human beings have biological, psychological, social, and spiritual components and needs, and we believe in holistic nursing, then our task is to assess and plan care for the whole individual under our care. There are also many factors that can affect the severity and progress of a mental health illness, biologically based or otherwise, and these same factors can affect a "normal person's" mental health as well. Some of these factors include available support systems, family influences, developmental events, cultural or subcul-

tural beliefs and values, health practices, and negative influences impinging upon an individual's life. If possible, these influences need to be evaluated and factored into an individual's plan of care. Figure 1–3 identifies some influences that can affect a person's mental health. In fact, the DSM-IV-TR states that there is evidence that suggests that the symptoms and causes of a number of DSM-IV-TR disorders are influenced by cultural and ethnic factors (APA 2000).

MEDICAL DIAGNOSIS AND NURSING DIAGNOSIS OF MENTAL ILLNESS

In order to carry out their professional responsibilities, clinicians and researchers need clear and accurate guidelines for identifying and categorizing mental illness. Such guidelines help clinicians plan and evaluate treatment for their clients. A necessary element for categorizing includes agreement regarding which behaviors constitute a mental illness.

Medical Diagnoses and the DSM-IV-TR

In *Diagnostic and Statistical Classification of Mental Disorders DSM-IV-TR*, each of the mental disorders is conceptualized as a clinically significant behavioral or psychological syndrome or pattern that occurs in an individual and is associated with present **distress** (e.g., a painful symptom) or **disability** (i.e., impairment in one or more important areas of functioning) or with a significantly increased risk of suffering death, pain, disability, or an important loss of freedom. This syndrome or pattern must not be merely an expected and culturally sanctioned response to a particular event, such as the death of a loved one. Whatever its original cause, it must currently be considered a manifestation of a behavioral, psychological, or biological dysfunction in the individual. Deviant behavior (e.g., political, religious, or sexual) and conflicts between the individual and society are not considered mental disorders unless the deviance or conflict is a symptom of a dysfunction in the individual.

A common misconception is that a classification of mental disorders classifies **people** when actually the DSM-IV-TR classifies disorders that people have. For this reason, the text of the DSM-IV-TR avoids the use of such expressions as "a schizophrenic" or "an alcoholic" and instead uses the more accurate, "an individual with schizophrenia" or "an individual with alcohol dependence."

Since the DSM-III appeared in 1980, the criteria for classification of mental disorders have been sufficiently detailed for clinical, teaching, and research purposes. See Box 1–1 for an example of how the DSM-IV-TR provides specific criteria for the diagnosis of generalized anxiety disorder.

Special efforts have been made in the DSM-IV-TR to incorporate an awareness that the manual is used in culturally diverse populations in the United States and internationally. Clinicians evaluate individuals from numerous ethnic groups and cultural backgrounds (including many who are recent immigrants). Diagnostic assessment can be especially challenging when a clinician from one ethnic or cultural group uses the DSM-IV-TR classification to evaluate an individual from a different ethnic or cultural group. For example, among certain cultural groups, certain religious practices or beliefs (e.g., hearing or seeing a deceased relative during bereavement) may be misdiagnosed as manifestations of a psychotic disorder; furthermore, a syndrome often takes different superficial forms in different cultures. Also, people from minority or migrant populations may have good reason to be distrustful, and it should not be assumed that these clients are suffering from paranoia or paranoid schizophrenia (Westmeyer 1986). Refer to Chapter 7 for more on culturally based syndromes.

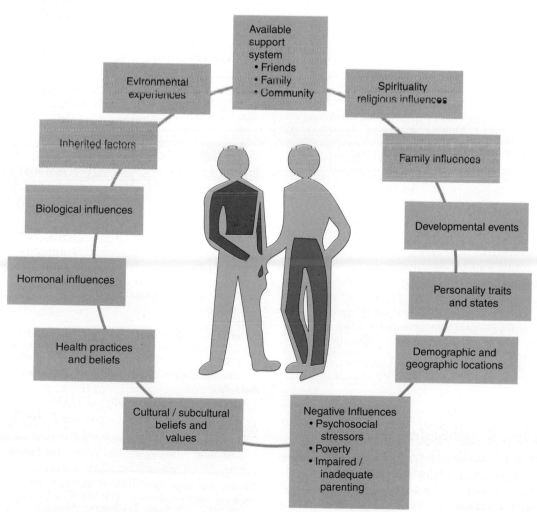

Figure 1–3 Influences that can have an impact on an individual's mental health.

Box 1–1 DSM-IV-TR *Criteria for Generalized Anxiety Disorder*

A. Excessive anxiety and worry (apprehensive expectation), occurring more days than not for at least 6 months, about a number of events or activities (such as work or school performance).

B. The person finds it difficult to control the worry.

C. The anxiety and worry are associated with three (or more) of the following six symptoms (with at least some symptoms present for more days than not for the past 6 months). Note: Only one item is required in children.
   (1) Restlessness or feeling keyed up or on edge
   (2) Being easily fatigued
   (3) Difficulty concentrating or mind going blank
   (4) Irritability
   (5) Muscle tension
   (6) Sleep disturbance (difficulty falling or staying asleep; or restless, unsatisfying sleep)

D. The focus of the anxiety and worry is not confined to features of an Axis I disorder, e.g., the anxiety or worry is not about having a panic attack (as in panic disorder), being embarrassed in public (as in social phobia), being contaminated (as in obsessive-compulsive disorder), being away from home or close relatives (as in separation anxiety disorder), gaining weight (as in anorexia nervosa), having multiple physical complaints (as in somatization disorder), or having a serious illness (as in hypochondriasis), and the anxiety and worry do not occur exclusively during posttraumatic stress disorder.

E. The anxiety, worry, or physical symptoms cause significant distress or impairment in social, occupational, or other important areas of functioning.

F. The disturbance is not due to the direct physiologic effects of a substance (e.g., a drug of abuse, a medication) or a general medical condition (e.g., hyperthyroidism) and does not occur exclusively during a mood disorder, a psychotic disorder, or a pervasive developmental disorder.

Diagnostic criteria from American Psychiatric Association, (2000). *Diagnostic and statistical manual of disorders,* (DSM-IV-TR) (4th ed., revised). Washington, DC: American Psychiatric Association. Reprinted with permission. Copyright 2000 American Psychiatric Association.

The DSM-IV-TR Axis System

The DSM-IV-TR axis system, by requiring judgments to be made on each of the five axes, forces the diagnostician to consider a broad range of information. Refer to Table 1–3.

Axis I refers to the collection of signs and symptoms that together constitute a particular disorder, e.g., schizophrenia, or a condition that may be a focus of treatment (refer to Appendix A for a list of all the DSM-IV-TR mental disorders). Axis II refers to personality disorders and mental retardation. Thus, axes I and II constitute the classification of abnormal behavior. Axes I and II were separated to ensure that the possible presence of long-term disturbance is considered when attention is directed to the current one. For example, a heroin addict would be diagnosed on axis I as having a substance-related disorder; this client might also have a long-standing antisocial personality disorder, which would be noted on axis II.

Although the remaining three axes are not needed to make the actual diagnosis, their inclusion in the DSM-IV-TR indicates recognition that factors other than a person's symptoms should be considered in an assessment. On axis III the clinician indicates any general medical conditions believed to be relevant to the mental disorder in question. In some individuals, a physical disorder (e.g., a neurological dysfunction) may be the cause of the abnormal behavior, whereas in others, it may be an important factor in their overall condition (e.g., diabetes in a child with a conduct disorder). Axis IV is for reporting psychosocial and environmental problems that may affect the diagnosis, treatment, and prognosis of a mental disorder. These may include occupational problems, educational problems, economic problems, interpersonal difficulties with family members, and a variety

Table 1–3 DSM-IV-TR *Multiaxial System of Evaluation*

Axis	Example
Axis I Clinical disorders Other conditions that may be a focus of clinical attention	Major depression (MM)
Axis II Personality disorders Mental retardation	Dependent personality disorder
Axis III General medical conditions	Diabetes *physical Health*
Axis IV Psychosocial and environmental problems	Divorce 3 months ago *mild → mood → Severe*
Axis V Global assessment of functioning	31 years old and unable to work or respond to family and friends

From American Psychiatric Association (2000). *Diagnostic and statistical manual of disorders* (DSM-IV-TR) (4th ed., revised). Washington, DC: American Psychiatric Association. Reprinted with permission. Copyright 2000 American Psychiatric Association.

of problems in other life areas. Finally, axis V, called global assessment of functioning (GAF), gives an indication of the person's best level of psychological, social, and occupational functioning during the preceding year, rated on a scale of 1 to 100 (from persistent danger of severely hurting oneself or others (1) to superior functioning in a variety of activities (100) at the time of the evaluation, as well as the highest level of functioning for at least a few months during the past year. See Box 1–2 for the

Box 1–2 *Global Assessment of Functioning (GAF) Scale*

Consider psychological, social, and occupational functioning on a hypothetical continuum of mental health–mental illness. Do not include impairment in functioning due to physical (or environmental) limitations. **Note:** Use intermediate codes when appropriate, e.g., 45, 68, 72.

Code

100 | **Superior functioning in a wide range of activities, life's problems never seem to get out of hand, is sought out by others because of his or her many positive**
91 | **qualities. No symptoms.**

90 | **Absent or minimal symptoms** (e.g., mild anxiety before an examination), **good functioning in all areas, interested and involved in a wide range of activities,**
81 | **socially effective, generally satisfied with life, no more than everyday problems or concerns** (e.g., an occasional argument with family members).

80 | **If symptoms are present, they are transient and expected reactions to psychosocial stressors** (e.g., difficulty concentrating after family argument); **no more than**
71 | **slight impairment in social, occupational, or school functioning** (e.g., temporarily behind in schoolwork).

70 | **Some mild symptoms** (e.g., depressed mood and mild insomnia) **OR some difficulty in social, occupational, or school functioning** (e.g., occasional truancy, or
61 | theft within the household), **but generally functioning pretty well, has some meaningful interpersonal relationships.**

60 | **Moderate symptoms** (e.g., flat affect and circumstantial speech, occasional panic attacks) **OR moderate difficulty in social, occupational, or school functioning**
51 | (e.g., few friends, conflicts with peers or co-workers).

50 | **Serious symptoms** (e.g., suicidal ideation, severe obsessional rituals, frequent shoplifting) **OR any serious impairment in social, occupational, or school func-**
41 | **tioning** (e.g., no friends, unable to keep a job).

40 | **Some impairment in reality testing or communication** (e.g., speech is at times illogical, obscure, or irrelevant) **OR major impairment in several areas, such as**
31 | **work or school, family relations, judgment, thinking, or mood** (e.g., depressed man avoids friends, neglects family, and is unable to work; child frequently beats up younger children, is defiant at home, and is failing at school).

30 | **Behavior is considerably influenced by delusions or hallucinations OR serious impairment in communication or judgment** (e.g., sometimes incoherent, acts
21 | grossly inappropriately, suicidal preoccupation) **OR inability to function in almost all areas** (e.g., stays in bed all day; no job, home, or friends).

20 | **Some danger of hurting self or others** (e.g., suicide attempts without clear expectation of death; frequently violent; manic excitement) **OR occasionally fails to**
11 | **maintain minimal personal hygiene** (e.g., smears feces) **OR gross impairment in communication** (e.g., largely incoherent or mute).

10 | **Persistent danger of severely hurting self or others** (e.g., recurrent violence) **OR persistent inability to maintain minimal personal hygiene OR serious suicidal**
1 | **act with clear expectation of death.**

0 | Inadequate information.

This rating scale highlights important areas in the assessment of functioning. Since many of the answers are subjective in nature, experienced clinicians use this tool as a guide when planning care, in addition to their knowledge of their clients.

TABLE 1-4   *Clinical Example Demonstrating DSM-IV-TR Axes*

Axis I
Schizophrenic disorder, paranoid

For the past 9 months, Michael, a 33-year-old sales representative, has suffered delusions of grandeur and persecution. Believing himself to be a genius, he became convinced that another salesman in his firm was trying to kill him because the other man could not tolerate Michael's superiority. In the past 2 weeks, Michael has become certain that this other man has had a pale green gas pumped into his office through the air-conditioning ducts, but there is no objective evidence of such gas or any other malfunctioning of the air-conditioning system.

Axis II
Paranoid traits, no personality disorder

Michael has always tended to be suspicious and distrustful of people. He looks constantly for evidence that others are trying to get the better of him or to harm him and his manner is guarded. He has trouble relaxing and others see him as cold and unemotional. He has no close friends and is considered a "loner." He was extremely jealous of his wife, from whom he is now separated, and often accused her, falsely, of having affairs with other men.

Axis III
Colitis

Michael sees a flare-up of his colitis (inflammation of the colon) as evidence that the salesman is poisoning him, even though Michael has had the same symptoms many times before.

Axis IV
Psychosocial and environmental problems
  a. Marital separation
  b. Loss of work responsibility
Rated severe

Michael left his wife 10 months ago. Two months ago, the president of Michael's firm reassigned one of Michael's important accounts to the salesman Michael now suspects of hostile intent. Michael thinks this was maneuvered by the other salesman, but in fact, the president acted because the quality of Michael's work was deteriorating. His work has slowed visibly, and co-workers complained that they could not perform their work properly when he was present.

Axis V
Highest level of adaptive functioning in last year (GAF)
Serious symptoms 45–50
Rated moderate to serious

Michael's functioning was adequate until he separated from his wife. At that point, he began to withdraw further from friends and acquaintances. He appeared to concentrate more on his job but actually spent his time checking and rechecking his work. When the firm's president reassigned his major account, Michael's work deteriorated further, and Michael began to air some of his suspicions about the partner who took over the account. When his colitis flared up 2 weeks ago, he requested an appointment with the president and accused the partner openly. Michael was fired.

GAF, global assessment of functioning.
Adapted from Altrocchi, J. (1980). *Abnormal behavior*. New York: Harcourt Brace Jovanovich.
Reprinted with permission from the *Diagnostic and statistical manual of disorders*, Fourth Edition, Text Revision. Copyright 2000 American Psychiatric Association.

GAF scale. Table 1–4 illustrates how the multiaxial system of classification might be applied to a hypothetical case.

Caution needs to be exercised in diagnosing or labeling, whether a medical diagnosis or a nursing diagnosis is being formulated. The premise that every society has its own view of health and illness and its own classification of diseases has long been observed by anthropologists, historians, and students of cross-cultural society (Klerman 1986). The process of psychiatric labeling can have harmful effects on an individual and family, especially if the

diagnosis was made on insufficient evidence and proves faulty.

An example of cultural and social bias influencing psychiatric diagnosis is the inclusion of homosexuality as a psychiatric disease in both the DSM-I and DSM-II. All research consistently failed to demonstrate that people with a homosexual orientation were any more maladjusted than heterosexuals, but despite the research data, change occurred in the medical community only when gay rights activists advocated an end to discrimination against lesbians and gay men. No longer is homosexuality classified as a mental disorder. Other instances of bias may extend to many minority groups, including blacks, elderly persons, children, and women. These biases are often reflected in our power structures and political systems. Awareness of the cultural bias and dangers in labeling have enormous implications for nursing practice, especially in the field of mental health, because nurses often take their cues from the medical structure.

Nursing Diagnoses and the DSM-IV-TR

Psychiatric mental health nursing includes the diagnosis and treatment of human responses to actual or potential mental health problems. The North American Nursing Diagnosis Association (NANDA) describes a nursing diagnosis as a clinical judgment about individual, family, or community responses to actual or potential health problems and life processes. Therefore, the DSM-IV-TR is used to diagnose a psychiatric disorder, while a well-defined nursing diagnosis provides the framework for identifying appropriate nursing interventions for dealing with the phenomena a client with a mental health disorder is experiencing, e.g., hallucinations, low self-esteem issues, ability to function (job/family), and so on. Refer to Appendix C for a list of NANDA-approved nursing diagnoses. The individual clinical chapters offer suggestions for potential nursing diagnoses for the behaviors and phenomena often encountered in specific disorders. A more thorough discussion of nursing diagnoses in psychosocial nursing is found in Chapter 9.

INTRODUCTION TO CULTURE AND MENTAL ILLNESS

What should society do with George? Over the past four months, George has struck and injured several dozen people, most of them he hardly knew. Two of them had to be sent to the hospital. George expresses no guilt, no regrets. He says he would attack every one of them again if he got the chance.

■ Send him to jail?
■ Commit him to a mental hospital?
■ Give him an award for being the best defensive lineman in the league?

Before you can answer, you must know the context of George's behavior. Behavior that seems nor-

mal at a party might seem bizarre at a business meeting. Behavior that earns millions for a rock singer might earn a trip to the mental hospital for a college professor. Behavior that is perfectly routine in one culture might be considered criminal in another.

Even when we know the context of someone's behavior, we may wonder whether it is normal. Suppose your Aunt Tillie starts to pass out $5 bills to strangers on the street corner and vows that she will keep on doing so until she has exhausted her entire fortune. Is she mentally ill? Should the court commit her to a mental hospital and turn her fortune over to you as her trustee?

A man claims to be Jesus Christ and asks permission to appear before the United Nations to announce God's message to the world. A psychiatrist is sure that he can relieve this man of his disordered thinking by giving him antipsychotic drugs, but the man refuses to take them and insists that his thinking is normal. Should we force him to take the drugs, just ignore him, or put his address on the agenda of the United Nations?

In determining the mental health or mental illness of the individual, we must consider the norms and influence of culture. Throughout history, people (including us) have interpreted health or sickness according to their own current views. People in the Middle Ages, for example, regarded bizarre behavior as a sign that the disturbed person was possessed by a demon. To exorcise the demon, priests resorted to prescribed religious rituals. During the 1880s, when the "germ theory" of illness was popular, physicians interpreted bizarre behavior as stemming from biological causes. A striking example of how cultural change influences the interpretation of mental illness is the diagnosis of hysteria, which is much less common today than it was in the nineteenth century; according to some authors, this is because of a less restrictive family atmosphere and more permissive child-rearing, especially in sexual areas.

Cultures differ not only in their views regarding mental illness but also in the types of behavior categorized as mental illness. For example, one form of mental illness recognized in parts of Southeast Asia is **running amok**, in which someone (usually a male) runs around engaging in furious, almost indiscriminate violent behavior. **Pibloktoq** is an uncontrollable desire to tear off one's clothing and expose oneself to severe winter weather; it is a recognized form of psychological disorder in parts of Greenland, Alaska, and the Arctic regions of Canada. In our own society, we recognize **anorexia nervosa** as a psychobiological disorder that entails voluntary starvation. That disorder is well known in

Europe, North America, and Australia, but unheard of in many other parts of the world. Refer to Chapter 7 for more on culture-based syndromes.

What is to be made of the fact that certain disorders occur in some cultures but are absent in others? One interpretation is that the conditions necessary for causing a particular disorder occur in some places but are absent in other places. Another interpretation is that people learn certain kinds of abnormal behavior by imitation. However, the fact that some disorders may be culturally determined does not prove that all mental illnesses are so determined. The best evidence suggests that schizophrenia and bipolar affective disorders are found throughout the world. The symptom patterns of schizophrenia have been observed among indigenous Greenlanders and West African villagers, as well as in our own Western culture.

The DSM-IV-TR includes information specifically related to culture in three areas:

1. A discussion of cultural variations for each of the clinical disorders
2. A description of culture-bound syndromes
3. An outline for cultural formulation for evaluating and reporting the impact of the individual's cultural context.

Refer to Chapter 7 for discussion of the differing ways people view the world and a review of discrete cultural syndromes, and Chapter 9 under psychosocial assessment.

SUMMARY

This chapter focuses on the difficulty in defining mental illness and identifies some of the myths people hold regarding mental illness. Five important aspects of mental health are proposed and contrasted with mental illness and some components of mental health are identified.

The reader is introduced to the terms epidemiology and prevalence rate and how the study of epidemiology can help identify high-risk groups and behaviors. In turn, this can lead to a better understanding of the etiologies of some disorders.

With the recognition that many common mental disorders are now biologically based, it is easier to see how these biologically based disorders can be classified as medical disorders as well. Many of the more prevalent mental disorders are placed on a Mental Health Continuum, which is used throughout the clinical chapters.

You were introduced to the Diagnostic and Statistical Classification of Mental Disorders (DSM-IV-TR) and the DSM-IV-TR Axis System and the Global Assessment of Functioning Scale (GAF). The five axes of the DSM-IV-TR make it possible for clinicians to make a more holistic and realistic assessment of their clients, thus allowing for more comprehensive and appropriate interventions. Influences that may affect the intensity or cause of a mental illness, as well as affect a normal person, are illustrated in Figure 1–3. The use of well-thought-out nursing diagnoses helps to target the symptoms and needs of clients in order that they may achieve a higher level of functioning and a better quality of life.

Lastly, we discussed the influence of culture on behavior and how symptoms may reflect a person's cultural patterns. At times, symptoms need to be understood in terms of a person's cultural background. **Caution is recommended for all health care professionals concerning the damage and disservice that stereotypes can cause in the lives of clients in need of medical/mental health services.** Lack of knowledge and ignorance on the part of health care professionals about people from backgrounds and cultures other than our own can result in lack of or inappropriate service to those under our care.

Visit the **Evolve** website at http://evolve.elsevier.com/Varcarolis for a post-test on the content in this chapter.

Visit the **Evolve** website at
http://evolve.elsevier.com/Varcarolis
for additional self-study exercises.

Critical Thinking and Chapter Review

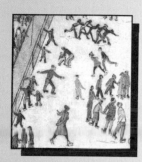

Critical Thinking

1. Timothy Harris is a college sophomore with a GPA of 3.4. He is brought to the emergency room after a suicide attempt. He has been extremely depressed after the death of his girlfriend five months ago when the car he was driving careened out of control and crashed. Timothy's parents have been very distraught since the accident. To compound things, the parent's religious beliefs include that taking one's own life will prevent a person from going to heaven. Timothy has epilepsy and has had increased seizures since the accident and refuses help because he says he should be punished for his carelessness and doesn't care what happens to him. He has not been to school and has not showed up for his part-time job of tutoring younger children in reading.

   A: Questions regarding Timothy and the use of the Multiaxis System

      1. What might be a possible DSM-IV-TR diagnosis for Axis I?
      2. What information should be included on Axis 3?
      3. What should be included on Axis 4?
      4. What might you evaluate Timothy's GAF (range)?

   B: Mental Health and Mental Illness

      1. What are some factors that you would like to assess regarding aspects of Timothy's overall mental health and other influences that can affect mental health before you plan your care?
      2. If an antidepressant medication could help him with his depression, explain why this alone would not meet his multiple needs. What issues do you think have to be addressed if Timothy was to receive a holistic approach to care?
      3. Formulate at least two potential nursing diagnoses for Timothy.
      4. How would Timothy's parents' religious beliefs factor into your plan of care? Would it?

2. Using Table 1–1, evaluate yourself and one of your clients in terms of mental health.

3. In a small study group, share experiences you have with others from unfamiliar cultural, ethnic, or racial backgrounds and identify two positive learning experiences from these encounters.

Chapter Review

Choose the most appropriate answer.

1. Which statement about mental illness is true? Mental illness

   1. is a matter of individual nonconformity with societal norms.
   2. is present when individual irrational and illogical behavior occurs.
   3. changes with culture, time in history, political system, and group doing the defining.

    4. is evaluated solely by considering individual control over behavior and appraisal of reality.

2. A nursing student new to psychiatric nursing asks a peer what resource can he or she use to find out what symptoms are part of the picture of a specific psychiatric disorder. The best answer would be

    1. NIC
    2. NOC
    3. NANDA
    4. DSM-IV-TR 2000

3. Why is it important for the nurse to be aware of the multiple factors that can impact on an individual's mental health?

    1. Rates of illness differ among various groups.
    2. The DSM-IV-TR 2000 cannot be used without this information.
    3. A holistic nursing assessment requires this awareness.
    4. The nurse must contribute this data for epidemiological research.

4. Epidemiological studies contribute to improvements in care for individuals with mental disorders by

    1. providing information about effective nursing techniques.
    2. identifying risk factors that contribute to the development of a disorder.
    3. identifying who in the general population will develop a specific disorder.
    4. identifying which individuals will respond favorably to a specific treatment.

5. A major difference between a DSM-IV-TR 2000 diagnosis and a nursing diagnosis is

    1. There is no functional difference between the two. Both serve to identify a human deviance.
    2. The DSM-IV-TR 2000 diagnosis disregards culture while the nursing diagnosis takes culture into account.
    3. The DSM-IV-TR 2000 is associated with present distress or disability, while a nursing diagnosis considers past and present responses to actual mental health problems.
    4. The DSM-IV-TR 2000 diagnosis impacts the choice of medical treatment, while the nursing diagnosis offers a framework for identifying interventions for phenomena a client is experiencing.

REFERENCES

Altrocchia, J. (1980). *Abnormal behavior*. New York: Harcourt Brace Jovanovich.

American Psychiatric Association (1987). *Diagnostic and statistical manual of mental disorders (DSM-III-R)* (3rd ed., revised). Washington, DC: American Psychiatric Association.

American Psychiatric Association (1994). *Diagnostic and statistical manual of mental disorders (DSM-IV)* (4th ed.). Washington, DC: American Psychiatric Association.

American Psychiatric Association (2000). *Diagnostic and statistical manual of mental disorders (DSM-IV-TR)* (4th ed.). Washington, DC: American Psychiatric Association.

Cambell, R.J. (1995). *Psychiatric dictionary* (7th ed.). New York: Oxford University Press.

Goldberg, R.J. (1998). *Practical guide to the care of the psychiatric patient* (2nd ed.). St. Louis: Mosby.

Kessler, R.C.: National Comorbidity Survey, 1990–1992 [Computer File]. Conducted by University of Michigan, Survey Research Center. ICPSR ed. Ann Arbor, MI: Inter-University Consortium for Political and Social Research [producer and distributor], 2000.

Klerman, G.L. (1986). *Contemporary directions in psychopathology: Toward the DSM-IV*. New York: Guilford Press.

Leff, J. (1981). *Psychiatry around the globe*. New York: Marcel Dekker.

NAMI (1999). *Federal legislation to provide full coverage for severe mental illness*. National Alliance for the Mentally Ill.

Peplau, H. E. (1952). *Interpersonal relations in nursing*. New York: G. P. Putnam's Sons.

Regier, D.A., and Burke, J.D., Jr. (1999). Epidemiology. In B.J. Sadock and V.A. Sadock (Eds.). *Kaplan and Sadock's Comprehensive textbook of psychiatry* (7th ed.). Philadelphia: Lippincott Williams & Wilkins.

Sadock, B.J. (1999). Signs and symptoms in psychiatry. In B.J. Sadock and V.A. Sadock (Eds.). *Kaplan and Sadock's Comprehensive textbook of psychiatry* (7th ed.). Philadelphia: Lippincott Williams & Wilkins.

Westmeyer, J. (1986). Cross cultural diagnosis. *Harvard Medical School Mental Health Letter*, 2(12):4.

Outline

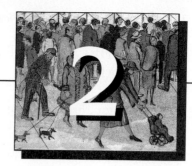

Relevant Theories and Therapies for Nursing Practice

JULIUS TRUBOWITZ

Key Terms and Concepts

The key terms and concepts listed here also appear in color where they are defined or first discussed in this chapter.

aversion therapy

behavior modification

behavioral therapy

cognitive therapy

conscious

countertransference

defense mechanisms

ego

id

interpersonal
    psychotherapy (IPT)

milieu therapy

modeling

operant conditioning

preconscious

psychodynamic
    psychotherapy

short-term dynamic
    psychotherapy

superego

systematic desensitization

transference

unconscious

Objectives

After studying this chapter, the reader will be able to

1. Compare and contrast the developmental stages of Freud, Erikson, Sullivan, and Piaget.

2. Evaluate the premise behind the approaches to the various therapeutic models discussed in this chapter.

3. Identify ways that each theorist contributes to the nurse's ability to assess client's behaviors.

4. Using examples from clinical experience, identify:
   a) two of Freud's defense mechanisms
   b) an example of countertransference within your relationship to a client
   c) a clinical incidence of selective-inattention or dissociation

5. Clarify the difference between the **art** and the **science** of nursing.

6. Identify Peplau's expectation of the nurse-patient relationship.

7. Choose the one therapeutic model you think would be most useful for you, if you had an issue you wanted to resolve. Which one would you recommend to a friend?

MAJOR THEORIES OF PERSONALITY

All people go through a series of stages in their development from infancy to old age. Each stage has its own character and offers its own unique opportunities for growth. The meaning of particular events and relationships is deeply influenced by the stage in the life cycle in which they occur. Although each of us is unique, we all go through the same basic stages of growth. Each has its own special contribution to the individual as a whole. Hebrew, Chinese, and Greek writings dating back more than 2000 years attest to our interest in and observation of the "stages of man." Each ancient writing has identified similar stages in the human life cycle.

Nurses draw on relevant theories of personality and human development as a basis for assessment, nursing diagnosis, planning, intervention, and evaluation. Different theorists view the life cycle through their own disciplines and individual theories of personality development. Hildegard Peplau's body of work, based in H.S. Sullivan, is only briefly covered here, but the concepts of the nurse-patient relationship, process recordings, interviewing, and theory of anxiety are covered further in subsequent appropriate chapters.

The contributions of Freud, Erikson, Sullivan, Peplau, Piaget, Maslow, and Kohlberg are discussed here.

Freud

Sigmund Freud (1856–1939), an Austrian psychiatrist and the founder of psychoanalysis, developed a complex theoretical formulation of the nature of the human personality. The major components of his theory discussed here include levels of awareness, personality structure, the concept of anxiety and defense mechanisms, and psychosexual stages of development.

Levels of Awareness

Essentially, Freud's levels of awareness provide a mental typography that is divided into three parts: the conscious, the preconscious, and the unconscious.

CONSCIOUS. The conscious includes all experiences that are within a person's awareness at any given time. For example, all intellectual, emotional, and interpersonal aspects of a person's behavior that he or she is aware of and is able to control are within conscious awareness. All information that is easily remembered and immediately available to an individual is in the conscious mind. The conscious mind is logical and, according to Freud, regulated by the reality principle.

PRECONSCIOUS. The preconscious includes experiences, thoughts, feelings, or desires that might not be in immediate awareness but can be recalled to consciousness. The preconscious (sometimes called **subconscious**) can help screen out extraneous information and can enhance concentration. It can censor certain wishes and thoughts and helps repress unpleasant thoughts or feelings.

UNCONSCIOUS. Although Freud cannot be credited with discovering the unconscious, it was he who developed the concept of the unconscious in clear, rich, and original terms. Freud described the mind as an iceberg to convey the relationship between the conscious and the unconscious. The water's surface represents the boundary between conscious and unconscious, with nine tenths of the mind submerged (Fig. 2–1).

The unconscious refers to all memories, feelings, thoughts, or wishes that are not available to the conscious mind. Often these repressed memories, feelings, thoughts, or wishes could, if made prematurely conscious, trigger enormous anxiety. However, unconscious material often does become manifest in dreams, slips of the tongue, or jokes; or through the use of hypnosis, therapy, or certain drugs (e.g., sodium pentothal and hallucinogens).

The unconscious exists comfortably with extreme contradictions and ambivalence (love and hate toward the same object), intense emotions, and strong sexual urges. The unconscious is not logical, has no conception of time, and is governed by what Freud calls the pleasure principle. Conscious, preconscious, and unconscious are not mental processes or systems. They are adjectives that describe unique psychological activity.

Personality Structure

Freud sought to describe what he called the "anatomy of the mental personality." He isolated three categories of experience—the id, the ego, and the superego—that represent a method of looking at the

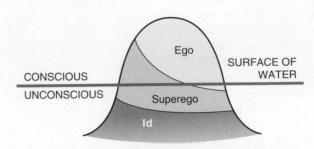

Figure 2–1 The mind as an iceberg.

way an individual functions. They are not separate entities or sections of the mind. Very roughly, they may be identified as biologically driven energy (id), ways of coping with reality (ego), and conscience (superego). The way the three interact, the conflicts they produce, and their blending provide a comprehensive picture of the behavior of the individual.

THE ID. The id is the "core of our being." It is the source of all drives and the reservoir of instincts. The id is the oldest and the first original function of the personality, and it is the basis out of which the ego and the superego develop. The id includes all our genetic inheritance, our reflexes, and our capacities to respond, including the instincts, basic drives, needs, and wishes that motivate us.

The id operates according to the pleasure principle and uses primary processes. The individual driven by the id cannot tolerate frustration and seeks to discharge the tension and return to a more comfortable, constant level of energy.

EGO. The ego emerges because the needs, wishes, and demands of the id require appropriate exchanges with the outside world of reality. Hungry people have to be able to seek, find, and eat food in order to meet their needs and survive. The ego emerges out of the id and acts as an intermediary between the id and the external world. The ego is said to begin its development during the fourth or fifth month of life. The ego distinguishes between things in the mind and things in the external world, whereas the id knows only the subjective reality of the mind. Reality testing is one function of the ego.

The ego follows the **reality principle** (i.e., realistic thinking). The aim of the reality principle is to satisfy the id's impulses in the external world with a suitable object. Whereas the id employs fantasies and wishes to satisfy a need, the ego uses the realistic thinking characteristic. Using problem-solving methods, the ego devises a plan and then tests it, usually by some kind of action, to see whether it will work. Problem solving, then, is another function of the ego.

Through the use of mental functions of judgment and intelligence, the ego selects the parts of the environment to which it will respond and decides which instincts will be satisfied, and in what fashion. Carrying out its executive function is not an easy task for the ego. The ego has to try to integrate the often-conflicting demands of its "three harsh masters": external reality, the id, and the superego.

THE SUPEREGO. The third and last system of personality to be developed is the superego, the internal representative of the values, ideals, and moral standards of society. From a system of rewards and punishments originally imposed on the child from without, the child internalizes the moral standards of parents and society. The superego is the moral arm of personality. It strives for perfection rather than pleasure and represents the ideal rather than the real.

The development of the superego is a necessary part of socialization because young children's egos are too weak to control their impulses. Parental "thou shalt nots" are needed for a time. However, a harsh superego can be uncompromising and may lead to blocking of necessary and reasonable satisfactions. Furthermore, a rigid superego can create feelings of inferiority (expressed as "I'm a bad person") when the individual fails to meet parental dictates. The superego is said to have its development between 3 and 5 years of age.

The three systems of the personality—the id, the ego, and the superego—are names for the psychological processes that follow different operating principles. In a mature and well-adjusted personality, they work together as a team under the administrative leadership of the ego. Too powerful an id or a superego may gain control, and imbalance and maladjustment may be the result.

Let us take a look at a hypothetical situation and consider the roles of the id, ego, and superego. A young person is out on a date with an attractive member of the opposite sex with whom there may be a wish to have a sexual relationship. The id would declare, "I want, I want!" while the superego might assert, "Thou shalt not!" The ego would be faced with the problem of meeting the id's demands within the limitations and standards of society. A solution might involve the young person's waiting until better acquainted with the other individual or until some other social norm is met.

Defense Mechanisms and Anxiety

Freud believed that anxiety was an inevitable part of living. The environment, physical and social, presents dangers and insecurities, threats and satisfactions. It can produce pain and increase tension or produce pleasure and decrease tension. The ego develops defenses, or defense mechanisms, to ward off anxiety by preventing conscious awareness of threatening feelings. Without defense mechanisms, anxiety might overwhelm and paralyze us and interfere with daily living.

Defense mechanisms share two common features: (1) they operate on an unconscious level (except suppression), so that we are not aware of their operation; and (2) they deny, falsify, or distort reality to make it less threatening. We cannot survive without defense mechanisms. However, if they become too extreme in distorting reality, interference with healthy adjustment and personal growth may occur. Table 2–1 includes an overview of some of the defense mechanisms and a brief description of their

TABLE 2–1   *Common Defense Mechanisms*

DEFENSE MECHANISMS	CHARACTERISTICS	EXAMPLE
Repression	Blocking a wish or desire from conscious expression.	You forget the name of someone for whom you have intense negative feelings.
Denial	A more serious form of repression. Person lives as though an unwanted piece of information or reality does not exist. There's a persistent refusal to be swayed by evidence.	An alcoholic states, "I do not have a problem with alcohol. I never drink before 5:00 PM. My stomach problems and liver problems are caused by something else."
Projection	Attributing an unconscious impulse, attitude, or behavior to someone else (blaming or scapegoating).	A man who is attracted to his friend's wife on an unconscious level accuses his wife of flirting with his friend.
Reaction-formation	An intense feeling regarding an object, person, or feeling is out of awareness and is unknowingly acted out consciously in an opposite manner.	You treat someone whom you unconsciously dislike intensely in an overly friendly manner.
Regression	Returning to an earlier level of adaptation when severely threatened.	A child resumes bed-wetting after having long since stopped when his baby brother is born and fussed over at home.
Rationalization	Unconsciously falsifying an experience by giving a contrived, socially acceptable, and logical explanation to justify an unpleasant experience or questionable behavior.	A student who did not study for an examination blames his failure on the teacher's poor lecture material and the unfairness of the examination.
Identification	Modeling behavior after someone else.	A 6-year-old girl dresses up in her mother's dress and high-heeled shoes.
Introjection	A more primitive form of identification. More closely relates to unconscious imitation.	A child who becomes irritable after angry interactions with a parent, the child takes in "swallows whole" and the image of the angry parent grows into him or herself.
Displacement	Discharging intense feelings for one person onto another object or person who is less threatening, thereby satisfying an impulse with a substitute object.	A child who has been scolded by her mother hits her doll with a hairbrush.
Sublimation	Rechanneling an impulse into a more socially desirable object.	A student satisfies sexual curiosity by conducting sophisticated research into sexual behaviors.

characteristics, with examples from daily living. A more complete list and fuller discussion of defense mechanisms is found in Chapter 13, where they are organized in a hierarchy of defenses and show relevance to nursing care.

Psychosexual Stages of Development

Freud believed that human development proceeds through a series of stages from infancy to adulthood. Each stage is characterized by the inborn tendency of all individuals to reduce tension and seek pleasure. During the first 5 years of life, each stage is defined by and named for the erogenous zone that produces the main source of gratification during that stage. Each stage is associated with a particular conflict that must be resolved before the child can move successfully to the next stage. Freud believed that the experiences during the early stages determine an individual's adjustment patterns and the personality traits that he or she has as an adult. In fact, Freud thought that personality was rather well formed by the time the child entered school, and that subsequent growth consisted of elaborating this basic structure.

The three early stages, collectively called the **pregenital stage,** are the oral, anal, and phallic stages. The child then enters a prolonged **latency period,** the quiet years in which the dynamics become more or less stabilized. With the arrival of adolescence, there is a burst of libidinal forces, primitive impulses from the id, which upset the stabilization of the latency period and gradually come under control as the adolescent moves into adulthood. The final developmental stage of adolescence and adulthood is the **genital stage.** Table 2–2 summarizes Freud's psychosexual stages of development and can be used to follow the narrative here.

ORAL STAGE (0 TO 1 YEAR). The first stage is the oral stage. The baby is "all mouth," getting most of his or her gratification from sucking. The erogenous zones are the lips and mouth, through which the infant receives nourishment, has the closest contact with the mother (in breast-feeding), and discovers information about the world.

During this stage, which Freud called **primary narcissism,** the infant is all id, concerned only with gratification of self. The ego begins to emerge during this time (fourth or fifth month of life), as the infant begins to see the self as separate from the mother; this is the beginning of the development of a "sense of self." When the infant experiences gratification of basic needs, a sense of trust and security begins.

ANAL STAGE (1 TO 3 YEARS). Freud's second psychosexual stage is the anal stage. Generally, toilet training occurs during this period. According to Freud, the child gains pleasure both from the elimination of feces and from their retention. Until this time, the infant has experienced few demands from others, but now there appear to be direct attempts by the parents to interfere with the pleasure obtained from the excretory functions. Thus, the conflict of this stage is between those demands from society in the person of the parents and the sensations of pleasure associated with the anus.

According to Freud, parents' reactions during this stage may have far-reaching effects on the formation of specific traits and values. If the mother is very strict and repressive in her approach, the child will develop a retentive character (i.e., the child will become stubborn and stingy, unwilling to give). Alternatively, under the pressure of coercive measures in toilet training, the child may vent rage by expelling the feces at the most inappropriate times. This can become the original model for all kinds of expulsive traits, including cruelty, malicious destructiveness, temper tantrums, and messy disorderliness. On the other hand, according to Freudian theorists, if the mother is warm and sensitive in her urging and extravagantly praises the child in toilet activity, this would be the basis for creativity and productivity. The child learns to delay immediate gratification (expelling feces) to obtain a future goal (parental approval).

PHALLIC STAGE (3 TO 6 YEARS). During this stage called the Oedipal phase, the child experiences both pleasurable and conflicting feelings associated with genital organs. At this time, children devote much energy to examining their genitalia, masturbating, and expressing interest in sexual matters. Children are curious about everything, including anatomical differences between the sexes and the origin of babies. Their ideas are frequently inaccurate and unrealistic, such as believing that a pregnant woman has swallowed her baby or that a baby is expelled through the mouth or the anus.

The pleasures of masturbation and the fantasy life of children set the stage for the Oedipus complex, the concept of which Freud considered to be one of his greatest contributions to the study of personality development. Freud's concept was suggested by the Greek tragedy of Sophocles in which King Oedipus unwittingly murdered his father and married his mother. To Freud, the Greek myth symbolized the unconscious psychological conflict that each child faces: the child's unconscious sexual attraction to, and wish to possess, the parent of the opposite sex; and the hostility toward, and desire to remove, the parent of the same sex; as well as subsequent guilt for these wishes. The conflict is resolved when the child identifies with the parent of the same sex.

Since these intense erotic and murderous impulses have no prospect of succeeding, children channel this emotional energy through the defense mechanisms of identification and introjection. As a result, children not only identify with the parent of the same sex but also incorporate into their own belief system the values and social standards of their parents and those of their culture and subculture.

LATENCY PERIOD (6 TO 12 YEARS). After the phallic stage, the child enters school and begins what Freud termed **latency.** This period, encompassing approximately 6 years between the phallic and genital stages, is marked by a tapering off of conscious biologic and sexual urges. The sexual impulses, which are unacceptable in their direct expression, are channeled and elevated into more culturally accepted levels of activity, such as sports, intellectual interests, and peer relations. Freud was relatively silent about the latency period. He did not consider it a genuine psychosexual stage but, rather, he viewed it as a period of transition and comparative sexual quiescence.

Today, Freud's view of latency has been questioned by most critics, who consider that a more accurate observation is that during this period children learn to hide their sexuality from disapproving adults.

GENITAL STAGE (12 YEARS OLD AND BEYOND). Freud's final stage is termed the **genital stage,** which emerges as adolescence with the onset of puberty, when the genital organs mature. The impulses of the pregenital period are narcissistic in character: i.e., the individual gains gratification from his or her own body. The child values other people

TABLE 2–2   *Freud's Psychosexual Stages of Development*

STAGE (AGE)	SOURCE OF SATISFACTION	PRIMARY CONFLICT	TASKS	DESIRED OUTCOMES	OTHER POSSIBLE PERSONALITY TRAITS
Oral (0–1 yr)	Mouth (sucking, biting, chewing)	Weaning	Mastery of gratification of oral needs; **beginning of ego development** (4–5 mo)	Trust in the environment develops with the realization that needs can be met	Fixation at the oral stage is associated with passivity, gullibility, and dependence; the use of sarcasm; and the development of orally focused habits (e.g., smoking, nail-biting)
Anal (1–3 yr)	Anal region (expulsion and retention of feces)	Toilet training	Beginning to gain a sense of control over instinctual drives; **learns to delay immediate gratification** to gain a future goal	Control over impulses	Fixation associated with anal retentiveness (stinginess, rigid thought patterns, obsessive-compulsive disorder) or anal expulsive character (messiness, destructiveness, cruelty)
Phallic (oedipal) (3–6 yr)	Genitals (masturbation)	Oedipus and Electra	Sexual identity with parent of same sex; **beginning of superego development**	Identification with parent of the same sex	Unresolved outcomes may result in difficulties with sexual identity and difficulties with authority figures
Latency (6–12 yr)	—	—	**Growth of ego functions** (social, intellectual, mechanical) and the ability to care about and relate to others outside the home (peers of the same sex)	The development of skills needed to cope with the environment	Fixations can result in difficulty in identifying with others and in developing social skills, resulting in a sense of inadequacy and inferiority
Genital (12 yr and beyond)	Genitals (sexual intercourse)	—	**Developing satisfying** sexual and emotional **relationships** with members of the opposite sex; **emancipation from parents—planning life goals** and gaining a strong **sense of personal identity**	The ability to be creative and find pleasure in "love and work"	Inability to negotiate this stage could result in difficulties in becoming emotionally and financially independent, lack of strong personal identity and future goals, and inability to form satisfying intimate relationships

Data from Gleitman, H. (1981). *Psychology*. New York: WW Norton.

because they satisfy his or her narcissistic pleasures. During adolescence, some of this self-love (narcissism) becomes redirected toward gratification involving genuine interaction with other people. Sexual attraction, socialization, group activities, vocational planning, and preparation for marrying and rearing a family begin to manifest themselves. By the end of adolescence, the person becomes transformed from what was originally a pleasure-seeking individual to a more reality-oriented, socialized adult.

According to Freud, a mature individual is one who has reached conventional genital sexuality; one who satisfies his or her needs in socially approved ways; and one who is able, in Freud's words, "to love and to work."

Although Freud differentiated five stages of personality growth, he did not assume that there were any sharp breaks or abrupt transitions in proceeding from one stage into another. The final organization of personality represents contributions from all stages.

Freud provides nursing with a framework for organizing behaviors into categories of experience (id, ego, superego) and evaluates to some degree how individuals function. The ego defenses are useful for categorizing defensive behavior. It should be noted that most defense mechanisms can be used in healthy as well as unhealthy ways. Having a system for categorizing defensive behaviors allows for assessment of maladaptive behaviors. The identification of defense mechanisms along with other nursing data provides nurses with important data in identifying overall objectives for further interactions.

Erikson's Psychosocial Stages of Development

Erik Erikson (1902–1994), an American psychoanalyst who was initially a follower of Freud, broadened Freud's theory of human development. **First,** Erikson stressed the role of the ego, or the rational part of the personality, whereas Freud had concentrated largely on the nonrational, instinctual parts of the personality (the id). **Second,** Erikson viewed the growing individual within the larger social setting of the family and its cultural heritage rather than in the more restricted triangle of mother-child-father. **Third,** Erikson's stages span the full life cycle, in contrast to Freudian theory, which views basic personality as established by 5 years of age. **Fourth,** Erikson differed from Freud in that he studied healthy personalities emphasizing strengths as well as weaknesses and pointing out that failures at one stage could be rectified by successes at later stages. The stages listed in Table 2–3 are the major stages

in the life cycle as described by Erikson. In summary, Erikson remolded Freud's psychosexual stages of development into eight psychosocial stages, from infancy to old age emphasizing the growth of individuals as they establish new ways of understanding and relating to themselves and their changing social world throughout the whole life cycle.

Erikson provides nursing with a developmental model that spans the entire life span. In working with all clients, nurses can assess difficulties with specific life tasks which, with other nursing data, help define potential interventions.

Sullivan's Interpersonal Theory

Harry Stack Sullivan (1892–1949), an American-born theorist in interpersonal psychiatry, used the Freudian framework early in his career. Later he developed a new concept of personality. Sullivan stopped trying to deal with what he considered unseen and private mental processes within the individual (Freud's intrapsychic processes) and began to focus on interpersonal processes that could be observed in a social framework. The basis of Sullivan's theory was the contention that personality can be observed and studied only when a person is actually behaving in relation to one or more other individuals. Thus, he defines personality as "the group of characteristic ways in which an individual relates to others" (Sullivan 1953). According to Sullivan, personality consists of behavior that can be observed.

Sullivan's theory is fundamentally one of needs and anxiety. Needs are defined as: (1) the need for satisfactions and (2) the need for security. **Satisfactions** refer to biologic needs, including sleep and rest, sexual fulfillment, food and drink, and physical closeness to other human beings. **Security** was used by Sullivan to refer to a state of well-being, belonging, and being accepted.

Anxiety and the Self-System

Anxiety is a key concept in Sullivan's interpersonal psychiatry that refers to any painful feeling or emotion. It comes from tension that arises from social insecurity or blocks to satisfaction (organic needs). According to Sullivan, there are a number of characteristics of anxiety. **First,** it is interpersonal in origin. Sullivan spoke of the "empathetic linkage" between the mothering one and the infant. For example, a mother's anxious feelings can be transmitted to a child. **Second,** anxiety can be described, and behaviors stemming from anxiety can be observed. The anxious person can tell how he or she feels, and behavior resulting from anxiety can be observed and studied. **Third,** individuals strive to reduce anxiety. For example, children learn that they can avoid anx-

TABLE 2–3   *Erikson's Eight Stages of Development*

APPROXIMATE AGE	DEVELOPMENTAL TASK	PSYCHOSOCIAL CRISIS	SUCCESSFUL RESOLUTION OF CRISIS	UNSUCCESSFUL RESOLUTION OF CRISIS
Infancy (0–1½ yr)	Attachment to mother, which lays foundations for later trust in others	Trust vs. mistrust	Sound basis for relating to other people; trust in people; faith and hope about environment and future	General difficulties relating to people effectively; suspicion; trust-fear conflict; fear of future
Early childhood (1½–3 yr)	Gaining some basic control of self and environment (e.g., toilet training, exploration)	Autonomy vs. shame and doubt	Sense of self-control and adequacy; will power	Independence-fear conflict; severe feelings of self-doubt
Late childhood (3–6 yr)	Becoming purposeful and directive	Initiative vs. guilt	Ability to initiate one's own activities; sense of purpose	Aggression-fear conflict; sense of inadequacy or guilt
School age (6–12 yr)	Developing social, physical, and school skills	Industry vs. inferiority	Competence; ability to work	Sense of inferiority; difficulty learning and working
Adolescence (12–20 yr)	Making transition from childhood to adulthood; developing sense of identity	Identity vs. role confusion	Sense of personal identity; fidelity	Confusion about who one is; identity submerged in relationships or group memberships
Early adulthood (20–35 yr)	Establishing intimate bonds of love and friendship	Intimacy vs. isolation	Ability to love deeply and commit oneself	Emotional isolation; egocentricity
Middle adulthood (35–65 yr)	Fulfilling life goals that involve family, career, and society; developing concerns that embrace future generations	Generativity vs. self-absorption	Ability to give and to care for others	Self-absorption; inability to grow as a person
Later years (65 yr to death)	Looking back over one's life and accepting its meaning	Integrity vs. despair	Sense of integrity and fulfillment; willingness to face death; wisdom	Dissatisfaction with life; denial of or despair over prospect of death

Data from Erikson, E. H. (1963). *Childhood and society.* New York: W. W. Norton; and Altrocchi, J. (1980). *Abnormal psychology* (p. 196). New York: Harcourt Brace Jovanovich.

iety that comes from punishment and the threat to their security by conforming to their parents' wishes.

Sullivan used the term **security operations** to describe those measures that the individual employs to reduce anxiety and enhance security. Collectively, all of the security operations an individual uses to defend him- or herself against anxiety and ensure self-esteem make up the **self-system**.

Sullivan identified three components of the self-system, which is based on the child's experiences with others early in life. These three components are:

1. **The good-me.** The good-me represents that part of the personality that develops in response to rewarding appraisals from others.
2. **The bad-me.** The bad-me develops in response to anxiety-producing appraisals from others. The child learns to avoid these feelings of discomfort and distress by altering certain behaviors.
3. **The not-me.** The not-me develops in response to overwhelming feelings of horror, dread, and loathing. In an effort to relieve anxiety, the child represses or dissociates these intense feelings. These feelings, now gone from awareness, become the not-me.

There are many parallels between Sullivan's notion of security operations and Freud's concept of defense mechanisms. Both are processes of which we are unaware, and both are ways in which we reduce anxiety. However, Freud's defense mechanism of repression is an **intrapsychic** activity, whereas Sullivan's security operations are **interpersonal** relationship activities that can be observed. Two examples of the observable manifestations of security operations are selective inattention, and dissociation.

SELECTIVE INATTENTION. Sullivan (1953) states that **selective inattention** refers to an individual who "doesn't happen to notice an almost infinite series of more-or-less meaningful details of one's living" that might cause anxiety. For example, a husband may not notice his wife's seductive behavior toward other men because it threatens his own self-esteem.

DISSOCIATION. Some things are so threatening to the security of the self that they cannot be faced by the individual. For example, abused children—needy, helpless, and dependent on the abusing parent—block out or dissociate themselves from the experience of hate or anger toward the parent. Such feelings are excluded from conscious awareness before they are able to trigger overwhelming and intolerable anxiety. Thus, **dissociation** is similar to the defense Freud referred to as repression.

Hildegard Peplau and Interpersonal Theory

Sullivan's interpersonal theory has had a great impact on the direction of nursing practice. Hildegard Peplau (1909–1999), influenced by the work of Sullivan and learning theory, developed the first systematic theoretical framework for psychiatric nursing in her groundbreaking book *Interpersonal Relations in Nursing* (1952). Peplau laid the foundation for the professional practice of psychiatric nursing and continued to enrich psychiatric nursing theory and the advancement of nursing practice.

Hildegard Peplau is internationally thought of as the mother of psychiatric nursing, a scholar, and a leader. Sills (2000) identifies Peplau's style of leadership as that of a teacher role modeler, and student of the data. She believes that knowledge changes behavior, that is, if people know more, they would act better or differently (Sills 2000).

Peplau spent a lifetime illuminating the science and art of professional nursing practice, which has had a profound effect on the nursing profession, nursing science, and the clinical practice of psychiatric nursing (Haber 1999). The art of nursing is the care, compassion and advocacy, and hands-on care that nurses provide to enhance comfort and well-being. "The art of communication (e.g., interviewing, problem solving, counseling, and health teaching) was positioned by Peplau (1952/1988) to highlight the importance of nursing intervention in facilitating achievement of quality patient outcomes, such as improved functioning, quality of life, relaxation, and self-understanding" (Haber 2000). The science component of nursing is knowledge applied for understanding a broad range of human problems and psychosocial phenomena (Haber 2000) and applying scientifically based knowledge and interventions to relieve clients' suffering and promote growth.

Peplau visualized nursing as a significant therapeutic and interpersonal process (Gauthier 2000). The crux of psychiatric nursing practice, which is caring, is central to the nurse-patient relationships. This one-to-one nurse-patient relationship has its power in our understanding of the interpersonal process as developed by Hildegard Peplau, drawing upon her work with H.S. Sullivan (Barker 1999).

Peplau (1952, 1988) described four phases of the interpersonal process (orientation, identification, working phase, and resolution). The idea of the interpersonal process between the nurse and the patient is basic to the therapeutic relationship and to Peplau's work. Peplau's influence on the practice of psychiatric nursing can be viewed by her expectations that the nurse patient relationship should have the following characteristics (Ryan 2000):

- The focus is on the patient
- The nurse uses participant observation rather than spectator observations
- The nurse has an awareness of role
- Nursing is primarily investigative
- The nurse will use theory (Peplau 1989a)

In her works Peplau constantly reminds nurses to look beyond the illness and to "care for the person as well as the illness" and "think exclusively of patients as persons" (Peplau 1995). Peplau's nurse-patient relationship and the phases of that relationship have been well documented, and are discussed further in Chapter 10.

Peplau's development of the one-to-one nursing relationship, the concept of therapeutic milieu, and her constant focus on the human experience of mental distress, are all basic to the process of psychiatric nursing (Barker 1999).

An important component of Peplau's work was derived from her use of process recordings, in which students described verbatim their interactions with patients. From these interactions, Peplau collected data about "phenomena" that go on between the nurse and the patient, as well as developed the art and science of interviewing (Ryan 2000). An example of a process recording is seen in Chapter 11 and a list of phenomena that psychiatric nurses address is explained further in Chapter 4.

Perhaps Peplau's most universal contribution to the everyday practice of psychiatric nursing is her application of Sullivan's theory of anxiety to the practice of nursing. She described the effects of different levels of anxiety (mild, moderate, severe, and panic levels) on perception and learning. She promoted interventions that would lower people's anxiety with the aim of improving the client's ability to think and to function at more satisfactory levels. More on the application of Peplau's theory of anxiety and interventions is discussed in Chapter 13. An excellent article by Church (2000) gives a well-researched and comprehensible overview of Peplau's achievement in the advancement of psychiatric nursing.

Piaget

Jean Piaget (1896–1980), after earning a doctorate in zoology in his homeland of Switzerland, went on to explore the field of psychology. Piaget believed that, just as other living organisms adapt to their environment biologically, so humans adapt to their environment **psychologically.** Piaget used the word **schema** to refer to categories that people form in their minds to organize and understand the world. At the beginning, the young child has only a few schemata with which to understand the world. Gradually, these are increased. Adults use a wide variety of schemata to comprehend the world.

Two complementary processes of adaptation help in the development of schemata: assimilation and accommodation. **Assimilation** refers to the ability to incorporate new ideas, objects, and experiences into the framework of one's thoughts. Through assimilation, the growing child will perceive and give mean-

TABLE 2–4 *Piaget's Stages of Cognitive Development*

PERIOD	CHARACTERISTIC OF THE PERIOD	MAJOR CHANGE OF THE PERIOD
Sensorimotor (0–2 yr)	Reflex activity only; no differentiation	
Stage 1 (0–1 mo)	Hand-mouth coordination; differentiation via sucking reflex	
Stage 2 (1–4 mo)	Hand-eye coordination; repeats unusual events	
Stage 3 (4–8 mo)	Hand-eye coordination; repeats unusual events	
Stage 4 (8–12 mo)	Coordination of two schemata; object performance attained	Development proceeds from reflex activity to representation and sensorimotor solutions to problems
Stage 5 (12–18 mo)	New means through experimentation—follows sequential displacements	
Stage 6 (18–24 mo)	Internal representation; new means through mental combinations	
Preoperational (2–7 yr)	Problems solved through representation; language development (2–4 yr); thought and language both egocentric; cannot solve conservation problems	Development proceeds from sensorimotor representation to prelogical thought and solutions to problems
Concrete operational (7–11 yr)	Reversibility attained; can solve conservation problems—logical operations developed and applied to concrete problems; cannot solve complex verbal problems	Development proceeds from prelogical thought to logical solutions to concrete problems
Formal operational (11 yr to adulthood)	Logically solves all types of problems—thinks scientifically; solves complex verbal problems; cognitive structures mature	Development proceeds from logical solutions to concrete problems to logical solutions to all classes of problems

From Wadsworth B.J. (1996). *Piaget's theory of cognitive and affective development.* (5th ed.). Needham Heights, MA: Allyn & Bacon. Reprinted/adapted by permission of Allyn & Bacon

ing to new information according to what is already known and understood. Assimilation is conservative, in that its main function is to make the unfamiliar familiar, to reduce the new to the old. In contrast, **accommodation** refers to the ability to change a schema in order to introduce new ideas, objects, or experiences. Whereas the process of assimilation molds the object or event to fit the child's existing frame of reference, accommodation changes the mental structure in order that new experiences may be added. These two processes are constantly working together to produce changes in the growing child's understanding of the world.

Children do not passively receive stimulation from the environment; they learn about the world through active encounters with it. The development of the child's thinking relies on changes made in the mental structure of the child as he or she interacts with the environment. The true measure of a child's intellectual growth depends on the ability to change old ways of thinking to solve new problems.

Piaget's Stages of Cognitive Development

The development of children's thinking progresses through a sequence of four major stages, each very different from the others: (1) the sensorimotor period (0 to 2 years), (2) the preoperational period (2 to 7 years), (3) the period of concrete operations (7 to 11 years), and (4) the period of formal operations (11 years to adulthood) (Table 2–4).

The sequence of these four stages and of the substages they comprise never varies; no stage is ever skipped, because each one further develops the preceding stage and lays the groundwork for the next. The stages are somewhat related to chronological age. As with all development, however, each individual reaches each stage according to his or her own timetable. For this reason—and also because there is considerable overlapping between the stages of retention, and some characteristics from preceding stages occur in those that follow—all age norms must be considered approximate.

Piaget's focus on cognitive development provides a broad base for cognitive intervention with people with negative self views. Refer to Table 2–5 to identify some ways to reframe dysfunctional thinking into more factual statements that can be positively acted upon.

Maslow

Abraham Maslow (1908–1970), one of the founders of humanistic psychology, introduced the concept of a "self-actualized personality," a better-than-merely-

TABLE 2–5   *Dysfunctional vs. Functional Thinking*

IRRATIONAL THOUGHTS THAT CAUSE DISTURBANCE	RATIONAL THOUGHTS THAT PROMOTE EMOTIONAL SELF-CONTROL
1. How *awful*.	This is disappointing.
2. I can't stand it.	I can put up with what I don't like.
3. I'm stupid.	What I *did* was stupid.
4. He stinks!	He's not perfect either.
5. This *shouldn't* have happened.	This should have happened because it did!
6. I am to be blamed.	I am at fault but am not to be blamed.
7. He has no right.	He has every right to follow his own mind though I wish he hadn't exercised that right!
8. I *need* him to do that.	I want/desire/prefer him to do that, but I don't have to have what I want.
9. Things *always* go wrong.	Sometimes—if not frequently—things will go wrong.
10. *Every time* I try I fail.	Sometimes—even often—I may fail.
11. Things *never* work out.	More often than I would like, things don't work out.
12. This is bigger than life.	This is an important part of my life.
13. This *should* be easier.	I wish this was easier, but often things that are good for me aren't—no gain without pain. Tough, too bad!
14. I *should* have done better.	I would have *preferred* to do better, but I did what I could at the time.
15. I am a failure.	I'm a person who sometimes fails.

From Bernard, M. E., and Wolfe, J. L. (Eds.). (1993). *The RET resource book for practitioners.* New York: Institute for Rational-Emotive Therapy.

normal personality, associated with high productivity and enjoyment of life (Maslow 1970). He believed that psychology has been too concerned with humanity's frailties, and not enough with its strengths—that in the process of exploring our sins we had neglected our virtues. Where is the psychology, Maslow asks, that takes into account such experiences as love, compassion, gaiety, exhilaration, and well-being to the same extent that it deals with hate, pain, misery, guilt, and conflict? Maslow has undertaken to supply the other half of the picture, the brighter, better half, and to round out a portrait of the whole person.

Maslow offers a theory of human motivation that assumes people to have a hierarchy of needs. He proposes that each person has five **basic needs,** which are arranged in hierarchical order. Maslow describes basic needs as physiological (food, drink) and psychological (security, love, esteem), and **meta-needs** as higher-level needs (desire to know, the appreciation of truth and beauty, and the tendency toward growth and fulfillment—qualities that define **self-actualization**).

Our needs are hierarchically arranged, says Maslow, in the sense that the metaneeds will not be attended to unless the basic needs have been reasonably well satisfied; that is, we pay attention to beauty, truth, and the development of our potential when we are no longer hungry or feel unloved.

Maslow made intensive clinical investigations of people who are, or were, in the truest sense of the word, self-actualizing; that is, they move in the direction of achieving and reaching their highest potentials. People of this sort are rare, as Maslow discovered when he was selecting his group. Some were historical figures (Lincoln, Jefferson, Harriet Tubman, Walt Whitman, Beethoven, William James, F. D. Roosevelt), while others were living at the time they were studied (Einstein, Eleanor Roosevelt, Albert Schweitzer, along with some personal acquaintances of the investigator). Upon studying healthy, self-actualizing individuals, Maslow was able to sort out some basic personality characteristics that distinguished them from what might be called ordinary people. This is not to suggest that each person he studied reflected all of these characteristics, but each did exhibit a greater number of these characteristics and in more different ways than might be expected in a less self-actualized person. Maslow (1962, 1970) identified some characteristics of the self-actualized person (SA) (Box 2–1).

Maslow's beliefs about humankind included that:

1. Humans are neither inherently good nor evil. We are born basically neutral, with a capacity for both good and evil. All of us have inherent drives toward self-actualization as well as drives

BOX 2–1 *Some Characteristics of Self-Actualized Persons*

1. Perceive reality accurately. Not defensive in their perceptions of the world.
2. An acceptance of themselves, others, and nature. The AA Serenity prayer. Acceptance not the same as happiness.
3. Spontaneity, simplicity, and naturalness. Do not live programmed lives.
4. Problem-centered rather than self-centered. Possibly the most important characteristic. SAs have a sense of mission to which they dedicate their lives.
5. Like privacy and detachment. Enjoy being alone; can reflect on events.
6. Freshness of appreciation. Don't take life for granted.
7. Mystic or peak experiences. A peak experience is a moment of intense ecstasy, similar to a religious or mystical experience, during which the self is transcended. More currently, Mihaly Csikzentmihalyi developed the term "flow experience" to describe times when people become so totally involved in what they are doing that they forget all sense of time and awareness of self.
8. Active social interest.
9. An unhostile sense of humor.
10. Democratic character structure. SAs display little racial, religious, or social prejudice.
11. Creative, especially in managing their lives.
12. Resistance to conformity (enculturation)—SAs are autonomous, independent, and self-sufficient.

From Maslow A. H. (1970). *Motivation and personality,* 2/e. New York: Harper & Row.

toward more regressive behaviors. Which direction an individual takes is a matter of choice. The choices of course can be influenced by interpersonal and social events.

"Basic human needs can be filled *only* by and through other human beings, e.g., society. The need for community (belongingness, contact, and groupiness) is itself a basic need. Loneliness, isolation, ostracism, rejection by the group—these are not only painful but pathogenic as well . . . Humanness and specieshood in the infant are only a potentiality and must be actualized by the society." (Maslow 1970b)

2. A person does the very best he or she can at the time.
3. When adequate information is given in a form that the person can use, a person will make a good decision for him- or herself.

"Yes, man is in a way his own project and he does make himself. But there are limits upon which what he can make himself into." (Maslow 1970b)

4. Man has a higher and transcendent nature, and this is part of his essence, for example, his biological nature as a member of a species that has evolved.

"The great lesson from the true mystics, from the Zen monks, and now also the—Humanistic and Transpersonal psychologists—that the sacred is *in* the ordinary, that it is to be found in one's daily life, in one's neighbors, friends, and family, in one's back yard, and that travel may be *flight* from confronting the sacred—this lesson can be easily lost. To be looking elsewhere for miracles is to me a sure sign of ignorance that *everything* is miraculous." (Maslow 1970b)

Critics have attacked Maslow's description on the grounds that it is based on his own choice of subjects and that it reflects the characteristics he himself admired. In any case, Maslow set a precedent for other attempts to define a healthy personality as something more than personality without disorder.

Maslow's positive view of human potential and inherent potential for dynamic personal growth provides nurses with a framework for holistic intervention. People have strengths, and potential for positive growth is always possible when people choose it. Maslow's view of humankind is uplifting.

Kohlberg

The provocative view of moral development in recent years was crafted by Lawrence Kohlberg (1958, 1976, 1986). He studied moral development by using the concept of a progression of stages that Piaget worked out in relation to cognitive development (Table 2–6). In the interviews with children Kohlberg presented them with a series of stories in which characters face moral dilemmas. The following is the most popular of the Kohlberg dilemmas:

In Europe a woman was near death from a special kind of cancer. There was one drug that the doctors thought might save her. It was a form of radium that a druggist was charging ten times what the drug cost him to make. He paid $200 for the radium and charged $2000 for a small dose of the drug. The sick woman's husband, Heinz, went to everyone he knew to borrow the money, but he could only get together $1000, which is half of what it cost. He told the druggist that his wife was dying and asked him to sell it cheaper or let him pay later. But the druggist said, "No, I discovered the drug, and I am going to make money from it." So Heinz got desperate and broke into the man's store to steal the drug for his wife. (Kohlberg 1969, p. 379)

After reading the story, interviewees answer a series of questions about the moral dilemma. Should Heinz have stolen the drug? Was stealing it right or wrong? Why? Is it a husband's duty to steal the drug for his wife if he can get it no other way? Would a good husband steal? Did the druggist have the right to charge that much when there was no law setting a limit on the price? Why?

On the basis of the answers interviewees gave for this and other moral dilemmas, Kohlberg concluded that three levels of moral development exist, each of which is characterized by two stages. A key concept in understanding moral development, especially for Kohlberg's theory, is **internalization**, the developmental change from behavior that is externally controlled to behavior that is controlled by internal, self-generated standards and principles. As children develop, their moral thoughts become more internalized.

Kohlberg believed that certain types of parent-child experiences can induce the child to think at more advanced levels of moral thinking. In particular, parents who allow or encourage conversation about value-laden issues promote more advanced moral thought in their children; however, many parents do not systematically provide their children with such perspective-taking opportunities. Nonetheless, in one study, children's moral development was related to their parents' discussion style, which involved questioning and supportive interaction (Walker and Taylor 1991). There is an increasing emphasis on the role of parenting in moral development (Eisenberg and Murphy 1995).

Kohlberg's theory has been criticized for placing too much emphasis on moral thought and not enough on moral behavior. Moral reasons can sometimes be a shelter for immoral behavior. For example, bank embezzlers and presidents may endorse the loftiest of moral virtues when commenting about moral dilemmas, but their own behavior may be immoral. No one wants a nation of cheaters and thieves who can reason at the postconventional level. The cheaters and thieves may know what is right, yet still do what is wrong.

Another critique of Kohlberg's theory of development comes from Gilligan (1982, 1990, 1991, 1992), who believes that Kohlberg's theory does not adequately reflect relationships and concern for others. In extensive interviews with girls 6 to 18 years of age, Gilligan and her colleagues found that girls consistently interpret moral dilemmas in terms of human relationships and base these interpretations on listening and watching other people (Gilligan 1990, 1992). Gilligan called this a care perspective specific to females and different from Kohlberg's findings with male subjects.

According to Gilligan, girls have the ability to

sensitively pick up different rhythms in relationships and can often follow the pathways of feelings. She believes that girls reach a critical juncture in their development when they reach adolescence. Usually around 11 to 12 years of age, girls become aware that their intense interest in intimacy is not prized by the male-dominated culture, even though society values women as caring and altruistic. The dilemma is that girls are presented with a choice that makes them look either selfish or selfless. Gilligan believes that, as adolescent girls experience this dilemma, they increasingly silence their distinctive voice.

Kohlberg offers nurses a very thoughtful framework for evaluating moral decisions and understanding the thinking of others regarding moral issues. Moral and immoral, right and wrong, can be viewed from a person's immediate situation and level of moral development.

TRADITIONAL THERAPEUTIC APPROACHES

Those therapies that have proven effective for the treatment of specific mental disorders will be addressed at length in the appropriate clinical chapters.

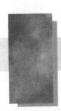

TABLE 2–6 *Kohlberg's Six Stages of Moral Reasoning*

LEVELS	STAGES OF REASONING	TYPICAL ANSWERS TO HEINZ'S DILEMMA
Level I: Preconventional (ages 4–10) Emphasis in this level is on external control. The standards are those of others, and they are observed either to avoid punishment or to reap rewards.	*Stage 1: Orientation toward punishment and obedience.* "What will happen to me?" Children obey the rules of others to avoid punishment. They ignore the motives of an act and focus on its physical form (such as the size of a lie) or its consequences (e.g., the amount of physical damage).	*Pro:* "He should steal the drug. It isn't really bad to take it. It isn't as if he hadn't asked to pay for it first. The drug he'd take is worth only $200; he's not really taking a $2000 drug." *Con:* "He shouldn't steal the drug. It's a big crime. He didn't get permission; he used force and broke and entered. He did a lot of damage, stealing a very expensive drug and breaking into the store, too."
	Stage 2: Instrumental purpose and exchange. "You scratch my back, I'll scratch yours." Children conform to rules out of self-interest and consideration for what others can do for them in return. They look at an act in terms of the human needs it meets, and differentiate this value from the act's physical form and consequences.	*Pro:* "It's all right to steal the drug because his wife needs it, and he wants her to live. It isn't that we want to steal, but that's what he has to do to get the drug to save her." *Con:* "He shouldn't steal it. The druggist isn't wrong or bad; he just wants to make a profit. That's what you're in business for—to make money."
Level II: Morality of conventional role conformity (ages 10–13) Children now want to please other people. They still observe the standards of others, but they have internalized these standards to some extent. Now they want to be considered "good" by those persons whose opinions are important to them. They are now able to take the roles of authority figures well enough to decide whether an action is good by their standards.	*Stage 3: Maintaining mutual relations, approval of others, the golden rule.* "Am I a good boy or girl?" Children want to please and help others, can judge the intentions of others, and develop their own ideas of what a good person is. They evaluate an act according to the motive behind it or the person performing it, and they can take circumstances into account.	*Pro:* "He should steal the drug. He is only doing something that is natural for a good husband to do. You can't blame him for doing something out of love for his wife. You'd blame him if he didn't love his wife enough to save her." *Con:* "He shouldn't steal. If his wife dies, he can't be blamed. It isn't because he's heartless or that he doesn't love her enough to do everything that he legally can. The druggist is the selfish or heartless one."

TABLE 2–6 *Kohlberg's Six Stages of Moral Reasoning* (Continued)

LEVELS	STAGES OF REASONING	TYPICAL ANSWERS TO HEINZ'S DILEMMA
	Stage 4: Social concern and conscience. "What if everybody did it?" People are concerned with doing their duty, showing respect for high authority, and maintaining the social order. They consider an act always wrong, regardless of motive or circumstances, if it violates a rule and harms others.	*Pro:* "You should steal the drug. If you did nothing, you'd be letting your wife die. It's your responsibility if she dies. You have to take it with the idea of paying the druggist." *Con:* "It's a natural thing for Heinz to want to save his wife, but it's still always wrong to steal. He knows that he is stealing and taking a valuable drug from the man who made it."
Level III: Morality of autonomous moral principles (age 13, or not until young adulthood, or never) This level marks the attainment of true morality. For the first time, the person acknowledges the possibility of conflict between two socially accepted standards and tries to decide between them. The control of conduct is now internal, both in the standards observed and in the reasoning about right and wrong. Stages 5 and 6 may be alternative methods of the highest level of moral reasoning.	*Stage 5: Morality of contract, of individual rights, and of democratically accepted law.* People think in rational terms, valuing the will of the majority and the welfare of society. They generally see these values best supported by adherence to the law. While they recognize that there are times when human need and the law conflict, they believe that it is better for society in the long run if they obey the law. *Stage 6: Morality of universal ethical principles.* People do what they as individuals think is right, regardless of legal restrictions or the opinions of others. They act in accordance with internalized standards, knowing that they would condemn themselves if they did not.	*Pro:* "The law wasn't set up for these circumstances. Taking the drug in this situation isn't really a right, but it's justified." *Con:* "You can't completely blame someone for stealing, but extreme circumstances don't really justify taking the law into your own hands. You can't have people stealing whenever they are desperate. The end may be good, but the ends don't justify the means." *Pro:* "This is a situation that forces him to choose between stealing and letting his wife die. In a situation where the choice must be made, it is morally right to steal. He has to act in terms of the principle of preserving and respecting life." *Con:* "Heinz is faced with a decision of whether to consider the other people who need the drug just as badly as his wife. Heinz ought to act not according to his particular feelings toward his wife, but considering the value of all the lives involved."

Adapted from Kohlberg L. (1969). Stage and sequence: The cognitive-developmental approach to socialization. In D. A. Guslin (Ed.), *Handbook of Socialization Theory and Research.* Chicago: Rand McNally; and Kohlberg L. (1976). Moral stages and moralization: The cognitive developmental approach. In T. Lickona (Ed.), *Moral Development and Behavior.* New York: Holt, Rinehart, and Winston.

Classical Psychoanalysis

Classical psychoanalysis is perhaps the least prevalent approach to therapy today, for many reasons: (1) it is extremely expensive, (2) it takes years and years, and (3) Freud's original premise that all mental illness is caused by early intrapsychic conflict is no longer thought to be valid.

In classical analysis the client lies on a couch while the analyst sits behind the client and out of view. The client is instructed to verbalize whatever comes to mind, that is, to free associate. A positive transference is developed in which the client experiences feelings toward the analyst originally held toward significant others in his or her life. The analyst gently assists the client in exploring these emotion-loaded areas by pointing out and interpreting the resistance in an effort to weaken the client's defenses and bring repressed conflicts into the open. The client re-experiences crucial episodes from childhood, including both insufficiently resolved traumatic events and (more important) inadequately resolved interpersonal relationships. The analyst's stance enables the client to work through these situations to a more satisfactory conclusion. Finally, the analyst assists the client in converting newly won insights into everyday existence and behavior.

Countertransference is the health care worker's

unconscious and personal response to the client and can be an important part of any relationship. Countertransference can be intense and enduring. It can appear as a reaction to the client's conscious or unconscious feelings and behaviors, and when countertransference goes unrecognized, it can hinder a therapeutic relationship. Refer to Chapter 10 for more on countertransference and the nurse-client relationship.

Psychodynamic/Psychoanalytic Psychotherapy

The **psychoanalytic model of psychotherapy** uses many of the tools of psychoanalysis, such as free association, dream analysis, transference, and countertransference, but the therapist is much more involved and interacts with the client more freely. Psychodynamic psychotherapy is oriented more to the here and now and there is less of an attempt to reconstruct the developmental origins of conflicts (Ursano and Silburman 1999).

Clinical nurse specialists, psychiatric social workers, and psychologists with special training at the master's level or above may undertake psychodynamic psychotherapy with clients. The therapist works with the client to uncover unconscious material that appears in the form of symptoms or unsatisfactory life patterns. This is done through an intimate professional relationship between the therapist and the client over a period of months to years.

Within the environment of the managed care behavioral health system, a revolution in treatment modalities has been gradually taking place.

Short-Term Dynamic Psychotherapy

It was once assumed that clients would spend many months, even years, in psychotherapy. However, most dynamic therapies last fewer than ten sessions. One of many reasons for the short duration of therapy is the growing reluctance of insurance companies to cover more than perhaps 25 psychotherapy sessions in a given calendar year, along with their limits on the amount of reimbursement provided. The emergence of cognitive and behavioral therapies over the past 20 to 30 years has also played a role; these approaches focus on discrete problems and avoid long-term therapy.

Another strand in the history of short-term dynamic psychotherapy grew out of the need to provide short-term treatment for the posttraumatic stress disorder of returning veterans from World War II and Vietnam.

The best candidate for brief psychotherapy is the relatively healthy and well-functioning individual, with a clearly circumscribed area of difficulty, who is intelligent, psychologically minded, and well motivated for change. Psychotic, severely depressed, and borderline clients, as well as individuals with severe character disorders, are often not appropriate for this type of treatment. Supportive therapies are useful for these clients. You will be introduced to a variety of supportive therapies in chapters about specific disorders (Ch. 14–21).

At the start of treatment, client and therapist agree on what the focus will be and concentrate their work on the area of focus. Sessions are held weekly, and the total number of sessions to be held (anywhere from 12 to 40) is determined at the outset of therapy. There is a rapid, back-and-forth pattern between client and therapist, both participating actively. The therapist intervenes constantly to keep the therapy on track, either by redirecting the client's attention or by interpreting deviations from the focus to the client.

Brief therapies share the following common elements:

1. Assessment tends to be rapid and early.
2. It is made clear right away to the client that therapy will be limited and that improvement is expected within a small number of sessions.
3. Goals are concrete and focused on the amelioration of the client's worst symptoms, on helping the client understand what is going on in his or her life, and on enabling the client to cope better in the future.
4. Interpretations are directed toward present life circumstances and client behavior rather than on the historical significance of feelings.
5. Some positive transference to the therapist is fostered in an effort to encourage the client to follow the therapist's suggestions and advice.
6. There is a general understanding that psychotherapy does not cure, but that it can help troubled individuals learn to deal better with life's inevitable stressors.

Interpersonal Psychotherapy

Interpersonal psychotherapy (IPT) is an effective psychotherapeutic modality. It derives more from the school of psychiatry that originated with Adolph Meyer and Harry Stack Sullivan. The focus is on reassurance, clarification of feeling states, improvement in interpersonal communication, and improvement of interpersonal skills, rather than on personality reconstruction (Ursano and Silburman 1999). Interpersonal psychotherapy has been found to be successful in the treatment of depression, and it is predicated on the notion that disturbances in important interpersonal relationships (or a deficit in the capacity to form those relationships) can play a role in initiating or maintaining clinical depression. In IPT the therapist identifies the nature of the problem to be resolved, and then selects strategies that are consistent with that area. Four types of problem areas have been identified (Hollon and Engelhardt 1997):

1. **Grief:** defined as complicated bereavement following the death or loss of a loved one.
2. **Role disputes:** defined as conflicts with a significant other.
3. **Role transition:** defined as problematic change in life status or social or vocational role, and
4. **Interpersonal deficit:** defined as an inability to initiate or sustain close relationships.

More recently IPT has been studied with adolescents (IPT-A). IPT-A focuses on increasing youths' sense of competence and resistance to the stressful impact of life events. The effort to decrease stress and improve their sense of self can help adolescents with negotiating the developmental issues that are related to affective regulations, such as, grieving, interpersonal deficits, interpersonal role disputes, and role transitions (Myers and McCauley 1997).

Cognitive Theory and Therapy

Aaron Beck's (Beck et al. 1979) approach to therapy for people suffering from depression illustrates the major components of cognitive therapy. This is an active, directive, time-limited, structured approach used to treat a variety of psychiatric disorders (e.g., depression, anxiety, phobias, pain problems). It is based on an underlying theoretical rationale that individuals' affect and behavior are largely determined by the way in which they structure the world (Beck 1967, 1976). Their **cognitions** (verbal or pictorial events in their stream of consciousness) are based on **schemata** (attitudes or assumptions) developed from previous experiences. For example, if a person interprets all experiences in terms of whether he or she is competent and adequate, thinking may be dominated by the schema "Unless I do everything perfectly, I'm a failure." Consequently, the person reacts to situations in terms of adequacy even when they are unrelated to whether he or she is personally competent. Albert Ellis (b. 1913), founder of rational emotive behavioral therapy (REBT), calls these dysfunctional thoughts irrational beliefs. Refer back to Table 2–5 for common dysfunctional or irrational thoughts or beliefs that many people are influenced by.

The therapeutic techniques of the cognitive therapist are designed to identify, reality-test, and correct distorted conceptualizations and the dysfunctional beliefs (schemata) underlying these cognitions. The cognitive therapist helps clients to think and act more realistically and adaptively about their psychological problems, and thus to reduce symptoms.

A variety of cognitive and behavioral strategies are utilized in cognitive therapy. For example, the depressed person's tendency to feel responsible for negative outcomes while consistently failing to take credit for their own success is identified and discussed. The therapy focuses on specific "target symptoms" (e.g., suicidal impulses). The cognitions supporting these symptoms are identified ("My life is worthless and I can't change it") and then subjected to logical and empirical investigation.

In cognitive therapy the client begins to incorporate many of the therapeutic techniques of the therapist. For example, clients frequently find themselves spontaneously assuming the role of the therapist in questioning some of their conclusions or predictions. Some examples of self-questioning are: What is the evidence for my conclusion? Are there other explanations? How serious is the loss? How much does it actually subtract from my life? What is the degree of harm to me if a stranger thinks badly of me? What will I lose if I try to be more assertive? Such self-questioning plays a major role in the generalization of cognitive techniques from the interview to external situations. Without such questioning, the depressed individual is pretty much bound by stereotyped automatic patterns, a phenomenon labeled "thoughtless thinking."

In contrast to those employing more traditional psychotherapies such as psychoanalytic therapy, the therapist applying cognitive therapy is continuously active and deliberately interacting with clients, exploring their psychological experiences, setting up schedules of activities, and making homework assignments. Unlike psychoanalytic therapy, the content of cognitive therapy is focused on "here and now" problems. Little attention is paid to childhood recollections except to clarify present observations. The major thrust is toward investigating clients' thinking and feeling during the therapy session and between the sessions. Interpretations of unconscious factors are not made.

Cognitive therapy contrasts with behavioral therapy in its greater emphasis on clients' internal (mental) experiences such as thoughts, feelings, wishes, daydreams, and attitudes. The overall strategy of cognitive therapy may be differentiated from the other schools of therapy by its emphasis on the empirical investigation of clients' automatic thoughts, inferences, conclusions, and assumptions. Clients' dysfunctional ideas and beliefs about themselves, their experience, and their future are formulated into hypotheses, and an attempt is made to test the validity of these hypotheses in a systematic way. Thus, almost every experience may provoke an opportunity for an experiment relevant to clients' negative views or beliefs. If clients believe, for example, that everybody they meet turns away from them in disgust, they are helped to set up a system for judging other people's reactions, and are motivated to make objective assignments of the facial expression and bodily movements of other people. Alternatively, for example, if clients believe that they are incapable of carrying out simple hygienic procedures, the therapist may jointly with the client de-

vise a checklist or graph that clients can use to record the degree of success in carrying out these activities.

The therapist's major task is to help the client think of reasonable responses to negative cognitions. The therapist's goal is to increase the client's objectivity about cognitions, unpleasant affect, and unproductive behavior and (most important) to differentiate between a realistic accounting of events and an accounting distorted by idiosyncratic meanings. The following is an example of this behavioral technique.

A 24-year-old nurse recently discharged from the hospital for severe depression presented this record (Beck et al. 1979):

EVENT	FEELING	COGNITIONS	OTHER POSSIBLE INTERPRETATIONS
While at a party, Jim asked me, "How are you feeling?" shortly after I was discharged from the hospital.	Anxious	Jim thinks I am a basket case. I must really look bad for him to be concerned.	He really cares about me. He noticed that I look better than before I went into the hospital and wants to know if I feel better too.

TABLE 2–7 *Comparison of Psychoanalytic, Interpersonal, and Cognitive Psychotherapies*

	PSYCHODYNAMIC/ PSYCHOANALYTIC PSYCHOTHERAPY	INTERPERSONAL PSYCHOTHERAPY	COGNITIVE PSYCHOTHERAPY
Treatment focus	Internal experience	Interpersonal relationships and social supports	Thoughts/cognitions
Primary diagnosis treated	Anxiety Depression Personality disorders	Depression Anxiety	Depression Anxiety
Skills needed by therapist	+ + + +	+ + + +	+ + + +
Therapeutic alliance	+ + + +	+ + + +	+ + + +
Nonjudgmental stance	+ + + +	+ + + +	+ + + +
Focus			
Cognitive	+ + + (defense mechanisms)	+	+ + + + (cognitive distortions)
Interpersonal	+ + + + (transference and past relationships)	+ + + + (interpersonal withdrawal, attachment and models)	+
Technique: Nondirective	+ + + +	+	+
Directive (interventions)	+	+ + + +	+ + + +

Note: Plus signs indicate degree, from small (+) to great (+ + + +).

From Ursano, R. J., and Norwood, A. E. (1999). Brief psychotherapy. In B. J. Sadock and V. A. Sadock (Eds.), *Kaplan & Sadock's comprehensive textbook of psychiatry* (7th ed.) (p. 168). Philadelphia: Williams & Wilkins.

Refer to Box 2–2 for an example of cognitive therapy and see Table 2–7, which compares and contrasts basic differences between psychodynamic psychotherapy, interpersonal psychotherapy, and cognitive psychotherapies.

Behavioral Theory and Therapy

Behavioral therapists work on the assumption that changes in maladapted behavior can occur without insight into the underlying cause. Behavioral therapy is based on learning theory. The basic premise of behavioral theory is that behavioral responses are learned and can be modified in a particular environment. Ivan Pavlov's (1849–1936) **classic conditioning** developed from his early work with dogs. He found that when a stimulus (e.g., bell) was repeatedly paired with another stimulus (food triggering salivation), eventually just the sound of the bell alone could elicit the salivation in the dogs (concept of stimulus and response). James Watson (1878–1958) placed emphasis on the role of social environment in shaping behavior. B.F. Skinner (1904–1990) added the behavioral theory base by introducing the concept of operant conditioning. Skinner added principles of learning that included motivation and

BOX 2–2 *Example of Cognitive Therapy*

The client was an attractive woman in her early twenties. Her depression of 18 months' duration was precipitated by her boyfriend's leaving her. She had numerous automatic thoughts that she was ugly and undesirable. These automatic thoughts were handled in the following manner.

Therapist: Other than your subjective opinion, what evidence do you have that you are ugly?

Client: Well, my sister always said I was ugly.

Therapist: Was she always right in these matters?

Client: No. Actually, she had her own reasons for telling me this. But the real reason I know I'm ugly is that men don't ask me out. If I weren't ugly, I'd be dating now.

Therapist: That is a possible reason why you're not dating. But there's an alternative explanation. You told me that you work in an office by yourself all day and spend your nights alone at home. It doesn't seem like you're giving yourself opportunities to meet men.

Client: I can see what you're saying, but still, if I weren't ugly, men would ask me out.

Therapist: I suggest we run an experiment: that is, for you to become more socially active, stop turning down invitations to parties and social events, and see what happens.

After the client became more active and had more opportunities to meet men, she started to date. At this point, she no longer believed she was ugly.

Therapy then focused on her basic assumption that one's worth is determined by one's appearance. She readily agreed this didn't make sense. She also saw the falseness of the assumption that one must be beautiful in order to attract men or be loved. This discussion led to her basic assumption that she could not be happy without love (or attention from men). The latter part of treatment focused on helping her to change this belief.

Therapist: On what do you base this belief that you can't be happy without a man?

Client: I was really depressed for a year and a half when I didn't have a man.

Therapist: Is there another reason why you were depressed?

Client: As we discussed, I was looking at everything in a distorted way. But I still don't know if I could be happy if no one was interested in me.

Therapist: I don't know either. Is there a way we could find out?

Client: Well, as an experiment I could not go out on dates for a while and see how I feel.

Therapist: I think that's a good idea. Although it has its flaws, the experimental method is still the best way currently available to discover the facts. You're fortunate in being able to run this type of experiment. Now, for the first time in your adult life you aren't attached to a man. If you find you can be happy without a man, this will greatly strengthen you and also make your future relationships all the better.

In this case, the client was able to stick to a "cold turkey" regimen. After a brief period of dysphoria, she was delighted to find that her well-being was not dependent on another person.

There were similarities between these two interventions. In both, the distorted conclusion or assumption was delineated and the client was asked for evidence to support it. An experiment to gather data was also suggested in both instances. However, in order to achieve the results, a contrasting version of the same experimental situation was required.

From Beck, A., et al. (1979). *Cognitive theory of depression.* New York: Guilford Press.

social reinforcement. Operant conditioning refers to the use of specific "reinforcers" to elicit desired behavior. The best known learning principle contributed by operant conditioning is the principle of **positive reinforcement**—the process by which certain consequences of behavior raise the probability that the behavior will occur again (Agras and Berkowitz 1999).

This theory works best when it is directed at specific problems and the goals are well defined. Behavioral therapy is effective in people with agoraphobia (graded exposure and flooding) and other phobias (desensitization), alcoholism (aversion therapy), schizophrenia (token economy), and many other conditions. Classical conditioning has played a prominent role in the way clinical disorders have been conceptualized and generated a variety of treatments. It plays a role in contemporary behavior therapy that has become more eclectic and theoretically broader than it was during its early origins (Agras and Berkowitz 1999).

Four types of **behavioral therapy** are discussed here: (1) modeling, (2) operant conditioning, (3) systematic desensitization, and (4) aversion therapy.

Modeling

In **modeling** the therapist provides a role model for specific identified behaviors, and the client learns through imitation. The therapist may do the modeling, provide another person to model the behaviors, or present a video for the purpose. Bandura and colleagues (1969) were able to help people reduce their phobias about nonpoisonous snakes by having them view both live and filmed close and successful confrontations between people and snakes. In an analogous fashion, some behavior therapists use role playing in the consulting room. They demonstrate to clients patterns of behaving that might prove more effective than those the clients usually engage in, and then have the clients practice them. For example, a student who does not know how to ask a professor for an extension on a term paper would watch the therapist portray a potentially effective way of making the request. The clinician would then help the student practice the new skill in a similar role-playing situation.

Operant Conditioning

Operant conditioning entails rewarding a person for desired behaviors and is the basis for **behavior modification**. In behavior modification, someone sets a specific behavior goal and then systematically reinforces the subject's successive approximations to it. Called **positive reinforcement,** it is thought to be

one of the best ways to increase desired behaviors. For example, when desired goals are achieved or behaviors are performed, clients are rewarded with "tokens." These tokens can be exchanged for food, small luxuries, or privileges. This reward system is known as **token economy**.

Operant conditioning has been useful in improving verbal behaviors of mute, autistic, and developmentally disabled children. In clients with severe and persistent mental illness, behavior modification has helped to increase levels of self-care, social behavior, attendance in group activities, and more.

We use positive reinforcement all the time in everyday life, whether we know it or not. Reinforcers can increase, decrease, or maintain a behavior. Here is an example of three ways in which behavior can be reinforced (Aldinger 1992). A mother takes her son to the market. The child starts acting out, wanting this and that, nagging, crying, and yelling:

ACTION	RESULT
1. The mother gives the child what he wants.	The child continues to use this behavior. This is positive reinforcement of negative behavior.
2. The mother scolds the child.	Acting out may continue because the child gets what he or she really wants—attention. This positively rewards negative behavior.
3. The mother ignores the acting out but gives attention to the child when he is acting appropriately.	The child gets a positive reward for appropriate behavior.

Systematic Desensitization

Systematic desensitization is another form of behavior modification therapy. For example, a client who has a fear of a particular situation or object (a phobia) will be introduced to short periods of exposure to the phobic object or situation while in a relaxed state. Gradually, over a period of time, exposure is increased until the anxiety about or fear of the object or situation has ceased. This is a common treatment for a variety of phobias (e.g., school phobia, fear of flying, fear of closed spaces).

Aversion Therapy

Aversive conditioning, or *negative reinforcement*, is another technique used to change behavior. In aversive conditioning, a stimulus attractive to the client is paired with an unpleasant event, such as shock to the fingertips, in hopes of endowing it with negative properties. One example of the use of aversion therapy is with people who have drinking problems. Each time the person takes a drink, he or she is given antabuse or an emetic. Over time, it is hoped that the taking of a drink will be associated with an unpleasant experience, which will eventually override the desire for a drink.

Biofeedback, which is also a form of behavioral therapy successfully used today, especially for controlling the body's physiological response to stress and anxiety, is discussed in Chapter 12.

Refer to Box 2–3 for an example of behavior therapy.

Milieu Therapy

In 1948, Bruno Bettelheim coined the term milieu therapy to describe his use of the total environment to treat disturbed children. Bettelheim created a comfortable, secure environment (or milieu) in which psychotic children were helped to form a new world. Staff members were trained to provide 24-hour support and understanding for each child on an individual basis. It was Bettelheim's goal "to create for (each child) a world that is totally different from the one he abandoned in despair, and moreover a world he can enter right now" (Bettelheim 1967). In 1953, Maxwell Jones wrote a book in Great Britain, *The Therapeutic Community*, that laid the

BOX 2–3   *Example of Behavior Therapy*

A 30-year-old married woman, mother of three boys, presented a complaint of anxiety and depression as a chronic state for several years. She became disheveled, hair and clothes in disarray, her walk a shuffling pace—all overt signs of psychomotor retardation.

An attempt was made to get details about the things that were disturbing her. She felt inadequate as a mother, and situations that involved making decisions concerning her three boys, ages 6, 5, and 2½, were distressing to her. In addition, she felt that her husband, to whom she had been married for 9 years, gave her no emotional support, constantly criticized her, and never gave her any positive advice, although he was quick to tell her about the things she did wrong.

The first interview was productive, primarily as an opportunity for her to unburden herself about the things she had not been able to talk about with anyone before, and it was felt by the therapist that an excellent working relationship had been established. It was possible to get some idea about the things that were distressing her, but more details were needed, because she reported being distressed all the time. So far, it was impossible to tell what situations made her feel either worse or better, so she was asked to do some homework: to keep records about any upsetting events that occurred during the ensuing week. In addition, she was asked to fill out and bring in a Fear Survey Schedule.

When she came back the next time, she brought in her homework assignment. She said, "I went to a movie and I became very upset." Only upon closer questioning about what specifically was happening at the time she became distressed did it become apparent that the disturbing scene was one in which people

were drinking. The second thing she noted was that her husband would withdraw when they were talking about emotionally laden things, when what she really needed was for him to put his arms around her and give her some comfort. The third event she noted was that she was very sensitive to the fact that her husband had asked her to make an appointment with the dentist that he had not kept. She felt as though the dentist wouldn't think her trustworthy. In some way, she felt she would be seen by the dentist as being less of a person; he would be critical of her. The fourth area that she brought up was that anytime her children were engaged in fighting or disagreement, she became upset. The fifth observation was that sudden noises distressed her.

In subsequent sessions the therapist went over each of these situations with the client to further clarify them. *Assertiveness training* was begun using a hierarchical approach, by giving her the instruction that between that session and the next session she was to go up and greet anyone that she knew even slightly. A list of people from whom she feared criticism was obtained; these were graded in terms of how distressing each might be to her.

Relaxation training was begun at this point to prepare for *systematic desensitization* in the areas of criticism and rejection. In subsequent sessions the assignments in assertiveness training were continued, as she was carrying them out effectively.

At termination, the client no longer looked depressed. A one-year follow-up indicated that she was continuing to function fully, no longer experiencing depression, and on the whole enjoying life.

From Goldstein, A. (1978). Behavior therapy. In R. Corsini (Ed.), *Current psychotherapies* (2nd ed.) (pp. 239–245). Itasca, IL: F. E. Peacock. Reproduced by permission of the publisher, F. E. Peacock Publishers Inc.

groundwork for the movement in the United States toward a therapeutic milieu and the nurse's role in this therapy.

There are certain basic characteristics of milieu therapy, whether the setting involves psychotic children, clients in a psychiatric hospital, drug abusers in a residential treatment center, or psychiatric clients in a day hospital. Milieu therapy, or therapeutic community, has as its locus a living, learning, or working environment. Such therapy may be based on any number of therapeutic modalities, from structured behavioral therapy to spontaneous, humanistically oriented approaches.

The concept of milieu therapy has also been extended to halfway houses. Because some people function too well to remain in a mental hospital, and yet are unable to function independently enough to live on their own or even within their own families, halfway houses have been established. These are protected living units, typically located in large, formerly private residences. Here, clients discharged from a mental hospital live, take their meals, and gradually return to ordinary community life by holding a part-time job or going to school. Living arrangements may be relatively unstructured; some houses set up money-making enterprises that help to train and support the residents. Depending on how well funded the halfway house is, the staff may include psychiatrists or clinical psychologists. The most important staff members are paraprofessionals, often graduate students in clinical psychology or social work who live in the house and act both as administrators and as friends to the residents. Group meetings, at which residents talk out their frustrations and learn to relate to others in honest and constructive ways, are often part of the routine.

Actually, nurses are constantly involved with assessing and providing for safe and effective milieus for their clients. Common examples include providing a safe environment for the suicidal client or a client with a cognitive disorder (i.e., Alzheimer's disease), referring abused women to safe houses, and advocating for children suspected of being abused in their home environment. In a sense, milieu therapy is a basic intervention in their practice.

Fringe Therapies

All health care professionals need to be aware of "fringe" therapies that are not only *not* researched or found to be effective, but can be harmful, even fatal. The recent tragic death of a 10-year-old girl subjected to a type of therapy called "rebirthing" is a dramatic example (April 2001). Clients should be urged to check out the qualifications of a prospective therapist, as well as be assured that the type of therapy they are seeking has been proven successful for other people with like problems (e.g., depression, relationship difficulties, and anxiety).

SUMMARY

Sigmund Freud advanced the first theory of personality development, parts of which still influence the thinking of many mental health workers today. He articulated levels of awareness (unconscious, preconscious, conscious) and demonstrated the influence of our unconscious behavior on everyday life, as evidenced by the use of defense mechanisms. Freud identified three psychological processes of personality (id, ego, superego) and described how they operate and develop. He proposed one of the first modern developmental theories of personality based on five psychosexual stages of human growth from infancy to adulthood.

Erik Erikson viewed the growth of the individual in terms of social setting (family, community, and culture). He expanded on Freud's developmental stages to include middle age through old age. Erikson called his stages psychosocial and emphasized the social aspect of personality development.

Harry Stack Sullivan proposed the interpersonal theory of personality development, which focuses on interpersonal processes that can be observed in a social framework. Anxiety is a key concept in Sullivan's theory, and he described certain security operations people use to decrease anxiety (e.g., sublimation, selective inattention, and dissociation).

Hildegard Peplau was influenced by Sullivan's interpersonal theory. Peplau's theoretical framework in psychiatric nursing has become the foundation of psychiatric nursing practice and her whole life was devoted to the development of professionalism in psychiatric mental health nursing. Her many contributions that are today fundamental to nursing include the interpersonal process in the one-to-one therapeutic relationship, the levels of anxiety and effect on perception and learning, and the clinical interview.

Jean Piaget added to the understanding of personality development by identifying four cognitive stages in an individual's development: (1) the sensorimotor period, (2) the preoperational period, (3) the period of concrete operations, and (4) the period of formal operations. All stages follow this sequence, and each stage lays the groundwork for the next stage. Lawrence Kohlberg applied Piaget's concept of stage development to the study of moral development.

Abraham Maslow, the founder of humanistic psychology offered the theory of human motivation that is basic to all nursing education today. He also described the features of a self-actualized person that can be used as another yardstick to measure mental health.

Kohlberg's view of moral development is important for bringing another dimension to growth and development; however, there is some criticism concerning his need for cultural consideration and his emphasis on thought, not behavior.

Finally, five basic therapy approaches have been discussed: psychodynamic psychotherapy, short-term dynamic therapy, interpersonal therapy (IPT), cognitive-behavioral therapy, and behavior modification.

Visit the **Evolve** website at
http://evolve.elsevier.com/Varcarolis
for a post-test on the content in this chapter.

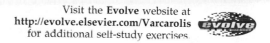

Visit the **Evolve** website at
http://evolve.elsevier.com/Varcarolis
for additional self-study exercises.

Critical Thinking and Chapter Review

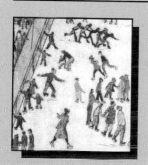

Critical Thinking

1. What influences can or do the theorists discussed in this chapter have on your practice of nursing?

   a. What defense mechanisms have you recognized in your clients and used in your assessment? (Freud)

   b. Are Erikson's psychosocial stages a sound basis for identifying disruptions in stages of development with some of your clients? Can you give a clinical example?

   c. What implications does Sullivan's self-system "good me, bad me, not me" have for your nursing assessment (e.g. client's strengths, appraisal of reality)?

   d. Which of Peplau's five expectations of the nurse-patient relationship is your strength. In which expectation do you plan to demonstrate self-growth?

   e. How does a theory of cognitive development (Piaget) lend itself to interventions with people who have negative self-views of themselves and their lack of hope for the future?

   f. Do you share any of Maslow's beliefs of humankind? If yes, how does it affect your understanding of clients and their behaviors?

   g. How would you have answered Kohlberg's dilemma presented in this chapter? Do you agree with him about where your answer would place you on his phases of moral dilemmas?

2. Which of the therapies described here do you think would be most helpful to you? What are the reasons you would choose this one over one of the other therapies discussed here?

Chapter Review

Choose the most appropriate answer.

1. Which of the following contributions to modern psychiatric nursing practice was not made by Freud?

1. Providing a framework for organizing behaviors into categories of experience.
    2. Providing a way of evaluating to some degree how individuals function.
    3. Providing a means for assessing and categorizing defensive behaviors.
    4. Providing a developmental model that includes the entire life span.

2. According to Piaget's theory of development, children progress from one stage to another

    1. in an orderly, invariant sequence.
    2. entirely on the basis of chronological age.
    3. when behavior is consistent with the final stage.
    4. when high levels of anxiety produce intrapsychic readiness.

3. The concepts at the heart of Sullivan's theory of personality are

    1. needs and anxiety.
    2. basic needs and metaneeds.
    3. schemata, assimilation and accommodation.
    4. developmental tasks and psychosocial crises.

4. The premise that an individual's behavior and affect are largely determined by the attitudes and assumptions one has developed about the world underlies

    1. modeling.
    2. milieu therapy.
    3. cognitive therapy.
    4. psychoanalytic psychotherapy.

5. Providing a safe environment for clients with impaired cognition, referring an abused spouse to a "safe house," and conducting a community meeting are nursing interventions that address aspects of

    1. milieu therapy.
    2. cognitive therapy.
    3. behavioral therapy.
    4. interpersonal psychotherapy.

REFERENCES

Addis, M.E. (1997). Brief psychotherapies. In D.L. Dunner (Ed.), *Current psychiatric therapy II*. Philadelphia: W.B. Saunders.

Agras, W. S., and Berkowitz, R.I. (1999). Behavior therapies. In R. E. Hales, S.C. Yadofsky, and J.A. Talbott (Eds.), *The American Psychiatric Press textbook of psychiatry*, (3rd ed.). Washington, DC: American Psychiatric Press.

Aldinger, B. (1992). Personal communication.

Bandura, A., Blahard, E.B., and Ritter, B. (1969). Relative efficacy of desensitization and modeling approaches for inducing behavioral, affective, and attitudinal changes. *Journal of Personality and Social Psychology*, 13:173–199.

Barker, P. (1999). *The philosophy and practice of psychiatric nursing*. London: Churchill Livingstone.

Beck, A. T. (1967). *Depression: Clinical, experimental and theoretical aspects*. New York: Harper & Row.

Beck, A. T. (1976). *Cognitive therapy and the emotional disorders*. New York: New American Library.

Beck, A. T., Rush, A. J., Shaw, B. F., and Emery, G. (1979). *Cognitive theory of depression*. New York: Guilford Press.

Bernard, M. E. (1991). *Using rational-emotive therapy effectively: A practitioner's guide*. New York: Plenum Press.

Bettelheim, B. (1967). *The empty fortress*. New York: Free Press.

Church, O. M. (2000). Hildegard E. Peplau's leadership and achievements in the advance of psychiatric nursing: The right person in the right time and place. *Journal of the American Psychiatric Nurses Association*, 6(l): 16–24.

Eisenberg, N., and Murphy, B. (1995). Parenting and children's moral development. In M. H. Bornstein (Ed.), *Children and parenting* (Vol. 4). Hillsdale, NJ: Erlbaum.

Gauthier, P. A. (2000). Use of Peplau's interpersonal relations model to counsel people with AIDS. *Journal of the American Psychiatric Nurses Association*, 6(4): 119–125.

Gilligan, C. (1982). *In a different voice*. Cambridge, MA: Harvard University Press.

Gilligan, C. (1990). Teaching Shakespeare's sister. In C. Gilligan, N. Lyons, and T. Hammer (Eds.), *Making connections: The relational worlds of adolescent girls at Emma Willard School*. Cambridge, MA: Harvard University Press.

Gilligan, C. (1991, April). How should "we" talk about development? Paper presented at the biennial meeting of the Society for Research in Child Development, Seattle.

Gilligan, C. (1992, May). Joining the resistance: Girls' development in adolescence. Paper presented at the Symposium on Development and Vulnerability in Close Relationships, Montreal.

Haber, J. (2000). Hildegard E. Peplau: The psychiatric nursing legacy of a legend. *Journal of the American Psychiatric Nurses Association*, 6(2):56–62.

Hollon, S.D., and Engelhardt, N. (1997). Review of psychosocial treatment of mood disorders. In D.L. Dunner (Ed.), *Current psychiatric therapy II*. Philadelphia: W.B. Saunders.

Jones, M. (1953). *The therapeutic community*. New York: Basic Books.

Kaplan, H. I., and Sadock, B. I. (Eds.). (1995). *Comprehensive textbook of psychiatry—VI* (6th ed.) (Vol. 2). Baltimore: Williams & Wilkins.

Kohlberg, L. (1958). *The development of modes of moral thinking and choice in the years 10 to 16*. Unpublished doctoral dissertation: University of Chicago.

Kohlberg, L. (1976). Moral stages and moralization: The cognitive developmental approach. In T. Lickona (Ed.), *Moral development and behavior*. New York: Holt, Rinehart and Winston.

Kohlberg, L. (1986). A current statement on some theoretical issues. In S. Modgil and C. Modgil (Eds.), *Lawrence Kohlberg*. Philadelphia: Palmer.

Kohlberg, L. (1969). Stage and sequence: The cognitive-developmental approach to socialization. In D. A. Guslin (Ed.), *Hand book of socialization theory and research*. Chicago: Rand McNally.

Maddi, S. R. (1972). *Personality theories: A comparative analysis* (Revised). Homewood, IL: Dorsey Press.

Maslow, A. H. (1970). *Motivation and personality* (2nd ed.). New York: Harper & Row.

Maslow, A. H. (1962). *Toward a psychology of living*. Princeton, N.J.: Van Nostrand.

Maslow A.H. (1964/1970). *Religions, values and peak experiences*. New York: The Viking Press Published by Penguin Books Limited.

Myers, K., and McCauley, E. (1997). Treatment of depressive disorders during adolescence. In D.L. Dunner (Ed.), *Current psychiatric therapy II*. Philadelphia: W.B.Saunders.

Peplau, H. E. (1952). *Interpersonal relations in nursing*. New York: G. P. Putnam's Sons.

Peplau, H.E. (1952/1988). *Interpersonal relations in nursing conceptual framework of reference for psychodynamic nursing*. New York: G.P. Putnam's Sons.

Peplau, H.E. (1986b). Theory: The professional dimension. Reprinted from *Proceedings of the First Nursing Theory Conference*, pp. 33–46. University of Kansas Medical Center, Department of Nursing Education, March 20–21, 1969. In A.W. O'Toole and S.R. Welt (Eds.) (1989). *Interpersonal theory in nursing practice: Selected works of Hildegard E. Peplau*. (p. 23). New York: Springer.

Peplau, H.E. (1995). Another look at schizophrenia from a nursing standpoint. In C.A. Anderson (Ed.), *Psychiatric nursing 1946–94: The state of the art*. St. Louis: Mosby Year Book.

Ryan, J.A., and Brooks, A.M.T. (2000). What effect has Dr. Peplau had on psychiatric nursing? *Journal of the American Psychiatric Nurses Association*, 6(l): 25–28.

Shapiro, T., and Hertzig, M.E. (1999). Normal child and adolescent development. In R. Hales, S.C. Yadofsky, and J.A. Talbott (Eds.). *The American Psychiatric Press textbook of psychiatry* (3rd ed.). Washington, D.C.: American Psychiatric Press.

Sills, G.M. (2000). Peplau and professionalism: The emergence of the paradigm of professionalism. *Journal of the American Psychiatric Nursing Association*, 6(1):29–34.

Snarey, J. (1987). A question of morality. *Psychology Today*, June:6–8.

Sullivan, H. S. (1953). *The interpersonal theory of psychiatry*. New York: W. Norton.

Ursano, R.J., and Norwood, A.E. (1999). Brief psychotherapy. In B.J. Sadock and V.A. Sadock (Eds.), *Kaplan & Sadock's comprehensive textbook of psychiatry* (7th ed.). Philadelphia: Williams & Wilkins.

Walker, L. J., de Vries, B., and Trevethan, S. D. (1987). Moral stages and moral orientation in real-life and hypothetical dilemmas. *Child Development*, 58:842–858.

Walker, L. J., and Taylor, J. H. (1991). Family interaction and the development of moral reasoning. *Child Development*, 62:264–283.

Yussen, S. R. (1977). Characteristics of moral dilemmas written by adolescents. *Developmental Psychology*, 12:162–163.

Outline

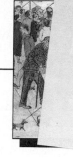

9. Brie
th

Biological Basis for Understanding Psychotropic Drugs

JOHN RAYNOR

Key Terms and Concepts

The key terms and concepts listed here also appear in color where they are defined or first discussed in this chapter.

acetylcholine

antagonists

antianxiety/anxiolytic drugs

anticholinesterase/ cholinesterase-inhibiting drugs

atypical antipsychotic drugs

atypical/novel antidepressants

basal ganglia

circadian rhythms

GABA

hypnotic

limbic system

lithium

mood-stabilizing drugs

monoamine oxidase

monoamine oxidase inhibitors

neurons

neurotransmitters

pharmacodynamics

pharmacokinetics

reuptake

receptors

reticular activating system (RAS)

selective serotonin reuptake inhibitors

synapse

standard (first-generation) antipsychotic drugs

therapeutic index

typical/standard antidepressants

Objectives

After studying this chapter, the reader will be able to

1. Discuss at least eight functions of the brain and how these functions can be altered by psychotropic drugs.

2. Describe the process of how a neurotransmitter functions as a neuromessenger.

3. Draw the three major areas of the brain and identify at least three functions of each.

4. Identify how specific brain functions are altered in certain mental disorders (e.g., depression, anxiety, schizophrenia).

5. Describe how the use of imaging techniques can be useful for understanding mental illness.

6. Apply to a medication teaching plan the knowledge gained from this chapter that the blockage of dopamine at the receptor site can result in motor abnormalities and hyperprolactinemia.

7. Describe the result of blockage to the muscarinic receptors and the alpha$_1$ receptors by the standard neuroleptics.

8. Contrast and compare the side-effect profile of the standard antipsychotics with those of (a) clozapine and (b) risperidone.

...ly identify the main neurotransmitters ...at are affected by the following psycho-tropic drugs:

    (a) standard (first-generation) antipsychotics

    (b) tricyclic antidepressants (TCAs)

    (c) selective serotonin reuptake inhibitors (SSRIs)

    (d) monoamine oxidase inhibitors (MAOIs)

    (e) antianxiety agents (benzodiazepines, buspirone)

    (f) anticholinesterase drugs

10. Apply knowledge of why a person on an MAOI would have special dietary and drug restrictions to a medications teaching plan.

*W*hether conscious or unconscious, focused on the logical or filled with fantasy, the locus of all mental activity is the brain. This implies that a primary goal of psychiatry is to understand both normal and abnormal mental processes in terms of brain function. Ultimately, we would like to be able to apply this understanding to the treatment of mental disease and the alleviation of mental suffering. Approached in terms of brain function, psychiatric problems are explained and treated in the same way as any other biological problems.

Implied in the biological approach to psychiatric illness is the idea that, while the origin of a psychiatric illness may be determined by any of a number of factors (genetics, neurodevelopmental factors, drugs, infection, psychosocial experience), there will eventually be an alteration in cerebral function that accounts for the disturbances in the client's behavior and mental experiences. These physiological alterations are the targets of the psychotropic drugs used to treat mental disease.

Reversal of these alterations is the goal of the use of psychotropic drugs in the treatment of these illnesses. During recent years there has been an explosion of information in this area. Earlier theories, such as the dopamine theory of schizophrenia and the monoamine theory of depression, are now seen as overly simplistic because a large number of other transmitters, hormones, and co-regulators are now thought to play important and complex roles. The importance of receptor subtypes and the role of these receptors in normal physiology, pathology, and pharmacology are also receiving increasing attention.

The goal of this chapter is to relate psychiatric disturbances and the psychotropic drugs used to treat these disturbances to normal brain structure and function. We will first look at the normal functions of the brain and how these functions are carried out from an anatomical and physiological perspective. We will then review current theories of the neuropsychological basis of various types of emotional and physiological dysfunctions. As will be seen, these theories focus primarily on neurotransmitters and their receptors. Finally, we will attempt to relate both the beneficial and the untoward effects of psychiatric drugs to their interaction with various transmitter-receptor systems.

Although the modern era of the treatment of mental illness with psychotropic drugs extends back almost half a century, a full understanding of how these drugs improve the symptoms of these illnesses continues to elude investigators. The focus of research is on neurotransmitters—their release from presynaptic cells and their actions on postsynaptic cells—and how psychotropic drugs interact with the physiology of these substances. In recent years many subtypes of receptors for the various neurotransmitters have been discovered, and the importance of long-term changes induced in postsynaptic cells has taken on increased significance. This information is becoming increasingly important for nurses to understand. It is particularly crucial for advanced practice psychiatric nurses who, in many states, have prescriptive authority.

Included in this chapter is an overview of the major drugs used to treat mental disorders and an explanation of how they work. Additional and detailed information regarding the side and toxic effects, dosage, nursing implications, and teaching tools are covered in appropriate clinical chapters.

In many ways all of this new information has clouded rather than cleared the water, leaving much to be clarified in understanding the complex ways in which the brain carries out its normal functions, is altered during disease, and is improved by pharmacological intervention. Upon completing this chapter, students should have a biological framework into which they can fit existing, as well as future, information about mental illness and its treatment.

Structure and Function of the Brain

FUNCTIONS OF THE BRAIN

The regulation of behavior and the carrying out of mental processes are important, but far from the only responsibilities of the brain. Box 3–1 summarizes some of the major activities for which the brain is responsible. Since all of these brain functions are carried out by similar mechanisms (interactions of neurons), and often in similar locations, it is not surprising that mental disturbances are often associated with alterations in other brain functions and that the drugs used to treat mental disturbances can also interfere with other activities of the brain.

The brain serves as the coordinator and director of the body's response to both internal and external changes. Appropriate responses require a constant monitoring of the environment, interpretation and integration of the incoming information, and control over the appropriate organs of response. The goal of these responses is to maintain homeostasis and thus to maintain life. Information about the external world is relayed from various senses to the brain by the peripheral nerves. This information, which is at first received as gross sensation (light, sound, touch), must ultimately be interpreted (a key, a train whistle, a hand on the back). Interestingly, a component of a major psychiatric disturbance (e.g., schizophrenia) is an alteration of sensory experience. Thus, the client may experience a sensation that does not originate in the external world. People with schizophrenia may hear voices talking to them (auditory hallucination), or they may misinterpret incoming information that does originate in the external world—for instances, thinking that a broom is a rifle (illusion). To some extent these types of phenomena are experienced by all of us, i.e., during the time we dream.

The brain not only monitors the external world but also keeps a close watch on the internal one.

Thus, information about blood pressure, body temperature, blood gases, and the chemical composition of the body fluids is continuously received by the brain so that it can direct the appropriate responses required to maintain homeostasis.

To respond to external changes, the brain must and does have control over the skeletal muscles. This control involves not only the ability to initiate contraction (e.g., to contract the biceps and flex the arm) but also the ability to fine-tune and coordinate contraction so that a person can guide his fingers to the correct keys on the piano. Unfortunately, both psychiatric disease and the treatment of psychiatric disease with psychotropic drugs are associated with disturbance of movement.

It is important to remember that the skeletal muscles controlled by the brain include the diaphragm, which is essential for breathing, and the muscles of the throat, tongue, and mouth, which are essential for speech. Thus, drugs that affect brain function can stimulate or depress respiration or lead to slurred speech.

Adjustments to changes within the body require that the brain exert control over the various internal organs. For example, if blood pressure drops, the brain must direct the heart to pump more blood and the smooth muscles of the arterioles to constrict. This increase in cardiac output and vasoconstriction allows the body to return blood pressure to its normal level.

The autonomic nervous system and the endocrine system serve as the communication links between the brain and the cardiac muscle, smooth muscle, and glands of which the internal organs are composed (Fig. 3–1). Thus, if the brain needs to stimulate the heart, it must activate the sympathetic nerves to the sinoatrial node and the ventricular myocardium, and if it needs to bring about vasoconstriction, it must activate the sympathetic nerves to the smooth muscles of the arterioles.

The linkage between the brain and the internal organs that allows for the maintenance of homeostasis may also serve to translate mental disturbances, such as anxiety, into alterations of internal function. For example, anxiety in some people can cause activation of parasympathetic nerves to the digestive tract, leading to hypermotility and diarrhea. Likewise, anxiety can activate the sympathetic nerves to the arterioles, leading to vasoconstriction and hypertension.

In addition to the connections formed via the autonomic nervous system, the brain exerts its influence over the internal organs by its regulation of the hormonal secretions of the pituitary gland, which in turn, regulate those of a number of other glands. A specific area of the brain, the hypothalamus, secretes hormones called releasing factors, which are carried

Box 3–1   *Functions of the Brain*

1. Monitor changes in the external world
2. Monitor the composition of the body fluids
3. Regulate the contractions of the skeletal muscles
4. Regulate the internal organs
5. Initiate and regulate the basic drives: hunger, thirst, sex, aggressive self-protection
6. Conscious sensation
7. Memory
8. Mood (affect)
9. Thought
10. Regulate sleep cycle
11. Language

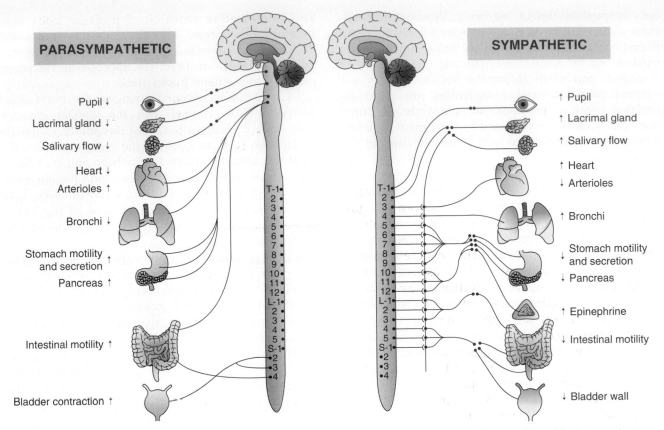

PARASYMPATHETIC

Pupil ↓
Lacrimal gland ↓
Salivary flow ↓
Heart ↓
Arterioles ↑
Bronchi ↓
Stomach motility and secretion ↑
Pancreas ↑
Intestinal motility ↑
Bladder contraction ↑

SYMPATHETIC

↑ Pupil
↑ Lacrimal gland
↑ Salivary flow
↑ Heart
↓ Arterioles
↑ Bronchi
↓ Stomach motility and secretion
↓ Pancreas
↑ Epinephrine
↓ Intestinal motility
↓ Bladder wall

Figure 3–1 The autonomic nervous system has two divisions: the sympathetic and parasympathetic. The sympathetic division is dominant in stress situations, such as fear and anger—known as the fight-or-flight response.

directly to the pituitary gland where they stimulate or inhibit the synthesis and release of pituitary hormones. These pituitary hormones, in turn, are carried in the general circulation where they can influence various internal activities. A classic example of this linkage is the release of gonadotropin-releasing hormone by the hypothalamus at the time of puberty. This hormone stimulates the release of the gonadotropins, follicle-stimulating hormone and luteinizing hormone, by the pituitary and consequent activation of the ovaries or testes. Not surprisingly, this linkage may explain why anxiety or depression in some women may lead to disturbances of the menstrual cycle.

The relationship among the brain, the pituitary, and the adrenal gland seems to play a particularly important role in normal and abnormal mental function. Specifically, the hypothalamic secretion **corticotropin-releasing hormone (CRH)** stimulates the pituitary to release corticotropin, which in turn stimulates the cortex of the adrenal gland to secrete the hormone cortisol. This system is activated as a normal component of the body's general response to a variety of mental and physical stresses. Among many other actions, all three hormones—CRH, cor-

ticotropin, and cortisol—influence the functions of the nerve cells of the brain. There is considerable evidence that in both anxiety and depression this system is overactive and does not respond to the normal limitations of negative feedback.

In attempting to understand the neurobiological basis of mental disease and its treatment, it is helpful to distinguish between the various types of brain activities that serve as the basis of mental experience and of behavior. An understanding of these activities focuses attention on where to look for disturbed function and what to hope for in treatment.

The brain, for example, is responsible for the basic drives, such as sex and hunger, that play a strong role in molding behavior. Disturbances of these drives (e.g., over- or under-eating, loss of sexual interest) can be an indication of an underlying psychological disease such as depression.

The entire cycle of sleep and wakefulness, as well as the intensity of alertness while the person is awake, is regulated and coordinated by various regions of the brain. Although we are far from a full understanding of the true homeostatic function of sleep, there is no question that it is essential for both physiological and psychological well-being. Sleep disturbances are often a symptom of psychological distress, and an assessment of sleep patterns is part of what is required to determine a psychiatric diagnosis.

When a person is awake, the degree of alertness and the ability to focus attention are regulated in complex ways by the brain. Disturbances in alertness and focus—hypervigilence in a person with paranoid schizophrenia or inability to concentrate in a person who is depressed—can be indications of mental disturbance.

Unfortunately, many of the drugs used to treat psychiatric problems interfere with the normal regulation of sleep and alertness. Drugs with a sedative-hypnotic effect can blunt the degree to which a person feels alert and is able to focus attention and can make the client feel drowsy and fall asleep. A sedative-hypnotic effect demands caution in using these drugs while engaging in activities that require a great deal of attention, such as driving a car or operating farm machinery. One way of minimizing the danger is to give such drugs at night just before the client goes to sleep. Alteration in this area may also form a component of the attention deficit disorder/hyperactivity (ADDH) syndrome in which a child or adult has difficulty maintaining their focus of attention on one source and is continuously in search of novel and intense stimuli.

The cycle of sleep and wakefulness is only one aspect of what we call circadian rhythms, the fluctuation of various physiological and behavioral parameters over a 24-hour cycle. Other variations include changes in body temperature, the secretion of hormone such as corticotropin and cortisol, and the secretion of neurotransmitters such as norepinephrine and serotonin. Both norepinephrine and serotonin are thought to be involved in mood (affect), whether normal or abnormal; thus, daily fluctuations of mood may be related in part to circadian variations in these transmitters. There is some evidence that the circadian rhythm of neurotransmitter secretion is altered in psychological disease, particularly in disorders that involve alteration of mood.

All aspects of conscious mental experience and sense of self must ultimately result from the neurophysiological activity of the brain. The most basic type of conscious mental activity is probably the loose, meandering stream of consciousness that can jump back and forth between thoughts of future responsibilities, past experience, fantasized activities, interpersonal grievances, and so on. Conscious mental activity must, of course, become much more organized when it is applied to problem solving and the interpretation of the external world. Both the random stream of consciousness and the ability to

interpret the environment can become extremely distorted in psychiatric illness. Thus, a person with schizophrenia can present with chaotic and seemingly incoherent speech and thought patterns (a jumble of unrelated words known as **word salad**, unconnected phrases and topics known as **looseness of association**) and delusional interpretations of personal interactions, such as beliefs about people or events that are not supported by data or reality.

An extremely important component of mental activity is memory, the ability to retain and recall past experience. From both an anatomical and physiological perspective, it is thought that there is a major difference in the processing of short- and long-term memory. Clinically, this can be seen dramatically in some forms of cognitive mental disorders such as dementia, in which a person has no recall of the events of the previous 8 minutes but may have vivid recall of events that occurred 80 years ago.

Conscious mental activity and memory become integrated in complex, and still unknown ways, in the process of learning. In some cases, learning the names of the states in the U.S., learning primarily involves memory storage and retrieval. In others, the analysis of a poem or the solution of a complex mathematical problem, in-depth thought processes (abstract, organizing, categorizing) must be applied along with the retrieval of facts.

A very important, and often neglected, aspect of learning involves the social skills that cement interpersonal relationships. In almost all types of mental illness, from mild anxiety to severe schizophrenia, difficulties in interpersonal relationships are an important part of the disorder and improvements in these relationships an important part of the cure. The relationship between brain activity and social behavior is an area of intense research. It involves basic genetic drives modified by individual experience. There is evidence that positive reward–based experiential learning and negative avoidance learning may involve different areas of the brain.

CELLULAR COMPOSITION OF THE BRAIN

The brain is composed of nerve cells, or **neurons**, that conduct electrical impulses and the various types of cells that surround these neurons. Traditionally it has been thought that the types of activities we have discussed thus far, the various functions carried out by the brain, result from the interactions of neurons. The surrounding cells have been thought to provide for the physical, metabolic, and immunological support of the neurons. However it may well be that the interactions of the various types of cells are more complex than was originally assumed.

Most functions of the brain, from regulation of blood pressure to the conscious sense of self, are thought to result from the actions of individual neurons and the interconnections between these neurons. Although neurons come in a great variety of shapes and sizes, all carry out the same three types of physiological actions: (1) they respond to stimuli, (2) they conduct electrical impulses, and (3) they release chemicals called neurotransmitters.

An essential feature of neurons is their ability to conduct an electrical impulse from one end of the cell to the other. This electrical impulse consists of a self-propagating change in membrane permeability that first allows the inward flow of sodium ions and then the outward flow of potassium ions. The inward flow of sodium ions changes the polarity of the membrane from positive on the outside to positive on the inside. Movement of potassium ions out of the cell returns the positive charge to the outside of the cell. Since these electrical charges are self-propagating, a change at one end of the cell is conducted along the membrane until it reaches the other end of the cell (Fig. 3–2). The functional significance of this propagation is that the electrical impulse serves as a means of communications between one part of the body and another.

Once an electrical impulse reaches the end of a neuron, a chemical called a neurotransmitter is released. A **neurotransmitter** is a chemical substance that functions as a neuromessenger. Neurotransmit-

ters are released from the axon terminal at the **presynaptic** neuron on excitation. This transmitter then diffuses across a narrow space, or synapse, to an adjacent **postsynaptic** neuron, where it attaches to specialized receptors on the cell surface and either inhibits or excites the postsynaptic neuron. It is the interaction between transmitter and receptor that allows the activity of one neuron to influence the activity of other neurons. Depending on the chemical structure of the transmitter and the specific type of receptor to which it attaches, the postsynaptic cell will be rendered either more or less likely to have an electrical impulse. As we shall see, it is the interaction between transmitter and receptor that is a major target of the drugs used to treat psychiatric disease. Table 3–1 lists some of the most important neurotransmitters and the types of receptors to which they attach. Also listed are the mental disorders that are associated with an increase or decrease in these neurotransmitters.

After attaching to a receptor and exerting its influence on the postsynaptic cell, the transmitters separates from the receptor and are destroyed. The process of transmitter destruction is illustrated in Box 3–2. As can be seen, there are two basic mechanisms by which transmitters are destroyed. Some transmitters (e.g., acetylcholine) are destroyed by specific enzymes at the postsynaptic cell. The specific enzyme that destroys acetylcholine is called **acetylcholinesterase**. Other transmitters (e.g., norepinephrine) are taken back into the presynaptic cell from which they were originally released by a process called cellular reuptake. Upon their return to these cells, the transmitters are either reused or destroyed by intracellular enzymes. In the case of the monoamine transmitters, the destructive enzyme is called **monoamine oxidase (MAO)**.

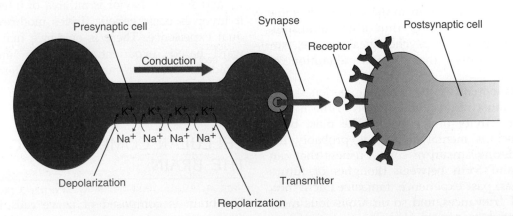

Figure 3–2 Activities of neurons. Conduction along a neuron involves the inward movement of sodium (Na$^+$) followed by the outward movement of potassium (K$^+$). When the current reaches the end of the cell, a neurotransmitter is released. The transmitter crosses the synapse and attaches to a receptor on the postsynaptic cell. The attachment of transmitter to receptor either stimulates or inhibits the postsynaptic cell.

TABLE 3-1 *Transmitters/Receptors*

TRANSMITTERS	RECEPTORS	EFFECTS/COMMENTS	ASSOCATION WITH MENTAL HEALTH
Monoamines			
Dopamine (DA)	D_1, D_2, D_3, D_4, D_5	■ Fine muscle movement ■ Integration of emotions and thoughts ■ Involved with decision making ■ Stimulates hypothalamus to release hormones (sex, thyroid, adrenals)	*Decrease:* ■ Parkinson's disease ■ Depression *Increase:* ■ Schizophrenia ■ Mania
Norepinephrine (NE)	Alpha$_1$, alpha$_2$, beta$_1$, beta$_2$	■ Level in brain affects mood ■ Stimulates sympathetic branch of ANS for "fight or flight"	*Decrease:* ■ Depression *Increase:* ■ Mania ■ Anxiety states ■ Schizophrenia
Serotonin (5-HT)	5-HT, 5-HT$_2$, 5-HT$_3$, 5-HT$_4$	■ Plays a role in sleep regulation, hunger, mood states, and pain perception ■ Plays a role in aggression and sexual behavior	*Decrease:* ■ Depression *Increase:* ■ Anxiety states
Amino Acids			
Gamma-aminobutyric acid (GABA)	GABA$_A$, GABA$_B$	■ Plays a role in inhibition; reduces aggression, excitation, and anxiety ■ May play a role in pain perception ■ Anticonvulsant and muscle-relaxing properties	*Decrease:* ■ Anxiety disorders ■ Schizophrenia ■ Huntington's chorea *Increase:* ■ Reduction of anxiety
Cholinergics			
Acetylcholine (ACh)	Nicotinic muscarinic (M_1, M_2, M_3)	■ Plays a role in learning, memory ■ Mood regulator: manic, sexual aggression ■ Affects sexual and aggressive behavior ■ Stimulates parasympathetic nervous system	*Decrease:* ■ Alzheimer's disease ■ Huntington's chorea ■ Parkinson's disease *Increase:* ■ Depression
Amino Acid Derivative			
Histamine	H_1, H_2w	■ Alertness ■ Inflammatory response ■ Stimulates gastric secretion	*Decrease:* ■ Depression

ANS, autonomic nervous system.

As a means of regulating the concentration of transmitters at the postsynaptic receptors, many of the transmitters exert a feedback inhibition of their own release. This inhibition is accomplished by the attachment of transmitters to what are called presynaptic receptors, at the synapse, and acts to inhibit the release of further transmitters.

In recent years it has become clear that the picture of a neuron releasing a specific transmitter that stimulates or inhibits a postsynaptic membrane receptor and acts via negative feedback on a presynaptic receptor is an accurate but far from complete picture of the interaction between nerve cells. It is now known that in many cases neurons release more than one chemical at the same time. Transmitters such as norepinephrine or acetylcholine, which have

BOX 3–2   *Destruction of Neurotransmitters*

A full explanation of the various ways in which psychotropic drugs alter neuronal activity requires a brief review of the manner in which neurotransmitters are destroyed after attaching to the receptors. As a means of avoiding continuous and prolonged action on the postsynaptic cell, the neurotransmitter is released shortly after attaching to the postsynaptic receptor. Once released, the transmitter is destroyed in one of two ways. *One* is the immediate inactivation of the transmitter at the postsynaptic membrane.

An example of this method of destruction is the action of the enzyme acetylcholinesterase on the neurotransmitter acetylcholine. Acetylcholinesterase is present at the postsynaptic membrane and destroys acetylcholine shortly after it attaches to nicotinic or muscarinic receptors on the postsynaptic cell.

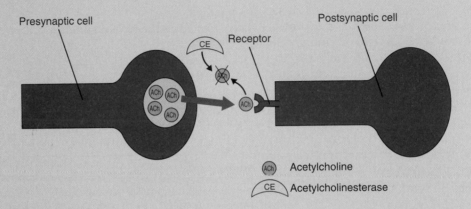

A *second* method of neurotransmitter inactivation is a little more complex. After interacting with the postsynaptic receptor, the transmitter is released and taken back into the presynaptic cell, the cell from which it was released. The process, referred to as the reuptake of neurotransmitter, is a common target for drug action. Once inside the presynaptic cell, the transmitter is either recycled or inactivated by an enzyme within the cell. The monoamine transmitters norepinephrine, dopamine, and serotonin are all inactivated in this manner by the enzyme monoamine oxidase.

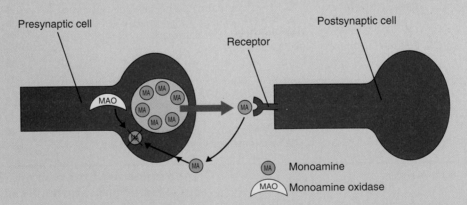

Looking at this second method, you might naturally ask what prevents the enzyme from destroying the transmitter before its release. The answer is that before release the transmitter is stored within a membrane and is thus protected from the degradative enzyme. After release and reuptake, the transmitter is either destroyed by the enzyme or reenters the membrane to be used once again.

immediate effects on postsynaptic membranes, are often joined by larger molecules, neuropeptides, that may initiate long-term changes in the postsynaptic cells. The changes may involve basic cell functions such as genetic expression and lead to modifications of cell shape and responsiveness to stimuli. Ultimately this means that the action of one neuron on another not only affects the immediate response of that neuron but its sensitivity to future influence. The long-term implications of this for neural development, normal and abnormal mental health, and the treatment of psychiatric disease are being intensely investigated.

It is also becoming increasingly clear that the communication between neurons at a synapse is not unidirectional. Neurotrophic factors are proteins and even simple gases such as carbon monoxide (CO) and nitrous oxide (NO) that are released by postsynaptic cells and influence the growth, shape, and activity of presynaptic cells. These factors are thought to be particularly important during the development of the brain *in utero*, guiding the growing brain to form the proper neuronal connections. However, it is now apparent that the brain retains anatomical plasticity throughout life and that internal and external influences can alter the synaptic network of the brain. There is much current investigation of the role that altered genetic expression or that environmental trauma can play in the action of these factors and the negative and positive consequences of these changes on mental function and psychiatric disease.

The development and responsiveness of neurons is not only dependent on chemicals released by other neurons but also on chemicals brought to the neurons by the blood, particularly the **steroid hormones**. Estrogen, testosterone, and cortisol can bind to neurons where they can cause short- and long-term changes in neuronal activity. A clear and tragic example of this is seen in the psychosis that can sometimes result from the hypersecretion of cortisol in Cushing's disease or from the use of prednisone in high doses to treat chronic inflammatory disease.

ORGANIZATION OF THE NERVOUS SYSTEM

The Brainstem

The central core of the brainstem regulates the internal organs and is responsible for such vital functions as the regulation of blood gases and the maintenance of blood pressure.

The hypothalamus, a small area in the ventral superior portion of the brainstem, plays a vital role in such basic drives as hunger, thirst, and sex. It also serves as a crucial link between higher brain activities such as thought and emotion and the functioning of the internal organs. It is a crucial psychosomatic link. The brainstem also serves as an initial processing center for sensory information that is then sent on to the cerebral cortex. Through projections of what is called the **reticular activating system** (RAS), the brainstem regulates the entire cycle of sleep and wakefulness and the ability of the cerebrum to carry out conscious mental activity.

A variety of other ascending pathways, referred to as mesolimbic and mesocortical pathways, seem to play a strong role in modulating the emotional value of sensory material. These pathways project to those areas of the cerebrum, collectively known as the limbic system, that play a crucial role in emotional status and psychological function. They use norepinephrine, serotonin, and dopamine as their neurotransmitters. Much attention has been paid to the role of these pathways in normal and abnormal mental activity. For example, it is thought that the release of dopamine from what is called the ventral tegmental pathway plays a role in psychological reward and drug addiction. As we shall see, the neurotransmitters released by these neurons are major targets of the drugs that are used to treat psychiatric disease.

The Cerebellum

Located posteriorly to the brainstem, the cerebellum (Fig. 3–3) is primarily involved in the regulation of skeletal muscle coordination and contraction and the maintenance of equilibrium. It plays a crucial role in coordinating contractions so that movement is accomplished in a smooth and directed manner.

The Cerebrum

The brainstem and cerebellum of the human brain are similar in both structure and function to these same structures in the brains of other mammals. The development of a much larger and more elaborate cerebrum is what distinguishes human beings from the rest of the animal kingdom.

The cerebrum, situated on top of and surrounding the brainstem, is responsible for mental activities and a conscious sense of being. Thus, the cerebrum is responsible for our conscious perception of the external world and of our own body, for emotional status, for memory, and for the control of the skele-

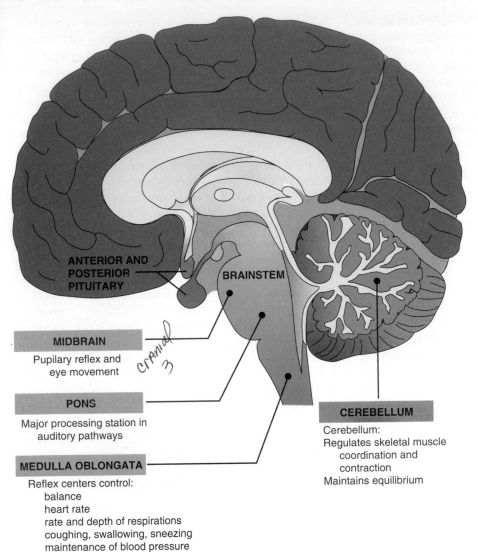

ANTERIOR AND
POSTERIOR
PITUITARY

BRAINSTEM

Cramal 3

MIDBRAIN

Pupilary reflex and
eye movement

PONS

Major processing station in
auditory pathways

MEDULLA OBLONGATA

Reflex centers control:
  balance
  heart rate
  rate and depth of respirations
  coughing, swallowing, sneezing
  maintenance of blood pressure
  vomiting

CEREBELLUM

Cerebellum:
Regulates skeletal muscle
  coordination and
  contraction
Maintains equilibrium

Figure 3–3 The functions of the brainstem and cerebellum.

tal muscles that allow the willful direction of movement. The cerebrum is also responsible for language and the ability to communicate.

Anatomically, the cerebrum consists of surface and deep areas of integrating gray matter (the cerebral cortex and basal ganglia) and of the connecting tracts of white matter that link these areas with each other and with the rest of the nervous system. The cerebral cortex, which forms the outer layer of the brain, is responsible for conscious sensation and the initiation of movement. It is organized in such a way that specific areas of the cortex are responsible for specific sensations: the parietal cortex is responsible for touch, the temporal cortex for sound, the occipital cortex for vision, and so on. Likewise, the initiation of skeletal muscle contraction is controlled by a specific area of the frontal cortex. Of course, all the areas of the cortex are interconnected so that an integral picture of the world can be formed and,

if necessary, linked to an appropriate response (Fig. 3–4).

Specialized areas of the cerebral cortex are responsible for language in both its sensory and motor aspects. Sensory language functions include the ability to read, to understand spoken language, and to know the names of objects that are perceived by the senses, whereas motor functions involve the ability to use muscles properly for speech and writing. In both neurological and psychological dysfunction, the use of language may become compromised or distorted. The change in linguistic ability may be a factor in determining a diagnosis.

In addition to forming the surface of the cerebrum, there are pockets of integrating gray matter deep within the cerebrum. Some of these, the basal ganglia, are involved in the regulation of movement. Others, the amygdala and hippocampus, are involved in the emotions, learning, memory, and basic drives. Significantly, there is an overlap of these various areas both anatomically and in the types of neurotransmitters employed. One consequence of this is that drugs used to treat emotional disturbances may cause movement disorders and that drugs used to treat movement disorders may cause emotional changes.

A variety of noninvasive imaging techniques are used to visualize brain structure, functions, and metabolic activity in clients experiencing various mental disorders. Table 3–2 identifies some common brain imaging techniques and some preliminary findings as they relate to psychiatry. There are basically two types of neuro-imaging techniques: structural and functional. **Structural** imaging techniques (e.g., CT and MRI scans) identify gross anatomical changes in the brain,. **Functional** imaging techniques (e.g., PET and SPECT) show physiological activity in the brain, as described in Table 3–2.

Positron-emission tomography (PET) scans are particularly useful in identifying physiological and biochemical changes as they occur in living tissue. Usually a radioactive "tag" is used to trace com-

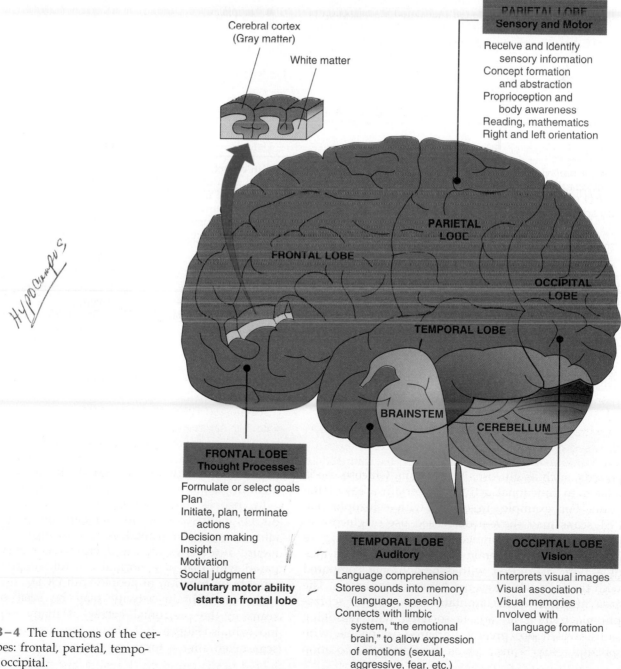

Figure 3–4 The functions of the cerebral lobes: frontal, parietal, temporal, and occipital.

TABLE 3–2 *Common Brain Imaging Techniques*

STRUCTURAL: Shows Gross Anatomical Details of Brain Structures

EXAM	TECHNIQUE	USES	PSYCHIATRIC RELEVANCE PRELIMINARY FINDINGS
Computed tomography (CT)	A series of x-rays are taken of the brain while a computer analysis produces "slices" providing a precise 3D-like reconstruction of each segment.	**Can detect:** ■ Lesions ■ Abrasions ■ Areas of infarct ■ Aneurysm	Schizophrenia ■ Cortical atrophy ■ Third ventricle enlargement ■ Cognitive disorders-abnormalities
Magnetic resonance imaging (MRI)	A magnetic field is applied to the brain. The nucleus of hydrogen absorbs and emits radio waves that are computerized and provide three-dimensional visualization of the brain's structure in sectional images.	**Can detect:** ■ Brain edema ■ Ischemia ■ Infection ■ Neoplasm ■ Trauma	Schizophrenia ■ Enlarged ventricles ■ Reduction in temporal lobe and prefrontal lobe
fMRI	A functional imaging approach that avoids exposure to ionizing radiation.		

FUNCTIONAL: Shows Some Activity of the Brain

EXAM	TECHNIQUE	USES	PSYCHIATRIC RELEVANCE PRELIMINARY FINDINGS
Positron-emission tomography (PET) (uses radioactive tracer)	Radioactive substance is injected and travels to the brain and shows up as bright spots on the scan. Data collected by the detectors are relayed to a computer which produces images of the activity and visualizes the CNS in three dimensions	**Can detect:** ■ Oxygen utilization ■ Glucose metabolism ■ Blood flow ■ Neurotransmitter-receptor interaction	Schizophrenia ■ Increased D_2, D_3 receptors in caudate nucleus ■ Abnormalities in limbic system Mood disorder ■ Abnormalities in temporal lobes Adult ADHD ■ Decreased utilization of glucose
Single photon emission computed tomography (SPECT) (uses radioactive tracer)	Similar to PET but SPECT uses radionuclides that emit gamma radiation (photons)	**Can detect:** Similar to PET	Measures various aspects of brain functioning and provides images of multiple layers of the CNS (as does PET)

pounds, such as glucose, in the brain. Glucose use is related to functional activity in certain areas of the brain. For example, in clients with schizophrenia, PET scans may show a decreased use of glucose in the frontal lobes of unmedicated individuals. Figure 3–5 shows reduced brain activity in the frontal lobe of a twin diagnosed with schizophrenia compared with the twin who does not have schizophrenia. The area affected in the frontal cortex of the schizophrenic twin is an area associated with reasoning skills, which are greatly impaired in people with schizophrenia. Scans such as these suggest a location in the frontal cortex as the site of functional impairment in people with schizophrenia.

In people with obsessive-compulsive disorder (OCD), increased brain metabolism shows up in certain areas of the frontal cortex during PET scans. Figure 3–6 shows increased brain metabolism compared with that of a normal control, suggesting altered brain function in people with OCD.

Decreased brain activity may be seen on PET scans in the prefrontal cortex of many depressed individuals. Figure 3–7 shows the results of a PET scan taken after a form of radioactively tagged glu-

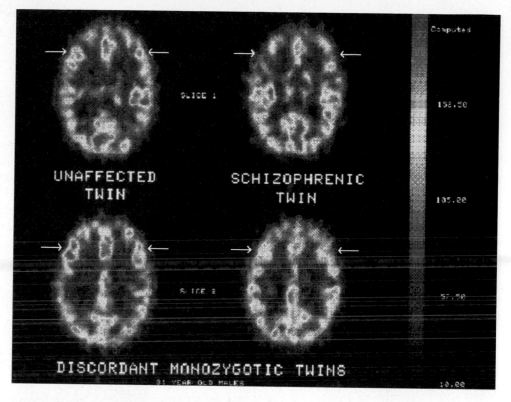

Figure 3–5 Positron-emission tomography (PET) scans of blood flow in identical twins, one of whom has schizophrenia, illustrate that individuals with this illness have reduced brain activity in their frontal lobes when asked to perform a reasoning task that requires activation of this area. Schizophrenic clients also perform poorly on the task. This suggests a site of functional impairments in schizophrenia (From Karen Berman, MD, courtesy of National Institute of Mental Health, Clinical Brain Disorders Branch.)

cose was used as a tracer to visualize brain activity. The depressed client shows reduced brain activity compared with a nondepressed control. Finally, see Figure 3–8 for three views of a PET scan of the brain in a client with Alzheimer's disease.

Modern imaging techniques have also become an important tool in assessing molecular changes in mental disease and marking the receptor sites of drug action.

From a psychiatric perspective, we would like to

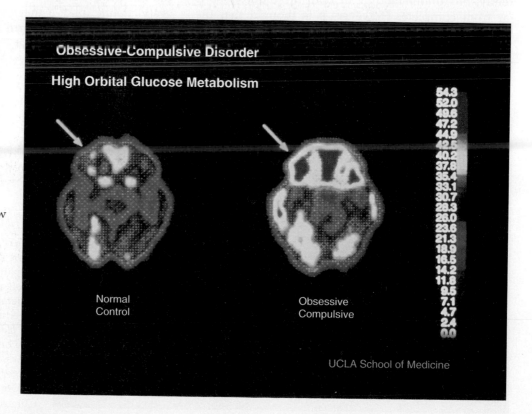

Figure 3–6 PET scans show increased brain metabolism *(brighter colors)*, particularly in the frontal cortex, in an obsessive-compulsive disorder (OCD) client, compared with a normal control. This suggests altered brain function in OCD. (From Lewis Baxter, MD, University of Alabama, courtesy of National Institute of Mental Health.)

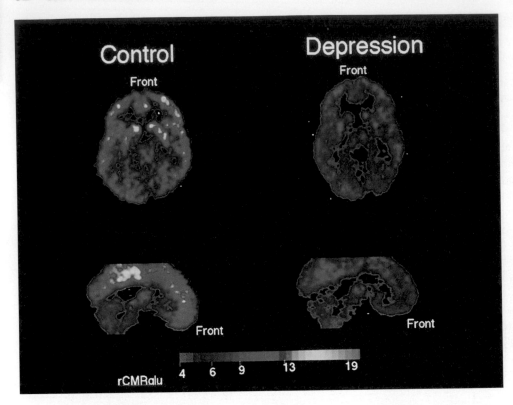

Figure 3–7 PET scans of a normal subject *(left)* and depressed client *(right)* reveal reduced brain activity *(darker colors)* during depression, especially in the prefrontal cortex. A form of radioactively tagged glucose was used as a tracer to visualize levels of brain activity. (From Mark George, MD, courtesy of National Institute of Mental Health, Biological Psychiatry Branch.)

be able to understand where in the brain the various components of psychological activity take place, and what are the types of neurotransmitters and receptors that underlie this activity physiologically. Currently, our understanding of both these questions is far from complete. However, it is thought that the limbic system—a group of structures that include parts of the frontal cortex, the basal ganglia, and the brainstem—is a major locus of psychological activity.

Within these areas the monoamine transmitters (norepinephrine, dopamine, and serotonin), the amino acid transmitters glutamate and gamma-aminobutyric acid (GABA), and the neuropeptides corticotropin-releasing hormone and endorphin, as well as acetylcholine, play a major role. Alterations in these areas are thought to form the basis of psychiatric disease and are the target for pharmacological treatment.

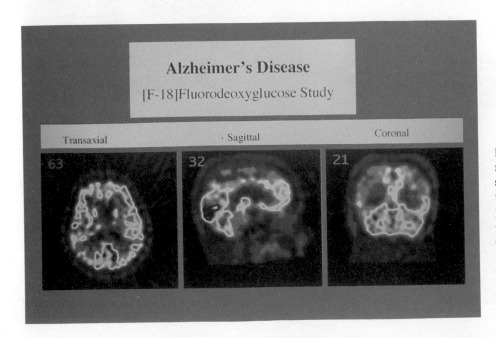

Figure 3–8 PET scan of Alzheimer's disease demonstrates a classic pattern for areas of hypometabolism in the temporal and parietal regions of the brain. Areas of reduced metabolism *(dark blue and black regions)* are very noticeable on the sagittal and coronal views. (Courtesy of PET Imaging Center, Department of Radiology, University of Iowa Hospitals and Clinics, Iowa City.)

DISTURBANCES OF MENTAL FUNCTION

Although in a limited number of clients the cause of mental dysfunction is known, most occurrences are of unknown origin. Among known causes are drugs (lysergic acid diethylamide [LSD], long-term use of prednisone), excess levels of hormones (thyroxine, cortisol), infection (encephalitis, AIDS), and physical trauma. However, even when the etiology is known, the link between the causative factor and the mental dysfunction is far from understood.

Results from numerous studies seem to indicate that there is at least in part a genetic component to psychological dysfunction. The incidence of both thought and mood disorders is higher in relatives of people with these diseases than in the general population. There is also a strong concordance, although certainly not 100%, among identical twins even when they are raised apart. Psychosocial stress, either in the family of origin or in contacts with society at large, increases the likelihood of mental problems, as does physical disease. Genetics and environment interact in complex ways so that some people are better able to cope with stress than others.

Researchers want ultimately to be able to understand mental dysfunction in terms of altered activity of neurons in specific areas of the brain; the hope is that such understanding could lead to better treatments and possible prevention of mental disorders. Current interest is focused on certain neurotransmitters and their receptors, particularly in the limbic system, which links the frontal cortex, basal ganglia, and upper brainstem. As mentioned, the transmitters that have been most consistently linked to mental activity are norepinephrine, dopamine, serotonin, GABA, glutamate, and CRH.

Although the underlying physiology is complex, in simple terms, it is thought that a deficiency of norepinephrine, or serotonin, or both may serve as the biological basis of depression. Figure 3–9 shows that an insufficient degree of transmission may be due to a deficient release of the transmitters by the presynaptic cell or to a loss of the ability of postsynaptic receptors to respond to the transmitters. Changes in transmitter release and receptor response can be both a cause and a consequence of intra-

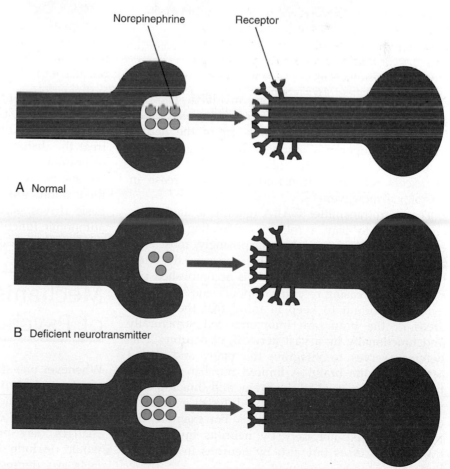

A Normal

B Deficient neurotransmitter

C Deficient receptor

Figure 3–9 Normal transmission of neurotransmitters (*A*). Deficiency in transmission may be due to deficient release of transmitter, as shown in *B*, or by reduction in receptors, as shown in *C*.

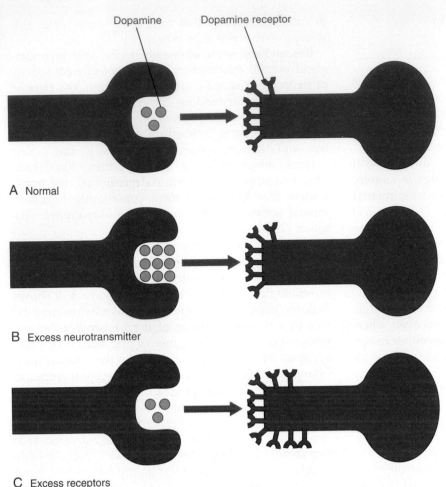

A Normal

B Excess neurotransmitter

C Excess receptors

Figure 3–10 Causes of excess transmission of neurotransmitters. Excess transmission may be due to excess release of transmitter, as shown in *B*, or by excess responsiveness of receptors, as shown in *C*.

cellular changes in the neurons involved. Thought disorders such as schizophrenia are associated physiologically with excess transmission of the neurotransmitter dopamine, among other changes. As illustrated in Figure 3–10, this may be due to either an excess release of transmitter or an increase in receptor responsiveness.

The neurotransmitter GABA (gamma-aminobutyric acid) seems to play a role in modulating neuronal excitability and anxiety. Not surprisingly, most antianxiety (anxiolytics) drugs act by increasing the effectiveness of this transmitter. This is accomplished primarily by increasing receptor responsiveness.

It is important to keep in mind that the various areas of the brain are interconnected structurally and functionally by a vast network of neurons. This network serves to integrate the many and varied activities of the brain. A limited number of neurotransmitters are used in the brain, and thus a particular transmitter is often used by different neurons to carry out quite different activities. For example, dopamine is used not only by neurons involved in thought processes but also by neurons involved in the regulations of movement.

As a result of the use of the same transmitter by different types of neurons, alterations in transmitter activity, either as the causative factor of a mental disturbance or brought about by the drugs used to treat the disturbance, can affect more than one area of brain activity. In order words, alterations in mental status, whether arising from disease or from medication, are often accompanied by changes in basic drives, sleep patterns, body movement, and autonomic functions.

Mechanisms of Action of Psychotropic Drugs

Whenever one studies drugs, the important concepts of pharmacodynamics and pharmacokinetics must be kept in mind. Pharmacodynamics refers to the actions of the drug on the person, the types of changes they produce. Pharmacodynamic changes would include both large-scale effects (the client feels less depressed) and molecular effects (the enzyme monoamine oxidase is inhibited).

The term pharmacokinetics refers to the actions of the person on the drug. How is the drug absorbed into the blood? How is it transformed in the liver? How is it excreted by the kidney? Pharmacokinetics determine the blood level of a drug and are used to guide the dosage schedule. They are also used to determine the type and amount of drug used in cases of liver and kidney disease.

Many drugs are transformed by the liver into active metabolites—chemicals which themselves have pharmacological actions. This knowledge is used by researchers in designing new drugs that make use of the body's own mechanisms to activate a chemical for pharmacological use.

An ideal psychiatric drug would relieve the mental disturbance of the client without inducing untoward cerebral (mental) or somatic (physical) effects. Unfortunately, in psychiatry, as in most areas of pharmacology, there are no drugs that are both fully effective and at the same time free of undesired side effects. Researchers work toward developing medications that target the symptoms with no or minimal side effects.

Since all the activities of the brain involve the actions of neurons, neurotransmitters, and receptors, these are the targets of pharmacological intervention. Most psychotropic drugs act by either increasing or decreasing the activity of certain transmitter-receptor systems. It is generally agreed that different transmitter-receptor systems are dysfunctional in different psychiatric conditions. These differences offer more specific targets for drug action. In fact, much of what is known about the relationship between specific transmitters and specific disturbances has been derived from a knowledge of the pharmacology of the drugs used to treat these conditions. For example, it was found that most agents that were effective in reducing the delusions and hallucinations of schizophrenia block the D_2 receptors for dopamine. From this information, it was concluded that delusions and hallucinations result from overactivity of dopamine at these receptors.

ANTIPSYCHOTIC DRUGS

Conventional/Standard Antipsychotics

Box 3–3 illustrates the proposed mechanism of action of the standard (first-generation) antipsychotic drugs: the phenothiazines, thioxanthenes, butyrophenones, and pharmacologically related agents. These drugs are strong antagonists of the D_2 receptors for dopamine. By attaching to these receptors and blocking the attachment of dopamine, they reduce dopaminergic transmission. It has been postu-

lated that an overactivity of the dopamine system in certain areas of the limbic system may be responsible for at least some of the symptoms of schizophrenia; thus, blockage of dopamine may reduce these symptoms. This is thought to be particularly true of the "positive" symptoms of schizophrenia, such as delusions (e.g., paranoid and grandiose ideas) and hallucinations (e.g., hearing or seeing things not present in reality) (refer to Chapter 20).

These drugs, however, are also antagonists (blocking the action), to varying degrees, at muscarinic receptors for acetylcholine, alpha$_1$ receptors for norepinephrine, and H$_1$ receptors for histamine. Although it is unclear if this antagonism plays a role in the beneficial effects of the drugs, it is certain that antagonism is responsible for some of the major side effects.

As summarized in Box 3–4, many of the untoward side effects of these drugs can be understood as a logical extension of their receptor-blocking activity. Thus, since dopamine in the basal ganglia plays a major role in the regulation of movement, it is not surprising that dopamine blockage can lead to motor abnormalities such as parkinsonism, akinesia, akathisia, dyskinesia, and tardive dyskinesia. Nurses and physicians often monitor clients for evidence of involuntary motor movement after administration of the standard antipsychotic agents. One popular scale is called the Abnormal Involuntary Movement Scale (AIMS), which is included in Chapter 20. You can practice with a classmate the administration of AIMS. These disturbances and others are discussed in Chapter 20, which details the clinical use of the antipsychotic drugs along with specific nursing interventions and client teaching strategies.

An important physiological function of dopamine is that it acts as the hypothalamic factor that inhibits the release of prolactin from the anterior pituitary gland; thus, blockage of dopamine transmission can lead to increased pituitary secretion of prolactin. In women this hyperprolactinemia can result in amenorrhea (absence of the menses) or galactorrhea (milk flow), and in men it can lead to gynecomastia (development of the male mammary glands).

Acetylcholine is the neurotransmitter released by the postganglionic neurons of the parasympathetic nervous system. Through its attachment to muscarinic receptors on internal organs, it serves to help regulate internal function. Blockage of the muscarinic receptors by phenothiazines and a wide variety of other psychiatric drugs can lead to a constellation of untoward effects predictable from a knowledge of the normal physiology of the parasympathetic nervous system. These side effects typically involve blurred vision, dry mouth, constipation, and urinary hesitancy.

In addition to blocking dopamine and muscarinic

BOX 3-3   *How the Standard (First-Generation) Antipsychotic Drugs Work*

It is thought that at least some of the symptoms of psychosis are due to an excess of the neurotransmitter dopamine in those areas of the brain involved in thought and in emotions. Most antipsychotic drugs (phenothiazines and related compounds) seem to produce many of their beneficial effects as well as some of their undesired side effects by blocking dopamine receptors and thus reducing dopamine-induced responses in the brain.

When a client takes an antipsychotic medication, even though excess dopamine may be released by presynaptic cells in the brain, it will not cause a corresponding response in the postsynaptic cells because the receptors to which dopamine must attach are blocked by the medication. Because dopamine is used as a neurotransmitter in many areas of the brain in addition to those involved in thought and emotion, blocking of these receptors can also lead to serious untoward effects. Specifically, dopamine is a neurotransmitter in the basal ganglia, where it is involved in modulating and fine-tuning motor activity. Blocking of dopamine

receptors in this area of the brain probably accounts for the disorders of movement (known as extrapyramidal effects), such as parkinsonian symptoms, that can result from the use of antipsychotic drugs. In fact, Parkinson's disease is thought to result from a deficiency of dopamine in the basal ganglia.

Dopamine also plays a normal physiological role as an inhibitor of prolactin release. Blocking of dopamine receptors by the antipsychotic drugs can therefore lead to elevated levels of prolactin in the blood. This abnormally high level of prolactin may induce disturbances such as galactorrhea in women and gynecomastia in men.

To understand more fully the pharmacology of the antipsychotic drugs, it is necessary to recognize that **these agents block other types of receptors in addition to those for dopamine. In particular, they can block the muscarinic receptors for acetylcholine and the alpha$_1$ receptors for norepinephrine.** The degree to which individual drugs block these receptors varies to a considerable extent.

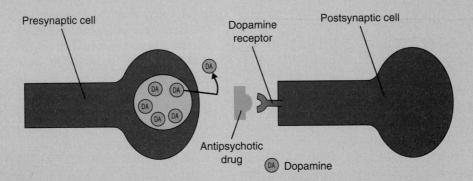

BLOCKING OF MUSCARINIC RECEPTORS

Because it is the attachment of acetylcholine to muscarinic receptors on smooth muscle, cardiac muscle, and exocrine gland cells that is responsible for the actions of the parasympathetic nervous system, it follows that blockage of these receptors will have antiparasympathetic effects. Included in these effects are blurred vision, tachycardia, constipation, and urinary retention.

BLOCKING OF ALPHA$_1$ RECEPTORS

Stimulation of alpha$_1$ receptors by norepinephrine is normally responsible for the vasoconstriction necessary to maintain blood pressure when a person is in the upright position. Therefore, the consequence of alpha$_1$-receptor blocking is often orthostatic hypotension.

receptors, many of the first-generation antipsychotic drugs act as antagonists at the alpha$_1$ receptors for norepinephrine. These receptors are found on smooth muscle cells that contract in response to norepinephrine from sympathetic nerves. For example, the ability of sympathetic nerves to constrict blood vessels is dependent on the attachment of norepinephrine to alpha$_1$ receptors; thus, blockage of these receptors can bring about vasodilation and a consequent drop

in blood pressure. Sympathetic-mediated vasoconstriction is particularly essential for maintaining normal blood pressure in the upright position; blockage of the alpha$_1$ receptors can lead to orthostatic hypotension.

Alpha$_1$ receptors are also found on the vas deferens and are responsible for the propulsive contractions leading to ejaculation. Blockage of these receptors can lead to a failure to ejaculate.

BOX 3–4 *Untoward Effects of Dopamine, Muscarinic, and Alpha₁ Antagonism*

Dopamine Blockage
Movement defects
  Parkinsonian symptoms
  Akinesia
  Akathisia
  Tardive dyskinesia
Increased prolactin
  Gynecomastia in men
  Galactorrhea-amenorrhea in women
Muscarinic Blockage
Blurred vision
Dry mouth
Constipation
Urinary difficulty
Alpha₁ Antagonism
Orthostatic hypotension
Failure to ejaculate

Finally, many of these antipsychotic agents, as well as a variety of other psychiatric drugs, block the H receptors for histamine. The two most significant side effects of blocking these receptors are sedation and substantial weight gain. The sedation may be beneficial in severely agitated clients.

Atypical Antipsychotics

The atypical antipsychotic drugs have few or no extrapyramidal symptoms and also target the negative as well as the positive symptoms of schizophrenia, as discussed in Chapter 20.

These newer drugs seem to show a difference in receptor binding profile from the older agents. They bind to dopamine receptors in the limbic system preferentially over those in the neostriatal areas of the basal ganglia and thus are able to exert psychiatric actions without motor side effects. They are also antagonists at the 5-HT₂ receptors for serotonin. This action may explain their efficacy on negative as well as positive symptoms in schizophrenia.

Clozapine

Clozapine (Clozaril), the first of the atypicals, is an antipsychotic drug that is relatively free of the motor side effects of the phenothiazines and other first-generation antipsychotics. It is thought that clozapine preferentially blocks the dopamine receptors in the limbic system rather than those in the neostriatal

area of the basal ganglia. This allows this agent to exert an antipsychotic action without leading to difficulties with movement.

Clozapine can have a possibly fatal side effect in about 1% to 2% of clients. This is due to its potential to suppress bone marrow and induce agranulocytosis. Any deficiency in white blood cells (WBC) renders a person prone to serious infection. For this reason, regular weekly measurement of WBC count is mandatory for any client taking clozapine.

Clozapine also has the potential for inducing convulsions in a small percentage (3%) of clients. This means that all clients taking the drug must be monitored closely.

The most common side effects of clozapine are drowsiness and sedation (40%), hypersalivation (30%), tachycardia (25%), and dizziness (20%). Because of these side effects, this drug is not used as a first choice. When it is used, the person's WBC count is monitored at frequent intervals for signs of granulocytosis. The other atypicals discussed here are all good first-line drugs for schizophrenia. Unfortunately, all the atypicals are much more expensive than the first-line agents, thereby putting them out of reach for many individuals.

Risperidone

Risperidone (Risperdal) is an antipsychotic drug that shares with clozapine the ability to treat psychotic symptoms of delusions and hallucinations without frequently inducing motor abnormalities, as many of the older drugs did. Unlike clozapine, it does not seem to have the potential for inducing agranulocytosis or convulsions. These advantages are offset, however, by the fact that at doses of risperidone only slightly higher than those that are effective, clients taking this drug may begin to experience motor difficulties. Because risperidone blocks alpha₁ and histamine-1 (H₁) receptors, it can cause orthostatic hypotension and sedation. Keep in mind that orthostatic hypotension can lead to falls, which are a serious problem among the elderly.

Quetiapine

Quetiapine (Seroquell) has a very broad receptor-binding profile; this drug binds to and antagonizes D₁, D₂, 5-HT₁, 5-HT₂, alpha₁, alpha₂, and H₁ receptors. Its strong blockage of H₁ receptors accounts for the sedation and weight gain associated with this drug. It causes moderate blockage of muscarinic and alpha₁ receptors and associated side effects. At normal doses it has not been associated with extrapyramidal symptoms.

Olanzapine

Olanzapine (Zyprexa) is chemically related to clozapine. It seems to have a similar receptor profile and efficacy, but to be free of the danger of bone marrow suppression. One of its major disadvantages is significant weight gain in some clients.

Please refer to Chapter 20 for a detailed discussion of the positive and negative symptoms in schizophrenia, and the indications for use of the standard and atypical antipsychotics, as well as side effects, toxic effects, dosage, nursing implications, and client and family teaching.

MOOD STABILIZERS

Lithium

Although the efficacy of lithium as a mood-stabilizing drug in bipolar (manic-depressive) clients has been established for many years, its mechanism of action is still far from understood. As a positively charged ion, similar in structure to sodium and potassium, it may well act by affecting electrical conductivity in neurons.

As we discussed earlier, an electrical impulse consists of the inward, depolarizing flow of sodium followed by an outward, repolarizing of potassium. These electrical charges are propagated along the neuron so that, if they are initiated at one end of the neuron, they will pass to the other end. Once they reach the end of a neuron, a transmitter is released.

It may be that an overexcitement of neurons in some parts of the brain underlies bipolar disorders and that lithium interacts in some complex way with sodium and potassium at the cell membrane to stabilize electrical activity. Even if not responsible for its beneficial effects, an alteration in electrical conductivity certainly explains some of the adverse effects and toxicity of lithium.

By altering electrical conductivity, lithium represents a potential threat to all body functions that are regulated by electrical currents. Foremost among these functions, of course, is cardiac contraction, so that lithium can induce cardiac dysrhythmias. Extreme alteration of cerebral conductivity can lead to convulsions. Alteration in nerve and muscle conduction can lead to tremor or more extreme motor dysfunction.

The fact that sodium and potassium play a strong role in regulating fluid balance and the distribution of fluid in various body compartments explains the disturbances in fluid balance that can

be caused by lithium. These include polyuria (the output of large volumes of water) and edema (the accumulation of fluid in the interstitial space). There seems to be some evidence that long-term use of lithium increases the risk of kidney and thyroid disease.

Primarily because of its effects on electrical conductivity, lithium has the lowest therapeutic index of all psychiatric drugs. The therapeutic index represents the ratio of the lethal dose to the effective dose, and thus the safety of a drug. A low therapeutic index means that the blood level of a drug that can cause death is not far removed from the blood level required for drug effectiveness. This means that the blood level of lithium needs to be monitored on a regular basis to be sure that the drug is not accumulating and rising to dangerous levels. Table 3–3 lists some of the adverse effects of lithium. Chapter 19 goes into more depth as to lithium levels as they relate to specific side and toxic effects, nursing implications, and client teaching plan.

Antiepileptic Drugs

Carbamazepine, valproic acid, and clonazepam were originally introduced as antiepileptic agents but are now being used to treat a variety of psychiatric conditions. Their anticonvulsant properties derive from the fact that they alter electrical conductivity in membranes; in particular, they reduce the firing rate of very-high-frequency neurons in the brain. It is possible that this membrane-stabilizing effect accounts for the ability of these drugs to reduce the mood swings that occur in bipolar clients. The drugs are particularly effective in reducing the excitement of the manic phase of this disease; thus, they are sometimes used to calm a manic client before long-term stabilization with lithium. When the client cannot tolerate lithium, carbamazepine or clo-

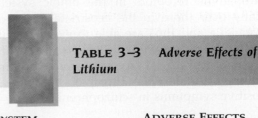

TABLE 3–3 *Adverse Effects of Lithium*

SYSTEM	ADVERSE EFFECTS
Nervous system and muscle	Tremor, ataxia, confusion, convulsions
Digestive	Nausea, vomiting, diarrhea
Cardiac	Arrhythmias
Fluid and electrolyte	Polyuria, polydipsia, edema
Endocrine	Goiter and hyperthyroidism

nazepam may be used for long-term maintenance therapy.

Carbamazepine

Carbamazepine (Tegretol) is structurally similar to the tricyclic antidepressants (TCAs) (see later discussion), although it is not clear if it shares the ability of these drugs to treat unipolar depression. Carbamazepine does, however, share the ability of TCAs to serve as a neurological analgesic. It is particularly effective in conditions such as trigeminal neuralgia that involve paroxysms (bursts) of severe pain. The efficacy of carbamazepine as an analgesic may be related to its ability to reduce the firing rate of overexcited neurons as well as to its ability to calm the accompanying psychological agitation associated with the pain.

Valproic Acid

Valproic acid/valproate (Depakote) is an anticonvulsant, structurally different from other anticonvulsants and psychiatric drugs, that shows efficacy in the treatment of manic depression. Both hepatic failure and birth defects have been associated with this drug, and liver function tests are required periodically.

Clonazepam

Clonazepam (Klonopin) is structurally a benzodiazepine, a type of antianxiety drug discussed later in this chapter. These drugs have strong sedating properties, which may in part account for the ability of clonazepam to calm a client rapidly in the manic phase of a bipolar disorder. Clonazepam is also increasingly being used as part of a multiple-drug regimen to treat clients who show a mixture of anxious and depressive symptoms concomitantly; these individuals are sometimes given both antidepressants and antianxiety agents.

Refer to Chapter 19 for a detailed discussion of the side effects, toxic effects, dosage, indications for use, nursing implications, and client and family teaching.

Antidepressant Drugs

Our understanding of the neurophysiological basis of mood disorders is far from complete. However, a great deal of evidence seems to indicate that the neurotransmitters norepinephrine and serotonin play a major role in regulating mood. It is thought that a transmission deficiency of one or both of these monoamines within the limbic system underlies depression. Figure 3–11 identifies the types of side effects that a person may experience when specific neurotransmitters are blocked or bound. One of the lines of evidence pointing in this direction is that all the drugs that show efficacy in the treatment of depression increase the synaptic level of one or both of these transmitters. Figure 3–12 illustrates the normal release, reuptake, and destruction of the monoamine transmitters. A grasp of this underlying physiology is essential for understanding the mechanisms by which the antidepressant drugs are thought to act.

Typical/Standard Antidepressants

TRICYCLIC ANTIDEPRESSANTS. Typical/standard antidepressants such as the TCAs (amitriptyline [Elavil], imipramine [Tofranil], and nortriptyline [Pamelor]) are thought to act primarily by blocking the reuptake of norepinephrine and, to a lesser degree, serotonin. As described in Box 3–5, this blocking prevents norepinephrine from coming into contact with its degrading enzyme, MAO, and thus increases the level of norepinephrine at the synapse. Similarly, the TCAs block the reuptake and destruction of serotonin and also increase the synaptic level of this type of transmitter. Exactly how the increased level of these transmitters alleviates depression is far from clear; however, many controlled scientific studies attest to the efficacy of these drugs.

To varying degrees, many of the tricyclic drugs also block the muscarinic receptors that normally bind acetylcholine. As discussed in the previous section, this blockage leads to typical anticholinergic effects such as blurred vision, dry mouth, tachycardia, and constipation. These adverse effects can be troubling to clients and can limit their compliance with the regimen.

Again to varying degrees, depending on the individual drug, these drugs can block H_1 receptors in the brain. Blockage of these receptors by any drug causes sedation and drowsiness, an unwelcome symptom in daily use.

Selective Serotonin Reuptake Inhibitors

As the name implies, the selective serotonin reuptake inhibitors (SSRIs), such as fluoxetine (Prozac), sertraline (Zoloft), paroxetine (Paxil), and citalopram (Celexa), preferentially block the reuptake and thus the destruction of serotonin, with little or no effect on the other monoamine transmitters. These drugs, as a group, also have less ability to block the muscarinic and H_1 receptors than do the tricyclic agents. As a result of their more selective action, they seem

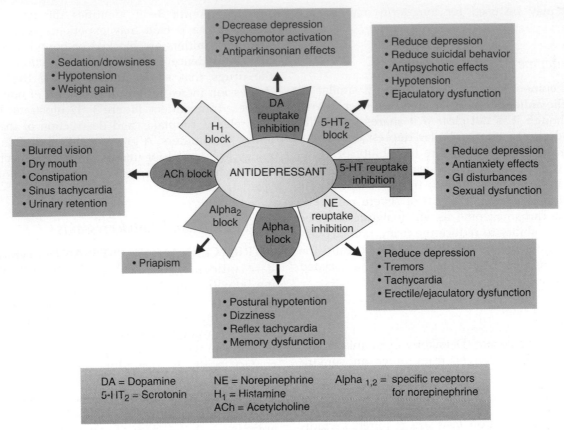

Figure 3–11 Possible effects of receptor binding.

to show comparable efficacy while not eliciting the anticholinergic and sedating side effects that limit client compliance (Box 3–6).

Monoamine Oxidase Inhibitors

The monoamine oxidase inhibitors are a group of antidepressant drugs that illustrate the principle that drugs can have a desired and beneficial effect in the brain, while at the same time having possibly dangerous effects elsewhere in the body. To understand the action of these drugs, keep in mind the following definitions:

Monoamines: a type of organic compound; includes the neurotransmitters norepinephrine, epinephrine, dopamine, and serotonin, as well as many different food substances and drugs

Monoamine oxidase (MAO): an enzyme that destroys monoamines.

Monoamine oxidase inhibitors (MAOIs): drugs that prevent the destruction of monoamines by inhibiting the action of MAO.

The monoamine neurotransmitters, as well as any monoamine food substance or drugs, are degraded (destroyed) by the enzyme MAO, which is located in neurons and in the liver. Antidepressant drugs

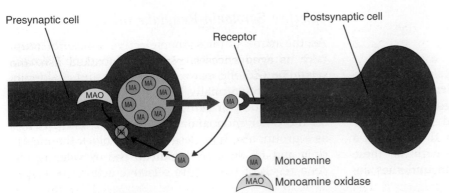

Monoamine

Monoamine oxidase

Figure 3–12 Normal release, reuptake, and destruction of the monoamine transmitters.

BOX 3–5 *How the Tricyclic Antidepressant Drugs Work*

Whether the original cause of depression is biological, psychological, or social, its symptomatic expression seems to be associated with a deficiency of either or both of the monoamine neurotransmitters norepinephrine and serotonin. The most commonly used pharmacological interventions for the treatment of depression are directed at increasing the activity of these transmitters. Tricyclic antidepressant drugs accomplish this task by blocking the reuptake of norepinephrine and, to a lesser degree of serotonin into the presynaptic cell, as illustrated.

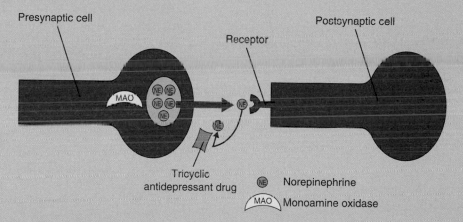

Presynaptic cell
Postsynaptic cell
Receptor
MAO
NE
Tricyclic antidepressant drug
NE Norepinephrine
MAO Monoamine oxidase

Blocking norepinephrine reentry into the presynaptic cell increases the concentration of this transmitter in the synaptic space and, presumably, its action on the postsynaptic cell. This explanation of the beneficial actions of tricyclic drugs is called into question somewhat by the fact that the blockage of transmitter reuptake occurs immediately, whereas the alleviation of depressive symptoms by these drugs usually takes 2 or 3 weeks. Although a number of theories attempt to explain this discrepancy, a proved and agreed explanation is not available at present.

The pharmacological actions of the tricyclic antidepressants are not limited to the blockade of monoamine reuptake and destruction. As is the case with the phenothiazines, these drugs can block muscarinic and alpha₁-adrenergic receptors. Many of these agents have quite strong muscarinic blocking ability and can produce the predictable antiparasympathetic responses of blurred vision, constipation, tachycardia, and urinary retention. Alpha₁ antagonism blocks the pressor response necessary to avoid orthostatic hypotension.

Although an antidepressant drug might be thought to be somewhat of a stimulant, this is not the case for the tricyclic drugs. In fact, many of these drugs have strong sedating properties. The sedating actions of tricyclic drugs are believed to be due to their ability to block histamine receptors in the brain.

In addition to those untoward effects attributable to known mechanisms of action, most drugs can also have undesirable actions for which there is no clear-cut explanation at present. The most serious toxic and life-threatening effects of tricyclic drugs at high doses are convulsions and the depression of cardiac conductivity and contractility. The therapeutic index (ratio of toxic dose to safe dose) of tricyclic drugs is low, and they are potential agents of accidental and deliberate death.

such as phenelzine (Nardil) and tranylcypromine (Parnate) are MAOIs; that is, they act by inhibiting the enzyme and interfering with the destruction of the monoamine neurotransmitters. This in turn increases the synaptic level of the transmitters (Box 3–7) and makes possible the antidepressant effects of these drugs.

The use of MAO-inhibiting drugs is complicated by the fact that the enzyme is also present in the liver and is responsible for degrading monoamine substances that enter the body via food or drugs.

Of particular importance is the monoamine tyramine, which is present in many food substances such as aged cheeses, pickled or smoked fish, and wine. Tyramine poses a threat of hypertensive crises because it can produce intense vasoconstriction, and thus an elevation in blood pressure, if allowed to circulate freely in the blood. Normally, this does not happen, because tyramine is destroyed by MAO as it passes through the liver before entering the general blood circulation. However, in the presence of MAOIs, tyramine is not destroyed by the liver and can cause serious, even life-threatening, hypertension.

A substantial number of drugs are chemically monoamines. The dosage of these drugs is determined by the rate at which they are destroyed by MAO in the liver. In a client on MAOIs, the blood level of monoamine drugs can reach high levels and cause serious toxicity.

Because of the dangers that result from destruction of hepatic MAO, clients on MAO-inhibiting drugs must be given a list of food and drugs high in tyramine that need to be avoided. Chapter 18 discusses the treatment of depression and contains a list of forbidden foods and foods to be taken in moderation, along with nursing measures and instructions for client teaching.

Atypical/Novel Antidepressants

A number of drugs seem to work by mechanisms less clearly defined than those of the TCAs, SSRIs, and MAOIs and are sometimes grouped under the heading of atypical antidepressants. Of these, we will briefly discuss trazodone, nefazodone, venlafaxine, mirtazapine, and bupropion.

Trazodone and nefazodone are chemically related compounds that affect the reuptake of serotonin and, to a lesser degree, norepinephrine. They differ from the TCAs and SSRIs in that they and their metabolites (chemicals formed from the drugs by the liver) can act directly on the 5-hydroxytryptamine (5-HT) postsynaptic receptors for serotonin. The complexity of relating the biological actions of a drug to its clinical effects is well illustrated by these agents, in that the drugs themselves can antagonize the receptors while their metabolites act as receptor agonists. Thus, we have drugs that increase the concentration of serotonin at the synapse by blocking its reuptake, that block serotonin at the receptor, and that form chemicals, thereby mimicking serotonin at the receptor. We are left with a question as to the overall physiological results of these drugs and how they relate to their proven efficacy in reducing depression.

TRAZODONE (DESYREL). Trazodone (Desyrel) is a very weak antagonist of muscarinic receptors that was originally introduced as an alternative to the TCAs, which have strong anticholinergic actions. It does, however, block alpha$_1$ and H$_1$ receptors and thus can cause orthostatic hypotension

Box 3–6 *How the Inhibitors of Serotonin Reuptake (SSRIs) Work*

Fluoxetine, sertraline, paroxetine, and related selective serotonin reuptake inhibitors (SSRIs) specifically block the reuptake of serotonin (5-hydroxytryptamine) into the presynaptic cell from which it was originally released. As a result of this blockage, in a fashion analogous to the action of tricyclic antidepressants on norepinephrine, the destruction of the transmitter is reduced and its concentration at the postsynaptic cell increased. Because these drugs are specific to serotonin and have little or no ability to block muscarinic and other receptors, they tend to have fewer untoward autonomic effects than the tricyclic drugs. In addition, they do not cause as much sedation or have cardiac toxicity. However, to the degree that depression involves norepinephrine deficiency and presents with symptoms of agitation, the serotonin blockers may have less efficacy than the tricyclic antidepressants. Untoward effects of the serotonin reuptake inhibitors include excessive stimulation and changes in body weight.

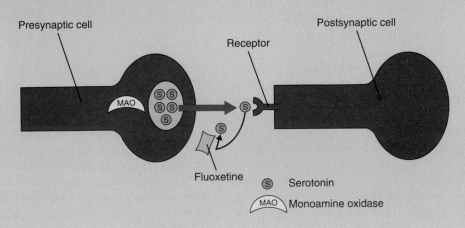

Box 3–7 *How the Monoamine Oxidase Inhibitors Work*

As illustrated, inhibitors of the enzyme monoamine oxidase (MAO) act by interfering with the ability of this enzyme to destroy the monoamines norepinephrine, dopamine, and serotonin (5-hydroxytryptamine). Enzyme inhibition eventually leads to an increase in the presynaptic, synaptic, and postsynaptic concentrations of these neurotransmitters. Increased postsynaptic activity of one or more of these transmitters would then account for the beneficial effects of these drugs in certain forms of depression. As with the tricyclic drugs, this explanation still leaves unsolved the problem of the 2 to 3 week time lag between enzyme inactivation and clinical improvement.

MAO is present in liver cells, as well as in mono-amine-releasing neurons. In the liver, this enzyme has the function of destroying circulating endogenous monoamines (e.g., the hormone epinephrine) and exogenous monoamines (e.g., tyramine), which are present in many foods and readily absorbed from the digestive tract. Inactivation of hepatic MAO by MAO-inhibiting drugs can lead to a potentially fatal interaction between these drugs and foods such as aged cheeses, which contain significant amounts of tyramine. This is because tyramine can trigger the release of norepinephrine from sympathetic nerve endings. Norepinephrine is a potent vasoconstrictor, and the sudden release of large amounts of norepinephrine in response to tyramine can produce a life-threatening hypertensive crisis. In the absence of MAO-inhibiting drugs, tyramine does not present a problem because it is destroyed by MAO when the absorbed food is brought to the liver by the blood passing through the hepatic portal system. To avoid the possibility of a hypertensive crisis, clients are given a list of foods that contain large amounts of tyramine and are to be eliminated from the individual's diet.

A large number of pharmacological agents, particularly sympathomimetic drugs, are monoamines and are broken down by hepatic MAO. The plasma level of such drugs resulting from a given dose may be vastly increased in the presence of MAO-inhibiting drugs. Thus these drugs must be used with great care, if at all, in a client who is also taking MAO inhibitors. **Because many of the monoamine drugs are sold over the counter, clients taking MAO inhibitors must be given a list of drugs as well as foods to be avoided.**

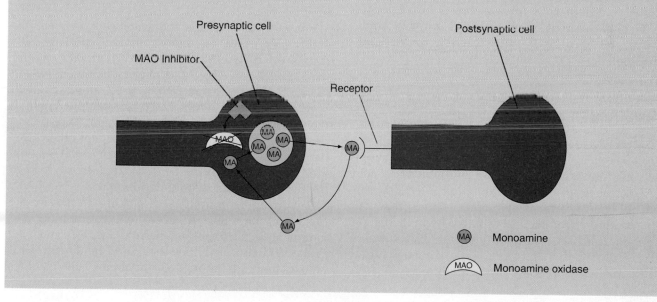

and sedation. These are very serious problems in the elderly, since they can increase the likelihood of falls and broken bones. Trazodone has also been associated with **priapism** in males; this is a painful, continuous erectile state unrelated to sexual desires or activity.

NEFAZODONE (SERZONE). Nefazodone (Serzone), a relative of trazodone, does not block alpha$_1$ and H$_1$ receptors, so it does not lead to orthostatic hypotension and sedation, and it has proved to be an effective antidepressant agent.

VENLAFAXINE (EFFEXOR). Venlafaxine (Effexor) blocks the reuptake of both norepinephrine and serotonin. Since it does not block muscarinic, alpha$_1$, or H$_1$ receptors, it is relatively free of the adverse effects that occur when these receptors are inhibited. It has been found particularly useful in the treatment of severely depressed and melancholic clients. For reasons not currently understood, it can cause some clients to feel heightened anxiety and the very uncomfortable sensations of nausea, vomiting, and dizziness. It has also been associated with abnormal ejaculation and impotence in males. Refer to Chapter 19 for the nursing implications, dosages, side effects, and toxic effects of each group of antidepressants, as well as teaching tools.

MIRTAZAPINE (REMERON). Mirtazapine (Remeron) acts on 5-HT$_2$ and alpha$_2$ presynaptic norepinephrine receptors. It is thought that the end result of these actions is to increase the firing of norepinephrine neurons. Unfortunately, this drug is also an antagonist at H$_1$ and muscarinic receptors, leading to the expected side effects of sedation, weight gain, dry mouth, and constipation. The antimuscarinic effects are not quite as strong as with some of the other antidepressants.

BUPROPION (WELLBUTRIN). Bupropion (Wellbutrin) is another antidepressant that provides efficacy by a mechanism that is far from understood. Unlike many other antidepressants, it rarely causes sedation, weight gain, or sexual dysfunction. The absence of these untoward effects can lead to greater patient acceptance. However, headache, insomnia, nausea, and restlessness are experienced as side effects by some clients.

Refer to Chapter 18 for a detailed discussion of the side effects, toxic effects, dosages, nursing implications, and client and family teaching for the antidepressants.

ANTIANXIETY/ANXIOLYTIC DRUGS

The neurotransmitter **gamma-aminobutyric acid (GABA)** seems to exert an inhibitory effect on neurons in many parts of the brain. Drugs that can enhance this effect exert a sedative-hypnotic action on brain function. Many drugs with this type of effect, called antianxiety/anxiolytic drugs, tend to reduce anxiety, and some are actually used as anti-anxiety agents. The most commonly used drugs of this group are the benzodiazepines.

Benzodiazepines

Figure 3–13 shows that benzodiazepines, e.g., diazepam (Valium), clonazepam (Klonopin), and alprazolam (Xanax), bind to specific receptors adjacent to the GABA receptors. Because of their ability to bind benzodiazepines, these receptors are called benzodiazepine receptors. Binding of benzodiazepines to these receptors at the same time as GABA allows GABA to inhibit more forcefully than it would if binding alone. The fact that benzodiazepines do not inhibit neurons in the absence of GABA limits the potential toxicity of these drugs.

Of the various benzodiazepines, some, such as flurazepam (Dalmane) and triazolam (Halcion), have a predominantly hypnotic (sleep-inducing) effect, whereas others, such as lorazepam (Ativan) and alprazolam (Xanax), reduce anxiety without being as soporific (sleep producing). Currently, there is no clear explanation for the differential effects of the various benzodiazepines. There seems to be some evidence that there are subtypes of the benzodiazepine receptors in different areas of the brain, and these subtypes differ in their ability to bind the different drugs.

The fact that the benzodiazepines potentiate the ability of GABA to inhibit neurons probably accounts for their efficacy as anticonvulsants and for their ability to reduce the neuronal overexcitement of alcohol withdrawal. When used alone, even at high doses, these drugs rarely inhibit the brain to the degree of respiratory depression, coma, and death. However, when combined with other CNS depressants, such as alcohol, opiates, or TCAs, the inhibitory actions of the benzodiazepines can lead to life-threatening respiratory depression.

Any drug that inhibits electrical activity in the brain can interfere with motor ability, attention, and judgment; a client taking benzodiazepines must be cautioned about activities that could be dangerous if reflexes and attention are impaired. This includes

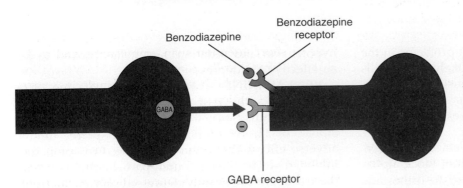

Figure 3–13 Action of **benzodiazepines.** The group of drugs called benzodiazepines attach to receptors adjacent to the receptors for the neurotransmitter GABA. Drug attachment to receptors results in a strengthening of the inhibitor effects of GABA. In the absence of GABA there is no inhibitory effect of benzodiazepines.

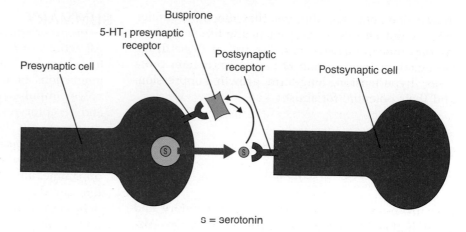

Figure 3–14 Action of **buspirone**. A proposed mechanism of action for buspirone is that it blocks feedback inhibition by serotonin. This leads to increased release of serotonin by the presynaptic cell.

s = serotonin

specialized activities such as working in construction on a tall building and more common activities such as driving a car. In the elderly, the use of benzodiazepines may contribute to falls and broken bones. Chapter 14 discusses the nursing considerations, indications, side and toxic effects, and teaching strategies for clients taking benzodiazepines.

Buspirone (BuSpar)

Buspirone (BuSpar) is a drug that reduces anxiety, without having strong sedative-hypnotic properties. Since this agent does not leave the client sleepy or sluggish, it is often much better tolerated than the benzodiazepines. It is also not a CNS depressant and thus does not represent as great a danger of interaction with other CNS depressants such as alcohol, nor is there the potential for addiction that exists with benzodiazepines.

Although at present the mechanism of action of buspirone is not clearly understood, one possibility is illustrated in Figure 3–14. Buspirone seems to act as an antagonist at presynaptic 5-HT$_1$ receptors. The normal function of these receptors is to monitor the synaptic level of serotonin; that is, serotonin released by the neurons binds not only to postsynaptic receptors to exert its effects on adjacent neurons but also to presynaptic receptors on the neuron from which it is released. Once bound to the presynaptic receptor, serotonin inhibits the further release of this transmitter; this release serves as negative feedback. Buspirone, by blocking these presynaptic receptors, prevents the negative feedback and allows more transmitter to be released. The end result is an increased synaptic level of serotonin that presumably accounts for the beneficial action of this drug.

Please refer to Chapter 14 for the side effects, toxic effects, dosages, nursing implications, and client and family teaching for the anxiolytic drugs.

ANTIDEPRESSION TREATMENT OF CONDITIONS ASSOCIATED WITH ANXIETY

A variety of psychiatric conditions involve symptom formation for which it is thought anxiety plays a major role. Included among these would be panic attacks, generalized anxiety disorder, phobias, obsessive-compulsive disorder, social anxiety, and possibly eating disorders. Although the etiologies of these conditions are far from understood, it has been found clinically that antidepressants often show efficacy in their treatment. Antidepressants from all the various classes are being investigated in the treatment of these conditions. There is some indication that specific classes, or drugs, show special efficacy in specific conditions. Thus, imipramine is often used to treat panic attack, SSRIs for obsessive-compulsive disorders, and sertraline in social phobias. The relationships of depression and the anxiety disorders is an area of active research.

TREATMENT OF ATTENTION DEFICIT DISORDER/ HYPERACTIVITY SYNDROME

Children and adults with this condition show symptoms of short attention span, impulsivity, and overactivity. Paradoxically, the mainstay of treatment for this condition in children, and increasingly in adults, is the administration of psychostimulant drugs. Both methylphenidate (Ritalin) and amphetamines such as Adderall seem to show efficacy in these conditions. These drugs seem to work by increasing the release and blocking the reuptake of monoamines. How this translates into clinical efficacy is far from understood, but it is thought that the monoamines may inhibit an overactive part of the limbic system. Among many concerns with the use of these drugs are agitation, exacerbation of psychotic thought processes, hypertension, long-term growth suppression, and their potential for abuse.

DRUG TREATMENT FOR ALZHEIMER'S DISEASE

The insidious and progressive loss of memory and other higher brain functions brought about by Alzheimer's disease is a great individual family and social tragedy. Since the disease seems to involve progressive structural degeneration of the brain, there are two major pharmacological directions in its treatments. The first is to attempt to prevent or slow the structural degeneration. Although actively pursued, this approach has so far not been successful. The second is to attempt to maintain normal brain function for as long as possible. Much of the memory loss in this disease has been attributed to dysfunction of neurons that secrete acetylcholine. Tacrine and donepezil are *anticholinesterase drugs*, or *cholinesterase inhibitors*, that show some efficacy in slowing the rate of memory loss and, in some clients, may even improve memory. The drugs work by interfering with the action of acetylcholinesterase. Inactivation of this enzyme leads to less destruction of the neurotransmitter acetylcholine and, therefore, a higher concentration at the synapse.

TACRINE (COGNEX). Tacrine (Cognex) was the first anticholinesterase approved by the Food and Drug Administration for the treatment of Alzheimer's disease. It has been shown to have moderate efficacy in some clients. Untoward effects include nausea, abdominal distress, tachycardia, and hepatic toxicity in some clients. Liver enzymes should be monitored on a regular basis.

DONEPEZIL (ARICEPT). This anticholinesterase shows clinical efficacy in some clients with Alzheimer's disease without the liver toxicity associated with tacrine. Untoward effects include nausea, diarrhea, and sedation.

Refer to Chapter 21 for appropriate nursing knowledge of these drugs and teaching strategies.

SUMMARY

All actions of the brain—sensory, motor, intellectual—are carried out physiologically through the interactions of nerve cells. These interactions involve impulse conduction, transmitter release, and receptor response. Alterations in these basic processes can lead to mental disturbances and physical manifestations.

In particular, it seems that excess activity of dopamine, among other factors, is involved in the thought disturbances of schizophrenia, and that deficiencies of norepinephrine, or serotonin, or both underlie the mood disturbances of depression. Insufficient activity of GABA seems to play a role in anxiety.

Pharmacological treatment of mental disturbances is directed at the suspected transmitter-receptor problem. Thus, antipsychotic drugs block dopamine receptors, antidepressant drugs increase synaptic levels of norepinephrine and/or serotonin, and antianxiety drugs increase the effectiveness of GABA.

Since the immediate target activity of a drug can result in many downstream alterations in neuronal activity, it has been found that drugs with a variety of chemical actions may show efficacy in the same clinical condition. Thus, in the treatment of schizophrenia, depression, and anxiety, newer drugs with novel mechanisms of action are being brought into use. This often makes understanding the pharmacology of mental disease more, rather than less, difficult. Unfortunately, as is the case for almost all pharmacological agents, the agents used to treat mental disease can also cause various undesired effects. Prominent among these can be sedation or excitement, motor disturbances, muscarinic blockage, alpha antagonism, sexual dysfunction, and weight gain. There is a continuing effort on the part of pharmacologists to develop new drugs that are effective as well as safe and comfortable for people suffering from emotional disorders.

Visit the **Evolve** website at
http://evolve.elsevier.com/Varcarolis
for a post-test on the content in this chapter.

Visit the **Evolve** website at
http://evolve.elsevier.com/Varcarolis
for additional self-study exercises.

Critical Thinking and Chapter Review

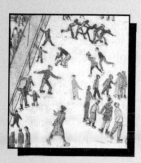

Critical Thinking

1. With an understanding that no matter where you practice nursing, many individuals under your care will be taking one psychotropic drug or another (especially an antidepressant, antianxiety medication, or even antimanic), how important is it for you in your nursing practice to understand the normal brain structure and function as they relate to mental disturbances and psychotropic drugs? Include in your answer:

   ■ Ways nurses can use the knowledge about how normal brain function (control of peripheral nerves, skeletal muscles, the autonomic nervous system, hormones, and circadian rhythms) can be affected by either psychotropic drugs or psychiatric illness
   ■ Ways brain imaging can help in understanding and treating people with mental disorders
   ■ Ways your understanding of how neurotransmitters work may affect your ability to assess your clients' responses to specific medications

2. What specific information could you include in your medication teaching for your client based on your understanding of what symptoms may occur with alterations of the following neurotransmitters?

   ■ Dopamine D_2 (as in phenothiazines and other drugs)
   ■ Blockage of muscarinic receptors (as in phenothiazines and other drugs)
   ■ Alpha$_1$ receptors (as in phenothiazines and other drugs)
   ■ Histamine (as in phenothiazines and other drugs)
   ■ MAO (as in an MAOI)
   ■ GABA (as in antianxiety drugs)

Chapter Review

Choose the most appropriate answer.

1. A nurse administering a benzodiazepine should understand that the therapeutic effect of benzodiazepines results from potentiating the neurotransmitter

   1. GABA
   2. dopamine
   3. serotonin
   4. acetylcholine

2. Fluoxetine (an SSRI) exerts its antidepressant effect by blocking the reuptake of

   1. GABA
   2. dopamine
   3. serotonin
   4. norepinephrine

3. The nurse administers each of the following drugs to various clients. The client who should be most carefully assessed for fluid and electrolyte imbalance is the one receiving

   1. lithium
   2. clozapine
   3. diazepam
   4. amitriptyline

4. Which drug group calls for nursing assessment for development of parkinsonian movement disorders among individuals who take therapeutic doses?

   1. SSRIs
   2. phenothiazines
   3. benzodiazepines
   4. tricyclic antidepressants

5. Which of the following effects cannot be attributed to a medication that blocks muscarinic receptors?

   1. dry mouth
   2. constipation
   3. hypotension
   4. blurred vision

REFERENCES

Abelson, J. L. and Curtis, G. C. (1996). Hypothalamic-pituitary-adrenal axis activity in panic disorder. *Archives of General Psychiatry.* 53:323–331.

American College of Neuropsychopharmacology. (1992). Suicidal behavior and psychotropic medication (consensus statement). *Neurophsychopharmacology,* 8:177.

Andersen, P.H. et al. (1990). Dopamine receptor subtypes. *Trends in Pharmacological Science,* 11:231.

Baldessarini, R. J., et al. (1990). Clozapine—a novel antipsychotic agent. *New England Journal of Medicine,* 324: 746.

Ballenger, J. C. (1995). Benzodiazepines. In A. F. Schatzberg and C. B. Nemeroff (Eds.), *Textbook of psychopharmacology.* Washington, DC: American Psychiatric Press.

Beare, R.G. and Myers J.L. (1994). *Principles and practices of adult health nursing,* (2nd ed.) (p. 1167). St. Louis: Mosby-Yearbook.

Boyer, W.E., and Feighner, J.P. (1991). The efficacy of selective serotonin uptake inhibitors in depression. In Feighner and W.E. Boyer (Eds.), *Selective serotonin uptake inhibitors.* Chichester, England: John Wiley.

Burman, R.M., et al. (1999). Principles of the pharmacotherapy of depression. In D.S. Charney, E.J. Nestler and B.S. Bunney (Eds), *Neurobiology of mental illness.* New York: Oxford University Press.

Byne, W., et al. (1999). The neurochemistry of schizophrenia. In D.S. Charney, E.J. Nestler and B.S. Bunney (Eds), *Neurobiology of mental illness.* New York: Oxford University Press.

Charney, D.S., et al. (1991). Current hypotheses of the mechanism of antidepressant treatment: Implications for the treatment of refractory depression. In J.S. Amsterdam (Ed.), *Advances in neuropsychiatry and psychopharmacology* (Vol. 2). New York: Raven Press.

Charney, D.S., and Bremmer J.D. (1999). The neurobiology of anxiety disorder. In D.S. Charney, E.J. Nestler and B.S. Bunney (Eds), *Neurobiology of mental illness.* New York: Oxford University Press.

Cole, J.O., and Yonkers, K.A. (1995). Nonbenzodiazepine anxiolytics. In A.F. Schatzberg and C.B. Nemeroff (Eds.), *Textbook of psychopharmacology.* Washington, DC: American Psychiatric Press.

Cooper, J.R., Bloom, F.E., and Roth, R.H. (1992). *The biochemical basis of neuropharmacology* (6th ed.). New York: Oxford University Press.

Dechant, K.L., and Cissold, S.P. (1991). Paroxetine. *Drugs,* 41:225.

Dentch, A. Y. and Roth, R. H. (1999). Neurochemical systems in the central nervous systems. In D. S. Charney, E.J. Nestler and B.S. Bunney (Eds), *Neurobiology of mental illness.* New York: Oxford University Press.

Duman, R.S. (1999). The neurochemistry of mood disorders: Preclinical Studies. In D.S. Charney, E.J. Nestler and B.S. Bunney (Eds), *Neurobiology of mental illness.* New York: Oxford University Press.

Faraona, S.V. and Biederman, J. (1999). The neurobiology of attention deficit hyperactivity disorder. In D.S. Charney, E.J. Nestler and B.S. Bunney (Eds), *Neurobiology of mental illness.* New York: Oxford University Press.

Fitton, A., and Heel, R.C. (1990). Clozapine—a review of pharmacological properties and therapeutic use in schizophrenia. *Drugs,* 40:722.

Gerlach, J. (1991). New antipsychotics: classification, efficacy and adverse effects. *Schizophrenia Bulletin,* 17(2):289.

Goddard, A.W., et al. (1999). Principles of the pharmacotherapy of the anxiety disorders. In D.S. Charney, E.J. Nestler and B.S. Bunney (Eds), *Neurobiology of mental illness.* New York: Oxford University Press.

Goodwin, F. K., and Jamison, K.R. (1990). *Manic-depressive illness.* New York: Oxford University Press.

Heninger, G. R. (1999). Special challenges in the investigation of the neurobiology of mental illness. In D. S. Charney, E.J. Nestler and B.S. Bunney (Eds), *Neurobiology of mental illness.* New York: Oxford University Press.

Hollister, L.E. (1995). Antipsychotic agents and lithium. In G.G. Katzung (Ed.), *Basic and clinical pharmacology.* Norwalk: Appleton & Lange.

Hyman, S. E. and Nestler, E. (1996). Initiation and adaptation: a paradigm for understanding psychotropic drugs' action. *American Journal of Psychiatry*, 153:151–162.

Krishnan, K.R. (1995). Monoamine oxidase inhibitors. In A.F. Schatzberg and C.B. Nemeroff (Eds.), *Textbook of psychopharmacology*. Washington, DC: American Psychiatric Press.

Lavin, M.R., and Rifkin, A. (1992). Neuroleptic induced parkinsonnism. In J.M. Kane and J.A. Lieberman (Eds.), *Adverse effects of psychotropic drugs*. New York: Guilford Press.

Manji, H.K., et al. (1991). Mechanisms of action of lithium. *Archives of General Psychiatry*, 48:505.

Mansour, A., et al. (1995). Biochemical anatomy: Insights into the cell biology and pharmacology of neurotransmitter systems in the brain. In A. F. Schatzberg and C. B. Nemeroff (Eds.), *Textbook of psychopharmacology*. Washington, DC: American Psychiatric Press.

Marin, D.B. (1999) Principles of the pharmacotherapy of dementia. In D.S. Charney, E.J. Nestler and B.S. Bunney (Eds), *Neurobiology of mental illness*. New York: Oxford University Press.

Modell, S., et al. (1997) Corticosteroid receptor function is decreased in depressed patients. *Neuroendocrinology*, 65:216–222.

Nestler, E. J., and Hyman, S. E. (1999). Mechanisms of neural plasticity. In D. S. Charney, E.J. Nestler and B.S. Bunney (Eds), *Neurobiology of mental illness*. New York: Oxford University Press.

Owens, M.J., and Rich, S.L. (1995). Atypical antipsychotics. In A.F. Schatzberg and C.B. Nemeroff (Eds.). *Textbook of psychopharmacology*. Washington, DC: American Psychiatric Press.

Perl, D.P. (1999). Abnormalities in brain structures on postmortem analysis of dementias. In D.S. Charney, E.J. Nestler and B.S. Bunney (Eds), *Neurobiology of mental illness*. New York: Oxford University Press.

Ray, W.A. (1992). Psychotropic drugs and injuries among the elderly: A review. *Journal of Clinical Psychopharmacology*, 12:386.

Risby, E.D., et al. (1991). The mechanisms of action of lithium. *Archives of General Psychiatry*, 48:513.

Risch, N., and Merileangas, K. (1996). The future of genetic studies of complex human disease. *Science*, 273:1516–1517.

Rudorfer, M.S. (1994). Comparative tolerability profiles of the newer versus the older antidepressants. *Drug Safety*, 10:18.

Seibyl, J. P. et al. (1999). Neuroimaging methodologies. In D. S. Charney, E.J. Nestler and B.S. Bunney (Eds), *Neurobiology of mental illness*. New York: Oxford University Press.

Siever, L.J., et al. (1991). Critical issues in defining the role of serotonin in psychiatric disorders. *Pharmacological Reviews*, 43: 509.

Snyder, S.H. (1990). The dopamine connection. *Nature*, 247:121.

Spencer, T.J., et al. (1996). Pharmacotherapy of ADHA across the life cycle: a literature review. *Journal of the American Academy of Child and Adolescent Psychiatry*, 32:1031–1037.

Stober, G., et al. (1996). Serotonin transporter gene polymorphism and affective disorder. *Lancet*, 347:1340–1341.

Tammings, C.A. (1999). Principles of the pharmacology of schizophrenia. In D.S. Charney, E.J. Nestler and B.S. Bunney (Eds), *Neurobiology of mental illness*. New York: Oxford University Press.

Theonen, H. (1995). Neurotrophins and neuronal plasticity. *Science*, 270: 593–598.

Tollefson, G.D. (1995). Selective serotonin reuptake inhibitors. In A. F. Schatzberg and C.B. Nemeroff (Eds), *Textbook of psychopharmacology*. Washington, DC: American Psychiatric Press.

Trevor, A.J., and Way, W.L. (1995). Sedative hypnotics. In G.G. Katzung (Ed.), *Basic and clinical pharmacology*. Norwalk: Appleton & Lange.

Wilcox, R. F., and Gonzales, R. A. (1995). Introduction to neurotransmitters, receptors, signal transaction, and second messengers. In A. F. Schatzberg and C. B. Nemeroff (Eds.), *Textbook of psychopharmacology*. Washington, DC: American Psychiatric Press.

Wileng, T. et al (1995). Pharmacotherapy of adult attention deficit/hyperactivity disorders: a review. *Journal of Clinical Psychopharmacology* 15:270–279.

Wyatt, R.J. (1991). Neuroleptics and the natural cause of schizophrenia. *Schizophrenia Bulletin*, 17:325.

*M*ost of you will probably never work on a psychiatric unit or in a mental health community center. However, all of you will be working with people who are going through crises, suffering periods of intense anxiety and fear, experiencing loss, or facing a life-altering event. Most of you will encounter clients who are experiencing feelings of hopelessness, helplessness, anxiety, anger, low self-esteem, or confusion. No matter what work setting you choose as a registered nurse, you will encounter people who are withdrawn, suspicious, elated, depressed, hostile, manipulative, suicidal, intoxicated, or withdrawing from a substance. Many of you have already come across people who are going through difficult times in their lives. At times you may have handled these situations skillfully, and at other times you may have wished you had additional skills and knowledge.

Basic concepts of psychosocial nursing will become central to your practice of nursing and increase your competency as a practitioner in all clinical settings. Your experience in the psychiatric nursing rotation can help you gain insight into yourself and greatly increase your insight into the experiences of others. This part of your nursing education can also give you guidelines and the opportunity to learn new skills for dealing with a variety of challenging behaviors. Therefore, psychosocial skills are relevant to anything you choose to do inside and outside your nursing profession. I hope this is an enjoyable, exciting, and gratifying experience for you. I hope some of you may even choose to become psychiatric nurses. This chapter presents a brief overview of what professional psychiatric nurses do, the scope of practice, their role in managed care, and the challenges and evolving roles that are present in the current managed care environment.

WHAT IS A PSYCHIATRIC MENTAL HEALTH NURSE?

Psychiatric mental health nurses work with children, adolescents, adults, and the elderly. Psychiatric mental health nurses work with healthy people in crisis or who are experiencing life problems, as well as those with long-term mental illness. Their clients may include people with dual diagnoses (a mental disorder and a co-existing substance disorder), homeless persons and families, people in jail (forensic nursing), people who have survived abusive situations, people with acquired immunodeficiency syn-

drome, and people in crisis. Psychiatric nurses work with individuals, couples, families, and groups. They work with clients in hospitals, in their homes, in halfway houses, in shelters, in clinics, in storefronts, on the street—virtually wherever there are people.

The *Scope and Standards of Psychiatric–Mental Health Nursing Practice* defines psychiatric mental health nursing as "the diagnosis and treatment of human responses to actual or potential mental health problems (p. 10)." Psychiatric mental health nursing is a specialized area of nursing practice "employing a wide range of explanatory theories of and research on human behavior as its science and purposeful use of self as its art (p. 10)." The theories are derived from nursing, as well as from the "biological, cultural, environmental, psychological, and sociological sciences (p. 10)," and "these theories provide a basis for psychiatric mental health nursing practice" (ANA, APNA, ISPN 2000, p. 11). Psychiatric mental health nurses, like all nurses, use both primary sources (client interview and client observation) and secondary sources (staff, chart, and family, friends, and others) to make their assessment and formulate their nursing diagnoses. Psychiatric mental health nurses also make use of the standard classifications of mental disorders such as the *Diagnostic and Statistical Manual of Mental Disorders* of the American Psychiatric Association (APA 2000). Many psychiatric mental health nurses also use the *International Classification of Disease* developed by the World Health Organization, the latest update of which was in 1993 (WHO 1993).

LEVELS OF PSYCHIATRIC MENTAL HEALTH CLINICAL NURSING PRACTICE

Psychiatric nursing did not enter the modern era of nursing until after World War II with the passage of the Mental Health Act in 1946. Hildegard Peplau formulated the first systematic theoretical framework in psychiatric nursing in 1952. Peplau's interpersonal theory of nursing is the cornerstone of psychiatric nursing practice. The advent of psychotropic drugs in the 1950s and the move to the community that resulted from the Community Mental Health Center (CMHC) Act in 1963 were two trends that stimulated the growth of the role of the psychiatric nurse in the community setting. Since that time psychiatric nursing has made remarkable advances in defining and expanding its scope of practice to meet the needs of society and the profession (Shea 1999).

Through the efforts of many leaders who have gone before and of the nurses who are presently active in the professional, political, and social arenas today, "psychiatric nurses are prepared to greet the future with a proud history, standards, credentials, advanced powers of observation, and communication skills" (McBride 1996, p. 3). An overview of psychiatric nursing leaders and the milestones in psychiatry is found in Appendix B.

Psychiatric mental health nurses are registered nurses (RNs) who are educated in nursing and are licensed to practice in their individual state. Psychiatric mental health nurses are qualified at two levels depending on educational preparation. The two levels are basic and advanced (ANA, APNA, ISPN 2000).

Basic Level

Psychiatric Mental Health Registered Nurse

At the basic level, the nurse has completed a nursing program and passed the state licensure examination (RN). Registered nurses practice psychiatric mental health nursing care for individuals with mental health problems in various settings and perform a variety of roles, such as staff nurses, case managers, nurse managers, and other nursing functions.

Psychiatric Mental Health Registered Nurse, Certified

The basic level psychiatric mental health nurse holds a baccalaureate (bachelor of science) degree in nursing and may become certified as a psychiatric mental health registered nurse, certified (RN,C) after acquiring experience and ongoing continuing education in this specialty. Certification demonstrates that the basic level nurse has met the profession's standards of knowledge and experience in the specialty, exceeding those of a beginning RN or a novice in the specialty (ANA, APNA, ISPN 2000). To designate the basic level certification status, the nurse would put a "C" after the RN (e.g., Tom Rogers, RN,C). This certification does not signify that the person is of advanced practice status.

Advanced Level

Advanced Practice Registered Nurse— Psychiatric Mental Health

The advanced practice registered nurse—psychiatric mental health (APRN-PMH) is a licensed RN who is educationally prepared at the master's degree level in psychiatric nursing (master of arts or science). The APRN-PMH applies knowledge, skills, and experience autonomously to complex psychiatric mental health problems. The term "APRN-PMH" applies to either the clinical nurse specialist or the nurse practitioner whose education and experience in psychiatric nursing practice meet criteria established by the profession (ANA, APNA, ISPN 2000).

Advanced Practice Registered Nurse— Psychiatric Mental Health, Certified Specialist

The term "certified specialist" indicates certified advanced practice in the specialty by either a psychiatric mental health clinical nurse specialist or psychiatric mental health nurse practitioner (NP). The advanced practice registered nurse, certified specialist, signifies this certification by adding a CS after the RN (e.g., Mary Thompson, RN,CS). The scope of practice in psychiatric mental health nursing continues to expand. In addition to the role of the APRN-PMH as psychotherapist, the advanced practice registered nurse may be eligible for prescriptive authority, inpatient admission privileges, third party reimbursement, and other specialty privileges (ANA, APNA, ISPN 2000).

WHAT DO PSYCHIATRIC NURSES DO?

The main focus of the psychiatric mental health nurse is to promote and maintain optimal mental functioning, to prevent mental illness (or prevent further dysfunction), and to help clients regain or improve their coping abilities. These goals are realized through a variety of nursing activities in all sorts of hospital and community settings.

The *Scope and Standards of Psychiatric–Mental Health Nursing Practice* (ANA, APNA, ISPN 2000) clearly defines nursing actions for the professional nurse, distinguishing between those nursing activities appropriate for the basic level psychiatric nurse and those for the advanced practice nurse specialist.

Essentially, the interventions of the **basic level psychiatric mental health registered nurse** (ANA, APNA, ISPN 2000) focus on

■ Counseling, including crisis intervention
■ Managing the therapeutic environment ("milieu management")

■ Assisting clients with self-care activities
■ Administering and monitoring psychobiological treatments
■ Health teaching, including psychoeducation
■ Psychiatric rehabilitation
■ Providing telehealth services
■ Working in community-based care and outreach activities
■ Providing culturally relevant health promotion and disease prevention strategies
■ Performing case management
■ Participating in advocacy

In addition to these nursing activities, the **advanced practice registered nurse—psychiatric mental health specialist** is qualified to provide

■ Psychotherapy (individual, group, family, and other therapeutic treatments)
■ Prescription of pharmacological agents, ordering and interpretation of diagnostic and laboratory testing
■ Consultation-liaison activities
■ Complementary interventions (e.g., relaxation, therapeutic touch, light therapy)
■ Clinical supervisory activities
■ Expanded advocacy activities

A list of interventions available to the various levels of psychiatric mental health nurses based on the *Scope and Standards of Psychiatric–Mental Health Nursing Practice 2000* is outlined on the page opposite the inside front cover. Refer to Table 4–1 for a more comprehensive understanding of the nursing activities provided by psychiatric mental health nurses as outlined in the *Scope and Standards*.

IN WHAT PHENOMENA DO PSYCHIATRIC MENTAL HEALTH NURSES INTERVENE?

Psychiatric mental health nurses plan intervention strategies through the nursing process. "Diagnosis of human responses to actual or potential mental health problems involves the application of theory to human phenomena, through the process of assessment, diagnosis, planning, intervention or treatment, and evaluation" (ANA, APNA, ISPN 2000, p. 11). Psychiatric mental health nurses plan interventions to target and ameliorate the painful, frightening, harmful, and dysfunctional phenomena their clients are experiencing. Specific phenomena can include the following (ANA, APNA, ISPN 2000):

■ Self-care limitations related to mental and emotional distress
■ Crisis or emotional stress
■ Self-concept changes
■ Problems related to emotions such as anxiety, anger, sadness, loneliness, and grief
■ Alterations in thinking and perceiving (hallucinations, delusions)
■ Difficulty relating to others
■ Self-violence (suicidal behaviors/thinking) or violence to others
■ Difficulty relating to others

Refer to Box 4–1 for psychiatric mental health nursing's phenomena of concern.

RECENT ISSUES AFFECTING PSYCHIATRIC MENTAL HEALTH NURSING

The 1990s have been called the "decade of the brain." The advent of numerous imaging techniques opened up a new world of understanding the neurophysiology and neuroanatomy of the brain. Neurobiological changes can now be observed and categorized in people with mental disorders. This knowledge has led to a revolution in the understanding of mental health, providing evidence that many of the most serious mental disorders should be viewed as "diseases of the brain." Today, many psychiatric disorders are now categorized as psychobiological diseases. Thus, there has been a major shift in the way to treat people with mental diseases, mainly through psychopharmacology.

In 1994 the American Nurses' Association (ANA) published the *Psychiatric–Mental Health Nursing Psychopharmacology Project*, a summary of the work of its psychopharmacology task force. The purpose of the project was to evaluate and advance the scope of psychiatric nursing practice with respect to psychopharmacology and related neuroscience. The ANA advocated that undergraduate programs prepare their nurses with a solid foundation of neuroscience and psychopharmacology as they relate to mental illness. Graduate programs should include advanced learning, clinical application, and research inquiry in these essential fields. The ANA task force on psychopharmacology proposed that the future should include "a refinement of levels of psychopharmacology practiced by psychiatric–mental health nurses, including appropriate credentials for psychiatric–mental health nurses in psychopharmacology" (ANA 1994b).

TABLE 4–1 *Psychiatric Mental Health Nursing Interventions as Defined by the Standards of Psychiatric Mental Health Nurses*

LEVEL	INTERVENTION	DESCRIPTION
Basic Level		

Psychiatric mental health nurse	A. Case management
	B. Counseling
	C. Health promotion and health maintenance
	D. Health teaching
	E. Milieu therapy
	F. Psychobiological intervention
	G. Self-care activities
	H. Promotion of self-care activities
		■ **In inpatient and outpatient settings**
		  a. Coordinates health and human services
		  b. Designs and evaluates the use of culturally appropriate services (refer to text)
		■ **Use of communication skills** and interviewing skills, problem-solving skills, crisis intervention, stress management, assertiveness training, and behavior modification
		  a. Conduct health assessments
		  b. Targets at-risk situations
		  c. Initial interventions
		    1. Assertiveness training
		    2. Stress management
		    3. Parenting classes
		    4. Health teaching
		  d. Use of Internet for communication and teaching purposes with client and family
		  e. Targets potential complications related to symptoms or treatment
		■ **Formal and informal information** regarding coping, interpersonal relationships, mental health problems, mental disorders, treatments and their effects on daily living, developmental needs, and more; information is given in gender, developmental, cultural, and educational appropriate levels
		■ **Provision of a therapeutic environment** (hospital, community, home) focusing on a wide range of factors such as physical environment, social structures interactions, and cultural setting
		■ **Administering and monitoring responses** to medications as well as emergency procedures, relaxation techniques, nutrition and diet regulations, exercise and rest schedules, and other somatic treatment

Advanced Level		
Advanced practice registered nurse—psychiatric mental health (APRN-PMH)	All of the above plus: I. Consultation J. Prescription authority and treatment K. Psychotherapy	■ **Encourages highest level of independent functioning** in areas such as personal hygiene, feeding, recreational activities, practical skills (e.g., shopping, using public transportation) ■ **Provides consultation** to health care providers and others as well as supervision to other mental health care providers and trainers ■ **May prescribe pharmacological agents (medications)** order and interpret laboratory tests ■ **Performs individual, group, family, child, and adolescent psychotherapy** ■ **Uses complementary therapies** ■ **Performs clinical supervisory activities** ■ **Has expanded advocacy role**

Data from American Nurses' Association (ANA), American Psychiatric Nurses Association (APNA), International Society of Psychiatry and Mental Health Nursing (ISPN). (2000). *Scope and standards of psychiatric–mental health clinical nursing practice—2000 edition.* Washington, D.C.: ANA.

Box 4–1 *Psychiatric Mental Health Nursing's Phenomena of Concern*

ACTUAL OR POTENTIAL MENTAL HEALTH PROBLEMS OF CLIENTS PERTAINING TO

■ Maintenance of optimal health and well-being and the prevention of psychobiological illness
■ Self-care limitations or impaired functioning related to mental and emotional distress
■ Deficits in the functioning of significant biological, emotional, and cognitive systems
■ Emotional stress or crisis components of illness, pain, and disability
■ Self-concept changes, developmental issues, and life process changes
■ Problems related to emotions such as anxiety, anger, sadness, loneliness, and grief
■ Physical symptoms that occur along with altered psychological functioning
■ Alterations in thinking, perceiving, symbolizing, communicating, and decision making
■ Difficulties relating to others
■ Behaviors and mental states that indicate the client is a danger to self or others or has a severe disability
■ Interpersonal, systematic, sociocultural, spiritual, or environmental circumstances or events that affect the mental and emotional well-being of the individual, family, or community
■ Symptom management, side effects/toxicities associated with psychopharmacological intervention and other aspects of the treatment regimen

From American Nurses' Association (ANA), American Psychiatric Nurses Association (APNA), International Society of Psychiatry and Mental Health Nursing (ISPN). (2000). *Scope and standards of psychiatric–mental health nursing practice—2000 edition.* Washington, D.C.: ANA.

Many nursing leaders, while applauding the strides taken in the amelioration of suffering for people with mental diseases, caution us not to lose sight of our identity and our unique strength as psychosocial and psychiatric nurses. A technician can be taught to be an expert in psychopharmacology—psychiatric nurses offer that expertise and a great deal more. Yes, we do need to educate ourselves and prepare future nurses to be competent regarding the growing body of information on the relationship among neuroanatomy, neurophysiology, mental diseases, and psychopharmacology. Psychotropics are powerful chemicals. They are frequently prescribed, but nurses know that they do not always work. Clients are not always compliant with medications when the medications cause discomfort or embarrassing side effects. In these cases, compliance should *not* be expected until the issues around noncompliance are addressed. Nurses need to listen to the consumer.

Although the emphasis on psychopharmacology is not misplaced, Billings (1993) cautioned that psychosocial nurses also need to continue to grow in their unique capacity to help people with the quality of their lives through psychoeducational approaches, clarification of verbal content, alteration of environmental stimuli, systems intervention within the family, or the classic application of a therapeutic nurse-client relationship.

Psychotropic drugs can have a profound and beneficial effect on cognition, mood, and behavior. However, they do not change the underlying process, which is often highly sensitive to intrapsychic and psychosocial stressors. Optimal benefits are achieved by simultaneously reducing symptoms and promoting the individual's capacity to adapt to the pressure and demands of life (Trubowitz 1994). Research substantiates that the combined treatment of psychopharmacology and psychotherapy for people with mental health problems is superior to either treatment alone.

What medicine and I do is complementary, and our combined approach is invaluable in the restoration of a productive life for the client. If I simply narrow my focus to the medical perspective, then the client is deprived of the rich potential that additional or alternative views could have provided. Naming the "human response" with a nursing diagnosis sanctions my prescription and provides the basis for my nursing intervention. In our society, it is the diagnosis that justifies the prescription and codes the service for payment. In the future, it may be the only means by which we [nurses] will be compensated for our work (Billings 1993, p. 176).

MENTAL HEALTH AND MANAGED CARE

Managed care programs attempt to provide care equal to or better in quality than the care that the client has received in the past, for less cost, and with more accountability to the payer. Changes in the relationship between provider and consumer are at the core of what managed mental health care seeks to accomplish. As part of an effort to conform systems, improve client outcomes, and control costs, health and mental health managers have implemented a number of strategies designed to monitor and assess treatment plans and outcomes that were, in the past, largely free from such oversight. These efforts have taken many forms, ranging from preadmission reviews to continuing treatment authorizations, concurrent reviews, and screen design (increasingly computerized) to determine the appropriateness of a treatment plan. With the growth of private health maintenance organizations (HMOs) and coverage by private insurance companies, the professional autonomy of providers has been significantly affected. Physicians and mental health personnel have been organized under strict treatment and financial guidelines. Changes have affected key areas such as provider income, system and client cost, provider control, and quality of care. The cornerstone of managed care for both physical and mental health is capitation. Capitation is an arrangement whereby a managed care program (e.g., an HMO) is given a fixed amount of money to provide all aspects of needed health care for a client (Lamb 1999).

The three most common forms of managed care plans are the

1. Health maintenance organization (HMO). HMOs contract to provide care at a fixed yearly rate (capitation). Health care for its members usually includes ambulatory care, preventive health care, hospitalization, and catastrophic care. The primary physician is the gatekeeper to specialty care. A patient's visit to a specialist must be deemed necessary by the primary physician.
2. Preferred provider organization (PPO). A PPO contracts with certain physicians and hospitals, and members are free to choose any provider they want within the PPO's network, for a set co-payment. If the member goes outside the network, the cost of treatment is usually considerably higher.
3. Point of service (POS). This plan shares similarities of HMOs and PPOs in that the member has freedom of choice.

Managed behavioral health care organization (MBHO) is the term that applies to managed care for mental health and substance abuse disorders. Many management products and services are offered by MBHOs to employers, health plans, unions, and state and federal agencies.

There has been a flood of criticism directed at HMOs and MBHOs to the effect that their entire philosophy of service is antithetical to the well-being of the client (often referred to as the consumer). Many observers have noted an explosion of complaints from psychologists who believe their clients are being shortchanged and a conflict of interest exists when nonclinicians decide how much therapy is warranted (Bush 1996; Goleman 1996; Korb 1996; Wolf 1996). Contrary to reports by Seligman (1995), who showed that clients who are in psychotherapy longer than 6 months fare better than those whose treatment period is shorter, the practice of managed care plans has been in many instances to cut back the number of sessions to 10 or fewer. HMOs experience maximum profit when services are limited: the less they provide, the bigger is the profit. Thus, managed care agencies (e.g., MBHOs and HMOs) exert a subtle pressure against the treatment that may be essential to the well-being of subscriber members. Similarly, participating physicians have been offered financial incentives to limit treatment or services; some HMOs award bonuses to physicians who use less than the allocated funds. This practice has come under review because such incentives might influence primary providers to refer fewer clients to specialists. Clearly, primary providers may feel undue pressure when making a decision that is in the client's interest rather than in the economic interest of the managed care agencies (HMOs and MBHOs).

Therefore, problems with managed care agencies have included difficulties for individuals finding and accessing services, denial of services to people who need them, lack of accountability and follow-up for consumers, absence of coordination among providers, and lack of continuity in treatment planning (Lamb 1999). Consequently, people with mental health problems often fail to receive appropriate treatment, are subject to needless tests and procedures, and consume an undue proportion of the limited resources of the primary care system.

Fortunately, recent legislation and pressure from health care consumers seem to have started a trend toward more responsible medical care, with an emphasis on quality. Some positive aspects of managed care include the initiation of many procedures that expand services to consumers of health care in the community, such as extended office hours, telephone triage, and telehealth services. Telehealth services include telephone consultation, fax, computers, e-mail, image transmission, and interactive video sessions, all with the purpose of maintaining a therapeutic relationship with a client by creating an alternative sense of the nurse's presence that may or may not occur in "real" time (ANA, APNA, ISPN 2000). See A Nurse Speaks, Unit VIII, for an example of an APRN-PMH who deals with HMOs within her own private practice.

THE ROLE OF PSYCHIATRIC MENTAL HEALTH NURSES IN MANAGED CARE

Both basic level and advanced practice psychiatric mental health nurses are uniquely qualified to serve directly and indirectly within the managed care system. Nurses at the basic level of preparation interact with managed care companies indirectly. However, their documentation of care is crucial. Nurses at the advanced level speak to managed care companies directly in providing clinical information (Shea 1999).

There is a great deal of variability of nursing activity based on various settings and on geographic location; however, the basic level nurse and the advanced practice nurse both can assume a number of roles in the managed care/behavioral managed care systems. See Table 4–2 for some examples of these roles and functions.

CHALLENGES AND EMERGING ROLES FOR NURSES

The spiraling costs of health care and the diminishing access to health care by large populations within our society have contributed to the need for radical reform. The intense demands being made on health care organizations and providers of care are increasingly complex and volatile. To trim costs, hospitals shorten the length of the clients' hospital stays and cut out available units and services (referred to as downsizing).

Shorter hospital stays have increased the need for community-based support for people with acute mental illness and those with prolonged mental illness (PMI)/serious mental illness (SMI). The acutely ill who are discharged to the community continue to need expert professional care and intensive case management. These changes in the environment of health care practices have posed many challenges for nurses. At the same time, the breaking up of static and ineffective patterns of health care delivery has paved the way for many exciting opportunities. For example, one direction for the practice of psychiatric mental health nursing is to provide primary and preventive care in community settings, including urban, rural, and school-based clinics. Another approach is to focus on the population with PMI, providing intervention with acute exacerbations, stabilization, and rehabilitative care. Nurses at the advanced practice level who are certified specialists are prepared to provide safe, efficient, and cost-effective

TABLE 4–2 *Roles of Nurses in Behavioral Health Care*

ROLE	FUNCTIONS WITHIN CONTRACTED FACILITIES AND PRACTICES
1. Clinical care manager/case manager	Nurses assess client needs, develop treatment plans, and make referrals to coordinate care. The care manager continuum of care over the episode of care includes rehabilitation as well as relapse prevention.
2. Assessment, evaluation, triage, and referral nurse	Nurses evaluate clients in person or via telephone to triage the client to the most appropriate level of care.
3. Client educator/family educator	Nurses assume responsibility for client and family teaching to improve compliance and self-management of symptoms.
4. Risk manager	Nurses are charged with decreasing the probability of diverse outcomes related to client care.
5. Chief quality officer	Nurses assume primary responsibility for formulating and implementing comprehensive quality management and improvement programs for managed care companies.
6. Utilization review nurse	Nurses focus on the current episode of care, serve as gatekeeper to behavioral health care services, and manage the mental health benefit.
7. Marketing and development specialist	Nurses work in growth area of sales, marketing, and program development. They interface with consumers, employers, providers, and regulators and make recommendations for furthering the goals of the managed care organization.
8. Corporate managers and executives	Nurses work in middle and senior management positions, participating in the development of corporate policy and strategic planning.

Data from Pelletier, L. R., and Beaudin, C. L. (1999). Mental health services and delivery and managed care. In C. A. Shea, et al. (Eds.), *Advanced practice nursing in psychiatric and mental health nursing*. St. Louis: C. V. Mosby. (pp. 66–67).

health care. As more nurses move into the community, they will need to possess astute assessment and evaluation skills as well as the ability to make independent decisions about client care (Christensen and Bender 1994).

A number of nursing care delivery models have evolved in an attempt to meet the challenge of maintaining high-quality care in a changing health care environment that places an emphasis on cost containment.

Creation of Mental Health Nursing Units

In the United States the community nursing center (CNC) is not a new concept. The Henry Street Nurses Settlement, one of the earliest nursing centers, was founded by Lillian Wald in 1893 in New York City. In 1916 Margaret Sanger opened the first birth control clinic, also in New York City. Throughout the 1980s, a number of nurse-managed centers were opened, including those that were academically based, hospital based, freestanding, and agencies for home health care (Knauth 1994). CNCs, or nurse-managed centers, are "organizations that provide direct access to professional nurses who offer holistic, client-centered health services for reimbursement" (Fehring et al. 1986, p. 63). Historically, CNCs have provided care to the poor and underserved populations. Today, CNCs are expanding to provide care in both rural and urban settings (Walker 1994).

For community centers that work primarily with people with mental health diseases, current and future trends in mental health nursing should concentrate on mentally healthy individuals undergoing a crisis and address the needs of those with severe and persistent mental health problems. In the community setting, nursing actions for those with PMI need to focus appropriately on teaching skills to empower their clients and contribute to their ability to live up to their potential for independence, social assimilation, and work performance. In so doing, psychiatric mental health nurses provide the chance for their clients to experience the optimal quality of life for themselves and their families.

It is apparent that the growth and progress of nursing go hand in hand with the political and social developments of the time. For nursing to take a leading role in the reformed health care of the future, it is imperative that more nurses become involved with legislative and policy initiatives. Nursing research showing that nurse-managed health care agencies do indeed provide high-quality care in a cost-effective manner can affect legislative decisions.

Trends in the profession of psychiatric mental health nursing are greatly influenced by trends in the social and political arenas. From this vantage point, we can try to predict how the present will affect the future.

Nurse as Case Manager

Case management is perhaps one of the most enduring of the many models of care that has emerged as a framework for quality client-centered nursing care. Many nurses are now finding that they need to redefine their primary function from providers of care to *managers* of care. Case management is an extension of the primary care model. However, in case management there is more deliberation in planning resources needed by the client and more emphasis on interdisciplinary collaboration (McCloskey et al. 1994).

"Nurses who are case managers take on the responsibility for a client or group of clients, arrange assessment of need, formulate a comprehensive plan of care, arrange for delivery of suitable services to address the individual client's needs, and assess and monitor the services delivered" (Marshall et al. 1995). Case management is becoming the recommended method for the treatment of severely and persistently mentally ill clients. This approach allows for optimal community adjustment for individuals with PMI by providing a link between the clients and the support services they require.

Forchuck and associates (1989) have formulated a case management model incorporating Peplau's theory. The authors identified the essential component of case management as that of the one-to-one, long-term, therapeutic nurse-client relationship. Within this relationship, the case manager plays a variety of roles, as dictated by the client's needs, including those of

- Counselor or therapist
- Client advocate
- Teacher
- Community organizer
- Coordinator of services

Figure 4–1 illustrates this case management model and helps outline the overall goals of the case manager.

Nurse as Client Advocate

Nurses play a critical advocacy role in protecting the rights of clients, especially those with psychiatric

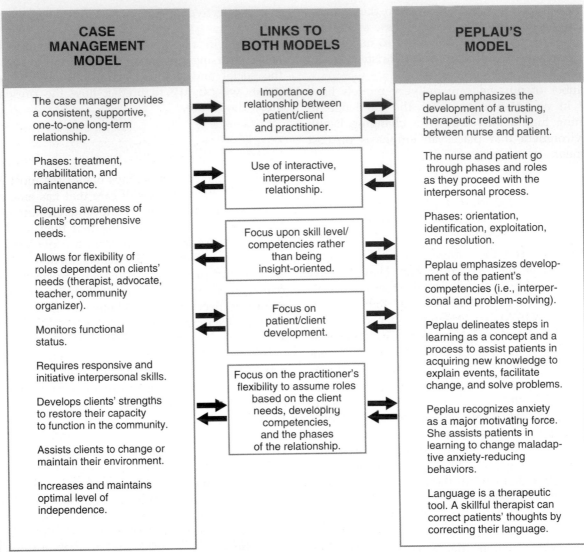

CASE MANAGEMENT MODEL

The case manager provides a consistent, supportive, one-to-one long-term relationship.

Phases: treatment, rehabilitation, and maintenance.

Requires awareness of clients' comprehensive needs.

Allows for flexibility of roles dependent on clients' needs (therapist, advocate, teacher, community organizer).

Monitors functional status.

Requires responsive and initiative interpersonal skills.

Develops clients' strengths to restore their capacity to function in the community.

Assists clients to change or maintain their environment.

Increases and maintains optimal level of independence.

LINKS TO BOTH MODELS

Importance of relationship between patient/client and practitioner.

Use of interactive, interpersonal relationship.

Focus upon skill level/ competencies rather than being insight-oriented.

Focus on patient/client development.

Focus on the practitioner's flexibility to assume roles based on the client needs, developing competencies, and the phases of the relationship.

PEPLAU'S MODEL

Peplau emphasizes the development of a trusting, therapeutic relationship between nurse and patient.

The nurse and patient go through phases and roles as they proceed with the interpersonal process.

Phases: orientation, identification, exploitation, and resolution.

Peplau emphasizes development of the patient's competencies (i.e., interpersonal and problem-solving).

Peplau delineates steps in learning as a concept and a process to assist patients in acquiring new knowledge to explain events, facilitate change, and solve problems.

Peplau recognizes anxiety as a major motivating force. She assists patients in learning to change maladaptive anxiety-reducing behaviors.

Language is a therapeutic tool. A skillful therapist can correct patients' thoughts by correcting their language.

Figure 4–1 Case management model. (Adapted from Forchuck, C., et al. [1989]. Incorporating Peplau's theory and case management. *Journal of Psychosocial Nursing*, 27[2]:36.)

disabilities. Nurses are also in a position to play an important role in identifying and reporting incidents of abuse and neglect. Five actions that pertain to the nurse's role of patient advocate are presented in Box 4–2.

Many nurses will be working as case managers in managed care settings such as HMOs and MBHOs. Many of these managed care facilities will be corporately managed, with an eye to cost-effective care; therefore, nurses will increasingly practice in corporate settings. Nurses working in these settings will be affected by corporate goals and rules, which could lead to ethical dilemmas for them and threaten the appropriateness and quality of client care. Mohr (1995) pointed out that the role of client advocate may become increasingly difficult in the health care environment as nurses are becoming cor-

porate employees or even "day laborers" dispatched from agencies.

The nursing code of ethics defines the nurse's primary commitment as being to the client. "Nurses are employed by institutions, but their allegiance is to the client and his or her welfare, rather than to a group of shareholders" (Mohr 1995, p. 31). The mission, goals, and values of the corporate health care system are not always consistent with those of nursing. Mohr further warned nurses not to be placated by temporary guarantees of material concessions or to allow the fear of dismissal to push aside their humanistic values of commitment to their clients. The ANA has published *Guidelines on Reporting Incompetent, Unethical, or Illegal Practices* (1994). All nurses should know about this publication and have a copy available for guidance, because these issues and concerns will follow us, and perhaps haunt us, throughout our career. Sines (1994) stated that the central concepts of nursing remain those of empowerment and advocacy and that the art of accurate empathy is a prerequisite for contemporary mental health care.

Domains of Psychiatric Mental Health Nursing Practice

It is not just that the locations where nurses work are undergoing radical changes; there are changes in the types of agencies for which they work. This reformed health care system is seeing more managed care facilities, and there is much more emphasis on proving the cost effectiveness of provider services. More and more nurses are working for corporations, in a move away from nonprofit or private hospital organizations, which is bringing obvious and subtle changes. One area of concern is that the values and philosophies of corporate medicine are not always compatible with those of nursing. The roles and practice settings for the psychiatric nurse are vast and are continually expanding.

A change in nursing education is needed to prepare mental health nurse practitioners for the future. Owen and Sweeney (1995) stated that the reliance on developing skills associated with problem "removal" should no longer be the focus for future practice. Current and future trends in mental health nursing education require a greater emphasis on the development of skills to empower clients in diverse settings, to help mentally healthy people during times of crisis, and to participate in long-term planning and treatment as well as rehabilitation for those with prolonged and severe mental health issues. A number of priorities in mental health services are evident. These priorities acknowledge the special needs of people from ethnic minority groups, people with severe and persistent mental health problems, people with problems associated with

Box 4–2 *Nurse's Role of Patient Advocate*

1. **Nurses need to improve their observation, listening, and communications skills.** Patients complain that some nurses are burned out, hide behind their desks, take the easy way out, and are quick to punish for infraction of rules rather than doing what is best for the patient. Nurses need to "ensure that a good nursing care plan exists, that activities of daily living and personal hygiene are addressed, and that bodily functions are monitored and assisted. . . . They need to be sensitive to assessing consumer's comfort levels regarding noise, temperature, lighting, and access to personal belongings" (p. 236).

2. **Nurses need to develop and implement policies and procedures that affect the client's quality of care.** These include the Patient's Bill of Rights; informed consent; policies addressing confidentiality, seclusion, and restraint; and policies for reporting and providing appropriate remedies for staff abuse.

3. **Nurses need to know that unaddressed, ongoing abusive or neglectful behaviors may be brought to the attention of a Protection and Advocacy (P&A) system from any source, including nurses.** Examples of such behaviors include assault, failure to provide appropriate mental health or medical diagnostic evaluation or treatment, financial exploitation, and failure to provide discharge planning. The P&A is authorized to investigate incidents of abuse and neglect of mentally ill individuals. "Unfortunately, the P&A cannot protect nurses from retaliation from employers, but reports can be made anonymously and systemic problems can be identified" (p. 237).

4. **Nurses can provide mental health consumers with the telephone number of the appropriate P&A system; it should be posted next to the patient's phone.**

5. **Nurses have a vital role in the administration of medication.** Mental health care consumers complain of being overmedicated, wrongly medicated, and poorly medicated. Nurses must take the responsibility for ensuring that the appropriate medication is administered at a dose that makes sense and that side effects are immediately noted, reported, and addressed. Nurses are responsible for seeing that patients are provided with understandable medication teaching plans. Patients are to be well informed of what medications they are getting, what side effects they might expect, any toxic effects, whom to contact when they suspect problems, and actions they can take to lessen side effects.

From Schauer C. (1995). Special report: Protection and advocacy: what nurses need to know. *Archives of Psychiatric Nursing,* 9(5): 233–239.

poverty, and people who are socially disadvantaged (Owen and Sweeney 1995).

SUMMARY

All nurses need to know, and must be able to apply, psychosocial concepts to give effective and competent care. However, some of you may go on to choose a career in psychiatric nursing. Psychiatric nurses work in a wide array of settings with people who have acute and prolonged mental health problems. They work with homeless persons and families; with people in jails; with people who have survived abusive situations; with people who are positive for human immunodeficiency virus; with people in crisis; and with children, adults, and the elderly.

Specific criteria must be met for a nurse to be qualified as either a psychiatric mental health registered nurse at the basic level or a psychiatric mental health registered nurse at the advanced practice level (APRN).

Psychiatric nurses are responsible for counseling clients, providing crisis intervention, managing the therapeutic environment, health and psychoeducational teaching, practicing case management, arranging psychiatric rehabilitation, planning community and health care, administering and monitoring of psychobiological treatments, and much more. The decade of the brain has brought not only great strides in the relief of mental anguish for many people with mental health diseases but also great opportunities for nurses. Nurses of the advanced level are trained to prescribe pharmacological treatment according to their state's Nurse Practice Act, perform psychotherapy (individual, group, family, and other forms), and carry out consultation and supervision with other health care providers; some may also have admitting privileges and therefore admit their clients to the hospital in times of crisis.

Psychiatric nursing has an important history that has grown out of the work of dedicated and gifted nurses who were innovators in their time. This history clearly reflects the social and political movements of the times. The advent of psychotropic drugs and the move to the community that resulted from the CMHC Act of 1963 were two trends that stimulated growth of the role of the psychiatric mental health nurse. These two trends provided exciting opportunities for psychiatric nursing that will continue to expand into the 21st century.

Health care reform is focused on cutting costs while maintaining quality of care. Shorter hospital stays mean that some clients are returning to the community before they are stabilized and are thus in greater need of supervision and community support. The managed care environment has posed many problems and dilemmas for both clients and health care professionals. On the other hand, it has led to increased opportunities for nurses. The requirement for orchestrating of support services to meet clients' needs once they are discharged into the community has increased the importance of the role of case manager.

The roles of the nurse in the managed care setting are discussed. Challenges and emerging roles are covered, including

■ Mental health nursing units
■ Case management
■ Client advocate
■ Domains of psychiatric nursing practice

Visit the **Evolve** website at **http://evolve.elsevier.com/Varcarolis** for a post-test on the content in this chapter.

Visit the **Evolve** website at
http://evolve.elsevier.com/Varcarolis
for additional self-study exercises.

Critical Thinking and Chapter Review

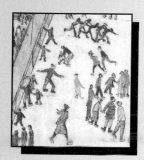

Critical Thinking

1. What level of nursing do you think would be most appropriate for some-one working in a nurse-managed community center? What would be some of the advantages for a nurse in such a setting? What are some of the concerns and questions you might have? What populations would be the best served? Talk about why you would or would not like to work in such a setting someday.

Chapter Review

Choose the most appropriate answer.

1. A nursing student asks the psychiatric nursing instructor, "What's the differ-ence in preparation between a basic level psychiatric nurse and an advanced practice psychiatric nurse?" The instructor should reply

   1. "The basic level psychiatric nurse needs to have only RN licensure, while the advanced practice psychiatric nurse holds a baccalaureate degree in nursing."
   2. "The basic level psychiatric nurse has a baccalaureate degree in nursing, and the advanced practice psychiatric nurse has a baccalaureate degree in nursing and holds certification in the specialty."
   3. "The basic level psychiatric nurse has a baccalaureate degree in nursing, and the advanced practice psychiatric nurse has a master's degree in psy-chiatric nursing."
   4. "The basic level psychiatric nurse has a master's degree in psychiatric nursing, and the advanced practice psychiatric nurse has a master's degree and certification in psychiatric nursing."

2. The intervention that can be practiced by an advanced practice registered nurse—psychiatric mental health that cannot be practiced by a basic level registered nurse—psychiatric mental health is

   1. Advocacy.
   2. Psychotherapy.
   3. Case management.
   4. Community-based care.

3. Only advanced practice psychiatric mental health nurses provide interventions pertaining to

   1. Self-care limitations.
   2. Self-concept changes.
   3. Alterations in thinking and perceiving.
   4. Prescribing psychopharmacological treatment.

4. A trend in psychiatric mental health nursing related to cost control imposed in the managed care environment is

   1. Approval of longer treatment periods.
   2. Decreased use of case management.
   3. Increased ease of access to treatment.
   4. Shift from inpatient care to community care.

5. An *emerging* role for psychiatric mental health nurses working with clients with prolonged mental illness (PMI) is

   1. Client and family empowerer.
   2. Giver of direct care.
   3. Manager of care.
   4. Counselor.

REFERENCES

American Nurses' Association (ANA). (1994). Guidelines on reporting incompetent, unethical, or illegal practices, pub. #NP-91. Washington, D.C.: ANA.

American Nurses' Association (ANA), American Psychiatric Nurses Association (APNA), International Society of Psychiatric–Mental Health Nurses (ISPN). (2000). *Scope and standards of psychiatric–mental health nursing practice—2000 edition.* Washington, D.C.: ANA.

American Nurses' Association (ANA), American Psychiatric Nurses Association (APNA), Association of Child and Adolescent Psychiatric Nursing (ACAPN), Society for Education and Research in Psychiatric–Mental Health Nursing (SERN). (1994a). *Statement on the scope and standards of psychiatric–mental health clinical nursing practice.* Washington, D.C.: ANA.

American Nurses' Association (ANA). (1994b). *Psychiatric–mental health nursing psychopharmacology project.* Washington, D.C.: ANA.

American Psychiatric Association (APA) (2000). Diagnostic and statistical manual of mental disorders 4th ed., revised, DSM-IV-TR. Washington, DC: APA.

Billings, C. V. (1993). Psychiatric–mental health nursing professional progress notes. *Archives of Psychiatric Nursing,* 7(3):174–181.

Bush, J. W. (1996). Long-term therapy may not survive managed-care model (letter to the editor). *New York Times,* January 26, p. A26.

Christensen, P., and Bender, L. H. (1994). Models of nursing care in a changing environment: Current challenges and future directions. *Orthopedic Nursing,* 13(2):64–70.

Fehring, R., Riesch, S., and Schulte, J. (1986). Toward a definition of nurse-managed centers. *Journal of Community Health Nursing,* 3(2):59–67.

Forchuck, C., et al. (1989). Incorporating Peplau's theory and case management. *Journal of Psychosocial Nursing,* 27(2):35–37.

Goleman, D. (1996). Critics say managed-care savings are eroding mental care. *New York Times,* January 24, p. C9.

Knauth, D. G. (1994). Community nursing centers: Removing impediments to success. *Nursing Economics,* 12(3).140–145.

Korb, L. J. (1996). Long-term therapy may not survive managed care model (letter to the editor). *New York Times,* January 26, p. A26.

Lamb, H. R. (1999). Public psychiatry and prevention. In R. F. Hales, S. C. Yudofsky, and J. A. Talbott (Eds.), *The American Psychiatric Press textbook of psychiatry.* Washington, D.C.: American Psychiatric Press.

Marshall, M., Lockwood, A., and Gath, D. (1995). Social services case-management for long-term mental disorders: A randomised controlled trial. Lancet, 345(8947): 409–412.

McBride, A. B. (1996). Psychiatric–mental health nursing in the twenty-first century. In A. B. McBride and J. K. Austin (Eds.), *Psychiatric–mental health nurse: Integrating the behavioral and biological sciences* (pp. 1–10). Philadelphia: W. B. Saunders.

McCloskey, J. C., et al. (1994). Nursing management innovations: A need for systematic evaluation. *Nursing Economics,* 12(1):35–44.

Mohr, W. K. (1995). Values, ideologies, and dilemmas: Professional and occupational contradictions. *Journal of Psychosocial Nursing and Mental Health Services,* 33(1):29–34.

Owen, S., and Sweeney, J. (1995). The future role of the mental health nurse. *Nurse Education Today,* 15(1):17–21.

Schauer, C. (1995). Special report: Protection and advocacy: What nurses need to know. *Archives of Psychiatric Nursing,* 9(5):233–239.

Seligman, M. E. P. (1995). The effectiveness of psychotherapy: The Consumer Reports study. *American Psychologist,* 50:965–974.

Shea, C. A. (1999). Careers in advanced practice psychiatric nursing. In C. A. Shea, et al. (Eds.), *Advanced practice nursing in psychiatric and mental health nursing.* St. Louis: C. V. Mosby.

Sines, D. (1994). The arrogance of power: A reflection on contemporary mental health nursing practice. *Journal of Advanced Nursing,* 20(5):894–903.

Stuart, G. W., and Laraia, M. T. (1998). *Principles and practices of psychiatric nursing* (6th ed.). St. Louis: C. V. Mosby.

Trubowitz, J. (1994). Personality theories and therapies. In E. Varcarolis (Ed.), *Foundations of psychiatric–mental health nursing* (2nd ed.) (pp. 29–64). Philadelphia: W. B. Saunders.

Walker, P. H. (1994). Dollars and sense in health reform: Interdisciplinary practice and community nursing centers. *Nursing Administration Quarterly,* 19(1).1–11.

Wolf, P. F. (1996). Long-term therapy may not survive managed-care model (letter to the editor). *New York Times,* January 26, p. A26.

World Health Organization (1993). International Statistical Classification of Diseases and Related Health Problems, Tenth Revision (ICD-10). Geneva: World Health Organization.

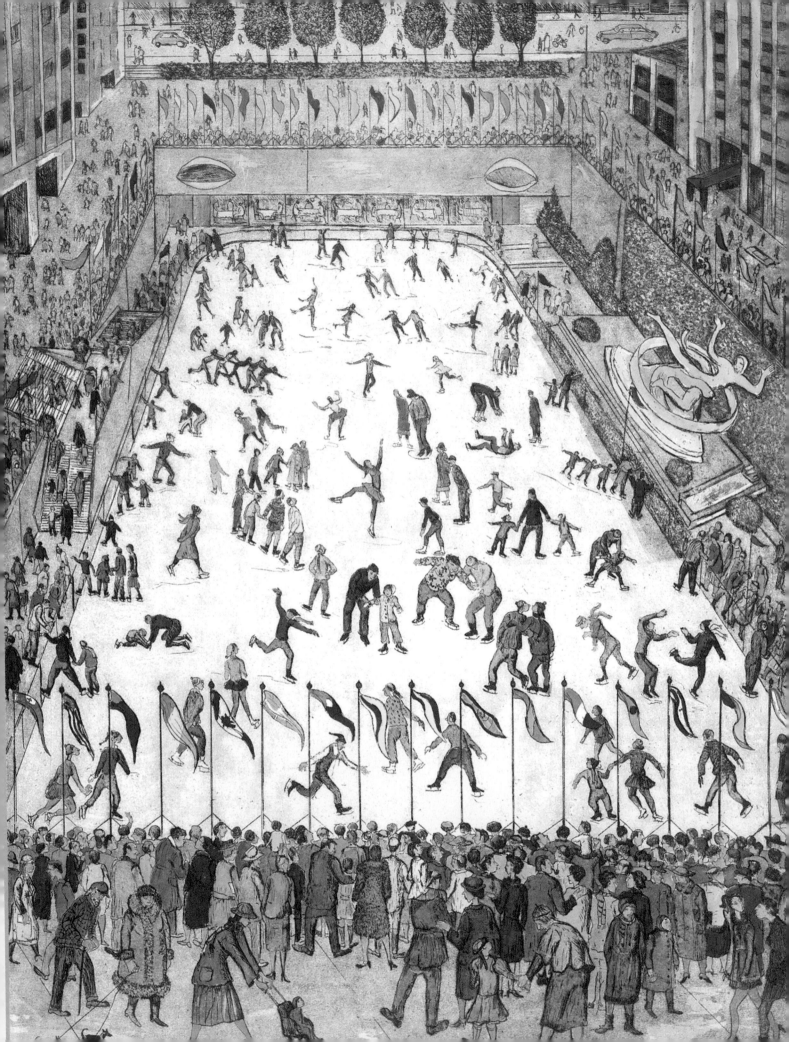

Unit

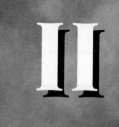

II

Foundations for Practice

When spiders unite, they can tie up
a lion.

ETHIOPIAN PROVERB

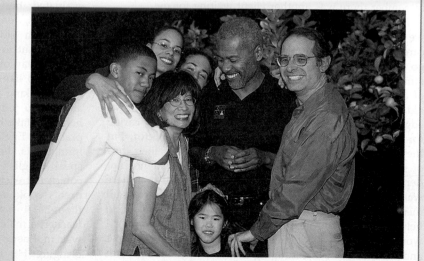

Outline

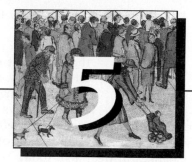

Mental Health Nursing in Acute Care Settings

MARGARET SWISHER
THOMAS WENZKA

Key Terms and Concepts

The key terms and concepts listed here also appear in color where they are defined or first discussed in this chapter.

behavioral health

case managers

codes

clinical pathways

elopement

health maintenance
  organization (HMO)

managed behavioral health
  care organization
  (MBHO)

managed care

preferred provider
  organization (PPO)

Objectives

After studying this chapter, the reader will be able to

1. Analyze the psychiatric hospital experience from the client's perspective.

2. Explain how the mental health team collaborates to plan and implement care for the hospitalized client.

3. Describe the role of the nurse as advocate and provider of care for the client.

4. Explain the interrelationships among the managed care system, the clinical pathways, and the role of the case manager.

5. Discuss the managerial and coordinating roles of nursing on an inpatient acute care unit.

6. Discuss the process for preparing clients to return to the community for ongoing care.

ospitalization remains one option for the treatment of patients with mental disorders and emotional crises. Although lengths of stay have decreased from weeks to days since the 1980s, the inpatient setting provides effective, focused treatment for crises stabilization of the acutely ill client. Changes in treatment today arise from the evolution of managed care, the principal model for delivery of health care services (Schreter et al. 1997).

MANAGED CARE

Managed care refers to a system of health insurance that integrates quality care and cost management. The health maintenance organization (HMO), preferred provider organization (PPO), managed behavioral health care organization (MBHO), and managed care options from government and private indemnity health insurance plans offer a managed care focus. The goals of managed care are to provide

- Coordinated and efficient care to control costs
- Appropriate utilization of care
- Increased access to preventive care
- Maintenance and improvement of quality care

Behavioral health, which includes mental health and substance abuse care, has been carved out of medical services into MBHOs. A continuum of care options available in MBHOs intended to meet managed care goals include outpatient therapy in clinics and private offices, home- and school-based services, partial hospitalization programs, community residential care, emergency crisis services, hospital-based alcohol and drug treatment, and acute inpatient treatment. Inpatient treatment is reserved for those conditions that cannot be safely treated in a less restrictive and less costly setting. Managed care health care reform has had a profound effect on how psychiatric treatment occurs in this country. Health care reform has resulted in decreasing lengths of hospitalization, thereby reducing staff levels and making traditional approaches to mental health care infeasible (McGihon 1999). Managed care and how it affects psychiatric nursing are addressed in Chapter 4.

Planned short hospital stays have proved in some cases to be effective as measured in a reduction of the so-called revolving door syndrome (Johnstone and Zolese 1999). Admission to the hospital must be justified by at least one of the following criteria:

- Clear risk of client danger to self or others
- Dangerous decompensation of a client under long-term treatment
- Failure of community-based treatment with a clearly demonstrable need for more intensive and structured treatment to avoid harmful consequences
- Medical need, either unassociated with psychiatric treatment (such as intractable pain experienced by a depressed person) or associated with treatment (such as serious adverse reactions to a psychotropic medication)

These criteria for acute care hospitalization are common to many third-party payers. Exceptions may occur with a few insurance companies or with clients who are paying for their own hospitalization. Currently, therefore, goals for acute psychiatric hospitalization tend to include

- Prevention of self-harm to the client
- Prevention of harm to others by the client
- Stabilization of crisis with a return to community-based services
- Initiation or modification of a psychotropic medication regimen for clients requiring careful titration or observation
- Brief, specific problem solving designed to enable the client to gain or regain a state of compensation
- Rapid establishment of a plan for outpatient therapy

Table 5–1 illustrates a process model for successfully achieving outcomes of inpatient psychiatric treatment (Delaney et al. 2000).

The following two vignettes demonstrate the application of these criteria.

Vignette

- *Allen G., a 49-year-old computer programmer, has arrived at the emergency mental health center in tears, stating that he has had suicidal thoughts after losing his job during corporate restructuring. He has been divorced for the past 6 months. The clinical nurse specialist who interviews him determines that his risk of suicide is not high at this time. (Refer to Chapter 23 for assessment of suicide risk.) Allen responds to crisis counseling and agrees to an appointment for the next morning at an outpatient facility. The nurse assists Allen to identify supports and to begin to recognize coping skills that he has used to survive past crises. No hospitalization is required.*

TABLE 5–1 **Six Processes and Outcomes of Inpatient Psychiatric Treatment**

OUTCOME	BASIC PROCESS LABEL	CLINICAL FUNCTION
Resolve crisis	Increase patient's perception of control Increase supports to patient's system Decrease patient's symptom activity	Support, safety, and symptom management
Normalize	Restore sleep pattern Re-engage in socialization	Structure
Thorough assessment	Comprehensive battery of diagnostic interviews and testing completed in a timely manner	Symptom management
Mutual goal setting	Ascertaining patient's goals Reaching understanding of what inpatient treatment can provide Assessing patient's attributions of illness and treatment	Support
Client understands presumed efficacy of medication, cognitive and behavioral techniques, and rationale for referrals	Outpatient treatment planning Guide patient and family through logic of basic cognitive and behavioral approaches Pharmacological recommendations and potentials of service agency referrals	Symptom management
Do no harm	Provide physically and psychologically safe milieu Handle milieu tension proactively Use least-restrictive methods in handling dyscontrol Demonstrate persistent effort to develop collaborative relationship with patient Adequately train staff to maintain safety, sustain structure, affect-attune with client, and understand symptom management techniques	Safety structure

From Delaney, K., Pitula, C., and Perrand, S. (2000). Psychiatric hospitalization and process description. *Journal of Psychosocial Nursing,* 38(3):7–13.

Vignette

■ *Jordan S., 31 years old, arrives at the emergency mental health center in the company of a law enforcement officer. Jordan is nearly mute, so the officer explains to the clinical nurse specialist that Jordan was stopped from jumping off a bridge. After establishing a relationship with Jordan, the nurse determines that he has been treated for a severe and persistent mental disorder for the past 14 years and that, until 3 months ago, he attended a partial hospital day program at a community mental health center. He lost contact with his family 2 years ago. Jordan continually states that "God wants me to liquidate myself." After consultation with the attending psychiatrist, the nurse specialist arranges for voluntary admission, and Jordan agrees.*

RIGHTS OF THE HOSPITALIZED CLIENT

People, although hospitalized, retain their rights as citizens. The psychiatric team has an obligation to balance the client's needs for safety with his or her rights as a citizen. All mental health facilities provide a written statement of these rights, often with copies of applicable state laws attached. Students are also advised to become familiar with the client's handbook and the policy and procedure manual on the unit. Each student should be familiar with the unit's procedures for (1) suicide precautions, (2) seclusion and restraints, and (3) client elopement. (Refer again to Chapter 8 for a full account of clients' legal rights.) Box 5–1 gives an overview of a patient's rights. A listing of these should be displayed prominently on the unit. In addition, clients are often given a copy of their rights.

Vignette

■ Helen Weaver, RN,C, is a certified psychiatric mental health nurse. She has just heard the morning report, learning about the conditions of all the clients on the unit and about the status of the treatment community. Four clients have been assigned to her care during the coming shift. When she hears that Jordan is to be readmitted to her acute care unit, she volunteers to conduct the admissions process, because Jordan had been one of her primary clients during his previous three hospital admissions. Ms. Weaver proceeds to interview Jordan. While her assessment priority is his risk for self-harm, she also gathers data regarding his physical, social, cognitive, and emotional status. The physician is contacted for orders based on these data. A plan of care is initiated.

On the basis of Ms. Weaver's assessment of Jordan's current ability to understand, she ensures that Jordan has freely consented to hospitalization and explains to him his rights as a hospitalized client. He is given a copy of the hospital's Patient's Bill of Rights and is shown where it is displayed on the unit. Jordan is oriented to the unit and to the schedule of activities. With the assistance of a client who is designated the "host," Ms. Weaver introduces Jordan to a few of the other clients. Because of Jordan's risk for self-harm, Ms. Weaver maintains a distance of no more than an arm's length from him during these activities. After Jordan demonstrates some degree of comfort with his new situation, Ms. Weaver delegates responsibility for keeping Jordan under close watch to another staff member. Ms. Weaver then documents her assessment and plan. This initial plan will guide Jordan's care until the treatment team meets to consider his needs.

Refer to Chapter 23 for suicide precautions.

INTERDISCIPLINARY TEAMWORK AND CARE MANAGEMENT

The client's care is planned and implemented by a team composed of nurses, social workers, counselors, psychologists, occupational and activities therapists, psychiatrists, medical physicians, mental health workers, pharmacists, and other members of the hospital's health care team, according to the client's needs. In many inpatient settings, nurses convene and lead planning meetings, which provides a

Box 5–1   *Sample Statement of Patient's Rights*

TYPICAL ITEMS INCLUDED IN HOSPITAL STATEMENT OF PATIENT'S RIGHTS

1. Right to be treated with dignity.
2. Right to be involved in treatment planning and decisions.
3. Right to refuse treatment, including medications.
4. Right to request to leave the hospital, even against medical advice.
5. Right to be protected against the possible impulse to harm oneself or others that might occur as a result of a mental disorder.
6. Right to the benefit of the legally prescribed process of an evaluation occurring over a limited period (in most states, 72 hours) in the event of a request for discharge against medical advice that may lead to harm to self or others.
7. Right to legal counsel.
8. Right to vote.
9. Right to communicate privately by telephone and in person.
10. Right to informed consent.
11. Right to confidentiality regarding one's disorder and treatment.
12. Right to choose or refuse visitors.
13. Right to be informed of research and to refuse to participate.
14. Right to the least restrictive means of treatment.
15. Right to send and receive mail and to be present during any inspection of packages received.
16. Right to keep personal belongings unless they are dangerous.
17. Right to lodge a complaint through a plainly publicized procedure.
18. Right to participate in religious worship.

comprehensive approach to care (Norton et al. 1999). This nursing leadership reflects the holistic nature of nursing as well as the fact that nursing is the discipline that is present on the unit at all times. See Box 5–2 for a brief description of the roles of other members of the health team.

Each discipline is responsible for gathering data and participating in the planning of care. For the newly admitted client, this can prove extremely stressful or threatening. The team, often on the recommendation of the nurse, must consider the need for timing. These assessments should balance the urgency of the need for data against the client's ability to tolerate the assessments. Often, the assessments of the intake worker and the nurse provide the basis

Box 5-2 *Other Members of the Health Team*

Social workers: Basic social workers assist the client to prepare a support system that will promote mental health on discharge from the hospital. This includes contacts with day treatment, employers, sources of financial aid, and landlords. Licensed clinical social workers are prepared in individual, family, and group therapies, often as primary care providers.

Counselors: Counselors, prepared in disciplines such as psychology, rehabilitation counseling, and addiction counseling, may augment the treatment plan by co-leading groups, providing basic supportive counseling, or assisting in psychoeducational and recreational activities.

Psychologists: According to their master's or doctoral degree preparation, psychologists conduct psychological testing, provide consultation for the team, and offer direct services such as specialized individual, family, or marital therapies.

Rehabilitation,
Occupational, recreational, art, music, and dance therapists: On the basis of their specialist preparations, these therapists assist the clients to gain skills that help them cope more effectively, to gain or retain employment, to use leisure time to the benefit of their mental health, and to express themselves in healthy ways.

Psychiatrists: Depending on their specialty of preparation, psychiatrists may provide in-depth psychotherapy or medication therapy or head a team of mental health providers functioning as a private service based in the community. As physicians, psychiatrists may be employed by the hospital or may hold practice privileges in the facility. Owing to their legal power to prescribe and to write orders, psychiatrists often function as leaders of the team in terms of the patients assigned to the individual psychiatrist.

Medical physicians: These physicians provide, on a consultation basis, medical diagnosis and treatments. Occasionally, a physician prepared as an addictionologist may serve in a more direct role on the unit that offers treatment for addictive disease.

Mental health workers: Like nursing assistants, mental health workers function under the direction and supervision of registered nurses. They provide assistance to clients in meeting basic needs and also help the community to remain supportive, safe, and healthy.

Pharmacists: In view of the intricacies of prescribing, coordinating, and administering combinations of psychotropic and other medications, the consulting pharmacist can offer a valuable safeguard. Physicians and nurses collaborate with the pharmacist regarding new medications, which are proliferating at a steady rate.

Difference: Psychiatrists
b/w *can prescribe meds*

Discharge Planners:

for initial care. In most settings the psychiatrist must assess and provide orders within a limited time frame. Medical problems are usually referred to a primary care physician or specialist, who assesses the client and consults with the unit physicians.

The various disciplines meet within 72 hours to formulate or select a plan of care that reflects the consensus of the team. The plan reflects nursing process or an interdisciplinary path–based approach to care. The latter approach may be in the form of a multidisciplinary treatment plan or a clinical pathway. Clinical pathways provide a predetermined method for guiding care and measuring the client's progress based on the client's psychiatric diagnosis (Beyea 1996). The team either composes the plan of care or selects the clinical pathway, revising the plan or making clinical decisions if the client's progress differs from the expected outcomes. A member of the case management department, often the social worker, participates in all treatment planning conferences and daily report meetings to monitor and facilitate the achievement of outcomes along the

clinical pathway. It is important for the student nurse to have an understanding of case management and clinical pathways, since both approaches are common in health care settings today.

Case Management

Case management services first emerged within mental health care in response to the de-institutionalization movement of the mid to late 1950s and are a core component for meeting the comprehensive needs of clients with chronic mental illness (Austin and McClelland 1996). **Case managers** are client advocates who interact with and assess clients and family members, coordinate services appropriate to the client, monitor the delivery of services, and evaluate the outcome for the client (Cohen and Cesta 1993). In the inpatient setting, case managers communicate daily or weekly with the client's insurer and provide the treatment team with guidance regarding the availability of resources. Although social

Initiation Date:

	DAY 1	DAYS 2–4	DAYS 5–7	DAYS 8–12*
Medical Interventions	H&P, MSE, thought process and content, psychomotor agitation, judgment, SI/HI. Substance abuse. Order laboratory studies: toxicology screen, ECG 40+, lithium, carbamazepine level. Admission orders. Drug screen. Restrict for 24 hr.	Complete treatment plan. Monitor side effects of medications and lithium level. Review laboratory results and any previous records. Reevaluate restriction.	Update treatment plan. Monitor symptoms, medications, and side effects. Initiate D/C plans for F/U.	Discharge instruction form. Discharge orders. Prescriptions and F/U appointment. Terminate therapy.
Nursing Interventions	Admission, assessment, documentation. Provide safety. Orient to unit, schedule and give ITP. Check VS and weight; monitor intake.	Assess adaptation to unit; monitor activity level, agitation, mood, sleep, appetite, and side effects of medications. Assess VS. Assist with grooming. Educate PT/family illness about medications.	Continue monitoring (see previous). Evaluate ability to participate in small group. Evaluate ADLs. Evaluate medication/illness teaching.	Continue monitoring and evaluation (see previous). Complete D/C summary. Reinforce medication/illness teaching.
Social Work Interventions	Emergency intervention	Assessment by third workday. Identify living situation, financial status, and support systems. Initiate D/C planning and family counseling.	Continue counseling PT/family. Review with PT/family available support systems.	Terminate counseling. Make outpatient appointments.
Psychology Interventions		Initial psychological testing	Review findings	
Recreational Therapy Interventions	Initial contact	Initial RT assessment completed. Begin attendance to specified groups.	Begin or continue leisure plan, including activities for energy release.	Complete leisure D/C plan(s).
Key Patient Outcomes	Accepts staff's verbal redirection and limits @ _____	Abides by unit rules @ _____ PT verbalizes feeling of safety @ _____ Maintains control @ _____ Attends assigned groups @ _____ Identifies current medications @ _____	Sleeps >5 hr @ _____ Eats 75% of meals @ _____ Participates in assigned groups @ _____ Reports improved mood @ _____	Decreased or cessation of symptoms of altered thought process; content, misperceptions, grandiosity, agitation @ _____ Improved behavioral control @ _____ Identifies D/C plan and F/U care with medications @ _____

*Within today's managed care environment, 8–12 hospital days are rare for most public or private hospitals.
@ = achievement data.
H&P, history and physical; MSE, mental status examination; F/U, follow-up; D/C, discharge; PT, patient; VS, vital signs; ECG, electrocardiogram; RT, recreational therapy; ADL, activities of daily living; SI/HI, suicidal ideation/homicidal ideation; ITP, interdisciplinary treatment plan.
Adapted from Veterans Administration Medical Center, 10 North Green Street, Baltimore, Maryland 21201.

workers and counselors may be case managers, nurses are recognized as being "in a key position to implement case management and managed care by virtue of their clinical skills and the nature of their interactions with clients and other members of the health care team" (Etheredge 1989, p. 13).

When case managers plan inpatient programs focused on short-term goals, followed by appropriate aftercare, research supports the feasibility of quality mental health care (McGihon 1999). Appropriate care for the hospitalized client within the managed care environment needs to focus on rapid assessment and stabilization, as well as discharge planning and appropriate follow-up within an integrated system.

Case management is recognized as an essential service in the community setting for those with severe and persistent mental illness (Austin and McClelland 1996). Multiple levels of intervention are available within case management services, ranging from daily assistance with medications to ongoing resolution of housing and financial issues. Case management fosters success and reduces recidivism by the client with long-term illness (the revolving door problem). Ideally, case managers establish enduring relationships with clients, facilitate their involvement in outpatient settings, and access resources, thereby helping to avoid the crises that result in readmission to the acute care hospital.

Clinical Pathways

Clinical pathways are tools that assist the multidisciplinary team in prospectively detailing the course of daily treatments and interventions for a particular psychiatric diagnosis or behavior problem. Beyea (1996, p. 3) defined clinical pathways as "interdisciplinary client care plans that delineate assessments, interventions, treatments, and outcomes for specific health-related conditions across a designated time line." Chan and Wong (1999) reported success with the use of clinical pathways in caring for schizophrenic clients because they enhance resource management and increase collaborative practice. Case managers rely on clinical pathways to monitor the timely progression of appropriate treatment and to communicate this progression to the client's insurer. Most hospitals customize their clinical pathways to meet their individual needs and may include a format to document completion of interventions and variances from the pathway on the clinical pathway tool. Some of the chapters in Units IV and V contain examples of actual clinical pathways that are used by members of the health care team (see Clinical Pathway 5–1 for an example here). We are moving fast in this age of managed care, and a cautious

and thoughtful approach to clinical pathways is advised.

Vignette

■ Jordan is approached by the nurse on the next shift as that nurse briefly assesses Jordan's mental status and suicide status. He notices that once again he is being asked about thoughts of harming himself. So far he has spoken with the intake nurse, with his primary nurse (Ms. Weaver), with his psychiatrist, with a counselor who conducts a group activity in conjunction with his nurse, and with a social worker who states that he will be meeting with Jordan tomorrow. He has been asked to take a medication that will "help you think more clearly and feel more secure."

■ After Jordan's admission and assessments by the nurse and the psychiatrist, the treatment team meets to discuss several people under the care of that psychiatrist. Ms. Weaver introduces the team to the data and initial list of Jordan's identified problems and needs. The case manager reports that Jordan is approved by his MBHO for 5 hospital days. Priorities are set and agreements are reached regarding what further data are needed and which members of the team will obtain these data. The team chooses a clinical pathway. They note that Jordan has already progressed in terms of a decreased risk for self-harm but has not yet met the expected criteria for a reduction in psychotic thinking. The team agrees on the use of prn medication, as ordered by the psychiatrist, and the gentle guidance of Jordan's thought processes during one-to-one contacts with staff and during simple group activities to reduce psychotic thinking. It is agreed that the nurses will report on Jordan's progress in gaining clarity of thought at the next treatment planning meeting.

NURSING ON THE INPATIENT UNIT

Management

Nurses assume the bulk of the management of the daily functioning of the inpatient mental health unit. Organizationally, an arrangement of nursing management with a parallel program manager or a clinical coordinator may exist. The program staff may provide social services, activities, occupational therapy, and specialized counseling services, among others. On the other hand, these services may be managed by a nursing manager.

In either case, the nurse manager is responsible for an awareness of the safety of the unit, its effectiveness in the delivery of services, and how well the components of the health care team integrate their services. The nurse manager, in conjunction with the program manager or clinical coordinator, plans a comprehensive schedule of therapeutic activities. The constraints of an inpatient environment, the physician's schedules, and the availability of staff influence the composition of the daily program. Nursing management must be able to campaign effectively to gain administrative support for the program's clinical goals.

Vignette

■ *Consistency and attentiveness are essential to Jordan's safety during the time that he poses a risk to his own safety. The system of staffing and shift-to-shift reporting on Ms. Weaver's unit provides for continuity of care by overlapping of shifts combined with both a tape-recorded report and an opportunity for face-to-face clarification by nurses and other staff members. (Refer to Chapter 23 for specific guidelines and suicide protocol.) By the end of the report, the staff knows its roles and responsibilities for the upcoming shift. While Jordan is at risk for self-harm, continuous one-to-one assignment of staff to his care is provided. A documentation sheet is maintained by the assigned staff member to indicate client status at frequent intervals.*

■ *Two days after his admission, a neurologist arrives on the unit to examine Jordan because of neurological symptoms that Ms. Weaver has reported to the psychiatrist. Because the neurologist arrives during a group therapy session in which Jordan is participating, the charge nurse informs the neurologist that Jordan's chart may be reviewed but that the physician must wait until the conclusion of group before Jordan can be examined. The neurologist accepts this restriction because of previous negotiations carried out by the nurse manager of the unit with the medical staff.*

Therapeutic Strategies

Psychiatric mental health nurses implement a major portion of the treatment plan. The plan is partly carried out in formal sessions with the client but is followed more frequently during informal contacts with individuals and with small groups of clients. Often, the effectiveness of the informal contacts can be viewed as more significant than the formal ones, because they occur during natural activities of daily and social living and are therefore based on reality.

Appropriate psychological counseling skills are the basis for all nursing interventions. Nurses are prepared educationally with psychosocial communication skills to assist clients to feel heard and sup-

ported, to develop trust and increased feelings of safety, to receive feedback, and to learn more adaptive coping skills. Nurses who have furthered their formal education, participated in workshops, and gained recognition as certified psychiatric mental health nurses or nurse specialists can conduct more intensive interpersonal or group therapies. Nurses continue to provide such therapeutic interventions as team members, sharing successes and difficulties with the team to provide for consistency of care and to gain feedback regarding timing and technique. Group work is typically co-led, with at least one of the co-leaders trained in such therapies. The co-leaders plan before sessions and evaluate the group process and their joint efforts afterward.

Vignette

■ *Jordan continues to experience difficulty trusting and relating to others. The plan is to build trust gradually and to introduce Jordan to increasingly complex interpersonal and group challenges. Ms. Weaver and the other nurses approach Jordan cautiously in a nonthreatening way. They offer empathetic comments regarding his nonverbal messages of distrust and discomfort. As Jordan shows increasing comfort with such one-to-one interactions, the nurses invite him to join in simple social activities on the unit, such as eating and talking with other clients. Ms. Weaver and a social worker co-lead a structured group therapy session for clients whose goals include organizing their thought processes and socializing at a basic level. Jordan participates in this activity, gradually extending trust to several other clients and allowing himself to laugh and talk briefly about his immediate experiences and thoughts. After the most recent session, Ms. Weaver and the social worker discuss how Ms. Weaver's role with Jordan is purposefully being reduced to encourage Jordan to interact more with others.*

Milieu

Group Activities

Experienced mental health nurses conduct specific, structured activities involving the therapeutic community, special groups, or families on most mental health units. Examples of these activities include morning goal-setting meetings and evening goal-review meetings. Community meetings may be held daily or at other scheduled times of the week. At these meetings, new clients are greeted and departing clients are given farewells, ideas for unit activities are discussed, community problems or successes are processed, and other business of the therapeutic community is conducted. Nurses also offer psycho-educational groups for clients and families on topics such as stress management, coping skills, grieving, management of medications, and communication skills. Groups for creative expression encourage client involvement in art projects, poetry, music, or story writing and support exploration of feelings in a noncompetitive environment (McGarry and Prince 1998). For a fuller discussion of unit groups led by nurses, refer to Chapter 34, Therapeutic Groups.

Vignette

■ *Helen Weaver and another nurse are conducting a morning goal-setting meeting of the community. A thought for the day is chosen by the two nurses, taking into account some of the common concerns of a number of the clients. One client volunteers to read the thought from an inspirational book, and Ms. Weaver encourages the clients to discuss the reading briefly. Clients and staff members then introduce themselves, and each states a goal that is specific and can realistically be accomplished that day. The two nurses assist community members to state realistic goals in measurable, concrete terms. They invite the other members of the community to offer words of encouragement. The meeting ends with the community's choice of another reading or with the ever-popular choice of the Serenity Prayer.*

Management of Milieu

On an inpatient unit, nursing is the discipline primarily responsible for maintenance of a therapeutic milieu. Each nurse, through the course of a workday, is constantly gathering data about the well-being of the therapeutic community. As noted earlier, reports from shift to shift attend to the status of the milieu.

To maintain an atmosphere in which healing and growth can take place, nurses strive to keep communications and interpersonal feedback open and constructively honest. Verbal messages must be clear or must be clarified as needed. Nonverbal messages must also be congruent with verbal messages. Ideally, staff and clients should be interacting often and be seen as sharing a number of community goals. Clients need to be involved in some decisions and given explanations for those decisions that must be left to the staff. Behavioral limits and rules should be plainly understood and consistently enforced by all staff. All clients and staff must be held responsible for their own behavior and for the well-being of the community.

The therapeutic milieu operates on the understanding that the community can serve as a real-life training ground for learning about self and for practicing communication and coping skills in preparation for a return to the community outside the hospital. Even events that seemingly distract from the program of therapies can be turned into valuable learning opportunities for the members of the community.

Vignette

■ *Sally K., 34 years old, is a client on the unit who is well known to both clients and staff. Her bright, intelligent, and outgoing manner has made her popular. Because of her leadership and knowledge, however, she has prompted a number of clients to begin to question the unit's rules, schedules, and therapies. One of the nurses, Bob Kay, notices that he has begun to feel uncomfortable among several clients with whom he formerly had good rapport. He thinks that they are avoiding him and withholding trust. He mentions this in his shift report. Ms. Weaver validates his feelings by noting that she had also experienced this but had assumed that it may have been her own personal reaction to being a member of a different sociocultural group. The nursing staff consults with the rest of the treatment team and decides to open the community meeting to questions regarding the unit's rules, schedules, and therapies. At the meeting, the airing of issues satisfies the client community. Several of the clients involved ask to speak privately with staff about their feelings of having been influenced by Sally. Sally herself speaks with her nurse about how she realizes that she was using the situation to avoid working on her own painful feelings and decisions.*

Safety

The psychiatric mental health nurse assumes a responsibility for ongoing vigilance regarding safety hazards. A high level of client acuity exists today on inpatient units that contributes to an increase in risk for danger. The nurse carries out a variety of measures designed to reduce this risk on a daily basis. Environmental threats, such as fire, may also occur. Nurses must be able to rapidly isolate or evacuate clients while remaining in control of clients' whereabouts and minimizing their sense of threat.

The nurse must supervise the unit's systems for tracking which clients are on or off the unit and for periodic or constant checks on those clients at risk of harm to self or others. The flow of visitors and objects being brought onto the unit must be managed. Procedures for the safe control of sharp objects must be implemented. Use of illegal drugs or alcohol and sexual activity between clients must be prevented. Violence and disruption must be minimized while retaining an atmosphere that promotes healthy and appropriate expression of anger and other feelings. Elopement (escape) of clients has to be prevented, but in a way that avoids an atmosphere of imprisonment. Routine nursing concerns related to safety issues such as slippery floors, client falls, and electrical hazards must be addressed.

Vignette

■ *Helen Weaver has woven concern for safety into her daily nursing practice. As she enters or leaves the unit, she is checking the unit's locks. She is alert to any potential electrical or fire hazards. Her eyes routinely scan the unit for possible sharp objects. She tracks the locations of clients as she moves about the unit. If she is aware that staff have not been present in certain locations, she is sure to include those places in her rounds. Ms. Weaver informs new clients of rules regarding sharp objects, smoking, medications from home, visitors, leaving the unit, and behavioral restrictions. She clearly advises clients against the possession of alcohol and illicit drugs. She supervises inspection of clients' personal items and of any medications brought from home. She will later document her findings in the client's medical record. She participates in community meetings during which staff provide clarification of these rules. When visitors arrive, she teaches them the rules and checks bags and other incoming items.*

Documentation

Documentation of client progress is the responsibility of the entire mental health team. Although communication among team members and coordination of services are the primary goals when choosing a system for charting, practitioners in the inpatient setting must also consider professional standards, legal issues, requirements for reimbursement by insurers, and accreditation by regulatory agencies. Information must also be in a format that is retrievable for quality assurance monitoring, utilization management, peer review, and research. For nursing, documentation of the nursing process is a guiding concern and is reflected in different formats that are commonly found in psychiatric hospitals. See Chapter 9 for and overview of documentation options. Study Chapter 8 for your legal responsibility in maintaining accurate client records; they are considered legal documents. Computerized clinical documentation is the common trend in inpatient settings today.

Psychopharmacological Responsibilities

Nurses on the inpatient acute care unit are responsible for addressing complex health problems in clients. Fifty percent of clients with psychiatric disabilities have a co-morbid medical condition, and 35% have an undiagnosed medical problem that may contribute to psychiatric symptoms (Felker et al. 1996). The physical health status of clients is compromised owing to life style habits such as physical inactivity, smoking, and poor nutrition (Farnam et al. 1999). Anxiety, lack of trust, or thought impairment may cause clients to resist procedures such as vital signs, blood glucose monitoring, and insulin administration. As the therapeutic relationship develops, clients become more tolerant of physical interventions.

The safe administration and monitoring of medications is a 24-hour responsibility for the nurse. Because of their active leadership during treatment planning, nurses often exert great influence regarding medication decisions on mental health units. Detailed knowledge of psychoactive medications and of the interactions and psychological side effects of other medications is expected of mental health nurses (see Chapter 3). The nurse's observations of the expected and adverse effects of medication regimens provide data necessary for efficient and accurate medication decisions by the psychiatrist and treatment team. The legal issues of resistance to taking medication and of noncompliance are dealt with in Chapter 8.

In most hospital settings, clients come to a central location for medication administration. This fosters client responsibility and involvement in the treatment process. Psychiatric mental health nurses often have numerous decisions to make about prn medications. These decisions must be based on a combination of factors: the client's request, the team's plan, attempts to use alternative methods of coping, and the nurse's judgments regarding timing and the client's behavior. Nurses consult with team members when possible to make the best prn decision.

Vignette

■ *Helen Weaver has provided the team with data leading to an accurate diagnosis and choice of medications for Jordan. This choice reflects Ms. Weaver's knowledge of how Jordan responded to medication regimens during previous hospitalizations. His current regimen includes orders for medications that reduce his disorganized thought processes and thereby reduce his risk for self-harm. On Ms. Weaver's day off, the nurse assigned to Jordan assesses that he hears voices "commanding me to cease living." The nurse refers to*

Jordan's chart. The plan directs the nurse to spend 15 minutes helping Jordan to recall that he has learned to understand that when he hears such voices, it is his mind's way of expressing his feeling of being overwhelmed. He is to use relaxation techniques, but if he does not obtain relief within 20 minutes, he may use his prn medication along with relaxation.

The nurse notes that Jordan has received his oral dose of medication (same as the prn) only 10 minutes before her assessment. On the basis of her knowledge of the time needed for the onset of action of this medication, she follows the plan of care. The relaxation, along with the onset of action of Jordan's usual dose, leads to relief of his symptoms at this time.

Crisis Management

Nurses anticipate, prevent, and manage emergencies and crises on the unit. These crises may be of a medical or behavioral nature. Mental health units, whether situated in a general hospital or independently, must be able to stabilize the condition of a client who experiences a medical crisis. Mental health or addictive disease units that manage detoxification (withdrawal from alcohol or other drugs) must anticipate several common medical crises associated with that process. Mental health units therefore store crash carts containing the emergency medications used to treat shock and cardiorespiratory arrest. Nurses must maintain their cardiopulmonary resuscitation skills and be able to use basic emergency equipment. To be effective and to practice at a high level of competency, nurses are advised to attend inservice sessions and workshops designed to teach and maintain current skills. Nurses must be able to alert medical support systems quickly and mobilize transportation to the appropriate medical facilities. For more on crisis theory and therapy, refer to Chapter 22.

Vignette

■ Lester D., age 55, a client with acute mania and hypertension, complains of chest pain. The nurse asks Lester to be seated and checks his vital signs, carefully listening to his apical pulse. Noting irregularities that were not observed on previous assessments, the nurse stays with Lester while asking another nurse to notify the physician and to ready the crash cart. The portable electrocardiogram (ECG) monitor is attached and the nurse observes erratic, irregular heart beats. Transportation is arranged, and Lester is transferred after an intravenous line is started and ECG

monitoring is set up. The emergency is managed within 25 minutes of the client's first complaint.

Behavioral crises can lead to violence toward oneself or others. Crises are usually, but not always, observed to escalate through fairly predictable stages. Crisis prevention and management techniques are practiced by staff in most mental health facilities. Many psychiatric hospitals have special teams made up of nurses, psychiatric aides, and other professionals who respond to psychiatric emergencies called codes. Each member of the team takes part in the team effort to defuse a crisis in its early stages. If preventive measures fail, each member of the team participates in a rapid, organized movement designed to immobilize, medicate, or seclude a client. The nurse is most often this team's leader, not only organizing the plan but also timing the intervention and managing the concurrent use of prn medications. The nurse can initiate such an intervention in the absence of a physician in most states but must secure a physician's order for restraint or seclusion within a specified time. (Refer to Chapters 8 and 19 for further discussions and protocols on restraints and seclusion.)

The nurse also advocates for clients by ensuring that their legal rights are preserved, no matter how difficult their behavior may be for the staff to manage.

Crises on the unit are upsetting and threatening to other clients in the therapeutic community. A staff member is usually reserved for the needs of the community. This person removes other clients from the area of crisis and helps them express their fears. Clients may be concerned for the involved client and may fear that they, too, might experience such a loss of behavioral control.

Vignette

■ Jordan appears upset as he approaches a mental health worker. Jordan reports that Anthony, another client, is angrily throwing objects at the staff person assigned on a one-to-one basis to Anthony. The mental health worker reports this to the charge nurse, who quickly assigns the worker to remove other clients from the area. The nurse organizes other staff and checks Anthony's prn orders. There is no order for restraints or seclusion. The team gathers at the far areas of the dayroom while the nurse and one other staff person use calm but limit-setting communication techniques: "Anthony, you are not to hurt yourself or anyone here. If you are having trouble controlling your impulses, we will help you." Because Anthony's *behavior continues to escalate toward violence, the charge nurse directs another nurse to prepare Anthony's prn medication while the rest of the staff prepares to direct Anthony to the seclusion room. The staff uses its numbers as a "show of force" to convince Anthony of the seriousness of this directive. Anthony agrees and also reluctantly takes the prn medication. The staff remains prepared to intervene safely but decisively to take Anthony to the seclusion room if he cannot agree to the directive. While the charge nurse telephones the physician to report the incident and to obtain orders for seclusion, another nurse gathers the community in the dayroom to allow for expression of feelings about the situation. The nurse is careful to avoid breaking Anthony's confidentiality during this activity.*

Careful, accurate documentation in Anthony's chart demonstrates the need for these measures and how the intervention was carried out. While Anthony is in seclusion, he will be monitored at frequent intervals by a staff member.

Preparation for Discharge to the Community

As members of the multidisciplinary team, nurses assist clients and their families to prepare for independent or assisted living in the community. Community-based programs provide clients with psychosocial rehabilitation that moves the mentally ill beyond stabilization toward a qualitative life style. This is especially important to the concept and practice of managed behavioral health care, aiming toward the goal of reducing the length and frequency of hospital stays by the client.

Nurses therefore focus on the precipitants of the crisis that led to hospital admission. Clients are assisted to learn coping skills and behaviors that will help them avert future crises. Psychoeducational groups, individual exploration of options and supports, therapeutic leaves, and on-the-spot instruction (such as during medication administration) offer the client numerous opportunities. Nurses, during the 24-hour day experienced by the client, use the everyday experiences of the client as a testing ground for new, more adaptive behaviors.

The care plan or clinical pathway chosen for the client should reflect this discharge planning emphasis as early as the day of admission. The client is expected to begin to progress toward a resolution of acute symptoms, personal responsibility, and improved interpersonal functioning. Clients with prolonged mental illness benefit most from a seamless transition to community services. This is facilitated by collaboration with the community mental health center and the case manager in that setting. Readiness for community re-entry should include preparation by the client's support system for their role in enhancing the client's mental health.

Vignette

■ *The unit's schedule reflects its commitment to success in the community. Once his condition permits, Jordan attends evening group sessions that present information about safe and consistent use of medications, the importance of regular attendance in a community care program, communication skills, cognitive restructuring, self-esteem building, use of spiritual supports, and healthy interaction with one's family. Jordan uses role playing to learn more comfortable communication and assertiveness skills. The social worker invites Jordan's case manager from the community mental health center to attend a treatment team meeting. Jordan agrees to return to daily participation in a partial hospital day program and have a monthly medication evaluation. An appointment time is scheduled for assessment and readmission to the day program. In the group session, Jordan's peers encourage him to contact his family. He says one morning that his goal for the day is to phone his parents. The group helps him decide how to communicate during the phone conversation and later encourages him to discuss the results.*

By the day of his discharge from the hospital, Jordan is arriving for his medications independently, has plans for his follow-up care, is ready to return to his apartment, and has been invited to lunch with his parents.

Policy Review and Revision

Mental health nurses are usually expected or invited to participate in decisions about the system of providing care and the working environment. Nurses may address issues such as problems of scheduling of activities, work schedules, assignments, opportunities to expand professional practice, and safety. Nurses may research novel approaches to these or other aspects of delivery of care. Committee work may offer the nurse the chance to participate in the management and future of the unit.

Vignette

■ *Ms. Weaver collaborates with other nurses and program staff to develop a system for monitoring clinical outcomes. This system, based on the clinical pathways, will enable the staff to argue more persuasively for insurance payments for clients. It will also provide data useful for contracting with large regional employers to provide mental health services for their employees. Ms. Weaver describes her enthusiasm about participating in research and expanding beyond her customary nursing roles.*

SUMMARY

Nursing on an inpatient acute care psychiatric unit calls for skills in management, communication, and collaboration with an interdisciplinary team. The mental health nurse assists the client to adjust to hospitalization and to benefit from the therapies available. The nurse provides direct services to the client but also participates in the team effort to create a safe, supportive, growth-enhancing environment for the client. With additional experience, education, and training, the nurse participates in advanced therapies. Recovery and skills for reintegration into the community are a focus of nursing support throughout the inpatient stay. The nurse advocates for the client and ensures that the client's rights are protected.

The beginning practitioner needs to gather information about the functioning of this unique form of treatment from the clinical orientation, the unit's handbook for clients, the policy and procedure books, and the Patient's Bill of Rights. Students are advised to maintain open communication with staff, managers, and clinical instructors. Staff and clients often welcome an interest by students because of their ability to provide clients with time and empathy. The students' fresh perspectives on the unit also can offer the staff valuable feedback about the quality of its services.

Because of the sense of community on the inpatient unit, the student must be alert to the possibility of unwittingly becoming involved in divisive maneuvers (manipulations) initiated by some clients. Frequent verbal reporting to staff and seeking of evaluative comments from staff help safeguard students from such pitfalls. Students are reminded to become familiar with plans of care or clinical pathways to join in the interdisciplinary team effort.

Visit the **Evolve** website at
http://evolve.elsevier.com/Varcarolis
for a post-test on the content in this chapter.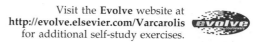

Visit the **Evolve** website at
http://evolve.elsevier.com/Varcarolis
for additional self-study exercises.

Critical Thinking and Chapter Review

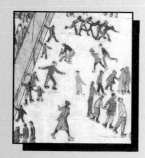

Critical Thinking

1. How does a nurse decide to place the clients' safety needs before their right to make decisions for themselves?
2. If nurses function as equal members of the multidisciplinary mental health team, what differentiates the nurse from the other members of the team?
3. Have managed behavioral health care organizations had a positive effect on the care of mentally ill clients? (http://www.surgeongeneral.gov/library/mentalhealth/home.html)
4. How is a community affected when clients with severe and persistent mental illness live in group homes?

Chapter Review

Choose the most appropriate answer.

1. The presence of which symptom will exert the greatest pressure to admit an individual to an inpatient psychiatric unit?

   1. Suicidal ideation
   2. Moderate anxiety
   3. Feelings of sadness
   4. Auditory hallucinations

2. When the mental health team meets initially to plan care for a client on an inpatient unit, the outcome should be

   1. Greater team cohesion
   2. Support for the psychiatrist
   3. Equal distribution of responsibility for the client among members of the staff
   4. An interdisciplinary care plan delineating assessments, interventions, treatments, and outcomes across a time line

3. Which goal should be evaluated as met prior to a client's discharge from an inpatient psychiatric unit?

   1. Family members are ready to accept the client.
   2. The client can return to productive work.
   3. The admission crisis is resolved.
   4. The client's illness is cured.

4. A therapeutic milieu for an inpatient psychiatric unit will be characterized by

   1. Few rules
   2. Staff control
   3. Open communication
   4. Conflict suppression

5. Of the several psychiatric inpatient unit staff activities listed below, which is most characteristically assumed by the discipline of nursing?

   1. Advocating for the legal rights of clients
   2. Compliance with documentation standards
   3. Creating an individualized client plan of care
   4. Leader of behavioral crisis management team

REFERENCES

Austin, C., and McClelland, R. (Eds.). (1996). *Perspectives in case management practice.* Milwaukee, Wisconsin: Families International.

Beyea, S. C. (1996). *Critical pathways for collaborative nursing care.* Menlo Park, California: Addison-Wesley Nursing.

Chan, S., and Wong, K. (1999). The use of critical pathways in caring for schizophrenic patients in a mental hospital. *Archives of Psychiatric Nursing,* 23(3):145–153.

Cohen, C. L., and Cesta, T. G. (1993). *Nursing case management: From concept to evaluation.* St. Louis: C. V. Mosby.

Daiski, I. (2000). The road to professionalism in nursing: Case management or practice based in nursing theory? *Nursing Science Quarterly,* 13(1):74–79.

Delaney, K., Pitula, C., and Perraud, S. (2000). Psychiatric hospitalization and process description. *Journal of Psychosocial Nursing,* 38(3):7–13.

Etheredge, M. L. S. (Ed.). (1989). *Collaborative care: Nursing case management.* Chicago: American Hospital Publishing.

Farnam, C., Zipple, A., Tyrrell, W., and Chittinanda, P. (1999). Health status risk factors of people with severe and persistent mental illness. *Journal of Psychosocial Nursing,* 37(6):16–21.

Felker, B., Yazel, J., and Short, D. (1996). Mortality and medical comorbidity among psychiatric patients: A review. *Psychiatric Services,* 47(12):1356–1363.

Gibson, D. (1999). Reduced rehospitalization and reintegration of persons with mental illness into community living. *Journal of Psychosocial Nursing,* 37(11):20–25.

Johnstone, P., and Zolesc, G. (1999). Systematic overview of the effectiveness of planned short hospital stays for mental health care. *British Medical Journal* 318(7195):1387–1390.

McGarry, T., and Prince, M. (1998). Implementation of groups for creative expression on a psychiatric inpatient unit. *Journal of Psychosocial Nursing*, 36(3):19–24.

McGihon, N. N. (1999). Psychiatric nursing for the 21st century: The PACED model. *Journal of Psychosocial–Mental Health Services*, 37(10):22–27.

Norton, J., Jones, R., Quarles, E., and Danielle, J. (1999). A nursing-centered treatment team in inpatient medical psychiatry. *Journal of Psychosocial Nursing*, 37(4):39–41.

Sauber, R. (Ed.). (1997). *Managed mental health care*. Bristol, Pennsylvania: Brunner/Mazel.

Schreter, R., Sharfstein, S., and Schreter, C. (Eds.). (1997). *Managing care, not dollars*. Washington, D.C.: American Psychiatric Press.

Wilbur, S., and Arns, P. (1998). Psychosocial rehabilitation nurses: Taking our place on the multidisciplinary team. *Journal of Psychosocial Nursing*, 36(4):33–41.

Outline

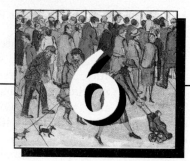

Mental Health Nursing in Community Settings

SUSAN CAVERLY

Key Terms and Concepts

The key terms and concepts listed here also appear in color where they are defined or first discussed in this chapter.

acculturation

de-institutionalization

ethical dilemma

trans-institutionalization

Objectives

After studying this chapter, the reader will be able to

1. Explain the evolution of the community mental health movement.

2. Distinguish between the goals and interventions of mental health nursing care in the hospital and the community setting.

3. Compare and contrast the levels of education and the roles and functions of the community mental health nurse.

4. Give examples of the psychiatric nurse's role as a member of a multidisciplinary team.

5. Summarize the role of the nurse and the goals of treatment for the following community resource facilities:
   - Community mental health centers
   - Homeless shelters
   - Mobile health care units
   - Forensic settings
   - Private practice settings
   - Home psychiatric mental health care
   - Outpatient chemical dependency treatment facilities
   - Telephone and Internet sites

6. Describe some of the ethical issues and conflicts a community mental health nurse might encounter.

7. Discuss how culture affects nurses and clients when formulating realistic and attainable health care goals in the community setting.

8. Assess how the future directions of health care in hospital and community settings could affect your career goals.

*T*he first psychiatric nurses working in the community setting were community health nurses who developed a specialty practice in mental health. They were able to move within the community, were comfortable meeting with clients in the home or neighborhood center, were competent to act independently, using professional judgment in sometimes unanticipated situations, and possessed knowledge of community resources. The heritage of these nurses began among European women who cared for the sick at home and American women who organized into religious and secular societies during the 1800s to visit the sick in their homes. By 1877, trained nurses worked as public health nurses visiting the homes of the poor in northeastern cities and generalist nurses engaged in community visits to rural areas for health promotion and care of the sick (Smith 1995).

THE CONTEXT FOR PSYCHIATRIC NURSING IN THE COMMUNITY

In 1963, President Kennedy signed into law the Community Mental Health Centers Act, thus solidifying the shift of mental health care from the institution to the community and heralding the era of de-institutionalization. Media focus raising public awareness regarding the horrors of psychiatric institutions, the mental health care needs presented by returning servicemen, and the advent of psychopharmacological agents all acted as catalysts for needed change in psychiatric treatment philosophy (Marcos 1990; Rochefort 1993).

The 1960s were also the time when federal entitlement programs proliferated: Social Security Disability, Supplemental Security Income, Medicaid, Medicare, housing assistance, and food stamps. These social programs provided the means for moving the mentally ill out of institutions and into the community. Talbott (1981) used the term trans-institutionalization to describe the process of providing institutional services in settings outside the institution. Policymakers of the time believed community care would be less expensive than the historic hospital-based care.

Caring for the severely and persistently mentally ill in the community is not without problems, and the community mental health system has been criticized for failing to serve those who are most severely ill. Funding is often inadequate to meet needs. Those who are most in need of psychiatric care are often the same clients who, for whatever reason, resist the use of available services. Despite these concerns, a second wave of de-institutionalization took place in the 1980s after President Carter's Commission on Mental Health highlighted the needs of the underserved and unserved chronically mentally ill. Concepts of de-institutionalization, rehabilitation, and long-term treatment of the severely and persistently mentally ill are embedded in the current mental health system and are the legacy of the Mental Health Services Act of 1980 (Bachrach 1994; Callahan 1994; Crosby 1987).

Community psychiatric mental health nurses have received similar criticism for having failed to adequately serve persons suffering from enduring mental illness, thereby relegating psychiatric specialty care to primary care practitioners. However, Barr (2000) found that persons identified as having a psychotic disorder were more likely than those with other disorders to be receiving psychiatric specialty care. Interestingly, this study found little difference in need, unmet need, and quality of life in relation to the specialty service contact. In recent years the locations where psychiatric nursing care is provided and the nursing specialties delivering psychiatric care have become more diverse (Kimball and Williams-Burgess 1995; Scales et al. 1993). Home health nurses often care for persons with undiagnosed mental or emotional disorders.

Nurses working in the criminal justice system provide mental health nursing care by default, if not by specialty; the Los Angeles County Jail has been recognized as the largest mental health institution in the United States. Jail diversion programs for mentally ill criminal offenders are becoming more and more common. These programs provide intensive mental health case management and offer psychiatric treatment to persons who would otherwise be incarcerated for crimes committed in part due to psychiatric illness. Psychiatric nurses are integral to such programs and often work directly with a designated mental health criminal court or a drug court to provide necessary and appropriate services to the individuals jointly served. The intent of these programs is to avoid incarceration, engage the client in care, and protect the interests of the community in the process.

School-based clinics are becoming more common in all communities, and as a consequence nurses trained to work with children and adolescents are currently providing mental health care. The list of both traditional and nontraditional community mental health care settings continues to increase. It is a challenge for nurses to meet this community need and for educators to ensure that nurses possess the knowledge and skills required to provide community psychiatric mental health nursing care. Box 6–1 lists some of the possible places in which nurses provide community psychiatric care.

Box 6-1 *Possible Community Mental Health Practice Sites (Nonexclusive List)*

- Community mental health centers
- Youth centers
- Private practice office
- Crisis centers
- Shelters (homeless, battered women, adolescent)
- Correction facilities, local jails, courts
- Primary care offices
- Chemical dependency program offices
- Client's home
- Schools and day care centers
- Nursing homes
- Day hospital facilities
- Group homes and adult foster homes or day care centers
- Work release housing
- Industry and business
- Emergency departments of community hospitals
- Outreach to multiple locations, including restaurants and shopping malls
- Churches, temples, synagogues, mosques
- Ethnic cultural centers
- Hospices and AIDS supportive living programs
- Client worksite

success at working in the community. Box 6–2 summarizes some of the attributes most helpful to the community psychiatric mental health nurse.

Community treatment hinges on enhancing client strengths in the same environment in which daily life must be maintained, thus making individually tailored psychiatric care imperative. The hospital represents a controlled setting and promotes stabilization, but strides made during hospitalization can be lost on return home. Treatment in the community permits clients and those involved in their support to learn new ways of coping with symptoms or situational difficulties. The result can be one of empowerment and self-management, to the extent possible given the client's disability. Research has shown that in many instances community psychiatric mental health nurses find that inpatient psychiatric nursing experience is not an essential prerequisite for work in the community setting and that in some instances such experience can create barriers to assuming an effective role in the community (Harris and Happell 1999).

Psychiatric Nursing Assessment Strategies

Assessment of the biopsychosocial needs and capacities of clients living in the community requires ex-

ASPECTS OF COMMUNITY NURSING

Psychiatric nursing in the community setting differs markedly from its hospital counterpart. The community setting requires that the psychiatric nurse possess knowledge about a broad array of community resources and be flexible in approaching problems related to individual psychiatric symptoms, family and support systems, and basic living needs such as housing and financial support. The setting is the realm of the client rather than of the health care provider; the nurse is in essence a guest or a consultant to the client, the housing manager, or the corrections officer who requested or agreed to psychiatric nursing intervention (Sullivan and Cohen 1990). Psychiatric nurses who have not previously worked in the community setting may find transition to this role difficult. It is an acculturation process, in which the nurse must revisit beliefs that there is a single definition of health or that professionals can or should control client behavior. A number of personal characteristics can ease the nurse's accommodation to the new role and enhance

Box 6–2 *Community Psychiatric Mental Health Nurse Attributes*

- Awareness of self; personal and cultural values
- Nonjudgmental attitude
- Flexibility
- Problem-solving skills
- Ability to cross service systems (e.g., to work with schools, corrections, shelters, health care providers, employers)
- Knowledge of community resources
- Excellent psychosocial and health assessment skills
- Excellent communications skills
- Knowledge of psychopharmacology
- Ability to recognize need for consultation
- Calm external manner
- Ability to see strength and ability in even the severely ill
- Willingness to work with the family or significant others identified by the client as support people
- Understanding of the social, cultural, and political issues that affect mental health and illness
- Knowledge of political activism

panding the general psychiatric nursing assessment. For the hospitalized client, the nurse must understand community living challenges and resources to assess presenting problems as well as to plan for discharge. The community psychiatric nurse must also develop a comprehensive understanding of the client's ability to cope with the demands of living in the community to be able to plan and implement effective treatment that will allow the client to stay in the community. Box 6–3 identifies the areas covered in a biopsychosocial assessment. Refer to Chapter 9 for a full assessment tool.

Among the key elements critical to the usefulness of this assessment are health status and interventions; mental status; psychiatric diagnoses (based on the *Diagnostic and Statistical Manual of Mental Disorders*, fourth edition, text revision [DSM-IV-TR]); somatic interventions for psychiatric symptoms; communication skills; support system availability and the client's willingness to accept support; community resource availability and the client's ability to gain access to these resources independently or with assistance; financial circumstances; ability to afford treatment and to purchase prescribed medication; availability of safe, affordable, habitable housing; access to and involvement in structured activity; ability to afford and prepare nutritious food; and possible legal entanglements.

Individual characteristics of clients have an effect on these areas of concern. For example, a person for whom Vietnamese is a primary language will require the nurse to consider the implications of language and culture as the psychiatric nursing assessment is undertaken. The use of an interpreter and cultural consultant is essential when the nurse and the client are not from the same culture and may speak different languages. Refer to Chapter 7 for more on cultural diversity applied to psychiatric nursing.

Psychiatric Nursing Intervention Strategies

In the hospital setting, the focus of care is on stabilization, as defined by staff. In the community setting, treatment goals and interventions are *negotiated* rather than imposed on the client. Community psychiatric nurses must approach interventions with flexibility and resourcefulness to meet the broad range of needs of those who manage their symptoms of mental illness in the community. The complexity of navigating the mental health system and the social service funding systems is often overwhelming to clients. Interventions cannot be directed only toward discrete psychiatric symptoms but must also facilitate client access to, and continuation of support for, basic needs such as housing and nutrition (Murray et al. 1995). Not unexpectedly, client outcomes with regard to mental status and functional level have been found to be more positive and cost effective when the community psychiatric mental health nurse integrates case management into the professional role (Chan et al. 2000a, 2000b).

An example of differences, in terms of treatment goals and nursing intervention strategies, between inpatient and community mental health settings is provided in Table 6–1. The table presents treatment approach, by setting, for clients who have established histories of mental illness and present with delusional thinking or hallucinatory experiences. Such clients are often fearful of care providers, resistant to taking medication, and reluctant to accept public assistance. They often have severely altered sleep patterns, racing thoughts, and poor concentration. The behavior of these individuals may be erratic or explosive when confronted even gently, and they may have difficulty caring for their own basic needs. However, those who use community mental

Box 6-3   Elements of Biopsychosocial Nursing Assessment

- Presenting problem and referring party
- Psychiatric history, including symptoms, treatments, medications, and most recent service utilization
- Health history, including illnesses, treatments, medications, and allergies
- Substance abuse history and current use
- Family history, including health and mental health disorders and treatments
- Psychosocial history, including
  Developmental history
  School performance
  Socialization
  Vocational success or difficulty
  Interpersonal skills or deficits
  Income and source of income
  Housing adequacy and stability
  Family and support system
  Level of activity
  Ability to care for needs independently or with assistance
  Religious or spiritual beliefs and practices
- Legal history
- Mental status examination
- Strengths and deficits of the client
- Cultural beliefs and needs relevant to psychosocial care

TABLE 6–1 *Characteristics, Treatment Goals, and Interventions by Setting*

SETTING	INPATIENT SETTING	COMMUNITY MENTAL HEALTH
Characteristics	■ Locked unit (possibly) ■ 24-hour supervision ■ Access to multidisciplinary team supports ■ Boundaries determined by staff ■ Food and housekeeping and security services ■ Milieu	■ Locked apartment ■ Boundaries determined by client ■ Client may refuse to take medication ■ Self-care, nutrition, and health care may be erratic ■ Social isolation
Goals	■ Stabilization of symptoms and return to community	■ Maintenance of stability in community ■ Client as an active member of treatment team ■ Improved ability to function
Intervention strategies	■ Boundaries enforced by seclusion and restraint if necessary ■ Develop short-term therapeutic relationship ■ Within limits of setting, develop and implement a plan of care that attends to sociocultural context of individual ■ Court-ordered medication ■ Monitor and assist self-care and nutrition ■ Health assessment and intervention as needed ■ Socialization activities provided and required as tolerated ■ Conferences with family or significant others and discharge planning activities related to long-term treatment and housing	■ Work with family or community resources such as police and landlord to gain access to apartment and client ■ Negotiate access and boundaries with client ■ Work with client and social support system to plan and implement care that is consistent with sociocultural belief system and context ■ Negotiate consent for and adherence to taking medications as prescribed ■ Establish, maintain, and use long-term therapeutic relationship ■ Intervene using creative strategies ■ Negotiate meaning of adequate self-care, nutrition, and health care with client and social support system (e.g., supply of fast food meal vouchers vs. home-cooked meals) ■ Assist client in assessing for needed services from those available in community

health services and those who care for those who use such services wish to have involvement in the process of individual care planning (Simpson 1999).

ROLES AND FUNCTIONS OF THE COMMUNITY PSYCHIATRIC NURSE

Psychiatric mental health nurses are educated at a variety of levels: associate, diploma, baccalaureate, masters, advanced practice, and doctoral. In addition to these levels of educational preparation, the specialty of psychiatric mental health nursing has access to a national certifying process through the American Nurses Association's Credentialing Center. There are two levels of certification: the psychiatric mental health nurse (generalist) and the psychiatric mental health clinical specialist (advanced practice nurse). The clinical specialist certification is the only national certification for master's prepared

advanced practice psychiatric mental health nurses. At this level, there is an option to subspecialize with a focus on children and adolescents or on adults (ANA 2000).

Combined education and expertise recognized by national certification provides a framework within which psychiatric nursing may determine the scope of practice. The American Nurses Association has published scope of practice statements for psychiatric mental health nursing and for psychiatric consultation and liaison nursing that further guide the differentiation among the levels of nursing practice (see Chapter 4).

Perhaps the most significant distinction among the multiple levels of preparation is the degree to which the nurse acts autonomously and provides consultation to other nurses, members of the treatment team, primary care practitioners, and providers outside the health care system. The Nurse Practice Acts of individual states grant nurses authority to practice. As the national patchwork of practice acts is expanded, in keeping with the increased knowledge held within the profession of nursing, prescriptive authority and hospital privileges are becoming a delineation point between advanced practice and general practice psychiatric nursing (Carson 1993; Caverly 1996; Krauss 1993). Table 6–2 presents information regarding the roles of psychiatric nurses relevant to their education.

The scope of nursing practice, as related to educational preparation, is influenced by the increased emphasis on standardization of care and management by outcome. These factors have reduced the amount of educational preparation considered necessary to provide routine care (e.g., not long ago a medical degree was required to operate the equipment that measured blood pressure). As new technology enters everyday life, we find that medications previously available only by prescription are sold over the counter and some basic health care interventions are performed by lay people. There-

fore, the descriptions provided in the following cases differentiating community psychiatric nursing roles in the treatment of clients with mental illness must be understood to have a certain fluidity and flexibility. The case study of Mr. Butler describes the assessment and case management roles of the community psychiatric nurse and the psychiatric nurse practitioner as they work to meet the biopsychosocial needs of a person who suffers from a severe and persistent mental illness.

Vignette

■ *Mr. Butler has previously been diagnosed as suffering from schizophrenia. He has a history of both voluntary and involuntary psychiatric hospitalization. He does not trust mental health professionals and only reluctantly takes psychiatric medication. He lives in a subsidized apartment and*

TABLE 6–2 *Community Psychiatric Nursing Roles Relevant to Educational Preparation*

ROLE	DOCTORAL PREPARATION	MASTERS PREPARATION	BACCALAUREATE PREPARATION	ASSOCIATE DEGREE OR DIPLOMA PREPARATION
Practice	Nurse practitioner or clinical nurse specialist; manage consumer care and prescribe or recommend interventions	Nurse practitioner or clinical nurse specialist; manage consumer care and prescribe or recommend interventions	Direct nursing care for consumer and assist with medication management as prescribed	Provide nursing care for consumer and assist with medication management as prescribed
Consultation	Consultant to staff about assessment, plan of care, and pharmacological or other interventions; consult with family and consumer about treatment options; consult with community to plan mental health services	Consultant to staff about plan of care, to consumer and family about options for care; collaborate with community agencies about service coordination and planning processes	Consult with staff about care planning, and work with nurse practitioner or physician to promote health and mental health care; collaborate with staff from other agencies	Consult with staff about care planning, and work with nurse practitioner or physician to promote health and mental health care; collaborate with staff from other agencies.
Administration	Administrative or contract consultant roles within mental health agencies or mental health authority	Administrative or contract consultant roles within mental health agencies or mental health authority	Administrative roles within mental health agency or treatment team	Leadership roles within mental health treatment team
Research and education	Act as a research or teaching liaison with local university school of nursing; mentor nurse researchers and educators at clinical level	Assume an educator or a research role within agency or mental health authority	Participate in research at agency or mental health authority; precept undergraduate nursing students	Participate in research at agency or mental health authority; precept undergraduate nursing students

receives intensive case management from staff at the local community mental health center. His family members are supportive in terms of financial help but are distant emotionally because of inability to predict the behavior they will encounter when they see him. His chief emotional tie was to an elderly cat, and the death of this pet has led to an increase in paranoid symptoms.

Before his most recent hospitalization, Mr. Butler was distressed because his landlord threatened eviction if his apartment was not cleaned and fumigated. Mr. Butler was unwilling to permit the landlord to enter his apartment, and when the issue was pressed by his case manager, he refused further contact with the case manager. Subsequently, Mr. Butler stopped taking his medication, refused to leave his apartment, and ran out of food. The landlord complained that he was disturbing other tenants by constant yelling at all hours. Attempts to suggest hospitalization were met with increased agitation.

The case manager followed steps to have Mr. Butler hospitalized involuntarily. Within 3 days after being hospitalized, Mr. Butler was restabilized on medication, interacting with staff and other clients in a socially comfortable manner, and was engaging in self-care activities. He was discharged back to the community 6 days after admission, with the plan that community mental health care would resume.

Within weeks, the community psychiatric nurse noted that Mr. Butler had begun to miss appointments for medication management. He had never been a regular member of the daily clubhouse program and was still suspicious of his case manager because of the involuntary hospitalization. The nurse telephoned Mr. Butler, without response. At the next team meeting, the nurse arranged with the case manager to visit Mr. Butler at home. On the day of the visit, Mr. Butler presented as sedated, somewhat confused, and fearful. During the outreach to Mr. Butler's apartment, the nurse discovered that he had not been taking his medication as prescribed (a total of five: an antipsychotic, an anticonvulsant, a side-effect medication, an antidiabetic medication, and an antihypertensive agent). All were to be taken at different times of the day. He had clearly missed multiple doses of each.

The psychiatric mental health nurse sat with Mr. Butler and asked general questions about his well-being. During this discussion, she was able to ascertain his mental state and assess a recent history of change in health status. He agreed that she could check his blood pressure, which was elevated. The nurse sorted Mr. Butler's medications and filled a reminder box with a 7-day supply divided into morning, afternoon, and evening doses. She and Mr. Butler contracted that he would take the medication in the box and she would keep the extra medication. The nurse also

learned that Mr. Butler had not purchased food since discharge, so she took him to the grocery store near his home. They selected food that required minimal preparation, and Mr. Butler agreed to eat at least once each day. He did have a large supply of coffee in the house, so they also problem-solved ways to reduce his daily consumption of 16 to 20 cups of coffee.

On return to the community mental health center, the nurse stored the medication in a locked box for safety. She consulted with the case manager and the psychiatric nurse practitioner responsible for prescribing Mr. Butler's medication, informing both of Mr. Butler's elevated blood pressure and fragile mental state. The plan of care was revised so that the nurse assumed the responsibility for home visits and for ensuring that Mr. Butler was able to keep appointments with his primary care provider. The psychiatric nurse practitioner requested laboratory tests, including fasting blood glucose level, 12-hour anticonvulsant blood level, liver enzymes, electrolytes, and serum ammonia level. She also scheduled appointments to meet with Mr. Butler weekly until he stabilized.

Member of Multidisciplinary Community Practice Team

The concept of using multidisciplinary treatment teams originated with the Mental Health Reform Act of 1963. The practice of psychiatric nursing was identified as one of the core mental health disciplines, along with psychiatry, social work, and psychology. This recognition permitted the allocation of resources to educate psychiatric nurses. It also acknowledged the particular contribution of psychiatric nursing. The team model provided a means of cross-fertilization among the disciplines. This led to enrichment and allowed for the development of a shared language among those providing mental health services (Chamberlain 1987; Peplau 1989).

In team meetings, each member is recognized for individual and discipline-specific expertise as the variety of professions represented on the multidisciplinary treatment team has grown. Generally, the configuration of the team reflects the availability of fiscal and professional resources in the community. Box 6–4 presents a list of disciplines that may be represented on a multidisciplinary treatment team. Note that deference is still given to the authority of the psychiatrist as a director of the mental health team. This is in part related to the demands of regulatory and legal authorities, which historically have recognized only those practitioners with medical degrees (Safriet 1994; Talley and Brooke 1992). Increasingly, advanced practice nurses are assuming roles

Box 6–4 *Multidisciplinary Treatment Team (Nonexclusive List)*

- Client
- Peer counselors
- Family members
- Employers
- Landlord
- Spiritual counselor
- Case manager
- Chemical dependency counselor
- Psychiatric nurse
- Psychiatric nurse practitioner
- Psychiatrist
- Psychiatric social worker
- Psychologist
- Occupational therapist
- Chiropractor
- Vocational rehabilitation therapist
- Nutritionist
- Primary care provider
- Recreation therapist
- Physical therapist

has led to rethinking and revision of titling. In the current health and mental health care environment, identification as a nurse or (in particular) as an advanced practice nurse is usually considered preferable to other titling alternatives. Furthermore, the community psychiatric mental health nurse of today better integrates the multidisciplinary perspective with a strong nursing identity. The role incorporates case management, assessment and intervention, client advocacy, somatic therapies, community interaction, and systems intervention (Talley and Caverly 1994). As a team member, the community psychiatric mental health nurse, at all levels, is in a critical position to link the biopsychosocial components relevant to mental health care and to do so in a manner that the client, significant others, and members of the treatment team can accept and understand. In particular, the management and administration of psychotropic medications have become a significant expectation of the community psychiatric mental health nurse, and there is evidence that this is most successfully accomplished when the nursing approach to drug therapy seeks to empower the individual client (Marland and Sharkey 1999).

Biopsychosocial Care Manager

The role of the community psychiatric mental health nurse includes the coordination of mental health, physical health, social service, educational service, and vocational realms of care for the mental health client. The reality of community mental health practice in the new millennium is that few clients present with uncomplicated symptoms of a single mental illness that can be either resolved or managed through brief psychotherapy and pharmacotherapy. The severity of illness with which individuals present, especially in the public sector, has increased and is correlated with increased substance abuse, poverty, and stress. In addition, there is well-documented evidence that the mentally ill not only experience greater risk for physical illness but also are less likely to receive timely and effective treatment (Farmer 1987; Talley 1988; Talley and Caverly 1994).

The 1980s brought increased emphasis on implementing case management, as a core mental health service and provider relationship, for the severely and persistently mentally ill in the community. In the private domain, case management, or care management, has also found a niche. The intent is to charge case managers with designing individually tailored treatment services for clients, tracking needs for care, and facilitating connection with the range of services. Case management implies attention to and coordination of necessary services for the client,

formerly considered the sole purview of medicine (Caverly 1996).

Recognition of the ability of nurses to have a voice in team treatment planning and to question the authority of other professionals was novel at the time it was implemented in community psychiatric practice; this level of professional performance was later modeled for the other nursing specialties. However, the multidisciplinary treatment team approach also led to some dilution of the nursing role embraced by psychiatric mental health nurses in the community. The autonomy of the role, the language of psychiatry and social services, and the respect available to the nurse in this setting created a professional dilemma. How could nurses in this actualized specialty of nursing (including entry educational levels) identify with nurses who functioned in institutional settings, followed physician orders, and received little recognition of their expertise?

In many cases, this conflict resulted in a schism between community psychiatric mental health nurses and their colleagues in other nursing specialties and settings. Community psychiatric mental health nurses in some parts of the United States sought job titles consonant with those of generic mental health practitioners in the community mental health system because of the perceived additional benefits. The improved lot of nursing in recent years

including client identification and outreach, individual assessment, service planning, linking with services, monitoring of service delivery, and client advocacy (Francis et al. 1995; Mellon 1994). Nursing and medicine are the only mental health disciplines possessing the knowledge, skill, ability, and legal authority to intervene in the full range of mental health care. This scope of practice, coupled with issues of personnel cost and availability, underscores the critical need for community psychiatric nurses to participate in coordination of care activities. Effective case management reduces unnecessary costly care by maintaining housing and providing creative alternatives to hospitalization (Bawden 1990; Francis et al. 1995; Mellon 1994).

Community tenure likewise increases when medications are taken as prescribed. Nurses are in a position to assist the client to manage medication, recognize side effects, and be aware of the interactions among drugs prescribed for physical illness and those for mental illness. Client education, and the efforts of prescribers to minimize both the number of medications and the frequency of daily dosing, increases the ability of clients to cooperate with treatment and to maintain stability (Meyer et al. 1991; Omori et al. 1991).

Psychiatric mental health nurses have not always valued their unique and important practice abilities. This is changing, and nursing is reclaiming direct care relationships with clients and embracing the advanced practice roles of the nurse practitioner in general and psychiatric specialties. This is a timely rediscovery, because health care reforms and realities of community funding are likely to have a significant impact on the role of psychiatric nurses in the community (Huch 1995, Peplau 1989). One example of a change in the work of the community psychiatric mental health nurse is assuming the gatekeeping role as the need for community mental health care taxes the system resources. Determining individual need and referring to the most appropriate service or provider require that the screening professional have a scope of expertise that permits a holistic assessment; the community psychiatric nurse is an ideal professional for this task. However, this administrative role creates some conflicts for the nurse, who becomes more clearly responsible for the distribution of mental health care resources as well as finding ways to meet individual needs (McEvoy 1999).

COMMUNITY RESOURCES

Community psychiatric mental health nurses originally practiced on site at a community mental health facility. As financial, health care, regulatory, cultural, and population changes have occurred, the location of practice has diversified. Nurses are providing primary mental health treatment at therapeutic day care centers, schools and school-based health centers, outpatient psychiatric hospital programs, and shelters. In addition to these more traditional environments for mental health care, psychiatric mental health nurses increasingly enter forensic settings as practitioners or consultants in drug and alcohol treatment centers, coroner's offices, and jails. Mobile mental health units have even been developed in some service areas. In a growing number of communities, mental health programs are collaborating with other health or community services to provide integrated approaches to treatment. A prime example of this is the growth of dual-diagnosis programming at both mental health and chemical dependency clinics. Technology has begun to contribute to the venues for providing community psychiatric mental health care; in some areas, telephone crisis counseling, telephone outreach, and even the Internet are being considered means for enhancing access to community mental health services (Wilson and Williams, 2000). The characteristics of the client population, the geography, the community resources, and the personnel available are perhaps the greatest determinants of where community mental health nurses will be recruited to practice. These factors also influence expectations regarding the extent of preparation for community psychiatric mental health nursing practice (Osborne and Thomas 1991; Worley 1995).

Community Mental Health Centers

Community mental health centers (Box 6–5) were created in the 1960s and have since taken center stage for those who have no access to private care. The range of services available at such mental health centers varies, but generally there are emergency services, adult services, children's services, and elder services. There may also be a psychopharmacology clinic staffed by psychiatric nurses, psychiatric nurse practitioners, and psychiatrists. Common components of mental health center services include groups such as life skills psychoeducational classes, supportive day treatment groups, vocational rehabilitation groups, and clubhouse programs. Increasingly, dual-diagnosis services for chemically dependent mentally ill clients are available at community mental health centers. Some organizations provide consultation services to nursing homes, manage adult residential facilities for the severely and persistently mentally ill, and provide emergency respite beds to prevent unnecessary hospitalization for cli-

BOX 6–5   *Community Mental Health Center*

Tim is a 31-year-old man who was diagnosed as having bipolar disorder when he was a 19-year-old college student. In subsequent years he self-medicated with alcohol and failed to stabilize on lithium carbonate. Tim was hospitalized a number of times. At the age of 28, he became sober and engaged in regular psychopharmacological management at the mental health center. He has now been employed full-time as a mechanic for more than a year. He is married and expecting a first child in 4 months. His wife is also bipolar, and because of the pregnancy she has chosen to remain off her medication. Her mood disorder has remained remarkably stable, and she continues to be monitored closely. Even so, the situation has been very stressful for Tim. He has been having trouble sleeping and has noticed that his thoughts are racing at times. He is worried because he knows he is responsible for the welfare of his new family. He admits that he has been working as much overtime as he can to save money to buy baby supplies. The couple has no support from family because of the troubles they caused their parents while they were unstable and abusing substances.

The nurse recognizes that Tim appears more pressured than usual. He states that he has been taking his medication regularly but that it seems not to be working as well as in the past. It is helpful for him to talk about the stress he is experiencing, and he does visibly calm during the interview; however, he is clearly in a hypomanic state.

Tim has been taking lithium carbonate, 1200 mEq, at bedtime for the past year and a half. He has not changed his diet during this time and has not experienced side effects. Tim's most recent 12-hour lithium level was determined 6 months ago, and at the time it was a relatively high 1.5 (normal range 0.8–1.2). The nurse determines that the dosage probably needs to be increased but would prefer to have a level drawn first. Since Tim took his medication at 10 PM last night and it is only 9 AM now, she sends him directly to the laboratory to have his blood drawn. She also increases the dose of lithium to 1500 mg at bedtime for the next week and reschedules to see Tim in 1 week. She plans to consult with his primary physician regarding her intervention.

Tim is comfortable with the plan and follows through with the intervention. Within a few days he notices that his thoughts are more collected and his sleep, while still disturbed, is much more restful. When he returns to the clinic the following week, he learns that his lithium level had dropped to 0.9. He appears more stable at the follow-up appointment. In spite of the improvement noted, the nurse schedules Tim to be seen every 2 weeks for the next month to ensure that he maintains his current stability.

1. Did the educational level of the nurse affect the nursing assessment or intervention with this client?
2. What additional considerations might be taken by the nurse in the future for this family?
3. What would you assess as the strengths of this family?

---

ents experiencing crisis (Broskowski and Eaddy 1994; Caverly 1991; Power 1991).

Vignette

■ Nina is a psychiatric nurse who works in a medication clinic at a state-funded community mental health center. She is responsible for managing medications for a large caseload of relatively stable public-sector clients. In monthly half-hour appointments with clients, she assesses the client's response to the medication, looks for previously unrecognized side effects, and determines whether there is continued need for the medication. She also discusses general health care needs and psychosocial concerns such as marital stress or work-related problems. At times, difficulties with parenting or other family issues result in a client's referral to another provider at the clinic for specialized assessment.

Most of the people Nina sees have known her for a long time and are open about their needs; some require careful probing about potential problem areas. It is essential that, when Nina refills a prescription, she feel confident it is a safe decision in the best interests of the client. She works using protocols established for the clinic. If she has concerns, Nina contacts the psychiatric nurse practitioner or the psychiatrist who is the primary prescriber for the client.

Treatment goals might include the following:

■ Assess response to prescribed medication and recognize side effects that will require intervention.
■ Promote stable functioning in the community.
■ Identify the need for additional services and assist the client to obtain them.

Homeless Shelters

Frequently, homeless shelters (Box 6–6) and community mental health centers affiliate to provide mental health services to those who otherwise would not be noticed or receive treatment. In some cities, model programs provide funding for mental health services in shelter sites; other cities use community networking to patch together needed services for the disenfranchised. Shelters are of many different configurations, offering many targeted services to specific homeless populations.

The mental health needs at shelter sites vary with the clients who receive homeless care. Primary needs include mental health, substance abuse, and physical health assessment as well as triage to community services. In some instances, there is a need for care to be delivered on site because the client is reluctant to go to a mental health center. At times, the shelter staff transport disorganized or paranoid clients to appointments to ensure that they receive care (Caverly 1991; First et al. 1995; Mowbray et al. 1993).

Vignette

■ Erin is a psychiatric nurse who works 4 hours each day at the downtown emergency service center and 4 hours at the women's day shelter. She is employed by the city's homeless project but is part of a team of mental health professionals affiliated with the local community mental health center. Erin spends her day meeting with shelter residents who need help with public assistance paperwork or have questions about obtaining regular mental health care. She also has a group of clients whom she sees weekly to help manage the medications prescribed for them by staff at the mental health center. Sometimes people come to her because they have health problems and do not know where to go; they have no money and are not registered for medical coupons. She either helps with these needs or arranges for appointments with providers who can help. Sometimes Erin

BOX 6–6   *Homeless Shelter*

Rose is a woman of unknown age. She is unkempt and communicates little with others. She uses the women's day shelter and sometimes sleeps at the main downtown shelter (when the weather is cold or wet). She is often seen talking to herself in a corner, and other residents give her wide berth because she has a history of slapping people if they get too close. Most of the time she just stays to herself; when staff offer her food, she will always eat. She leaves without a word when the day shelter closes and returns regularly in the morning. Staff like her, but since they realize that she doesn't want to get too involved with them, they also give her a great deal of space.

The request for a psychiatric assessment came as a surprise, because the psychiatric nurse knew Rose would refuse to speak with her. The previous night, Rose was forced to leave the shelter because she became loud and unruly, screaming that the devil was eating her feet. She apologized for being profane, but no one heard her use profanity. She refused to be quiet. Once evicted, Rose remained in the street, walking back and forth and loudly complaining about her feet. Shelter staff considered calling the police or having her taken to the emergency department, but she left before the intervention could take place. Still, the behavior was not usual for Rose, and it was of concern.

The nurse found Rose the next morning sitting at her regular spot in the corner. Rose was still complaining under her breath about the devil eating her feet. The nurse decided that rather than ask Rose about her mental state, she would ask to see her feet. Rose appeared nervous about this but consented, saying she was in great discomfort. With the wet shoes and socks removed, it became apparent that Rose's feet were darkly mottled and cold and had several open wounds where there was pressure from her shoes. The nurse offered Rose the opportunity to bathe her feet in warm water and found some clean socks. She asked Rose when her foot pain began, and Rose indicated it had been quite some time, but only recently the pain was so severe she was unable to stop thinking about her feet. The nurse contacted a health care clinic where free indigent care was available and arranged to take Rose to the clinic. In the course of this supportive work, Rose confided to the nurse that she had also been hearing voices more often lately and wondered if she should tell someone. The nurse suggested that they first take care of Rose's feet and then focus on the voices, and that there was probably something that would help quiet the voices. Rose looked grateful that someone understood.

1. Identify a positive approach this nurse took when assessing Rose's situation.
2. What lesson(s) did you learn from this case study that you might apply in your practice?

actually drives residents to appointments to ensure their arrival on time. She is more likely to help change a bandage or check a wound than are the nurses at the mental health center. The residents appreciate her willingness to be flexible about her role. Erin practices good personal and professional boundaries but is comfortable with a broad definition of her practice.

Treatment goals might include the following:

- Develop a trusting relationship with residents of the shelter to determine their needs for mental health care, physical health care, or social service intervention.
- Provide mental health and other health or social services on site to clients who need immediate intervention or who resist other services.
- Secure necessary services for clients who otherwise would not be likely to attain them.
- Assist residents to use their own resources as well as those offered to stabilize psychiatric symptoms.

Mobile Mental Health Care Units

Mobile outreach units (Box 6–7) have sprung up in various areas throughout the United States to respond to those mentally ill clients who cannot effectively use traditional outpatient mental health services. Primm and Houck (1990) described Johns Hopkins Hospital Community Support Treatment and Rehabilitation (COSTAR), a mobile treatment unit serving inner city Baltimore. Professional staff

pursue, "woo," and support treatment in whatever setting clients find themselves or feel comfortable in: at home, in a public place, in a comfortable clinic, or in jail. Clients might be assessed and treated in fast food restaurants, receive fluphenazine decanoate (Prolixin Decanoate) injections in restaurant bathrooms, and at the close of a "session" be offered milkshakes and meals as rewards. If adherence to a prescribed medication schedule or dosing is a problem related to understanding rather than resistance, medications are packaged and labeled with the time and date to be taken. Creative problem solving and intervention planning are hallmarks of the care provided by mobile mental health care teams.

In such a program, experienced nurses triage somatic complaints; monitor physical illnesses; provide psychoeducation on topics such as substance abuse, nutrition, hygiene, sexual relations, and safer sex; and assist clients to manage symptoms of mental illnesses. Housing is ensured through active community case management coupled with a protective payee system to manage the client's funds. Intervention and psychoeducational efforts are directed toward both clients and those who make up their support systems. Recreation and social groups are valued as a means of developing social skills and a step toward pre-employment training. Other pre-employment activities include vocational rehabilitation and work training. In keeping with the philosophical base of such a program, case management staff is available by pager to clients and families or significant others (e.g., landlords, employers) 24 hours a day to permit emergency intervention or to avert a crisis.

BOX 6–7 *Mobile Care Setting*

A 37-year-old woman presents with a complaint of low energy, sadness, and poor concentration. She has a bruise on her face, and her arm is bandaged, but she refuses to have the wound evaluated. She is accompanied by her husband, who appears quite concerned. He is reluctant to leave her alone during the interview and she is adamant that he remain. He responds to questions directed to her and she defers to him. She shows signs of anxiety and hyperalertness when asked about her marriage and support system. A request that her husband leave the room creates a great deal of agitation, but he does leave. The woman is then asked direct questions about domestic violence.

Her only family is her husband, and she says he is a good man whom she will not speak against. She only wishes to feel better so that he won't be angry with

her. The nurse acknowledges the woman's dilemma. She also confronts her regarding the need to be safe. The nurse provides education regarding domestic violence and the community resources available, should she wish to reach them. An appointment is scheduled for the following week when the mobile unit will again be in town. Before the woman's discharge, the nurse completes a risk assessment.

1. What are some of the ethical dilemmas presented in this case?
2. In situations such as these, what are some of the personal issues (self-assessment) you might want to look at when working with clients in similar situations? (See Chapter 25 for guidelines.)

Vignette

■ *Jennifer provides emergency psychiatric evaluations and individual counseling as a member of a mobile treatment program. She and two primary health care providers travel in a van to rural areas of the state. In addition, there is a psychiatrist who travels with the team 1 week each month. The psychiatrist prescribes medications for the clients who receive mental health care and case management from Jennifer throughout the month. She practices autonomously and provides consultation services to the family nurse practitioners with whom she works. Many of the individuals for whom she provides care are migrant workers. Jennifer speaks fluent Spanish and can effectively interview clients when interpreters are not available. Many of the people she sees are separated from their families and homesick. They are often living in austere circumstances, and depression is a common diagnosis. She is careful to evaluate for substance abuse disorders during all her assessments.*

Often Jennifer attempts to secure other social services for clients and their family members. Sometimes an intervention may be as simple as locating a source of infant formula for a mother who is unable to breast-feed. At other times, Jennifer must evaluate whether psychotic symptoms are due to a mood disorder, schizophrenia, or substance abuse. Jennifer has access to an on-line computer for literature and pharmacotherapy reference and consults with the psychiatrist as necessary by telephone. She has standing orders that permit her to initiate pharmacological intervention in psychiatric emergencies.

Treatment goals might include the following:

■ Provide assessment and intervention for psychiatric and psychosocial disorders to a population that would otherwise have little or no access to mental health care.
■ Provide differential diagnoses, recommend and enhance access to appropriate treatment by nonpsychiatric health care practitioners.
■ Manage medications prescribed by another practitioner.
■ Enhance individual client and family's ability to function productively in the community.

Forensic Settings

A small but growing number of nurses work with mentally ill offenders. Society has increased its efforts toward social control; consequently, we are seeing an increased use of correctional facilities to house the mentally ill. De-institutionalization has evidenced a so-called hydraulic effect (i.e., as people are discharged from state mental hospitals, they en-

ter the correctional institutions) (Reeder and Meldman 1991). Psychiatric mental health nurses are faced with a number of challenges, not least of which is the conflict arising around the provision of mental health care in an environment where the intent is punitive. Correction staff (from administrators to correction officers) often devalue or even resent the care the psychiatric nurse provides to the inmate. The inmate requesting mental health services is often viewed as enjoying an undeserved privilege or using manipulative behavior to seek drugs that will help make incarceration tolerable. The nurse is at the heart of this struggle, often needing to make difficult assessments both about inmates' needs and about the motivations behind individual requests for service. The psychiatric nurse, to work successfully in a forensic setting (Box 6–8),

BOX 6–8 Forensic Setting

Julia has been arrested for possession with intent to sell narcotics. She has recently used heroin and is fearful of detoxifying. Other prescribed medications include methadone maintenance and venlafaxine (Effexor), an antidepressant with a short half-life and withdrawal agitation. She informed the corrections officer that she would find a way to kill herself unless she could continue to receive the methadone and the Effexor. The nurse received a request to evaluate Julia the morning after she was incarcerated. At that time, she was irritable, impatient, sweating, and complaining of gastrointestinal distress. Her mood had become more labile than it had been at booking, and she was not amenable to being interviewed.

The nurse aborted the interview, ordered a toxicology screen, and contacted the practitioners who had been prescribing methadone and Effexor. It was established that Julia was truthful regarding her medication, and the nurse was then able to obtain medical orders for continued treatment during her incarceration. Julia was informed that she would receive her required medications and immediately contracted to remain safe from self-inflicted harm while incarcerated.

1. In what way would you have approached the same problem in a similar setting?
2. In another setting, would a different approach be more appropriate?
3. What personal issues might you want to be aware of (nurse's self-assessment) before assessing and intervening with (a) forensic clients or (b) clients with substance abuse problems in the community setting?

must come with a background in crisis intervention and apply "a creative approach using a humanist, nonjudgmental philosophy" (Reeder and Meldman 1991).

The advocacy role of nursing is tested in this setting; there is a need to educate and collaborate with correction staff while integrating the agenda of care with that of incarceration. The necessity of a psychiatric nursing presence in correctional facilities cannot be overemphasized. As with any underserved and vulnerable population, there is a humanistic mandate to provide access to care, and in this circumstance there is an accompanying imperative need that care providers have a high level of expertise, including the ability to engage in a process to determine which problems require intervention.

Forensic psychiatric mental health nurses often find roles outside the confines of the correctional institution. Examples of such roles are seen in nurses who act as investigators for medical examiners or coroners, clinical forensic nurses who collect evidence from victims, nurses who provide competency evaluations, those who provide therapy to criminal defendants in pretrial settings or to persons who have recently returned to the community from an incarcerated setting, and nurses who intervene after unexpected deaths to review evidence and care for survivors (Lynch 1993). Psychiatric nurses are also among the professionals working in publicly funded programs intended to divert persons with mental illness or substance dependence from being incarcerated for crimes considered to be related to one of these disorders. As the presence of the forensic psychiatric mental health nurse becomes more prevalent, there has been more exploration about the stress the nurse in this circumstance experiences. These nurses are likely to identify the lack of resources for forensic psychiatric clients in the community as the chief cause of burnout in this field of nursing (Coffey 1999).

Vignette

■ *Robert is a nurse who provides care to clients who are incarcerated at the county jail. It is his responsibility to respond to referrals made by corrections and nursing staff for inmates who present with symptoms of psychiatric disorder or who have reported on entry to the jail that they are currently taking a psychiatric medication. He is not a nurse practitioner, but jail protocols permit him to contact psychiatric providers for the inmate and accept orders for the continuation of medication. Robert also has access to standing orders that allow certain psychiatric medications to be dispensed as needed to inmates. Often the referrals he receives are for assessment of suicide risk in a newly incar-*

cerated individual. He performs a standard risk assessment and a mental status examination and also attempts to gather relevant psychosocial history if the inmate is cooperative.

The challenges of Robert's work include distinguishing inmates who adopt psychiatric symptoms as a means of being removed to more private housing within the jail from those who are in need of psychiatric intervention, recognizing drug-seeking behavior and substance withdrawal symptoms before problems arise, and dealing with conflict between the agendas of care and punishment that separate him from the corrections staff with whom he works.

Treatment goals might include the following:

■ Assess the psychiatric status of inmates who present with psychiatric symptoms or are at risk for self-harm, and enhance access to routine or emergency psychiatric services as needed.
■ Recommend appropriate placement within the facility to ensure the safety of inmates with psychiatric impairment and of those around them.
■ Maintain medications and stable psychiatric status for inmates who have a psychiatric history.

Private Practice Settings

The advent of managed mental health care, and the expansion of legal scope for advanced practice psychiatric mental health nurses in many states, has encouraged a subgroup of nurses to enter the arena of private community practice (Box 6–9). The setting for this entrepreneurial practice varies, depending on the interest of the nurse, community need, and the characteristics of the community and client population. As third-party payers and other clients become familiar with the services offered by advanced practice psychiatric mental health nurses, there is a growing appreciation for the flexible, all-encompassing, biopsychosocial approach the advanced practice nurse brings to community mental health care. This is not to imply that all insurers recognize advanced practice; a number of reimbursement barriers continue to exist (Safriet 1994). The psychiatric mental health nurse serves a varied population of clients in a general psychiatric practice using a broad array of approaches from family and individual psychotherapy to pharmacotherapy. Subspecialization is increasingly common, and some nurses choose to work with a specific population such as survivors of trauma, children with learning disorders, persons suffering from chronic mental illness, or those with both physical and psychiatric illnesses. Advanced practice nurses in the field of psychiatric mental

BOX 6–9   *Nursing Home and Private Practice Nursing Consultation*

Mr. Thomas is a 77-year-old man who has resided in a nursing care facility for 3 years after hip surgery following the death of his wife. He is pleasant and gregarious in spite of having had repeated health problems. His current diagnoses include congestive heart failure, transient ischemic attacks, adult-onset diabetes, and severe osteoarthritis. He is receiving medications for each of these disorders but is seen only quarterly by the general practitioner at the nursing home. Within the past 2 months he has become increasingly confused and has been belligerent at times toward staff and residents. He becomes especially disturbed at night, but the staff has also noticed a change in his level of functioning throughout the day. There is speculation that he is depressed because his grandson left for college 3 months ago. Until then, this grandson had visited Mr. Thomas every Sunday.

The psychiatric nurse practitioner was asked to meet with Mr. Thomas to assess his mental state and assess his presenting problems. Mr. Thomas appreciated the attention but became obstreperous when asked about the change in his behavior; however, he glowed when the topic of his grandson was broached. Review of the chart revealed the increased confusion, episodes of which were associated with loss of balance and visual disturbance. His blood glucose level was last checked 5 months previously when his medication was changed. Also, his arthritis medication has been changed and there has been no neurological evaluation in the past year. He has been complaining of physical discomfort more often since the medication change, and his sleep has been less consistent.

The nurse consultant's report recommended that Mr. Thomas receive a comprehensive physical assessment, including laboratory work-up and neurological examination. In the event of negative findings, the next step would be to try to engage Mr. Thomas in the available social activities at his resident community rather than immediately prescribing an antidepressant or antipsychotic medication. Mr. Thomas agreed to this plan.

1. In what way would you approach the same problem in a similar setting? Would your consult include recommendations for additional medication protocols?
2. Was the setting important to the decision-making process of the nurse?
3. What would be one concern for this client's future care? How could you address this concern?

---

health have also begun to form and administer privately run multidisciplinary agencies (Caverly 1996; Caverly and Talley 1997).

Vignette

■ Carolyn is a psychiatric nurse practitioner with prescriptive authority. She has a full-time private practice serving persons who have mild to moderate mental illness and who either are able to pay for services or are insured by the companies for which she is a preferred provider of psychiatric specialty care. She is thinking about discontinuing her relationship with the managed care organizations because she has concerns about the level of personal information they require her to provide regarding her clients. Her only reservation is that such a decision may result in the termination of long-standing relationships with clients because they would need to pay out-of-pocket for her services.

Discomfort with this ethical dilemma has led Carolyn to create a sliding fee scale and cultivate a clientele who prefer to pay independently for services. In addition to the clients who see her for therapy, she provides medication management for individuals who receive therapy from nonprescribing providers.

Carolyn works primarily in her own office, but one afternoon each week she sees clients at a local AIDS residence facility. She has developed expertise in providing both pharmacological and psychotherapeutic intervention to persons with AIDS. She also occasionally visits a nursing home to provide mental health assessment of residents who are exhibiting psychiatric symptoms.

Carolyn has a strong biopsychosocial background and conducts comprehensive assessments before she considers potential intervention strategies. She often orders laboratory or psychometric testing to ascertain the client's diagnosis and capacity to tolerate medication. She has a relationship established with two community laboratories and admitting privileges at the local psychiatric hospital. Since a large percentage of her practice consists of persons with both physical and mental health disorders, she has established consulting relationships with a family nurse practitioner and with an internist. She usually obtains preliminary laboratory results before sending clients to one of these consultants for follow-up on a health-related concern. Among the routine laboratory tests she requests are those for thyroid-stimulating hormone, blood cell count, electrolytes, and liver enzymes.

Treatment goals might include the following:

■ Evaluation and diagnosis of general psychiatric and mental health complaints.
■ Psychotherapeutic or pharmacological intervention to stabilize or resolve psychiatric symptoms.
■ Assistance to providers in planning and delivering care in a manner appropriate for the client.

Outpatient Chemical Dependency Treatment Facilities

The incidence of mental illness among those who are also substance abusing is greater than 50% by most estimates. Identification of the dual-diagnosed mentally ill chemical abuser has led to the development of treatment services to accommodate these clients in both the mental health and chemical dependency treatment settings (Box 6–10). However, because of different funding streams and treatment philosophies, there have often been significant gaps between the two systems. Psychiatric mental health nurses who have expertise in treatment of substance abuse have the ability to provide care and consultation that integrates the benefits of the two models.

Vignette

■ *Kathryn is a psychiatric nurse who has also worked at an inpatient psychiatric facility and a chemical detoxification center. She currently works for an outpatient chemical dependency program, providing individual case management, counseling, and group therapy to clients who are both chemically dependent and mentally ill. She assists other*

Box 6–10   Outpatient Chemical Dependency Treatment Setting

Roberta is a pregnant woman addicted to heroin who entered methadone treatment to decrease the risk to her unborn child. She is motivated to stay clean and sober. She is an adult survivor of incest and physical abuse; the pregnancy has brought these to the surface, causing significant depression. She currently has no housing and lives with her husband in single-room-occupancy hotels when they have money. He has a history of being physically abusive; Roberta is fearful he may harm her and the baby while she is pregnant, but she needs him to protect her on the streets and is ambivalent about leaving the relationship. She had an opportunity to stay at a women's shelter but chose not to leave her husband on the streets alone. She now regrets that decision.

The pregnancy is at month 7 and has been difficult. Roberta is fatigued and unable to sleep because of discomfort and inconsistent shelter. She has recurrent suicidal ideation but readily denies intention to hurt herself or her child. She has an earlier child, now 3 years old, who was taken by child protective services shortly after birth because of Roberta's heroin abuse during pregnancy. Her one focus now is on having a healthy baby and the opportunity to be a mother.

The nurse assessed Roberta's strengths and problem areas. Despite her motivation to be clean and sober, several circumstances threaten her ability to do so. Roberta exhibits symptoms of depression, but it is not clear whether these arise from psychiatric illness or situational factors. There is no concern that Roberta will volitionally harm herself or her baby, but her husband might. Priorities are identified as securing a stable place to live and arranging for consistent prenatal care. The nurse works with Roberta to develop a list of problems, identify means of approaching them, and look at available resources. Roberta is given the task of using a phone at the facility to call the organizations that may have services she needs.

Antidepressant medication is discussed, but, given the primacy of daily living needs, together they decide it is premature to consider medication before situational factors are addressed. Finally, the nurse confronts the issue of domestic violence. Roberta makes it clear that she has no intention of permitting her husband to hurt her while she is pregnant and that if he does she will immediately contact a women's shelter. She is given the shelter hotline number and encouraged to keep it where it will not be accessible to her husband. Plans are made for Roberta to enter the high-risk pregnancy program, to meet with her case manager twice a week, and to attend group sessions twice weekly as she feels physically able.

1. What are some of the ethical issues the nurse might encounter in this situation? Which one would you grapple with first?
2. Are there cultural contradictions or ethical questions you might have (self-assessment) for you to plan and implement the best care for this client?
3. What other concerns would you have for this client?
4. What might you plan with Roberta in the future if she were to stay involved with the health care system?

counselors when they have questions about the medications their clients take or about possible physical problems related to substance abuse. She does not have responsibility for medication dispensing or management; there are other nurses who work in a more traditional role dispensing methadone and naltrexone hydrochloride but have no counseling responsibilities. Kathryn sometimes works with probation officers or jail health personnel, and she has frequent contact with child protective services because she works with the mothers of small children. Occasionally she helps clients to find housing or to negotiate agreements with landlords to prevent eviction. Kathryn often finds herself in the position of enforcing the rules of the program, including termination of treatment when ongoing substance abuse is established through the use of drug testing.

Treatment goals might include the following:

■ Maintenance of sobriety.
■ Stabilization of psychiatric symptoms and appropriate use of psychiatric resources.
■ Stabilization of life style, including housing, family structure, and work or school.

Home Psychiatric Mental Health Care

Despite historical precedent, home health care (Box 6–11) is now considered an innovative treatment (Daudell-Strejc and Murphy 1995). Provision of community psychiatric nursing is closely linked to home health nursing, yet it has been rare for community psychiatric nurses to make home visits. Psychiatric nursing in the home has been viewed as a costly service and restricted to homebound, severely disabled clients. Clients who receive such care are usually elderly, physically impaired, or nonparticipators in traditional center-based community mental health care (Kimball and Williams-Burgess 1995). These individuals often have long-term severe mental problems as well as chronic physical problems (e.g., arthritis, diabetes). As community mental health agencies and bureaus become accountable for inpatient as well as outpatient costs of care, there is increased interest and willingness on the part of the organizations to provide this service as a means of reducing inpatient treatment days.

The mentally ill within the community are often vulnerable. They may lack family support, work skills, the ability to use public resources, and the

Box 6–11 *Home Health Care Setting*

Mrs. Avery is an 88-year-old woman who lives alone. She has recently had difficulty managing her diabetes, especially in taking her insulin appropriately. Her house is cluttered with stacks of old newspapers and there was a pan melted to the electric burner on the stove when the visiting nurse came for a regular visit. Apparently, Mrs. Avery's limited olfactory sensation prevented her smelling the enamel burning on the pan, but she refuses to take it seriously and won't agree to have someone stay at her home to assist her. Recently, she has called the police frequently to report crimes; when the police respond, they find no one in the vicinity and no evidence of damage. Mrs. Avery is hopeful the nurse consultant can help her rectify the problems with her neighbors by forcing them to move.

Mrs. Avery is alert and oriented. Her fund of knowledge is adequate and her thought processes are intact, although she is preoccupied with the perceived troubles her neighbors are causing. She shows no evidence of responding to internal stimuli, but she appears to have beliefs about her neighbors that are not reality-based and becomes angry when these are challenged. Her insight and judgment are poor.

When her health status is discussed, Mrs. Avery proudly displays her new blood glucose monitoring device, but she doesn't know how to use it. Her insulin dosing has been erratic. A quick look in Mrs. Avery's refrigerator reveals a quart of milk, a bunch of celery, and a box of sweet rolls.

Mrs. Avery agrees to have the nurse meet with her neighbors to discuss her complaints. She also agrees to have the nurse arrange for more in-home assistance with blood glucose monitoring and diet management. Mrs. Avery remains socially isolated with the exception of her contact with police and home health nurses. She agrees to meet someone from the local senior center, so long as the first meeting occurs with the home health nurse present. The assessment and plan are provided to the home health agency and to the general practitioner who care for Mrs. Avery.

1. What are the ethical implications of the nurse's behavior?
2. How was the setting important in the decision-making process with Mrs. Avery?
3. Would the educational level of the nurse affect the nursing assessment or interventions?

cognitive or affective capacity to cope with daily living. Murphy and colleagues (1995) found that clients believed that community-based care meant increased personal freedom, self-selection of diet, greater mobility, more self-management, fewer prescribed medications, and less pressure to interact with people.

A client's resistance to coming to a clinic for mental health care may be due to symptoms of psychiatric illness: the apathy or withdrawal of depression, the ambivalence or paranoid ideation associated with schizophrenia, or the anxiety related to agoraphobia. The downside of community-based care is the often difficult process of ensuring that those who need psychiatric services have access to them. Home mental health care improves the potential for many to receive treatment, but there will continue to be those who are reluctant to permit care providers into their homes (Sullivan and Cohen 1990). A practice of having family members (or neighbors) of clients who are homebound or reclusive accompany professionals when they visit the client increases the probability that the professional will be granted access to the client's home (Peternelji-Taylor and Hartley 1993). The environment in which a person chooses to live provides rich information about that person's culture, values, level of functioning, resources, and needs. Many aspects of assessment and intervention are facilitated through an outreach to the home. The realities with which an individual client must contend cannot be adequately appreciated when information is gleaned only through an interview at a mental health facility or an inpatient setting. The information obtained during a home visit can result in medication regimens being negotiated rather than merely ordered. Differential diagnoses are more easily made in the home because of the degree to which evidence of adaptive ability or dysfunction is present. For example, the depressed client's home may be organized but barren, whereas the organically impaired client's home may present random disorganization.

The concept of the professional as a guest in the home of the client requires nurses to rethink the manner in which the business of nursing is conducted. Bowers (1992) studied the community psychiatric nurse's interaction in a home visit and found it to be associated with a change in the dynamics of power and control. The client is firmly in charge, and the nurses must use nonauthoritarian strategies, such as persuasion and negotiation, to intervene. Matters directed by the professional in the office (e.g., where to sit, whether there is music or television) must be worked out with clients when in their homes. The nurse must acknowledge that "because [clients are] on home ground, [they lay] down the rules, decide upon actions, and direct the visit"

(Bowers 1992). Determining the areas in which it is appropriate to establish and exert oneself as the expert or to offer consultation and guidance is a skill nurses must develop.

Boundaries become important, albeit less clear, in the home setting, where there is inherently a greater degree of intimacy between nurse and client. It may be important for the psychiatric home health nurse to begin a visit by reinforcing or developing an informal relationship with the client. Efforts to accomplish this might include accepting refreshment offered by the client. This interaction can be a strain for the nurse who struggles to maintain distance and professional formality. However, there is great significance to the interaction that occurs during a home visit, and the therapeutic use of self in such a circumstance incorporates establishing connectedness, comfort, and emotional warmth through chatting about family issues or helping with small chores (e.g., mailing letters). The manner in which the nurse responds in a client's home is likely to be keenly observed and to have profound meaning to that individual or family, both positive and negative (Daudell-Strejc and Murphy 1995).

Vignette

■ *Linda provides consultation to the city's Visiting Nurse Service (VNS). She is a psychiatric clinical specialist with a subspecialization in geropsychiatry. The local VNS predominantly serves an elderly, homebound, physically compromised population. This includes both rural and urban clients, because the county is quite large and diverse. She may be asked to assess whether an elderly man is capable of remaining in his home after having threatened the building manager with a golf club, to evaluate an elderly woman's complaint of abuse by a home living attendant, or to determine the ability of a confused elderly woman to continue to live independently in her own home.*

The variety of her work is what appeals to Linda. She is sometimes able to establish ongoing relationships with clients; at other times, she provides consultation only intended to help home health care nurses and their assistants to deliver appropriate care. She does not prescribe medication but does recommend pharmacological interventions to general practitioners. In most cases, there is no other psychiatric practitioner involved in the client's care; her assessments and recommendations are accepted by both nursing and medical providers.

Treatment goals might include the following:

■ Assess the psychiatric and functional status of the client.

■ Determine the safety of the living situation.

■ Ascertain the need for additional resources or redistribution of existing resources.

■ Assess the need for, or response to, psychopharmacological intervention.

■ Implement or recommend a psychosocial treatment plan.

■ Enhance the client's ability to function independently and safely in the community setting.

ETHICAL ISSUES

As community psychiatric nurses assume greater autonomy and accountability for the care they deliver, ethical concerns become more of an issue. Ethical dilemmas are common in disciplines and specialties that care for the vulnerable and disenfranchised. Nurses who choose to become community psychiatric nurses have an obligation to develop a model for assessing the ethical implications of the clinical decisions required of them. In many cases, there is dissonance between what is best for the individual and what is in the best interest of the community or the general client milieu. State laws require reporting of some behaviors (e.g., child abuse), but often the information obtained from a client during psychiatric treatment is considered to be privileged. Psychiatric mental health nurses have an obligation to communicate clearly with clients about categories of information that fall beyond personal or professional understanding of privilege and that will not remain confidential. This standard is best communicated to the client before sensitive information is disclosed.

Each incident requiring ethical assessment is somewhat different, and the individual nurse brings personal insights to each situation. The role of the nurse is to act in the best interests of the client and of society, to the degree that this is possible. It is never acceptable for the nurse to seek self-gain from the relationship with a client, and there is most certainly an expectation of honesty in the relationship the nurse enters with the client. However, elements of justice, beneficence, and nonmaleficence are affected by the parameters of the nurse-client relationship and by the others who are a part of the equation. Ethical dilemmas arise in situations where there *is* no clear-cut ethical response. The nursing profession must find improved ways of supporting individual nurses as they struggle to find the best response to these difficult situations. Organized nursing has assisted in this process by addressing ethical dimensions in published practice standards and guidelines.

Ethical problems have been discussed in the literature, most often in relation to hospital settings. As psychiatric mental health nurses increasingly practice in independent home and community settings, important ethical concerns await identification and reflection. Forchuk (1991) identified and studied three ethical problem areas experienced by community psychiatric nurses: moral uncertainty, dilemma, and moral distress. Ethical issues identified by Forchuk include doing good, autonomy, maintaining client confidentiality, and avoiding deception. Community psychiatric mental health nurses indicated a belief in the client as decision maker, yet described an ownership for nursing actions.

The issue of social control and the associated role of community mental health professionals in maintaining social control represents an important and constant ethical conflict for community psychiatric mental health nurses. The mentally ill are cared for in the community so long as they are able to maintain social standards of acceptable behavior. The community funds public sector mental health care, and as such the community is the customer purchasing community mental health services. This is problematic for those who work in the public sector, because the desires of the community may not be consistent with the wishes of the individual client who is mentally ill. Like the public health model from which it has evolved, the health—or, in this case, the mental health and safety—of the community seems to supersede that of the individual. At the same time, community psychiatric mental health nurses are educated and socialized to care for individuals with mental illness. The power of the nurse in this dynamic process, and the often unacknowledged, secondary agenda of community safety cannot but affect the nature and experience of the relationship between the nurse and the client.

In the acute care setting the power differential inherent in psychiatric treatment is generally clear. In the community setting the nurse must consciously assess the effect of power and control on the long-term therapeutic relationship between nurse and client. Regulations have evolved to restrict the rights and privileges of those who suffer from mental illness. Each state has some version of an involuntary treatment act that permits professionals, sometimes community psychiatric nurses, to hospitalize and medicate persons against their will when sufficient grounds are evident. Key grounds for detention tend to be danger to self and to others (Whitley 1991). Refer to Chapter 8 for legal precedents. The following case presents a dilemma faced by the psychiatric nurse and shows one path that might be taken to resolve conflict. It is understood that, while the decision-making process may be explicit and consistent, the definition of ethical dilemma implies the lack of a clear right or wrong solution. Each nurse must weigh the issues and chart an action within an ethical frame of reference. It is important that the community psychiatric mental health nurse consider the impact of factors such as ethnicity, social status, and client gender and the impact of client behavior on significant others or the community (including involvement with the police) on the decision process when involuntary detention is at issue. Clark and Bowers (2000) have addressed these factors as they relate to social control and disenfranchisement, and have questioned the assumption that client psychiatric symptoms and behavioral dyscontrol are the primary drivers when an individual is compulsorily hospitalized.

Ethical Conflict

Vignette

■ *Sharon is a 34-year-old woman recently hospitalized after a suicide attempt. She has suffered from depression since the age of 14 and has experienced only rare, brief episodes of euthymic (normal) mood since that time. Sharon has been cooperative in taking antidepressant medications in spite of discomforts associated with side effects such as dry mouth, psychomotor stimulation, and blurred vision. Within the last year, she has been divorced, lost custody of her two young children, and become unemployed because she complained of workplace abuse.*

Sharon has recently been diagnosed with multiple sclerosis and has significant muscle weakness and pain attributed to this illness. The increased severity of Sharon's depressive symptoms, including fatigue and suicidal intent, are considered to be directly related to the prognosis of her physical illness. Her general practitioner has become frustrated because Sharon is failing to follow through on treatment recommendations and physical therapy. He is also uncomfortable with her refusal to commit to a contract not to harm herself (refer to Chapter 23 for setting up a no-suicide contract). He has begun to disengage, and Sharon describes feeling hurt by this in spite of understanding the practitioner's reasons.

As the primary mental health care provider for Sharon, the nurse feels an obligation to help Sharon clarify her own wishes for psychiatric treatment and to attempt to pursue mutually agreed-on treatment goals. This has become more difficult since Sharon expresses almost constant suicidal thoughts. Sharon has promised that she will not overdose on the medications she receives from the mental health clinic because she does not want the nurse to feel responsible for her death. She is clear, however, that she does intend to complete a successful suicide attempt at some undisclosed time.

Sharon's thoughts are clear, she has made arrangements for her children to receive her belongings and has written them loving letters. She has also compiled albums that include their preschool report cards and pictures of the children and their mother together. In spite of her refusal to contract to be safe, she gives no indication that she is in immediate danger. She directly states that she appreciates the mental health care she is receiving and values her relationship with the nurse but, frankly, does not wish to continue living. She asks that the nurse respect her decision.

The fact that Sharon is so clearly considering her death, has a realistic understanding of her life circumstance, and has made what she believes to be an informed decision causes the nurse to feel uncomfortable, assuming that Sharon's decision is an indication of psychiatric impairment. The mental health center standard is that when clients refuse to contract to be safe from self-harm they must be hospitalized. If the individual declines a voluntary admission, the court-appointed mental health professionals are asked to detain the person.

The nurse is aware that this is the treatment plan the agency expects her to pursue and realizes that a history of depression, with past suicide attempts plus current suicidal ideation, is adequate grounds for a request that Sharon be detained. However, she chooses not to take this approach because she believes that such action will further distance Sharon from care. Also, Sharon says she would find involuntary treatment dehumanizing and that it would exacerbate her wish to die; she indicates she would wait to be discharged and then complete her suicide plans. Given this knowledge, the nurse does not refer Sharon for an evaluation. She believes that she does not have the power to prevent Sharon from an ultimate decision to commit suicide but that perhaps Sharon can be helped to consider alternatives and to create a series of reasons to delay taking action, thus allowing her to benefit from individual, group, and pharmacological interventions in such a manner that might result in a decision to continue living.

Instead of seeking hospitalization for Sharon, the nurse increases the frequency of their appointments. She tries to reestablish a regular visitation schedule for Sharon and her children to strengthen Sharon's relationship with them and to intervene with Sharon's ex-husband to ensure his cooperation (if not understanding). In conversations about the children or about parental suicide, the nurse comments about the wonderful qualities possessed by Sharon's children and the emotional trauma known to occur when a child's parent commits suicide. She offers to assist with transportation to physical therapy and health care appointments. While doing these things, she is careful to be honest in communicating her motives to Sharon. She expresses both concern and caring when she does this and states that she personally values Sharon. At no time does the nurse promise not to seek involuntary psychiatric hospitalization; rather, she bases nursing actions, including commitment, on frequent assessment of imminent danger. She is also careful to evaluate for any indication that Sharon's desire to end her life is extended to the lives of her children and has clearly documented a plan for immediate intervention in the event of any indication that the lives or welfare of Sharon's children are at risk.

ETHNIC AND CULTURAL CONSIDERATIONS

Culture is a concept that transcends mere ethnic diversity; its definition can include, but is not limited to, such elements as ethnicity, race, nationality, region, language, class, sexual orientation, and gender. Obviously, culture can be of tremendous significance when nurse and client are from different backgrounds; thus, psychiatric nurses are in great need of cultural awareness regarding their own biases and beliefs as they embark on community practice. It is a basic requirement that nurses become comfortable working with individuals, families, and communities who have diverse life experiences and understandings. Refer to Chapter 7.

Community work frequently involves engagement with people who, because they are not acculturated, may have failed to secure services at a clinic or hospital. Migration and social change are considered the two primary stresses affecting the mental health of the world population (Lin 1986). Thus, it is not infrequent that immigrants suffer significant mental health disorders. Culturally sensitive and culturally competent assessment and intervention are necessary for effective mental health treatment, whether or not the practitioner is intimate with a given culture. The following case provides insight into ways culturally naive practitioners who have flexibility are able to seek out cultural brokers to assist in providing psychiatric care that is helpful to the client.

Cultural Context

Vignette

■ *Sara is a community psychiatric nurse who works as a liaison practitioner with the local refugee clinic. She is experienced working with interpreters and is comfortable*

with clients from other cultures. Sara has requested an interpreter for her first appointment with an Eritrean client who is new to the clinic. She has no specific knowledge of Eritrea. The only available interpreter is Ethiopian. Unfortunately, Sara is not aware that there is significant struggle between the two African nations and that animosity also exists between their nationals who are living in the United States. Worse, the Eritrean people generally distrust the Ethiopians.

As the interview progresses, it becomes clear that the interpreter is unable to develop a relationship with the client. Either the client appears not to comprehend the questions or the answers are curt. Tension mounts in the room. Finally, the interpreter tells Sara that the situation is untenable. The interpreter is not interested in further victimizing the client by forcing him to reveal inadequacies to someone he perceives to be an enemy.

Sara is grateful for the information, which helps her understand why this interview was unproductive and the context for the client's presenting problems. She terminates the session, rescheduling at a time a non-Ethiopian interpreter will be available.

Treatment goals might include the following:

■ Use the interpreter as a cultural broker to learn about the Eritrean culture.
■ Assess presenting psychiatric symptoms in the context of the client's culture.
■ Plan intervention strategies that fit the client's cultural context.
■ Use culturally relevant or available resources in implementing mental health care.

To be effective, the nurse must understand the client's culturally acceptable ways to resolve dysfunction. Kagawa-Singer and Chung (1994) suggested that therapists must do more than just "know the client's culture." The culture of the individual prescribes and defines not only what constitutes the healthy self but also the intrapersonal and interpersonal ways in which the person achieves and maintains integrity and self-worth.

There are no cultural universals—each member of a culture has a personal interpretation of the cultural experience. Presumption of culturally appropriate care on the basis of stereotypes is never acceptable practice. Expression of disease varies with cultural identity and experience (Tabora and Flaskerud 1994). Psychiatric mental health nurses are accountable for understanding how the symptoms of an illness are expressed culturally and, conversely, what the meaning of a symptom is within the context of culture (Westermeyer 1985).

Interventions at a community level also need to be culturally competent; it is important that the intervention not be implemented using a template based on the dominant culture (Marin 1993). Sensitivity to clients includes consideration of their cultural values as well as an understanding of their culture's attitudes toward the identified needs and expected outcomes. Community interventions are most successful when approached from a collaborative, mutually respectful model.

Physiological and somatic differences between racial and ethnic groups are important considerations for those who prescribe or manage somatic therapies. Medications are prescribed in all cultures, but there are important differences in effective dosage levels and the potential for unwanted side effects (Lin 1986). In some instances, it is important to target physical rather than affective symptoms when recommending medications. For example, a woman may come to a clinic believing that the pain in her stomach and head is the problem; once domestic violence is ruled out, psychiatric and physical assessments suggest a diagnosis of posttraumatic stress disorder with depression and somatic symptoms. The pharmacotherapeutic intervention of choice is an antidepressant medication. However, if the woman must first accept depression as her primary problem, she may either decline treatment or accept medication but fail to take it; it also becomes more likely that she will fail to return for future care. A more effective approach might be to offer medication that will help with the stomach pains and headache. The name of the drug, the side effects, and the benefits can be addressed in a routine fashion; the diagnosis of depression is downplayed. Treatment is then acceptable to the client, and both the physical symptoms and the psychiatric disorder improve.

THE CHANGING HEALTH CARE ENVIRONMENT

Community psychiatric nursing, like all the health care professions, will be affected by the changing health care environment. Health care spending has continued to grow, and some predict that it will reach 32% of the U.S. gross domestic product in the year 2030. Health care purchasers (both private and public) press for revisions in health insurance that will compress costs associated with new and expensive technology, an aging population, and inefficient

use and distribution of health care resources. Managed care as a way to distribute financial and health care resources favors outpatient services and a focus on prevention and wellness, rather than inpatient care (McLaughlin 1994). Policymakers demand greater proof of the effectiveness of a health care service before funding programs, yet are often isolated from the direct provision of mental health care, thus reinforcing fiscal aspects of mental health reforms to the possible detriment of the human aspects (Mechanic 1993, 1994).

Managed Care

The changing health care environment is a product of a number of forces: the globalization of our economy; the lack of state and local control in setting up many of the federally subsidized programs (e.g., Medicare and Medicaid) and the pressure on them to provide more care to the severely mentally ill; the efforts of the National Institute of Mental Health to direct its research focus toward biological understandings of mental illness; and a current mandate to focus once more on prevention. The National Alliance for the Mentally Ill emerged in the 1980s as a powerful voice for the mentally ill at state, local, and federal levels.

Within the health care delivery system, the array of health care provider disciplines has broadened. Health care management, through utilization reviews, put forth the concept that appropriate care is given in the appropriate setting by the appropriate provider. Geographical distribution of the health care workforce is changing the overall nature of the health care delivery system (McLaughlin 1994; Safriet 1994). Racial and ethnic minority groups are still under-represented among health care providers; given the growing U.S. minority population, schools of nursing must grapple with the need to increase student and faculty diversity.

Previously, cost was driven by treatment decisions determined by the health care providers, who were paid directly by the insurance company or government program (e.g., Medicare, Medicaid) for the care or service provided to the client. The insurance company in turn approached the employers, who purchased the insurance for their employees.

The current health care environment embraces a managed care approach in which services are determined, provided, and monitored by a network of providers who are part of a health care company. Managed care companies define practice guidelines that frame the limits of services for which health care providers can receive reimbursement, and even dictate which medications will be provided for the client. Health care providers become just one part of the treatment triangle (client, provider, insurer) yet retain the responsibility for achieving good treatment outcomes in a cost-effective, timely manner. Currently, there are a multitude of community psychiatric nursing opportunities and not nearly an adequate supply of nurses prepared to meet the challenges inherent in this dynamic environment.

Future Models

Future models of psychiatric mental health care suggest a separation between mental illness and mental health care. Mental illness will be addressed under the category of neurological disorders, along with Parkinson's disease, strokes, and schizophrenia. This new model encompasses a brain disease concept, with care being conceptualized and delivered on a neurological continuum that incorporates concepts of chronicity, persistence, and severity. Separating mental health and mental illness places diseases such as schizophrenia, bipolar disorder, and obsessive-compulsive disorder with other neurological diseases such as Parkinson's disease and multiple sclerosis. This model supports arguments for insurance parity for psychiatric disorders.

Mental health prevention and treatment will be designated social services; psychotherapy; stress management; preventive mental health care; and family, child, and adolescent behavioral and marital therapy delivered by persons working in social services. Psychiatric mental health nurses will be educated in either social services or neurological treatment. Psychiatric mental health service delivery will focus on the social networks necessary to support the level of function a client is capable of achieving.

Nurses at every level will have a larger role to play as this new model unfolds. There may be greater necessity for subspecialization in the area of brain disorders and somatic interventions or psychotherapy modalities. Nursing has enjoyed a long history of caring for the client in the home; with the shift to community-based care and home health care, the nurse is in an obvious position to play a crucial role (Mellon 1994). However, as nurses increase their presence in the field in general, and in home health care in particular, they need to become increasingly progressive, autonomous, and active in designing their role in the delivery of home health care (Bunn 1995; Worley 1995).

Interdisciplinary teams, as we know them today, may not exist in years to come because there will be no strict disciplines to define teams. All health care provider education may begin with a single core curriculum; the focus will be on outcome competencies rather than on degrees. Problem-based learning outlines a new approach to health care professional education that organizes curricula around problems, not disciplines; integrates theory and clinical learning; and emphasizes critical thinking skills as well as basic knowledge. Future professionals will be required to skillfully adapt to change, reason critically, and treat holistically in an integrated approach to health care (Bruhn 1992).

To meet the challenge of the 21st century, Price and Capers (1995) suggested that for the associate degree nurse "educators must increase their focus on leadership development, include principles of home health nursing, increase content on gerontology, and introduce basic community health concepts". Those nurses who elect to work with geropsychiatric clients will be more and more in demand as the population ages and the health care needs of the geropsychiatric clients are increasingly complex (Hedelin and Svensson, 1999). Primary care geriatric practitioners and general psychiatric practitioners and home care providers will likely rely heavily on community psychiatric mental health nurses with this subspecialty. Those who use community psychiatric mental health nursing services and those who care for them (both family caregivers and non-nursing professionals) are increasing expressing interest in having voice with regard to the education of nurses who will work in community psychiatric mental health settings. Nurses are pressed to consider partnerships with professional and nonprofessional providers of services to the mental health client as well as individual and organizations of community psychiatric mental health clients (Forrest et al. 2000). A relatively new role for the community psychiatric mental health nurse may be that of a consultant to the primary health care practitioners who fill the gap in existing community mental health services (Walker et al. 2000). Bunn (1995) stated that "the emphasis on community-based mental health care will require not only a paradigm shift in the way educators and practicing nurses think but also result in a role transformation for nurses". Knowledge, skill, and increased role presence of all health professionals will be necessary as we enter the 21st century.

SUMMARY

The community psychiatric mental health nurse has a history of home health nursing that dates back to the 1800s, when trained nurses visited homes in both urban and rural communities. A revolution in community mental health occurred after World War II and was in great part due to the combined effect of new psychotropic medications, a raised level of awareness and conscience about the conditions of institutions, and the normalization of mental health problems (as the armed services rejected or traumatized a great number of men). In response, mental health treatment began to shift to the community setting.

Community psychiatric mental health nurses have become service brokers for clients. In the community, clients direct their own lives, and thus treatment is a negotiated process. The nurse acts as a consultant to the client and the client's extended social support network.

The characteristics of treatment goals and intervention strategies within the community setting are consistent with hospital-based mental health nursing, except that a great deal more flexibility may be called for, as well as a constant demand for creative problem-solving skills. Nurses must demonstrate a number of personal attributes, such as an awareness of self as a therapeutic agent; flexible, creative problem-solving ability; calm presentation under stress; and the requisite knowledge and skills appropriate to the position. Community practice opportunities are varied, limited only by creativity, resources, the needs of the client population, the geography, and the community.

As mental health treatment becomes increasingly standardized, psychotropic medication is better understood to be an effective treatment. In the era of managed care, treatment has shifted to the community and into the homes of those afflicted with psychiatric mental health disorders. It is predicted that psychiatric mental health nurses will become increasingly visible and viable as the emphasis in mental health treatment embraces the full biopsychosocial spectrum of disorders. The necessity for the psychiatric nursing profession to practice comfortably in neighborhood settings and community treatment agencies is becoming critical as health care resources become more limited. Entering the home of a client as a visitor/guest/clinician requires conscious preparation and ongoing reflection on the part of the community psychiatric mental health nurse. Treatment can be expected to incorporate innovative interventions, new psychotropic medications, the application of communication technology, and assertive outreach treatment modalities. Psychiatric mental health nursing beyond the confines of the hospital represents a tremendous challenge and an extraordinary opportunity for the discipline and specialty. The capacity to adapt and assume a flexible approach to the role plus a commitment to delivering appropriate and relevant care to clients will permit nurses without community expertise to assume and develop new psychiatric mental health nursing roles for the 21st century.

Visit the **Evolve** website at
http://evolve.elsevier.com/Varcarolis
for a post-test on the content in this chapter.

Visit the **Evolve** website at
http://evolve.elsevier.com/Varcarolis
for additional self-study exercises.

Critical Thinking and Chapter Review

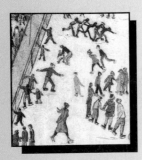

Critical Thinking

1. You are a community psychiatric mental health nurse working at a local mental health center. You have been assigned a male client new to the agency and find that there are a multitude of factors affecting his life. You are not certain that you have enough information to accurately diagnose his psychiatric condition but are aware that he has significant distress. He reports that he has not been sleeping and that his thoughts seem to be "all tangled up." He informs you that he is hoping you will help him today because he doesn't know how much longer he can go on feeling the way he does. He does not make any direct reference to suicidal intent. He is disheveled and has been

either staying at the local shelter or sleeping outside. He has little interaction with his family and he starts to become agitated when you suggest that it might be helpful for you to contact them. He has not agreed to sign any release of information forms but does report recent inpatient psychiatric care at the local Veterans Hospital, reasons for this treatment remaining vague. You recognize one of the facilities at which he received treatment as a dual-diagnosis program, yet he vehemently denies any history of drug or alcohol abuse. In addition to his mental health problems, he is undergoing treatment for HIV infection and is on antiviral medications he cannot remember the names of.

■ What are your immediate concerns as you assess this client?
■ What do you believe to be essential information you need to care for this client?
■ How might you proceed to gather necessary information, and also develop a relationship with the client?
■ What systems do you need to include in the treatment planning for this client, how would you initiate necessary collaboration?
■ What services do you find to be essential that your agency provide for this client? Are any of these services needed immediately or in an emergency basis?
■ Do you feel you need to obtain consultation from any other staff at your agency before proceeding or having the client leave the office? If so, who do you need to consult with, and for what purpose?
■ Do any ethical dilemmas present for you in this situation as described?
■ Would you approach this client differently if he were deaf, non-English speaking, wheel-chair bound?
■ Do you believe you would provide differential services depending on ethnicity, race, age or gender?

Chapter Review

Choose the most appropriate answer.

1. A significant influence allowing for psychiatric treatment to move from hospital to community was

    1. Television.
    2. The discovery of psychotropic medication.
    3. Identification of external causes of mental illness.
    4. The use of a collaborative approach by clients and staff focusing on rehabilitation.

2. For psychiatric nurses a major difference between caring for clients in the community and caring for clients in the hospital is

    1. Negotiating treatment versus imposing treatment.
    2. Encountering fewer ethical dilemmas in the community setting.
    3. The lesser importance of cultural considerations during treatment in the community.
    4. The focus in the community setting is solely on managing symptoms of mental illness.

3. A typical treatment goal for a client with mental illness being treated in a community setting is that the client will

    1. Experience destabilization of symptoms.
    2. Demonstrate optimal level of independent functioning.
    3. Learn to live with dependency and decreased opportunities.
    4. Accept guidance and structure of significant others.

4. Assessment data that would be considered least relevant to developing an understanding of a persistently mentally ill 65-year-old client's ability to cope with the demands of living in the community are

1. Strengths and deficits of the client.
2. School and vocational performance.
3. Client health history and current mental status.
4. Client home environment and financial status.

5. Which action on the part of a community psychiatric nurse visiting the home of a client would be considered inappropriate?

1. Turning off an intrusive TV program without client permission.
2. Facilitating client access to a community kitchen for two meals a day.
3. Going beyond professional role boundary to hang curtains for an elderly client.
4. Arranging to demonstrate use of public transportation to a mental health clinic.

REFERENCES

American Nurses Association (2000). *A statement on psychiatric–mental health clinical nursing practice and standards of psychiatric–mental health clinical nursing practice.* Washington, D.C.: American Nurses Publishing.

American Psychiatric Association. (2000). *Diagnostic and Statistical Manual of Mental Disorders* (4th ed., text revision). Washington, D.C.: Author.

Bachrach, L. L. (1994). The chronic patient: The Carter Commission's contributions to mental health service planning. *Hospital and Community Psychiatry,* 45(6):527–528, 543.

Barr, W. (2000). Characteristics of severely mentally ill patients in and out of contact with community mental health services. *Journal of Advanced Nursing,* 31(5):1189–1198.

Bawden, E. L. (1990). Reaching out to the chronically mentally ill homeless. *Journal of Psychosocial Nursing,* 28(3):9–13.

Bowers, L. (1992). Ethnomethodology: II. A study of the community psychiatric nurse in the patient's home. *International Journal of Nursing Studies,* 29(1):69–79.

Broskowski, A., and Eaddy, M. (1994). Community mental health centers in a managed care environment. *Administration and Policy in Mental Health,* 21(4):335–351.

Bruhn, J. G. (1992). Problem-based learning: An approach toward reforming allied health education. *Journal of Allied Health,* 2(3):161–173.

Bunn, H. (1995). Preparing nurses for the challenge of the new focus on community mental health nursing. *Journal of Continuing Education in Nursing,* 26(2):55–59.

Callahan, D. (1994). Setting mental health priorities: Problems and possibilities. *Milbank Quarterly,* 72(3):451–470.

Carson, W. (1993). Prescriptive practice in the 1990s: A crazy quilt of overregulation. Unpublished manuscript. Washington, D.C.: Nurse Practice Council, American Nurses Association.

Caverly, S. (1991). Coordinating psychosocial nursing care across treatment settings. *Journal of Psychosocial Nursing and Mental Health Services,* 29(8):26–29.

Caverly, S. (1996). The role of the psychiatric nurse practitioner. *Nursing Clinics of North America,* 31(3):449–463.

Caverly, S., and Talley, S. (1997). Roles and functions of psychiatric nurses in the community. In N. K. Worley (Ed.), *Mental health nursing in the community.* St. Louis: Mosby–Year Book.

Chamberlain, J. G. (1987). Update on psychiatric–mental health nursing education at the federal level. *Archives of Psychiatric Nursing,* 1(2):132–138.

Chan, S., Mackenzie, A., and Jacobs, P. (2000a). Cost-effectiveness analysis of case management versus a routine community care

organization for patients with chronic schizophrenia. *Archives of Psychiatric Nursing,* 14(2):98–104.

Chan, S., Mackenzie, A., Tin-Fu, D., and Leung, J. K. (2000b). An evaluation of the implementation of case management in the community psychiatric nursing service. *Journal of Advanced Nursing,* 31(1):144–156.

Clark, N., and Bowers, L. (2000). Psychiatric nursing and compulsory psychiatric care. *Journal of Advanced Nursing,* 31(2):389–394.

Coffey, M. (1999). Stress and burnout in forensic community mental health nurses: An investigation of its causes and effects. *Journal of Psychiatric and Mental Health Nursing,* 6(6):433–443.

Crosby, R. L. (1987). Community care of the chronically mentally ill. *Journal of Psychosocial Nursing,* 25(1):33–37.

Daudell-Strejc, D., and Murphy, C. (1995). Emerging clinical issues in home health psychiatric nursing. *Home Healthcare Nurse,* 13(2):17–21.

Farmer, S. (1987). Medical problems of chronic patients in a community support program. *Hospital and Community Psychiatry,* 38:745–749.

First, R. J., Wheeler, D. P., Belcher, J. R., and Johnson, D. (1995). Redefining the health care needs of persons who are homeless and mentally ill: Implications for diagnosis and treatment. *Journal of Applied Social Sciences,* 19(1):1–9.

Forchuk, C. (1991). Ethical problems encountered by mental health nurses. *Issues in Mental Health Nursing,* 12:375–383.

Forrest, S., Risk, I., Masters, H., and Brown, N. (2000). Mental health service user involvement in nurse education: Exploring the issues. *Journal of Psychiatric and Mental Health Nursing,* 7(1):51–57.

Francis, P., Merwin, E., and Fox, J. (1995). Relationship of clinical case management to hospitalization and service delivery for seriously mentally ill clients. *Issues in Mental Health Nursing,* 16:257–274.

Harris, D. M., and Happell, B. (1999). Hospital-based psychiatric experience before community-based practice for nurses: Imperative or dispensable? *Issues in Mental Health Nursing,* 20(5):495–503.

Hedelin, B., and Svensson, P. (1999). Psychiatric nursing for promotion of mental health and prevention of depression in the elderly: A case study. *Journal of Psychiatric and Mental Health Nursing,* 6(2):115–124.

Huch, M. H. (1995). Nursing and the next millennium. *Nursing Science Quarterly,* 8(1):38–44.

Kagawa-Singer, M., and Chung, R. C. (1994). A paradigm for culturally based care in ethnic minority populations. *Journal of Community Psychology,* 22:192–208.

Kimball, M. J., and Williams-Burgess, C. (1995). Failure to thrive: The silent epidemic of the elderly. *Archives of Psychiatric Nursing,* 9(2):99–105.

Krauss, J. B. (1993). Health care reform: Essential mental health services. Washington, D.C.: American Nurses' Association.

Lin, T. Y. (1986). Multiculturalism and Canadian psychiatry: Opportunities and challenges. *Canadian Journal of Psychiatry*, 31(7): 681–690.

Lynch, V. A. (1993). Forensic nursing: Diversity in education and practice. *Journal of Psychosocial Nursing and Mental Health Services*, 31(11):7–14.

Marcos, L. R. (1990). The politics of deinstitutionalization. In N. L. Cohen (Ed.), *Psychiatry takes to the streets: Outreach and crisis intervention for the mentally ill* (pp. 3–15). New York: Guilford Press.

Marin, G. (1993). Defining culturally appropriate community interventions: Hispanics as a case study. *Journal of Community Psychology*, 21:149–161.

Marland, G. R., and Sharkey, V. (1999). Depot neuroleptics, schizophrenia, and the role of the nurse: Is practice evidence based? A review of the literature. *Journal of Advanced Nursing*, 30(6):1255–1262.

McEvoy, P. (1999). Drawing the line: Gatekeeping access to the community mental health team. *Mental Health Care*, 2(8):266–269.

McLaughlin, C. J. (1994). Health workforce issues and policymaking roles. In P. F. Larson, et al. (Eds.), *Health workforce issues for the 21st century* (pp. 1–22). Washington, D.C.: Association of Academic Health Centers.

Mechanic, D. (1993). Mental health services in the context of health insurance reform. *Milbank Quarterly*, 71(3):349–364.

Mechanic, D. (1994). Establishing mental health priorities. *Milbank Quarterly*, 71(3):501–514.

Mellon, S. K. (1994). Mental health clinical nurse specialist in home care for the 90s. *Issues in Mental Health Nursing*, 15:229–237.

Meyer, T. J., Van Kooten, D., Marsh, S., and Prochazka, A. V. (1991). Reduction of polypharmacy by feedback to clinicians. *Journal of General Internal Medicine*, 6(2):133–136.

Mowbray, C. T., Cohen, E., and Bybee, D. (1993). The challenge of outcome evaluation in homeless services: Engagement as an intermediate outcome measure. *Evaluation and Program Planning*, 16:337–346.

Murphy, L. N., Gass-Sternas, K., and Knight, K. (1995). Health of the chronically mentally ill who rejoin the community: A community assessment. *Issues in Mental Health Nursing*, 16:239–256.

Murray, R., et al. (1995). Components of an effective transitional residential program for homeless mentally ill clients. *Archives of Psychiatric Nursing*, 9(3):152–157.

Olson, D. P. (1994). The ethical considerations of managed care in mental health treatment. *Journal of Psychosocial Nursing and Mental Health Services*, 32(3):25–32.

Omori, D. M., Potyk, R. P., and Kroenke, K. (1991). The adverse effects of hospitalization on drug regimens. *Archives of Internal Medicine*, 151:1562–1564.

Osborne, O. H., and Thomas, M. D. (1991). On public sector psychosocial nursing: A conceptual framework. *Journal of Psychosocial Nursing and Mental Health Services*, 29(8):13–18.

Peplau, H. E. (1989). Future directions in psychiatric nursing from the perspective of history. *Journal of Psychosocial Nursing and Mental Health Services*, 27(2):18–28.

Peternelji-Taylor, C. A., and Hartley, V. L. (1993). Living with mental illness: Professional/family collaboration. *Journal of Psychosocial Nursing and Mental Health Services*, 31(3):23–28.

Power, J. (1991). Expanding the role of community mental health nurses. *Canadian Nurse*, 5:20–21.

Price, C. R., and Capers, E. S. (1995). Associate degree nursing education: Challenging premonitions with resourcefulness. *Nursing Forum*, 30(4):26–29.

Primm, A. B., and Houck, J. (1990). COSTAR: Flexibility in urban community mental health. In N. L. Cohen (Ed.), *Psychiatry takes to the streets: Outreach and crisis intervention for the mentally ill* (pp. 107–120). New York: Guilford Press.

Reeder, D., and Meldman, L. (1991). Conceptualizing psychosocial nursing in the jail setting. *Journal of Psychosocial Nursing and Mental Health Services*, 29(8):40–44.

Regier, D. A., et al. (1993). The de facto U.S. mental and addictive disorders service system. *Archives of General Psychiatry*, 50:85–94.

Rochefort, D. A. (1993). From poorhouses to homelessness: Policy analysis and mental health care. Westport, Connecticut: Auburn House.

Safriet, B. J. (1994). Impediments to progress in health care workforce policy: License and practice laws. *Inquiry*, 31:310–317.

Scales, C. J., Mitchell, J. L., and Smith, R. D. (1993). Survey report on forensic nursing. *Journal of Psychosocial Nursing*, 31(11):39–44.

Simpson, A. (1999). Creating alliances: The views of users and careers on the education and training needs of community mental health nurses. *Journal of Psychiatric and Mental Health Nursing*, 6(5):347–356.

Smith, C. M. (1995). Origins and future of community health nursing. In C. M. Smith and F. A. Maurer (Eds.), *Community health nursing: Theory and practice* (pp. 30–52). Philadelphia: W. B. Saunders.

Sullivan, A. M., and Cohen, N. L. (1990). The home visit and the chronically mentally ill. In N. L. Cohen (Ed.), *Psychiatry takes to the streets: Outreach and crisis intervention for the mentally ill* (pp. 42–60). New York: Guilford Press.

Tabora, B., and Flaskerud, J. H. (1994). Depression among Chinese Americans: A review of the literature. *Issues in Mental Health Nursing*, 15:569–584.

Talbott, J. A. (Ed.). (1981). *The chronic mentally ill*. New York: Human Sciences Press.

Talley, S. (1988). Basic health care needs of the mentally ill: Issues for psychiatric nursing. *Issues in Psychiatric Nursing*, 9:409–423.

Talley, S., and Brooke, P. S. (1992). Prescriptive authority for psychiatric clinical specialists: Framing the issues. *Archives of Psychiatric Nursing*, 6(2):71–82.

Talley, S., and Caverly, S. (1994). Advanced-practice psychiatric nursing and health care reform. *Hospital and Community Psychiatry*, 45(6):545–547.

Walker, L., Barker, P., and Pearson, P. (2000). The required role of the psychiatric–mental health nurse in primary health care: An augmented Delphi study. *Nursing Inquiry*, 7(2):91–102.

Westermeyer, J. (1985). Psychiatric diagnosis across cultural boundaries. *American Journal of Psychiatry*, 142:798–805.

Whitley, M. P. (1991). Treatment dilemma: A political science perspective. *Journal of Psychosocial Nursing*, 29(8):35–39.

Wilson, K., and Williams, A. (2000). Visualism in community nursing: Implications for telephone work with service users. *Qualitative Health Research*, 10(4):507–520.

Worley, N. K. (1995). Community psychiatric nursing care. In G. W. Stuart and S. J. Sundeen (Eds.), *Principles and practice of psychiatric nursing* (5th ed.) (pp. 831–849). St. Louis: Mosby-Year Book.

Visit the **Evolve** website at
http://evolve.elsevier.com/Varcarolis
for a pre-test on the content in this chapter.

Outline

**RELEVANCE OF CULTURE IN
PSYCHIATRIC NURSING**

**INDEPENDENT AND
INTERDEPENDENT WORLD VIEWS**

The Self and Culture

**CULTURE AS A MULTIDIMENSIONAL
AND DYNAMIC PROCESS**

World View

Explanatory Models of Disease and
Mental Illness

Nursing Implications

Political and Economic Factors

Nursing Implications

Practice or Behavioral Dimension

Idioms of Distress

Help Seeking and Healing Options

Nursing Implications

**CULTURALLY COMPETENT
PSYCHIATRIC NURSING PRACTICE**

Cultural Competence

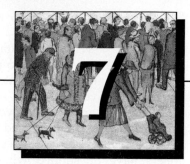

7

Culturally Relevant Mental Health Nursing

DENISE SAINT ARNAULT

Key Terms and Concepts

The key terms and concepts listed here also appear in color where they are defined or first discussed in this chapter.

cultural competence

cultural ideology

cultural translator

culture broker

environmental causes of
  illness

ethnocentrism

ethnorelativism

explanatory models

harmony

idioms of distress

imbalance

independent world view

interdependent world view

political-economic aspects
  of culture

spiritual causes of illness

world view

Objectives

After studying this chapter, the reader will be able to

1. Analyze the relationship between dominant American cultural values and Western psychological theory and practice.

2. Compare and contrast conceptions of the self within the Interdependent and Independent world views.

3. Evaluate the psychiatric nursing implications of using culture in planning care.

4. Apply the concepts of culture to psychiatric mental health nursing assessment and practice.

*P*sychiatric mental health nurses are often required to provide skilled assessment and intervention for people very different from themselves. Standard practice around the world has been to use psychological theories derived from the Western tradition. However, for decades, non-Western practitioners have questioned whether Western theories can be applied universally. As the people of non-Western nations have increased their access to advanced education and high technology, they are also not as likely to accept Western thinking as authoritative, choosing instead to work from their own models of understanding the world and the human condition. These views can differ substantially from those of Eastern psychological theories about the nature of self and mental illness.

The challenge to contemporary Western psychiatric nurses is to recognize that our theories and methods are themselves part of a cultural tradition. Only in doing so can we then appreciate the vast differences among the world's peoples and evaluate how these differences can profoundly affect our assessment of psychiatric nursing phenomena (e.g., family functioning, experience of and expression of feelings, and behavioral modes). In addition, we must begin to develop theories of mental health that incorporate a variety of world views and traditions.

This chapter offers a brief sketch of Western and non-Western conceptions of the self, conceptualizing the self as the place where societal norms and expectations become internalized, acted on, and evaluated. Next, it explores a dynamic cultural framework that allows analysis of people with regard to the cultural aspects of their health beliefs and behaviors as a starting point for cross-cultural analysis of mental health. Finally, it suggests some assessment and intervention strategies that arise from these cross-cultural understandings.

RELEVANCE OF CULTURE IN PSYCHIATRIC NURSING

For the last two decades, medical and nurse anthropologists and critical feminist nursing scholars have examined the relationship between the white, English-speaking, middle class that dominates American society and the rest of the diverse U.S. population (Barbee 1992; Singer 1986; Singer et al. 1992). While there is considerable debate about whether we can even speak about a single culture when referring to such a multicultural mix of peoples, many scholars agree that there is an American culture and that this culture has its roots in Western tradition (Fiske et al. 1998; Sahlins 1996). This culture, with its beliefs and traditions, enjoys a dominant status in the United States, and is reflected in the primary use of English, the predominance of Christianity, and the reinforcement of its ideals in every person's daily life. Values and practices are upheld within the legal, educational, and medical systems of the United States. Within American nursing, there has also been growing concern regarding how expectations about and differences among customs, languages, and traditions might affect the usefulness or relevance of the care provided. The assumption that one's own beliefs and practices are the best, preferred, or only way of being is referred to as ethnocentrism. Ethnocentrism causes barriers to access for minorities, and also prevents nurses from assessing and appreciating diversity and variety in health-related beliefs and practices.

Many attempts have been made within nursing and other health care professions to catalog the infinite varieties of understandings and traditions held by the peoples whom nurses may encounter in the health care settings (Andrews and Boyle 1999; Dienemann 1997; Geissler 1994; Giger and Davidhizar 1995; Kavanaugh 1995; Kleinman 1988; Koenig 1998; Lefley 1999; Leighton 1998; Lewis-Fernandez and Kleinman 1995; MacLachlan 1997; Mezzich et al. 1996, 1999; Okasha 1999; Pierce et al. 1999; Spector 1996, 2000). Unfortunately, cultural handbooks have tended to ignore intracultural differences. Handbooks may perpetuate stereotyping groups who may have vast differences in language, social status, gender, religion, involvement with technology, ethnicity, migration trajectory, and a host of other variables that shape health beliefs and behaviors. Second, cultural handbooks tend to continue the perception that non–Euro-Americans are different, strange, exotic, and difficult to understand. Many handbooks have given less emphasis to how *all* persons are part of some culture and that all cultural processes include beliefs, expectations, and power dynamics. Understanding the universality of cultural processes allows nurses to recognize their own culture as well as that of others. In addition, nurses can recognize the beliefs, values, and power that are part of their subculture of nursing. This new awareness can change the nurse-client encounter so that it is one of equal power, in which each party is attempting to understand the other. Indeed, each party, the nurse and the client, must clearly verbalize his or her expectations and ideals. Finally, the handbook approach to culture may mask the processes in which nursing is part of the larger culture of the health care system and science. These social institutions have beliefs about health and social norms that can exclude or silence nondominant groups (Table 7–1). Evidence of these barriers is exemplified in the small numbers of nondominant groups' access to and use of health care except in emergencies.

In the fields of cultural psychology, anthropology, and transcultural nursing, scholars have called into question the relevance of psychological theories derived from Western tradition about the nature of the personality in non-Western peoples. These writers have also challenged the limited attention paid to the influence of cultural processes on personality development. This research has documented diversity in personality characteristics such as emotional expression, ego boundaries, and interpersonal and intrapersonal perceptions. However, the current challenge for nurses has been in how to apply these findings in practice. This chapter will review some of these findings and suggest nursing strategies to incorporate these into nursing care.

TABLE 7–1 *Culture-Based Theories of Health and Illness*

SYSTEM	CONCEPTS	VALUES	CAUSATION BELIEFS	HEALING PRACTICES
Western biomedicine	Germs Genetics Neurotransmitters Organs Function Technology	Objectivity Science Logic	Malfunction Inheritance Biochemical imbalance Organic defects Germ invasion	Surgery Antibiotics Medication Targeted cellular destruction
Western psychology	Maturity Ego Conflicts Conditioning Anxiety Emotions	Independence Verbal expression Self-esteem Productivity	Ego failure Developmental immaturity Enmeshment Weak identity formation Low self-esteem	Psychotherapy Behavioral therapy Art and play therapy
Chinese medicine	Chi (energy, breath or life force) Meridians Ying/cold/inner Yang/hot/outer Elements	Harmony with forces of nature and social environment	Imbalance or disharmony Energy blockage	Acupuncture Massage Chi kung Breathing Herbalism
Ayurvedic medicine	Mind/body or constitutional types Energy flow Chakras Natural law	Harmony between mind/body, energy and environment Self-knowledge	Imbalance between daily routine, diet, and constitutional type	Astrology Pure metals Gemstones Herbs Meditation Yoga
Shamanic healing	All things have spirit Winds/directions (forces, life's requirements) Levels of existence or worlds Linkages to ancestors and unborn	Self-knowledge Self-control Recognize and validate spirit Recognize one's place in human and natural worlds Modesty	Disconnection with spirit Immodesty, jealousy and greed Ignorance	Protective rituals Divination Restoration of connection Restoration of social/spiritual order Cleansings Prayer
Spiritual healing	Supernatural Ancestors Souls	Appropriate relationship with supernatural and ancestral spirits	Spirit invasion Soul loss Weakness/vulnerability Jealousy/envy	Protective ritual Divination Witchcraft/voodoo Cleansings Prayer

INDEPENDENT AND INTERDEPENDENT WORLD VIEWS

Nurses learning about mental health, psychology, and psychiatry throughout the world are generally schooled in the classic personality and developmental theories of Freud, Erikson, Maslow, Piaget, and other Europeans and Americans. Although these theories may be applicable to people who share their world view, they have been challenged as being unable to explain or predict behavior and mental health across diverse populations. It is important for psychiatric nurses to understand the beliefs and values that are embedded in these theories before attempting to provide culturally relevant psychiatric nursing care. In America, these Western cultural ideals have become the standard for the mental health of people regardless of their cultural background. Individuals may be considered emotionally and developmentally immature if the Western culturally valued abilities of autonomy, individuation, and clear self-control are lacking. (See the classic works of Erikson [1968], S. Freud [1923] and A. Freud [1936], Kernberg [1976], Mahler and associates [1975], and Rapaport [1960]. For further discussion of these ideas, see Bellah [1985], Geertz [1975], Hsu [1983], Johnson [1995], Sampson [1988], Shweder and Borne [1984], and Spindler and Spindler [1987].)

The Self and Culture

The self is a central feature in Western psychological theories. Traditional psychoanalytic theory conceptualized the self as the ego (see Chapter 2). The ego is the psychological structure that moderates the conflict between the biological drives of the individual and the internalized social mandates for conformity and self-restraint (A. Freud 1936; S. Freud 1923; Levan 1992; Rapaport 1960). The ego is where individuals define who they are in relation to others. In many of the world's non-Western cultures, however, the ego or self is articulated in terms of roles and obligations and defined in terms of similarities to others in the social sphere (Triandis et al. 1988) (Fig. 7–1). Indeed, research within American society has shown that definitions of the self differ from male to female; for example, white women in the dominant society are more likely than white men to see themselves as part of a social system and operating in relation to the social context. (For more about the self and gender, see Gergen and Gergen [1988], Gergen [1992], Gilligan [1986], Lykes [1985], and Lyons [1983].) The self, from this perspective, is inseparable from the social context in which it emerges. Indeed, perception may be guided by gender (Cross and Markus 1993; Markus and Oyserman 1989). Some authors in cultural and gender psychology have focused on how the different socialization and acculturation experiences of people could theoretically account for variations in the organization or content of the ego or self (Chodorow 1978; Stoller 1985).

As stated earlier, the ideal of the self-determined, emancipated individual is rooted in European and American values (Gergen 1992; Kleinman 1988). This world view has also been described as the *independent world view* (individualistic or ideocentric) and has been broadly differentiated from cultures that have an *interdependent world view* (collectivist or sociocentric) (Fiske et al. 1998; Kagitcibasi 1989; Markus and Kitayama 1991; Triandis et al. 1988). People from sociocentric cultures experience their selfhood and their life as part of an interdependent web of relationships and expectations. Their concept of the self is better described in terms of roles, responsibilities, and relationships. Personal feelings and desires, although certainly present, are a much less relevant piece of information in understanding behavior. Authority, group needs, and family obligations carry more weight (Dien 1992; Espin 1985; Johnson 1995; Kleinman 1988; Roland 1988; Shweder and Miller, 1991). People within these sociocentric cultures have personality styles and behavioral norms unlike those in the West. These broad categorizations of world views are only for initial contrasting of overarching themes within the world's major philosophical and cultural ideologies and may not necessarily fit any particular group. Differences between and within groups evolve throughout time because of intercultural contact, economic and material conditions, and both immigration and migration into vastly different ecological regions.

"The self" is the place through which individuals understand and organize their responses to the world around them. In that way, all aspects of the social, physical, emotional, and mental life are understood through the self. The self—who one is in the world—is partly shaped by culture. The possibilities are limited, and the ways to perceive, feel, and act are given. However, individuals are active agents in that they select or construe their self from within that range of options, such that within any given culture, there is considerable variation—people within any culture are more or less shy, adventuresome, attentive to others, anxious, athletic, and so forth. The understanding of perceptions and emotional life from the cultural perspective requires a recognition that there is a general range of normal or desired within a given cultural sphere as well as a specific individual variation among members of the same group.

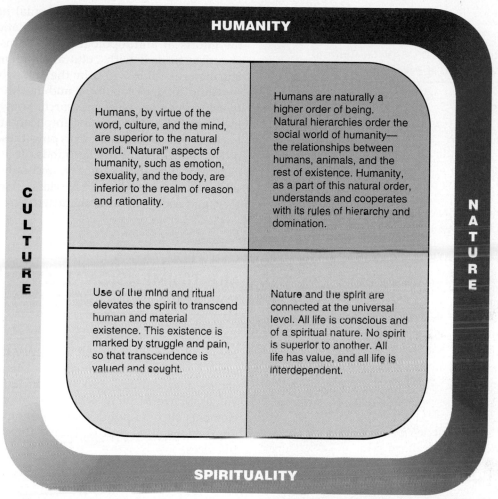

HUMANITY

CULTURE

Humans, by virtue of the word, culture, and the mind, are superior to the natural world. "Natural" aspects of humanity, such as emotion, sexuality, and the body, are inferior to the realm of reason and rationality.

Humans are naturally a higher order of being. Natural hierarchies order the social world of humanity—the relationships between humans, animals, and the rest of existence. Humanity, as a part of this natural order, understands and cooperates with its rules of hierarchy and domination.

NATURE

Use of the mind and ritual elevates the spirit to transcend human and material existence. This existence is marked by struggle and pain, so that transcendence is valued and sought.

Nature and the spirit are connected at the universal level. All life is conscious and of a spiritual nature. No spirit is superior to another. All life has value, and all life is interdependent.

SPIRITUALITY

Figure 7–1 The self across cultures: Major world views along experiential dimensions. (Inspired by T. S. Lebra, 1992.) Because of natural and forced migration, colonization, and human expansion, cultures around the world have historically exchanged language and traditions. Any culture represents a hybrid of life ways and—to a much less extent—world views. For example, Mesoamerican and South American cultures represent a blend of indigenous nature-based/spiritual world views with the humanity/culture world view imposed by Spanish colonization in the early 1400s. Similarly, the culture/spirit world view is represented by Hindu and Buddhist traditions in India and the surrounding nations. However, Buddhism has been exported to, and is widely practiced in, China, Japan, and other Asian countries. Moreover, in Japan these world views are superimposed on the nature-based ideology of the Shinto religion, which might more clearly fit with the spirit/nature quadrant of this grid.

The self also plays a central role in the cultural definition of illness and mental illness. People do not all experience depression, anxiety, perceptual problems, and behavioral problems in the same way. Just as cultures give a person a range of options within which to construe a self, so, too, culture defines for individuals what to focus on, what the appropriate emotion is in a given situation, or what the meaning of a situation is for the people involved. In that way, culture shapes what kinds of factors or events cause concern, illness, or distress, and how that illness or distress will be experienced and expressed.

Diverse modes of mental illness experience and expression may not conform closely to those de-scribed in the *Diagnostic and Statistical Manual of Mental Disorders* (DSM). The DSM was based on studies with a predominately white American sample. Only recently have research efforts begun to document the incredible diversity of forms of mental illness. Toward this end, cross-cultural research is concerned with the experience of psychological distress in its broadest form. It seeks to document the kinds of factors or events that people understand to cause distress. These are referred to as etiological factors, or **explanatory models**. In addition, researchers are documenting the forms of experience and expression that distress takes. Since these are understood only in their cultural context, they are referred to as **idioms of distress**.

Box 7–1 DSM-IV-TR *Cultural Foundation of Psychiatric Diagnosis*

CLINICAL HISTORY

■ Patient information
■ History of present illness
■ Psychiatric history and previous treatment
■ Social and developmental history
■ Family history
■ Course and outcome of illness
■ Diagnostic formulation (DSM-IV)

CULTURAL FORMULATION

Cultural identity

■ Cultural reference group
■ Language
■ Involvement in culture of origin
■ Involvement in host culture

Cultural explanation of illness

■ Predominant idioms of distress
■ Meaning and severity of symptoms in relation to cultural norms
■ Perceived causes and explanatory models
■ Help-seeking experiences and plans

Cultural factors related to psychosocial environment and levels of functioning

■ Social stressors
■ Social supports
■ Levels of functioning and disability

Cultural elements of the clinician-client relationship
Overall cultural assessment

Data from American Psychiatric Association. (2000). *Diagnostic and statistical manual of mental disorders* (4th ed., Text Revision). Washington, D.C.: American Psychiatric Press; and American Psychiatric Association. (2000). *Practice guidelines for the treatment of psychiatric disorders*. Washington, D.C.: American Psychiatric Press.

This research has prompted the American Psychiatric Association to examine the cultural biases in their psychiatric diagnoses. While falling short of revision of these diagnostic formulations, a panel of cross-cultural psychologists, psychiatrists, and medical and psychological anthropologists developed a guide to understanding illness in its cultural context. This is included in an appendix of the DSM-IV-TR (APA 2000; Mezzich et al. 1999). Unfortunately, while this is an attempt describe illnesses in the client's own terms, there is still no resolution to

questions about the nature of mental health and illness across cultures. Still, this formulation represents the efforts of anthropologists and transcultural psychiatrists to deal with cultural differences in a systematic way (Box 7–1). In the following section, a dynamic model of culture and health is presented that incorporates recent research, suggesting assessment strategies and nursing implications. The reader is cautioned to avoid stereotyping these data across others with similar backgrounds. It is essential to generalize this data carefully, and only with groups who share language, social class, regional, migratory, and socioeconomic characteristics.

CULTURE AS A MULTIDIMENSIONAL AND DYNAMIC PROCESS

The model presented in Figure 7–2 applies anthropological and sociological concepts to the nursing care of culturally diverse clients. This model understands that cultural processes include beliefs and values, or world view, which are enforced by power elements such as political and economic factors, and are demonstrated and replicated through behavioral practices.

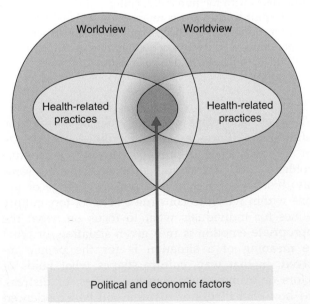

Figure 7–2 Cultural model of cross-cultural health care encounter.

World View

The beliefs and values held by people within a given culture about what is good, right, and normal are referred to as their **cultural ideology,** or **world view.** The ideology or world view of a culture refers to the available symbols, meanings, and values about what is important and what behaviors are right and correct. These beliefs and values are convictions about how a person should be, what is the appropriate way to behave, and how one should be in the world. They are the rules for living provided by society, and as such, serve as a model or ideal way of being. Of course, they are only guides, so that the average person rarely achieves them. Yet they are selectively internalized into the individual personality or self, and act as individual guides to self-evaluation, motivation, and behavior. This is the link between the larger world view of a culture and the individual psychological functioning of any given person. Mental health can be said to be the degree to which a person is able to fulfill the cultural expectations of his or her society (Fiske et al. 1998; Markus and Kitayama 1991; Saint Arnault 1998).

Vignette

■ *An American television commercial depicts a 2- to 3-year-old toddler in a high chair. The announcer describes that this child is at the point in her life where she is learning to make choices. The video shows the mother offering the toddler a choice of two different juices to drink. The commercial then shows her making a choice, depicting at some length her pleasure in drinking the juice that she selected.*

This vignette illustrates that it is a value within American society to determine our desires, needs, and preferences. The dominant American culture values exploring inner selves to get a clear sense of who one is and what one needs. In the commercial, the toddler is being taught the values held within her culture—that this ability to choose is an important ability to have. It also conveys to the viewer that this is an important skill to provide to children. The media, as an agent of culture, is instructing mothers that choice making is an ideal behavior in a child. The mother in American society learns that it is her task to assist her children in the full development of this ability if they are to become competent members of American society.

However, these kinds of intrapersonal awareness, self-directed behaviors, and interpersonal autonomy are not the only preferred way.

Vignette

■ *[In a day care center in Japan] each item of the menu is served on a separate plate or bowl for each child. . . . Each teacher brings food for his or her children on several trays from the kitchen to the classroom. For the younger children (ages 1 to 4), teachers set the table for the children. However, among the oldest children, a boy and a girl are assigned this duty each day. These children are called* toban. *They serve the plates and bowls, which are already filled with food, from the trays to each child. Meanwhile the other children are supposed to sit quietly. When the children on duty finish serving, they stand in front of everyone and say* itadakimasu *(I will gratefully receive this food) and the others follow. . . . Every child has an equal opportunity to be a* toban. *. . . Each child knows when his or her turn comes next. . . . Each one takes pride in being responsible and also in being able to do the task as well as the other children do (Fujita and Sano, 1988, p. 82.)*

This vignette demonstrates another set of cultural values. This time, the values lie in doing well in other's eyes and fulfilling responsibilities and obligations with pride. The children are excited about the opportunity to be "in charge," but the role of being in charge carries with it a responsibility to do one's best and to do well for the others who are dependent on them. At another time, the children will practice gratefulness for being attended.

Mental health is defined by the culture, and deviance from cultural expectations is considered by others within the culture to be a problem. The culture defines what types of differences are still within the range of normal (mentally healthy) and which ones are outside the range of normal (mentally ill). In the examples given earlier, there is a range within which the American toddler would be considered mentally healthy. For example, it is still considered normal for her to want her mother to choose or to resist choice altogether and refuse to eat (the so-called "terrible two's"). However, it might be considered mentally unhealthy for the child to have tantrums at every mealtime or for her to be unable to initiate any action on her own. In the Japanese example, it might be considered normal for a child to take excessive pride in being the *toban,* to be very shy in front of others, or to be afraid of making a mistake. It might be considered mentally unhealthy for the child to refuse to help or to be selfish or ungrateful. It might also be unhealthy for a Japanese child to focus on self-needs to the exclusion of those of others or to be unable to allow others to do for them (Johnson 1995).

In a discussion of the role of culture in the socialization of children, and the misapplication of Western-derived psychological theory across cultures, Turkish researcher Kagitcibasi (1989) wrote:

> To illustrate the point, I shall refer to the maternal regulation strategies of the Japanese mother. . . . Here is the contrast between two meaning systems that render the same pattern normal or abnormal. The Japanese mother's message to the child, "I am one with you, and we can be of the same mind," . . . is exactly the definition of a "symbiotic" relationship, an expression of pathological "enmeshment" in the Western family, as interpreted by Western psychology (p. 155).

Explanatory Models of Disease and Mental Illness

Illness and disease occur within a cultural and social context. Culture provides the frameworks within which the meaning of the illness, and the necessary care or cure, are determined. The types of mental illness seen within a given culture reflect the way that culture understands the self and its relationship to society; the ways people within the culture understand themselves in the world; and the way they express grief, fear, anxiety, and depression. In summarizing the impact of culture on the expression of mental illness, Kleinman (1980) contrasted the experience of depression in the Western client and that of neurasthenia in the Chinese client. He encouraged health care providers to understand the cultural meaning of the illness experience; the roles of the client, family, and community regarding the illness; and the expectations the client and family have in the health care encounter. Kleinman referred to these as explanatory models. These models are the way that people within a given culture understand the factors that cause and cure illnesses (Fig. 7–3).

Explanatory models are the ways that the people explain the source of distress or the cause of the illness. One such explanation for problems are the concepts of imbalance and harmony. Physical, social, emotional, and spiritual imbalance can be caused by a variety of factors. The balance between one's diet and one's current biological state is important in some cultures. For them, physical states

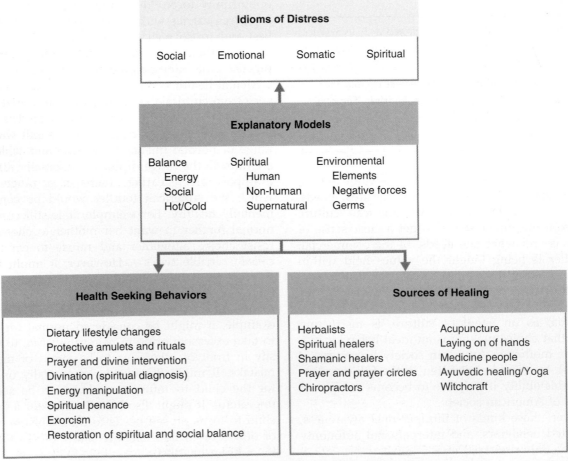

Figure 7–3 Effects of explanatory models on illness experience and practice.

such as menstruation, childbirth, and illness represent changes in the heat of the body. In cases such as these, dietary or environmental changes are warranted to restore balance. Social behaviors can also cause social imbalance. Immodesty, excessive sex or drinking, jealousy, and greed can upset the social balance and are believed to cause illness. Finally, energy can become blocked or concentrated, or both, creating an imbalance in energy flow.

There are other important beliefs about the **spiritual causes of illness.** Spiritual sources can be further subdivided into those involving human spirits or souls, nonhuman spirits, and supernatural forces. There are many different cultural beliefs about the nature, location, and character of the human spirit or soul. Some cultures believe that the soul or souls can be captured, dislodged, or lost. These spiritual events can occur because of witchcraft or as a result of some kind of traumatic experience. Nonhuman spirits include the spiritual nature of plants, animals, mountains, water, and other nonhuman forms. Many non-Western healing systems consider respect for and recognition of these nonhuman spiritual forces essential for health. Disrespect and disconnection from them can lead to illness. Supernatural forces or spirits can include ancestors. They might also be gods, which may be benevolent, evil, or changing. Often, humans are called on in these systems to give offerings to ancestors or supernatural spirits, to act in ways that are pleasing to them, or to protect the soul from capture with rituals or amulets. In most of these cases, there is a relationship between social conduct and spiritual sources of illness, such that people need to maintain good relationships with other people and the spirits.

Environmental causes of illness, which are external forces, might be bad winds, ghosts, negative energies, germs, and elements such as cold, impurities, or negative or jealous thoughts. People holding these beliefs feel that inner strength, resistance, and purity are important protections against invasion from these outside forces. This set of beliefs is related to the balance concept described earlier because imbalance can make one vulnerable or weak, and therefore susceptible to these outside forces. In addition, sometimes the outside forces are spiritual in nature, such that the outside threat is a negative or evil spirit that enters the body and causes illness.

The believed cause of the illness is related to the choice of treatment. These practices are discussed in more detail later but might include ceremonies, restitution, cleansings, rest, dietary changes, and the like. Therefore, people seek help based on the believed cause. However, it has often been noted that people select assistance and help from a variety of sources. Political and economic forces also play a role in the choices of healing people choose (also

discussed later). For example, people who do not speak English, are unfamiliar with technology, and who live outside of urban areas might not choose biomedical care because they feel more comfortable and have better access to folk treatments, which they also better understand.

Nursing Implications

Examination of what is normal and healthy as well as what is abnormal and unhealthy depends on the social norms and expectations. This also requires that you clearly understand that most of the beliefs, values, and treatments provided in nursing have been adapted from Western science and psychology. The importance of knowing yourself as a cultural product cannot be overstated. You should evaluate whether these theories are relevant for the persons you are attempting to help. Andrews and Boyle (1999) have suggested that this perspective is **ethnorelativism**, which is essential for providing care that is not bound by Western culture.

The second implication for nurses is the importance of assessing the beliefs held by the person and their family. Accurately assessing health-related beliefs and values often necessitates the collaboration with a **cultural translator.** Cultural translators do more than translate language. They can assist the nurse in understanding the health-related concepts that are specific to that culture. The cultural translator should also closely resemble the patient with regard to geographical region, social class, and gender.

Using information gained from work with clients, families, and cultural translators, you can use concepts of health and illness to understand the meaning of the illness to the person and their community. Often, beliefs about the causes of illness reveal feelings of failure, concerns about social problems, spiritual distress, or other negatively sanctioned problems. These are not easy for the person and their family to reveal because they may feel stigmatized. In addition, although treatment of the symptoms is usually the immediate need for the family and the client, there are often other types of protections, reparation, or social ceremonies that are warranted to restore harmony with spirits or others in the community.

Political and Economic Factors

Another important and often overlooked element of culture is the political-economic dimension. The **political-economic aspects of culture** include the social structure of the society, including how families, groups, and political institutions distribute resources, divide labor, and acquire and distribute wealth. These elements of culture are found any time there is power and control asserted. The political-economic dimension is related to ideation in that it is defined by the rules about what is right and good. These are the ways that people organize themselves, who has the power to control whom, and who should have less or more. The political-economic dimension of culture, therefore, incorporates cultural beliefs and values about "good" and "right" to justify who will hold power over whom. In addition, people can use their power to punish or ostracize someone who does not conform to their ideals. This aspect of culture includes how those in power define proper social conduct and how public behavior is regulated.

Stigma is an example of the use of social structure to uphold an ideal. In many cultures, a person with mental illness is considered frightening and abnormal. However, if one examines the cultural values more closely, one finds on what basis society defines abnormal, immoral, or unnatural. In American society, for example, the mentally ill were historically seen as those who were controlled by evil forces, morally weak, and economically unproductive. Therefore, these people were feared, stigmatized, and ostracized. These beliefs about the mentally ill have also historically been seen in the public's treatment of people with tuberculosis, cholera, syphilis, and acquired immunodeficiency syndrome.

Other aspects of political and economic dimensions include social power. Social power is reflected in the dominant language used. People who are unable or unwilling to use the dominant language are shut out of avenues of power. They may not be able to work, use needed services, read public information, shop, drive, bank, obtain legal representation, and obtain health care. Another cultural feature of daily life is the familiarity with technology. Besides the additional information and conveniences that technology can afford, people may feel that technologies are against their traditions or may not access health-related services because of the strange and frightening technological use. While many young people from diverse cultures may be interested in technologies, older people are often less so. Combining an unknown language with an environment that is dominated by technology can make accessing health care an impossibly frightening and alien experience. Finally, the infrastructure of a region may make use of technology impossible. If electricity, phone lines, or passable roads are not available, it is unlikely that one will seek out or value technological advances.

The political-economic aspects of culture are related to the cultural world view of any given people. The institutional organizations do not stand outside the values of the people but rather enforce them. Institutions include social organizations at the grand scale, and examples of these are the legal, educational, and medical systems—they are systems in that they are integrated into every facet of our daily lives. The political-economic dimensions of culture are the enactments of the ideals of a culture at the institutional or macro level. Within the political-economic sphere of culture, cultural ideology is used to justify inequities within the society, including social class and gender. Examples of the overlap of ideology and political-economic dimensions of culture include social and gender roles, which are both defined by ideation and politically enforced.

Nursing Implications

Language and communication are central in the accessibility of health care. The choice of language affects the perception of the people, including some and excluding others. For example, the use of Spanish may seem to the nurse to be the best language for communication with an indigenous Mexican group, but on further investigation, he or she may find that Spanish implies power and privilege and that the preferred language is an indigenous tongue. As stated earlier, it is important that the translator speak not only the same language but also share cultural characteristics such as region, social status, and gender.

The second implication is the need for nurses to minimize barriers to direct access of health care. Nurses can work on behalf of the community to translate materials, make videotaped materials for those who cannot read, provide translators, and create health care settings that include familiar symbols and objects that are delivered in a familiar and understandable environment.

Practice or Behavioral Dimension

The final aspect of culture is the **practice dimension of culture** or behavioral aspect. The practice domain includes the rituals, spatial organization, and interpersonal behaviors used in a culture. The practice aspect of culture includes both power and ideas—these two forces are acted out in even the smallest gestures, speech patterns, manner of dress, social distances, food choices, and so forth. Practice is the embodiment of tradition. Thus, cultural practices are the enactments of the cultural ideology at the personal or small group level. In some ways, practice is the easiest or the first thing one sees about cultural differences. The two primary ways that illness is practiced is in the idioms of distress used, and in the help seeking and healing options used. These are described in the following sections.

Idioms of Distress

Since illness and health are culturally defined and made meaningful within social contexts, it is necessary to document the varieties of illness and distress experiences and expressions. This type of research often examines the symptoms or syndromes that are common in a region or among certain groups. The researcher tries to discover the kinds of problems people seek help for, where they go for what type of help, and the way that they express suffering. The phrase idioms of distress captures the common, local, or typical way that distress or suffering is experienced and communicated without imposing labels or illness categories onto them prematurely. This research also discovers some of the beliefs about the causes of the illness. Research of this type often selects samples of people who present to either dominant medical practitioners or traditional healers. The research sometimes examines the interaction between the healer and the patient to understand how symptoms are communicated by the patient and which symptoms the healer attends to and which they do not. Another line of research is to explore the symptoms as they are experienced by the patient, attempting to understand what symptoms occur together, what are accompanying life events, what the sufferer thinks caused them, and what these symptoms mean about them and their world. Kirmayer and associates (1998) defined idioms of distress as modes of expression that explicitly refer to indigenous theories of mind, self, and emotion. When the concept of person differs substantially between cultures, psychological idioms of distress also differ. Cultures have their own theories of what basic emotions and emotion-producing situations are important, how these are expressed, and what the appropriate social response is to them. Illness is therefore experienced and expressed in different combinations of physical, emotional, and social terms.

Vignette

■ Han is a form of regret or resentment syndrome in Korea. It may be experienced with or without a sensation of obstruction by a lump in the epigastric region, and dysphoric affect, such as self-pity. . . . Hwabyung, commonly known as bodily disorder, has been described as an anger syndrome that encompasses elements of depression, resentment, somatic illness, and neurotic symptoms. . . . Shingyungshayak, an emotional, psychic, and bodily disorder, is characterized by impaired functioning in interpersonal relationships and often by fatigue, depression, feelings of inadequacy, headaches, hypersensitivity to sensory stimulation, and psychosomatic symptoms such as digestive disturbances and insomnia (Pang 1998, pp. 96–97).

In this research, Pang (1998) found that illness for the Korean elderly in her sample was a kind of emotional/physical/interpersonal complex, with references to emotion as the cause of malfunctioning of organs, and the source of the emotions as arising from remorse, hurts, resentments, and unexpressed anger. She encouraged health care practitioners to recognize the holistic interrelationship of the mind (emotions and thoughts) with one's interpersonal life. Often, as is the case worldwide, the body is the place where these troubles are experienced and expressed.

In another classic study, Nichter (1981) documented the experiences of distress in 100 women in Gopal, India, who presented for medical treatment in a local clinic. He documented that 39% of the women had leukorrhea. Leukorrhea is loosely translated from bili hoguvudu, or "white going," and is a syndrome that is associated with complex cultural meanings. It is culturally understood as caused by loss of dhatu, which is a vital bodily essence that regulates body heat, vitality, and emotions. Loss of this bodily essence creates a physical imbalance that is experienced as weakness, back pain, and poor concentration and a feeling of being overheated. Another 29% of the women's complaints focused on menstrual problems, which, within their culture, is understood to convey concerns about feelings of distance from the family, unstable emotions, rumination about interfamily conflict, marriage anxiety, anxiety about childbearing, and the transition from daughter to wife (Nichter 1981).

Vignette

■ Ataques de nervios is an idiom of distress used by Puerto Ricans and other Latinos to express dislocations in the social world of the family. The experience of ataques de nervios involves a loss of control in several important domains of experience: emotional expressions (including screaming, crying, depression, fearfulness, anguish, and anger), bodily sensations (including trembling, palpitations, chills, headache, stomach upset, and seizures), action dimensions (including aggression toward self and others, and suicide attempts), and alterations in consciousness (including fainting, dizziness, amnesia, and hallucinations). That loss of control is closely linked to important social contexts relating to major life problems and the experience of suffering (Guarnaccia et al. 1996).

As in the other research examples, people with *ataques de nervios* also experience illnesses that are characterized as interpersonal in source and emotional-physical in nature. The concept of idioms of distress allows nurses interested in psychological health to document the full range of experiences patients have and to assess the meaning of these for the patient, family, and community.

Help Seeking and Healing Options

The type of healing a person seeks depends largely on one's beliefs about the cause of the illness. The practice of healing aims to remove the cause of illness or protect people from these causes. Since these causes are culturally defined, so, too, are the health-related practices of the ill person, their family, and the healer. Table 7–1 shows some major health-related systems. These systems have core concepts, values, and beliefs about the causes of illness and provide experiences necessary to restore health. These systems are overlapping in many countries. Therefore, people may choose to use elements from many traditions. Indeed, people may subscribe to more than one set of beliefs. Before the reader concludes that this is irrational, consider the white American middle class, which may use meditation, yoga, psychotherapy, and medication to heal anxiety. People select from the variety of options that they perceive as available and useful.

Political-economic factors might limit the perception of availability. As discussed earlier, when healing is provided in a known language, the healer uses familiar symbols, and the environment is familiar, people may prefer that healing regardless of its ultimate efficacy. In addition, sometimes the preferred therapy or healing is cost prohibitive, inaccessible, or simply unavailable.

Vignette

■ *In a rural area of Mexico, in a village that is heavily populated by an indigenous Indian tribe, a Western hospital facility is annexed by a traditional health care center. The decor of the traditional center is familiar to the locals, and treatment is provided in both the indigenous and Spanish languages. Villagers may receive surgeries, medication, or radiation in the Western facility, then go next door for a spiritual cleansing and protective rituals, prayers, and herbal remedies. Women may have their baby delivered with a traditional midwife, and if complications occur, be transported into the hospital for medical intervention.*

In this example, people in the village combine healing traditions with radically different world views. However, there was a long history of political-economic struggling and concessions for this arrangement to take place. Prior to the development of the collaborative system, villagers had to choose which system to access and had to pay out of their meager pockets for the folk system, while feeling disenfranchised by the Western system they felt was being forced onto them.

Nursing Implications

Most cultures do not separate physical, social, and emotional symptoms in the way that is common in biomedicine. Therefore, nursing assessment must be sensitive to the common ways that distress is experienced and communicated. In addition, the cultural translator can help the nurse investigate the beliefs behind certain symptom clusters. These beliefs often prompt the typical strategies used to alleviate the symptoms. It is also important to assess carefully the social conditions surrounding the symptoms and to delineate beliefs about social causes. Nurses are in a unique position to assess these factors fully since they use a biopsychosocial-spiritual approach.

The second implication is to determine relevant aspects of folk or traditional healing that can be incorporated into nursing care. Based on beliefs about spiritual causes, for example, the appropriate spiritual healer should attend to the spiritual aspects of the illness without sanction or evaluation by the nurse. This is more than respect for diverse traditions but rather an incorporation of other methods of healing into the biopsychosocial-spiritual care of the client and the family in much the same way as calling in a priest or rabbi. In addition, the safety and compatibility of folk remedies and therapies must be evaluated. For example, herbal remedies often contain biochemicals with powerful pharmacological effects. If the patient is using herbal remedies, these may interact with medical therapies.

The ways that families care for each other and the sick roles of clients are culturally defined and enacted. Caregiving roles of various family members must be ascertained and incorporated in all aspects of care, from acute care to outpatient care. The nurse can designate the appropriate recipient for teaching based on family roles in the caregiving process.

Community health promotion centers around working with the intersection of beliefs, recognizing political and economic forces, and helping community members alter or enact health-related practices. For example, dietary practices of American Indians were altered through contact with whites that have had consequences to the overall health of the population. Through a complex interplay of political-economic forces and enculturation in Western values, traditional dietary customs have been abandoned, resulting in a high incidence of diabetes in some American Indian communities. Some of these communities are working with Western care providers, traditional healers, and key community members to re-enact health-related dietary practices. In this way, health promotion efforts can use this model to design health promotion strategies that remove barriers and incorporate both cultural values and Western health-related goals.

CULTURALLY COMPETENT PSYCHIATRIC NURSING PRACTICE

As the discussion in the previous section indicates, psychiatric nurses cannot apply a standard model of assessment, diagnosis, and intervention to all clients with equal confidence. Using only the Western-de-

rived model creates the possibility that interpersonal and intrapersonal characteristics may be poorly assessed and misdiagnosed, leading to culturally irrelevant interventions. The United States is an amalgam of cultural values that presents a special challenge to caregivers. Complete understanding of all the possible self-structures, world views, and approaches to health and illness is impossible. Since people come to the therapeutic arena with differing adherence to traditional world views, socioeconomic situations and practices, assessment must include all of these areas (Box 7–2).

Psychiatric nursing care is a culturally derived set of interventions designed to promote verbalization of feelings, teach individually focused coping skills, and assist clients with behavioral and emotional self-control consistent with Western cultural ideals. However, consideration should be given to providing psychiatric nursing care that is not bound to specific cultural ideologies but aimed at general mental health goals. In an early effort to analyze

Box 7–2   *Assessment Dimensions and Nursing Implications*

CULTURAL DIMENSION	SAMPLE ASSESSMENT QUESTIONS	RATIONALE
Beliefs and values	■ What does someone in your community (culture, religion) call this illness? ■ What do people believe caused this illness? ■ Do people shun or avoid someone who has this illness? ■ What does a mature person act like—how do they conduct themselves?	■ Recognize self as a cultural being ■ Recognize practice as based in Western beliefs and practices ■ Collaborate with cultural translator to assess explanatory models ■ Determine meaning of illness to person and family/community
Political/Economic	■ What are the social classes, ethnic or racial categories used by the people? ■ How does being a woman or a man affect someone with this illness? ■ Who makes decisions about what needs to be done for the ill person? ■ Source and availability of income ■ Familiarity with technology ■ Accessibility of preferred type of health care and of dominant health care ■ Language spoken. Language of dominant health care. Language barriers to access to health care ■ Transportation and infrastructure	■ Match translator with region, ethnicity, social class and gender whenever possible ■ Minimize language and environmental barriers ■ Remove environmental aspects that cause illness ■ Combat and eliminate racism and oppression
Practice	■ How do people communicate with each other (space, gestures, mannerisms, voice tone)? ■ What is done for the sick, and by whom? ■ What dietary practices or restrictions are used when one has this illness? ■ Are there any ceremonies, special prayers, or other protections used to treat this illness, or protect people from it? Who performs these? Have they been seen? Result?	■ Assess idioms of distress and their meanings and expression ■ Determine preferred or commonly used healing methods ■ Determine caregiving strategies and roles: work with appropriate family members ■ Community-based health promotion

how cross-cultural psychotherapy might be developed, Kleinman (1988) conducted an analysis of the curative factors of local or folk healing worldwide and developed the following list of factors that these healing systems have in common:

■ Healing integrates the physical symptoms with the symbolic system of the culture.
■ The explanatory models of the client and the healer are congruent.
■ The healer has characteristics of charisma and confidence.
■ Both the healer and the client conceptualize the illness in cultural terms.
■ There are elements of confession, or moral witnessing, especially in an emotionally charged or cathartic way.
■ There is emotional arousal and faith in the healing method, both within the client and within the community.
■ The healer, the family, and the community use social persuasion.
■ Healing techniques use rhetorical devices such as irony and paradox.

Consideration of these commonalties suggests that the psychiatric nurse should collaborate with cultural translators and engage in extensive involvement with the family and the community when delivering education and making treatment plans. For example, it is within the community that understanding of the cultural meaning of the disease is formed and the illness itself is dealt with. Family members and the community are primary factors in the success of a treatment plan, based on whether they agree with the diagnosis and whether they support compliance with the treatment (Kleinman, 1980).

Box 7–3 *Culturally Competent Clinical Services*

■ **Bicultural staffing**—matched with predominant patient populations according to social class, gender, language preferences, ethnic and religion divisions, and migratory history or cultural region
■ **Coverage for all encountered languages**—available translation and cultural interpretation for patient populations that are not numerous enough to have as permanent staff
■ **Family involvement**—recognize that all family members have a role in the patient's care and delineate what those roles are. Together, designate one or two key family members who will be the staff contact and liaison between the staff and the rest of the family
■ **Cultural formulation included in assessment** (see Box 7–2)—staff should focus on idioms of distress, explanatory models, and help-seeking behaviors in day-to-day interactions. These should be clearly marked in the client's chart and in staff-to-staff communication about the client's condition
■ **Use cultural interpreters, designated family members, and community liaison work** to gain a full understanding; retain this information, along with relevant social class, gender, language preferences, ethnic and religion divisions, and migratory history or cultural region information to begin to develop a cultural resource library that is specific to cultural subpopulations in your area

■ **Biological response to medication**—examine medication profiles for people from the specific genetic phenotype, if available, in formularies, drug company trials, and other pharmaceutical databases
■ **Stigma related to psychiatric diagnosis**—recognize that all cultures have not normalized emotional distress in the same way that we have in the dominant white American culture (where child psychology is actively discussed and it can be chic to be "in therapy"). Mental illness is understood in social terms and may indicate a lack of harmony, social disruption, lack of personal strength, failure to perform roles, and the like
■ **Community linkages with predominant non-Western and non-white American populations**—attend public functions, fairs, support groups, and so forth; be visible as a delegate from your treatment agency; and designate interest groups among staff to divide up the tasks involved
■ **Get your primary materials translated** and leave them in appropriate public areas such as community centers, beauty salons, grocery stores, and schools
■ **Relevant symbols**—use symbols, translated signs, and informational documents in caregiving areas; recognize holidays, accommodate religious traditions such as prayer times, and assess and accommodate food restrictions; consider allowing food to be brought by family

Data from Gee, K. K., Du, N., Akiyama, K., and Lu, F. (1999). The Asian Focus Unit at UCSF: An 18-year perspective. In J. Herrera, W. B. Lawson, and J. J. Sramek (Eds.), *Cross cultural psychiatry* (pp. 275–285). Chichester, England: John Wiley & Sons; and Guarnaccia, P. J. (1999). Anthropological issues on ethnic units. In J. Herrera, W. B. Lawson, and J. J. Sramek (Eds.), *Cross cultural psychiatry* (pp. 303 312). Chichester, England: John Wiley & Sons.

Cultural Competence

Literature regarding multicultural counseling and cultural competence has focused on three main areas: (1) awareness of one's own personal world views and how one is the product of cultural conditioning, (2) knowledge of the world views of culturally different clients, and (3) skills necessary for work with culturally different clients (Holcomb-McCoy and Myers 1999). However, most education in health-related fields has focused on the first two factors. It has been much more difficult to ascertain how to provide care in a culturally competent way. In nursing, cultural competence has been defined as the nurses' ability to achieve ethnorelativism so as to work within the cultural context of clients and to know, assess, and integrate the beliefs, values, practices, and problem-solving strategies of the patients' cultures in the care provided to patients (Campinha-Bacote 1994; St. Clair and McKenry 1999). The Campinha-Bacote model defines cultural competence as the process in which the health care provider continuously strives to achieve the ability to effectively work within the cultural context of a client (individual, family, or community). This process requires health care providers to see themselves as *becoming* culturally competent rather than being culturally competent. This model views cultural awareness, cultural knowledge, cultural skill, and cultural encounters as constructs of cultural competence. However, an additional construct has been added: cultural desire. These five constructs have an interdependent relationship with each other, and no matter where health care providers enter this process, all five constructs eventually must be experienced or addressed (Campinha-Bacote 1999).

A related concept focusing on nursing intervention is that of the nurse as a culture broker (Tripp-Reimer and Brink 1985). This framework incorporates advocacy, negotiation, mediation, and sensitivity to clients' and families' needs. Culture brokerage, as a nursing intervention, is a strategy that is intended to assist nurses to bridge the gap between the orthodox health care system and the health belief systems of clients and their families who are from different cultures (Box 7–3).

nursing has the special challenge of defining mental health and providing behavioral control. Western ideas of normalcy have been applied universally to quite different cultures, and little research has been done historically about the role of culture in shaping psychological functioning. Recent research is only beginning to delineate these differences, and culturally relevant psychological care is still at the experimental stage. However, authors agree that the current model of Western psychotherapy must be used cautiously, and our definition of mental health must be expanded to include a broader range of behaviors.

Before making any cross-cultural encounter, nurses must be aware of personal values and beliefs, expose themselves to cultural diversity, challenge their own ethnocentrism, and dispel cultural myths. Understanding world views can help the nurse categorize and understand assessment data and promote critical thinking about culture and mental health. While forming a therapeutic relationship with a client, family, or community of another culture, the nurse should conduct a relevant cultural assessment. General assessment data about cultural aspects of mental health include beliefs, behaviors, and political and economic factors that affect social relationships; modes of emotional experience and expression; understanding the self and the world; developmental maturity; conceptions of mental health and illness; and health-related practices. Finally, cultural psychology data suggest that interdependent cultural models stress roles, relationships, interpersonal harmony, and authority. These values can inform nursing practice when the nurse incorporates the sociocultural factors into the plan of care. Curiosity, negotiation, compromise, and flexibility are attributes that can help the nurse provide culturally relevant care.

Future research is needed to test psychiatric nursing assessment tools. International psychiatric nursing models need to be developed that focus on general mental health goals along a continuum of normalcy. Finally, psychiatric nursing must develop and test goals and interventions that assist all clients to achieve culturally relevant outcomes.

SUMMARY

All nursing care needs to accommodate cultural diversity; however, psychiatric mental health

Visit the **Evolve** website at
http://evolve.elsevier.com/Varcarolis
for a post-test on the content in this chapter.

Visit the **Evolve** website at
http://evolve.elsevier.com/Varcarolis
for additional self-study exercises.

Critical Thinking and Chapter Review

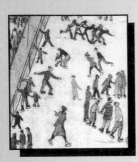

Critical Thinking

1. Define the phrase "explanatory models of health and illness" and discuss how this affects therapeutic goals and interventions.
2. Define the phrase "idioms of distress" and give at least three examples.
3. Differentiate between "the self" of the individualist and collectivist societies. Relate this to psychiatric nursing practice.
4. A Chinese woman has recently moved to America. She is a wife and the mother of two small children and lives in a tight-knit Chinese community with her husband's parents. She comes to an emergency department with complaints of fatigue, headache, and stomach pain. Diagnostic tests are unrevealing. Inquiry by the nurse reveals that the woman wants to be more like an American woman and has been trying to "speak her mind" to her husband's parents. She has received increasing pressure from her husband and the family to "be a good wife." Using understandings about cultural variations of the self:

   (a) What are the symbolic or cultural meanings of her symptoms?
   (b) What are the cultural expectations for this client and the possible cultural explanations for her suffering?
   (c) What might the family and her community recommend for her, and how does this contrast with the typical psychiatric nursing approach to her problems?
   (d) How might a culturally relevant approach modify these? and
   (e) What can a culturally competent psychiatric nurse do for this client?

Chapter Review

Choose the most appropriate answer.

1. Providing culturally relevant mental health nursing requires nurses to

   1. Assume Western psychological theories can be applied to non-Western clients.
   2. Recognize the superiority of Western cultural values, beliefs about relationships, and world views.
   3. Understand the values and beliefs embedded within one's own culture and medical practices.
   4. Educate clients on language and culture so they are not offended by Western customs and terminology.

2. Use of a cultural handbook by a nurse caring for a client of different cultural background

   1. Will prevent stereotyping the client.
   2. Is an excellent way to learn about a new culture.
   3. May mislead by not recognizing subgroup differences.
   4. Will provide understanding of the universality of cultural processes.

3. One possible negative result of applying Western psychological theories when assessing individuals of other cultures is

  1. Identifying client idioms of distress.
  2. Identifying cognitive deficit where none exists.
  3. Recognizing individual variation among group members.
  4. Seeing a sociocentric individual as developmentally immature.

4. Culturally relevant psychiatric nursing practice includes

  1. Understanding all self-structures, world views, and explanatory models of illness.
  2. Seeking clarification of the client's health-related beliefs.
  3. Applying a standard model of assessment to all clients.
  4. Using standard interventions for all clients.

5. Which action on the part of the nurse is least useful in promoting delivery of culturally relevant psychiatric nursing care?

  1. Working within the cultural context of the client.
  2. Providing a culturally relevant client assessment.
  3. Using direct eye contact and touch to facilitate communication.
  4. Bridging the gap between the U.S. health care system and the health belief system of the client.

REFERENCES

Abu-Lughod, L. (1986). *Veiled sentiments*. Berkeley, CA: University of California Press.

Alarcon, R. D., Westermeyer, J., Foulks, E. F., and Ruiz, P. (1999). Clinical relevance of contemporary cultural psychiatry. *Journal of Nervous and Mental Disease,* 187(18):465–471.

American Psychiatric Association. (2000). *Diagnostic and statistical manual of mental disorders* (4th ed., Text Revision). Washington, D.C.: American Psychiatric Press.

American Psychiatric Association. (2000). *Practice guidelines for the treatment of psychiatric disorders*. Washington, D.C.: American Psychiatric Press.

Andrews, M., and Boyle, J. (1999). *Transcultural concepts in nursing care* (2nd ed.). Philadelphia: J. B. Lippincott.

Barbee, E. L. (1992). African American women and depression: A review and critique of the literature. *Archives of Psychiatric Nursing,* 6(5):257–265.

Bellah, R. N. (1985). *Habits of the heart: Individualism and commitment in American life*. Berkeley, CA: University of California Press.

Bhui, K., and Olajide, D. (1999). *Mental health service provision for a multicultural society*. London: W. B. Saunders.

Campinha-Bacote, J. (1999). A model and instrument for addressing cultural competence in health care. *Journal of Nursing Education,* 38(5):203–207.

Campinha-Bacote, J. (1994). Cultural competence in psychiatric mental health nursing: A conceptual model. *Nursing Clinics of North America,* 29(1):1–8.

Chodorow, N. (1978). *The reproduction of mothering: Psychoanalysis and the sociology of mothering*. Berkeley, CA: University of California Press.

Chrisman, N. J. (1991). Cultural systems. In S. Baird, R. McCorkle, and M. Grant (Eds.), *Cancer nursing: A comprehensive textbook* (pp. 45–54). Philadelphia: W. B. Saunders.

Cross, S. E., and Markus, H. R. (1993). Gender in thought, belief, and action: A cognitive approach. In A. E. Beall and J. Sternberg (Eds.), *The psychology of gender* (pp. 55–98). New York: Guilford Press.

Derne, S. (1992). Beyond institutional and impulsive conceptions of the self: Family structure and the socially anchored real self. *Ethos,* 20(3):259–288.

Dien, D. S. (1992). Gender and individuation: China and the west. *Psychoanalytic Review,* 79(1):105–119.

Dienemann, J. A. (Ed.). (1997). *Cultural diversity in nursing: Issues, strategies, and outcomes*. Washington, D.C.: American Academy of Nursing.

Edwards, C. P., and Kumru, A. (1999). Culturally sensitive assessment. *Child and Adolescent Psychiatric Clinics of North America,* 8(2):409–424.

Erikson, E. H. (1968). *Identity, youth, and crisis*. New York: Norton.

Espin, O. M. (1985). Psychotherapy with Hispanic women: Some considerations. In P. B. Pedersen (Ed.), *Handbook of cross-cultural counseling and therapy* (pp. 165–171). Westport, CT: Greenwood Press.

Fiske, A. P., Kitayama, S., Markus, H. R., and Nisbett, R. E. (1998). The cultural matrix of social psychology. In D. T. Gilbert, S. T. Fiske, G. Lindzey (Eds.), *The handbook of social psychology* (4th ed.) (pp. 915–981). Boston: McGraw-Hill.

Freud, A. (1936). *The ego and mechanisms of defense*. New York: International Universities Press.

Freud, S. (1923). *The ego and the id*. London: Hogarth.

Fujita, M., and Sano, T. (1988). Children in American and Japanese day care centers: Ethnographic and reflective cross-cultural interviewing. In H. T. Trueba and C. Delgado-Gaitan (Eds.), *School and society: Learning content through culture* (pp. 76–89). New York: Praeger.

Gee, K. K., Du, N., Akiyama, K., & Lu, F. (1999). The Asian Focus

Unit at UCSF: An 18-year perspective. In J. Herrera, W. B. Lawson, and J. J. Sramek (Eds.), *Cross cultural psychiatry.* (pp. 275–285). Chichester, England: John Wiley & Sons.

Geertz, C. (1975). On the nature of anthropological understanding. *American Scientist*, 63:53–67.

Geissler, E. M. (1994). *Pocket guide to cultural assessment.* St. Louis: Mosby.

Gergen, K. J. (1991). *The saturated self: Dilemmas of identity in contemporary life.* New York: Basic Books..

Gergen, K. J., and Gergen, M. M. (1988). Narrative and the self as relationship. In L. Berkowitz (Ed.), *Advances in experimental social psychology* (Vol. 21). New York: Academic Press.

Giger, J., and Davidhizar, R. (1995). *Transcultural nursing: Assessment and intervention.* St. Louis: Mosby–Year Book.

Gilligan, C. (1986). Remapping the moral domain: New images of the self in relationship. In T. C. Heller, M. Sosna, and D. E. Wellbery (Eds.), *Reconstructing individualism: Autonomy, individuality, and the self in Western thought* (pp. 237–252). Stanford, CA: Stanford University Press.

Guarnaccia, P. J. (1999). Anthropological issues on ethnic units. In J. Herrera, W. B. Lawson, and J. J. Sramek (Eds.), *Cross cultural psychiatry* (pp. 303–312). Chichester, England: John Wiley & Sons.

Guarnaccia, P. J., Rivera, M., Franco, F., and Neighbors, C. (1996). The experiences of *ataques de nervios*: Towards an anthropology of emotions in Puerto Rico. *Culture, Medicine, and Psychiatry,* 20(3):343–367.

Holcomb-McCoy, C. C., and Myers, J. E. (1999). *Journal of Counseling and Development* 77(3):294–302.

Hsu, F. L. K. (1983). *Rugged individualism reconsidered.* Knoxville, TN: University of Tennessee Press.

Hughes, C. C., and Okpaku, S. O. (1998). Culture's role in clinical psychiatric assessment. In S. O. Okpaku (Ed.), *Clinical methods in transcultural psychiatry* (pp. 213–232). Washington, D.C.: American Psychiatric Press.

Jacob, K. S. (1999). Mental disorders across cultures: The common issues. *International Review of Psychiatry*, 11(2/3):111–115.

Jenkins, J. H., Kleinman, A., and Good, B. J. (1991). Cross-cultural studies of depression. In J. Becker and A. Kleinman (Eds.), *Psychosocial aspects of depression* (pp. 67–99). Hillsdale, NJ: Lawrence Erlbaum Associates.

Johnson, F. (1995). *Dependency and Japanese socialization.* New York: New York University Press.

Juss, S. S. (1999). Cultural competence and the law of mental health. In *Service provision for multicultural society.* Philadelphia: W. B. Saunders.

Kagitcibasi, C. (1989). Family and socialization in cross cultural perspectives: A model of change. In J. Berman (Ed.), *Nebraska symposium on motivation* (Vol. 37). Lincoln, NE: University of Nebraska Press.

Kavanaugh, K. (1995). Transcultural perspectives in mental health. In M. Andrews and J. Boyle (Eds.), *Transcultural concepts in nursing care* (2nd ed.) (pp. 153–285). Philadelphia: J. B. Lippincott.

Kernberg, O. (1976). *Object relations theory and clinical psychoanalysis.* New York: Jacob Aronson.

Kirmayer, L. J., Dao, T. H. T., and Smith, A. (1998). Somatization and psychologization: Understanding cultural idioms of distress. In S. O. Okpaku (Ed.), *Clinical methods in transcultural psychiatry* (pp. 233–265). Washington, D.C.: American Psychiatric Press.

Kleinman, A. (1987). Anthropology and psychiatry: The role of culture in cross-cultural research on illness. *British Journal of Psychiatry*, 151:447–454.

Kleinman, A. (1980). *Patients and healers in the context of culture.* Berkeley, CA: University of California Press.

Kleinman, A. (1988). *Rethinking psychiatry: From cultural category to personal experience.* New York: Free Press.

Koenig, H. G. (Ed.). (1998). *Handbook of religion and mental health.* San Diego, CA: Academic Press.

Lebra, T. S. (1992 June). *Culture, self, and communication.* Paper presented at the University of Michigan, Ann Arbor.

Lefley, H. P. (1999). Mental health systems in cross-cultural context. In A. V. Horwitz and T. L. Scheid (Eds.), *A handbook for the study of mental health: Social contexts, theories, and systems* (pp. 566–584). New York: Cambridge University Press.

Leighton, A. H. (1998). Recollections of culture and personality. In S. O. Okpaku (Ed.), *Clinical methods in transcultural psychiatry* (pp. 18–41). Washington, D.C.: American Psychiatric Press.

Levan, J. D. (1992). *Theories of the self.* Washington, D.C.: Taylor & Frances.

Lewis-Fernandez, R., and Kleinman, A. (1995). Cultural psychiatry: Theoretical, clinical, and research issues. *Psychiatric Clinics of North America*, 18(3):433–448.

Lykes, M. B. (1985). Gender and individualistic versus collectivist notions about the self. In A. J. Stewart and M. B. Lykes (Eds.), *Gender and personality: Current perspectives on theory and research* (pp. 269–295). Durham, NC: Duke University Press.

Lyons, N. P. (1983). Two perspectives: On self, relationships, and morality. *Harvard Educational Review*, 53(2):125–145.

MacLachlan, M. (1997). *Culture and health.* Chichester, England: John Wiley & Sons.

Mahler, M., Pine, F., and Bergman, A. (1975). *The psychological birth of the human infant: Symbiosis and individuation.* New York: Basic Books.

Markus, H., and Kitayama, S. (1991). Culture and the self: Implications for cognition, emotion, and motivation. *Psychological Review*, 98(2):224–253.

Markus, H., and Oyserman, D. (1989). Gender and thought: The role of the self-concept. In M. Crawford and M. Gentry (Eds.), *Gender and thought: Psychological perspectives* (pp. 100–127). New York: Springer-Verlag.

Mezzich, J. E., et al. (1999). The place of culture in DSM-IV. *Journal of Nervous and Mental Disease*, 187(18):457–464.

Mezzich, J. E., Kleinman, A., Fabrega, H., Jr., and Parron, D. L. (Eds.). (1996). *Culture and psychiatric diagnosis: A DSM-IV perspective.* Washington, D.C.: American Psychiatric Press.

Nichter, M. (1981). Idioms of distress: Alternatives in the expression of psychological distress. *Culture, Medicine, and Psychiatry*, 5:379–408.

Okasha, A. (1999). Mental health in the middle east: An Egyptian perspective [Special Issue: Mental health issues in Middle East societies]. *Clinical Psychology Review*, 19(8):917–933.

Pang, K. Y. C. (1998). Symptoms of depression in elderly Korean immigrants: Narration and the healing process. *Culture, Medicine, and Psychiatry*, 22(1):93–122.

Pierce, C. M., et al. (1999). Psychiatry and society. In A. M. Nicholi (Ed.), *The Harvard guide to psychiatry* (3rd ed.) (pp. 735–823). Cambridge, MA: Belknap Press/Harvard University Press.

Rapaport, D. (1960). On the psychoanalytic theory of motivation. In *Nebraska Symposium on Motivation* (pp. 173–247). Lincoln, NE: University of Nebraska Press.

Roland, A. (1988). *In search of the self in India and Japan: Toward a cross-cultural psychology.* Princeton, NJ: Princeton University Press.

Sahlins, M. (1996). Personal communication.

Saint Arnault, D. (1998). *Japanese company wives living in America: Culture, social relationships, and self* [Unpublished dissertation]. Detroit: Wayne State University.

Sampson, E. E. (1988). The debate of individualism: Indigenous psychologies of the individuals and their role in personal and social functioning. *American Psychologist*, 43:15–22.

Shweder, R. A., and Borne, E. J. (1984). Does the concept of person vary cross-culturally? In R. A. Shweder and R. A. LeVine (Eds.), *Culture theory: Essays on mind, self, and emotion* (pp. 158–199). Cambridge, England: Cambridge University Press.

Shweder, R. A., and Miller, J. G. (1991). The social construction of the person: How is it possible? In R. A. Shweder (Ed.), *Thinking through cultures: Expeditions in cultural psychology* (pp. 156–185). Cambridge, MA: Harvard University Press.

Singer, M. (1986). Toward a political-economy of alcoholism: The missing link in the anthropology of drinking [Special Issue: Toward a critical medical anthropology]. *Social Science and Medicine*, 23(2):113–130.

Singer, M., Valentin, F., Baer, H., and Jia, Z. (1992). Why does Juan Garcia have a drinking problem? The perspective of critical medical anthropology [Special Issue: The application of theory in medical anthropology]. *Medical Anthropology*, 14(1):77–108.

Spector, R. E. (1996). *Guide to heritage assessment and health traditions.* Stamford, CT: Appleton & Lange.

Spector, R. E. (2000). *Cultural diversity in health and illness* (5th ed.). Upper Saddle River, NJ: Prentice Hall Health.

Spindler, G., and Spindler, L. (1987). *Interpretive ethnography of education at home and abroad.* Hillsdale, NJ: Lawrence Erlbaum Associates.

St. Clair, A., and McKenry, L. (1999). Preparing for culturally competent practitioners. *Journal of Nursing Education,* 38(5):228–234.

Stoller, R. (1985). *Presentations of gender.* New Haven, CT: Yale University Press.

Triandis, H., et al. (1988). Individualism and collectivism: Cross-cultural perspectives on self in group relationships. *Journal of Personality and Social Psychology,* 54:323–338.

Tripp-Reimer, T., and Brink, P. J. (1985). Culture brokerage. In G. M. Bulechek and J. C. McCloskey (Eds.), *Nursing interventions* (pp. 352–364). Philadelphia: W. B. Saunders.

Worley, N. (1994). *Mental health nursing in the community* (unit 1). Providence, RI: Project ADEPT.

*T*hrough licensure, a state confers on the registered nurse (RN) the privilege of practicing the profession of nursing in that state. Nursing practice is regulated through licensure. A growing number of states specifically license psychiatric nurses as advanced practice registered nurses in psychiatric mental health (APRN-PMH). "An APRN-PMH is a licensed registered nurse who is educationally prepared either as a clinical nurse specialist or as a nurse practitioner at least at the master's degree level in the specialty of psychiatric–mental health nursing" (ANA, APNA, ISPN 2000, p. 17). Prescriptive authority licenses are also granted in some states to psychiatric nurse specialists and nurse practitioners. Implicit in this right to practice psychiatric nursing is the responsibility to practice safely and competently and in a manner consistent with state laws and regulations.

Each state has a licensing agency, a state board of nursing composed of experts in nursing as well as members of the public who are there to bring up public concerns. The state board of nursing establishes rules and regulations that specifically define the Nurse Practice Act of its state, and it is charged with the implementation of the Nurse Practice Act. The board also serves as the hearing panel in disciplinary matters.

This chapter introduces you to current legal and ethical issues that may be encountered in the practice of psychiatric nursing. Because the law is dynamic and evolving, it does not always lend itself to clear answers. Accordingly, in situations in which the law is not clearly stated by statute, regulation, or court decision, the nurse often encounters an *ethical dilemma* (a situation that requires a choice between morally conflicting alternatives).

The fundamental concept in any legal or ethical issue confronting the nurse in a psychiatric setting is striking the balance between the rights of the individual client and the rights of society at large. This chapter is designed to assist you in identifying competing ethical or legal interests involved in various nursing interventions and to help you consider their impact on decision making.

You are encouraged to be aware of the mental health statutes in your own state. These state codes are available through the State Department of Professional Licensure via State Boards of Nursing and often available on Websites.

LEGAL AND ETHICAL DILEMMAS IN MANAGED CARE

During the last decade **managed care** has become a household word in America. There are proponents and opponents of this new concept of how organizations manage the care of groups of patients. Some believe that the caregiver-patient relationship is threatened because the power is shifted to the organization through the control of resources that are expended on patient care. Some claim that ethical dilemmas are created when the cost of providing care becomes of prime importance versus the Hippocratic ideal that encourages care providers to put their client's welfare before the least costly alternative. The concerns that have been raised by managed care have resulted in both legal issues and compliance regulations as well as ethical dilemmas for providers who must practice within the guidelines and protocols of the managed care organization that pays for the patient's care.

On the other hand, proponents of managed care have pointed out the positive potential for nurses and patients as the shift of power is away from individual physicians and toward larger organizations for which nurses work. It is possible that nurses will have a greater influence on patient care through this reorganization of power. Additionally, more preventive care may be likely when a patient's health is being managed by an organization that wishes to see the patient remain healthy. For example, prenatal care and diabetic screening are an expectation of membership in most managed care organizations. The legal issues that have been most prominent since managed care became a way of life in our American society include the gatekeeping of resources available to the caregiver. Too frequently, health care resources have not been made available to the patient, which has been to the detriment of the patient's health. Also, the question of physicians receiving bonuses when costs are contained at the expense of patient care has been a legal challenge to managed care organizations. The current trend is away from having referrals to specialists so closely guarded by managed care agencies. The American public is demanding that they be treated more fairly by their health maintenance organization. The Patient's Bill of Rights Plus Act has been under consideration by the U.S. Congress in the latter part of the 1990s and into 2002. This consumer protection act promotes standards for more than 48 million Americans covered by self-funded group health plans. The act would also provide more information to the public regarding insurance plans as well as internal and external appeal rights for Americans covered by both self-insured and fully insured group health plans. The act would also attempt to protect the insurability of persons who have a predictive genetic diagnosis. Additionally, deductibility of health insurance fees and a focus on quality for health care policy and research are included in the proposed act (Volunteer Trustees 2000).

The major consumer protection elements of the Patient's Bill of Rights Plus Act include the "prudent layperson" standard for determining whether a patient's plan would be required to cover an emergency department visit out of his or her network for screening and stabilization. Plans would also be required to offer the option of allowing insured persons to purchase point of service coverage. This coverage would allow the insured more options outside of the plan's limited network. Continuity of care and access to specialists and medication are also important elements of the proposed act. Psychiatric mental health specialists and prescription drugs that are in the best interest of the patient will be affected by these proposed plans. If specialists are not available within the managed care plan's network, then it would be necessary to have a contractual arrangement with specialists outside the network to provide the needed care. The proposed act would prohibit gag rules that restrict providers from communicating with patients about their treatment options. Finally, plans that offer behavioral health services would be prohibited from barring a participant from self-paying for behavioral health care services. All plans would also have a grievance and appeals process in place for determining lack of medical necessity or experimental treatment by a provider who has expertise in the field involved. Enrollees and their authorized providers could also appeal to independent external medical reviewers for amounts above a significant financial threshold or where the enrollee's health is in jeopardy based on medical necessity.

ETHICAL CONCEPTS

Ethics is the study of philosophical beliefs about what is considered right or wrong in a society. Discussions of ethical practice in nursing involve the topics of morals and values. The term bioethics is used in relation to ethical dilemmas surrounding client care. Bioethics in psychiatric mental health nursing is the application of ethical principles within the scope of the psychiatric nursing practice setting.

The five principles of bioethics are discussed in the following list:

1. Beneficence is the duty to benefit or promote the good of others, for example, the decision to remain by the bedside of an extremely anxious client to be supportive, even if the shift has ended, until a replacement can be found.
2. Autonomy is the right to make one's own decisions and respect the rights of others to make their own decisions, for example, acknowledging the client's right to make decisions that do not conform with the recommendation of the staff.
3. Justice is the treating of others fairly and equally.
4. Fidelity (nonmaleficence) is the observance of loyalty and commitment to the client and doing no wrong to the client, for example, the commitment of the nurse to clinical expertise through participation in continuing education.
5. Veracity refers to one's duty to always tell the truth. Clients have the right to know about their diagnosis, treatment, and prognosis. There are times when limitation may be justified (when the truth would be knowingly harmful to a client).

Ethical decisions involve morals and values that may differ widely among decision makers. Therefore, it is important to respect and protect the client's autonomy and the client's right to be the ultimate decision maker about decisions that affect his or her life. You must avoid trying to impose personal values on the client. Your life experiences may be dramatically different from those of the client, and part of becoming a professional is developing the ability to recognize and accept the client's right to have an opinion that differs from your own.

At times, your values may be in conflict with the value system of the institution. This situation further complicates the decision-making process and necessitates careful consideration of the client's desires. For example, you may experience a conflict in a setting in which there is abundant use of tranquilizers for the treatment of an elderly or a depressed client. Whenever one's value system is challenged, increased stress results.

Within today's technological revolution, nurses and clients have more choices than ever, and ethical decisions are more complex than ever before. When faced with tough ethical decisions, you should use a number of resources, alone or in combination, that can help with the problem-solving process. These resources include the following (Dunn 1994):

- Legal advice
- American Nurses' Association (ANA) Code of Ethics
- Nurse Practice Acts
- Hospital and organizational policies
- Patient's Bill of Rights
- Colleagues
- Clergy
- Examination of one's own ideals and morals

Ethical standards, although lacking the clarity and power of law, do serve as a field guide for decision making. As each generation advances in knowledge and technology, society inherits increased options.

American Nurses' Association Code of Ethics

The ANA code (Box 8–1) provides helpful general guidelines for nurses dealing with ethical dilemmas. The distinction between legal and ethical issues is often vague. However, there is an important distinction when you rely on ethical guiding principles instead of the guiding principles of law. You are bound to comply with the laws, and even though you may feel morally obligated to follow ethical guidelines, these guiding principles should not override laws. For example, if you are aware of a statute, or of a specific rule or regulation created by the state board of nursing, that prohibits certain behavior (e.g., restraining clients against their will) and you feel you have an ethical obligation to protect the client by using restraints, you would be wise to follow the law. Laws override ethical principles, which do not have the same legal strength. However, ethical dilemmas can influence laws when society is concerned enough to take specific ethical issues to the courts or to the legislature.

Ethical issues become legal issues through court case decisions or when the legislature has heard from many people that a law is needed to protect certain rights.

BOX 8–1 *American Nurses' Association Code of Ethics for Nurses*

1. The nurse provides services with respect for human dignity and the uniqueness of the client unrestricted by considerations of social or economic status, personal attributes, or the nature of health problems.
2. The nurse safeguards the client's rights to privacy by judiciously protecting information of a confidential nature.
3. The nurse acts to safeguard the client and the public when health care and safety are affected by the incompetent, unethical, or illegal practice of any person.
4. The nurse assumes responsibility and accountability for individual nursing judgments and actions.
5. The nurse maintains competence in nursing.
6. The nurse exercises informed judgment and uses individual competence and qualifications as criteria in seeking consultation, accepting responsibilities, and delegating nursing activities to others.
7. The nurse participates in activities that contribute to the ongoing development of the profession's body of knowledge.
8. The nurse participates in the profession's efforts to implement and improve standards of nursing.
9. The nurse participates in the profession's efforts to establish and maintain conditions of employment conducive to high-quality nursing care.
10. The nurse participates in the profession's effort to protect the public from misinformation and misrepresentation and to maintain the integrity of nursing.
11. The nurse collaborates with members of the health professions and other citizens in promoting community and national efforts to meet the health needs of the public.

Modified from *Code for Nurses With Interpretive Statements,* © 1985. American Nurses Publishing, American Nurses Foundation/American Nurses Association, Washington, DC.

Mental Illness and the Social Norm

Social norms are known to every society, and most members of society conform to these norms. However, some members of society do not conform. What happens to them? Must all people conform? Does society need the nonconformist (the artist, the scientist, the inventor)? Does the majority have the right to impose its will on the individual?

What about the freedom of individuals to do what they want to do when they want to do it? When is the right of the individual curtailed for the benefit of society? Take, for example, the street lady who for years has been unobtrusively pilfering from trash containers every evening. This behavior, although not desirable, is acceptable. Eventually, she starts rummaging after midnight, and as the noise level escalates, the community responds by notifying authorities of the violation of the peace. What was once tolerable behavior becomes unacceptable.

What constitutes desirable or acceptable behavior of the individual is decided by the group (society) that establishes the norms. Methods of changing human behavior include behavior modification techniques and psychotherapy. Psychotropic drugs can also dramatically alter behavior and must therefore be prescribed carefully. Freedom of expression is a fundamental value of our society, a right embodied in the U.S. Constitution. Some hold the view that many psychiatric treatment modalities alter the individual's thought processes and thus challenge our fundamental societal values.

Responsibilities of the Therapeutic Relationship

The psychotherapeutic relationship carries with it serious ethical and legal obligations to the client. The psychotherapist becomes extremely important to the client and must assume this role conscientiously. Termination of the psychotherapeutic relationship can be traumatic to clients if the break is not handled skillfully. Nurse clinicians also have a legal and ethical obligation to the client and to society not to abuse the power that can exist when a client relies on them.

Protection of the client when he or she is in a vulnerable state of mind must be considered. Sadly, many therapeutic relationships are in the news because of sexual abuse of clients by therapists. This misuse of the therapeutic relationship constitutes grounds for losing a license and violates the ethical duty of fidelity to the client. Pennington and associates (1993) reported sexual intimacy as the primary boundary issue studied and reported among nurses in the literature, although it is not directly addressed in the ANA Code of Ethics. Boundary issues are covered in more depth in Chapter 10.

Protection of the confidentiality and privacy of the client's disclosures during therapeutic communication is also vitally important. Because of the complexity of human behavior, therapeutic relations may be long-lasting and complicated. Skilled nurse clinicians must have great insight into their own behavior as well as the client's behavior. Without self-awareness, nurses risk imposing their own value system upon the client. Issues of confidentiality are covered in more depth in Chapter 11.

MENTAL HEALTH LAWS

Laws have been enacted in each state to regulate the care and treatment of the mentally ill. Many of these laws have undergone major revision since 1963, reflecting a shift in emphasis from state institutional care of the mentally ill to community-based care. This was heralded by the enactment of the Community Mental Health Center Act of 1963 under President John Kennedy.

Along with this shift in emphasis has come the more widespread use of psychotropic drugs in the treatment of mental illness—enabling many people to integrate more readily into the larger community—and an increasing awareness of the need to provide the mentally ill with humane care that respects their civil rights.

Client's Civil Rights

Persons with mental illness are guaranteed the same rights under federal and state laws as any other citizen. Included in these are the right to treatment provided by the least restrictive means; the right to prompt medical care and treatment; the right to be free from hazardous procedures; and the right to dignity, privacy, and humane care.

The determination of legal competency is not necessarily the function of the psychiatric staff. Often the physician or another member of the health care team performs an assessment at the time consent is requested in consultation with other health professionals if there is an obvious mental disorder or a disease that affects the patient's mental functioning. Although courts hold a strong presumption of a patient's continued competency, the court may appoint a legal guardian or representative who is legally responsible for giving or refusing consent for a person the court has found to be incompetent. Court-appointed guardians must always consider the patient's wishes, if they are known, when the patient was still fully competent. For a legal guardian to be appointed, the court must first declare that the patient is incompetent and then appoint a guardian either temporarily or permanently. Guardians are usually selected from family members. The order of selection is usually (1) spouse, (2) adult children or grandchildren, (3) parents, (4) adult brothers and sisters, and (5) nieces and nephews. This order of selection has been supported by both state laws and court decisions (*Farber v Olkon* 1953 and *Mississippi Code Annotated* 1972).

The single most important action nurses can take to protect a client's rights is to be aware of the state laws regarding the care and treatment of the mentally ill in the state in which they practice. This includes knowledge of their institution's policies, as well as the Patient's Bill of Rights.

Patient's Bill Of Rights

CIVIL RIGHTS. Most states specifically prohibit any person from depriving a recipient of mental health services of his or her civil rights, including the right to vote; the right to civil service ranking; the rights related to granting, forfeit, or denial of license; and the right to make purchases and to enter contractual relationships (unless the client has lost legal capacity by being adjudicated incompetent). The psychiatric client's rights include the right to humane care and treatment. The medical, dental, and psychiatric needs of the client must be met in accordance with the prevailing standards accepted in these professions. The mentally ill in prisons and jails are afforded the same protections.

The right to religious freedom and practice, the right to social interaction, and the right to exercise and recreational opportunities are also protected.

CLIENT CONSENT. Proper orders for specific therapies and treatments are required and must be documented in the client's charts. Consent for surgery, electroconvulsive treatment, or the use of experimental drugs or procedures must be obtained. Clients have the right to refuse participation in experimental treatments or research and the right to voice grievances and recommend changes in policies or services offered by the facility, without fear of punishment or reprisal.

COMMUNICATION. Clients have the right to communicate fully and privately with those outside the facility. They have a right to have visitors, to have reasonable access to phones and mail, and to send as well as receive unopened correspondence. Clients may seek, at their own expense, consultation with other mental health professionals or attorneys. Clients may not be forced to work for the hospital, with the exception of being assigned routine duties that are developed to enhance their living abilities outside the agency. The rules and regulations of the hospital need to be explained to the client, and the client needs to have reasonable access for communicating with persons outside the hospital.

FREEDOM FROM HARM. Most state laws also provide for the right to be free from harm, which includes freedom from unnecessary or excessive physical restraint, isolation, medication, abuse, or neglect. Use of medications for staff convenience, as a punishment, or as a substitute for treatment programs is explicitly prohibited.

DIGNITY AND RESPECT. Clients in psychiatric hospitals have the right to be treated with dignity and respect. These rights are not only ethically important but also legally protected. Clients have the right to be free from discrimination on the basis of ethnic origin, gender, age, disability, or religion.

CONFIDENTIALITY. Confidentiality of care and treatment is also an important right for all clients, particularly psychiatric clients. The client's records must be treated as confidential by the staff. Photographs may not be taken without the client's written consent. The client's privacy is protected along with the confidentiality of the treatment. Any discussion or consultation involving a client should be conducted discreetly and only with individuals who have a need and a right to know this privileged information. Discussions about a client in public places such as elevators and the cafeteria, even when the client's name is not mentioned, can lead to disclosures of confidential information and liabilities for you and the hospital.

The client's permission must be given to share information with persons who are not directly involved in his or her care. These protections also apply to the client's medical record, which should be read only by individuals directly involved in the client's treatment or in monitoring the quality of care given. Clients must issue a written authorization to allow others to read their medical record. They have a right to expect that all communications and other records relating to treatment are treated as confidential. Institutions that use computerized records must safeguard against intrusion into their client record systems. This issue of client confidentiality is discussed in more detail later in the chapter.

PARTICIPATION IN THEIR PLAN OF CARE. Additional rights the psychiatric client enjoys include a written individualized treatment plan that is reviewed regularly and that involves the client in the planning decisions. Clients are also entitled to a discharge plan that includes follow-up care or continuing care requirements. The treatment plan needs to include the least restrictive treatment environment that is appropriate. Reasonable safety is an expectation of this environment. If the client is unable to make these decisions, the person legally authorized to act on the client's behalf must be consulted.

Clients have the right to be informed by their physician of the benefits, risks, and side effects of all medications and treatment procedures used. **They cannot be subjected to any procedure or treatment without their consent, or a battery will have occurred.** (Assault is the threat of harm or putting a person in a state of apprehension; battery is the actual contact with the person. These principles are discussed in greater detail later in this chapter.) Refer to Chapter 5 for a sample copy of a Patient's Bill of Rights.

ADMISSION, COMMITMENT, AND DISCHARGE PROCEDURES

Due Process in Civil Commitment

The courts have recognized that involuntary civil commitment to a mental hospital is a "massive curtailment of liberty" (*Humphrey v. Cady* 1972, p. 509) requiring due process protections in the civil commitment procedure. This right derives from the Fifth Amendment of the U.S. Constitution, which states that "no person shall . . . be deprived of life, liberty, or property without due process of law." The Fourteenth Amendment explicitly prohibits states from depriving citizens of life, liberty, and property without due process of law. State civil commitment statutes, if challenged in the courts on constitutional grounds, will have to afford minimal due process protections to pass the court's scrutiny.

In most states, a client can institute a court proceeding to seek a judicial discharge. This is referred to as a *writ of habeas corpus*, meaning, "free the person." The writ of habeas corpus is the procedural mechanism used to challenge unlawful detention by the government.

The writ of habeas corpus and the *least restrictive alternative doctrine* are two of the most important concepts applicable to civic commitment cases. The least restrictive alternative doctrine mandates that the least drastic means be taken to achieve a specific purpose.

Admission to the Hospital

All students are encouraged to become familiar with the important provisions of the laws in their own states regarding admissions, discharges, client's rights, and informed consent. Either voluntary or involuntary admission to a mental facility does not determine whether patients are capable of making informed decisions about the health care they may need to receive. The involuntarily committed patient is considered to be capable of consenting to treatment, unless a judicial determination has been made or the patient lacks the capacity to understand the implications of his or her decision. Involuntary commitment also requires that the patient retain freedom from unreasonable bodily restraints and the right to refuse medications, including psychotropic or antipsychotic medications.

A medical standard or justification for admission should exist. A well-defined psychiatric problem must be established, based on current *Diagnostic and Statistical Manual of Mental Disorders, Fourth Edition*, Text Revised (DSM-IV-TR) illness classifications. The presenting illness should also be of such a nature that other less restrictive alternatives are inadequate or unavailable or cause an immediate crisis situation. There should also be a reasonable expectation that the hospitalization will improve the presenting problems.

Voluntary Admission

Generally, *voluntary admission* is sought by the client or the client's guardian through a written application to the facility. Voluntary clients have the right to demand and obtain release. If the client is a minor, the release may be contingent on the consent of the parents or guardian. However, few states require voluntary clients to be notified of the rights associated with their status. In addition, many states require that a client submit a written release notice to the facility staff, who re-evaluate the client's condition for possible conversion to involuntary status according to criteria established by the state law.

Involuntary Admission (Commitment)

Involuntary admission is made without the client's consent. Generally, involuntary admission is necessary when a person is a danger to self or others, is in need of psychiatric treatment, or is unable to meet his or her own basic needs. Three different commitment procedures are commonly available: judicial determination, administrative determination, and agency determination. Additionally, a specified number of physicians must certify that a person's mental health status justifies detention and treatment.

Involuntary hospitalization can be further categorized by the nature and purpose of the involuntary admission. It may be emergency, observational or temporary, or indeterminate or extended.

■ **Emergency involuntary hospitalization.** Most states provide for emergency involuntary hospitalization or civil commitment for a specified period (1 to 10 days on average) to prevent dangerous behavior that is likely to cause harm to self or others. Police officers, physicians, and mental health professionals may be designated by statute to authorize the detention of mentally ill persons who are dangers to themselves or others.

■ **Observational or temporary involuntary hospitalization.** Civil commitment for observational or temporary involuntary hospitalization is of longer duration than emergency hospitalization. The primary purpose of this type of hospitalization is the observation, diagnosis, and treatment of persons who suffer from mental illness or pose a danger to themselves or others. The length of time is specified by statute and varies markedly from state to state. Application for this type of admission can be made by a guardian, family member, physician, or other public health officer. States vary as to their procedural requirements for this type of involuntary admission. Medical certification by two or more physicians that a person is mentally ill and in need of treatment or a judicial or administrative review and order is often required for involuntary admission.

■ **Long-term or formal commitment.** Long-term commitment for involuntary hospitalization has as its primary purpose extended care and treatment of the mentally ill. Like clients who undergo observational involuntary hospitalization, those who undergo extended involuntary hospitalization are committed solely through judicial or administrative action or medical certification. States that do not require a judicial hearing before commitment often provide the client with an opportunity for a judicial review after commitment procedures. This type of involuntary hospitalization generally lasts 60 to 180 days, but it may be for an indeterminate period.

Clients who are involuntarily committed do not lose their right of informed consent. Clients must be considered legally competent until they have been declared incompetent through a legal proceeding. Competency is related to the capacity to understand the consequences of one's decisions. If the psychiatric nurse believes a client lacks this ability, action should be initiated to have a legal guardian appointed by the court.

Release from the Hospital

Release from hospitalization depends on the client's admission status. Clients who sought informal or voluntary admission, as previously discussed, have the right to demand and receive release. Some states, however, do provide for conditional release of voluntary clients, which enables the treating physician or administrator to order continued treatment on an outpatient basis if the clinical needs of the client warrant further care.

Conditional Release

Conditional release usually requires outpatient treatment for a specified period to determine the client's compliance with medication protocols, ability to meet basic needs, and ability to reintegrate into the community. Generally, a voluntary client who is conditionally released cannot be re-institutionalized without consent unless the institution complies with the procedures for involuntary hospitalization. However, an involuntary client who is conditionally released may be re-institutionalized while the commitment is still in effect without recommencement of formal admission procedures.

Discharge

Discharge, or unconditional release, is the termination of a client-institution relationship. This release may be court ordered or administratively ordered by the institution's officials. Generally, the administrative officer of an institution has the discretion to discharge clients.

CLIENT'S RIGHTS UNDER THE LAW

Right to Treatment

With the enactment of the Hospitalization of the Mentally Ill Act in 1964, the federal statutory right to psychiatric treatment in public hospitals was created. The statute requires that "a person hospitalized in a public hospital for a mental illness shall, during his hospitalization, be entitled to medical and psychiatric care and treatment."

Although state courts and lower federal courts have decided that there may be a federal constitutional right to treatment, the U.S. Supreme Court has never firmly grounded the right to treatment in a constitutional principle. The evolution of these cases in the courts provides an interesting history of the development and shortcomings of our mental health delivery system. Through the decision of a number of early court cases, treatment must meet the following criteria:

■ The environment must be humane
■ Staff must be qualified and sufficient to provide adequate treatment
■ The plan of care must be individualized

The initial cases presenting the psychiatric client's right to treatment arose in the criminal justice system. An interesting case regarding a person's right to treatment is *O'Connor v. Donaldson* (1975) (Box 8–2).

The U.S. Supreme Court, in declining to affirm the lower court's finding of damages and a broad constitutional right to treatment, narrowly defined the issue for consideration: whether or not a finding of mental illness alone can justify the state's indefinite custodial confinement of a mentally ill person against his or her will. The Court held that a "state cannot constitutionally confine a nondangerous individual who is capable of surviving safely in freedom by himself or with the help of willing and responsible family members or friends" (*O'Connor v. Donaldson* 1975, p. 576).

Right to Refuse Treatment

A corollary to the right to consent to treatment is the right to withhold consent. A client may also withdraw consent at any time. Retraction of consent previously given must be honored, whether it is a verbal or written retraction. However, the mentally ill client's right to refuse treatment with psycho-

Box 8–2 *Right to Treatment:* O'Connor v. Donaldson (1975)

In 1957, Mr. Donaldson was involuntarily committed, on his father's initiation, to a Florida state hospital for care, treatment, and maintenance. For 14 years before his commitment, he was gainfully employed. Despite the fact that Mr. Donaldson posed no danger to himself or others, his requests for ground privileges, occupational training, and an opportunity to discuss his case with the superintendent, Dr. O'Connor, or others were denied. During his 15 years of confinement, he was not provided with any treatment.

Mr. Donaldson frequently requested his release, which the superintendent was authorized to grant even though Mr. Donaldson was lawfully confined, because even if he continued to be mentally ill, he posed no danger to himself or others. Between 1964 and 1968, Mr. Donaldson's friend requested on four separate occasions that he be released into his custody. These requests, and requests made by a halfway house on Mr. Donaldson's behalf, were all denied by Dr. O'Connor, who believed that Mr. Donaldson should be released into his parents' custody. Dr. O'Connor further believed that Mr. Donaldson's parents were too old and infirm to care for him adequately.

The court found that Mr. Donaldson's care was merely custodial because he received no treatment. He was not dangerous, community alternatives were available for him, and the physician's refusal to release him was "malicious." The Federal Court of Appeals ruled that Mr. Donaldson had a constitutional right to treatment and awarded him $38,000 in damages.

tropic drugs has been debated in the courts, turning partly on the issue of mental clients' competency to give or withhold consent to treatment and their status under the civil commitment statutes. These early cases, initiated by state hospital clients, consider principles of constitutional law, balancing competing state interests and societal interests against the client's interest in autonomy and self-determination, in the face of the often permanent and disfiguring side effects of psychotropic drugs. The analyses in these cases included medical, legal, and ethical considerations, such as basic treatment problems, the doctrine of informed consent, and the bioethical principle of autonomy. For a summary of the evolution of one landmark case regarding the client's right to refuse treatment, see Table 8–1.

In instances in which forcible medication is sought to prevent violence to third persons, to prevent suicide, or to preserve security, the court noted that the medication is being used as a chemical restraint, and the justification for medication thus changes from individual treatment to public protection. Accordingly, the infringement on a person's liberty is at least equal to that with involuntary commitment. In this circumstance, the noninstitutionalized, incompetent, mentally ill client has the right, through substituted judgment, to determine whether to be involuntarily committed or to be medicated.

In New Jersey, involuntarily committed psychiatric clients also brought a suit in federal court alleging violation of their constitutional rights through forcible administration of antipsychotic drugs. See Table 8–2 for a summary of the evolution of the *Rennie v. Klein* (1979) case.

An interesting study by Schwartz and colleagues (1988) of patients' attitudes after involuntary medication concluded that the decision to refuse treatment was based more on symptoms of the patients' illness rather than autonomous functioning.

Cases involving the right to refuse psychotropic drug treatment are still evolving. Without clear direction from the Supreme Court, there will be different case outcomes in different jurisdictions.

In the 1989 case of *State of Washington v. Harper*, the Supreme Court addressed the issue of whether mentally ill prisoners' refusal of medication can be overridden by administrative procedures or whether a full judicial hearing is required. The court held that the State of Washington Department of Corrections policy provided adequate due process protections and that prisoners were not entitled to a separate judicial hearing on the right to refuse medication. The court did not address the rights of involuntarily committed mentally ill clients.

A 1999 case, *Rabenberg v. Rigney*, held that a mental health facility had the authority to involuntarily medicate a patient who had been diagnosed with chronic paranoid schizophrenia. The patient was unable to make a competent, informed, and voluntary decision about his need for medication. He suffered from delusions and his perceptions of reality, emotional process, judgment, and behavior had been impaired because of his mental illness. The patient had refused to attend treatment team meetings or to discuss medication needs. The court in this case stated that the medication determinations and treatment plans are best left to the appropriate professionals, not the court.

The numerous cases on the right to refuse medication have illustrated the complex and difficult task of translating social policy concerns into a clearly articulated legal standard.

TABLE 8−1 *Right to Refuse Treatment: Evolution of Massachusetts Case Law to Present Law*

CASE	COURT	DECISION
Rogers v. Okin, 478 F Supp 1342 (D Mass 1979)	Federal District Court	Involuntary mental patients are competent and have the right to make treatment decisions. Forcible administration of medication is justified in an emergency if needed to prevent violence and if other alternatives have been ruled out. A guardian may make treatment decisions for an incompetent client.
Rogers v. Okin, 634 F2nd 650 (1st Cir 1980)	Federal Court of Appeals	Affirmed that involuntary mental patients are competent and have the right to make treatment decisions. The staff has substantial discretion in an emergency. Forcible medication is also justified to prevent the client's deterioration. A client's rights must be protected by judicial determination of incompetency.
Mills v. Rogers, 457 US 291 (1982)	U.S. Supreme Court	Set aside the judgment of the Court of Appeals with instructions to consider the effect of an intervening state court case.
Rogers v. Commissioner of the Department of Mental Health, 458 NE 2d 308 (Mass 1983)	Massachusetts Supreme Judicial Court answering questions certified by Federal Court of Appeals	Involuntary clients are competent and have the right to make treatment decisions unless they are judicially determined to be incompetent.

TABLE 8−2 *Right to Refuse Treatment: Evolution of New Jersey Case Law to Present Law*

CASE	COURT	DECISION
Rennie v. Klein, 476 F Supp 1294 (D NJ 1979)	Federal District Court	Involuntary mental patients have a qualified constitutional right to refuse treatment with antipsychotic drugs. Voluntary clients have an absolute right to refuse treatment with antipsychotic drugs under New Jersey law.
Rennie v. Klein, 653 F2d 836 (3rd Cir 1981)	Federal Court of Appeals	Involuntary mental patients have a constitutional right to refuse antipsychotic drug treatment. The state may override a client's right when the client poses a danger to self or others. Due process protections are required before forcible medication of clients in nonemergency situations.
Rennie v. Klein, 454 US 1078 (1982)	U.S. Supreme Court	Set aside the judgment of the Court of Appeals with instructions to consider the case in light of the U.S. Supreme Court decision in *Youngberg v. Romeo*.
Rennie v. Klein, 720 F2d 266 (3rd Cir 1983)	Federal Court of Appeals	Involuntary mental patients have the right to refuse treatment with antipsychotic medication. Decisions to forcibly medicate must be based on "accepted professional judgment" and must comply with due process requirements of the New Jersey regulations.

Right to Informed Consent

The principle of informed consent is based on a person's right to self-determination, as enunciated in the landmark case of *Canterbury v. Spence* (1972, p. 780).

> The root premise is the concept, fundamental in American jurisprudence, that every human being of adult years and sound mind has a right to determine what shall be done with his own body. . . . True consent to what happens to one's self is the informed exercise of choice, and that entails an opportunity to evaluate knowledgeably the options available and the risks attendant on each.

For consent to be effective legally, it must be informed. Generally, the informed consent of the client must be obtained by the physician or other health professional to perform the treatment or procedure. Clients must be informed of the nature of their problem or condition, the nature and purpose of a proposed treatment, the risks and benefits of that treatment, the alternative treatment options, the probability that the proposed treatment will be successful, and the risks of not consenting to treatment.

Because psychiatric mental health nursing procedures are generally noninvasive and are commonly understood by the client, the need for you to obtain informed consent does not occur as frequently as it does in the setting of medical treatment. Many procedures that nurses perform have an element of implied consent attached. For example, if you approach the client with a medication in hand and the client indicates a willingness to receive the medication, implied consent has occurred. A general rule for you to follow is that the more intrusive or risky the procedure, the higher is the likelihood that informed consent must be obtained. The fact that you may not have a legal duty to be the person to inform the client of the associated risks and benefits of a particular medical procedure does not excuse you from clarifying the procedure to the client and ensuring his or her expressed or implied consent.

Rights Regarding Restraint and Seclusion

Legally, behavioral restraint and seclusion are authorized as an intervention

- When the particular behavior is physically harmful to the client or a third party
- When the disruptive behavior presents a danger to the facility

- When alternative or less restrictive measures are insufficient in protecting the client or others from harm
- When a decrease in sensory overstimulation (seclusion only) is needed
- When the client anticipates that a controlled environment would be helpful and requests seclusion

As indicated, most state laws prohibit the use of unnecessary physical restraint or isolation. The use of seclusion and restraint is permitted only (Simon 1999)

- On the written order of a physician
- When orders are confined to specific time-limited periods (e.g., every 2 to 4 hours)
- When the client's condition is reviewed and documented regularly (e.g., every 15 minutes)
- When the original order is extended after review and reauthorization (e.g., every 24 hours) and specifies the type of restraint

Only in an emergency may the charge nurse place a client in seclusion or restraint and obtain a written or verbal order as soon as possible thereafter. Federal laws require the consent of the client unless an emergency situation exists in which an immediate risk of harm to the client or others can be documented. The client must be removed from restraints when safer and quieter behavior is observed. While in restraints, the client must be protected from all sources of harm. Document the behavior leading to restraint or seclusion and the time the client is placed in and released from restraint. Assess the client in restraint at regular and frequent intervals (e.g., every 15 to 30 minutes) for physical needs (food, hydration, toileting), safety, and comfort, and also document these observations (every 15 to 30 minutes).

Restraint and seclusion should never be used as punishment or for the convenience of the staff. For example, if the unit is short staffed, restraining clients to protect them while you pass medications is an inappropriate use of restraints.

The least restrictive means of restraint for the shortest duration is always the general rule. Verbal interventions are the first approach; restraints are used only to prevent harm or to provide benefit to the client. Chemical restraints are more subtle than physical restraints but can have a greater impact on the client's ability to relate to the environment. The psychiatric mental health nurse must be aware of the severe and powerful impact of chemical restraints on psychiatric clients. The client's personality and ability to relate to others is greatly controlled by chemical restraints. The practice of secluding a client is comparable with the practice of

Box 8–3   *Contraindications to Seclusion and Restraint*

1. Extremely unstable medical and psychiatric conditions*
2. Delirious or demented patients unable to tolerate decreased stimulation*
3. Overly suicidal patients*
4. Patients with severe drug reactions or overdoses or those patients requiring close monitoring of drug dosages*
5. Punishment or for convenience of staff

---

*Unless close supervision and direct observation are provided.
From Simon, R. I. (1992). *Concise guide to clinical psychiatry and law for clinicians* (3rd ed.) Washington, D.C.: American Psychiatric Press. Copyright 1992, American Psychiatric Press, Inc., p. 117.

sedating a client until the client is secluded within himself or herself.

An example of the misuse of chemical restraints is a case in which a verbally abusive or pacing client is deeply sedated and placed in his or her room to control the unit's environment. You must always be able to document professional judgment regarding the use of physical or chemical restraint, as well as the use of seclusion.

With recent changes in the law regarding the use of restraint and seclusion that require a client's consent to be restrained, agencies have revised their policies and procedures, greatly limiting these practices of the past. Most agencies have found no negative impact associated with the reduced use of restraints and seclusion. Alternative methods of therapy and cooperation with the client have been successful.

Nurses also need to know in which circumstances seclusion and restraints are contraindicated. Refer to Box 8–3 for specific examples.

TORT LAW APPLIED TO PSYCHIATRIC SETTINGS

Torts are civil wrongs for which money damages are collected by the injured party (the plaintiff) from the wrongdoer (the defendant). The injury can be to persons, property, or reputations. Because tort law has general applicability to nursing practice, this section may contain a review of material previously covered elsewhere in your nursing curriculum.

In a psychiatric setting, nurses are more likely to encounter provocative, threatening, or violent behavior. Such behavior may require the use of restraint or seclusion until a client demonstrates quieter and safer behavior. Accordingly, the nurse in the psychiatric setting should understand the intentional torts of battery, assault, and false imprisonment, described more fully later in this chapter

Common Liability Issues

Protecting Clients

Legal issues common in psychiatric nursing relate to the failure to protect the safety of clients. If a suicidal client is left alone with the means to harm himself or herself, the nurse who has a duty to protect the client will be held responsible for the resultant injuries. Leaving a suicidal client alone in a room on the sixth floor with an open window is an example of unreasonable judgment on the part of the nurse. Precautions to prevent harm must be taken whenever a client is restrained. Miscommunications and medication errors are common in all areas of nursing, including psychiatric care. A common area of liability in psychiatry revolves around abuse of the therapist-client relationship. Issues of sexual misconduct during the therapeutic relationship have become a source of concern among the psychiatric community. Misdiagnosis is also frequently charged in legal suits.

Defamation of Character

Charges of defamation of character, either written (libel) or oral (slander), can be brought if confidential information regarding clients is divulged that harms their reputation. The privacy protections afforded all clients by the law are especially protective of the rights of psychiatric clients.

Supervisory Liability

Supervisory liability may be incurred if nursing duties are delegated to persons who cannot safely perform these duties. The nurse who does not verify that the assistive personnel can safely and appropriately provide the care being delegated will be held vicariously liable for any harm or injury the client suffers. Supervision of assistive personnel is essential. Supervisors are no longer protected under the National Labor Relations Act because of a ruling that held they were closely aligned with employers in these roles and therefore fell outside the bargaining units of organized unions. This ruling makes it even more important that nurses who delegate tasks to others clarify whether or not they will be considered supervisors and therefore outside the protections of the employee bargaining unit.

Short-Staffing Issues

Short-staffing issues have raised concerns about client safety as well as of delegation to assistive personnel. A study by the ANA **(ANA 1996)** found that hospitalized patients have better outcomes in hospitals with higher ratios of RNs. "RN care makes the difference in reducing complications and allowing patients to be discharged . . . on the path to recovery."

If you believe that a staffing pattern is not allowing appropriate and reasonable care, a written appeal to the nurse's supervisor and the institution will document your concerns. Nurses should not perform tasks for which they are not prepared, including the assumption of responsibility for the safety and care of an unreasonable number of clients. If the institution is unwilling to correct an unsafe situation, you must determine whether you wish to remain employed and incur possible liability if a client for whom you are ultimately responsible is injured. Proper channels of appeal must be followed to avoid charges of insubordination and possible firing. Institutional policies should outline the correct procedure for voicing a reasonable grievance.

However, note that the ANA believes that nurses should reject assignments that put patients or themselves in serious immediate jeopardy, even when there is not a specific legal protection for rejecting such an assignment (ANA 1996).

There are constant changes in the health care system and in those who use it. One area of concern is that in many parts of the United States nurses are often asked to work outside the scope of their license because of decreased hiring of RNs and an increase in hiring of unlicensed personnel and licensed practical nurses (LPNs). It is important for nurses to keep in mind that they must not work outside the scope of their license. In many states an LPN license is forfeited when the nurse becomes an RN. If the nurse is hired in an LPN position, even though an RN license is held, it is likely that the nurse will be held to the standards of care of an RN. This situation may place nurses in the position of working beyond the scope of their present employment. This is a conflict that must be resolved by the nurse, the state board of nursing, and the employer on a state-by-state basis.

Some guidelines for avoiding liability include the following:

1. Always put the client's rights and welfare first.
2. Observe the hospital's or agency's policy manual.
3. Practice within the scope of the Nurse Practice Act.
4. Maintain current understanding and knowledge of established practice standards.
5. Keep accurate, concise, and timely nursing records.

Forensic Nursing

Forensic means pertaining to the law or the science of augmentation and debate. Forensic nurses provide direct service to individual crime victims as well as those accused of or incarcerated for crimes and law enforcement agencies. In collaboration with physicians, health care providers, and the police, forensic nurses work within the justice system dealing with trauma, death investigations, and stress disorders. Forensic nurses may serve as medical examiners or death investigators who assist with autopsies and exhumations in some states.

The application of forensic and nursing sciences to the legal process primarily relates to violence, sexual assault, abuse, or criminal activities. Forensic nurses are educated to recognize patterns of injuries as well as to collect evidence such as DNA and human bite marks. Forensic nurses provide documentation through photographs and also provide psychological intervention to assess trauma at crime scenes and disaster sites (Lynch 1995).

A forensic nurse can serve as an expert witness regarding the defendant's competency to stand trial if an insanity plea is entered. The court must decide whether the accused was competent to understand the consequences of his or her actions and that he or she were committing a crime. The insanity plea (*not guilty by reason of insanity*) has been supplemented in many states with a plea of *guilty but mentally ill*. The reason for this new plea alternative where a crime has been committed, yet the accused has been found to be not competent to understand the ramifications of his or her behavior, is to protect society from potentially violent person while at the same time protecting the rights of the accused who has been found guilty but insane. Previously, the *insanity defense* protected the accused from facing incarceration; now these pleas of guilty but mentally ill result in having the defendant placed in a secured facility where treatment is available and society is kept safe.

Several colleges of nursing throughout the country offer forensic nursing courses. A multidisciplinary faculty including forensic pathologists, psychologists, physicians, forensic nurses, criminologists, law enforcement officers, and attorneys are involved as faculty members in these nursing programs. The American Association of Nursing (ANA) recognized forensic nursing as a specialty at the Congress of Nursing Practice in 1997. Forensic nursing has been identified as one of the four critical areas for development in nursing education, practice, and research (Marullo 1996). Along with the role as a sexual assault examiner, forensic nurses are involved in identifying and investigating human rights violations. Increasingly, forensic nurses are working to help governments promote justice, including international crime prevention (Weaver and Lynch 1998). The epidemic of violence in our society, which is increasingly being recognized as a major public health problem, will increase the need for forensic nurses (Lynch 1996). Refer to Chapter 32 for additional discussion on forensic nursing and Unit VII A Nurse Speaks.

Intentional Torts

Torts are a category of civil law that commonly applies to health care practice. Some torts can also carry criminal penalties. **An intentional tort requires a voluntary act and an intent to bring about a physical consequence.** In the most basic terms, a voluntary act is a voluntary movement of the body. The requirement for intent is met when the defendant acts purposefully to achieve a result or is substantially certain that the result will occur. If the injured party consents to participate in an act, there can be no intentional tort. Likewise, self-defense and defense of others are privileges that can be used to defend successfully against a court action for intentional torts. Reckless behavior may be classified as intentional or negligent. Malpractice actions typically result from negligent behavior. For example, the foreseeability that a suicidal client will harm himself or herself if left alone with sharp objects or an open window is great enough for negligence to be found on the part of the nurse, who has a duty to protect the client. If the nurse left the client alone, knowing of the likelihood of self-harm, an intentional decision could be argued. It would not be a wise nursing judgment to test the suicidal client's ability to be left alone with dangers in the immediate environment.

Assault and Battery

An **assault** is an act resulting in a person's apprehension of an immediate harmful or offensive touching (battery). In an assault, there is no physical contact. The aggressor's act must amount to a threat to use force, although threatening words alone are not enough. The aggressor must also have the opportu-

nity and the ability to carry out the threatened act immediately. A **battery** is a harmful or offensive touching of another's person. For example, the nurse approaches the client with a restraint in hand. The client fearfully pleads not to be restrained. If the nurse proceeds to apply the restraints, both an assault and a battery may be charged against the nurse.

False Imprisonment

False imprisonment is an act with the intent to confine a person to a specific area. The use of seclusion or restraint that is not defensible as being necessary and in the client's best interest may result in false imprisonment of the client and liability for the nurse. As another example, if a psychiatric client wants to leave the hospital and the nurse prohibits the client from leaving, the nurse may have falsely imprisoned the client if the client was voluntarily admitted and if there are no agency or legal policies for detaining the client. On the other hand, if the client was involuntarily admitted or had agreed to an evaluation before discharge, the nurse's actions would be reasonable.

Punitive Damages

Punitive damages may be recoverable by an injured party in an intentional tort action. Because these damages are designed to punish and make an example, punitive damage awards can be very large. Often, the plaintiff's actual damages are insignificant, and nominal damages may be awarded in the sum of $1.00. However, intentional acts are not covered by malpractice insurance, which makes intentional torts a less attractive theory of liability for injured clients to pursue against health professionals and hospitals. The case of *Plumadore v. State of New York* (1980) (Box 8–4) illustrates the use of intentional tort in the psychiatric setting.

Violence

Violent behavior is not acceptable in our society. Nurses must protect themselves in both institutional and community settings. Employers are not typically held responsible for employee injuries due to violent client behavior. Nurses have placed themselves knowingly in the range of danger by agreeing to care for unpredictable clients. It is therefore important for nurses to protect themselves by participating in setting policies that create a safe environment. Good judgment means not placing oneself in a potentially violent situation. Nurses, as citizens, have

BOX 8–4 *False Imprisonment and Negligence:* Plumadore v. State of New York (1980)

Mrs. Plumadore was admitted to Saranac Lake General Hospital for a gallbladder condition. Her medical work-up revealed emotional problems stemming from marital difficulties, which had resulted in suicide attempts several years before her admission. After a series of consultations and tests, she was advised by the attending surgeon that she was scheduled to have gallbladder surgery later that day. After the surgeon's visit, a consulting psychiatrist who examined her directed her to dress and pack her belongings because he had arranged to have her admitted to a state hospital at Ogdensburg.

Subsequently, two uniformed state troopers handcuffed her and strapped her into the back seat of a patrol car. She was also accompanied by a female hospital employee and was transported to the state hospital. On arrival, the admitting psychiatrist recognized that the referring psychiatrist lacked the requisite authority to order her involuntary commitment. He therefore requested that she sign a voluntary admission form, which she refused to do. Despite Mrs. Plumadore's protests regarding her admission to the state hospital, the psychiatrist assigned her to a ward without physical or psychiatric examination and without the opportunity to contact her family or her medical doctor. The record of her admission to the state hospital noted an "informed admission," which is the patient-initiated voluntary admission in New York.

The court awarded $40,000 to Mrs. Plumadore for false imprisonment, negligence, and malpractice.

the same rights as clients not to be threatened or harmed. Appropriate security support should be readily available to the nurse practicing in an institution. When you work in community settings, you must avoid placing yourself unnecessarily in dangerous settings, especially when alone at night. You should use common sense and enlist the support of local law enforcement officers when needed. A violent client is not being abandoned if placed safely in the hands of the authorities.

The psychiatric mental health nurse must also be aware of the potential for violence in the community when a patient is discharged following a short-term stay. The duty of the nurse to protect both the patient as well as others who may be threatened by the violent client is discussed in the section Duty to Warn and Protect Third Parties later in this chapter. The nurse's assessment of the patient's potential for

violence must be documented and acted on if there is legitimate concern for discharge of a patient who is discussing or exhibiting potentially violent behavior. The psychiatric mental health nurse must communicate his or her observations to the medical staff when discharge decisions are being considered.

There may be situations in which your duty is to protect not only the patient but also, indirectly, third parties, when the patient, because of his or her mental or physical condition, presents a risk of harm to that third party.

Negligence

Negligence is an act or an omission to act that breaches the duty of due care and results in or is responsible for a person's injuries. The five elements required to prove negligence are (1) duty, (2) breach of duty, (3) cause in fact, (4) proximate cause, and (5) damages. Foreseeability of harm is also evaluated.

Duty is measured by a standard of care. When nurses represent themselves as being capable of caring for psychiatric clients and accept employment, a duty of care has been assumed. The duty is owed to psychiatric clients to understand the theory and medications used in the specialty care of these clients. Persons who represent themselves as possessing superior knowledge and skill, such as psychiatric nurse specialists, are held to a higher standard of care in the practice of their profession. The staff nurse who is assigned to a psychiatric unit must be knowledgeable enough to assume a reasonable or safe duty of care to the clients.

If you are not capable of providing the standard of care that other nurses would be expected to supply under similar circumstances, you have breached the duty of care. **Breach of duty** is the conduct that exposes the client to an unreasonable risk of harm, through either commission or omission of acts on the part of the nurse. If you do not have the required education and experience to provide certain interventions, you have breached the duty by neglecting or omitting to provide necessary care. You can also act in such a way that the client is harmed and can thus be guilty of negligence through acts of commission.

Cause in fact may be evaluated by questioning: But for what the nurse did, would this injury have occurred? **Proximate cause**, or legal cause, may be evaluated by determining whether there have been any intervening actions or persons that were, in fact, the causes of harm to the client. **Damages** include actual damages (e.g., loss of earnings, medical expenses, and property damage) as well as pain and suffering.

DETERMINING A STANDARD OF CARE

Professional standards of practice determined by professional associations differ from the minimal qualifications set forth by state licensure for entry into the profession of nursing. The ANA has established standards for psychiatric mental health nursing practice and credentialing for the psychiatric mental health RN (RN-PMH) and the advanced practice RN in psychiatric mental health nursing (ANA, APNA, ISP MHN (2000)).

Standards for psychiatric mental health nursing practice differ markedly from minimal state requirements because the primary purposes for setting these two types of qualifications are different. The state's qualifications for practice provide consumer protection by ensuring that all practicing nurses have successfully completed an approved nursing program and passed the national licensing examination. The professional association's primary focus is to elevate the practice of its members by setting standards of excellence. The ANA Standards of Psychiatric and Mental Health Nursing Practice are provided inside the front cover of this book.

Nurses are held to the standard of care exercised by other nurses possessing the same degree of skill or knowledge in the same or similar circumstances. In the past, community standards existed for urban and rural agencies. However, with greater mobility and expanded means of communication, national standards have evolved. Psychiatric clients have the right to receive the standard of care recognized by professional bodies governing nursing, whether they are in a large or a small, a rural or an urban, facility. Nurses must participate in continuing education courses to stay current with existing standards of care.

Hospital policies and procedures set up institutional criteria for care, and these criteria, such as the frequency of rounds on clients in seclusion, may be introduced to prove a standard that the nurse met or failed to meet. The shortcoming of this method is that the hospital's policy may be substandard. For example, the state licensing laws for institutions might set a minimal requirement for staffing or frequency of rounds on certain clients, and the hospital policy might fall below that minimum. **Substandard institutional policies do not absolve the individual nurse of responsibility to practice on the basis of professional standards of nursing care.**

Like hospital policy and procedures, custom can be used as evidence of a standard of care. For example, in the absence of a written policy on the use of restraint, testimony might be offered regarding the customary use of restraint in emergency situations in which the combative, violent, or confused client poses a threat of harm to self or others. Using custom to establish a standard of care may result in the same defect as in using hospital policies and procedures: custom may not comply with the laws, accrediting body recommendations, or other recognized standards of care. Custom must be carefully and regularly evaluated to ensure that substandard routines have not developed. Substandard customs do not protect you when a psychiatric client charges that a right has been violated or that harm has been caused by the staff's common practices.

Guidelines for Nurses Who Suspect Negligence

It is not unusual for a student or practicing nurse to suspect negligence on the part of a peer. In most states, nurses have a legal duty to report such risks of harm to the client. It is also important that you document clear and accurate evidence before making serious accusations against a peer. If you question a physician's orders or actions, or those of a fellow nurse, it is wise to communicate these concerns directly to the person involved. If the risky behavior continues, you have an obligation to communicate these concerns to a supervisor, who should then intervene to ensure that the client's rights and well-being are protected. If you suspect a peer of being chemically impaired or of practicing irresponsibly, you have an obligation to protect not only the rights of the peer but also the rights of all clients who could be harmed by this impaired peer. If, after you have reported suspected behavior of concern to a supervisor, the danger persists, you have a duty to report the concern to someone at the next level of authority. It is important to follow the channels of communication in an organization, but it is also important to protect the safety of the clients. If the supervisor's actions or inactions do not rectify the dangerous situation, you have a continuing duty to report the behavior of concern to the appropriate authority, such as the state board of nursing.

A useful reference for nurses is the ANA's *Guidelines for Reporting Incompetent, Unethical, and Illegal Practices* (1994).

Guidelines for Issues of Understaffing

The issue of understaffing has become an issue for all nurses, including psychiatric mental health nurses. If a student or a practicing nurse is asked to assume the duty of care for a psychiatric population without proper support services, it is important for the student or nurse to bring the understaffing issue to the supervisor's attention. Once you have assumed the duty of responsibility, you may be charged with abandonment if you do not follow through with the care of the patient population. It is, therefore, important to document the need for adequate staffing and to follow through with communication to the supervisor that the standards of care cannot be met with inadequate staffing of a unit.

California became the first state to require all patient care units in hospitals to meet fixed minimum nurse-to-patient care ratios (Health Benchmarks 1999). ANA's president, Beverly L. Malone, was quoted as saying that "cutting the number of RNs and substituting unlicensed aides for registered nursing is exactly the wrong move" (p. 138). Refer to A Nurse Speaks in the Unit V opening, for a nurse manager's experience with this serious concern.

DUTY TO INTERVENE AND DUTY TO REPORT

The psychiatric mental health nurse has a duty to intervene when the safety or well-being of the client or another person is obviously at risk. A nurse who follows an order that is known to be incorrect or that the nurse believes will harm the client is responsible for the harm that results to the client. **If you have information that leads you to believe that the physician's orders need to be clarified or changed, it is your duty to intervene and protect the client.** It is important that you communicate with the physician who has ordered the treatment to explain the concern. If the treating physician does not appear willing to consider your concerns, you should carry out the duty to intervene through other appropriate channels.

It is important for you to express concerns to the supervisor to allow the supervisor to communicate with the appropriate medical staff for intervention in the physician's treatment plan. As the client's advocate, you have a duty to intervene to protect the client; at the same time, you do not have the right to interfere with the physician-client relationship.

It is also important to follow agency policies and procedures for communicating differences of opinion. If you fail to intervene and the client is injured, you may be partly liable for the injuries that result because of failure to use safe nursing practice and good professional judgment.

The legal concept of **abandonment** may also arise when a nurse does not leave a client safely back in the hands of another health professional before discontinuing treatment. Abandonment issues arise when accurate, timely, and thorough reporting has not occurred or when follow-through of client care, on which the client is relying, has not occurred. The same principles apply for the psychiatric mental health nurse who is working in a community setting. For example, if a suicidal client refuses to come to the hospital for treatment, you cannot abandon the client but must take the necessary steps to ensure the client's safety. These actions may include enlisting the assistance of the law in temporarily involuntarily committing the client.

The duty to intervene on the client's behalf poses many legal and ethical dilemmas for nurses in the workplace. Institutions that have a chain-of-command policy or other reporting mechanisms offer some assurance that the proper authorities in the administration are notified. Most client care issues regarding physicians' orders or treatments can be settled fairly early in the process by nurses' discussing their concerns with the physician. If further intervention by the nurse is required to protect the client, the next step in the chain of command can be initiated. Generally, the nurse then notifies the immediate nursing supervisor; the supervisor thereupon discusses the problem with the physician, and then with the chief of staff of a particular service, until a resolution is reached. If there is no time to resolve the issue through the normal process because of the life-threatening nature of the situation, the nurse must act to protect the client's life.

Unethical or Illegal Behaviors

The issues become more complex when a professional colleague's conduct, including that of a student nurse, is criminally unlawful. Specific examples include the diversion of drugs from the hospital and sexual misconduct with clients. Increasing media attention and the recognition of substance abuse as an occupational hazard for health professionals have led to substance abuse programs for health care workers in many states. These programs provide appropriate treatment for impaired professionals to protect the public from harm and to rehabilitate the professional.

The problem previously discussed—of reporting impaired colleagues—becomes a difficult one, particularly when no direct harm has occurred to the client. Concern for professional reputations, damaged careers, and personal privacy rather than public protection has generated a code of silence regarding substance abuse among health professionals.

Several states now require reporting of impaired or incompetent colleagues to the professional licensing boards. Without this legal mandate, the questions of whether to report and to whom to report become ethical ones. You are again urged to use the ANA's *Guidelines for Reporting Incompetent, Unethical, and Illegal Behavior* (1994). Chapter 27 deals more fully with issues related to the chemically impaired nurse.

The duty to intervene includes the duty to report known abusive behavior. Most states have enacted statutes to protect children and the elderly from abuse and neglect. Psychiatric mental health nurses working in the community may be mandated by the law to report unsafe relationships they discover.

DOCUMENTATION OF CARE

Purpose of Medical Records

The purpose of the medical record is to provide accurate and complete information about the care and treatment of clients and to give health care personnel responsible for that care a means of communicating with each other. The medical record allows for continuity of care. A record's usefulness is determined by evaluating, when the record is read later, how accurately and completely it portrays the client's behavioral status at the time it was written.

Timeliness in recording nursing actions and observations is as important as the accuracy of the information shared. Clients' safety is compromised when their high-risk behavior or statements are not immediately communicated. Miscommunications and delays in sharing pertinent information are major causes of legal liability. If a member of the health care team relies on old information because you have not recently charted new data and the client is harmed, you share the responsibility for the resultant injury.

For example, if a psychiatric client describes to a nurse a plan to harm himself or herself or another person and that nurse fails to document the information, including the need to protect the client or the identified victim, the information will be lost when the nurse leaves work and the client's plan may be carried out. The harm caused could be linked directly to the nurse's failure to communicate this important information. Even though documentation takes time away from the client, the importance of communicating and preserving the nurse's memory through the medical record cannot be overemphasized.

Accrediting agencies, such as the Joint Commission on Accreditation of Healthcare Organizations, and state regulatory agencies require health care facilities to maintain records on clients' care and treatment. Noncompliance with record-keeping responsibilities may result in fines, loss of accreditation, or both.

Facility Use of Medical Records

The medical record has many other uses aside from providing information on the course of the client's care and treatment to health care professionals. A retrospective chart review can provide valuable information to the facility on the quality of care provided and on ways to improve that care. A facility may conduct reviews for risk management purposes, to determine areas of potential liability for the facility, and to evaluate methods used to reduce the facility's exposure to liability. For example, documentation of the use of restraints and seclusion for psychiatric clients may be reviewed by risk managers. Accordingly, the chart may be used to evaluate care for quality assurance or peer review. Utilization review analysts review the chart to determine appropriate use of hospital and staff resources consistent with reimbursement schedules. Insurance companies and other reimbursement agencies rely on the medical record in determining payments they will make on the client's behalf.

Medical Records as Evidence

From a legal perspective, the chart is a recording of data and opinions made in the normal course of the client's hospital care. It is deemed to be good evidence because it is presumed to be true, honest, and untainted by memory lapses. Accordingly, the medical record finds its way into a variety of legal cases for a variety of reasons. Some examples of its use include determining (1) the extent of the client's damages and pain and suffering in personal injury cases, such as when a psychiatric client attempts suicide while under the protective care of a hospital; (2) the nature and extent of injuries in child abuse or elder abuse cases; (3) the nature and extent of physical or mental disability in disability cases; and (4) the nature and extent of injury and rehabilitative potential in workers' compensation cases.

Medical records may also be used in police investigations, civil conservatorship proceedings, competency hearings, and commitment procedures. In states that mandate a mental health legal services or clients' rights advocacy program, audits may be performed to determine the facility's compliance with state laws or violation of clients' rights. Finally, medical records may be used in professional and hospital negligence cases.

During the discovery phase of litigation, the medical record is a pivotal source of information for attorneys in determining whether a cause of action exists in a professional negligence or hospital negligence case. Evidence of the nursing care rendered will be reflected in what the nurse charted at the time. Incomplete or poor notes raise suspicion about the quality of care delivered.

Nursing Guidelines for Charting

Accurate, descriptive, and legible nursing notes serve the best interests of the client, the nurse, and the institution. As computerized charting becomes more widely available, it will also be important for psychiatric mental health nurses to understand how to protect the confidentiality of these records. Institutions must also protect against intrusions into the privacy of the client record systems.

Computerized charting is becoming common practice across our country. Concerns for the privacy of the legitimate patient's records have been addressed legally by federal laws that provide guidelines for agencies who use computerized charting. These guidelines include the recommendation that staff be assigned a password for entering patients' records to identify which staff have gained access to the patient's confidential information. There are penalties, including grounds for firing the staff, if they enter a record for which they are not authorized. Only those staff who have a legitimate need-to-know information about the patient are authorized to enter a patient's computerized chart. It is important for you to keep your password private and never to allow someone else to enter a record under your password. You are responsible for all entries into records using your password.

Your charting should reflect factual observations and not contain generalized opinions. For example, if the notation is made that the client "had a good night," does this indicate merely that you were not bothered by the client during the night? More appropriate notations would indicate the times that the client was checked on and what, specifically, you observed.

The various systems used allow specific time frames within which the nurse must make any necessary corrections if a charting error is made. The information charted assists those on the following shift to understand the client's current status. Information on whether the psychiatric client slept through the night or continued to pace the hallway has significant treatment implications. **It is important never to obliterate or erase previous charting.** A presumption of fraud will be made if it appears that an error is being hidden. Instead, a line drawn through the error with correct information provided in the next available space will maintain the integrity of the record.

Any charting method that improves communication between care providers should be encouraged. Courts assume that nurses and physicians read each other's notes on client progress. Many courts reflect the attitude that if care is not documented, it did not occur. Your charting also serves as a valuable memory refresher if the client sues years after the care is provided. In providing complete and timely information on the care and treatment of clients, the medical record enhances communication among health professionals. Internal, institutional audits of the record can improve the quality of care rendered. Nurses' charting is improved by following the guidelines in Box 8–5. Chapter 9 identifies four common charting forms and gives examples as well as the pros and cons of each.

MAINTAINING CLIENT CONFIDENTIALITY

Ethical Considerations

The ANA Code for Nurses states that "the nurse safeguards the client's right to privacy by judiciously protecting information of a confidential nature" (ANA 1985). The applicable interpretive statement provides further explanation for maintaining client confidentiality and recognizes the distinction between legal and ethical obligations. The interpretive statement follows:

> The right of privacy is an inalienable right of all persons, and the nurse has a clear obligation to safeguard any confidential information about the client acquired from any source. The nurse-client relationship is built on trust. This relationship could be destroyed and the client's welfare and reputation jeopardized by injudicious disclosing of information provided in confidence. Since the concept of confidentiality has legal as well as ethical implications, an inappropriate breach of confidentiality may also expose the nurse to liability.

Legal Considerations

The psychiatric client's right to have treatment and medical records kept confidential is legally protected. The fundamental principle underlying the ANA code on confidentiality is a person's constitutional right to privacy. Generally, your legal duty to maintain confidentiality is to act to protect the client's right to privacy. Therefore, you may not, without the client's consent, disclose information ob-

BOX 8–5   *Do's and Don'ts of Charting*

DO'S

- Chart, in a timely manner, all pertinent and factual information.
- Be familiar with the nursing documentation policy in your facility and make your charting conform to this standard. The policy generally states the method of charting, the frequency, pertinent assessments, interventions, and outcomes. If your agency's policies and procedures do not encourage or allow for quality documentation, bring the need for change to the administration's attention. (Refer to Chapter 9 for four charting methods.)
- Chart legibly in ink.
- Chart facts fully, descriptively, and accurately.
- Chart what you see, hear, feel, and smell.
- Chart a total patient assessment on admission, discharge, and transfer and in between when pertinent.
- Chart pertinent observations: psychosocial observations, physical symptoms pertinent to the medical diagnosis, and behavior pertinent to the nursing diagnosis.
- Chart follow-up care provided when a problem has been identified in earlier documentation. For example, if a patient has fallen and injured a leg, describe how the wound is healing.
- Chart fully the facts surrounding unusual occurrences and incidents, *but do not note in the chart that an incident report was filed.* This form is generally a privileged communication between the hospital and the hospital's attorney. Describing it in the chart may destroy the privileged nature of the communication.
- Chart *all* nursing interventions, treatments, and outcomes, including teaching efforts and patient responses, and safety and patient protection interventions.
- Chart the patient's expressed subjective feelings.
- Chart each time you notify a physician, the reason for notification, what was communicated, the accurate time, the physician's instructions or orders, and the follow-up activity.
- Chart physician visits and treatments.
- Chart discharge medications and instructions given for use, as well as all discharge teaching performed and which family members were included in the process.

DON'TS

- Do *not* chart opinions that are not supported by the facts.
- Do *not* defame clients by calling them names or by making derogatory statements about them (e.g., "an unlikable client who is demanding unnecessary attention").
- Do *not* chart before an event occurs.
- Do *not* chart generalizations, suppositions, or pat phrases (e.g., "client in good spirits").
- Do *not* obliterate, erase, alter, or destroy a record. If an error is made, draw one line through the error, write "mistaken entry" or "error," and initial. Follow your agency's guidelines closely.
- Do *not* leave blank spaces for chronological notes. If you must chart out of sequence, chart "late entry." Identify the time and date of the entry and the time and date of the occurrence.

tained from the client or information in the medical record to anyone except those necessary for implementation of a client's treatment plan.

Client's Employer

For example, your release of information to the client's employer about the client's condition, without the client's consent, is a breach of confidentiality that subjects you to liability for the tort of invasion of privacy. On the other hand, discussion of clients' history with other staff members to ascertain a consistent treatment approach is not a breach of confidentiality.

Generally, to create a situation in which information is privileged, a client–health professional relationship must exist, and the information must relate to the care and treatment of the client. The health professional may refuse to disclose information to protect the client's privacy. However, the right to privacy is the client's right, and health professionals cannot involve confidentiality for their own defense or benefit.

Rights After Death

A person's reputation can be damaged even after death. **It is therefore important not to divulge information after a person's death that could not have been legally shared before the death.** The Dead Man's Statute protects confidential information about people when they are not alive to speak for themselves.

A legal privilege of confidentiality is enacted legislatively and exists to protect the confidentiality of professional communications (e.g., nurse-client, physician-client, attorney-client). The theory behind such privileged communications is that clients will not be comfortable or willing to disclose personal information about themselves if they fear that the nurses will repeat their confidential conversations.

In some states in which the legal privilege of confidentiality has not been legislated for nurses, you must respond to a court's inquiries regarding the client's disclosures even if this information implicates the client in a crime. In these states, the confidentiality of communications cannot be guaranteed. If a duty to report exists, you may be required to divulge private information shared by the client.

Client Privilege and Human Immunodeficiency Virus

Some states have enacted mandatory or permissive statutes that direct health care providers to warn a

spouse if a partner is positive for human immunodeficiency virus (Table 8–3). Nurses must understand the laws in their jurisdiction of practice regarding privileged communications and warnings of infectious disease exposure.

Exceptions to the Rule

Duty to Warn and Protect Third Parties

The California Supreme Court, in its 1976 landmark decision *Tarasoff v. Regents of University of California,* ruled that a psychotherapist has a duty to warn the client's potential victim of potential harm. This decision created much controversy and confusion in the psychiatric and medical communities over breach of client confidentiality and its impact on the therapeutic relationship in psychiatric care and on the ability of the psychotherapist to predict when a client is truly dangerous. This trend continues as other jurisdictions have adopted or modified the California rule despite the psychiatric community's objections. These jurisdictions view public safety to be more important than privacy in narrowly defined circumstances.

The *Tarasoff* case acknowledged that generally there is no common law duty to aid third persons. An exception is when special relationships exist, and the court found the client-therapist relationship sufficient to create a duty of the therapist to aid Ms. Tarasoff, the victim. The duty to protect the intended victim from danger arises when the therapist determines—or, pursuant to professional standards, should have determined—that the client presents a serious danger to another. Any action reasonably necessary under the circumstances, including notification of the potential victim, the victim's family, and the police, discharges the therapist's duty to the potential victim.

In 1982, the California Supreme Court issued a second ruling in the case of *Tarasoff v. Regents of University of California* (now known as *Tarasoff II*). This ruling broadened the earlier ruling, the duty to warn, to include the **duty to protect**.

The psychologist's diagnostic function, a professional service rendered within the legal scope of practice, was central to the California Supreme Court's ruling in *Hedlum v. Superior Court of Orange County* (1983). The court stated that the duty to warn was composed of two elements: (1) the duty to diagnose and predict the client's danger of violence and (2) the duty to take appropriate action to protect the identified victim. The court stated that "a negligent failure to diagnose dangerousness in a *Tarasoff* action is as much a basis for liability as is a negligent failure to warn a known victim once

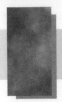

TABLE 8–3 *Legal Issues Involving Human Immunodeficiency Virus (HIV) and Psychiatric Mental Health Nursing*

ISSUE	THE LAW
1. Involuntary HIV testing of psychiatric patients	1. Consent from the psychiatric patient must be sought to test blood for HIV. Substitute decision making applies only to children age 13 or younger and to involuntarily committed adult psychiatric patients (Lo, 1989).
2. Involuntary confinement of a psychiatric patient who is HIV positive and having sex with other patients	2. Knowing transmission of HIV through sexual contact is prohibited by law. The institution has the legal means to prohibit such contact. The Illinois Supreme Court held that a statute prohibiting a person from knowingly transmitting HIV was constitutional (*Illinois v. Russel*, 1994).
3. Duty to warn the partner of a psychiatric patient who is HIV positive	3. In 1988, New York and California enacted laws permitting notification of contacts of HIV persons. These laws require that the informant persuade the patient to allow notification without disclosing the identity of the patient. Alternatively, public health officials may be asked to notify contacts. Recent statutes, however, do not require notification, encouraging voluntary notification (Lo, 1989).
4. Disclosure of a psychiatric patient's HIV status by the nurse to an unauthorized person	4. The Arkansas Supreme Court held that a nurse who disclosed information about a man's HIV test to an unauthorized third party did not constitute medical malpractice (*Wyatt v. St. Paul Fire & Marine Ins. Co.*, 1994).
5. Psychiatric nurses' refusal to care for an HIV-positive psychiatric patient	5. In general, nurses have no legal duty to care for HIV-positive psychiatric patients. However, moral obligation, employment contracts, and professional and ethical standards may impose some authority to obligate the nurse to care for HIV-positive patients.
6. Psychiatric nurses' duty to inform employer of HIV status	6. While HIV-positive psychiatric nurses have a moral obligation to inform their employer of their HIV status, their right to privacy should be balanced with the risk of infection to co-workers or patients who come under their care.
7. Nurses' claims for emotional distress caused by exposure to AIDS or needlestick	7. In *Tischler v. Dimenna* (1994), a New York court recognized claims for emotional distress caused by exposure to AIDS. Moreover, the Montana Supreme Court held that the State Worker's Compensation Act provided the exclusive remedy for a former employee who developed a fear of AIDS after being punctured by a needle (*Blythe v. Radiometer America, Inc.*, 1993).

AIDS, acquired immunodeficiency syndrome.
From Constantino, R. E. B. (1996). Legal issues in psychiatric–mental health nursing. In S. Lego (Ed.), *Psychiatric nursing: A comprehensive reference* (2nd ed.). Philadelphia: J. B. Lippincott.

such a diagnosis has been made" (p. 695) (*Hedlum* 1983).

Most states currently have similar laws regarding the duty to warn third parties of potential life threats. The duty to warn usually includes

■ Assessing and predicting the client's danger of violence toward another
■ Identifying the specific persons being threatened
■ Taking appropriate action to protect the identified victims

NURSING IMPLICATIONS. As this trend toward making it the therapist's duty to warn third persons of potential harm continues to gain wider acceptance, it is important for students and nurses to understand its implications for nursing practice. Although none of these cases has dealt with nurses, it is fair to assume that in jurisdictions that have adopted the *Tarasoff* doctrine, the duty to warn third

persons will be applied to clinical psychiatric nurse specialists in private practice who engage in individual therapy.

However, if a staff nurse who is a member of a team of psychiatrists, psychologists, psychiatric social workers, and other psychiatric nurses does not report client threats of harm against specified victims or classes of victims to the team of the client's management psychotherapist for assessment and evaluation, this failure is likely to be considered substandard nursing care.

So, too, the failure to communicate and record relevant information from police, relatives, or the client's old records might also be deemed negligent. Breach of client-nurse confidentiality should not pose ethical or legal dilemmas for nurses in these situations, because a team approach to the delivery of psychiatric care presumes communication of pertinent information to other staff members to develop a treatment plan in the client's best interest.

Child and Elder Abuse Reporting Statutes

Because of their interest in protecting children, all 50 states and the District of Columbia have enacted child abuse reporting statutes. Although these statutes differ from state to state, they generally include a definition of child abuse, a list of persons required or encouraged to report, and the governmental agency designated to receive and investigate the reports. Most statutes include civil penalties for failure to report. Many states specifically require nurses to report cases of suspected abuse.

There is a conflict between federal and state laws with respect to child abuse reporting when the health care professional discovers child abuse or neglect during the suspected abuser's alcohol or drug treatment. Federal laws and regulations governing confidentiality of client records, which apply to almost all drug abuse and alcohol treatment providers, prohibit any disclosure without a court order. In this case, federal law supersedes state reporting laws, although compliance with the state law may be maintained

■ If a court order is obtained, pursuant to the regulations

■ If a report can be made without identifying the abuser as a client in an alcohol or drug treatment program

■ If the report is made anonymously (some states, to protect the rights of the accused, do not allow anonymous reporting)

As reported incidents of abuse to other persons in society surface, states may require health professionals to report other kinds of abuse. A growing number of states are enacting elder abuse reporting statutes, which require RNs and others to report cases of abuse of the elderly. The elderly are defined as adults 65 years of age and older. These laws also apply to dependent adults—that is, adults between 18 and 64 years of age whose physical or mental

limitations restrict their ability to carry out normal activities or protect themselves—when the RN has actual knowledge that the person has been the victim of physical abuse.

Under most state laws, a person who is required to report suspected abuse, neglect, or exploitation of a disabled adult who willfully does not do so is guilty of a misdemeanor crime. Most state statutes state that anyone who makes a report in good faith is immune from civil liability in connection with the report.

You may also report knowledge of, or reasonable suspicion of, mental abuse or suffering. Both dependent adults and elders are protected by the law from purposeful physical or fiduciary neglect or abandonment. **Because state laws vary, students are encouraged to become conversant with the requirements of their state.**

SUMMARY

The states' power to enact laws for public health and safety and for the care of those unable to care for themselves often pits the rights of society against the rights of the individual. The complexities of these relationships can manifest as legal and ethical dilemmas in the psychiatric setting. Increasingly, nurses encounter problems requiring ethical choices. The nurse's privilege to practice nursing carries with it responsibility to practice safely, competently, and in a manner consistent with state and federal laws. Knowledge of the law and the ANA Code for Nurses and standards of psychiatric mental health nursing practice will enhance the nurse's ability to provide safe, effective psychiatric nursing care and will serve as a framework for decision making when the nurse is presented with complex problems involving competing interests.

Visit the **Evolve** website at
http://evolve.elsevier.com/Varcarolis
for a post-test on the content in this chapter.

Visit the **Evolve** website at
http://evolve.elsevier.com/Varcarolis
for additional self-study exercises.

Critical Thinking and Chapter Review

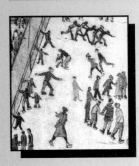

Critical Thinking

1. Two nurses, Joe and Beth, have worked on the psychiatric unit for 2 years. During the past 6 months, Beth has confided to Joe that she has been going through a particularly difficult marital situation. Joe has noticed that for 6 months Beth has become increasingly irritable and difficult to work with. He notices that minor tranquilizers are frequently missing from the unit dose cart on the evening shift. He complains to the pharmacy and is informed that the drugs were stocked as ordered. Several clients state that they have not been receiving their usual drugs. Joe finds that Beth has recorded that the drugs have been given as ordered. He also notices that Beth is diverting the drugs. What action, if any, should Joe take?

   ■ Should Joe confront Beth with his suspicions?
   ■ If Beth admits that she has been diverting the drugs, should Joe's next step be to report Beth to the supervisor or to the board of nursing?
   ■ Should Joe make his concern known to the nursing supervisor directly by identifying Beth, or should he state his concerns in general terms?
   ■ Legally, must Joe report his suspicions to the board of nursing?
   ■ Does the fact that harm to the clients is limited to increased agitation affect your responses?

2. Nurse A has worked in a psychiatric setting for 5 years, since she was licensed as a registered nurse by the state. She arrives at work on her unit and is informed that the nursing office has requested a nurse from the psychiatric unit to assist the intensive care unit staff in caring for an agitated car accident victim with a history of schizophrenia. Nurse A works with Nurse B in caring for the client. While the client is sleeping, Nurse B leaves the unit for a coffee break. Nurse A, unfamiliar with the telemetry equipment, fails to recognize an arrhythmia, and the client has a cardiopulmonary arrest. The client is successfully resuscitated after 6 minutes but suffers permanent brain damage.

   ■ Can Nurse A legally practice? (That is, does her license permit her to practice in the intensive care unit?)
   ■ Does the ability to practice legally in an area differ from the ability to practice competently in that area?
   ■ Did Nurse A have any legal or ethical grounds to refuse the assignment to the intensive care unit?
   ■ What are the risks in accepting an assignment to an area of specialty practice in which you are professionally unprepared to practice?
   ■ What are the risks in refusing an assignment to an area of specialty practice in which you are professionally unprepared to practice?
   ■ Would there have been any way for Nurse A to minimize the risk of action for insubordination by the employer had she refused the assignment?
   ■ What action could Nurse A have taken to protect the client and herself when Nurse B left the unit for a coffee break?
   ■ If Nurse A is negligent, is the hospital liable for any harm to the client caused by Nurse A?

3. A 40-year-old man who is admitted to the emergency department for a severe nosebleed has both nares packed. Because of his history of alcoholism and the probability of ensuing delirium tremens, the client is transferred to the psychiatric unit. He is admitted to a private room, placed in restraints, and checked by a nurse every hour per physician order. While unattended, the client suffocates, apparently by inhaling the nasal packing, which had become dislodged from the nares. On the next 1-hour check, the nurse finds the client without pulse or respiration.

   A state statute requires that a restrained client on a psychiatric unit be assessed by a nurse every hour for safety, comfort, and physical needs.

   ■ If standards are not otherwise specified, do statutory requirements set forth minimal or maximal standards?
   ■ Does the nurse's compliance with the state statute relieve him or her of liability in the client's death?
   ■ Does the nurse's compliance with the physician's order relieve him or her of liability in the client's death?
   ■ Was the order for the restraint appropriate for this type of client?
   ■ What factors did you consider in making your determination?
   ■ Was the frequency of rounds for assessment of client needs appropriate in this situation?
   ■ Did the nurse's conduct meet the standard of care for psychiatric nurses? Why or why not?
   ■ What nursing action should the nurse have taken to protect the client from harm?

4. Assume that there are no mandatory reporting laws for impaired or incompetent colleagues in the following clinical situation. In a private psychiatric unit in California, a 15-year-old boy is admitted voluntarily at the request of his parents because of violent, explosive behavior that seems to stem from his father's recent remarriage after his parents' divorce. A few days after admission, while in group therapy, he has an explosive reaction to a discussion about weekend passes for Mother's Day. He screams that he has been abandoned and that nobody cares about him. Several weeks later, on the day before his discharge, he elicits from the nurse a promise to keep his plan to kill his mother confidential.

   Consider the ANA code of ethics on client confidentiality, the principles of psychiatric nursing, the statutes on privileged communications, and the duty to warn third parties in answering the following questions:

   ■ Did the nurse use appropriate judgment in promising confidentiality?
   ■ Does the nurse have a legal duty to warn the client's mother of her son's threat?
   ■ Is the duty owed to the client's father and stepmother?
   ■ Would a change in the admission status from voluntary to involuntary protect the client's mother without violating the client's confidentiality?
   ■ Would your response be different depending on the state where the incident occurred? Why or why not?
   ■ What nursing action, if any, should the nurse take after the disclosure by the client?

See answers to these questions at end of Appendix E.

Chapter Review

1. Which resource will be the least authoritative help for a psychiatric mental health nurse faced with a client care ethical dilemma?

    1. Standards of Psychiatric Mental Health Nursing Practice.
    2. Federal and state laws.
    3. ANA Code of Ethics.
    4. Peer opinion.

2. The single most important action nurses can take to protect the rights of a psychiatric client is to

    1. Be aware of that state's laws regarding care and treatment of the mentally ill.
    2. Refuse to participate in imposing restraint or seclusion.
    3. Document concerns about unit short staffing.
    4. Practice the five principles of bioethics.

3. To provide appropriate care for a client who has been admitted involuntarily to a psychiatric unit, the nurse must be aware of the fact that the client has the right to

    1. Refuse psychotropic medications.
    2. Be treated by unit staff of his/her choice.
    3. Be released within 24 hours of making a written request.
    4. Consultation with other mental health professionals at the hospital's expense.

4. In which situation might the psychiatric mental health nurse incur liability?

    1. Placing a client with annoying behavior in seclusion.
    2. Reporting the substandard practice of a nurse peer.
    3. Reporting threats against a third party to the treatment team.
    4. Discussing an unclear medical order with the physician.

5. Observing the client's right to privacy permits the psychiatric mental health nurse to

    1. Freely disclose information in the medical record to the client's employer.
    2. Use information about the client when preparing a journal article.
    3. Discuss observations about the client with the treatment team.
    4. Disclose confidential information after the client's death.

REFERENCES

American Nurses' Association. (1985). *Code for nurses.* Kansas City, Missouri: Author.

American Nurses' Association. (1994). *Guidelines for reporting incompetent, unethical, and illegal behaviors.* Kansas City, Missouri: Author

American Nurses' Association. (1996). Position statement: The rights to accept or reject an assignment. *Pulse,* 33(1):4–5, 11.

American Nurses' Association. (1990). Suggested state legislation: *Nursing Practice Act, Nursing Disciplinary Act, Prescriptive Authority Act* (pp. 1–46). (Publication NP-78). Kansas City, Missouri: Author.

American Nurses Association, American Psychiatric Nurses Association, and International Society of Psychiatric Mental Health Nurses (2000). *Scope and Standards of Psychiatric Mental Health Practice.* Washington, DC: American Nurses Publishing.

Beck, J. C. (1987). The psychotherapist's duty to protect third parties from harm. *Mental Health and Physical Disability Law Reporter,* 2(2):2.

Blythe v. Radiometer America, Inc. 866 P.2d 218 (Mont. Sup. Ct. 1993).

Brakel, S. J., Parry, J., and Weiner, B. A. (1985). *Mentally disabled and the law* (2nd ed.). Chicago: American Bar Foundation.

California Department of Mental Health. (1985). *Patients' rights advocacy manual.* Sacramento, California: California Department of Mental Health.

Canadian Nurses' Association. (1996). Quality and cost effective care: A nursing solution. *Sexual Assault Nurse Examiners: S.A.N.E. Care for Sexual Assault.* (Flyer) Ottawa: Author.

Canterbury v. Spence, 464 F2d 722 (DC Cir 1972), quoting *Schloendorf v. Society of NY Hosp,* 211 NY 125 105 NE2d 92, 93 (1914).

Cole, R. (1981). Patients' rights to refuse antipsychotic drugs. *Law, Medicine, and Health Care,* 9(4):1.

Darling v. Charleston Community Memorial Hospital, 211 NE2d 253 (Ill. 1965).

Decisions and Reports. (1995). *Human Rights Law Journal,* 16(10–12):403–419.

Dunn, D. G. (1994). Bioethics in nursing. *Nursing Connections,* 7(3): 43–51.

Feuntz, S. A. (1987). Preventive legal maintenance. *Journal of Nursing Administration,* 17(1):8–10.

George, S., and Young, W. B. (1990). Baccalaureate entry into practice: An example of political innovation and diffusion. *Nursing Outlook,* 29(8):341–345.

Gittins, P. (1996). NPs and psychiatry: A winning combination. *Newsline for Nurse Practitioners,* 5(4):4–7.

Goldstein, A. S., Perdew, S., and Pruitt, S. S. (1989). *The nurse's legal advisor: Your guide to legally safe practice.* Philadelphia: J. B. Lippincott.

Guido, G. W. (1988). *Legal issues in nursing: A source book for practice* (pp 80–87, 146, 209–216). Norwalk, Connecticut: Appleton & Lange.

Health Benchmarks. (1999). *Nurse staffing law may herald benchmarks.* Author, 6(12):137–138.

Hedlum v. Superior Court of Orange County, 34 C3d 695 (1983).

Hessler v. Osawatomie State Hospital, 97, P2d 1169 (Kan 1999).

Humphrey v. Cady, 405 US 504 (1972).

Illinois v. Russel, 630 NE2nd 794 (Ill. Sup. Ct. 1994).

In re guardianship of Roe, 421 NE2d 40 (Mass 1981).

In re Oakes, 8 Law Rep 122 (Mass 1845).

Jablonski v. United States, 712 F2d 391 (9th Cir 1983).

Large v. Superior Court, 714 P.zd 399 (Arizona 1986).

Laughlin, S. D. (2000). Nursing case law update—Failure to monitor (2000). *Journal of Nursing Law,* 6(4):55–59.

Lo, B. (1989). Clinical ethics and HIV-related illnesses: Issues in treatment and health services. In W. Le Vee (Ed.), *New perspectives on HIV-related illnesses: Progress in health services research* (pp. 170–179). Bethesda, Maryland: U. S. Department of Health and Human Services.

Lynch, V. (1995). Clinical forensic nursing: A new perspective in the management of crime victims from trauma to trial. *Critical-Care Nursing Clinics of North America,* 7(3):489–507.

Lynch, V. (1996). Forensic nursing. *The Prosecutor,* November/December, p 13.

Marullo, G. (1996). Keynote address by the executive director of the American Nurses' Association at the 1996 Meeting of the International Association of Forensic Nurses, St. Louis, Missouri, as reported in Weaver, J. D., and Lynch V. (1998). Forensic nursing: Unique contributions to international law. *Journal of Nursing Law,* 5(4):24–25.

McHugh, J. (1997). Standards of forensic nursing practice. *On the Edge,* 3:1.

Millenson, M. (1997). *Demanding medical excellence: Doctors and accountability in the information age.* Chicago: University of Chicago Press.

Miller, R., and Fiddleman, P. (1984). Outpatient commitment: Treatment in the least restrictive environment? *Hospital and Community Psychiatry,* 35(2):147.

Mills v. Rogers, 457 US 291 (1982).

O'Connor v. Donaldson, 422 US 563 (1975).

Pennington, S., Gafner, G., Schelit, R., and Bechtel, B. (1993). Addressing ethical boundaries among nurses. *Nurse Manager,* 24(6):36–39.

Pisel v. Stamford Hospital, 430 A2d 1 (Conn 1980).

Plumadore v. State of New York, 427 NYS2d 90 (1980).

President's Advisory Commission on Consumer Protection and Quality in Health Care Industry. (1998). *Quality first: Better healthcare for all Americans* (pp. 11–15). Washington, D.C.: U. S. Government Printing Office.

Price, D. M. (1998). Doesn't everyone want an efficient nurse? *Journal of Nursing Law,* 5(1):51–55.

Price, D. M. (1998). Evaluating managed care: An ethical perspective. *Journal of Nursing Law,* 5(3):476–480.

Rabenberg v. Rigney, 597 NW2d 424 (S.D. 1999).

Rennie v. Klein, 476 F Supp 1294 (DNJ 1979).

Rennie v. Klein, 653 F2d 836 (3rd Cir 1981).

Rennie v. Klein, 454 US 1078 (1982).

Rennie v. Klein, 720 F2d 266 (3rd Cir 1983).

Rhoden, N. (1985). The presumption for treatment: Has it been justified? *Law, Medicine, and Health Care,* 13(2):65.

Rogers v. Commissioner of the Department of Mental Health, 458 NE2d 308 (Mass 1983).

Rogers v. Okin, 478 F Supp 1342 (D Mass 1979).

Rogers v. Okin, 634 F2d 650 (1st Cir 1980).

Rouse v. Cameron, 373 F2d 451 (DC Cir 1966).

Saunders, J., and DuPlessis, D. (1985). A historical view of right to treatment. *Journal of Psychosocial Nursing,* 23(9):12.

Schmid, D., Applebaum, P., Roth, L., and Lidz, C. (1983). Confidentiality in psychiatry: A study of the patients' view. *Hospital and Community Psychiatry,* 34(4):353.

Schwartz, H., Vingiano, W., and Perez, C. (1988). Autonomy and the right to refuse treatment: Patient's attitudes after involuntary medication. *Hospital and Community Psychiatry,* 39:1049.

Simon, R. I. (1999). The law and psychiatry. In R. E. Hales, S. C. Yadofsky, and J. A. Talbott (Eds.), *Textbook of psychiatry* (3rd ed). Washington, D.C.: American Psychiatric Press.

State of Washington v. Harper, 489 US 1064 (1989).

Tarasoff v. Regents of University of California, 17 C3d 425 (1976).

Thomas v. County of Alameda, 27 C3d 741 (1980).

Vitek v. Jones, 445 US 480 (1980).

Volunteer Trustees of Not-for-Profit Hospitals. (1995). *Issue update: New privacy rule for health information* (pp. 1–3). Washington, D.C.

Volunteer Trustees of Not-for-Profit Hospitals. (2000). *Issue update: Patient Bill of Rights gains political currency: Election-year pressure on Congress to act* (pp 1–3). Washington, D.C.

Wampler, D. M. (1995). *Elder mistreatment recognition, prevention, and reporting requirements for Utah healthcare providers* (Masters Project, Attachment I, p 21). University of Utah College of Nursing, Salt Lake City, Utah.

Weaver, J. D., and Lynch, V. (1998) Forensic nursing: Unique contributions to international law. *Journal of Nursing Law,* 5(4):p 23–34.

Wyatt v. Stickney, 325 F Supp 781 (MD Ala 1971).

Wyatt v. St. Paul Tire & Marine Ins. Co., 868 S. W. 2d 505 (Ark. Sup. Ct. 1994).

Youngberg v. Romeo, 457 US 307 (1982).

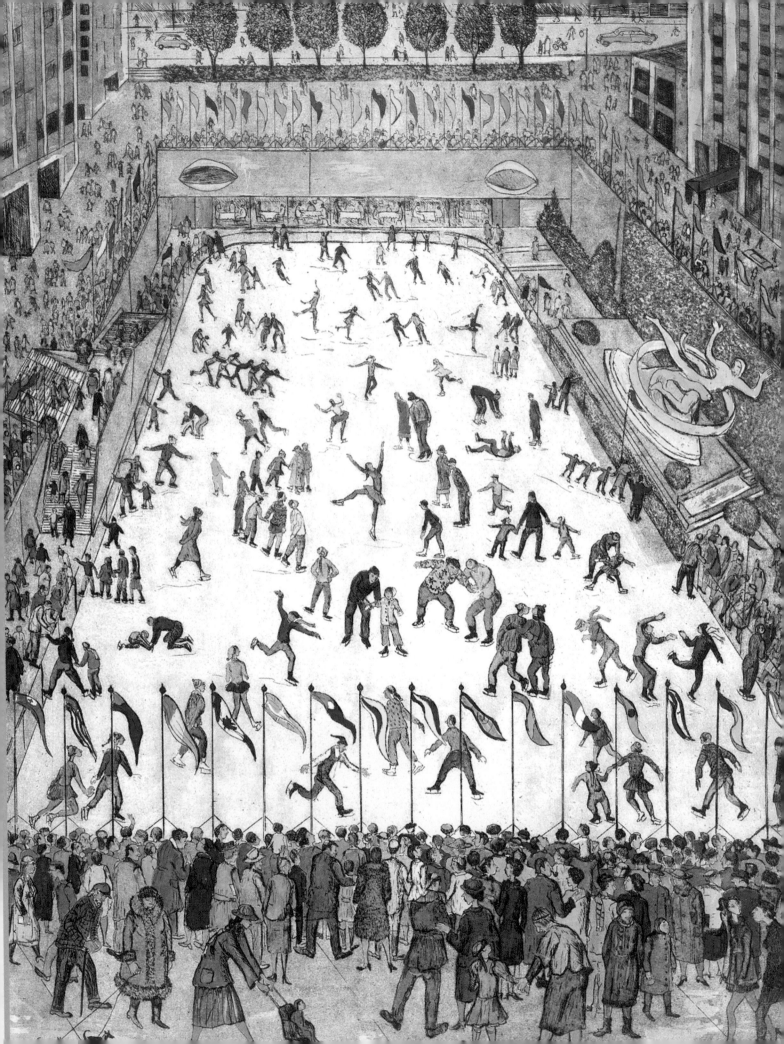

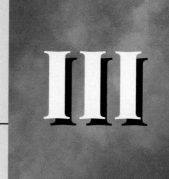
Psychosocial Nursing Tools

I do not try to dance better than anyone else. I only try to dance better than myself.

MIKHAIL BARYSHNIKOV

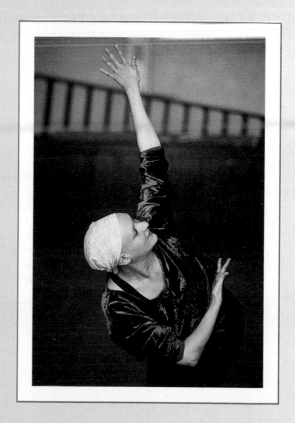

A Nurse Speaks

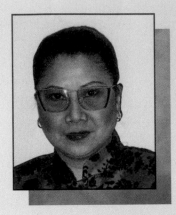

ELORA AFICIONADO ORCAJADA

I went to nursing school to become a nurse. It never dawned on me to become a teacher; nursing and teaching were two different things, I thought. Even a Master's degree at Columbia University did not fan the fires of teaching in me. I knew I was a nurse, a real dedicated nurse. I was, still am.

Right after nursing school, I was hired as a clinical instructor at the hospital I trained at. At that time a lot of medical doctors taught at the nursing school, and we worked, hand in hand with them. I believed I was equipped with the necessary skills and knowledge and I passed these to the next batch of Florence Nightingales, who not only equated nursing as a respectable profession but also primarily shared Florence's genuine concern for the infirm. Teaching and nursing grew simultaneously in me. They became synonymous in the practice of my profession when I started teaching at a community college, and I realized I had the passion and joy of teaching. Seeing our students metamorphose from being shy and passive to responsible and professional nurses became a source of pride and fulfillment. Years of working in different roles and different settings served as my solid groundwork for my vast knowledge and experience.

As teachers, how do we hone and whet the blunt blades of student nurses who come into our fold? How do we transform a tiny and ordinary pebble into a beautiful and expensive pearl but through constant and rigid friction?

Students enrolled in the Associate Degree Nursing Program never fail to amaze me. A small percentage of them are young but most of them are older, mature, working, and have families to take care of while they take the step to upgrade themselves.

Lena is a working mother with a teenage daughter and an 80-year-old father who although is still alert and independent is now showing signs of aging. Lena stated that being a nurse will allow her to take care of her loved ones and herself when illness affect the family. She claimed her knowledge will help her better understand those afflicted with diseases.

Mimi, a single mother of a 2-year-old son, stated that she is doing a payback to the nurses who took good care of her ill child in the hospital. She observed how these nurses were so committed in helping her son return to health.

Fe has chosen nursing as a profession because of the "ideal figure" she saw in the hospital and can never forget who was holding her grandmother's hand until she gasped her last breath on this earth.

Some go back to school with goal of nursing as a second profession or the fulfillment of a dream that was set aside for various reasons. A big percentage of the population are minorities, struggling to make a productive contribution while taking care of their own needs and their families' future in an increasingly productive multicultural society.

During the orientation program, student's handbooks or handouts are distributed. We make them aware of the college's expectations, requirements, rules and routine, etc.

Felnor, a working woman in her mid twenties and an A student in her preclinical courses, experienced a shocking revelation when she reached the clinical stage of nursing. She was astonished that she barely made a B in her first semester course. However, she had the desire to improve her grades; she came to me for advice. She was able to figure out that she has to improve her study habits and possibly request a change of shift and off days from her work. She learned to structure her time, set priorities in terms of short- and long-term goals. She graduated with honors.

Our practice of meeting each student individually on a one-to-one initial interview makes us aware of their problems and needs as well as their strengths, which we tap in several ways. We reiterate our expectations and ask them what they expect from us in return. Again, we internalize the value of self-discipline and perseverance. We also emphasize the importance of skill and safe practice in the care of clients.

Cultural diversity of our students can work to their

advantage, but can likewise pose problems. Cultural diversity can be a positive springboard for open-mindedness, critical thinking, and empathy for students when they become licensed nurses, or as student nurses in the clinical areas where clients are also culturally different. However, this diversity can put them in the midst of a maze of confusion and misunderstanding.

The college is affiliated with several teaching hospitals for our students' clinical experience. This is where they put their learned theory into practice, this is where they see and feel the real world of nursing. At the beginning as well as on the last day of every clinical experience the students are required to evaluate themselves in how they have done, their reactions and feelings about their experience and see venues for improvement. Often, one can see the difference in how they conceptualize as well as the changes in their attitude towards mental illness.

Marie, a student of mine in psychiatric nursing, was terribly upset and scared prior to going to the clinical area because we were on a locked unit. Further exploration revealed a traumatic experience in the past. While she was visiting a friend in a psychiatric unit, a patient became so violent that he was placed in the seclusion room. I encouraged her to share her feelings and apprehension not only with me but with the whole group during our pre-conference. This gave her and her peers an honest opportunity to look into their own thoughts, biases, and fears and also helped them gain insight into what necessary coping skills and defense mechanisms to employ. She was empowered by allowing her to take some control over her emotions. She was permitted to go out of the locked unit when she got too anxious. She expressed feeling relieved on the last clinical day. She also felt proud seeing the evidence of her good work when her withdrawn and depressed patient became verbally expressive and participated in the unit activities.

Many students see the evidence of their metamorphosis, especially during the last clinical day when the self evaluation is made. They realize how effective their therapeutic interaction skills are in decreasing patients' hallucinations and delusions.

Gina felt proud of herself when her patient claimed he was able to break away from "the so-called voices." It was just a matter of putting theory into correct practice.

Students realize that each client is unique. Each one has his own coping skills. This basic fact teaches us all that we have similarities and differences as well.

Romeo, a bright nursing student with a prior degree in psychology, expressed his concern, "I feel I experience similar problems with my clients as I study mental illness. I experience the same signs and symptoms when I am feeling overwhelmed."

Paolo, a young man, married with two kids, says he feels the same way. However he learned that there are different ways of coping that can differ in intensity, frequency, and duration of use. Also, he feels that a good supportive wife and family makes a lot of difference in dealing with life's stressors. Learning mental health/illness made him more aware of his strengths and limitations.

All of our students experience a change in themselves. They state they know more about mental health/illness after finishing the course. Therefore they can offer more to make a difference in their patients' return to the same or higher level of functioning. I always remind them that what they learned belongs to them and that they can also pass it on to others.

Teddy said, "My knowledge about mental illness changed my outlook about the mentally ill when I see them in the streets. They too are human beings and mental illness affected their lives just as physical illness affected mine. I learn that a lot of factors contribute to their predicament and possibly with treatment they will be able to function again as someone with a medical condition may remain stable with the proper treatment."

My students teach me how to be a better teacher. Likewise, our clients can offer us important learning experiences.

Nursing educators come and go but teaching is here to stay. As nursing educators, we are faced with the constant challenge of curriculum change, fast improving technology, demographics, racial diversity, new emerging diseases, alternative therapies, and the cycle of nursing shortages or downsizing and restructuring in the health arena. However, the invitation is always open. Be a NURSE but be a TEACHER too.

Visit the **Evolve** website at
http://evolve.elsevier.com/Varcarolis
for a pre-test on the content in this chapter.

Outline

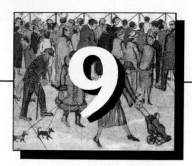

9

Assessment Strategies and the Nursing Process

ELIZABETH M. VARCAROLIS

Key Terms and Concepts

The key terms and concepts listed here also appear in color where they are defined or first discussed in this chapter.

assessment

counseling

health teaching

milieu therapy

nursing interventions
    classification (NIC)

nursing outcomes
    classification (NOC)

outcome criteria

self care activities

Objectives

After studying this chapter, the reader will be able to

1. Perform a mental health assessment on a client agreed upon with your instructor.
2. Explain three principles the nurse follows in planning actions to reach agreed upon outcome criteria.
3. Construct a plan of care for a client with a mental health problem.
4. Identify three advanced practice psychiatric nursing interventions.
5. Demonstrate one of the basic nursing interventions (with your instructor's guidance) and evaluate your care using your stated outcome criteria.

he nursing process continues to be the basic framework for nursing practice and has been used as a basis for the following:

1. Criteria for certification
2. Legal definition of nursing, as reflected in many states' nurse practice acts
3. The National Council of State Boards of Nursing licensure examination (NCLEX-RN) format

The nurse uses the nursing process when evaluating the client at any point on the health–illness continuum. A client may be an individual, a family, a group, or a community. Assessment is made on many levels: physical, social, emotional, intellectual, spiritual, and cultural. Psychiatric mental health nursing practice bases nursing judgments and behaviors on an accepted theoretical framework. The importance of a theoretical framework has been supported by the Scope and Standards of Psychiatric and Mental Health Nursing Practice, developed by the American Nurses' Association (2000 revised) (see inside front cover). Figure 9–1 depicts psychiatric mental health nursing through the nursing process.

ASSESSMENT

Although high levels of anxiety and maladaptive behaviors are commonly seen by psychiatric nursing practitioners, these phenomena are encountered in all areas in the health care setting. Depression, suicidal thoughts, anger, disorientation, delusions, and hallucinations may be encountered in medical-surgical units, obstetrical and intensive care units, outpatient settings, extended care facilities, emergency departments, clinics, and pediatric settings. The assessment of the client's psychosocial status is a part of any nursing assessment, along with assessment of the client's physical health.

Assessment is ongoing and continues throughout the planning, intervention, and evaluation phases. The initial assessment often clarifies the client's immediate needs. As the nurse works further with the client, the database is enlarged and other problems may become evident.

The assessment interview or intake interview may be conducted in a psychiatric inpatient setting, but most likely, it will take place in a variety of other settings such as emergency departments, medical-surgical units, intensive care units, crisis units, community mental health centers, private practice, homes, and schools. The time given for the interview varies, depending on the clinical setting and the circumstances of the client. During emergencies,

immediate intervention is often based on a minimal amount of data. A scheduled psychiatric interview and psychosocial assessment in a structured setting allows more time for an elaborate assessment. At times, completing the assessment process may involve many interviews.

The purpose of the psychiatric assessment is to

■ Establish a rapport
■ Obtain an understanding of current problem
■ Assess the person's current level of psychological functioning
■ Identify what the client and family hope to gain from treatment (goals)
■ Perform a mental status examination
■ Identify what behaviors, beliefs, or other areas of client life need to be modified to effect positive change
■ Formulate a plan of care

The nurse's primary source for data collection is the client; however, there may be times when the client is unable to assist with the assessment. For example, if the client is severely delusional, mute, comatose, or extremely confused, secondary sources should be used. Such sources include members of the family, friends, neighbors, police, other members of the health team, medical records, and laboratory results. Both primary and secondary sources may need to be used during assessment.

Considerations Regarding the Psychiatric Nursing Assessment

Assisting a person toward optimal functioning is accomplished through three levels of nursing intervention:

1. Primary—preventive, fostering mental health
2. Secondary—treating illness
3. Tertiary—rehabilitative

Underlying these three levels of nursing intervention are certain premises (Bower 1982):

■ Individuals have the right to decide their destiny and to be involved in decisions that affect them.
■ Nursing intervention is designed to assist individuals to meet their own needs or to solve their own problems.
■ The ultimate goal of all nursing action is to assist individuals to maximize their independent level of functioning.

During the initial interview, the nurse and the client are essentially strangers. Both experience anxi-

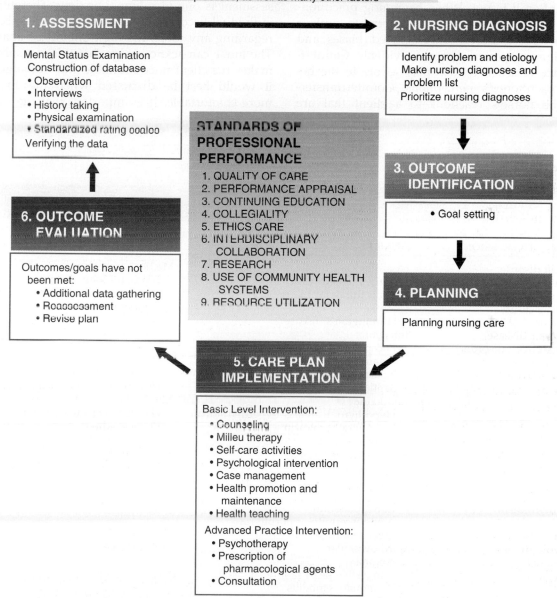

NURSING ASSESSMENT

The assessment interview requires culturally effective communication skills, and encompasses a large database: e.g., significant support system; family; cultural, and community system; spiritual and philosophical values, strengths, and health beliefs and practices; as well as many other factors

1. ASSESSMENT

Mental Status Examination
Construction of database
• Observation
• Interviews
• History taking
• Physical examination
• Standardized rating scales
Verifying the data

2. NURSING DIAGNOSIS

Identify problem and etiology
Make nursing diagnoses and problem list
Prioritize nursing diagnoses

STANDARDS OF PROFESSIONAL PERFORMANCE

1. QUALITY OF CARE
2. PERFORMANCE APPRAISAL
3. CONTINUING EDUCATION
4. COLLEGIALITY
5. ETHICS CARE
6. INTERDISCIPLINARY COLLABORATION
7. RESEARCH
8. USE OF COMMUNITY HEALTH SYSTEMS
9. RESOURCE UTILIZATION

3. OUTCOME IDENTIFICATION

• Goal setting

6. OUTCOME EVALUATION

Outcomes/goals have not been met:
• Additional data gathering
• Reassessment
• Revise plan

4. PLANNING

Planning nursing care

5. CARE PLAN IMPLEMENTATION

Basic Level Intervention:
• Counseling
• Milieu therapy
• Self-care activities
• Psychological intervention
• Case management
• Health promotion and maintenance
• Health teaching

Advanced Practice Intervention:
• Psychotherapy
• Prescription of pharmacological agents
• Consultation

Figure 9–1 The nursing process in psychiatric mental health nursing.

ety, as in any other meeting between strangers. The interviewer's anxiety may stem from the client's perception of the interviewer's ability (or inability) to help the client. If the interviewer is a nursing student, anxiety regarding the instructor's evaluation becomes an added dimension. Clients' anxiety centers on their problems, the nurse's view of them, and what is ahead for them in treatment.

Both client and nurse bring to their relationship their total background experiences. These experiences include cultural beliefs and biases, religious attitudes, educational background, and occupational and life experiences, as well as attitudes regarding sexual roles. These attitudes, beliefs, and values influence the nurse's interactions with clients. It is important for nurses, through examining their personal beliefs and clarifying their values, to be aware of their biases and values and not feel compelled to impose their personal beliefs on others.

Although the nurse shares perceptions and alternatives with the client, the goal is to work with the client so that decisions and actions taken are the right ones for the client. Theoretically, this sounds easy, but often it is not. When beginning practitioners share their perceptions and thoughts with a more experienced nurse, unrecognized biases and value judgments often become evident. **Countertransference** issues may also play a role in the beginning practitioner's perceptions. Countertransference is the nurse's reactions to a client that are based on the nurse's unconscious needs, conflicts, problems, or view of the world. These reactions are inappropriate in the nurse-client relationship. Experience and supervision help a nurse separate what is important to the client from any bias that might impede mutually agreed goals.

The best atmosphere in which to conduct an assessment is one of minimal anxiety. Therefore, if an individual becomes upset, defensive, or embarrassed regarding any topic, the topic should be abandoned. The nurse can acknowledge that this is a subject that makes the client uncomfortable and can suggest that it would best be discussed when the client feels more comfortable. It is important that the nurse not

TABLE 9–1 *Some Medical Conditions That May Mimic Psychiatric Illness*

DEPRESSION	ANXIETY	PSYCHOSIS
Neurological disorder	Neurological disorders	Medical conditions
Cerebrovascular accident (stroke)	Alzheimer's disease	Temporal lobe epilepsy
Alzheimer's disease	Brain tumor	Migraine headaches
Brain tumor	Stroke	Temporal arteritis
Huntington's disease	Huntington's disease	Occipital tumors
Epilepsy (seizure disorder)	Infections	Narcolepsy
Multiple sclerosis	Encephalitis	Encephalitis
Parkinson's disease	Meningitis	Hypothyroidism
Cancer	Neurosyphilis	Addison's disease
Infections	Septicemia	Human immunodeficiency virus (HIV)
Mononucleosis	Endocrine	Medications
Encephalitis	Hypothyroidism and hyperthyroidism	Hallucinogens (e.g., LSD)
Hepatitis	Hypoparathyroidism	Phencyclidine
Tertiary syphilis	Hypoglycemia	Alcohol (withdrawal)
Human immunodeficiency virus	Pheochromocytoma	Stimulants
Endocrine	Carcinoid	Cocaine
Hypothyroidism and hyperthyroidism	Metabolic	Corticosteroids
Cushing's syndrome	Low calcium	
Addison's disease	Low potassium	
Parathyroid disease	Acute intermittent porphyria	
Gastrointestinal	Liver failure	
Liver cirrhosis	Cardiovascular	
Pancreatitis	Angina	
Cardiovascular	Congestive heart failure	
Hypoxia	Pulmonary embolus	
Congestive heart failure	Respiratory	
Respiratory	Pneumothorax	
Sleep apnea	Acute asthma	
Nutritional	Emphysema	
Thiamine deficiency	Medications	
Protein deficiency	Stimulants	
B_{12} deficiency	Sedative (withdrawal)	
B_6 deficiency	Lead, mercury	
Folate deficiency		
Collagen vascular		
Lupus		
Rheumatoid arthritis		

probe, pry, or push for information that is difficult for the client to discuss. However, recognize that increased anxiety about any subject is data in itself. The nurse can note this in the assessment without obtaining any further information.

Age Consideration

All clients, regardless of age or circumstance, need to have a thorough physical examination completed before a diagnosis is made. See Table 9–1 for examples of physical conditions that may mimic psychiatric disorders.

Assessment of an Elderly Client

Elderly clients often need special attention. The nurse needs to be aware of any physical limitations, that is, sensory (difficulty seeing or hearing), motor (difficulty walking or maintaining balance), or medical condition (cardiac or refractory) that could cause increased anxiety, stress, or physical discomfort for the client.

It is wise to identify any physical needs the client may have at the onset of the intervention and make accommodations for them. For example, if the client is hard of hearing, speak in clear, loud tones and have the client seated close to you.

Assessment of Children

The assessment of children is covered in Chapter 31. Use of story telling, dolls, drawing, games, and a lot more can be useful in assessing critical concerns and painful issues a child may have. Usually, a clinician with special training in child and adolescent psychiatry works with young children.

Assessment of an Adolescent Client

Assessment tools and strategies for the child and adolescent are discussed in Chapter 31; however, some points are given here. All people need to feel safe during a psychiatric interview and assessment. This is particularly true for children and adolescents. All clients are concerned with confidentiality. This is especially true for adolescents. Adolescents may fear that anything they may say to the nurse will be repeated to their parents. The adolescent needs to know that the nurse will not give out information without informing the adolescent in advance. Discussion about feelings can be kept confidential; however, threats of suicide, homicide, use of illegal drugs, or issues of abuse have to be shared with other professionals as well as the parents. Since identifying risk factors is one of the key objectives

	TABLE 9–2 The HEADSSS **Psychosocial Interview Technique**
H	Home environment (e.g., relations with parents and siblings)
E	Education/employment (e.g., school performance)
A	Activities (e.g., sports participation, afterschool activity, peer relations)
D	Drug, alcohol, or tobacco use
S	Sexuality (e.g., whether the patient is sexually active; whether he or she uses condoms or contraception)
S	Suicide risk or symptoms of depression or other mental disorder
S	'Savagery' (e.g., violence or abuse in home environment or in neighborhood)

when assessing adolescents, it is helpful to use a brief structured interview technique called the *H-E-A-D-S-S-S Interview* (Table 9–2).

The Psychiatric Nursing Assessment

Gathering Data

The use of a standardized nursing assessment tool facilitates the assessment process. Many assessment forms are available. Most health care systems and schools of nursing have their own assessment tool; however, even though an assessment tool is used, it is best to gather information from the client in an informal fashion, with the nurse clarifying, focusing, and exploring pertinent data with the client. This method allows clients to state their perceptions in their own words and enables the nurse to observe a wide range of nonverbal behaviors. When the order and the questions on the assessment tool are too rigidly applied, spontaneity is reduced. Assessment is a skill that is learned over time. The development of this skill is enhanced by practice, supervision, and patience. A personal style of interviewing congruent with the nurse's personality develops as comfort and experience increase.

The basic components of the psychiatric nursing assessment include the client's history and mental and emotional status. Throughout the assessment, the nurse attempts to identify the client's

■ Strengths as well as weaknesses
■ Usual coping strategies
■ Cultural beliefs and practices that may affect implementing traditional treatment

■ Spiritual beliefs or practices that are an integral part of your client's lifestyle

Table 9–3 is an example of a comprehensive nursing assessment tool. These terms are defined in the Glossary in the back of the text.

The client's history is most often the *subjective* part of the assessment. The focus of the history is the client's perceptions and recollections in three broad areas: presenting problem, current life style, and life in general (family, friends, education, work experience).

The mental and emotional status is the *objective* part of the assessment. The nurse observes the person's physical behavior and nonverbal communication, appearance, speech patterns, thought content, and cognitive ability. Objective data are measurable.

The assessment covers the social, physical, emotional, cultural, cognitive, and spiritual aspects of an individual. It elicits information about the systems in which a person operates. To conduct such an assessment, you should have fundamental knowledge of growth and development and of basic cultural and religious practices, as well as pathophysiology, psychopathology, and pharmacology.

After you have concluded the assessment, it is useful to summarize pertinent data with the client. This summary provides clients with reassurance that they have been heard and it allows them the opportunity to clarify any misinformation. They should be told what will happen next. For example, if the initial assessment takes place in the hospital, you should tell the client who else the client will be seeing. If the initial assessment was conducted by a psychiatric nurse in a mental health clinic, you will let the client know when and how often they will meet to work on the client's problems. If you believe a referral is necessary (e.g., to a psychiatrist, social worker, or physician), you will discuss this with the client.

Verifying Data

It is necessary that you validate data obtained from the client with secondary sources. Whenever possible, family members should be a part of the assessment. Is there anything going on in the family that is affecting the family? How does the family define the problem? How do the client's problems affect the family?

Family, friends, and neighbors may verify or contradict the client's self-perception and actions or may add information. Often, police officers are the ones who bring clients into the psychiatric emergency departments. You must know as much as possible about what the client was doing that warranted police intervention.

Other members of the health team are important sources of information and data verification. Many members of the health team will have contact with the client on admission to the hospital. The psychiatrist or psychologist, social worker, psychiatric nurse, recreation therapist, therapy aides, and student nurses can add to your database. If, however, there is no one to verify the client's information, you need to document this.

Old charts and medical records can help validate information you already have or add new information. In many communities, client records have been computerized. Medical history can aid in assessing physical losses and stress and can alert the staff to potential medical problems. If the client has been admitted to a psychiatric unit in the past, information about the client's previous level of functioning and behavior gives you a baseline for making clinical judgments. A consent may need to be signed to obtain information for this purpose.

Laboratory reports can provide useful information. When the body's chemistry is abnormal, personality changes and violent behaviors can result. For example, abnormal liver enzyme levels can explain irritability, depression, and lethargy. People who have chronic renal disease often suffer from the same symptoms when their blood urea nitrogen and electrolyte levels are abnormal. People with endocrine diseases such as diabetes can have changes in mood and level of consciousness related to glucose and insulin levels. A toxicology screen for the presence of either prescription or illegal drugs may also provide useful information.

Special Areas to Assess

SPIRITUAL ASSESSMENT. The importance of religion and spirituality to the American public has been increasingly highlighted by the media, opinion polls, and empirical studies (Mytko and Knight 1999). This includes all Americans from all cultures, with a wide diversity of religious and spiritual beliefs. Kendall (1999) stated that nurses who use a holistic paradigm are ethically obligated to support spiritual aspects of care, just as they do biophysical elements. A study by Charters (1999) highlighted the necessity for mental health nurses and allied clinical staff to be conscious that their clients may have spiritual and religious needs. This area of assessment is often overlooked in all areas of health care. It is believed by a growing number of nurses and other health care providers that religious and spiritual needs all should be a part of assessments and that multidisciplinary liaison and utilization of spiritual and religious resources should be available to all those who need them (Charters 1999). Perhaps you have heard of the power of prayer, or experienced it

TABLE 9–3 *Comprehensive Nursing Assessment Tool*

1. Client History
  I. GENERAL HISTORY OF CLIENT
  Name _____ Age _____ Sex _____
  Racial and ethnic data _____
  Marital status _____
  Number and ages of children/siblings
  Living arrangements
  Occupation
  Education
  Religious affiliations
  II. PRESENTING PROBLEM
  A. Statement in the client's own words concerning why he or she is hospitalized or seeking help
  B. **Recent difficulties**/alterations in
    1. Relationships
    2. Usual level of functioning
    3. Behavior
    4. Perceptions or cognitive abilities
  C. **Increased feelings of**
    1. Depression
    2. Anxiety
    3. Hopelessness
    4. Being overwhelmed
    5. Suspiciousness
    6. Confusion
  D. **Somatic changes,** such as
    1. Constipation
    2. Insomnia
    3. Lethargy
    4. Weight loss or gain
    5. Palpitations
  III. RELEVANT HISTORY—PERSONAL
  A. **Previous hospitalizations and illnesses** _____
  B. **Educational background** _____
  C. **Occupational background** _____
    1. If employed, where? _____
    2. How long at that job? _____
    3. Previous positions and reasons for leaving _____
    4. Special skills _____
  D. **Social patterns**
    1. Describe friends _____
    2. Describe a usual day _____
  E. **Sexual patterns**
    1. Sexually active? _____
    2. Sexual orientation _____
    3. Sexual difficulties _____
  F. **Interests and abilities**
    1. What does the client do in his or her spare time? _____
    2. What is the client good at? _____
    3. What gives the client pleasure? _____
  G. **Substance use and abuse**
    1. What psychotropic drugs does the client take? _____
      How often? _____ How much? _____
    2. How many drinks of alcohol does the client take per day? _____
      Per week? _____
    3. Does the client identify use of drugs as a problem? _____
  H. **How does the client cope with stress?** _____
    1. What does the client do when he or she gets upset? _____
    2. Whom can the client talk to? _____

Table continued on following page

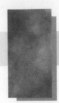

TABLE 9–3 *Comprehensive Nursing Assessment Tool (Continued)*

3. What usually helps to relieve stress? _____
4. What did the client try this time? _____

IV. RELEVANT HISTORY—FAMILY

A. **Childhood**
1. Who was important to the client growing up? _____
2. Was there physical or sexual abuse? _____
3. Did the parents drink or use drugs? _____
4. Who was in the home when the client was growing up? _____

B. **Adolescence**
1. How would the client describe his or her feelings in adolescence? _____
2. Describe the client's peer group at that time. _____

C. **Use of drugs**
1. Was there use or abuse of drugs by any family member? _____
   Prescription _____ Street _____ By whom? _____
2. What was the effect on the family? _____

D. **Family physical or mental problems**
1. Who in the family had physical or mental problems? _____
2. Describe the problems. _____
3. How did it affect the family? _____

E. Was there an unusual or outstanding event the client would like to mention? _____

2. Mental and Emotional Status

A. **Appearance**
Physical handicaps _____
Dress appropriate _____ Sloppy _____
Grooming neat _____ Poor _____
Eye contact held _____ Describe posture _____

B. **Behavior**
Restless _____ Agitated _____ Lethargic _____
Mannerisms _____ Facial expressions _____ Other _____

C. **Speech**
Clear _____ Mumbled _____ Rapid _____ Slurred _____
Constant _____ Mute or silent _____ Barriers to communications _____
Specify (e.g., client has delusions or is confused, withdrawn, or verbose) _____
_____

D. **Mood**
What mood does the client convey? _____
_____

E. **Affect**
Is the client's affect bland, apathetic, dramatic, bizarre, or appropriate? _____
Describe _____

F. **Thought process**
1. Characteristics
   Describe the characteristics of the person's responses: Flights of ideas _____
   Looseness of association _____ Blocking _____ Concrete _____
   Confabulation _____
   Describe _____
2. Cognitive ability
   Proverbs: Concrete _____ Abstract _____
   Serial sevens: How far does the client go? _____ Can the client do simple math? _____
   What seems to be the reason for poor concentration? _____
   Orientation to time(?), place(?), person(?) _____

G. **Thought content**
1. Central theme: What is important to the client? _____
   Describe _____
2. Self-concept: How does the client view himself or herself? _____
   What does the client want to change about himself or herself? _____
3. Insight: Does the client realistically assess his or her symptoms? _____
   Realistically appraise his or her situation? _____
   Describe _____

TABLE 9–3 *Comprehensive Nursing Assessment Tool (Continued)*

4. Suicidal or homicidal ideation? _____ What is suicide potential? _____
   Family history of suicide or homicide attempt or successful completion? _____
   Explain _____
5. Preoccupations. Does the client have hallucinations? _____ Delusions? _____
   Obsessions? _____ Rituals? _____ Phobias? _____ Grandiosity? _____
   Religiosity? _____ Sense of worthlessness? _____ Describe _____

H. **Spiritual Assessment**
   1. What importance does religion or spirituality have in your life? _____
   2. Do your religious or spiritual beliefs influence the way you take care of yourself or your illness? How? ____
   3. Who or what supplies you with hope? _____

I. **Cultural Influences**
   1. With what cultural group do you identify? _____
   2. Have you tried any cultural remedies or practices for your condition? If so what? _____
   3. Do you use any alternative or complementary medicines/herbs/practices? _____

in your own lives. For some clients, prayer or religious or spiritual practices are an important part of the quality of their lives and can give them hope, comfort, and support in healing. As nurses, whatever our personal feelings are regarding spiritual or religious beliefs, we are wise to support those beliefs of our clients and use appropriate referral services when agreed on by clients. Some questions we can ask to help with a spiritual assessment are

■ What role does religion or spirituality play in your life?
■ Does your faith help you in stressful situations?
■ Do you pray or meditate?
■ Who or what supplies you with strength and hope?
■ Has your illness affected your religious practices?
■ Do you participate in any religious activities?

RESEARCH FINDINGS

Spirituality and Psychiatric Assessment

The following is a summary of the study entitled, "Spiritual High versus High on Spirits: Is religiosity/spirituality, related to adolescent alcohol and drug abuse?" *

Study

Investigate the relationship between alcohol and drug abuse and frequency of religious/spiritual service attendance in the southeast United States

Population

Data obtained from 217 adolescents, aged 12 to 19, from both clinical and nonclinical settings

Method

Data obtained from surveys

Results

Results from both groups (clinical and nonclinical) showed that as attendance at religious services increased, alcohol and drug abuse decreased

Implications

Future study warranted to determine if the inclusion of spirituality could enhance recovery or reduce recidivism in alcohol or drug treatment programs

*Pullen, L., Modrcin-Talbott, M. A., West, W. R., and Muenchen, R. (1999). Spiritual high vs. high on spirits: Is religiosity/spirituality related to adolescent alcohol and drug abuse? *Journal of Psychiatric and Mental Health Nursing,* 6(1):3–8.

TABLE 9–4 *Standardized Rating Scales**

USE	SCALE
Depression	Beck Inventory
	Hamilton Depression Scale
	Zung Self-Report Inventory
Anxiety	Modified Spielberger State Anxiety Scale
	Hamilton Anxiety Scale
Substance use disorders	Addiction Severity Index (ASI)
	Recovery Attitude And Treatment Evaluator (RAATE)
	Brief Drug Abuse Screen Test (B-DAST)
Obsessive-compulsive behavior	Yale-Brown Obsessive-Compulsive Scale (Y-BOCS)
Mania	Mania Rating Scale
Schizophrenia	Scale for Assessment of Negative Symptoms (SANS)
	Brief Psychiatric Rating Scale (BPRS)
Abnormal movements	Abnormal Involuntary Movement Scale (AIMS)
	Simpson Neurological Rating Scale
	CLAMPS Abnormal Movement Scale
General psychiatric assessment	Brief Psychiatric rating Scale (BPRS)
	Global Assessment of Functioning Scale (GAF)
Cognitive function	Mini-Mental State Examination
	Alzheimer's Disease Rating Scale (ADRS)
	Memory and Behavior Problem Checklist
Family assessment	McMaster Family Assessment Device
Eating disorders	Eating Disorders Inventory (EDI)
	Body Attitude Test
	Diagnostic Survey for Eating Disorders

*These rating scales highlight important areas in psychiatric assessment. Since many of the answers are subjective in nature, experienced clinicians use these tools as guides when planning care, in addition to their knowledge of their clients.

■ Do you have a spiritual advisor or member of the clergy (priest, rabbi, minister) readily available?
■ Is there anyone I can contact to help put you back in touch with your church/synagogue/place of worship/prayer?

A nursing study (see Research Findings Box) investigated the relationship between attendance at religious services and change in drug and alcohol use.

CULTURAL AND SOCIAL ASSESSMENT. Because nurses are increasingly faced with caring for culturally diverse populations, there is an increasing need for nursing assessment, nursing diagnoses, and subsequent care to be planned around unique cultural health care beliefs, values, and practices. Burr and Chapman (1998) advocated that mental health nurses need a thorough understanding of the complexity of the cultural and social factors that influence health and illness. Awareness of individual cultural beliefs and health care practices can help nurses minimize labeling of clients. Some questions we can ask to help with a cultural and social assessment are

■ What is your primary language? Would you like an interpreter?
■ How would you describe your cultural background?
■ Who are you close to? Who do you seek in times of crisis?
■ Who do you live with?
■ Who do you seek when you are medically ill? Mentally upset or concerned?
■ What do you do to get better when you are medically ill? Mentally ill?
■ What are the attitudes toward mental illness in your culture?
■ How is your mental health problem viewed by your culture? Is it seen as a problem to fix a disease? A taboo? A fault or curse?
■ Are there special foods that you eat?
■ Are there special health care practices within your culture that address your particular mental health problem?
■ What economic resources are available to your family?

Use of Rating Scale

There are a number of standardized rating scales that are useful for psychiatric evaluation and monitoring. Rating scales are often administered by a clinician (nurse, psychologist, social worker, psychiatrist), but many are self-administered. Table 9–4 gives an example of some of the common ones in use. Many of the clinical chapters include a rating scale.

NURSING DIAGNOSIS

A nursing diagnosis has three structural components:

1. Problem (unmet need)
2. Etiology (probable cause)
3. Supporting data (signs and symptoms)

The *problem*, or unmet need, describes the state of the client at present. Problems that are within the nurse's domain to prescribe and treat are termed *nursing diagnoses.* The nursing diagnostic title states what should change, for example, *hopelessness.*

Etiology, or probable cause, is linked to the diagnostic title with the words "related to." Stating the etiology or probable cause tells what needs to be done to effect the change and identifies causes that the nurse can treat through nursing interventions.

Hopelessness: related to long-term stress

Supporting data, or signs and symptoms, state what the condition is like at present.

Supporting data (defining characteristics) that validate diagnosis include

- Client states "It's no use, nothing will change."
- Lack of involvement with family and friends.
- Lack of motivation to care for self or environment.

Here we will follow a client, Mr. Saltzberg, through the nursing process (see Fig. 9–1).

Vignette

- Mr. Saltzberg is a 47-year-old married man, the father of two boys, 7 and 9 years of age. He is admitted to the hospital because of depression and suicidal threats. Two months ago his business failed. Mr. Saltzberg states, "I built that business up from nothing; now I am left with nothing." He states he has been feeling depressed and "I just want to be alone."

He has been anorexic and has lost 12 pounds in the past 2 months. He weighs 140 pounds and is 10 pounds under his range for normal body weight (150 to 165 pounds). He has no interest in sex or any other activity. Family history reveals that his father suffered from depression and attempted suicide at age 60.

Mr. Saltzberg appears unkempt—his clothes are wrinkled and he has not shaved for 3 days. He sits slumped in the chair with his head down, facing the interviewer but seldom making eye contact. His speech is slow and his mood depressed. His thinking has slowed and he says, "I can't think."

He admits that he is preoccupied with suicidal thoughts. His wife says that he just sits and stares into space all day, keeping to himself. She states that this is the first time she has ever known him to react like this and that his behavior is a constant concern for the whole family. Mrs. Saltzberg says she feels overwhelmed without his help and support. The children are confused and miss doing things with their father. The family has not gone to temple, the movies, or sports activities—all of which are important events for this family—for 2 months.

Mr. Saltzberg was seen by the psychiatrist on the unit and was given the Diagnostic and Statistical Manual of Mental Disorders (APA 2000) diagnosis of major depression.

The nurse meets with Mr. Saltzberg and makes an initial assessment. She speaks with Mrs. Saltzberg, verifies her assessment, and adds it to the database. The nurse also shares information with other staff and members of the health team in conference.

Formulating a Nursing Diagnosis

After the nurse assesses Mr. Saltzberg, the data are organized into problems and placed in order of priority. Three major problem areas are identified, as follows:

1. Risk of suicide
2. Inadequate nutrition
3. Disrupted family functioning

From these problem areas, three nursing diagnoses are formulated:

Risk for suicide: possible suicidal behavior related to multiple losses

Supporting data that validate diagnosis

- Business is failing.
- The client says "I have nothing left to live for."
- Difficulty with activities of daily living (ADLs) and lowering of mood lasting 2 months.
- Father attempted suicide at age 60.
- Client states he has thoughts of killing himself.

Imbalanced nutrition: less than body requirements, related to apathy and poor self-concept

Supporting data that validate diagnosis

- Client has sustained a 12-pound weight loss in 2 months.
- He is 10 pounds less than his recommended weight range.
- He refuses to eat prepared meals.
- He says he has no appetite.

Interrupted family process: related to an ill family member

Supporting data that validate diagnosis

- Since client's illness, the family has not participated in usual family activities.
- Wife and husband have not shared usual activi-

ties involving companionship or sex since the onset of illness.

■ Wife says she feels overwhelmed without the husband's help and support.

■ Children are upset and confused over father's behavior.

Refer to Appendix C for a list of all current nursing diagnoses.

OUTCOME CRITERIA

Determining the Desired Outcomes

Outcomes are the measurable behaviors or situations that are the result of treatment and nursing intervention. Outcome criteria are the hoped-for outcomes that reflect the maximal level of client health that can realistically be reached by nursing interventions.

Changes in the delivery and finances of the present health care system have put increased pressure on the psychiatric mental health care system to be more accountable to consumers, insurance companies, and policy makers (Smith 1999) (Advanced Practice). The Nursing Outcomes Classification (NOC) (Johnson et al. 2000) has developed a total of 260 standardized outcomes based on research and clinical practice. NOC provides standardized language for outcomes used in the nursing process for all settings and clinical specialists. For nurses to work effectively with managed care organizations to improve quality and reduce costs, nurses must be able to measure and document patient outcomes influenced by nursing care (Phoon et al. 1996). See Table 9–5 for NOC-suggested outcomes for suicide self-restraint.

TABLE 9–5   *Nursing Outcomes Classification: Suicide Self-Restraint*

Nursing Outcomes: some or all may be appropriate outcome measures depending on the nursing assessment
Definition: ability to refrain from gestures and attempts at killing self

INDI-CATORS	SUICIDE SELF-RESTRAINT	NEVER DEMON-STRATED	RARELY DEMON-STRATED	SOME-TIMES DEMON-STRATED	OFTEN DEMON-STRATED	CONSIS-TENTLY DEMON-STRATED
1	Express feelings	1	2	3	4	5
2	Maintains connectedness in relationships	1	2	3	4	5
3	Seeks help when feeling self-destructive	1	2	3	4	5
4	Verbalizes suicidal ideas if present	1	2	3	4	5
5	Verbalizes control of impulses	1	2	3	4	5
6	Refrains from gathering means for suicide	1	2	3	4	5
7	Does not give away possessions	1	2	3	4	5
8	Does not require treatment for suicidal attempts	1	2	3	4	5
9	Refrains from using mood-altering substance(s)	1	2	3	4	5
10	Discloses plan for suicide if present	1	2	3	4	5
11	Upholds suicide contract	1	2	3	4	5
12	Maintains self-control without supervision	1	2	3	4	5
13	Does not attempt suicide	1	2	3	4	5
14	Other _____ (specify)	1	2	3	4	5

From Johnson, M., Maas, M., and Moorehead, S. (2000). *Nursing outcomes classification (NOC)* (2nd ed.). St. Louis: Mosby.

Goals should be realistic and acceptable to both client and nurse. An appropriate goal meets the following criteria:

■ It is stated in observable or measurable terms.
■ It indicates client outcomes.
■ It sets a specific time goal for achievement.
■ It is short and specific.
■ It is written in positive terms.

Referring to the nursing diagnoses formulated for Mr. Saltzberg, the nurse sets outcome criteria and short-term goals.

Risk for Self-Directed Violence: Possible Suicide Behaviors Related to Multiple Losses

OUTCOME CRITERION	SHORT-TERM GOAL
1. Refrains from attempting suicide	1. Client will remain free of injury with the aid of staff
	2. Client will speak to nurse, wife, rabbi when feeling overwhelmed or self-destructive

PLANNING

Planning consists of identifying nursing interventions that will help meet the outcome criteria and are appropriate to the client's level of functioning. The nurse writes a set of interventions appropriate for reaching each goal. Each stated goal should include nursing interventions, which should be seen as instructions for all people working with the client. These written plans aid in the continuity of care for the client and are points of information for all members of the health team. More and more units, both inpatient and community-based facilities, use standardized care plans or clinical pathways for clients with specific diagnoses. Other units are devising individual plans of care. The nurse considers specific principles when planning care. Nursing interventions planned for meeting a specific goal need to be

■ *Safe.* They must be safe for the client as well as for other clients, staff, and family.
■ *Appropriate.* They must be compatible with other therapies and with the client's personal goals and cultural values, as well as with institutional rules.

■ *Effective.* They should be based on scientific principles.
■ *Individualized nursing care.* They should be realistic: (1) be within the capabilities of the client's age, physical strength, condition, and willingness to change; (2) be based on the number of staff available; (3) reflect actual available community resources; and (d) be within the student's or nurses' capabilities.

The Nursing Interventions Classification (NIC) (McCloskey and Bulecheck 2000) is a research-based standardized language of nearly 500 interventions that the nurse can use to plan care. In all settings nurses can use NIC's standardized classification of nursing interventions to support quality patient care and validate the breadth and value of nursing practice (La Duke 2000).

The nurse plans the interventions to meet the goals set for Mr. Saltzberg. The development of one goal follows:

Nursing diagnosis: *Risk for suicide* related to multiple losses

Outcome Criteria: *Refrains from Attempting Suicide*

SHORT-TERM GOAL	NURSING INTERVENTION
1. Client will remain free of injury while in the hospital, with the aid of staff	1a. Remove all items that could potentially be used as weapons (e.g., belts, ties, shoelaces, razors, plastic bags).
	1b. Assess immediate degree of suicidal risk, and ask client if he is thinking of killing himself.
	1c. Check client every 15 minutes and keep him in view at all times.
	1d. Make a "no suicide contract" with the client stating he will not harm himself. (See Chapter 24 for specifics.)
	1e. Spend time with client for 15 minutes, three times a day.
	1f. Encourage client to express thoughts and feelings.
	1g. Encourage client to engage in unit activities even though he may resist and be withdrawn.
	1h. Document all assessments, interactions, and interventions.

BOX 9–1   *Communication and Counseling Intervention*

Short-term goal: Client will name three personal strengths that have worked for him in the past.

INTERACTION	RATIONALE
Nurse: You mentioned everything coming down on you when your business began to fail.	Placing the event in time and sequence, validating the precipitating event
Client: Yes. . . . Everything I had worked for was lost. That business was my whole life. Everything I did was for my business. It was my baby.	
Nurse: You lost a great deal. You said it was like your baby?	Reflecting and showing empathy Restating
Client: Yeah, well, I had dreamed of it for years. My brother lent me some money, but it was my idea, and I did most of the work to get it going.	
Nurse: It seems to me that building up a business from scratch takes a lot of work and know-how.	Pointing out realities and assisting to clarify strengths
Client: Oh yes, I was never afraid of hard work. I used to be good at figuring my way out of a tight spot. Now . . . I don't know. . . . Ever since that automated shop came in, I couldn't keep up with those prices. Everything caved in. . . . It doesn't seem to matter anymore.	
Nurse: What doesn't seem to matter?	Clarifying
Client: Me . . . being a success . . . being somebody. I guess now I'll never be anybody.	
Nurse: Are you saying that you equate what happens in business with your personal worth?	Validating the client's perception
Client: Yes . . . I mean . . . no, I just felt so awful when everything caved in . . . I felt so responsible.	
Nurse: Responsible?	Restating
Client: Yeah. . . . Responsible to my family.	
Nurse: How did your family react?	Giving broad openings
Client: Well . . . I really didn't say too much to them. I didn't want to worry them. . . . I guess I was afraid.	
Nurse: Afraid?	Restating
Client: Yeah. That they would think I was no longer a success now that the business was failing.	
Nurse: You were afraid they would see you as a failure if the business ran into trouble?	Reflecting
Client: I don't know. . . . The business was such a great success in the beginning.	
Nurse: What do you think made the shop so successful in the beginning?	Encouraging the client to realistically appraise his strengths
Client: Well, I worked very hard . . . and I am good at knowing what people want. Everyone says I have a unique way of marketing and advertising.	
Nurse: You are conscientious, observant of others, and creative.	Restating what the client has said. At this point the client can agree or clarify what he meant Encourage the client to problem solve
Client: Well . . . yes, but what does that matter now?	
Nurse: In what other ways could you use these qualities?	

BOX 9–1 *Communication and Counseling Intervention (continued)*

INTERACTION	RATIONALE
Client: Huh . . . I hadn't thought about other ways. . . . [*silence*]. Sam Cohn . . . well . . . Sam, he always wanted me to come in with him. I always wanted my own place though.	
Nurse: Well, that is one possibility. We talked this morning about some of your strengths and maybe this afternoon we can talk some more about other ways you can use these strengths in the future.	Summarizing and encouraging collaboration
Client: Yeah . . . some other possibilities.	

IMPLEMENTATION

The *Scope and Standards of Psychiatric–Mental Health Nursing Practice* (ANA 2000) identify 10 areas for intervention. Seven of these areas of intervention are at the basic level. Recent graduates and practitioners new to the psychiatric setting will participate in many of these activities with the guidance and support of more experienced health care professionals. Interventions at the basic level include

- Counseling
- Milieu therapy
- Promotion of self-care
- Psychobiological interventions
- Health teaching
- Case management
- Health promotion and health maintenance

Three other areas are specific for the advanced level. The psychiatric mental health advanced practice registered nurse is prepared at the master's level or beyond. Advanced practice interventions include

- Psychotherapy
- Prescription authority and treatment
- Consultations

Counseling

Counseling is usually carried out by a nurse minimally prepared at the basic level in psychiatric mental health nursing. The nurse is skilled in basic techniques of therapeutic communication. Some of the interventions include reinforcing healthy patterns of behavior; employing problem solving, interviewing, and communication skills; crisis intervention; stress management; relaxation techniques; conflict resolution; and behavior modification. The dialogue in Box 9–2 illustrates the use of communication and counseling skills during a nurse-client interaction with Mr. Saltzberg.

Health Teaching

Health teaching includes identifying health education needs of the client and teaching basic principles of physical and mental health, such as giving information about coping, mental health problems, mental disorders and treatments, and their effects on daily living. The following vignette illustrates health teaching.

Vignette

- *While working with Mr. Saltzberg on creating alternatives to his present solution, the nurse notes that family communications seem to break down when the client is faced with an issue that threatens his self-image. Mr. Saltzberg says that the family is usually able to talk about personal concerns. However, when the business started to falter, Mr. Saltzberg began to think of himself as a failure. He felt ashamed and impotent, and he isolated himself from his family emotionally, hiding his feelings.*

  The nurse intervenes to suggest alternative interpersonal communication skills Mr. Saltzberg can use within the family to minimize feelings of hopelessness and helplessness when problems arise. The nurse suggests to Mr. Saltzberg that the family and nurse meet together so that he can "practice" sharing personal feelings. Illness or problems of one family member usually affect all family members. By having the family meet together and work on important issues with some degree of safety and guidance, problems can be minimized, provide a variety of alternative actions, and decrease feelings of isolation and helplessness. The family may also identify outside resources that could prove helpful, for example, religious counseling and sympathetic relatives and friends.

Self-Care Activities

Self-care activities assist the client in assuming personal responsibility for ADLs and are aimed at improving the client's functional status when appropriate.

The nursing interventions aimed at increasing Mr. Saltzberg's physical care center on nutrition. See the following vignette.

Vignette

■ *The short-term goal is that Mr. Saltzberg will eat at least three quarters of his three meals a day, plus one snack. Getting an anorexic person to eat takes creative thinking and patience. In implementing the plan of care for Mr. Saltzberg, the nurse first finds out whether there are any religious or medical dietary restrictions. Mr. Saltzberg states that he eats only kosher foods and that he does have food preferences. These preferences are special dishes his wife makes for him at home.*

Kosher foods are requested for his hospital stay and Mrs. Saltzberg agrees to make foods her husband especially likes and that she feels will tempt him to eat once he is discharged. The importance of follow-up care, community resources, and suicide prevention centers is also a vital part of Mr. Saltzberg's total care. The nurse in charge of case management is involved in Mr. Saltzberg's discharge planning.

Psychobiological Interventions

One of the nurse's functions is the administration of medications to clients. Nurses are responsible for observing the therapeutic, as well as any untoward, effects of the drug. They are expected to know the intended action, therapeutic dose, and blood levels and to monitor these when appropriate (e.g., blood levels with lithium). The nurse is expected to discuss with the client and family both drug action and side effects and to provide time for questions.

Vignette

■ *Mr. Saltzberg is taking the antidepressant paroxetine hydrochloride (Paxil). The nurse discusses the purpose of the drug with him and potential side effects that he might experience at home. Mr. Saltzberg will have written instructions about potential side effects, toxic effects, and whom to contact in case of difficulty once he is discharged to the community.*

Milieu Therapy

Milieu therapy is an extremely important consideration for the nurse working with a client. The client should feel comfortable and safe and be assured that help is available. Milieu management includes reteaching activities that meet the client's physical and mental health needs. In the hospital setting and day-hospital setting, recreational, occupational, and dance therapists are often available to create appropriate activities for clients and give structure to their day. At times, milieu management might mean setting limits (restraints, seclusion, time out). In Mr. Saltzberg's case, milieu management includes certain environmental restrictions that can protect him from self-destructive behavior.

A safe environment for Mr. Saltzberg is the highest priority when he is first admitted to the unit. A person who is feeling overwhelmed and who is in a great deal of emotional pain often has difficulty figuring out ways to solve problems. Sometimes suicide appears to be the only solution. Mr. Saltzberg has suffered a great loss, is a man, and is older than 45 years of age; his father had attempted suicide at age 60; Mr. Saltzberg is clinically depressed. He has also disengaged himself from the support of his family and friends, and is not attending to ADLs (eating, dressing, appearance). All these factors place him at risk for suicide. (See Chapter 23 for assessing a person's suicide risk.)

A safe environment is arranged by providing Mr. Saltzberg with close observation and by setting limits. All potential weapons are removed, and he is put on suicide precautions, which entail checking the client every 15 minutes and keeping him in view at all times. He is also observed for any behaviors that might indicate thoughts of suicide, such as a sudden sense of well-being, giving away possessions, or making out a will.

The process is providing the presence of a person who is interested in the client's situation, is willing to work on issues in a nonjudgmental and nonthreatening manner, and is able to provide important resources when needed.

Continuing Data Collection

Data collection is an ongoing process throughout all the phases of the nursing process. While observing Mr. Saltzberg, one nurse noted that he had difficulty sharing problems with his family when his self-esteem was threatened. During these times, family communications broke down, and family members became confused and isolated. The added data directed future nursing intervention.

EVALUATION

Evaluation is often the most neglected part of the nursing process. Ideally, evaluation should be part of each phase in the process.

Evaluating Outcome Criteria

There are three possible outcomes when goals are evaluated: goal met, goal not met, goal partially met. The nurse develops the statement of evaluation and documents the client's behavior to determine whether the goal has been met. Diagrammatically, evaluation of goal achievement appears as follows:

EVALUATION
1. Goal met
2. Goal not met
3. Goal partially met

Whether the goal is met or only partially met, actual client behaviors should be added as evidence. For example, evaluation of the goals set by the nurse for

Risk for Suicide Related to Multiple Losses

SHORT-TERM GOAL	EVALUATION
1. Client will remain free of injury with the aid of staff	1. **Goal met.** By 2nd day client stated he had options and that he wanted to live.
2. Client will speak with nurse, wife, or rabbi when feeling overwhelmed or self-destructive	2. **Goal met.** Client stated he felt less embarrassed to discuss his feelings with his wife and stated he can talk of these things with his rabbi.

Vignette

■ *Mr. Saltzberg was discharged 3 days after he was admitted. By the second day he was taken off suicide precaution and stated, "I really do want to live. I feel a little better knowing there are some options." He was still feeling depressed but no longer hopeless. He understood that the medication might take up to 3 weeks to work. He also understood that, if this medication failed to work, or if the side effects interfered too much in his life, there were other types of medication to try. He readily agreed to be followed up in the clinic for medication monitoring, but told the caseworker that his rabbi was the person he would rather go to for guidance.*

DOCUMENTATION

Documentation could be considered the seventh step in the nursing process. Besides the evaluation of stated outcomes, the chart should reflect changes in client condition, informed consents (medications, treatments), reaction to medication, documentation of symptoms (verbatim when appropriate), and concerns of client and any untoward incidences in the health care setting. Documentation of client progress is the responsibility of the entire mental health team. Although communication among team members and coordination of services are the primary goals when choosing a system for charting, practitioners in all settings must also consider professional standards, legal issues, requirements for reimbursement by insurers, and accreditation by regulatory agencies. Information must also be in a format that is retrievable for quality assurance monitoring, utilization management, peer review, and research. For nursing, documentation of the nursing process is a guiding concern and is reflected in different formats that are commonly used in health care settings. See Table 9–6 for an overview of charting methods. Computerized clinical documentation is becoming the common trend in inpatient as well as outpatient settings today. Refer to Chapter 8 regarding legal guidelines for clinical documentation.

SUMMARY

The nursing process is an adaptation of the problem-solving process used by many professions. The *primary source* of assessment is the client. *Secondary sources* of information include the family, neighbors, friends, police, and other members of

TABLE 9–6   *Charting Methods*

	NARRATIVE	PROBLEM-ORIENTED CHARTING (SOAPIE)
Characteristics	A descriptive statement of client status written in chronological order throughout a shift. Used to support assessment finding from a flow sheet. In charting by exception, narrative notes are used to indicate significant symptoms, behaviors, or events that are exceptions to norms identified on an assessment flow sheet	Developed in the 1960s for physicians to reduce inefficient documentation. Intended to be accompanied by a problem list. Originally SOAP, with IE added later. The emphasis is on problem identification, process, and outcome S: Subjective data (patient statement) O: Objective data (nurse observations) A: Assessment (nurse interprets S and O and describes either a problem or a nursing diagnosis) P: Plan (proposed intervention) I: Interventions (nurse's response to problem) E: Evaluation (client outcome)
Example	Date/time/discipline Client was agitated in the morning and pacing in the hallway Blinks eyes, muttering to self, and looking off to the side States he hears voices Verbally hostile to another client Offered 2 mg haloperidol (Haldol) prn and sat with staff in quiet area for 20 minutes Client returned to community lounge and was able to sit and watch television	Date/time/discipline S: "I'm so stupid. Get away, get away." "I hear the devil telling me bad things." O: Client pacing the hall, mumbling to self, and looking off to the side. Shouted derogatory comments when approached by another client. Watching walls and ceiling closely A: Client is having auditory hallucinations and increased agitation P: Offer client haloperidol prn. Redirect client to less stimulating environment I: Client received 2 mg Haldol PO prn; sat with client in quiet room for 20 minutes E: Client calmer. Returned to community lounge, sat and watched television
Advantages	Narrative writing is a common form of expression Can address any event or behavior Explains flow sheet findings Multidisciplinary ease of use	Structured Consistent organization of data Easy to retrieve data for quality assurance and utilization management Contains all elements of nursing process Minimizes unnecessary data Multidisciplinary ease of use
Disadvantages	Unstructured Organization of information may vary from note to note Difficult format for retrieval of quality assurance and utilization management data Elements of nursing process frequently omitted Unnecessary and subjective information commonly included	Time/effort to structure the information Limits entries to problems Data about progress may be lost Not chronological Negative connotation

	Problem-Oriented Charting (PIE or APIE)	Focus Charting (DAR)
Characteristics	Either APIE or PIE. Intended to parallel nursing process. Problem is described by nursing diagnosis. Assessment is either included in the progress note or referenced from an assessment flow sheet A: Assessment P: problems (nursing diagnosis) I: Interventions E: Evaluation	Uses key words to indicate the primary subject of the note. May be a symptom, event, behavior, or nursing diagnosis. Has replaced SOAP notes in many hospitals D: Data (information pertinent to the focus) A: Action (intervention) R: Response (client outcome)

TABLE 9–6 *Charting Methods* (Continued)

	PROBLEM-ORIENTED CHARTING (PIE OR APIE)	FOCUS CHARTING (DAR)
Example	Date/time **A:** Client at severe level of anxiety, muttering to self and looking off to the side. Making verbal threats, has psychomotor agitation, states he hears voices **P:** Anxiety related to internal auditory stimulation **I:** Client received 2 mg haloperidol PO prn; sat with client in quiet room for 20 minutes **E:** Client calmer. Returned to community lounge, sat and watched television	Date/time/focus Agitated behavior **D:** Client pacing the hall, mumbling to self and looking off to the side; states he hears voices, verbal hostility **A:** Given 2 mg haloperidol PO prn; sat with client in quiet room for 20 minutes **R:** Client calmer. Returned to community lounge, sat and watched television
Advantages	Structured Consistent organization of data Easy to retrieve data for quality assurance and utilization management Contains all elements of nursing process Minimizes unnecessary data	Structured Consistent organization of data Easy to retrieve data for quality assurance and utilization management Fosters use of the nursing process Not necessarily problem oriented Includes a variety of data on client status
Disadvantages	Time/effort to structure the information Specific for nursing Limits entries to problems Data about progress may be lost Not chronological Negative connotation	Time/effort to structure the information Not chronological

the health team. Both the nurse's and the client's anxiety levels need to be acknowledged, as do personal biases and value judgments. The assessment interview includes gathering subjective data (client history) and objective data (mental or emotional status). An assessment tool is provided. The student is urged to practice taking a client history using this assessment guide. Assessment tools and standardized rating scales that may be used to evaluate and monitor a client's progress are useful and can help the nurse focus the interview. When the nurse develops skill and becomes more comfortable in this role, the interview becomes less formal without sacrificing important data. Refer to Chapter 8 regarding legal guidelines for clinical documentation.

The nursing diagnosis is a crucial phase in the nursing process. It performs a number of functions: it defines the practice of nursing, improves communication between staff, assists in accountability for care, differentiates nursing from medicine, and so forth. A nursing diagnosis consists of (1) an unmet need or problem, (2) an etiology or probable cause, and (3) supporting data.

Outcome criteria are established that are realistic and within the client's ability. Short- and long-term goals can be used as steps in accomplishing the final outcome criteria. The NOC provides standardized outcomes. Planning involves determining desired outcomes and goals. A goal should be measurable, indicate the desired outcome, have a set time for achievement, and be short and specific. Goals identify the direction for nursing care.

Planning nursing action to achieve the goals includes the use of specific principles: the plan should be (1) safe, (2) based on scientific rationale, (3) realistic, and (4) compatible with other therapies. The NIC provides all nurses with standardized nursing interventions in use for all settings.

Practice in psychiatric nursing encompasses seven basic level interventions: counseling, milieu therapy, self-care activities, psychobiological interventions, health teaching, case management, and health promotion and management.

Advanced practice skills are carried out by a nurse who is educated at the master's level and higher. Nurses certified for advanced practice-psychiatric mental health nursing can practice psychotherapy, prescribe certain medications, and perform consulting work.

The evaluation of care is done by determining if the outcome criteria (short- and long-term goals) have been achieved. The nurse judges the goal to be met, not met, or partially met. Supporting data are included to clarify the evaluation. If the goals have not been met, the nurse decides whether priorities in diagnosis need changing; new diagnoses need to be added; new interventions are required to meet goals; and whether diagnosis, goals, interventions, and plans are currently appropriate.

Documentation of client progress through evaluation of the outcome criteria is crucial. The chart is a legal document and should accurately reflect the client's condition, medications, treatment, tests, responses to these, and any untoward incidences.

Visit the **Evolve** website at
http://evolve.elsevier.com/Varcarolis
for a post-test on the content in this chapter.

Visit the **Evolve** website at
http://evolve.elsevier.com/Varcarolis
for additional self-study exercises.

Critical Thinking and Chapter Review

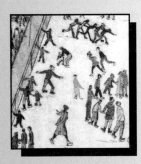

Critical Thinking

Ms. Jamison is a 25-year-old woman who came to the hospital because voices told her to kill herself and she became very frightened. She appears tense. Her posture is rigid, her respiration is rapid, and she says she has not eaten for 3 days. When asked what she usually does when she gets upset, she says that she used to talk to her mother, but her mother died a year ago. Since then, she has been extremely lonely. She tells the nurse she does not have any friends and works part-time as a temporary secretary. She says her voices started a week after her mother died. "They used to be friendly voices, but now they want me to die." She has an aunt and a brother but is hesitant to contact them. She states "They really don't need my problems . . . they have busy lives." She says she is frightened about the voices and is afraid she might obey them. She asks the nurse to help her.

Questions 1 to 4 refer to this situation. They are organized according to the steps of the nursing process.

1. There are a number of diagnoses the nurse could choose. Formulate one nursing diagnosis for Ms. Jamison. (Refer to Appendix C for a list of current nursing diagnoses.) Include the problem statement, probable etiology, and supporting data.

   A. The diagnostic title: What should change? _____
   B. The etiology or possible cause related to _____
   C. Supporting data to validate diagnosis: _____

2. State one outcome criterion (long-term goal) and two short-term goals for the diagnosis in question 1, using all four criteria.

    A. *Outcome criteria*: _____
    B. *Short-term goal*: _____
    C. *Short-term goal*: _____

3. When planning nursing care for Ms. Jamison, list four principles you would consider.

    A. _____
    B. _____
    C. _____
    D. _____

    Ms. Jamison is to be discharged tomorrow. She tells the nurse that the voices no longer tell her to kill herself and do not seem as threatening. She says she would like to continue seeing the nurse therapist in the clinic and plans to continue visiting her brother on weekends, but she does not feel up to trying any other activity at this time, although she completes her self-care. As to her medication, she is able to explain to the nurse the dose and time of the medications and possible side effects.

4. For the following goals, state whether the goal was met, not met, or partially met, and give the supporting data.

Outcome criterion: By discharge, client will state she no longer hears threatening or frightening voices.

    A. Goal: Supporting data: _____

Short-term goal: Within 2 weeks, client will be able to name three sources of support (church, community health center, women's groups, relatives, neighbors) that she is comfortable using.

    B. Goal: Supporting data: _____

Short-term goal: Client will complete self care while in the hospital, with the aid of medication and a daily therapy session with the nurse.

    C. Goal: Supporting data: _____

5. Discuss three positive outcomes for having standardized nursing outcomes classification (NOC) and standardized interventions classification (NIC) systems. Think in terms of the managed care environmental supporting quality care for clients in all settings.

Chapter Review

Choose the most appropriate answer.

1. Which statement by a nurse suggests an undesirable outcome of a psychiatric assessment interview conducted by the psychiatric nurse?

    1. "I think I was able to establish good rapport with the client."
    2. "I believe the client understands that my values differ from his."
    3. "I was able to obtain a good understanding of the client's current problem."
    4. "I was able to perform a complete assessment of the client's level of psychological functioning."

2. Assessment of an elderly client will be facilitated if the nurse

1. Identifies and accommodates client physical needs early.
2. Pledges complete confidentiality of all topics to the client.
3. Adheres strictly to the order of questions on the standardized assessment tool.
4. Interprets data without regard to client spiritual and cultural beliefs and practices.

3. A nurse tells a peer, "I place greatest weight on the subjective data I obtain during client assessment." From this the peer can infer that the nurse depends more on

1. Data obtained from secondary sources than data obtained from the primary source.
2. The client's perceptions of the presenting problem than on data obtained from the mental status examination.
3. Data obtained from the mental status examination than on information elicited during history taking.
4. Gut-level hunches about client strengths and weaknesses than on data obtained from rating scales.

4. Which statement about nursing diagnosis is correct?

1. A nursing diagnosis has three structural components: a problem, the etiology of the problem, and supporting data that validate the diagnosis.
2. A nursing diagnosis is complete when the problem statement reflects an unmet need and the etiology given reflects a probable cause.
3. An accurate nursing diagnosis requires a problem statement that identifies causes the nurse can treat via nursing interventions.
4. A nursing diagnosis must always be based on objective data measured by the nurse; subjective data may be used only as supporting data to validate the diagnosis.

5. What is the relationship between goals and nursing interventions?

1. Nursing interventions are instructions for staff aimed at facilitating goal attainment.
2. Goals reflect realistic expectations for client's progress while nursing interventions suggest best nursing practices.
3. Nursing interventions are guidelines for meeting nursing standards and do not relate directly to client goals.
4. Goals are required as part of interdisciplinary treatment plans while nursing interventions as specific to the discipline of nursing.

REFERENCES

American Nurses' Association. (2000). *Scope and standards of psychiatric mental health nursing practice*. Washington, D.C.: Author.

American Psychiatric Association. (2000). *Diagnostic and statistical manual of mental disorders* (4th ed., Text Revision). Washington, D.C.: Author.

Bower, F. L. (1982). *The process of planning nursing care*. St. Louis: Mosby.

Burr, J. A., and Chapman, T. (1998). Some reflections on cultural and social considerations in mental health nursing. *Journal of Psychiatric and Mental Health Nursing*, 5(6):431–437.

Charters, P. J. (1999). The religious and spiritual needs of mental health clients. *Nursing Standards*, 13(26):34–36.

Kendall, M. L. (1999). A holistic nursing model for spiritual care of the terminally ill. *American Journal of Hospice Palliative Care*, 16(2):473–476.

Johnson, M., Maas, M., and Moorehead, S. (2000). *Nursing outcomes classification (NOC)*. St. Louis: Mosby.

La Duke, S. (2000). NIC puts nursing into words. *Nursing Management*, 31(2):43–44.

McClosky, J. C., and Bulechek, G. M., (2000). *Nursing interventions classification (NIC)*. St. Louis: Mosby.

Mytko, J. J., and Knight, S. J. (1999). Body, mind, and spirit: Towards the integration of religiosity and spirituality in cancer quality of life research. *Psycho-oncology*, 8(5):439–450.

Phoon, J., Corder, K., and Barter, M. (1996). Managed care and total quality management: A necessary integration. *Journal of Nursing Care Quality*, 10(2):25–32.

Smith, G. B. (1999). Practice guidelines and outcome evaluation. In C. A. Shae, L. R. Pelletier, E. C. Poston, et al. (Eds.), *Advanced practice nursing in psychiatric and mental health care*. St. Louis: Mosby.

Outline

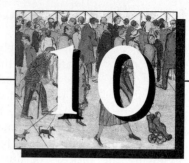

Chapter 10

Developing Therapeutic Relationships

Elizabeth M. Varcarolis

Key Terms and Concepts

The key terms and concepts listed here also appear in color where they are defined or first discussed in this chapter.

confidentiality

congruence

contract

countertransference

empathy

intimate relationship

orientation phase

social relationship

termination phase

therapeutic encounter

therapeutic relationship

transference

values

values clarification

working phase

Objectives

After studying this chapter, the reader will be able to

1. Contrast and compare the purpose, focus, communications styles, and goals for (a) a social relationship, (b) an intimate relationship, and (c) a therapeutic relationship.

2. Define and discuss the role of empathy, genuineness, and positive regard on the part of the nurse in a nurse-client relationship.

3. Identify two attitudes and four actions that may reflect the nurse's positive regard toward a client.

4. Analyze what is meant by boundaries and the influence of transference and countertransference on boundary blurring.

5. Assess five of your most important values using a values clarification exercise.

6. Contrast and compare the three phases of the nurse-client relationship.

7. Discuss the four areas of concern you will address during your first interview with a client.

8. Explore aspects that foster a therapeutic nurse-client relationship and those that are inherent in a nontherapeutic nursing interactive process according to Forchuk and associates (2000).

9. Identify four testing behaviors a client may demonstrate and discuss possible nursing interventions for each behavior.

*D*oes helping help? The answer is yes, no, and sometimes. When helping is done by skilled and socially intelligent people, it can do a great deal of good (Egan 1994). However, helping is a powerful process that can be mismanaged. Egan said that "helping is not neutral; it is for better or worse." In reviewing the process of human change, Mahoney (1991) suggested three fundamental questions:

1. Can humans change?
2. Can humans help humans change?
3. Are some forms of helping better than others?

Mahoney answered yes to all three questions. So, we see that helping can be, and often is, useful; unfortunately, sometimes it is not. Helping a person with a medical or emotional problem is rarely a straightforward task, and assisting a person to gain or regain physiological and functional normality can be a difficult goal to reach (Parsons and Wicks 1994).

UNDERSTANDING THE HELPFUL NURSE-CLIENT RELATIONSHIP

Types of Relationships

The nurse-client relationship is often loosely defined, but a therapeutic relationship incorporating principles of mental health nursing is more clearly defined and differs from other relationships. A helpful (or therapeutic) nurse-client relationship has specific goals and functions. Goals in a therapeutic relationship include

■ **Facilitating** communication of distressing thoughts and feelings
■ **Assisting** a client with problem solving to help facilitate activities of daily living
■ **Helping** clients examine self-defeating behaviors and test alternatives
■ **Promoting** self-care and independence

A relationship is an interpersonal process that involves two or more people. Throughout life, we meet people in a variety of settings and share a variety of experiences. With some individuals we develop long-term relationships; with others the relationship lasts only a short time. Naturally, the kinds of relationships we enter into vary from person to person and by situation. Generally, they may be defined as (1) social, (2) intimate, or (3) therapeutic in nature.

Social Relationships

A social relationship can be defined as a relationship that is primarily initiated for the purpose of friendship, socialization, enjoyment, or accomplishment of a task. Mutual needs are met during social interaction (e.g., participants share ideas, feelings, and experiences). Communication skills used in social relationships may include giving advice and (sometimes) meeting basic dependency needs, such as lending money and helping with jobs. Often the content of the communication remains superficial. During social interactions, roles may shift. Within a social relationship, there is little emphasis on the evaluation of the interaction.

Intimate Relationships

An intimate relationship occurs between two individuals who have an emotional commitment to each other. Those in an intimate relationship usually react naturally to each other. Often the relationship is a partnership wherein each member cares about the other's needs for growth and satisfaction. Within the relationship, mutual needs are met and intimate desires and fantasies are shared. Short- and long-range goals are usually mutual. Information shared between these individuals may be personal and intimate. People may want an intimate relationship for many reasons, such as procreation, sexual or emotional satisfaction, economic security, social belonging, and reduced loneliness. Depending on the style, level of maturity, and awareness of both parties, evaluation of the interactions may or may not be ongoing.

Therapeutic Relationships

The therapeutic relationship between nurse and client differs from both a social and an intimate relationship in that the nurse maximizes inner communication skills, understanding of human behaviors, and personal strengths to enhance the client's growth. The focus of the relationship is on the client's ideas, experiences, and feelings. Inherent in a therapeutic (helping) relationship is the nurse's focus on significant personal issues introduced by the client during the clinical interview. The nurse and the client identify areas that need exploration and periodically evaluate the degree of change in the client. **Although the nurse may assume a variety of roles** (e.g., teacher, counselor, socializing agent, liaison), **the relationship is consistently focused on the client's problem and needs.** Health care workers must get their needs met outside the relationship. When nurses begin to want the client to "like them," "do as they suggest," "be nice to them," or "give them recognition," the needs of the client cannot be adequately met and the interaction could be detrimental to the client. Working under supervision is an excellent way to keep the focus and boundaries clear. Communication skills and knowledge of the stages and phenomena occurring in a therapeutic relationship are crucial tools in the formation and maintenance of that relationship. Within the context of a helping relationship,

- The needs of the client are identified and explored.
- Alternate problem-solving approaches are taken.
- New coping skills may develop.
- Behavioral change is encouraged.

Staff nurses as well as students may struggle with requests by clients to "be my friend." When this occurs, the nurse should make it clear that the relationship is a therapeutic (helping) one. This does *not* mean that the nurse is not friendly toward the client at times. It does mean, however, that the nurse follows the stated guidelines regarding a therapeutic relationship; essentially, the focus is on the client, and the relationship is not designed to meet the nurse's needs. The client's problems and concerns are explored and potential solutions are discussed by both client and nurse, and solutions are implemented by the client.

FACTORS THAT ENHANCE GROWTH IN OTHERS

Rogers and Truax (1967) identified three personal characteristics that help promote change and growth in clients: (1) genuineness, (2) empathy, and (3) positive regard. These personal characteristics continue to be regarded as crucial ingredients in effective helpers.

Genuineness

Rogers (1967) used the word congruence to signify genuineness, or self-awareness of one's feelings as they arise within the relationship, and the ability to communicate them when appropriate. Essentially, genuineness is the ability to meet person to person in a therapeutic relationship. It is conveyed by actions such as not hiding behind the role of nurse, listening to and communicating with others without distorting their messages, and being clear and concrete in communications with clients. Congruence connotes the ability to use therapeutic communica-

tion tools in an appropriately spontaneous manner, rather than rigidly or in a parrot-like fashion.

Genuine helpers do not take refuge in the role of nurse or therapeutic counselor. "People who are genuine are at home with themselves, and therefore can comfortably be themselves in all their interactions" (Egan 1994, p. 55).

Empathy

Empathy is the ability to see things from the other person's perspective and to communicate this understanding to the other person. Empathy denotes understanding and acceptance of the client and his or her situation. Myrick and Erney (1984) stated that the term *empathy* is often used as a substitute for the term *understanding*. Empathy means that one understands the ideas expressed, as well as the feelings that are present in the other person. LaMonica (1980), a nurse researcher who developed a valid empathy instrument, says that empathy signifies a central focus and feeling with and in the client's world. It involves

- Accurate perception of the client's world by the helper
- Communication of this understanding to the client
- The client's perception of the helper's understanding

People often confuse the term empathy with sympathy. Being empathetic and being sympathetic are two different things. Egan (1994) stated that sympathy has more to do with feelings of compassion, pity, and commiseration. Although these are human traits, they may not be particularly useful in a counseling situation. When people express sympathy, they express agreement with another, which may in some situations discourage further exploration of a client's thoughts and feelings. Sympathy is the actual sharing of another's feelings, and consequently experiencing the need to reduce one's own personal distress. When a helping person is feeling sympathy with another, objectivity is lost, and the ability to assist the client in solving a personal problem ceases. For example, a friend tells you that her mother was just diagnosed with inoperable cancer. Your friend then begins to cry and pounds the table with her fist.

- **Sympathetic response:** "I know exactly how you feel. My mother was hospitalized last year and it was awful. I was so depressed. I still get upset just thinking about it." You go on to tell your friend about the incident.

Sometimes, when nurses try to be sympathetic, they are in danger of projecting their own feelings onto the client's, thus limiting the client's range of responses (Morse et al. 1992). A more useful response might be as follows:

■ **Empathetic response:** "How upsetting this must be for you. Something similar happened to my mother last year. What thoughts and feelings have you had?" You continue to stay with your friend and listen to his or her thoughts and feelings.

In the practice of psychotherapy or counseling, it is believed by many that empathy is an essential ingredient both for the better-functioning client and for the client who functions at a more primitive level (Book 1988). However, if a nurse feels empathetic toward a client and his or her situation, is therapeutic empathy *always* an effective or helpful response? Morse and associates (1992) questioned the use of therapeutic empathy in *all* nurse-client relationships. Although therapeutic empathy may be appropriate in community, psychiatric, and rehabilitation settings or with long-term clients, it might not be so in all nursing situations or settings. One example might be the case of acute and sudden illness. During this crisis phase, clients and families are learning to cope with discomfort and learning to accept their radically changed reality. This is a phase that must be "experienced before reaching the phases in which adaptation and change [personal growth] are important, relevant or possible" (Morse et al. 1992, p. 277). The authors concluded that responses that facilitate clients' and families' acceptance of their crisis situations are perhaps more appropriate and useful. Such facilitating responses include sympathy, compassion, consolation, and commiseration.

Positive Regard

Positive regard implies respect. It is the ability to view another person as being worthy of caring about and as someone who has strengths and achievement potential. Respect is usually communicated not directly in words but indirectly by actions.

Attitudes

One attitude through which a nurse might convey respect is willingness to work with the client. That is, the nurse takes the client and the relationship seriously. The experience is viewed not as "a job," "part of a course," or "time spent talking" but as an opportunity to work with people to help them develop their own resources and actualize more of their potential in living.

Actions

Some actions that manifest an attitude of respect are attending, suspending value judgments, and helping clients develop their own resources.

ATTENDING. This term refers to an intensity of presence, or being with the client (Egan 1994). At times, simply being with another person during a painful time can make a difference. Some nonverbal behaviors that reflect the degree of attending are the nurse's body posture (leaning forward toward the client, arms comfortably at sides), degree of eye contact, degree of relaxation during the interaction, and evaluating the client's response to such nurse behaviors.

SUSPENDING VALUE JUDGMENTS. Nurses are more effective when they guard against using their own value systems to judge a client's thoughts, feelings, or behaviors. For example, if a client is taking drugs or is sexually promiscuous, you might recognize that these behaviors are hindering the client from living a more satisfying life or from developing satisfying relationships. However, labeling these activities as bad or good is not useful. Rather, focus on exploring the behavior of the client and work toward identifying the thoughts and feelings that influence this behavior. Judgmental behavior on the part of the nurse will most likely interfere with further exploration.

The first steps in eliminating judgmental thinking and behaviors are to (1) identify its presence, (2) identify how or where you learned these responses to the client's behavior, and (3) reconstruct alternative ways to view the client's thinking and behavior. Just denying judgmental thinking will only compound the problem. Egan (1994, p. 53) cited the following example:

Client: I am really sexually promiscuous. I give in to sexual tendencies whenever they arise and whenever I can find a partner. This has been going on for at least 3 years.

A judgmental response would be

Nurse A: Immature sex hasn't been the answer, has it? It's just another way of making yourself miserable. These days it's just asking for AIDS.

A more helpful response would be

Nurse B: So, letting yourself go sexually is part of the picture also. You sound as if you're not happy about this.

In this example, Nurse B focuses on the client's behaviors and the possible meaning they might have to the client. Nurse B does not introduce personal value statements or prejudices regarding promiscuous behavior, as does Nurse A. Empathy and positive regard are essential qualities in a successful nurse-client relationship. See the discussion of the results of Forchuk and associates' study (2000) later in this chapter.

Helping Clients Develop Resources

The nurse becomes aware of clients' strengths and encourages them to work at their optimal level of functioning. The nurse does not act for clients unless absolutely necessary, and then only as a step toward helping them act on their own.

Client: This medication makes me so dry. Could you get me something to drink?

Nurse: There is juice in the refrigerator. I'll wait here for you until you get back.

or

I'll walk with you while you get some juice from the refrigerator.

Client: Could you ask the doctor to let me have a pass for the weekend?

Nurse: Your doctor will be on the unit this afternoon. I'll let her know that you want to speak with her.

Consistently encouraging clients to use their own resources helps minimize the clients' feelings of helplessness and dependency and also validates their potential for change.

ESTABLISHING BOUNDARIES

The nurse's role in the therapeutic relationship is theoretically rather well defined. The client's needs are separated from the nurse's needs, and the client's role is different from that of the nurse. Therefore, the boundaries of the relationship seem to be well stated. In reality, boundaries are at risk for blurring, and a shift in the nurse-client relationship may lead to nontherapeutic dynamics. Philette and associates (1995) described the following two common behaviors that may occur and blur boundaries:

■ When the relationship slips into a social context
■ When the nurse's behavior reflects getting the personal needs met at the expense of the client's needs

Resultant actions by the nurse may be manifested in specific groups of behaviors (Philette et al. 1995), although these violations are mostly unwitting, subtle, and unconscious. These behaviors include

■ **Overhelping:** going beyond the wishes or needs of the client
■ **Controlling:** asserting authority and assuming control of clients "for their own good"
■ **Narcissism:** having to find weakness, helplessness, and/or disease in clients to feel helpful, at the expense of recognizing and supporting the client's healthier, stronger, and more competent features

Role blurring (Philette et al. 1995) may take the form of

■ What is too helpful?
■ What is not helpful enough?

Table 10–1 points out certain behaviors that identify role boundary blurring when nursing behaviors

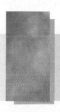

TABLE 10–1 *Client's and Nurse's Behaviors That Reflect Blurred Boundaries*	
WHEN THE NURSE IS OVERLY INVOLVED	**WHEN THE NURSE IS NOT INVOLVED**
The client more frequently requests assistance, which causes increased dependency on the nurse	The client's increased verbal or physical expression of isolation (depression)
Inability of the client to perform tasks of which he or she is known to be capable prior to the nurse's help, which causes regression	Lack of mutually agreed goals
Unwillingness on the part of the client to maintain performance or progress in the nurse's absence	Lack of progress toward goal
Expressions of anger by other staff who do not agree with the nurse's interventions or perceptions of the client	The nurse avoiding spending time with the client
The nurse keeping secrets about the nurse-client relationship	The nurse not following through on agreed interventions

Data from Philette, P. C., et al. (1995). Therapeutic management of helping boundaries. *Journal of Psychosocial Nursing and Mental Health Services*, 33(1):40–47.

reflect being too helpful and not helpful enough. When situations such as these arise, the relationship has ceased to be a helpful one and the phenomenon of control becomes an issue. Role blurring is often a result of unrecognized transference or countertransference.

Transference

Transference is a phenomenon originally identified by Sigmund Freud when using psychoanalysis to treat clients. Transference is the process whereby a person unconsciously and inappropriately displaces (transfers) onto individuals in his or her current life those patterns of behavior and emotional reactions that originated with significant figures from childhood. Although the transference phenomenon occurs in all relationships, transference seems to be intensified in relationships of authority. Because the process of transference is accelerated toward a person in authority, physicians, nurses, and social workers all are potential objects of transference. It is important to realize that the client may experience thoughts, feelings, and reactions toward a health care worker that are realistic and appropriate; these are *not* transference phenomena.

Common forms of transference include the desire for affection or respect and the gratification of dependency needs. Other transferential feelings the client might experience are hostility, jealousy, competitiveness, and love. Requests for special favors (e.g., cigarettes, water, extra time in the session) are concrete examples of transference phenomena.

Countertransference

Countertransference refers to the tendency of the nurse clinician to displace onto the client feelings caused by people in the therapist's past. Frequently, the client's transference to the nurse evokes countertransference feelings in the nurse. For example, it is normal to feel angry when attacked persistently, annoyed when frustrated unreasonably, or flattered when idealized. A nurse might also feel omnipotent or important when depended on exclusively by a client (Bonnivien 1992).

If the nurse feels either a strongly positive or a strongly negative reaction to a client, the feeling may signal a countertransferential process in the nurse. One common sign of countertransference in the nurse is overidentification with the client. In this situation the nurse may have difficulty recognizing or understanding problems the client has that are similar to the nurse's own. For example, a nurse who is struggling with an alcoholic family member may feel disinterested, cold, or disgusted toward an alcoholic client. Other indications of countertransference occur when the nurse gets involved in power struggles, competition, or arguing with the client. Table 10–2 identifies some common reactions and gives some suggestions for self-intervention.

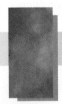

TABLE 10-2 *Common Countertransference Reactions*

As a nurse, you will sometimes experience countertransference feelings. Once you are aware of them, use them for self-analysis to understand those feelings that may inhibit productive nurse-client communication.

NURSE'S REACTION TO CLIENT	CHARACTERISTIC NURSE BEHAVIOR	SELF-ANALYSIS	SOLUTION
Boredom (indifference)	■ Inattention ■ Frequently asking client to repeat statements ■ Inappropriate responses	■ Is the content of what the client presents uninteresting? Or is the style of communication? Does the client exhibit an offensive style of communication? ■ Have you anything else on your mind that may be distracting you from the client's needs? ■ Is the client discussing an issue that makes you anxious?	■ Redirect client if he or she provides more information than you need or goes "off the track." ■ Clarify information with client. ■ Confront ineffective modes of communication.

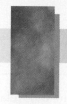

TABLE 10–2   *Common Countertransference Reactions* (Continued)

NURSE'S REACTION TO CLIENT	CHARACTERISTIC NURSE BEHAVIOR	SELF-ANALYSIS	SOLUTION
Rescue	<ul><li>Reaching for unattainable goals</li><li>Resisting peer feedback and supervisory recommendations</li><li>Giving advice</li></ul>	<ul><li>What behavior stimulates your perceived need to rescue the client?</li><li>Has anyone evoked such feelings in you in the past?</li><li>What are your fears or fantasies about failing to meet the client's needs?</li><li>Why do I want to rescue this client?</li></ul>	<ul><li>Avoid secret alliances.</li><li>Develop realistic goals.</li><li>Do not alter meeting schedule.</li><li>Let client guide interaction.</li><li>Facilitate client problem solving.</li></ul>
Overinvolvement	<ul><li>Coming to work early, leaving late</li><li>Ignoring peer suggestions, resisting assistance</li><li>Buying the client clothes or other gifts</li><li>Accepting client's gifts</li><li>Behaving judgmentally at family interventions</li><li>Keeping secrets</li><li>Calling client when off-duty</li></ul>	<ul><li>What particular client characteristics are attractive?</li><li>Does the client remind you of someone? Who?</li><li>Does your current behavior differ from your treatment of similar clients in the past?</li><li>What am I getting out of this situation?</li><li>What needs of mine are being met?</li></ul>	<ul><li>Establish firm treatment boundaries, goals, and nursing expectations.</li><li>Avoid self-disclosure.</li><li>Avoid calling client when off-duty.</li></ul>
Overidentification	<ul><li>Special agenda, secrets</li><li>Increased self-disclosure</li><li>Feelings of omnipotence</li><li>Physical attraction</li></ul>	<ul><li>With which of the client's physical, emotional, cognitive, or situational characteristics do you identify?</li><li>Recall similar circumstances in your own life. How did you deal with the issues now being created by the client?</li></ul>	<ul><li>Allow client to direct issues.</li><li>Encourage a problem-solving approach from client's perspective.</li><li>Avoid self-disclosure.</li></ul>
Misuse of honesty	<ul><li>Withholding information</li><li>Lying</li></ul>	<ul><li>Why are you protecting the client?</li><li>What are your fears about the client learning the truth?</li></ul>	<ul><li>Be clear in your responses and aware of your hesitation; do not "hedge."</li><li>If you can provide information, tell client and give your rationale.</li><li>Avoid keeping secrets.</li><li>Reinforce client about interdisciplinary nature of treatment.</li></ul>
Anger	<ul><li>Withdrawal</li><li>Speaking loudly</li><li>Using profanity</li><li>Asking to be taken off case</li></ul>	<ul><li>What client behaviors are offensive to you?</li><li>What dynamic from your past may this client be recreating?</li></ul>	<ul><li>Determine origin of anger (nurse, client, or both).</li><li>Explore roots of client anger.</li><li>Avoid contact with client if anger is not understood.</li></ul>
Helplessness or hopelessness	<ul><li>Sadness</li></ul>	<ul><li>Which client behaviors evoke these feelings in you?</li><li>Has anyone evoked similar feelings in the past? who?</li><li>What past expectations were placed on you (verbally and nonverbally) by this client?</li></ul>	<ul><li>Maintain therapeutic involvement.</li><li>Explore and focus on client's experience rather than on your own.</li></ul>

This identification of and working through various transference and countertransference issues is crucial for the nurse's professional and clinical growth and for positive change in the client. These issues are best dealt with by the use of supervision, either by a more experienced professional or by a peer. Regularly scheduled supervision sessions provide the nurse with the opportunity to increase self-awareness, clinical skills, and growth, as well as allow for progression of growth in the client.

Self-Check on Boundary Issues

It is helpful for all of us to take time out to be reflective and try to be aware of our thoughts and actions with clients, as well as colleagues, friends, and family. Table 10–3 can be a useful self-test you can use throughout your career, no matter what area of nursing you choose.

UNDERSTANDING SELF AND OTHERS

Relationships are complex. We bring into our relationships a multitude of thoughts, feelings, beliefs and attitudes—some rational and some irrational. It is helpful, even crucial, that we have an understanding of our own personal values and attitudes so that we may become aware of these beliefs or attitudes that we hold that may interfere with the establishment of positive relationships with those under our care.

Values

More and more we are working, living, and caring for people from diverse cultures and subcultures whose life experiences and life values may be quite

TABLE 10–3   Nursing Boundary Index Self-Check

Please rate yourself according to the frequency that the following statements reflect your behavior, thoughts, or feelings within the past 2 years while providing patient care.*

1. Have you ever received any feedback about your behavior being overly intrusive with patients and their families?	Never ___	Rarely ___	Sometimes ___	Often ___
2. Do you ever have difficulty setting limits with patients?	Never ___	Rarely ___	Sometimes ___	Often ___
3. Do you ever arrive early or stay late to be with your patient for a longer period?	Never ___	Rarely ___	Sometimes ___	Often ___
4. Do you ever find yourself relating to patients or peers as you might a family member?	Never ___	Rarely ___	Sometimes ___	Often ___
5. Have you ever acted on sexual feelings you have for a patient?	Never ___	Rarely ___	Sometimes ___	Often ___
6. Do you feel that you are the only one who understands the patient?	Never ___	Rarely ___	Sometimes ___	Often ___
7. Have you ever received feedback that you get "too involved" with patients or families?	Never ___	Rarely ___	Sometimes ___	Often ___
8. Do you derive conscious satisfaction from patients' praise, appreciation, or affection?	Never ___	Rarely ___	Sometimes ___	Often ___
9. Do you ever feel that other staff members are too critical of "your" patient?	Never ___	Rarely ___	Sometimes ___	Often ___
10. Do you ever feel that other staff members are jealous of your relationship with your patient?	Never ___	Rarely ___	Sometimes ___	Often ___
11. Have you ever tried to "match-make" a patient with one of your friends?	Never ___	Rarely ___	Sometimes ___	Often ___
12. Do you find it difficult to handle patients' unreasonable requests for assistance, verbal abuse, or sexual language?	Never ___	Rarely ___	Sometimes ___	Often ___

*Any item that is responded to with "sometime" or "often" should alert the nurse to a possible area of vulnerability. If the item is responded to with "rarely," the nurse should determine if it is an isolated event or a possible pattern of behavior.

From Pilette, P., Berck, C., and Achber, L. (1995). Therapeutic management. *Journal of Psychosocial Nursing*, 33(1), 45.

different from our own. Values are abstract standards and represent an ideal, either positive or negative. For example, in the United States, to create a social order in which people can live peaceably together and feel secure in their persons and property, two of society's values are a respect for one another's liberty and working cooperatively for the common goal. Not all the nation's people live up to these ideals all the time, and there may exist for some a dichotomy between theory and practice. For example, some people may pay lip service to the values of authority or the culture, while their behavior contradicts these values. For example, they may stress honesty and respect for the law, yet cheat on their taxes and in their business practices. They may love their neighbors on Sunday and demean or downgrade them for the rest of the week. They may declare themselves patriots, yet deny freedom of speech to any dissenters whose concept of patriotism is different from theirs.

A person's value system greatly influences both everyday and long-range choices. Values and beliefs provide a framework for the life goals people develop and for what they want their life to include. Our values are usually culturally oriented and influenced in a variety of ways through our parents, teachers, religious institutions, workplaces, peers, and political leaders and through Hollywood and the media. All these influences attempt to instill their values and to form and influence ours (Simon et al. 1995).

We also form our values through the example of others. **Modeling** is perhaps one of the most potent means of value education because it presents a vivid example of values in action (Simon et al. 1995). We all need role models to guide us in negotiating life's many choices. Young people in particular are hungry for role models and will find them among adults or their peers. As nurses, parents, bosses, coworkers, friends, lovers, teachers, spouses, singles, or whatever, we are constantly (in either a positive or negative manner) providing a role model to others.

One of the steps in the nursing process is represented by the planning outcome criteria (long-range and short-range goals). We emphasize that the client and the nurse identify realistic and measurable goals together. What happens when your beliefs and values are very different from those of a client? For example, the client wants an abortion, which is against the nurse's values (or vice versa). The client is sexually promiscuous, and that is against the nurse's values. The client puts material gain and objects far ahead of loyalty to friends and family, in direct contrast with a nurse's values. The client's life style includes the taking of illicit drugs, and sub-

stance abuse is against the nurse's values. The client is deeply religious, and the nurse is a nonbeliever who shuns organized religion. Can a nurse develop a working relationship and help a client solve a problem when the values and the goals of the client are so different from his or her own?

As nurses, it is useful for us to understand that our values and beliefs are not necessarily right, and certainly not right for everyone. It is helpful for us to realize that our values (1) reflect our own culture, (2) are derived from a whole range of choices, and (3) are those we have *chosen* for ourselves from a variety of influences and role models. These chosen values guide us in making decisions and taking the actions we hope will make our lives meaningful, rewarding, and full. Personal values may change over time; indeed, personal values may change many times over the course of a lifetime. Self-awareness requires that we understand what we value and those beliefs that guide our behavior. It is critical that as nurses we not only understand and accept our own values but also are sensitive to and accepting of the unique and different values of others.

Values Clarification

Values clarification is a process that helps people understand and build their value system, addressing some questions in the process. For example, "Where do we learn whether to stick to the old moral and value standards or try new ones? How do we learn to relate to people whose values differ from our own? What do we do when two important values are in conflict?" (Simon et al. 1995).

A popular approach to values clarification has been formulated by Louis Raths (1966). In his framework, a value has three components: emotional, cognitive, and behavioral. We do not just hold our values, we *feel* deeply about them and will stand up for them and affirm them when appropriate. We *choose* our values from a variety of choices after weighing the pros and cons, including the consequences of these choices and positions. And, ultimately, we *act* up our values. Our values determine how we live our lives. Values, according to Raths (1966), are composed of seven subprocesses:

PRIZING ONE'S BELIEFS AND BEHAVIORS (EMOTIONAL)

1. Prizing and cherishing
2. Publicly affirming, when appropriate

CHOOSING ONE'S BELIEFS AND BEHAVIORS (COGNITIVE)

3. Choosing from alternatives
4. Choosing after consideration of consequences
5. Choosing freely

ACTING ON ONE'S BELIEFS (BEHAVIORAL)

6. Acting
7. Acting with a pattern, consistency, and repetition

Simon and associates (1995) have added that part of the values clarification process should be to attend to the needs and rights of others. They suggested questions such as "What affect will this choice have on others around me? What is the ethical thing to do? If everyone followed my example, what kind of world would this become?" Box 10–1 is a values clarification exercise that you can use to identify and prioritize those things that are impor-

Box 10–1 *Values Clarification*

Your values are your ideas about what is most important to you in your life—what you want to live by and live for. They are the silent forces behind many of your actions and decisions. The goal of values clarification is for their influence to become fully conscious, for you to explore and honestly acknowledge what you truly value at this time in your life. You can be more self-directed and effective when you know which values you really choose to keep and live by as an adult and which ones will get priority over others. First, identify your values, and then rank your top three or five.

- Being with people
- Being loved
- Being married
- Having a special partner
- Having companionship
- Loving someone
- Taking care of others
- Having someone's help
- Having a close family
- Having good friends
- Having things in control
- Having self-control
- Being emotionally stable
- Having self-acceptance
- Having pride or dignity
- Being well organized
- Being competent
- Learning and knowing a lot
- Achieving highly
- Making a contribution to the world
- Fighting injustice
- Living ethically
- Being a good parent (or child)
- Being a spiritual person
- Having a relationship with God
- Having peace and quiet
- Making a home
- Being free from pain
- Avoiding boredom
- Having fun
- Enjoying sensual pleasures
- Looking good

- Being physically fit
- Being healthy
- Having prized possessions
- Being a creative person
- Not getting taken advantage of
- Being liked
- Being popular
- Getting someone's approval
- Being appreciated
- Being treated fairly
- Being admired
- Being independent
- Being courageous
- Being productively busy
- Having enjoyable work
- Having an important position
- Making money
- Striving for perfection
- Preserving your roots
- Having financial security
- Holding on to what you have
- Being safe physically
- Having it easy
- Being comfortable
- Having deep feelings
- Growing as a person
- Living fully
- "Smelling the flowers"
- Having a purpose

From Bernard, M. E., and Wolfe, J. L. (Eds.) (1993). *The RET resource book for practitioners*. New York: Institute for Rational-Emotive Therapy.

tant to you; you might also find this useful when counseling clients. There are many values clarification exercises that can help clients, individuals, partners, friends, and groups identify important values in their lives and compare values with others in a friendship, partnership, or group situation.

PHASES OF THE NURSE-CLIENT RELATIONSHIP

The ability of the nurse to engage in interpersonal interactions in a goal-directed manner for the purpose of assisting clients with their emotional or physical health needs is the foundation of nursing practice (Hagerty 1984).

The nurse-client relationship is synonymous with a professional helping relationship. Behaviors that have relevance to health care workers, including nurses, are as follows:

- **Accountability.** The nurse assumes responsibility for the conduct and consequences of the assignment and his or her actions.
- **Focus on client needs.** The interest of the client, not that of other health care workers or of the institution, is given first consideration. The nurse's role is that of client advocate.
- **Clinical competence.** The criteria on which the nurse bases his or her conduct are principles of knowledge and appropriateness to the specific situation. This involves awareness and incorporation of the latest knowledge made available from research.
- **Supervision.** Validation of performance quality is through regularly scheduled supervisory sessions. Supervision is conducted either by a more experienced clinician or through discussion with the nurse's peers in professionally conducted supervisory sessions (peer review).

Nurses interact with clients in a variety of settings, such as emergency departments, medical-surgical units, obstetric and pediatric units, clinics, community settings, schools, and clients' homes. Nurses who are sensitive to the client's needs and have effective assessment and communication skills can significantly help the client confront current problems and anticipate future choices.

Sometimes, the type of relationship that occurs may be informal and not extensive, such as when the nurse and client meet for only a few sessions. However, even though it is brief, the relationship may be substantial, useful, and important for the client. This limited relationship is often referred to

as a therapeutic encounter. When the nurse really is concerned with another's circumstances (has positive regard, empathy) even a short encounter with an individual can make a powerful impact on that individual's life.

At other times, the encounters may be longer and more formal, such as in inpatient settings, mental health units, crisis centers, and mental health centers. This longer time span allows the development of a therapeutic nurse-client relationship, which is the medium through which the nursing process is implemented (Hagerty 1984).

Hildegard Peplau introduced the concept of the nurse-client relationship in 1952 in her book, *Interpersonal Relations in Nursing*. This model of the nurse-client relationship is well accepted in the United States and Canada and has become an important tool for all nursing practice. Peplau proposed that the nurse-client relationship "facilitates forward movement" for both the nurse and the client (Peplau, 1952, p. 12). Peplau's interactive nurse-client process is designed to facilitate the client's boundary management, independent problem solving, and decision making that promotes autonomy (Haber, 2000, p. 60).

It is most likely that in the brief period you have for your psychiatric nursing rotation, these phases will not have time to develop. However, it is important for students to be aware of these phases since it will be important for you to recognize and use them later.

Peplau (1952, 1999) described the nurse-client relationship as evolving through interlocking, overlapping phases. The following distinctive phases of the nurse-client relationship are generally recognized:

- The orientation phase
- The working phase
- The termination phase

Although various phenomena and goals are identified for each phase, they often overlap from phase to phase. Even before the first meeting, the nurse may have many thoughts and feelings related to the first clinical session. This is sometimes referred to as the preorientation phase.

Preorientation Phase

Beginning health care professionals who are new to the psychiatric setting usually have many concerns and experience a mild to moderate degree of anxiety on their first clinical day. One common concern involves fear of physical harm or violence. Your instructor usually discusses this common concern in your first preconference. There are unit protocols for intervening with clients who have poor impulse control, and staff and unit safeguards should be constantly in place to help clients gain self-control. Although such disruptions are not common, the concern is valid. Most unit staff are trained and practice interventions for clients who are having difficulty with impulse control. Hospital security is readily available to give the staff support.

Some of you may be concerned with saying the wrong thing, using the client as a guinea pig, feeling inadequate about new and developing communication skills, feeling vulnerable without the uniform as a clear indicator of who is the nurse and who is the client, and feeling vulnerable as you relate to your own earlier personal experiences or crises. These are universal and valid feelings; if they were not discussed in class, they will be brought up on the first clinical day, either by you or by your instructor. Chapter 11 deals with a variety of clinical concerns student nurses have when beginning their psychiatric nursing rotation (e.g., what to do if clients do not want to talk, if they ask the nurse to keep a secret, if they cry). Usually after the first clinical day your anxiety is much lower, and it is easier to focus on clinical issues with the support of your instructor and classmates. The preorientation phase revolves around planning for the first interaction with the client.

Orientation Phase

The orientation phase can last for a few meetings or can extend over a longer period. This first phase may be prolonged in the case of severely and persistently ill mental health clients. Forchuk's study (1992) found that lengthy hospitalization patterns were related to a lengthy orientation phase. In this study the length of the orientation phase was 6 months or longer.

The first time the nurse and the client meet, they are strangers to each other. When strangers meet, whether or not they know anything about each other, they interact according to their own backgrounds, standards, values, and experiences. This fact—that each person has a unique frame of reference—underlies the need for self-awareness on the part of the nurse.

As the relationship evolves through an ongoing series of reactions, each participant may elicit in the other a wide range of positive and negative emotional reactions (Bonnivien 1992). Remember that the "stirring up" of feelings in the client by the nurse is referred to as transference, and the stirring up of feelings in the nurse or therapist by the client is referred to as countertransference. As discussed earlier, the nurse is responsible for identifying these two phenomena and maintaining appropriate boundaries.

Establishing Trust

A major emphasis during the first few encounters with the client is on providing an atmosphere in which trust can grow. As in any relationship, trust is nurtured by demonstrating genuineness (congruence) and empathy, developing positive regard, showing consistency, and offering assistance in alleviating the client's emotional pain or problems. This may take only a short time, but in many instances it may take a long time before a client feels free to discuss painful personal experiences and private thoughts.

During the orientation phase, four important issues need to be addressed:

1. The parameters of the relationship
2. The formal or informal contract
3. Confidentiality
4. Termination

THE PARAMETERS OF THE RELATIONSHIP. The client needs to know about the nurse (who the nurse is and what his or her background is) and the purpose of the meetings. For example, a student might furnish the following information:

> **Student:** Hello, Mrs. James. I am Nancy Rivera from Orange Community College. I am in my psychiatric rotation, and I will be coming to York Hospital for the next six Thursdays. I would like to spend time with you each Thursday if you are still here. I'm here to be a support person for you as you work on your treatment goals.

THE FORMAL OR INFORMAL CONTRACT. A contract emphasizes the client's participation and responsibility because it shows that the nurse does something *with* the client rather than *for* the client (Collins 1983). The contract, either stated or written, contains the place, time, date, and duration of the meetings. During the orientation phase, the client may begin to express thoughts and feelings, identify problems, and discuss realistic goals. Therefore, the mutual agreement on goals is also part of the contract. If the goals are met, the client's level of functioning will return to a previous level, or at least improve from the present level. If fees are to be paid, the client is told how much they will be and when the payment is due.

> **Student:** Mrs. James, we will meet at 10 AM each Thursday in the consultation room at the clinic for 45 minutes, from September 15th to October

27th. We can use that time for further discussion of your feelings of loneliness and anger with your husband and to explore some things you could do to make things better for yourself.

CONFIDENTIALITY. The client has a right to know who else will know about the information being shared with the nurse. He or she needs to know that the information may be shared with specific people, such as a clinical supervisor, the physician, the staff, or other students in conference. The client also needs to know that the information will *not* be shared with his or her relatives, friends, or others outside the treatment team, except in extreme situations. Extreme situations include (1) information that may be harmful to the client or others, (2) when the client threatens self-harm, and (3) when the client does not intend to follow through with the treatment plan. If information must be given to others, this is usually done by the physician, according to legal guidelines (refer to Chapter 8). The nurse must be aware of the client's right to confidentiality and must not violate that right.

> **Student:** Mrs. James, I will be sharing some of what we discuss with my nursing instructor, and at times I may discuss certain concerns with my peers in conference or with the staff. However, I will *not* be sharing this information with your husband or any other members of your family or anyone outside the hospital without your permission.

TERMINATION. Termination begins in the orientation phase. It may also be mentioned when appropriate during the working phase if the nature of the relationship is time limited (e.g., six or nine sessions). The date of the termination phase should be clear from the beginning. In some situations the nurse-client contract may be renegotiated when the termination date has been reached. In other situations, when the therapeutic nurse-client relationship is an open-ended one, the termination date is not known.

> **Student:** Mrs. James, as I mentioned earlier, our last meeting will be on October 27th. We will have three more meetings after today.

During the orientation phase and later, clients often unconsciously employ testing behaviors that may be used to test the nurse. The client wants to know if the nurse will

- Be able to set limits when the client needs them.
- Still show concern if the client acts angry, babyish, unlikable, or dependent.
- Still be there if the client is late, leaves early, refuses to speak, or is angry.

Table 10–4 identifies some testing behaviors and possible responses by nurses.

In summary, the initial interview includes the following:

- The nurse's role is clarified and the responsibilities of both the client and the nurse are defined.
- The contract containing the time, place, date, and duration of the meetings is discussed.
- Confidentiality is discussed and assumed.
- The terms of termination are introduced throughout the orientation phase and beyond.
- The nurse becomes aware of transference and countertransference issues and discusses them in conference/supervision.
- An atmosphere where trust can grow is established.
- Articulation of client problems and mutually agreed goals are established.

Working Phase

Moore and Hartman (1988) identified specific tasks of the working phase of the nurse-client relationship, such as to

- Maintain the relationship
- Gather further data
- Promote the client's problem-solving skills, self-esteem, and use of language
- Facilitate behavioral change
- Overcome resistance behaviors
- Evaluate problems and goals and redefine them as necessary
- Practice and express alternative adaptive behaviors

During the working phase, the nurse and client together identify and explore areas in the client's life that are causing problems. Often, the client's present ways of handling situations stem from earlier ways of coping devised to survive in a chaotic and dysfunctional family environment. Although certain coping methods may have worked for the client at an earlier age, they now interfere with the client's interpersonal relationships and prevent him or her from attaining current goals. The client's dysfunctional behaviors and basic assumptions about the world are often defensive in nature and the client is usually unable to change the dysfunctional behavior at will. Therefore, most of the problem behaviors or thoughts continue because of unconscious motivations and needs that are out of the client's awareness.

The nurse can work with the client to identify these unconscious motivations and assumptions that

TABLE 10–4   *Testing Behaviors Used by Clients*

CLIENT BEHAVIOR	CLIENT EXAMPLE	NURSE RESPONSE	RATIONALE
Shifts focus of interview *to* the nurse, *off* the client	"Do you have any children?" or "Are you married?"	"This time is for you." If appropriate, the nurse should add: 1. "Do you have any children?" or "What about your children?" 2. "Are you married?" or "What about your relationships?"	The nurse refocuses back to the client and client's concerns. The nurse sticks to the contract.
Tries to get the nurse to take care of him or her	"Could you tell my doctor?"	"I'll leave a message with the unit clerk that you want to see him" or "You know best what you want him to know. I'll be interested in what he has to say."	1. The nurse validates that the client is able to do many things for himself or herself. This aids in increasing self-esteem. 2. The nurse always encourages the person to function at the highest level, even if he or she doesn't want to.
	"Should I take this job?"	"What do you see as the pros and cons of this job?"	
Makes sexual advances toward the nurse, e.g., touching the nurse's arm, wanting to hold hands with or kiss the nurse	"Would you go out with me? . . . Why not?" or "Can I kiss you? . . . Why not?"	"I am not comfortable having you touch (kiss) me." The nurse briefly reiterates the nurse's role: "This time is for you to focus on your problems and concerns." If the client stops: "I wonder what this is all about?" 1. Is the client afraid the nurse will not like him or her? 2. Is the client trying to take the focus off the problems? If the client continues: "If you can't cease this behavior, I'll have to leave. I'll be back at (time) to spend time with you then."	1. The nurse needs to set clear limits on expected behavior. 2. Frequently restating the nurse's role throughout the relationship can help maintain boundaries. 3. Whenever possible, the meaning of the client's behavior should be explored. 4. Leaving gives the client time to gain control. The nurse returns at the stated time.
Continues to arrive late for meetings	"I'm a little late because (excuse)."	The nurse arrives on time and leaves at the scheduled time. (The nurse does not let the client manipulate him or her or bargain for more time.) After a couple of times, the nurse can explore behavior, e.g., "I wonder if there is something going on you don't want to deal with?" or "I wonder what these latenesses mean to you?"	1. The nurse keeps the contract. Clients feel more secure when "promises" are kept, even though clients may try to manipulate the nurse through anger, helplessness, and so forth. 2. The nurse does not tell the client what to do, but the nurse and the client need to explore the meaning of the behavior.

keep the client from finding satisfaction and reaching potential. Describing, and often re-experiencing, old conflicts generally awakens high levels of anxiety in the client. Clients may use various defenses against anxiety and displace their feelings onto the nurse. Therefore, during the working phase, intense emotions such as anxiety, anger, self-hate, hopelessness, and helplessness may surface. Behaviors such as acting out anger inappropriately, withdrawing, intellectualizing, manipulating, and denying are to be expected.

During the working phase, strong transferential feelings may appear. The emotional responses and behaviors in the client may also awaken strong countertransferential feelings in the nurse. **The nurse's awareness of personal feelings and reactions to the client is vital for effective interaction with the client.** Common transferential feelings, the reactions that nurses experience in response to different behaviors and situations, are discussed in the planning component of each of the clinical chapters.

The development of a strong working relationship can allow the client to experience increased levels of anxiety and demonstrate dysfunctional behaviors in a safe setting, and to try out new and more adaptive coping behaviors.

Termination Phase

Termination is discussed during the first interview. During the working stage, the fact of eventual termination may also be raised at appropriate times. Reasons for terminating the nurse-client relationship include

- Symptom relief
- Improved social functioning
- Greater sense of identity
- More adaptive behaviors in place
- Accomplishment of the client's goals
- Impasse in therapy that the nurse is unable to resolve

In addition, forced termination may occur, such as when the student completes the course objectives or a nurse leaves the hospital or clinical setting and there is a change of staff. Forchuk (1992) pointed out that, for the long-term mentally ill client, sudden termination with the nurse the client has been working with may trigger a return to the orientation phase with a new nurse or counselor. The termination phase is the final phase of the nurse-client relationship. Important reasons for the student/nurse counselor to address the termination phase are as follows:

1. Termination is an integral phase of the therapeutic nurse-client relationship, and without it the relationship remains incomplete.
2. Feelings are aroused in both the client and the nurse with regard to the experience they have had; when these feelings are recognized and shared, clients learn that it is acceptable to feel sadness and loss when someone they care about leaves.
3. The client is a partner in the relationship and has a right to see the nurse's needs and feelings about their time together and the ensuing separation.
4. Termination can be a learning experience; clients can learn that they are important to at least one person.
5. By sharing the termination experience with the client, the nurse demonstrates caring for the client.
6. This may be the first successful termination experience for the client.

Termination often awakens strong feelings in both nurse and client. Termination of the relationship between the nurse and the client signifies a loss for both, although the intensity and meaning of termination may be different for each. If a client has unresolved feelings of abandonment or loneliness, or feelings of not being wanted or of being rejected by others, they may be reawakened during the termination process. This process can be an opportunity for the client to express these feelings, perhaps for the first time.

It is not unusual to see a variety of client behaviors that indicate defensive maneuvers against the anxiety of separation and loss. For example, a client may withdraw from the nurse and not want to meet for the final session or may become outwardly hostile and sarcastic—for instance, accusing the student of using the client for personal gains ("like a guinea pig") as a way of deflecting the awakening of anger and pain that are rooted in past separations. Often, a client will deny that the relationship had any impact or that ending the relationship evokes any emotions whatsoever. Regression is another behavioral manifestation; it may be seen as increased dependency on the nurse or a return of earlier symptoms.

It is important for the nurse to work with the client to bring into awareness any feelings and reactions the client may be experiencing related to separations. If a client denies that the termination is having an effect (assuming the nurse-client relationship was strong), the nurse may say something like "Goodbyes are difficult for people. Often they remind us of other goodbyes. Tell me about another separation in the past." If the client appears to be displacing anger, either by withdrawing or by being overtly angry at the nurse, the nurse may use generalized statements such as "People may experience anger when saying goodbye. Sometimes they are angry with the person who is leaving. Tell me how you feel about my leaving." New practitioners and students new to the psychiatric setting need to give thought to their last clinical experience with their client and to work with their supervisor or instructor to facilitate communication during this time.

Summarizing the goals and objectives achieved in the relationship is part of the termination process. Reviewing situations that occurred during the time spent together and exchanging memories can help validate the experience for both nurse and client and facilitate closure of that relationship.

A common response of beginning practitioners is feeling guilty about terminating the relationship. These feelings may be manifested in students' giving the client their telephone number, making plans to get together for coffee after the client is discharged, continuing to see the client afterward, or exchanging letters. Beginning practitioners need to understand that such actions may be motivated by their own sense of guilt or by misplaced feelings of responsibility, not by concern for the client. Indeed, part of the termination process may be to explore, after discussion with the client's case manager, the client's plans for the future: where to go for help in the future, which agencies to contact, and which specific resource persons may be available.

During the student affiliation, the nurse-client relationship exists for the duration of the clinical course only. The termination phase is just that. Thoughts and feelings the student may have about continuing the relationship are best discussed with the instructor or shared in conference with peers, because these are common reactions to the student's experience.

WHAT HINDERS AND WHAT HELPS THE NURSE-CLIENT RELATIONSHIP

Not all nurse-client relationships follow the classic phases as outlined by Peplau. Some nurse-client relationships start in the orientation phase but move to a mutual frustrating phase, and finally to mutual withdrawal (Fig. 10–1).

Forchuk and associates (2000) conducted a qualitative study of the nurse-client relationship. They studied the phases of both the therapeutic and nontherapeutic relationship. From this study, they iden-

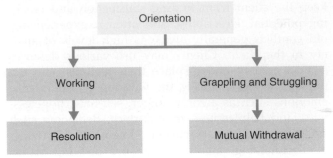

Figure 10–1 Phases of therapeutic and nontherapeutic relationships. (From Forchuk, C., et al. [2000]. The developing nurse-client relationship: Nurse's perspectives. *Journal of the American Psychiatric Nurses Association*, 6(1):3–10.)

tified certain behaviors that were beneficial to the progression of the nurse-client relationship as well as those that hampered the development of these relationships. The study emphasized the importance of consistent, regular, and private interactions with clients as essential to the development of therapeutic relationships. Nurses in this study stressed the importance of listening, pacing, and consistency.

Specifically, Forchuk and associates (2000) identified the following behaviors that are inherent in the nurse-client relationship that progressed in a mutually satisfying manner:

1. **Consistency** includes having a nurse always assigned to the same client and the client having a regular routine for activities. Interactions are facilitated when they are frequent and regular in duration, format, and location. Consistency also applies to the nurse being honest and consistent (congruent) in what is said to the clients.
2. **Pacing** includes letting the client set the pace and letting the pace be adjusted to fit the client's moods. A slow approach helps reduce pressure, and at times it is necessary to step back and realize that a strong relationship may take a long time.
3. **Listening** includes letting the client talk when this is the client's need. The nurse becomes a sounding board for the client's concerns and issues.
4. **Initial impressions,** especially positive initial attitudes and preconceptions, are significant considerations on how the relationship will progress. Preconceived negative impressions and feelings toward the client usually bode poorly for the positive growth of the relationship. In contrast, nurses who find their clients "interesting" or a "challenge" and have positive attitudes about the relationship usually reflect positively on the developing relationship.

5. **Comfort and control,** that is, promoting client comfort and balancing control, usually reflect caring behaviors. Control refers to keeping a balance in the relationship: not too strict and not too lenient.
6. **Client factors** that seem to enhance the relationship include trust on the part of the client and active participation in the nurse-client relationship.

In relationships that did not progress to therapeutic levels, there seemed to be some specific factors that hampered the development of positive relationships. These include

1. **Inconsistency and unavailability** on the part of the nurse and client, as well as lack of contact (infrequent meetings, meetings in the hallway, and client reluctance or refusal to spend time with the nurse) on the part of the nurse or the client, or both, plays a key role (mutual avoidance).
2. **Nurses' feelings and awareness** are significant factors. Major themes that contribute to the lack of progression of positive relationships were the lack of self-awareness on the part of the nurse and the nurses' own feelings. Negative preconceived ideas about the client and negative feelings (e.g., discomfort, dislike of clients, fear, and avoidance) seem to be a constant in relationships that ended in frustration and mutual withdrawal. This is in contrast with more successful relationships in which the nurse's attitude is that of positive regard and interest in understanding the client's story.

SUMMARY

The nurse-client relationship is well defined, and the role of the nurse and the client must be clearly stated. It is important that the nurse be aware of the differences between a therapeutic relationship and a social or intimate relationship. In a therapeutic nurse-client relationship, the focus is on the client's needs, thoughts, feelings, and goals. The nurse is expected to get personal needs met outside this relationship, in other professional, social, or intimate arenas. Genuineness, positive regard, and empathy are personal strengths in the helping person that foster growth and change in others.

Even though the boundaries of the nurse-client relationship are clearly defined, the blurring of these boundaries can be insidious and may occur on an unconscious level. Usually, transference and countertransference phenomena are operating when boundaries are blurred. An indication of blurred boundaries might be identified when the nurse is too helpful or not helpful enough. It is important to have a grasp of common countertransferential feelings and behaviors, along with the nursing actions to counteract these phenomena.

The importance of supervision cannot be overemphasized. Supervision aids in the professional growth of the nurse, as well as in safeguarding the integrity of the nurse-client relationship. It enhances the progression of the nurse-client relationship, allowing the client's goals to be worked on and met.

The phases of the nurse-client relationship include the orientation, working, and termination phases. At the first interaction of the orientation phase, certain issues need to be brought up: (1) setting the parameters of the relationship—who the nurse is and the purpose of the meetings; (2) the contract—who, what, where, when, and for how long, (3) the issues of confidentiality; and (4) the date of termination, if known. During the orientation phase (and at times throughout the relationship), a number of common client testing behaviors may arise that will require specific nursing interventions.

Forchuck and associates (2000) identified six specific nurse behaviors that seem to be inherent in a successful nurse-client relationship, and two that may foreshadow an unsuccessful relationship.

Visit the **Evolve** website at
http://evolve.elsevier.com/Varcarolis
for a post-test on the content in this chapter.

Visit the **Evolve** website at
http://evolve.elsevier.com/Varcarolis
for a pre-test on the content in this chapter.

Outline

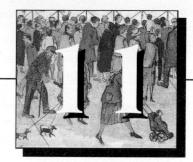

The Clinical Interview and Communication Skills

ELIZABETH M. VARCAROLIS

Key Terms and Concepts

The key terms and concepts listed here also appear in color where they are defined or first discussed in this chapter.

active listening

Berlo's communication model

clarifying techniques

clinical supervision

cultural filters

excessive questioning

exploring

feedback

giving advice

giving approval

nontherapeutic (nonhelpful) techniques

nonverbal behaviors

nonverbal communication

paraphrasing

process recordings

reflecting

restating

therapeutic (helpful) techniques

use of silence

verbal communication

"why" questions

Objectives

After studying this chapter, the reader will be able to

1. Identify and give rationales for suggested (a) setting, (b) seating, and (c) beginning of the nurse-client interaction.

2. Explain to a classmate the importance of clinical supervision and how it works.

3. Identify four client behaviors a nurse can anticipate, and discuss possible nursing interventions for each behavior.

4. Identify three personal factors that can impede accurate communication.

5. Identify two environmental factors that can impede accurate communication.

6. Discuss the differences between verbal and nonverbal communication and identify five areas of nonverbal communication.

7. Relate potential problems that can arise when nurses are insensitive to cultural differences in clients' communication styles.

8. Compare and contrast the range of nonverbal and verbal behaviors of different cultural groups in the areas of (a) communication style, (b) eye contact, and (c) touch. Give examples.

9. Describe four techniques that can enhance communication, and discuss what makes them effective.

10. Explain four techniques that can obstruct communication, and discuss what makes them ineffective.

*T*he clinical interview is not a random meeting between nurse and client. It is a systematic attempt to understand those problems in clients' lives that interfere with meeting their goals and to help them improve their skills or learn alternative ways of dealing effectively with their problems.

THE CLINICAL INTERVIEW

The clinical interview differs from the intake interview, or the assessment interview, which is described in Chapter 9, as part of the nursing process. In most instances, when a nurse meets a client for the first time, the intake interview has already been recorded. In the hospital setting the intake interview is often recorded in the chart by the physician or (in some places) a psychiatric mental health nurse. In the community setting the physician or nurse clinician is often the person doing the intake interview. However, during the clinical rotation, it is not uncommon for the student to obtain important data from the client that can be added to the client database.

The content and direction of the clinical interview are decided by the client. The client leads. The nurse employs communication skills and active listening (identifying what the client says as well as what the client does not say) to better understand the client's situation. The nurse also observes how congruent the content (what the client says) is with the process (what the client does). During the clinical interview, the nurse provides the opportunity for the client to reach specific goals, such as to

■ Identify and explore problems relating to others
■ Discuss healthy ways of meeting emotional needs
■ Experience a satisfying interpersonal relationship
■ Feel understood and comfortable

Communication and interviewing techniques are acquired skills. Nurses learn to increase their ability to use communication and interviewing skills through practice and supervision by a more experienced clinician. The second half of this chapter outlines ways you can increase your ability to use effective communication skills.

Health care practitioners new to the psychiatric setting often say they feel overwhelmed by the severity of some of the clients' problems and that they feel responsible for doing something to positively affect the emotional health of clients. It may help to know that numerous studies show the strength of the therapist-client relationship to be more important for a successful therapeutic outcome than a variety of other factors. Nicholi (1988) stated that studies bear out that the "therapist's ability to convey an intrinsic interest in the client has been found to be more important than . . . position, appearance, reputation, clinical experience, training, and technical or theoretical knowledge." This finding does not negate the importance of clinical training, skill, or experience. It does, however, emphasize the need for the nurse to convey genuine interest in another human, without being patronizing or condescending.

Anxiety during the first interview is to be expected, as in any meeting between strangers. Clients may be anxious about their problems, about the nurse's reaction to them, or about their treatment. Students may be anxious about the client's reaction to them, their ability to provide help, what the instructor will think of them, and how they will do compared with their peers.

Students have many concerns when beginning their psychiatric experience. Two common concerns are (1) how to begin the interview and (2) what to do in response to specific client behaviors. The following section offers some basic guidelines for the first interview, identifies some common problems in clinical situations, and offers possible solutions.

How to Begin the Interview

Helping a person with an emotional or medical problem is rarely a straightforward task. The goal of assisting a client to regain psychological or physiological functional normality can be difficult to achieve. Extremely important to any kind of counseling is permitting the client to set the pace of the interview, no matter how slow the progress happens to be (Parsons and Wicks 1994).

SETTING. Effective communication can take place almost anywhere. However, because the quality of the interaction—whether in a clinic, a clinical unit, an office, or the client's home—depends on the degree to which the nurse and client feel safe. Establishing a setting that enhances feelings of security can be important to the helping relationship. A health care setting, a conference room, or a quiet part of the unit that has relative privacy but is within view of others is ideal. When the interview takes place in the home, it offers the nurse a valuable opportunity to assess the person in the context of everyday life.

SEATING. In all settings, chairs need to be arranged so that conversation can take place in normal tones of voice and eye contact can be comfortably maintained or avoided. For example, a nonthreatening physical environment for nurse and client would involve

■ Assuming the same height—either both sitting or both standing

■ Avoiding a face-to-face stance when possible—a 90-degree angle or side by side may be less intense

■ Making sure that the door is easily accessible to both client and nurse

■ Avoiding a desk barrier between nurse and client

INTRODUCTIONS. In the orientation phase, students tell the client who they are and the name of their school, the purpose of the meetings, and how long and at what time they will be meeting with the client. The issue of confidentiality is also covered at some point during the initial interview. The nurse can then ask the client how he or she would like to be addressed. This question accomplishes a number of tasks (Shea 1998). For example,

■ It conveys respect.

■ It gives the client direct control over an important ego issue. (Some clients like to be called by their last names; others prefer being on a first-name basis with the nurse.)

HOW TO START. Once introductions have been made, the nurse can turn the interview over to the client by using one of a number of open-ended statements (MacKinnon and Michels 1971; Shea 1998), such as

■ "Where should we start?"

■ "Tell me a little about what has been going on with you."

■ "What are some of the stresses you have been coping with recently?"

■ "Tell me a little about what has been happening in the past couple of weeks."

■ "Perhaps you can begin by letting me know what some of your concerns have been recently."

■ "Tell me about your difficulties."

Communication can be facilitated by the appropriate use of **offering leads** (e.g., "Go on"), **statements of acceptance** (e.g., "Uh-huh"), or other conveyances of the nurse's interest.

TACTICS TO AVOID. The nurse needs to avoid some behaviors (Moscato 1988). For example,

■ Do not argue with, minimize, or challenge the client.

■ Do not praise the client or give false reassurance.

■ Do not interpret to the client or speculate on the dynamics of the client's problem.

■ Do not question the client about sensitive areas.

■ Do not try to sell the client on accepting treatment.

■ Do not join in attacks the client launches on his or her mate, parents, friends, or associates.

■ Do not participate in criticism of another nurse or any other staff member.

HELPFUL GUIDELINES. Some guidelines for conducting the initial interviews are offered by Meier and Davis (1989), such as

■ Speak briefly.

■ When you don't know what to say, say nothing.

■ When in doubt, focus on feelings.

■ Avoid advice.

■ Avoid relying on questions.

■ Pay attention to nonverbal cues.

■ Keep the focus on the client.

Clinical Supervision and Process Recordings

Communication and interviewing techniques are acquired skills. Nurses learn to increase their ability to use communication and interviewing skills through practice and through clinical supervision by a more experienced clinician. In clinical supervision, the focus is on the nurse's behavior in the nurse-client relationship. During clinical supervision, the nurse and the supervisor examine and analyze the nurse's feelings and reactions to the client and how they affect the nurse-client relationship. Farkas-Cameron (1995, p. 44) stated that "the nurse who does not engage in the clinical supervisory process stagnates both theoretically and clinically, while depriving him- or herself of the opportunity to advance professionally." She went on to observe that clinical supervision can be a therapeutic process for the nurse. During the process, feelings and concerns are ventilated as they relate to the developing nurse-client relationship. The opportunity to examine your interactions, obtain insights, and devise alternative strategies for dealing with various clinical issues enhances your clinical growth and minimizes frustration and burnout. Clinical supervision is a necessary professional activity that fosters professional growth and helps minimize the development of nontherapeutic nurse-client relationships.

The best way to increase communication and interviewing skills is to review clinical interactions exactly as they occur. This process offers students the opportunity to identify themes and patterns in their own, as well as their client's, communication. The student also learns to deal with the variety of situations that arise in the clinical interview.

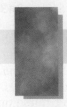

TABLE 11–1   *Segment of a Process Note*

NURSE	CLIENT	COMMENTS	FEELINGS
"Good morning Mr. L."		*Therapeutic.* Giving recognition. Acknowledging a client by name can enhance self-esteem and communicates that the client is viewed as an individual by the nurse.	
	"Who are you and where the devil am I?" *Looks around with a confused look on his face—quickly sits on the edge of the bed*		
"I am Mrs. V. I am a student nurse from [X] college, and you are at Mt. Sinai Hospital. I would like to spend some time with you today."		*Therapeutic.* Giving information. Informing the client of facts needed to make decisions or come to realistic conclusions. *Therapeutic.* Offering self. Making oneself available to the client.	
	"What am I doing here? How did I get here?" *Spoken in a loud, demanding voice.*		
"You were brought in by your wife last night after swallowing a bottle of aspirin. You had to have your stomach pumped."		*Therapeutic.* Giving information. Giving needed facts so that the client can orient himself and better evaluate his situation.	
	"Oh . . . yeah." *Silence for 2 minutes. Shoulders slumped, Mr. L. stares at the floor and drops his head and eyes.*		
"You seem upset, Mr. L." "What are you thinking about?"		*Therapeutic.* Making observations. He looks sad. *Therapeutic.* Giving broad openings in an attempt to get at his feelings.	
	"Yeah, I just remembered . . . I wanted to kill myself." *Said in a low tone almost to himself.*		
"Oh Mr. L., you have so much to live for. You have such a loving family."		*Nontherapeutic.* Defending. *Nontherapeutic.* Introducing an unrelated topic.	I felt overwhelmed. I didn't know what to say—his talking about killing himself made me nervous. I could have said, "You must be very upset" (verbalizing the implied) or "Tell me more about this" (exploring).
	"What do you know about my life? You want to know about my family? . . . My wife is leaving me, that's what." *Faces the nurse with an angry expression on his face and speaks in loud tones.*		
"I didn't know. You must be terribly upset by her leaving."		*Therapeutic.* Reflective. Observing the angry tone and content of the client's message and reflecting back the client's feelings.	

Perhaps the best way of reviewing nurse-client interactions is to view a videotape, which reveals the nonverbal as well as the verbal communications between both parties. The second-best method of capturing the interaction between nurse and client is through an audiotape recording. Unfortunately, these methods are often not possible. The most common form of evaluating the interactions in academic settings is through process recordings.

The use of process recordings is a popular way to identify patterns in the student's and the client's communication. Process recordings are written records of a segment from the nurse-client session that reflects as closely as possible the verbal and nonverbal behaviors of both client and nurse. Process recordings have some disadvantages because they rely on memory and are subject to distortions. However, they can be a useful tool for identifying communication patterns. It is usually best if the student can write notes verbatim (word for word) in a private area immediately after the interaction has taken place. Sometimes, a clinician takes notes during the interview. This practice also has disadvantages. One disadvantage is that it may be distracting for both interviewer and client; another is that some clients (especially those with a paranoid disorder) may resent or misunderstand the nurse's intent. Table 11–1 shows a segment of a process note. Nurses record their words and the client's words, identify whether the responses are therapeutic, and recall their emotions at the time.

What to Do in Response to Specific Client Behaviors

Often, students new to the mental health setting are concerned about being in situations that they may not know how to handle. These concerns are universal and often arise in the clinical setting. Table 11–2 identifies common client behaviors (e.g., crying, asking the nurse to keep a secret, threatening to commit suicide, gift giving). The table gives an example of an appropriate response, the rationale for the response, and a possible verbal statement. Read Table 11–2, paying particular attention to the rationales for responses. The exact words depend on the situation, but understanding the rationale will aid you in applying the information later on.

COMMUNICATION SKILLS

Beginning practitioners who are new to a psychiatric setting are often concerned that they may say the wrong thing, especially when initially learning to apply therapeutic techniques. *Will* you say the wrong thing? The answer is, yes, you probably will. That is how we all learn to find more useful and effective ways of helping clients reach their goals. Will saying "the wrong thing" be harmful to the client? This is doubtful, especially if your intent is honest, your approach is respectful, and you have a genuine concern for the client. We know that special skills (e.g., communications skills) and methods have been identified through scientific investigations that can aid people to become more effective helpers. However, knowledge of skills and techniques is not enough. Being an effective communicator, whether in nursing or in any other area of life, is not just a matter of knowing what techniques to use.

The idea of using techniques is "sometimes met with skepticism because it can imply that someone is deliberately and consciously trying to manipulate someone else" (Myrick and Erney 1984). Mechanical or forced use of communication skills is not helpful. However, when such skills are a genuine part of the helping process, applied with concern and respect for the other person, communication techniques can be a dynamic tool in working effectively with people, in any setting. As you continue to practice and evaluate the use of these techniques, you will develop your own style and rhythm, and eventually they will become a part of the way you communicate with others.

The Communication Process

Simply put, communication is the process of sending a message to one or more persons. One way of thinking about the process of communication is a communication model, which identifies the parts of an interaction. One example is Berlo's communication model, which has five parts: stimulus (referent), sender, message, medium (channel), and receiver (Berlo 1960).

The **stimulus** begins communication. For example, the stimulus can be a need for information, comfort, or advice. A stimulus in a nurse might be the perception that the client is feeling discomfort or confusion. A stimulus in a client could be the experience of anxiety, despair, or pain.

The **sender** initiates interpersonal contact. The **message** is the information sent or expressed to another. The clearest are those that are well organized and expressed in a manner familiar to the receiver. The message can be sent through a variety of **mediums**. A message can be sent through an auditory (hearing), a visual (seeing), or a tactile (touch) medium. For example, a person may send a clear message through silence, body language, or a hug, as well as through the stated word.

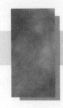

TABLE 11–2   *Common Client Behaviors and Nurse Responses*

POSSIBLE REACTIONS BY NURSE	USEFUL RESPONSES BY NURSE
What to Do if the Client Cries	
The nurse may feel uncomfortable and experience increased anxiety or feel somehow responsible for making the person cry.	The nurse should stay with the client and reinforce that it is all right to cry. Often, it is at that time that feelings are closest to the surface and can be best identified. ■ "You seem ready to cry." ■ "You are still upset about your brother's death." ■ "What are you thinking right now?" ■ The nurse offers tissues when appropriate.
What to Do If the Client Asks the Nurse to Keep a Secret	
The nurse may feel conflict because the nurse wants the client to share important information but is unsure about making such a promise.	The nurse *cannot* make such a promise. The information may be important to the health or safety of the client or others. ■ "I cannot make that promise. It might be important for me to share it with other staff." The client then decides whether to share the information or not.
What to Do If the Client Leaves before the Session Is Over	
The nurse may feel rejected, thinking it was something that he or she did. The nurse may experience increased anxiety or feel abandoned by the client.	Some clients are not able to relate for long periods without experiencing an increase in anxiety. On the other hand, the client may be testing the nurse. ■ "I will wait for you here for 15 minutes, until our time is up." During this time, the nurse does not engage in conversation with any other client or even with the staff. When time is up, the nurse approaches the client, tells him or her the time is up, and restates the day and time he or she will see the client again.
What to Do if Another Client Interrupts During Time with Your Selected Client	
The nurse may feel a conflict. The nurse does not want to appear rude. Sometimes the nurse tries to engage both clients in conversation.	The time the nurse had contracted with a selected client is that client's time. By keeping their part of the contract, nurses demonstrate that they mean what they say and that they view the sessions as important. ■ "I am with Mr. Rob for the next 20 minutes. At 10 AM, after our time is up, I can talk to you for 5 minutes."
What to Do if the Client Says He Wants to Kill Himself	
The nurse may feel overwhelmed or responsible to "talk the client out of it." The nurse may pick up some of the client's feelings of hopelessness.	The nurse tells the client that this is serious, that he or she does not want harm to come to the client, and that this information needs to be shared with other staff. ■ "This is very serious, Mr. Lamb. I do not want any harm to come to you. I will have to share this with the other staff." The nurse can then discuss with the client the feelings and circumstances that led up to this decision. (Refer to Chapter 23 for strategies in suicide intervention.)

TABLE 11–2 *Common Client Behaviors and Nurse Responses (Continued)*

POSSIBLE REACTIONS BY NURSE	USEFUL RESPONSES BY NURSE
What to Do if the Client Says He Does Not Want To Talk	
The nurse new to this situation may feel rejected or ineffectual.	At first, the nurse might say something to this effect: ■ "It's all right. I would like to spend time with you. We don't have to talk." The nurse might spend short, frequent periods (e.g., 5 minutes) with the client throughout the day. ■ "Our 5 minutes is up. I'll be back at 10 AM and stay with you 5 more minutes." This gives the client the opportunity to understand that the nurse means what he or she says and is back on time consistently. It also gives the client time between visits to assess the nurse and perhaps feel less threatened.
What to Do if the Client Seeks to Prolong the Interview	
Sometimes, clients open up dynamic or "juicy" topics just before the interview time is up. This is often to test or manipulate the nurse. The nurse might feel tempted to extend scheduled time or might not want to hurt the client's feelings.	The nurse sets limits and restates and reinforces the original contract. The nurse states that they will use the issues for the next session. ■ "Our time is up now, Mr. Jones. This would be a good place to start at our next session, which is Wednesday at 10 AM."
What to Do if the Client Gives the Nurse a Present	
The nurse may feel uncomfortable when offered a gift. The meaning needs to be examined. Is the gift (1) a way of getting better care? (2) a way to maintain self-esteem? (3) a way of making the nurse feel guilty? (4) a sincere expression of thanks? or (5) a cultural expectation?	*Possible guidelines:* If the gift is expensive, the best policy is to perhaps graciously refuse. If it is inexpensive and (1) given *at the end* of hospitalization when a relationship has developed, graciously accept; (2) given *at the beginning* of the relationship, graciously refuse and explore the meaning behind the present. ■ "Thank you, but it is our job to care for our clients. Are you concerned that some aspect of your care will be overlooked?" If the gift is money, it may be best to graciously refuse.
What to Do if the Client Asks You a Personal Question	
The nurse may think that it is rude not to answer the client's question. *or* A new nurse might feel relieved to put off having to start the interview. *or* The nurse may feel put on the spot and want to leave the situation. New nurses are often manipulated by a client to change roles. This keeps the focus off the client and prevents the building of a relationship.	The nurse may or may not answer the client's query. If the nurse decides to answer a natural question, he or she answers in a word or two, then refocuses back on the client. **Client:** Are you married? **Nurse:** Yes, do you have a spouse? **Client:** Do you have any children? **Nurse:** This time is for you—tell me about yourself. **Client:** You can just tell me if you have any children. **Nurse:** This is your time to focus on your concerns. Tell me something about your family.

The **receiver** receives and interprets the message. Often the message from the sender may act as a stimulus to the receiver. The receiver may then respond to the sender by giving feedback to the sender. The nature of the feedback often indicates whether the meaning of the message sent by the sender has been correctly interpreted by the receiver. Validating the accuracy of the sender message is extremely important. An accuracy check may be obtained by simply asking the sender "Is this what you mean?" or "It seems you are saying . . ." (Parsons and Wicks 1994). Feedback in a counseling situation may entail pointing out certain observed behaviors and giving your impression or reaction. "I notice you turn away when we talk about your going back to college. Is there a conflict there?" When the receiver gives feedback to the sender, communication becomes reciprocal. Communication is most effective when the message sent is the same as the message received.

Figure 11–1 shows this simple model of communication. However, communication is a complex process involving a variety of personal and environmental factors that can distort both the sending and the receiving of messages.

Factors that May Affect Communication

Personal factors that can impede accurate transmission or interpretation of messages include emotional factors (e.g., mood, knowledge levels, language use) and social factors (e.g., previous experience, differences in culture, language).

Environmental factors include physical factors (e.g., background noise, lack of privacy, uncomfortable accommodations) and societal factors (e.g, the presence of others, the expectations of others).

Effective communication in helping relationships depends on nurses knowing what they are trying to convey (the purpose of the message), communicating what is really meant to the client, and comprehending the meaning of what the client is intentionally or unintentionally conveying (Collins 1983).

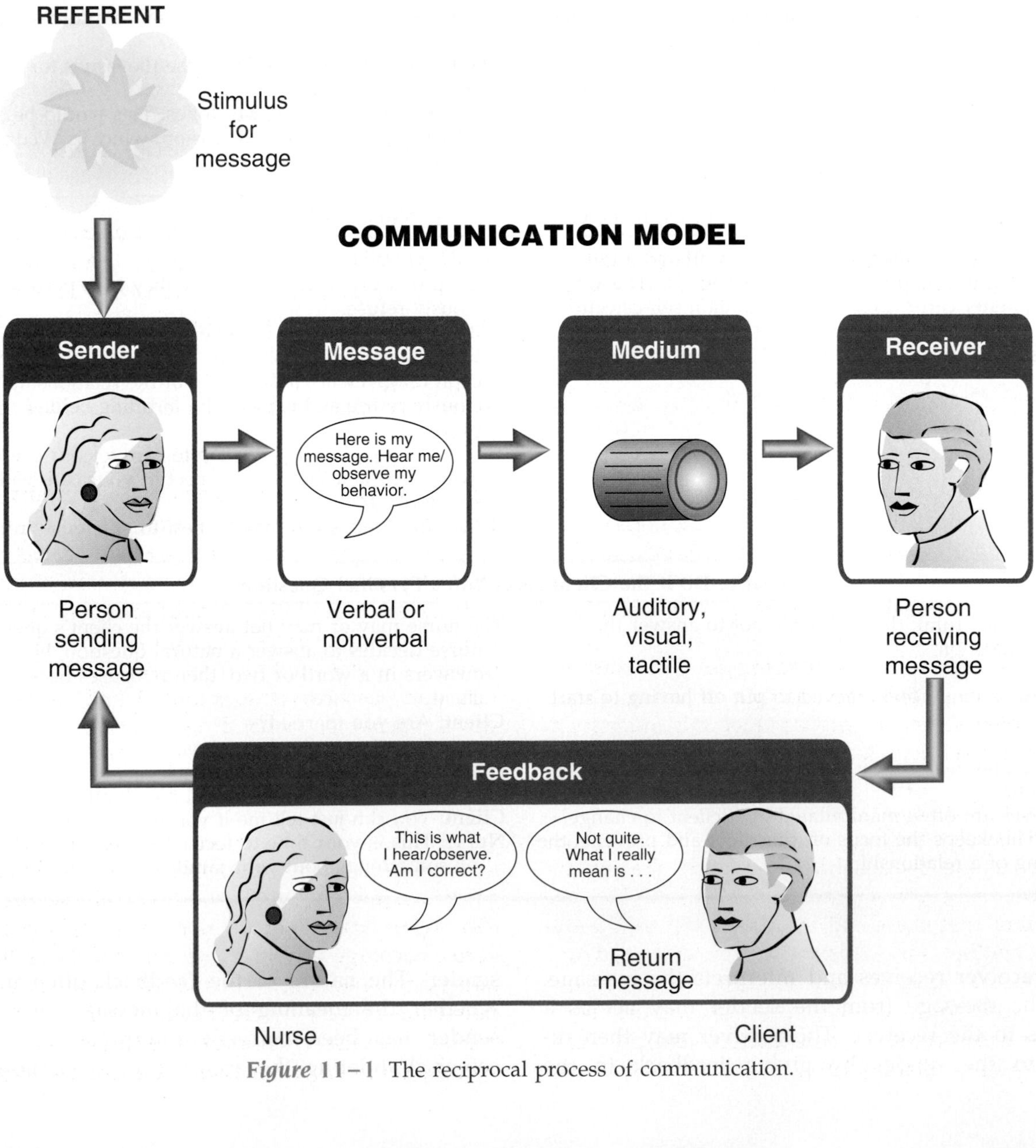

Figure 11–1 The reciprocal process of communication.

Peplau (1952, p. 290) identified two main principles that can guide the communication process during the nurse-client interview: (1) **clarity,** wherein the meaning of the message is accurately understood by both parties "as the result of joint and sustained effort of all parties concerned"; and (2) **continuity,** which promotes connections among ideas "and the feelings, events, or themes conveyed in those ideas."

Communication consists of verbal and nonverbal elements. Shea (1998) stated that communication is roughly 10% verbal and 90% nonverbal. Therefore, learning to be an effective communicator means using both verbal and nonverbal cues.

Verbal Communication

Verbal communication consists of all words a person speaks. We live in a society of symbols, and our supreme social symbol is words. Talking is our most common activity—our public link with one another, the primary instrument of instruction, a need, an art, and one of the most personal aspects of our private life. When we speak, we

■ Communicate our beliefs and values
■ Communicate perceptions and meanings
■ Convey interest and understanding *or* insult and judgment
■ Convey messages clearly *or* convey conflicting or implied messages
■ Convey clear, honest feelings *or* disguised, distorted feelings

Even if the nurse and client have the same cultural background, the mental image they have of a word may not be exactly the same. Although they believe they are talking about the same thing, the nurse and client may actually be talking about two quite different things. Words are the symbols for emotions as well as for mental images. For example, the word **trip** shows the manner in which differences in mental images can produce misunderstanding. If a nurse says to a client "I heard you had some trip!" the client will define **trip** according to the images that he or she has formed of the word from speaking, reading, writing, and listening. Depending on the client's life experience, the nurse's statement could convey interest or insult. Did the nurse think that the client stumbled and fell? Traveled to another city? Experimented with a drug? Reflecting the rapid and widespread changes in our society, words often change meanings and are therefore best interpreted in accordance with the company they keep (Collins 1983).

Nonverbal Communication

Nonverbal behaviors are the behaviors displayed by an individual in contrast with the actual content of speech. Tone of voice and the manner in which a person paces speech are examples of nonverbal communication. Other common examples of nonverbal communication (often called **cues**) are facial expressions, body posture, amount of eye contact, eye cast (emotion expressed in the eyes), hand gestures, sighs, fidgeting, and yawning. Table 11–3 identifies key components of nonverbal behaviors. Nonverbal behaviors need to be observed and interpreted in light of a person's culture, class, gender, age, sexual orientation, and spiritual norms.

Interaction of Verbal and Nonverbal Communication

Communication thus involves two radically different but interdependent kinds of symbols. The first type involves the **spoken word,** which represents our public selves. Verbal assertions can be straightforward comments or can be skillfully used to distort, conceal, deny, and generally disguise true feelings. The second type, **nonverbal behaviors,** covers a wide range of human activities, from body movements to responses to the messages of others. How a person listens and uses silence and sense of touch may also convey important information about the private self that is not available from conversation alone, especially when viewed through a cultural perspective.

Some nonverbal communication, such as facial expressions, seems to be inborn and is similar across cultures. Dee (1991) cited studies that found a high degree of agreement in spontaneous facial expressions or emotions across 10 different cultures. In public, however, some cultural groups (e.g., the Japanese) may control their facial expressions when observers are present. Other types of nonverbal behaviors, such as how close people stand to each other when speaking, depend on cultural conventions. Some nonverbal communication is formalized and has specific meanings (e.g., the military salute, the Japanese bow).

Therefore, an interaction consists of both verbal and nonverbal messages. Often, people have more conscious awareness of their verbal messages and less awareness of their nonverbal behaviors. The verbal message is sometimes referred to as the **content** of the message, and the nonverbal behavior is called the **process** of the message. When the content (verbal message) is congruent with (agrees with) the process (nonverbal behavior), the communication is

TABLE 11–3   *Nonverbal Behaviors*

POSSIBLE BEHAVIORS	EXAMPLE
Body Behaviors	
Posture, body movements, gestures, gait	The client is slumped in a chair, puts her face in her hands, and occasionally taps her right foot.
Facial Expressions	
Frowns, smiles, grimaces, raised eyebrows, pursed lips, licking lips, tongue movements	The client grimaces when speaking to the nurse; when alone, he smiles and giggles to himself.
Eye Cast	
Angry, suspicious, and accusatory looks	The client's eyes harden with suspicion.
Voice-Related Behaviors	
Tone, pitch, level, intensity, inflection, stuttering, pauses, silences, fluency	The client talks in a loud sing-song voice.
Observable Autonomic Physiological Responses	
Increase in respirations, diaphoresis, pupil dilation, blushing, paleness	When the client mentions discharge, she becomes pale, her respirations increase, and her face becomes diaphoretic.
General Appearance	
Grooming, dress, hygiene	The client is dressed in a wrinkled shirt and his pants are stained; his socks are dirty and he wears no shoes.
Physical Characteristics	
Height, weight, physique, complexion	The client appears grossly overweight and his muscle tone appears flabby.

more clearly understood and is considered healthy. For example, if a student says, "It's important that I get good grades in this class," that is **content**. If the student has bought the books, takes good notes and has a study buddy, that is **process**. Therefore, the content and process are congruent and straightforward and there is a "healthy" message. If, however, the verbal message is not reinforced or is in fact contradicted by the nonverbal behavior, the message is confusing. For example, if the student says, "It's important that I get good grades in this class," that is **content**. If the student does not have the books, skips several classes, and does not study, that is **process**. Here the student is sending out two different messages.

Conflicting messages are known as **double (mixed) messages**. Dee (1991) suggested that one way a nurse can respond to verbal and nonverbal incongruity is to reflect and validate the client's feelings. "You say you are upset that you did not pass this semester, but I notice that you look more relaxed and less conflicted than you have all semester. Do you want to share with me some of the pros and cons of not passing the course this semester?"

With experience, nurses become increasingly aware of a client's verbal and nonverbal communication. Nurses can compare the clients' dialogue with their nonverbal communication to gain important clues about the real message. What persons do may either express and reinforce, or contradict, what they say. As in the saying "actions speak louder than words," actions often reveal the true meaning of a person's intent, whether it is conscious or unconscious.

Raingruber's (2001) studies of the nonverbal rapport between nurse psychotherapists and clients found some important nonverbal behaviors that helped establish a rapport and create a comfortable sense of timing. These include such behaviors as emotional congruence, physical mirroring of gestures, postures, and expressions.

Negotiating Cultural Communication Barriers

Ethnic minorities are the most rapidly growing segment of the American population. Health care professionals are gradually becoming aware of the need to become more familiar with the verbal and nonverbal communications of the diverse multicultural populations using the health care system.

The nurse's awareness of the cultural meaning of certain verbal and nonverbal communications in initial face-to-face encounters with a client can lead to the formation of positive therapeutic alliances with culturally diverse populations (Siantz 1991).

Unacknowledged differences between aspects of the cultural identities of client and nurse can result in assessment and interventions that are not optimally respectful of the client and can be inadvertently biased or prejudiced (Lu et al. 1995). Lu and colleagues further emphasized that health care workers need to have not only knowledge of various clients' cultures but also awareness of their own cultural identity. Especially important are nurses' attitudes and beliefs toward ethnic minorities, because these will affect their relationships with clients. Siantz (1991) identified the following three areas that may prove problematic for the nurse interpreting specific verbal and nonverbal messages of the client:

1. Communication styles
2. Use of eye contact
3. Perception of touch

Communication Styles

People from some ethnic backgrounds may communicate in an intense and highly emotional manner. For example, Hispanic Americans may appear to use dramatic body language when describing their emotional problems, from the perspective of a non-Hispanic person. For clinicians from a non-Hispanic background, such behavior may be perceived as out of control and thus viewed as having a degree of pathology that is not actually present. However, from within the Hispanic culture, intensely emotional styles of communication often are culturally appropriate and are to be expected (Siantz 1991). French and Italian Americans also demonstrate animated facial expressions and expressive hand gestures during communication that can be mistakenly interpreted by others.

Conversely, in other cultures, a calm facade may mask severe distress. For example, in Asian cultures, expression of either positive or negative emotions is a private affair, and open expression of emotions is considered to be in bad taste and possibly a weakness. A quiet smile by an Asian American may express joy, an apology, stoicism in the face of difficulty, or even anger (Poole et al. 1995). German and British Americans highly value the concept of self-control and may show little facial emotion in the presence of great distress or emotional turmoil.

Ingram (1991) and others believe it is important to understand an ethnic minority in light of the historical context from which it evolved and its relationship to the dominant culture. For example, the African American, whose historical background in the United States is one of slavery and oppression, is likely to be aware of a basic need for survival. As a result of their experience, many African Americans have become highly selective and guarded in their communication with those outside their cultural group. Therefore, a tendency toward guarded and selective communication among African American clients may represent a healthy cultural paranoia (Grier and Cobbs 1968; Ingram 1991).

Eye Contact

Culture also dictates a person's comfort or lack of comfort with direct eye contact. Some cultures consider direct eye contact disrespectful and improper. For example, Hispanics have traditionally been taught to avoid eye contact with authority figures such as nurses, physicians, or other health care professionals. Avoidance of direct eye contact is seen as a sign of respect to those in authority. To nurses or other health care workers from non-Hispanic backgrounds, this lack of eye contact may be wrongly interpreted as disinterest in the interview or even taken as a lack of respect. Conversely, the nurse is expected to look directly at the client when conducting the interview (Siantz 1991). Similarly, in Asian cultures, respect is shown by avoiding eye contact. For example, in Japan, direct eye contact is considered a lack of respect and a personal affront; preference is for shifting or downcast eyes. With many Chinese, gazing around and looking to one side when listening to another is considered polite. However, when speaking to the elderly, direct eye contact is used (Geissler 1993). Philippine Americans may try to avoid eye contact; however, once it is established, it is important to return and maintain eye contact. Many Native Americans also believe it is disrespectful to engage in direct eye contact, especially if the speaker is younger. Direct eye contact by members of the dominant culture in the health care system can and does cause discomfort for some clients (Poole et al. 1995).

Among German Americans, direct and sustained eye contact indicates that the person listens, trusts, is somewhat aggressive, or in some situations is sexually interested. Russians also find direct, sustained eye contact the norm for social interactions. In Haiti, it is customary to hold eye contact with everyone but the poor (Geissler 1993). French, British, and many African Americans maintain eye contact during conversation; avoidance of eye contact by another person may be interpreted as disinterest, not telling the truth, or avoiding the sharing of important information. In some Arab cultures, a woman making direct eye contact with a man may imply a sexual interest or even promiscuity. In Greece, staring in public is acceptable (Geissler 1993).

Touch

The therapeutic use of touch is a basic aspect of the nurse-client relationship and is normally perceived as a gesture of warmth and friendship. However, touch can be perceived as an invasion of privacy or an invitation to intimacy by some clients (Dee 1991). The response to touch is often culturally defined. For example, many Hispanic Americans are accustomed to frequent physical contact. For some Hispanics, holding the client's hand in response to a distressing situation or giving the client a reassuring pat on the shoulder may be experienced as supportive and thus help facilitate openness early in the therapeutic relationship (Ramirez 1989). However, the degree and extent of comfort conveyed by touch in the nurse-client relationship are dependent on the country of origin. People from Italian and French cultural backgrounds may also be accustomed to frequent touching during conversation (Geissler 1993). In the Russian culture, touch is also an important part of nonverbal communication. In other cultures, personal touch within the context of an interview might be experienced as patronizing, intrusive, aggressive, or sexually inviting. For example, among German, Swedish, and British Americans, touch practices are infrequent, although a handshake may be common at the beginning and end of an interaction. In India, men may shake hands with other men but not with women; an Asian Indian man may greet a woman by nodding and holding the palms of his hands together but not touching the woman. In Japan, handshakes are acceptable; however, a pat on the back is not. Chinese Americans may not like to be touched by strangers. Some Native Americans extend their hand and lightly touch the hand of the person they are greeting rather than shake hands (Geissler 1993). Even among people of the same culture, the use of touch has clear interpretations and rules between people of different genders and class. **Students are urged to check the policy manual of their facility since some facilities have a "no touch" policy, particularly with adolescents and children who may have experienced inappropriate touch and would not know how to interpret the touch of the health care worker.**

So we see that there are numerous ways to interpret verbal and nonverbal communications for each cultural and subcultural group. Even if a nurse is aware of how a specific cultural group responds to touch, for example, the nurse could still be in error when dealing with an individual within that cultural group. Ingram (1991) proposed that a basic guiding principle when working with clients from various cultures is to recognize and use the client as the primary source of information.

> When approached from a posture of respect and compassion, clients of all cultures are the most accurate source of information about their own culturally specific behavior. Hence it is the task of nurses to identify and explore the meaning of nonverbal and verbal behavior with the clients with whom they interact (p. 40).

See Box 11–1 for some strategies that may increase nurses' awareness of culturally specific verbal and nonverbal behaviors.

Box 11–1   *Strategies to Increase Cultural Awareness*

1. Engage in personal and professional workshops and training seminars that facilitate awareness of biases and prejudices toward people who are culturally different.
2. Once trust has been established in a nurse-client relationship, share your observations with the client. Seek clarification and validate your perceptions with the client.
3. Explore the meaning of the behavior with the client, being careful not to inject preconceived notions.
4. Acquire knowledge outside your professional practice through participation in culturally diverse activities and through nonprofessional contacts.
5. Read history and literature written by members of the cultural group with whom you are working.
6. Engage in discussion of racial issues when they emerge in the context of your interaction with clients, peers, and others outside your work setting.
7. Gain an appreciation for how your own culture communicates and what you observe as different in others (e.g., foods, celebrations, issues of trust, expressions of joy or fear).

Data from Ingram, C. A. (1991). How can we become more aware of culturally specific body language and use this awareness therapeutically? *Journal of Psychosocial Nursing*, 29(11):40–41.

EFFECTIVE COMMUNICATION SKILLS

The art of communication (e.g. interviewing, problem solving, counseling, and health teaching) was positioned by Peplau to highlight the importance of nursing interventions in facilitating achievement of quality patient criticisms and quality of life (Haber 2000). Therefore, as previously stated, the goals of the nurse in the mental health setting are to help the client

■ Identify and explore problems relating to others
■ Discover healthy ways of meeting emotional needs
■ Experience satisfying interpersonal relationships
■ Feel understood and comfortable

Once specific needs and problems have been identified, the nurse can work with the client on increasing problem-solving skills, learning new coping behaviors, and experiencing more appropriate and satisfying ways of relating to others. To do this, nurses need to have a sound knowledge of communication skills. Therefore, nurses need to become more aware of their own interpersonal techniques, eliminating nontherapeutic (nonhelpful) techniques and applying additional responses that maximize nurse-client interactions and increase the number of therapeutic (helpful) techniques. Appropriate techniques are neither therapeutic nor nontherapeutic in themselves. They can, when used in the context of respect and genuine interest, greatly facilitate open communication.

Degree of Openness

Any question or statements can be classified as (1) open-ended verbalizations, (2) focused questions, or (3) closed-ended verbalizations. Furthermore, any questions or statement can be classified along the **continuum of openness**. There are three variables that influence where verbalization sits on this openness continuum (Shea 1998), including

1. The degree to which the verbalization tends to produce spontaneous and lengthy response
2. The degree to which the verbalization does not limit the client's answer set
3. The degree to which the verbalization opens up a moderately resistant client

Refer to Table 11-4 during the following discussion.

Open-Ended Questions

Open-ended questions require more than one-word answers, (i.e., as a "yes" or "no"). Even with a client who is sullen, resistant, or guarded, open-ended questions can encourage lengthy information on experiences, perceptions of events, or responses to a situation. Examples of an open-ended question include

■ "What are some of the stresses you are grappling with?"
■ "What do you perceive to be your biggest problem at the moment?"
■ " Tell me something about your family."

Shea (1998) encouraged the use of frequent open-ended questions or gentle inquiries (e.g., "Tell me about . . . " or "Share with me . . . "). This is especially helpful when beginning a relationship and in the early interviews. Although the initial responses may be short, over time the responses often become more informative as the client becomes more at ease. This is an especially valuable technique for clients who are resistant or guarded, but it is a good rule for opening phases of any interview, especially in the early phase of establishing a rapport with an individual.

Closed-Ended Questions

Closed-ended questions, in contrast, are questions that ask for specific information (dates, names, numbers, "yes" or "no" information). These are closed-ended questions because they limit the client's freedom of choice. For example,

■ "Is your mother alive?"
■ "When were you born?"
■ "Did you seek therapy after your first suicide attempt?"
■ "Do you think the medication is helping you?"

Closed ended questions give specific information when needed, such as during an initial assessment or intake interview, or to ascertain results, as in "Are the medications helping you?" They are usually answered by "yes," "no," or a short answer. When closed-ended questions are used frequently during a counseling session, or especially during an initial interview, they can close an interview down rapidly. This is especially true with a guarded or resistant client.

Other useful tools for nurses when communicating with their clients are (1) clarifying/validating techniques, (2) the use of silence, and (3) active listening.

Clarifying Techniques

Understanding depends on clear communication, which is aided by verifying with a client the nurse's interpretation of the client's messages. The nurse must request feedback on the accuracy of the message received from both verbal and nonverbal cues. The use of clarifying techniques helps both participants identify major differences in their frame of reference, giving them the opportunity to correct misperceptions before they cause any serious misunderstandings. The client who is asked to elaborate on or to clarify vague or ambiguous messages needs to know that the purpose is to promote mutual understanding.

Paraphrasing

For clarity, we might use paraphrasing, which means to restate in different (often fewer) words the

TABLE 11–4   *Degree of Openness Continuum*

VERBALIZATION	EXAMPLE
Open Ended	These questions are to be stated with a gentle tone of voice while expressing a genuine interest. They invite the client to share personal experiences. They cannot be answered with a "yes" or "no."
1. Open-ended questions (giving broad openings)	1. What would you like to discuss? 2. What are your plans for the future? 3. How will you approach your father? 4. What are some of your thoughts about the marriage?
2. Gentle commands (encouraging descriptions of perceptions, clarifying)	1. Tell me something about your home life. 2. Share with me some of your hopes about your future. 3. Describe for me the problem with your boss. 4. Give me an example of your being "no good."
Focused	These questions represent a middle ground with regard to openness. When the relationship is strong, these questions can result in spontaneous lengthy speech. Used with a resistant client, these questions can be answered tersely.
1. Exploring/focusing	1. Can you describe your feelings? 2. Can you tell me a little about your boss? 3. Can you say anything positive about your marriage? 4. Can you tell me what the voices are saying?
2. Qualitative questions	1. How's your appetite? 2. How's your job going? 3. How's your mood been?
3. Statements of inquiry (restating, reflecting, paraphrasing, clarifying)	1. You say you were fifth in your class? 2. So you left the marriage after 3 years? 3. So when she cries you feel guilty? 4. You seem to be saying that you're viewed as the bad guy in the family?
4. Empathetic statements (making observations, sharing perceptions, seeking clarification)	1. It sounds like a troubling time for you. 2. It's difficult to end a marriage after 10 years. 3. It looks like you're feeling sad. 4. You seem very disappointed about . . . 5. I notice you are biting your lip.
5. Facilitatory statements (accepting, offering general leads)	1. Uh-huh 2. Go on. 3. I see
Closed Ended	These techniques tend to decrease a client's response length. However, they can be effective in focusing a wandering client. Closed-ended questions help obtain important facts or ask for specific details. Closed-ended statements give information or explanations or have an educational slant.
1. Closed-ended questions (seeking information)	1. How long have you been hearing voices? 2. Are you feeling happy, sad, or angry? 3. What medications is he taking?
2. Closed-ended statements (giving information)	1. Anxiety can be helped with behavioral therapies. 2. This test will determine. . . . 3. I read in your chart that you tried suicide once before. 4. We will begin by taking a blood sample to check your medication level.

Adapted from Shea, S. C. (1998). *Psychiatric interviewing: The art of understanding.* Philadelphia: W. B. Saunders.

basic content of a client's message. Using simple, precise, and culturally relevant terms, the nurse may readily confirm interpretation of the client's previous message before the interview proceeds. By prefacing statements with a phrase such as "I am not sure I understand" or "In other words, you seem to be saying . . . ," the nurse helps the client form a clearer perception of what may be a bewildering mass of details. After paraphrasing, the nurse must validate the accuracy of the restatement and its helpfulness to the discussion. The client may confirm or deny the perceptions through nonverbal cues or by directly responding to a question such as "Was I correct in saying . . . ?" As a result, the client is made aware that the interviewer is actively involved in the search for understanding.

Restating

With **restating**, the nurse mirrors the client's overt and covert messages; thus, this technique may be used to echo feeling as well as content. Restating differs from paraphrasing in that it involves repetition of the same key words the client has just spoken. If a client remarks "My life is empty . . . , it has no meaning," additional information may be gained by restating, "Your life has no meaning?" The purpose of this technique is to explore more thoroughly subjects that may be significant. However, too frequent and indiscriminate use of restating might be interpreted by clients as inattention, disinterest, or worse. It is easy to overuse this tool and become mechanical. Inappropriately parroting or mimicking what another has said may be perceived as poking fun at the person, making this nondirective approach a definite drawback to communication. To avoid overuse of restating, the nurse can combine restating with direct questions that encourage descriptions: "What does your life lack?" "What kind of meaning is missing?" "Describe one day in your life that appears empty to you."

Reflecting

Reflection is a means of assisting people to better understand their own thoughts and feelings. **Reflecting** may take the form of a question or a simple statement that conveys the nurse's observations of the client when sensitive issues are being discussed (Parsons and Wicks 1994). The nurse might then describe briefly to the client the apparent meaning of the emotional tone of the client's verbal and nonverbal behavior. For example, to reflect a client's feelings about his or her life, a good beginning might be, "You sound as if you have had many disappointments." Sharing **observations** with a client shows acceptance. The nurse helps make the client aware of inner feelings and encourages the client to own them. For example, the nurse may tell a client, "You look sad." Perceiving the nurse's concern may allow a client spontaneously to share feelings. The use of a question in response to the client's question is another reflective technique (Parsons and Wicks 1994, p. 92). For example,

Client: Nurse, do you think I really need to be hospitalized?
Nurse: What do you think, Jane?
Client: I don't know, that's why I'm asking you.
Nurse: I'll be glad to share my impression with you at the end of this first session. However, you've probably thought about hospitalization and have some feelings about it. I wonder what they are.

Exploring

A technique that enables the nurse to examine important ideas, experiences, or relationships more fully is **exploring**. For example, if a client tells the nurse that he does not get along well with his wife, the nurse will want to further explore this area. Possible openers might include

■ *"Tell me* more about your relationship with your wife."
■ *"Describe* your relationship with your wife."
■ *"Give me an example* of you and your wife not getting along."

Asking for an example can greatly clarify a vague or generic statement made by a client.

Mary: No one likes me.
Nurse: Give me an example of one person who doesn't like you.

or

Jim: Everything I do is wrong.
Nurse: Give me an example of *one* thing you do that you think is wrong.

Use of Silence

In many cultures in our society, and in nursing, there is an emphasis on action. In communication, we tend to expect a high level of verbal activity. Many students and practicing nurses find that when the flow of words stops, they become uncomfortable. The effective **use of silence**, however, is a useful communication technique.

Silence is not the absence of communication. Silence is a specific channel for transmitting and receiving messages. The practitioner needs to understand that silence is a significant means of influencing and being influenced by others.

In the initial interview the client may be reluctant to speak because of the newness of the situation, the fact that the nurse is a stranger, self-consciousness, embarrassment, or shyness. Talking is highly individualized; some find the telephone a nuisance, whereas others believe they cannot live without it. The nurse must recognize and respect individual differences in styles and tempos of responding. How else can nurses learn of another's nature and their own but by courtesy, care, and time? People who are quiet, those who have a language barrier or speech impediment, the elderly, and those who lack confidence in their ability to express themselves may be communicating through their silences a need for support and encouragement in acts of self-expression (Collins 1983).

Although there is no universal rule concerning how much silence is too much, silence has been said to be worthwhile only as long as it is serving some function and not frightening to the patient (Schulman 1974). Knowing when to speak during the interview is largely dependent on the nurse's perception about what is being conveyed through the silence. Icy silence may be an expression of anger and hostility. Being ignored or given the silent treatment is recognized as an insult and is a particularly hurtful form of communication. Ingram (1991) pointed out that silence among some African American clients may relate to anger, insulted feelings, or acknowledgment of a nurse's lack of cultural sensitivity.

Silence may provide meaningful moments of reflection for both participants. It gives each an opportunity to contemplate thoughtfully what has been said and felt, to weigh alternatives, to formulate new ideas, and to gain a new perspective of the matter under discussion. If the nurse waits to speak and allows the client to break the silence, the client may share thoughts and feelings that could otherwise have been withheld. Nurses who feel compelled to fill every void with words often do so because of their own anxiety, self-consciousness, and embarrassment. When this occurs, the nurse's need for comfort tends to take priority over the needs of the client.

Conversely, prolonged and frequent silences by the nurse may hinder an interview that requires verbal articulation. Although the untalkative nurse may be comfortable with silence, this mode of communication may make the client feel like a fountain of information to be drained dry. Moreover, without feedback, clients have no way of knowing whether what they said was understood.

Active Listening

People want more than just physical presence in human communication. Most people are looking for the other person to be there for them psychologically, socially, and emotionally (Egan 1994). Active listening includes

- Observing the client's nonverbal behaviors
- Listening to and understanding the client's verbal message
- Listening to and understanding the person in the context of the social setting of his or her life
- Listening for "false notes" (e.g., inconsistencies or things client says that need more clarification)
- Providing clients feedback about themselves of which they might not be aware

We have already noted that effective interviewers must become accustomed to silence. It is just as important, however, for effective interviewers to learn to become active listeners when the client is talking, as well as when the client becomes silent. During active listening, nurses carefully note what the client is saying verbally and nonverbally, as well as monitoring their own nonverbal responses (Parsons and Wicks 1994). Using silence effectively and learning to listen on a deeper, more significant level to both the client and your own thoughts and reactions are both key ingredients in effective communications. Both these skills take time, profit from guidance, and can be learned.

Cultural Caution

It is important for all of us to recognize that it is impossible to listen to people in an unbiased way. In the process of socialization we develop cultural filters through which we listen to ourselves, others, and the world around us (Egan 1994). Cultural filters are a form of cultural bias or cultural prejudice.

> One of the functions of culture is to provide a highly selective screen between man and the outside world. In its many forms, culture therefore designates what we pay attention to and what we ignore. This screening provides structure for the world (Hall 1977, p. 85).

Egan (1994) stated that we need these cultural filters to provide structure for ourselves and to help us interpret and interact with the world. However, unavoidably, these cultural filters also introduce various forms of bias in our listening, since they are bound to influence our personal, professional, familial, and sociological values and interpretations. Egan also gave an example of how strong cultural filters can influence the likelihood of bias with multicultural clients. For instance, he used the example of a white, middle-class helper who would tend to use white, middle-class filters when listening. These cultural filters may not interfere with, and could even facilitate, working with someone from a white, middle-class background. However, if the awareness of our own cultural filters goes unacknowledged, the likelihood is great that they will distort our perceptions and interpretations of multiethnic clients. Therefore, the white, middle-class helper, if not cognizant of personal cultural biases, could easily introduce bias when working with, for example, a well-to-do Asian client with high social status in the community; an African American mother from the urban ghetto; or a poor white subsistence farmer (Egan 1994). We all need a frame of reference to help us function in our world. The trick is to understand that people use many other frames of reference to help them function in their world. Acknowledging that others view the world quite differently, and trying to understand other people's ways of experiencing and living in the world, can go a long way toward minimizing our personal distortions in listening. Building acceptance and understanding of those culturally different from ourselves is a skill, too.

Active listening helps strengthen the client's ability to solve personal problems. By giving the client undivided attention, the nurse communicates that the client is not alone; rather, the nurse is working along with the client, seeking to understand and help. This kind of intervention enhances self-esteem and encourages the client to direct energy toward finding ways to deal with problems. Serving as a sounding board, the nurse listens as the client tests thoughts by voicing them aloud. This form of interpersonal interaction often enables the client to clarify thinking, link ideas, and tentatively decide what should be done and how best to do it (Collins 1983).

OBSTRUCTIVE TECHNIQUES TO MONITOR AND MINIMIZE

A number of techniques that can interfere with communication are listed in Table 11–5. Although people may use these techniques in their daily lives, they can become problematic when one is working with clients who are attempting to cope with disruptions in their life. Two other techniques, excessive questioning and giving approval/disapproval, are discussed in the following sections. Giving advice and "why" questions are discussed in more detail.

Asking Excessive Questions

Excessive questioning, especially **closed-ended** questions, puts the nurse in the role of interrogator, demanding information without respect for the client's willingness or readiness to respond. This approach conveys lack of respect and sensitivity to the client's needs. Excessive questioning controls the range and nature of response and can easily result in a therapeutic stall or a shut-down interview. It is a controlling tactic and may reflect the interviewer's lack of security in letting the client tell his or her own story. It is better to ask more open-ended questions and follow the client's lead. For example,

EXCESSIVE QUESTIONS
■ "Why did you leave your wife?" "Did you feel angry at her?"

■ "What did she do to you?" "Are you going back to her?"

BETTER TO SAY
■ "Tell me about the situation between you and your wife."

Giving Approval/Disapproval

"You look great in that dress." "I am proud of the way you controlled your temper at lunch." "That's a great quilt you made." What could be bad about giving someone a pat on the back once in a while? Nothing, if it is done without involving a judgment (positive or negative) by the nurse. We often give our friends and family approval when they do something well. However, in a nurse-client situation, giving approval often becomes much more complex. A client may be feeling overwhelmed; experiencing low self-esteem; feeling unsure of where his or her life is going; and very needy of recognition, approval, and attention. Yet, when people are feeling vulnerable, a value comment might be misinterpreted. For example,

> **Nurse:** You did a great job in group telling John just what you thought about how rudely he treated you.

Implied in this message is that the nurse was pleased by the manner in which the client talked to John. The client then sees this response as a way to please the nurse, by doing the right thing. To continue to please the nurse (and get approval), the client may continue the behavior. The behavior might be useful behavior for the client, but when a behavior is being done to please another person, it is not coming from the individual's own volition or conviction. Also, when the other person whom the client needs to please is not around, the motivation for the new behavior might not be there either. Thus, it really is not a change in behavior as much as a ploy to win approval and acceptance from another person. Giving approval also cuts off further communication. It is a statement of the observer's (nurse's) judgment on another person's (client's) behavior. A more useful response would be the following:

> **Nurse:** I noticed you spoke up to John in group yesterday about his rude behavior. How did it feel to be more assertive?

This opens the way for finding out if the client was scared, was comfortable, wants to work more on assertiveness, or something else. It also suggests that this was a self-choice the client made. The client is given recognition for the change in behavior, and the topic is also open for further discussion.

TABLE 11–5 *Obstructive Communications*

TECHNIQUE	EXAMPLE	DISCUSSION	MORE HELPFUL RESPONSE
Premature Advice	**"Get out of this situation immediately."**	Assumes "nurse knows best" and clients can't think for themselves. Inhibits problem solving and fosters dependency.	■ "What are the pro's and con's of your situation?" ■ "What were some of the actions you thought you might take?" ■ "What are some of the ways you have thought of to meet your goals?" **Encourage problem solving**
Minimizing Feelings	**Client:** I wish I were dead. **Nurse:** Everyone gets down in the dumps. **Nurse:** I know what you mean. **Nurse:** I know how you feel. **Nurse:** You should feel happy you're getting better. **Nurse:** Things get worse before they get better.	The nurse is unable to understand or empathize with the client. Here the client's feelings or experiences are being belittled, and can cause the client to feel "small" or "insignificant."	"You must be feeling very upset. Are you thinking of hurting yourself?" **Empathize and explore**
False Reassurance	**Nurse:** I wouldn't worry about that. **Nurse:** Everything will be alright. **Nurse:** You will do just fine, you'll see.	Underrates a person's feelings and belittles a person's concerns. May cause clients to stop sharing feelings if they think they will be ridiculed or not taken seriously.	**Nurse:** What specifically are you worried about? **Nurse:** What do you think could go wrong? **Nurse:** What are you concerned might happen? **Clarifying client's messages**
Nonverbal Signs of Boredom or Resentment	Nurse frequently checks his or her watch, rustles papers, avoids eye contact, does not respond to client's concerns, looks annoyed at something client is doing or has said.	Clients quickly pick up the nurse's disapproval or boredom and may think nurse disapproves or is bored with them. Clients experience diminished self-esteem and can feel demeaned.	Nurses need to be alert to personal feelings toward client. If client's behavior is bothering the nurse (e.g., smoking in a non-smoking room) the nurse needs to deal with the issue, and not remain angry. If the nurse is feeling bored, it may be a clue to what is going on with the client that needs exploring. If there is something going on with the nurse, the nurse should make it clear to the client that it is the nurse who is distracted and has nothing to do with the client. **Self-assessment**
Value Judgments	**Nurse:** How come you still smoke when your wife has lung cancer?	Moralizing prevents problem solving. Moralizing can make clients feel guilty, angry, misunderstood, not supported, and/or anxious to leave.	**Nurse:** I notice you are still smoking even though your wife has lung cancer. Is this a problem? **Making observations**
"Why" Questions	**Nurse:** Why did you stop taking your medication?	Implies criticism; often has the effect of making the client feel defensive.	**Nurse:** Tell me some of the reasons that led up to you not taking your medications. **Open ended—broad opening**

TABLE 11–5 *Obstructive Communications* (Continued)

TECHNIQUE	EXAMPLE	DISCUSSION	MORE HELPFUL RESPONSE
Asking Excessive Questions	**Nurse:** How's your appetite? Are you losing weight? Are you eating enough? **Client:** No.	Client does not know what question to answer. Can be confused as to what is being asked.	**Nurse:** Tell me about your eating habits since you've been depressed. **Clarifying**
Giving Approval, Agreeing	**Nurse:** I'm proud of you for applying for that job. **Nurse:** I agree with your decision.	Implies the client is doing the *right* thing—and not doing it is wrong. Client may focus on pleasing the nurse/ clinician; denies client the opportunity to change his or her mind or decision.	**Nurse:** I noticed that you applied for that job. What factors will lead up to you changing your mind? **Making observations** **Nurse:** What led up to that decision? **Open ended—broad opening**
Disapproving, Disagreeing	**Nurse:** You really should have shown up for the medication group. **Nurse:** I disagree with that.	Make a person defensive.	**Nurse:** What was going through your mind when you decided not to come to your medication group? **Nurse:** That's one point of view. How did you arrive at that conclusion?
Changing the Subject	**Client:** I'd like to die. **Nurse:** Did you go to AA like we discussed?		**Client:** I'd like to die. **Nurse:** This sounds serious. Have you thought of harming yourself? **Validating and exploring**

Disapproving is moralizing and implies that the right to judge the client's thoughts or feelings. Again, make an observation instead.

Nurse: You really should not have an abortion, even if you were assaulted.

A more useful comment would be

Nurse: What do you think the pro's and con's of an abortion are in these circumstances?

Advising

Although we ask for and give advice all the time in daily life, giving advice to a client is rarely helpful. Often, when we ask for advice, our real motive is to discover if we are thinking along the same lines as someone else or whether they would agree with us. When the nurse gives advice to clients who are having trouble assessing and problem solving conflicted areas of their life, the nurse is interfering with their ability to make personal decisions. When we offer clients solutions, they eventually begin to think that the nurse does not view them as capable of making effective decisions. People often feel inadequate when they are given no choices over decisions in their life. Giving advice to clients can foster dependency ("I'll have to ask the nurse what to do about . . . "). Giving people advice can undermine their sense of competence and adequacy. It also keeps the nurse in control and feeling like the strong one, although this might be unconscious on the nurse's part. However, people do need information to make informed decisions. Often, the nurse can help the client define a problem and identify what information might be needed to come to an informed decision. A more useful approach would be "What do you see as some possible actions you can take?" It is much more constructive to encourage problem solving by the client. At times, the nurse can suggest several alternatives that a client might consider (e.g., "Have you ever thought of telling your friend about the incident?") Clients are then free to say yes or no and make their own decision from among the suggestions.

"Why" Questions

"Why did you come late?" "Why did you change your hair?" "Why didn't you study for the exam?"

Very often a "why" question implies criticism. We may ask our friends or family such questions and, in the context of a solid relationship, the "why" may be more understood as "what happened?" With people we do not know—especially an anxious person who may be feeling overwhelmed—a "why" question from a person in authority (nurse, physician, teacher) can be experienced as intrusive and judgmental, which serves only to make the person defensive. Most of the time we do not know why we do things, although when confronted by a "Why did you . . . ?" we may make up all sorts of responses on the spur of the moment.

It is much more useful to ask *what* is happening rather than *why* it is happening. Questions that focus on who, what, where, and when often elicit important information that can facilitate problem solving and further the communication process.

EVALUATION OF CLINICAL SKILLS

After you have had some introductory clinical experience, you may find the facilitative skills checklist

in Figure 11–2 useful for evaluating your progress in interviewing skills. Note that some of the items might not be relevant with some of your clients (e.g., numbers 11 to 13 may not be possible with a person who is highly psychotic). Self-evaluation of clinical skills is a way to focus on therapeutic improvement. The use of role play can be an effective tool for preparation for the clinical experience as well as a practice toward maturity in acquiring effective and professional communication skills.

SUMMARY

The clinical interview is a key component of psychiatric mental health nursing. Presented are the considerations needed for establishing a safe setting and planning for the following:

■ Seating
■ Introduction
■ How to start

Tactics to avoid and helpful guidelines are also presented.

Whether you are working in a psychiatric unit

FACILITATIVE SKILLS CHECKLIST

Instructions: Periodically during your clinical experience, use this checklist to identify areas needed for growth and progress made. Think of your clinical patient experiences. Indicate the extent of your agreement with each of the following statements by marking the scale: SA, strongly agree; A, agree; NS, not sure; D, disagree; SD, strongly disagree.

1. I maintain good eye contact.	SA	A	NS	D	SD
2. Most of my verbal comments follow the lead of the other person.	SA	A	NS	D	SD
3. I encourage others to talk about feelings.	SA	A	NS	D	SD
4. I am able to ask open-ended questions.	SA	A	NS	D	SD
5. I can restate and clarify a person's ideas.	SA	A	NS	D	SD
6. I can summarize in a few words the basic ideas of a long statement made by a person.	SA	A	NS	D	SD
7. I can make statements that reflect the person's feelings.	SA	A	NS	D	SD
8. I can share my feelings relevant to the discussion when appropriate to do so.	SA	A	NS	D	SD
9. I am able to give feedback.	SA	A	NS	D	SD
10. At least 75% or more of my responses help enhance and facilitate communication.	SA	A	NS	D	SD
11. I can assist the person to list some alternatives available.	SA	A	NS	D	SD
12. I can assist the person to identify some goals that are specific and observable.	SA	A	NS	D	SD
13. I can assist the person to specify at least one next step that might be taken toward the goal.	SA	A	NS	D	SD

Figure 11–2 Facilitative skills checklist. (Adapted from Myrick D., and Erney, T. [1984]. *Caring and sharing* [p. 154]. Copyright © 1984 by Educational Media Corporation, Minneapolis, Minnesota.)

or a clinic or in the client's home, you will be confronted with an array of behaviors during your student experience. It is useful to be somewhat prepared for specific client behaviors (e.g., clients cry, ask you to keep a secret, or say they want to kill themselves). Potentially problematic client behaviors during the interview are addressed with guidelines for nursing interventions.

Communication is the foundation for any nurse-client relationship. When effective communication skills are a genuine part of the helping process and are applied with concern and respect for the other person, they can be a dynamic tool in working effectively with people. Berlo's model has five parts: stimulus, sender, message, medium, and receiver. Feedback is a vital component in the communication process for validating the accuracy of the sender's message.

A number of factors can minimize or enhance the communication process. For example, differences in culture, language, and knowledge levels; noise; lack of privacy; the presence of others; and the expectations of others all can influence communication.

There are verbal and nonverbal elements in communication; the nonverbal often plays the larger role in identifying a person's message. Verbal communication consists of all words a person speaks. Nonverbal communication consists of the behaviors displayed by an individual in contrast with the actual content of speech.

Communication also has two levels: One is the content level (verbal) and the other the process level (nonverbal behavior). When content is congruent with process, the communication is said to be healthy. When the verbal message is not reinforced by the communicator's actions, the message is ambiguous; we call this a double (or mixed) message.

Cultural backgrounds (as well as individual differences) have a great deal to do with what nonverbal behavior means to different individuals. The degree of eye contact and the use of touch are two nonverbal behaviors that can be misunderstood across cultures.

There are a number of **effective counseling and communication techniques** that nurses can use to enhance their nursing practice. Most nurses are most effective when they use nonthreatening and open-ended communication techniques with clients during everyday encounters.

Effective communication is a skill that develops over time and is a crucial tool for all nurses in all settings all the time. There are also a number of **obstructive messages** that nurses can learn to avoid to enhance their effectiveness with people.

Visit the **Evolve** website at
http://evolve.elsevier.com/Varcarolis
for a post-test on the content in this chapter.

Visit the **Evolve** website at
http://evolve.elsevier.com/Varcarolis
for additional self-study exercises.

Critical Thinking and Chapter Review

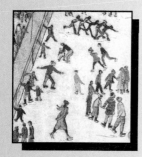

Critical Thinking

1. You are attempting to conduct a clinical interview with a very withdrawn client. You have tried silence and open-ended statements to engage the client, but all you get is one-word answers. What other actions could you take at this time?

2. You have been spending time with a client for 5 weeks, twice a week, at a community mental health center. Your client has been upset over the diagnosis that her son has AIDS, and you and she have been spending a lot of time discussing many of the painful issues she is presently dealing with. She is

going away for 3 weeks to visit her son in Seattle, and she brings you a leather-covered notebook "to keep your client notes in." How would you handle this situation? If she had brought you the "present" during the first week, how would you have handled it?

3. Keep a log for 30 minutes a day of your communication pattern (a tape recorder is ideal). Pick out four effective techniques that you notice you use frequently. Identify two techniques that are "obstructive." In your log, rewrite those obstructive techniques and replace them with statements that would better facilitate discussion of thoughts and feelings. Share your log and discuss the changes you are working on with one other classmate.

Chapter Review

Choose the most appropriate answer.

1. Paraphrasing, restating, reflecting, and exploring are techniques used for the purpose of

    1. Clarifying.
    2. Summarizing.
    3. Encouraging comparison.
    4. Placing events in time and sequence.

2. Which communication technique would yield positive results within the context of a therapeutic relationship?

    1. Advising.
    2. Giving approval.
    3. Active listening.
    4. Asking "why" questions.

3. When the client makes the statement, "I get all balled up when I try to talk to him," and the nurse responds, "Give me an example of getting all balled up," the nurse is using the technique called

    1. Exploring.
    2. Reflecting.
    3. Interpreting.
    4. Paraphrasing.

4. When beginning a relationship with a client, which advice will be helpful in establishing rapport?

    1. Fill any silences the client leaves.
    2. When in doubt, focus on feelings.
    3. Rely on direct questions to explore sensitive areas.
    4. Pay more attention to verbal than nonverbal communication.

5. Which statement by the nurse to a client would be considered nontherapeutic?

    1. "I know exactly how you feel."
    2. "I'm not sure I understand what you mean."
    3. "Tell me more about what happened when you resigned."
    4. "I see that you are wringing your hands as we talk about the job interview."

REFERENCES

Berlo, D. K. (1960). *The process of communication.* San Francisco: Reinhart Press.

Collins, M. (1983). *Communication in health care: The human connection in the life cycle* (2nd ed.). St. Louis: Mosby.

Dee, V. (1991). How can we become more aware of culturally specific body language and use this awareness therapeutically? *Journal of Psychosocial Nursing,* 29(11):39–40.

Egan, G. (1994). *The skilled helper: A problem-management approach* (5th ed.). Pacific Grove, California: Brooks/Cole.

Farkas-Cameron, M. M. (1995). Clinical supervision in psychiatric nursing. *Journal of Psychosocial Nursing and Mental Health Services,* 33(2):40–47.

Geissler, E. M. (1993). *Pocket guide to cultural assessment.* St. Louis: Mosby.

Grier, W. H., and Cobbs, P. M. (1968). *Black rage.* New York: Basic Books.

Haber, J. (2000). Hildgard E. Peplau: The psychiatric nursing legacy of a legend. *Journal of the American Psychiatric Nursing Association,* 6(2):56–62.

Hall, E. T. (1977). *Beyond culture.* Garden City, New Jersey: Anchor Press.

Ingram, C. A. (1991). How can we become more aware of culturally specific body language and use this awareness therapeutically? *Journal of Psychosocial Nursing,* 29(11):40–41.

Lu, F. G., et al. (1995). Issues in the assessment and diagnosis of culturally diverse individuals. In J. M. Oldhan and M. B. Riba (Eds.), *Review of Psychiatry* (Vol. 14) (pp. 477–510). Washington, D.C.: American Psychiatric Press.

MacKinnon, R. A., and Michels, R. (1971). *The psychiatric interview in clinical practice.* Philadelphia: W. B. Saunders.

Meier, S. T., and Davis, S. R. (1989). *The elements of counseling* (2nd ed.). Pacific Grove, California: Brooks/Cole.

Moscato, B. (1988). The one-to-one relationship. In H. S. Wilson and C. S. Kneisel (Eds.), *Psychiatric nursing* (3rd ed.). Menlo Park, California: Addison-Wesley.

Myrick, R. D., and Erney, T. (1984). *Caring and sharing.* Minneapolis, Minnesota: Educational Media Corporation.

Nicholi, A. M. (1988). The therapist-patient relationship. In A. M. Nicholi (Ed.), *The new Harvard guide to psychiatry.* Cambridge, Massachusetts: Belknap Press of Harvard University.

Parsons, R. D., and Wicks, R. J. (1994). *Counseling strategies and intervention techniques for human services* (4th ed.). Needham Heights, Massachusetts: Allyn & Bacon.

Peplau, H. E. (1952). *Interpersonal relations in nursing.* New York: G. P. Putnam.

Peplau, H. E. (1962). Interpersonal techniques: The crux of psychiatric nursing. *American Journal of Nursing,* 62:50.

Poole, V. C., et al. (1995). Cultural aspects of psychiatric nursing. In N. L. Kneltner, et al. (Eds.), *Psychiatric nursing* (2nd ed.) (pp. 185, 190).

Raingruber, B. J. (2001). Settling into moving in a climate of care: Styles and patterns of interaction between nurse psychotherapists and clients. *Perspectives in Psychiatric Care,* 37(1): 15–27.

Ramirez, D. (1989). Mexican American children and adolescents. In J. Gibbs, et al. (Eds.), *Children of color: Psychological interventions with minority youth.* San Francisco: Jossey-Bass.

Schulman, E. D. (1974). *Intervention in human services.* St. Louis: Mosby.

Shea, S. C. (1998). *Psychiatric interviewing: The art of understanding* (2nd ed). Philadelphia: W. B. Saunders.

Siantz, M. L. (1991). How can we become more aware of culturally specific body language and use this awareness therapeutically? *Journal of Psychosocial Nursing,* 29(11):38–39.

Outline

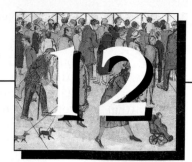

12

Understanding Stress and Holistic Approaches to Stress

ELIZABETH M. VARCAROLIS

Key Terms and Concepts

The key terms and concepts listed here also appear in color where they are defined or first discussed in this chapter.

assertiveness training

Benson's relaxation techniques

biofeedback

cognitive reframing

coping styles

distress

eustress

guided imagery

humor

journal keeping

meditation

physical stressors

progressive muscle relaxation (PMR)

psychological stressors

restructuring and setting priorities

stress

Objectives

After studying this chapter, the reader will be able to

1. Recognize the short- and long-term physiological consequences of stress.

2. Identify the relationship between stress and anxiety.

3. Analyze the ways in which culture can affect a person's perception and reaction to stress and give examples.

4. Assess life change units in a client's life using the Life-Changing Event Questionnaire.

5. Differentiate among four categories of coping and give at least two examples of each.

6. Teach a classmate or client two simple behavioral techniques to help lower stress and anxiety.

7. Explain how cognitive techniques can help lower a person's level of stress.

 tress is a universal experience and a component in all our lives, yet it is defined differently by different scholars. Selye (1993) defines **stress** as "the nonspecific (that is, common) result of any demand upon the body." Other definitions of stress describe the "occasions of sympathetic nervous system arousal, as well as the noxious nature of the stress stimulus and the attempts to remove it" (Mandler 1993). Stress may be chronic (e.g., poverty), transitory (e.g., noise), or highly individual (e.g., a bad relationship with a significant other).

STRESS

Hans Selye in 1956 popularized a physiological version of stress as **general adaptation syndrome.** It is now believed that general adaptation syndrome occurs in two stages: (1) an initial adaptive response (fight or flight) or acute stress, and (2) the eventual maladaptive consequences of prolonged stress. Stress produces a wide array of psychological and physiological responses. Table 12–1 gives an overview of some of the body's responses to acute stress and prolonged (chronic) stress. The body reacts physiologically in the same manner, whether the stress is real or perceived and whether it is of a physical, psychological, or social nature.

Figure 12–1 portrays the short-term (initial adaptive response) and long-term (eventual maladaptive consequences) **physiological** effects of stress on the hypothalamus (brain)-pituitary (endocrine) and the sympatho-adreno-medullary systems. A variety of chronic physical disorders (e.g., hypertension, diabetes) and numerous physical diseases have been linked to long-term, sustained stress.

In 1974 Selye distinguished between the **psychological** reactions of **distress** and **eustress.** According to Selye, **distress** is destructive to health. Selye's distress concept included three types: harm/loss, threat, and challenge. **Eustress** is demonstrated by a person's confidence in the ability to master given demands or tasks with success. Eustress is not harmful to a person's health and may even enhance a sense of well-being (Selye 1974). "Psychological stress focuses on the negative emotions, though the positive emotions of eustress often serve as breathers, . . . sustainers and restorers that replenish damaged resources" (Lazarus et al. 1980).

Selye's psychological reactions can be further described as follows:

■ **Distress**: negative, draining energy (anxiety, depression, confusion, helplessness, hopelessness, fatigue)

TABLE 12–1   *Reactions to Acute and Prolonged (Chronic) Stress*

ACUTE STRESS CAN CAUSE	PROLONGED STRESS CAN CAUSE
Uneasiness and concern	Anxiety and panic attacks
Sadness	Depression or melancholia
Loss of appetite	Anorexia or overeating
Suppression of the immune system	Lowered resistance to infections, leading to increase in opportunistic viral and bacterial infections
Increased metabolism and use of body fats	Insulin-resistant diabetes Hypertension
Infertility	Amenorrhea or loss of sex drive Impotence, anovulation
Increased energy mobilization and use	Increased fatigue and irritability Decreased memory and learning
Increased cardiovascular tone	Increased risk for cardiac events, e.g., heart attack, angina, and sudden heart-related deaths Increased risk of blood clots and stroke
Increased cardiopulmonary tone	Increased respiratory problems

■ **Eustress**: positive, motivating energy (happiness, hopefulness, peacefulness, purposeful movement)

Stressors

A variety of dissimilar situations (e.g., emotional arousal, fatigue, fear, loss, humiliation, loss of blood, and even great and unexpected success) all are capable of producing stress and triggering the stress response (Selye 1993). There are no factors that can be singled out as the cause of stress reaction; however, stressors can be divided into two categories: physical and psychological.

Physical stressors include environmental conditions such as trauma and excessive cold or heat, as well as physical conditions such as infection, hemorrhage, hunger, and pain.

Psychological stressors include divorce, loss of a job, unmanageable debt, death of a loved one, and retirement, as well as changes we might consider to be positive, such as marriage or unexpected success.

In 1967, Holmes and Rahe published a social readjustment rating scale. This life-change scale is a

THE STRESS RESPONSE

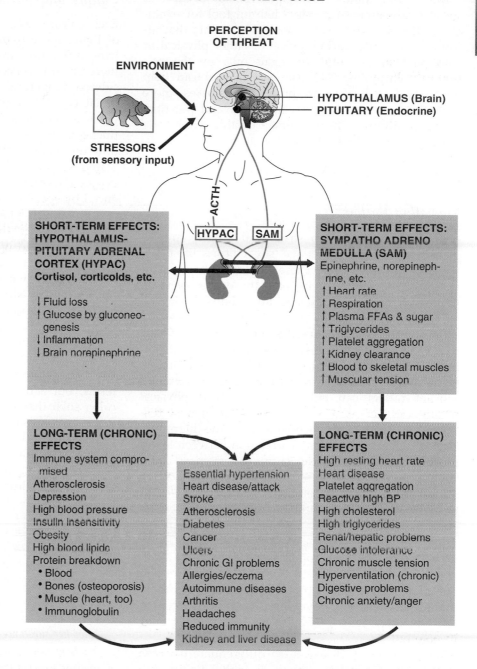

Figure 12–1 The stress response. ACTH, adrenocorticotropic hormone; BP, blood pressure; FEAs, free fatty acids; GI, gastrointestinal. (From Brigham, D. D. [1994]. *Imagery for getting well: Clinical applications of behavioral medicine.* New York: W. W. Norton.)

means of monitoring the level of stressful life events over a given period (1 year). The scale has been used extensively to evaluate people's situations and their susceptibility to physical and mental illness. Table 12–2, later in the chapter, presents the latest 1997 rescaling by Miller and Rahe.

Subsequent to Holmes and Rahe's contribution, a variety of scales have been devised to measure stressful life events that are conceptualized in different ways. These scales also show stressful life events to be related to a wide variety of physical and mental disorders (Brown and Harris 1989; Dohrenwend and Dohrenwend 1974, 1983; Lazarus and DeLongis 1983).

Researchers have looked at the degree to which various life events upset a specific individual. They found that it is more the *perception* of a recent life event that determines the person's emotional and psychological reactions to it (Rahe 1995). A man in his 40s who has a new baby, has just purchased a home, and is laid off with 6 months' severance pay may feel the stress of the event (lost job) more intensely than a man who is 62 years of age, financially secure, and asked to take an early retirement.

Miller and Rahe's 1997 updated life event and social readjustment scale is a helpful tool for evaluating clients in crisis and looking at events that affect a client's life during a time of either physical or emotional stress. Often we focus only on the presenting symptoms. The use of this tool can help nurses and all health care professionals assess more accurately a person's stress threshold and potential for future illness. Check yourself on this stress scale when you come to Table 12–2.

Stress and Coping

Mediating Factors

Behavioral responses to stress and anxiety are affected by factors such as age, sex, culture, life experiences, and life style. These all are elements that may work to lessen or increase the degree of emotional or physical influence and the sequelae to stress.

Social support, however, is one mediating factor that has been heavily researched and has significant implications for nurses and other health care professionals. The fact that strong social support from significant others can enhance mental and physical health and act as a significant buffer against distress has been well documented in the literature. Studies have found strong correlation between lower mortality rates and intact support systems (Fawzy 1995).

The proliferation of self-help groups attests to the need people have for social supports, and the explosive growth of a great variety of support groups reflects the effectiveness of such groups for many people. Many of the support groups currently available are for people going through similar stressful life events, such as the prototype Alcoholics Anonymous, Gamblers Anonymous, Reach for Recovery (for cancer patients), and Parents Without Partners, to note but a few.

It is important, however, to differentiate between social support relationships of high quality and those of low quality. Low-quality support relationships may, and often do, negatively affect a person's coping effectiveness in a crisis. High-quality relationships have been linked with less loneliness, more supportive behavior, and greater life satisfaction (Hobfall and Vaux 1993). High-quality emotional support is a critical factor in enhancing a person's sense of control and rebuilding feelings of self-esteem and competency. Supportive relationships of high quality have the following characteristics (Hobfall and Vaux 1993): (1) they are relatively free from conflict and negative interactions, and (2) they are close, confiding, and reciprocal.

Culture and Stress

Each culture not only emphasizes certain problems of living more than others but also interprets problems differently from other cultures. For example, there are differences across cultures in what is considered dangerous, how to manage violations of the social code, and what reactions are permissible in given experiences. These sociocultural variations influence how a stressful event is appraised as well as how the emotion produced by such an event is regulated (Lazarus 1993). So how, and to what extent, people interpret an event as stressful is greatly influenced by specific cultural variables.

Culture also plays a role in how people experience stressors in their life and how that experience dictates the kind of interventions that will be useful. For example, the idea that stress leads to an emotional state that may result in somatic discomfort is not necessarily shared by the rest of the world. The Western European and North American cultures subscribe to a psychophysiological view of stress and somatic distress. However, the overwhelming majority of Asians, Africans, and Central Americans "not only express subjective distress in somatic terms, but actually experience this distress somatically, such that psychological interpretations of suffering may not be much use cross-culturally" (Gonzalez et al. 1995). The authors also said that psychotherapeutic principles can and do apply cross-culturally, but an astute therapist must be mindful of cultural differences. The following vignette illustrates this point.

Vignette

■ A 62-year-old Puerto Rican woman was referred for evaluation of incapacitating abdominal pain for the previous 9 months, since a medical diagnostic evaluation of this pain was negative. The pain had begun approximately 1 month after her substance-abusing son had been jailed for killing his lover, whom the patient loved "like a daughter." The patient expected that the psychiatrist would prescribe medication that would take her pain away, and she was initially distressed to learn that she was expected to talk about her life. While not ruling out the use of medication, the therapist explained to her that her pain might be related to the wrenching emotional ordeal of the past year. The therapist made it a point to validate her pain and took great care not to imply that the pain was "merely" the expression of unacknowledged emotion. In particular, he told her that he understood her pain to be very real and that he did not expect her pain to be gone overnight. This approach allowed the patient to engage in a course of brief psychotherapy during which her conflicted feelings about her substance-

abusing offspring were examined, though these feelings were never specifically identified as the cause of her pain. Eventually the patient felt strong enough to make drastic changes in her role as enabler of her children, at which point she reported that her pain was much improved (Gonzalez et al., 1995, p. 60.)

Fulford (1999) makes the point that it is time for the health care workers to go from culturally sensitive to culturally confident.

Spirituality and Stress

There are many religious and spiritual beliefs that are helpful for many people in coping with stress. These deserve closer scientific investigation (Loenthal 1999). Studies have demonstrated that spiritual practices can enhance the immune system and sense of well-being (O'Neill and Kenny 1998). Some scholars propose that spiritual well-being helps people deal with health issues primarily because spiritual beliefs help people deal with issues of living (Warda 1999). People who include spiritual solutions to physical or mental distress often gain a sense of comfort and support that could aid in healing and lowering stress.

ASSESSING STRESS AND COPING STYLES

Measuring Stress

Physicians and others throughout the centuries have associated adverse life events with illness. The evidence for stress actually causing illness has not been proven. However, there is strong evidence that stress triggers illness in individuals when underlying illness is latent or subclinical. For instance, even discussing emotional conflicts can elicit life-threatening arrhythmias in vulnerable individuals (Dimsdale et al. 1999).

Holmes and Rahe (1967) developed a checklist of life change units called the "Recent Life Change Questionnaire." This questionnaire has subsequently been rescaled twice, first in 1978 and then again in 1994. An interesting recent finding (Miller and Rahe 1997) is that life stress over the last 35 years appears to have increased markedly. These findings have significance for modern-day stress and illness research (Miller and Rahe 1997).

Another finding from Miller and Rahe's studies (1997) is that there is a gender difference. Women,

LIFE CHANGE EVENT	LIFE CHANGE UNIT†
Health	
An injury or illness that	
Kept you in bed a week or more, or sent you to the hospital	74
Was less serious than above	44
Major dental work	26
Major change in eating habits	27
Major change in sleeping habits	26
Major change in your usual type and/or amount of recreation	28
Work	
Change to a new type of work	51
Change in your work hours or conditions	35
Change in your responsibilities at work	
More responsibilities	29
Fewer responsibilities	21
Promotion	31
Demotion	42
Transfer	32
Troubles at work	
With your boss	29
With coworkers	35
With persons under your supervision	35
Other work troubles	28
Major business adjustment	60
Retirement	52
Loss of job	
Laid off from work	68
Fired from work	79
Correspondence course to help you in your work	18
Home and Family	
Major change in living conditions	42
Change in residence	
Move within the same town or city	25
Move to a different town, city or state	47
Change in family get-togethers	25
Major change in health or behavior of family member	55
Marriage	50
Pregnancy	67
Miscarriage or abortion	65
Gain of a new family member	
Birth of a child	66
Adoption of a child	65
A relative moving in with you	59
Spouse beginning or ending work	46
Child leaving home	
To attend college	41
Due to marriage	41

TABLE 12–2 *Life-Changing Event Questionnaire**

Table continued on following page

TABLE 12–2 *Life-Changing Event Questionnaire* (Continued)*

LIFE CHANGE EVENT	LIFE CHANGE UNIT†
Home and Family	
For other reasons	45
Change in arguments with spouse	50
In-law problems	38
Change in the marital status of your parents	
Divorce	59
Remarriage	50
Separation from spouse	
Due to work	53
Due to marital problems	76
Divorce	96
Birth of grandchild	43
Death of spouse	119
Death of other family member	
Child	123
Brother or sister	102
Parent	100
Personal and Social	
Change in personal habits	26
Beginning or ending school or college	38
Change of school or college	35
Change in political beliefs	24
Change in religious beliefs	29
Change in social activities	27
Vacation	24
New, close, personal relationship	37
Engagement to marry	45
Girlfriend or boyfriend problems	39
Sexual differences	44
"Falling out" of a close personal relationship	47
An accident	48
Minor violation of the law	20
Being held in jail	75
Death of a close friend	70
Major decision regarding your immediate future	51
Major personal achievement	36
Financial	
Major change in finances	
Increased Income	38
Decreased income	60
Investment and/or credit difficulties	56
Loss or damage of personal property	43
Moderate purchase	20
Major purchase	37
Foreclosure on a mortgage or loan	58

*Six-month totals ≥300 LCUs, or 1-year totals ≥500 LCU, are considered indications of high recent life stress.
†LCU = Life change unit
From Miller, M. A., and Rahe, R. H. (1997). Life changes scaling for the 1990s. *Journal of Psychosomatic Research*, 43(3):279–292.

for example, score significantly higher for finances (a growing concern for women), pregnancy, miscarriage or abortion, and death of a child. In fact, women assess and react to life stress events at a higher level than men (Miller and Rahe 1997). These findings lend support for the more recent interest in assessing and treating women based on findings regarding women's health needs and concerns.

Men, on the other hand, seemed to underrate life change units by about 17%, thus underscoring the need to break down denial and carefully assess the stress in the life of some male clients (Miller and Rahe 1997). Table 12–2 presents the current rating for measuring stress in terms of life change units. Take a minute out to assess your stress level for the past 6 to 12 months.

Assessing Coping Styles

Just realize that the only way to survive our stressful existence is to recognize that we have choices and options in the way we live and respond to stress.
Edward Creagon, MD, Mayo Clinic

People use a variety of ways to cope with life stressors, and a number of factors can act as mediators for stress in our lives, such as life satisfaction (work, family, hobbies, humor) and social supports. Rahe (1995) identified four categories of coping styles that people use as stress buffers:

1. Health-sustaining habits (e.g., medical compliance, proper diet, relaxation, pacing one's energy)
2. Life satisfactions (e.g., work, family, humor, spiritual solace, arts, nature)
3. Social supports
4. Response to stress

Evaluating these four coping categories can help nurses identify areas to target for improving their client's and their own quality of life. Table 12–3 looks at some positive and some negative responses to stress.

Most people, when faced with stressful life events of a mild to moderate nature, use a variety of psychological defenses briefly and go on to other successful coping strategies as outlined earlier. However, when defense mechanisms do not lower our anxiety and stress levels, a number of psychophysiological responses may come into play. These psychophysiological defenses are divided into responses that are (1) in our own awareness, such as headache or muscle tension, and (2) out of our awareness, such as increased blood pressure or an increase in

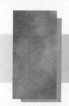

POSITIVE STRESS RESPONSES	NEGATIVE STRESS RESPONSES
1. **Problem solving**—figuring out how to deal with the situation	1. **Avoidance**—choosing not to deal with the situation, letting negative feelings and situations fester and continue to become chronic
2. **Using social support**—calling in others who are caring and may be helpful	2. **Self-blame**—blaming self keeps the focus on minimizing one's self-esteem and prevents positive action toward resolution or working through the feelings related to the event.
3. **Reframing**—redefining the situation to see positive as well as the negative sides and how to use the situation for one's advantage	3. **Wishful thinking**—a form of denial that involves thinking things will resolve by themselves and that "everything will be fine."

TABLE 12–3 *Positive and Negative Responses to Stress*

Adapted from Lazarus, R. S., and Folkman, S. (1984). *Stress, appraisal, and coping.* New York: Springer.

lipid levels. Other responses may be psychophysiological in nature, such as depression (Rahe 1995). Refer to Figure 12–2 for an operational definition of stress.

A person is at an elevated risk for near-future illness, however, if he or she is experiencing overwhelming or multiple stressors or using inadequate coping skills, or if there are other exacerbating circumstances (Rahe 1995).

HOLISTIC APPROACHES TO STRESS

Most nurses have learned a great variety of stress and anxiety reduction techniques and teach their clients alternative ways of handling anxiety and stress. Some of the benefits of stress reduction have been compiled by Varcarolis (1996):

■ Alter the course of certain medical conditions such as high blood pressure, arrhythmias, arthritis, cancer, and peptic ulcers
■ Decrease the need for medications such as insulin, analgesics, and antihypertensives
■ Diminish or eliminate the need for unhealthy and destructive behaviors such as smoking, addictions to drugs, insomnia, and overeating

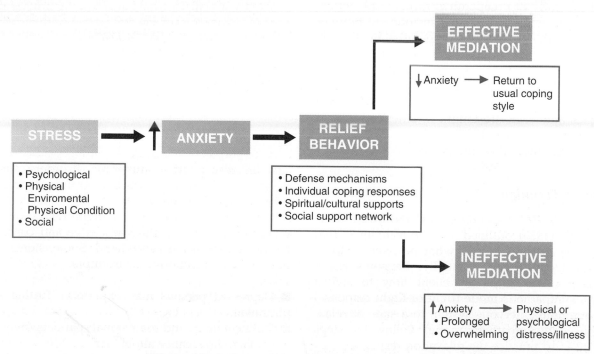

Figure 12–2 Stress and anxiety operationally defined.

■ Increase cognitive functions such as learning, concentration, and study habits
■ Break up static patterns of thinking and allow fresh and creative ways of perceiving life events
■ Increase the sense of well-being through endorphin release

Behavioral Approaches

Cognitive behavioral methods are the most effective ways to reduce stress. There is no one cognitive-behavioral technique that is right for everyone, and employing a mixture of cognitive-behavioral techniques together brings the best results. All are useful in a variety of situations for specific individuals. Given the fixed nature of many stressors (loss of loved one, chronic illness, pressure at work) cognitive-behavioral therapy, which teaches new ways of responding to stress, may be the most effective method of permanently relieving stress in an everyday life (CBS Health Watch 2000). Essentially there are stress-reducing techniques for every personality type, situation, and level of stress.

Behavioral methods include a number of relaxation techniques (meditation, guided imagery, and breathing exercises). Techniques that require special training include progressive muscle relaxation (PMR), eye movement desensitization and biofeedback.

Nurses use relaxation techniques in all areas of nursing practice, as well as in dealing with their own home or workplace stressful environments. For example, a study of preoperative cardiac catheterization patients showed that relaxation techniques could reduce the amount of preoperative medication (diazepam) [Valium] needed (Warner et al. 1992). Relaxation techniques are used successfully by nurses in critical care areas to help patients cope with their symptoms and treatment (Heath 1992). Relaxation techniques and PMR are taught to elderly clients to help treat areas of anxiety, altered comfort, or sleep pattern disturbances (Weinberger 1991).

Relaxation Techniques

BENSON'S RELAXATION TECHNIQUES. Herbert Benson (1985) outlined specific techniques that enable most people to elicit what he referred to as the *relaxation response*. Essentially, Benson's relaxation techniques teach the client how to switch from the sympathetic mode (fight-or-flight response) of the autonomic nervous system to a state of relaxation (the parasympathetic mode). Follow the steps in Box 12–1 to practice the relaxation response.

Benson's relaxation techniques have been used successfully in conjunction with meditation and vi-

BOX 12–1   *Benson's Relaxation Technique*

The nurse instructs the client as follows:

1. Choose any word or brief phrase that reflects your belief system, such as "love," "unity in faith and love," "joy," "shalom," "one God," "peace."
2. Sit in a comfortable position.
3. Close your eyes.
4. Deeply relax all your muscles, beginning at your feet and progressing up to your face. Keep them relaxed.
5. Breathe through your nose. Become aware of your breathing. As you breathe out, say your word or phrase silently to yourself. For example, breathe IN . . . OUT, "phrase," IN . . . OUT, "phrase," and so forth. Breathe easily and naturally.
6. Continue for 10 or 20 minutes. You may open your eyes and check the time, but do not use an alarm. When you finish, sit quietly for several minutes, at first with your eyes closed and then with your eyes open. Do not stand up for a few minutes.
7. Do not worry about whether you are successful in achieving a deep level of relaxation. Maintain a passive attitude and permit relaxation to occur at its own pace. When distracting thoughts occur, try to ignore them by not dwelling on them, and return to repeating your word or phrase. With practice, the response should come with little effort. Practice the technique once or twice daily, but not within 2 hours after any meal, since the digestive process seems to interfere with the elicitation of the relaxation response.

From Benson, H. (1985). *The relaxation response* (2nd ed.). New York: William Morrow.

sual imagery to treat numerous disorders, such as diabetes, high blood pressure, migraines, cancer, and peptic ulcers, to name a few.

Any client who is to be taught relaxation techniques should obtain the knowledge and consent of his or her physician beforehand. Some clients could have adverse reactions. For example,

■ Depressed persons may experience further withdrawal.
■ Hallucinating and delusional patients may lose contact with reality altogether.
■ The toxic effects of some medications may be enhanced.

■ Some patients in pain may have a heightened experience of pain corresponding to the increase in body awareness.

MEDITATION. Meditation follows the basic guidelines described for the relaxation response. It is a discipline for training the mind to develop greater calm and then using that calm to bring penetrative insight into one's experience. Meditation can be used to help people reach their deep inner resources for healing, calm the mind, and operate more efficiently in the world. It can help people develop strategies to cope with stress, make sensible adaptive choices under pressure, and feel more engaged in life (Kabat-Zinn 1993). Meditation elicits a relaxation response by creating a hypometabolic state of quieting the sympathetic nervous system. Some people meditate using a visual object or a sound to help them focus. Others may find it useful to concentrate on their breathing while meditating. There are many meditation techniques, some with a spiritual base, such as Siddha meditation or prayer. Meditation is easy to practice anywhere.

GUIDED IMAGERY. Used in conjunction with the relaxation response, guided imagery is a process whereby a person is led to envision images that are both calming and health enhancing. The content of the imagery exercises is shaped by the person helping with the imagery process. If a person has dysfunctional images, he or she can be helped to generate more effective and functional coping images to replace the depressogenic or anxiety-producing ones. For example, athletes have discovered that the use of positive coping and successful images can lead to an increase in performance (Freeman and Reinecke 1993).

Imagery tapes are commonly found in many kinds of stores (e.g., music, book); however, people can make their own tapes, using soothing music in the background. A common imagery technique used for deep relaxation is to lead the individual into a positive sensory experience. For example, a person will pick a favorite spot, one that is beautiful and quiet and that gives the person joy (e.g., a beach). It can be a real or imaginary place. The person is then asked to *see* in his or her mind the soft blue of the sky, *feel* the warm sand under the back, *smell* the fresh salty ocean breeze, and *feel* it brush the face and hair while *hearing* the soothing sounds of the waves in the background. Refer to Box 12–2.

Imagery techniques are an effective tool used for many medical conditions. They are an effective means of relieving pain for many people. Pain is reduced by producing muscle relaxation, focusing the person away from the pain; for some, imagery techniques are healing exercises in that they not only relieve the pain but in some cases diminish the

Box 12–2 *Script for Guided Imagery*

Imagine releasing all the tension in your body . . . letting it go.

Now, with every breath you take, feel your body drifting down deeper and deeper into relaxation . . . floating down . . . deeper and deeper.

Imagine your peaceful scene. You're sitting beside a clear, blue mountain stream. You are barefoot, and you feel the sun-warmed rock under your feet. You hear the sound of the stream tumbling over the rocks. The sound is hypnotic, and you relax more and more. You see the tall pine trees on the opposite shore bending in the gentle breeze. Breathe the clean, scented air, each breath moving you deeper and deeper into relaxation. The sun warms your face.

You are very comfortable. There is nothing to disturb you. You experience a feeling of well-being.

You can return to this peaceful scene by taking time to relax. The positive feelings can grow stronger and stronger each time you choose to relax.

You can return to your activities now, feeling relaxed and refreshed.

source of the pain (Matassarin Jacobs 1993). Guided imagery is used with cancer patients to help them reduce their chronic high levels of cortisol, epinephrine, and catecholamines (which prevent the immune system from functioning effectively) and produce beta-endorphins (which increase pain thresholds and enhance lymphocyte proliferation) (Brigham 1994). Guided imagery is used for all sorts of healing. Often tapes are made specifically for clients and their specific situation. However, there are many healing tapes available to clients and to health care workers.

BREATHING EXERCISES. Within the past several years, there has been increasing evidence that respiratory retraining, usually in the form of learning abdominal (diaphragmatic) breathing, has some definite merits in the modification of stress and anxiety reactions (Stoyva and Carlson 1993). One breathing exercise that has proved helpful for many clients with anxiety disorders is in two parts, as described in Box 12–3).

The second part helps clients interrupt trains of thought, thereby quieting mental noise. With increasing skill, this becomes a tool for dampening the cognitive processes likely to set off stress and anxiety reactions. In clinical work with people who have

---

Box 12–3 *Deep Breathing Exercise*

First, shift to relaxed, abdominal breathing. Breathe in by the mouth, hold for 3 seconds, and breathe out slowly through the nose.

Second, with every breath, turn attention to the muscular sensations that accompany the expansion of the belly.

---

performance anxiety, 50% reported breathing exercises to be useful during the feared situation (Stoyva and Carlson 1993).

Behavioral Techniques that Require Special Training

PROGRESSIVE MUSCLE RELAXATION. Progressive muscle relaxation (PMR) is a technique that can help patients achieve deep relaxation. The premise behind PMR is that deep relaxation can occur when muscle contraction is almost completely eliminated. Jacobson (1974), who first developed PMR, devised a program of instruction wherein systematic tensing and releasing of various muscles, and learning to discriminate between sensations of tension and relaxation, occur. The technique can be learned and practiced in hospitals as well as in the community for patients with a variety of conditions.

Many training sessions are usually needed for mastery of PMR. For best results the student should receive live instruction and proceed only with the approval of a physician.

BIOFEEDBACK. Biofeedback is usually thought to be most effective in people with low to moderate hypnotic ability. For people with hypnotic ability, meditation, PMR, and other cognitive-behavioral therapy techniques produce the most rapid reduction in clinical symptoms (Wickramasekera 1999). By using sensitive instrumentation, biofeedback gives a person prompt and exact information, otherwise unavailable, on muscle activity, brain waves, skin temperature, heart rate, blood pressure, and other bodily functions. This particular internal physiological process is detected and amplified by a sensitive recording device. It is assumed that a person can achieve greater voluntary control over phenomena once considered to be exclusively involuntary, if he or she knows instantaneously, through an auditory or visual signal, whether a somatic activity is increasing or decreasing.

With the increasing recognition of the role of stress in a variety of medical illnesses, including diseases affected by immune dysfunction, biofeedback has emerged as one of the strategies used in stress management. Although it is uncertain whether it is necessary to use complex instrumentation required for proper biofeedback of minute levels of muscle tension or certain patterns of electroencephalographic activity, it has been confirmed that teaching people to relax deeply and to apply these skills to real-life stressors can be helpful in lowering stress levels.

Cognitive Approaches

A number of cognitive techniques are discussed here that many nurses employ in their practices: journal keeping, priority restructuring, cognitive reframing, and assertiveness training.

Journal Keeping

Journal keeping is an extremely useful and surprisingly simple initial method of identifying what makes a person stressed. Keeping an informal diary of daily events and activities can reveal surprising information on sources of daily stress. It need not be a chore, or a painstaking exercise, but noting which activities put a strain on energy and time, those that trigger anger or anxiety, or those that precipitate a negative physical experiences (headache, backache, fatigue), can be an important first step in actual stress reduction. A few words accompanying a time or date can be sufficient reminders of significant events or activities (CBS Health Watch 2000).

After a week or two, the stressed individual identifies two or three events or activities that have been significantly upsetting or overwhelming.

After identifying these events or activities, priorities and goals are then carefully examined. Are the stressful activities meeting ones own goals or someone else's? Are the stressful tasks ones that can be reasonably accomplished? Which tasks are within one's control and which are not?

Dellasega's excellent article (2001) identifies a variety of studies in which daily writing about traumatic events can significantly reduce health problems (see Research Findings Box).

Priority Restructuring

The next step is restructuring and setting priorities, shifting the balance from stress-producing to stress-reducing activities. A recent study indicated that daily pleasant events had a positive effect on the immune system. In fact, adding pleasurable events has more benefit than simply reducing stressful or negative ones (CBS Health Watch 2000).

Essentially, learn to replace time-consuming chores that are not really necessary with activities that are pleasurable or interesting. Making time for recreation is as essential for healthy living as paying bills or shopping for groceries (CBS Health Watch 2000).

Cognitive Reframing

Cognitive reframing has been found to be positively correlated with greater positive affect and higher self-esteem (Fawzy 1995). Cognitive restructuring includes the restructuring of irrational beliefs, replacing the worried self-statement ("I can't pass this course, I can't pass this course") with more positive self-statements ("If I choose to study, I will increase my chances of success"). Cognitive restructuring and cognitive reframing are techniques commonly used in cognitive therapies.

Reframing is a healthy stress-reduction tool and a technique used by some counselors for a variety of purposes. When used to reduce stress, imagery may be used along with cognitive reframing. The goal of reframing is to change a participant's perceptions of stress through cognitive restructuring. Essentially, reframing is reassessing a situation. Most situations we can learn by asking ourselves

- "What positive came out of the situation or experience?"
- "What did I learn in this situation?"
- "What would I do in a different way?"

The desired result is to restructure a disturbing event or experience to one that is less disturbing and in which the client can have a sense of control. When the perception of the disturbing event is changed, there is less stimulation to the sympathetic nervous system, which in turn reduces the secretion of cortisol and catecholamines that destroy the balance of the immune system (Brigham 1994).

Cognitive distortions often include overgeneralizations ("He always . . ." or "I'll never . . .") and should statements ("I should have done better" or

RESEARCH FINDINGS

Reducing Stress by Writing: A Health Promotion Tool

Objective

Inhibiting or holding back one's thoughts, feelings, or behaviors is associated with long-term stress and disease. Actively confronting upsetting experiences can reduce the negative effects of inhibition. This study describes a unique approach to help people deal with psychologic and emotional issues that they must often face.

Method

Forty-one of the 81 university employees who were part of a wellness program were chosen for this study. Through random selection, subjects were assigned to write about either nontraumatic topics or personal traumatic experiences for 20 minutes once a week for four consecutive weeks.

Results

People who wrote about traumatic personal experiences showed significant decreases in selected blood measures compared with those who wrote about nontraumatic topics. During the four weeks that they wrote, the individuals who wrote about traumatic personal topics showed a 28.6% decrease in work absentee rates relative to the eight months before the experiment compared with a 48.5% increase in work absentee rates among individuals who wrote about nontraumatic topics. The people with low inhibition showed the greatest reductions in absentee rates following their writing about traumatic personal experiences compared with those with high emotional inhibition.

Conclusion

The strategy of writing about traumatic personal experiences offers a unique tool for health promotion.

Source: Francis, M. E., and Pennebaker, J. W. (1992). Putting stress into words: The impact of writing on physiological, absentee, and self-reported emotional well-being measures. *American Journal of Health Promotion*, 6(4):280–287.

"He shouldn't have said that"). Table 12–4 shows some examples of cognitive reframing of anxiety-producing thoughts (Ellis and Harper 1975). Often, cognitive restructuring is done along with progressive relaxation.

The use of humor is a good example of how a stressful situation can be "turned upside down" through cognitive restructuring. The intensity attached to a stressful thought or situation can be dissipated when made to appear absurd or comical. Essentially, the bee loses its sting.

Assertiveness Training

Assertiveness is a learned behavior that includes standing up for one's rights without violating the rights of others. Assertiveness training has proved to be a successful way of decreasing stress, anxiety, and conflict resulting from stressful interpersonal relationships, although some may experience the initial training and practice as somewhat stressful (Beare and Myers 1998). It has been demonstrated

TABLE 12–4 *Reframing Anxiety-Producing Thoughts*

IRRATIONAL BELIEFS	POSITIVE STATEMENTS
1. I'll never be happy until I am loved by someone I really care about.	1a. If I do not get love from one person, I can still get it from others and find happiness that way.
	1b. If someone I deeply care for rejects me, that will seem unfortunate, but I will hardly die.
	1c. If the only person I truly care for does not return my love, I could devote more time and energy to winning someone else's love and probably find someone better for me.
	1d. If no one I care for ever cares for me, I can still find enjoyment in friendships, in work, in books, and in other things.
2. He should treat me better, after all I do for him.	2. I would like him to do certain things to show that he cares. If he chooses to continue to do things that hurt me after he understands what those things are, I am free to make choices about leaving or staying in this hurtful relationship.

Adapted from Ellis, A., and Harper, R. A. (1975). *A new guide to rational living.* North Hollywood, California: Wilshire.

that stress and anxiety are considerably lowered when people openly and honestly express their needs, feelings, and desires while respecting the feelings and rights of others.

The concept of assertiveness is different from that of aggressiveness or passivity. Aggressively expressing feelings is more in line with venting frustration on workers or subordinates, boring friends with emotional minutiae, wallowing in self-pity, or driving mindlessly and recklessly endangering one's own life or the lives of others. When people are aggressive, their behavior escalates; their voice becomes loud; they interrupt others; and physiologically their heart rate, blood pressure, and levels of certain stress-related hormones are elevated. This sequence in turn can escalate stress and anxiety in others so that it becomes impossible to effectively problem solve or come together in a respectful, understanding manner toward a solution. In extreme situations, escalating anger can lead to physical violence. On the other hand, when people suppress their feelings or are passive, they may suffer high levels of anxiety, discomfort, and depression or develop physical problems. Brigham (1994) identified four situations and formulas for assertiveness communications, as outlined in Table 12–5.

More Effective Stress Reducers

Box 12–4 identifies some known stressbusters that can be incorporated into our lives with little effort. The positive effects of music, pets, and exercise are discussed in more detail and warrant deeper understanding.

Music

Music and emotion may share certain essential characteristics, allowing music to resonate with that of emotional experience. Music is common to all people and cultures. Certain impressions and emotions are often communicated more successfully through music than through the spoken word. In fact, simultaneous singing and rhythmic movement facilitate the initiation and fluency of speech (Borchgrevink 1993).

Music is used as an alternative channel of communication in aphasia and developmental disorders, as well as in psychotherapy. Gerdner and Swanson (1993), in a sample of elderly clients, found that music can be used successfully as an alternative approach to management of confusion and agitation. By altering affective, cognitive, and sensory processes, music therapists as part of multidisciplinary hospice teams use music to promote the quality of

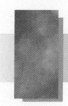

TABLE 12–5 *Formulas for Assertive Communication*

FORMULAS	EXAMPLES
Formula 1 (Simple Assertion)	
a. It is simply an open, honest, direct statement of a request, an opinion, a question, a feeling, or a need.	"No, I don't think that is the best plan of action." "Right now, I need some help with this." "Yes, I do like the way she handled that situation."
Formula 2 (Empathetic Assertion)	
a. Show understanding and recognition of the other person's feelings, *yet* b. Assertively state what one needs.	a. "I know you are concerned that I will be hurt by this decision, b. but I need to make this decision myself."
Formula 3 (Feeling Assertive)	
a. Nonaccusingly describe the situation or behavior in question. b. State one's feelings (not opinions), *and* c. Ask for a change.	a. "When I am criticized in front of others, b. I feel embarrassed and hurt, c. I'd prefer that if you need to tell me something, you do it in private."
Formula 4 (Confrontational Assertive)	
a. Ask for private time to talk. b. Point out the facts in a nonaccusing manner.	a. "I need to talk to you privately. b. It seems to me that our communication is not what it has been in the past. I notice that you watch TV while I am telling you things that are important to me.
c. Check areas in which you may not understand the situation. d. Ask for the changes you need.	c. It seems to me that we just aren't as close. Am I off-base? d. I'd like to find out what the problem is so we can get our relationship back on track."

Data from Brigham, D. D. (1994). *Imagery for getting well: Clinical applications of behavioral medicine.* New York: W. W. Norton.

life for terminally ill clients and their family members (Mandler 1993; Trauger-Querry and Haghighi 1999). The need to cope with disease, psychosocial integration, and promotion of positive resources for self-healing are all regarded as indications for music therapy (Escher et al. 1993; Kumar et al. 1999).

Pets

Peaceful contact with beloved pets can bring joy, laughter, and stress reduction, a fact known to all pet owners. Pets make us feel happy. They provide an outlet for the expression of warm and affection-

BOX 12–4 *More Effective Stressbusters*

SLEEP

1. Chronically stressed people are often fatigued, so go to sleep 30 to 60 minutes earlier each night for a few weeks.
2. If still fatigued, try going to bed another 30 minutes earlier.
3. Sleeping later in the morning is not helpful and can throw off body rhythms.

EXERCISE (AEROBIC)

1. Exercise can dissipate chronic and acute stress.
2. It is recommended at least for 30 minutes, three times a week.
3. It is best to do at least 3 hours before bedtime.

LOWER OR STOP CAFFEINE INTAKE

1. Such a simple thing can lead to more energy and fewer muscle aches and help you feel more relaxed.
2. Slowly wean off coffee, tea, colas, and chocolate drinks.

MUSIC (CLASSICAL OR SOFT MELODIES OF CHOICE)

1. Listening to music increases your sense of relaxation.
2. Increased healing effects may result.

PETS

1. Pets can bring joy and stress reduction.
2. They can be an important social support.
3. Pets can reduce medical problems aggravated by stress.

MASSAGE

1. This technique can slow down the heart and relax the body.
2. Alertness may actually increase.

ate feelings toward a safe and trusting being. The use of pets in nursing homes has long been known to bring out withdrawn individuals and aid socialization. Pets soothe us, so it is not surprising that spending time with them can help reduce high blood pressure in some individuals. A study by Friedmann and Thomas (1995) supported previous findings that pet ownership and social supports are significant predictors of survival among clients with coronary artery disease. For many, being around pets greatly improves their quality of life.

Exercise

Regular exercise is a great stressbuster for many people. High levels of epinephrine can be drained off physically instead of being internalized onto visceral targets (stomach, intestine) or affecting somatic functions (gastric secretion, vasoconstriction). Exercise helps reduce muscle tension and may also increase endorphin release. It has long been known that, for some depressed people, a brisk walk or other form of enjoyable exercise can help increase endorphin production and thus improve mood. There are a great deal of data that indicate a positive correlation between physical exercise and lowered levels of acute measures of anxiety, depression, and sensitivity to stress (Salmon 2001). In clinical work with clients who have performance anxiety, about 33% said that exercise was the single most useful maneuver during their encounter with anxiety-arousing situations (Stoyva and Carlson 1993).

Yoga and tai chi, which are slow-moving and nonvigorous forms of exercise, can aid in the attainment of deep psychological and physical relaxation. Tai chi is one of the best known of China's martial arts. When practiced seriously, tai chi and yoga affect a large part of a person's thoughts and behavior, and with increasing skill the experience becomes one of meditation in action.

SUMMARY

Stress is a universal experience. Selye popularized the now-famous general adaptation syndrome. Stress elicits an initial adaptive response (defense mechanisms or relief actions of some sort), and most of the time these suffice to lower people's stress levels so that they can continue with their lives. However, stress can lead to chronic psychological and physiological responses (eventual maladaptive consequences) when not mitigated at an earlier stage. There are basically two categories of stressors: physical (heat, hunger, cold, noise, trauma) and psychological (death of a loved one, loss of job, school, humiliation).

Age, sex, culture, life experience, and life style all are important in identifying the degree of stress a person is experiencing. However, perhaps the most important factor to assess is a person's support system. Studies have shown that social and intimate supports of high quality can go a long way to minimize the long-term effects of stress.

Cultural differences exist in the ways people perceive an event as stressful and in the appropriate behaviors to deal with a stressful event. Spiritual practices have been found to lead to enhanced immune systems and a sense of well-being. There are a variety of stress coping models; the one used in this chapter is that of Rahe.

Stress can be psychological, social, or biological. The body reacts the same if the threat is real or perceived. Physiologically, the body reacts to anxiety and fear by the arousal of the sympathetic nervous system. Specific symptoms include rapid heart beat, increased blood pressure, diaphoresis, peripheral vasoconstriction, restlessness, repetitive questioning, feelings of frustration, and difficulty concentrating.

Nurses are being trained in a great variety of holistic, noninvasive approaches to relieve people's stress. It is well accepted through replicated studies that the reduction of chronic stress is beneficial in many ways. For example, lowering the effects of chronic stress can alter the course of many physical conditions; decrease the need for some medications; diminish or eliminate the need for unhealthy and destructive behaviors such as smoking, insomnia, and drug addiction; and increase a person's cognitive functioning. Cognitive behavioral holistic approaches to stress are discussed with ways to implement these techniques for either the self or clients. Some techniques need special training.

Visit the **Evolve** website at
http://evolve.elsevier.com/Varcarolis
for a post-test on the content in this chapter.

Visit the **Evolve** website at
http://evolve.elsevier.com/Varcarolis
for additional self-study exercises.

Critical Thinking and Chapter Review

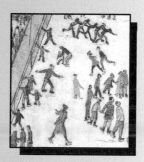

Critical Thinking

1. Assess your level of stress using the life events scale found in Table 12–2 and evaluate your potential for illness in the coming year. Identify stress reduction techniques, described toward the end of the chapter, that you think would be useful for you to learn.

2. Teach a classmate the breathing technique identified in this chapter.

3. Assess a classmate's coping styles. Have the same classmate assess yours. Discuss the relevance of both of your findings.

4. Using Figure 12–1, explain to a classmate the short-term effects of stress on the sympatho-adreno-medulla system, and if the stress is not relieved, identify three long-term effects. Have the classmate summarize what you have just told him or her.

5. Have a classmate explain to you, using Figure 12–1, the short-term effects of stress on the hypothalamus-pituitary-adrenal cortex, and if the stress becomes chronic, the eventual long-term effects. Summarize to your classmate your understanding of what was just presented.

6. Discuss in post-conference one patient you have cared for in the hospital who had one of the stress-related diseases identified in Figure 12–1. See if you can identify some stressors in that person's life and possible ways that that person could lower his or her chronic stress levels.

Chapter Review

Choose the most appropriate answer.

1. Which statement best contrasts the short-term and long-term physiological consequences of stress?

   1. Acute stress produces an initial adaptive response and prolonged stress produces maladaptive consequences.
   2. Acute stress produces maladaptive consequences and prolonged stress invokes adaptive responses.
   3. Acute stress produces immune system compromise and prolonged stress results in increased muscular tension and gluconeogenesis.
   4. Acute stress produces hypertension, anxiety, and depression and prolonged stress results in hyperlipidemia, glucose intolerance, and heart disease.

2. What statement about the influence of culture on stress can serve to guide nursing assessment, planning, and intervention?

   1. Client appraisal of a stressful event is little influenced by culture.
   2. Culture dictates the kind of interventions the client will find helpful.
   3. Culture rarely regulates the expression of emotion produced by a stressful event.
   4. Nursing interventions that promote adaptive behavior are the same across cultures

3. Which should the nurse assess as being the LEAST helpful for mediating a client's stress?

1. Psychophysiological responses within client awareness.
2. Health-sustaining habits such a proper diet.
3. Life satisfactions such as work or family.
4. Social supports from significant others.

4. A useful tool for assessing an individual's susceptibility to physical and mental illness is

1. Biofeedback.
2. Rational Living Survey.
3. Life-Changing Event Questionnaire.
4. General Adaptation Syndrome Assessment.

5. Which intervention has been shown to be most effective in reducing stress?

1. Avoidance.
2. Interpersonal confrontation.
3. Cognitive-behavioral therapy.
4. Psychopharmacological interventions.

REFERENCES

Beare, P. G., and Myers, J. L. (1998). *Adult health nursing* (3rd ed.). St. Louis: Mosby.

Benson, H. (1985). *The relaxation response* (2nd ed.). New York: William Morrow.

Borchgrevink, H. M. (1993). Music, brain and medicine. *Yidsskrift forden Norske Laegeforening,* 133(30):3733.

Brigham, D. D. (1994). *Imagery for getting well: Clinical applications of behavioral medicine.* New York: W. W. Norton.

Brown, G. W., and Harris, T. (1989). *Social virgins of depression: A study of psychiatric disorders in women.* New York: Free Press.

CBS Health Watch by Medscape 3/27/00. Http://cbshealthwatch.health.aol.com. RecId=202426 plus content type=Library.

Dellasega, C. A. (2001). Using structural writing experience to promote mental health. *Journal of Psychosocial Nursing,* 39(2):14–23.

Dimsdale, J. E., Keefe, F. J., and Stein, M. B. (1999). Stress and psychiatry. In Sadock and Sadock (Eds), *Kaplan and Sadock's Comprehensive Textbook of Psychiatry* (7th ed.) (Vol. 2.) Philadelphia: Lippincott, Williams and Wilkins.

Dohrenwend, B. S., and Dohrenwend, B. P. (1974). *Stressful life events: Their nature and effects.* New York: John Wiley.

Dohrenwend, B. S., and Dohrenwend, B. P. (1983). Life stress and illness: Formulation of the issues. In B. S. Dohrenwend and B. P. Dohrenwend (Eds.), *Stressful life events and their contexts.* New Brunswick, New Jersey: Rutgers University Press.

Ellis, A., and Harper, R. A. (1975). *A new guide to rational living.* North Hollywood, California: Wilshire.

Escher, J., et al. (1993). Music therapy and internal medicine. *Schweizerische Rundshau fur Medizin Praxis,* 82(36):957.

Fawzy, F. I. (1995). Behavior and immunity. In H. I. Kaplan and B. J. Sadock (Eds.), *Comprehensive textbook of psychiatry* (6th ed.) (Vol. 2, pp. 1559–1570). Baltimore: Williams & Wilkins.

Freeman, A., and Reinecke, M. A. (1993). *Cognitive therapy of suicidal behavior: A manual for treatment.* New York: Springer.

Friedmann, E., and Thomas, S. A. (1995). Pet ownership, social support, and one-year survival after acute myocardial infarction in the Cardiac Arrhythmia Suppression Trial. *American Journal of Cardiology,* 76(17):1213.

Fulford, K. W. M. (1999). From culturally sensitive to culturally competent. In K. Bhui and D. Olajide (Eds), *Mental Health Service for a Multi-cultural Society.* Philadelphia: W. B. Saunders.

Gerdner, L. A., and Swanson, E. A. (1993). Effects of individualized music on confused and agitated elderly patients. *Archives of Psychiatric Nursing,* 7(5):284.

Gonzalez, C. A., Griffith, E. E. H., and Ruiz, P. (1995). Cross-cultural issues in psychiatric treatment. In G. O. Gabbard (Ed.), *Treatment of psychiatric disorders* (2nd ed.) (Vol. 1, pp. 55–74). Washington, D.C.: American Psychiatric Press.

Ham, R. J. (1999). Evolving standards in patient and caregiver support. *Alzheimer's Disease and Associated Disorders,* 13(November; Suppl 2):S27–S35.

Health, A. H. (1992). Imagery: Helping ICU patients control pain and anxiety. *Dimensions of Critical Care Nursing,* 11(1):57.

Hobfall, S. E., and Vaux, A. (1993). Social support: Social resources and social context. In L. Goldberger and S. Breznitz (Eds.), *Handbook of stress: Theoretical and clinical aspects* (2nd ed.) (pp. 685–705). New York: Free Press.

Holmes, T. H., and Masuda, M. (1972). Life events and social readjustment scale: Psychosomatic medicine. *Psychology Today,* April, p. 71.

Holmes, T. H., and Rahe, R. H. (1967). The social readjustment rating scale. *Journal of Psychosomatic Research,* 11:213.

Jacobson, E. (1974). *Progressive relaxation* (3rd ed.). Chicago: University of Chicago Press.

Kabat-Zinn, J. (1993). Meditation. In B. Moyers (Ed.), *Healing and the mind* (pp. 115–144). New York: Doubleday.

Kumar, A. M., et al. (1999). Music therapy increases serum melatonin levels in patients with Alzheimer's disease. *Alternative Therapeutic Health Medicine,* 5(6):49–57.

Lazarus, R. S. (1991). *Emotion and adaptation.* New York: Oxford University Press.

Lazarus, R. S. (1993). Why we should think of stress as a subset of emotion. In L. Goldberger and S. Breznitz (Eds), *Handbook of Stress: Theoretical and clinical aspects.* (2nd ed.) pp. 31–39. New York: Free Press.

Lazarus, R. S., and DeLongis, A. (1983). Psychological stress and coping in aging. *American Psychologist,* 38:245.

Lazarus, R. S., and Folkman, S. (1984). *Stress, appraisal, and coping.* New York: Springer.

Lazarus, R. S., Kanner, A. D., and Folkman, S. (1980). A cognitive-phenomenological analysis. In R. Pluchik and H. Kellerman (Eds.), *Theories of emotion. Vol. 1: Emotion: theory, research, and experience.* New York: Academic Press.

Loewenthal, K. M. (1999). Religious issues and their psychological aspects. In Kamaldeep Bhui and Dele Olajide (Eds). *Mental Health Services for Multi-Cultural Society.* Philadelphia: W. B. Saunders.

Mandler, G. (1993). Thought, memory, and learning: Effects of emotional stress. In L. Goldberger and S. Breznitz (Eds.), *Handbook of stress: Theoretical and clinical aspects* (2nd ed.) (pp. 40–55). New York: Free Press.

Matassarin-Jacobs, E. (1993). Pain assessment and intervention. In J. M. Black and E. Matassarin-Jacobs (Eds.), *Luckmann and Sorensen's medical-surgical nursing: A psychopharmologic approach* (4th ed.) (pp. 311–358). Philadelphia: W. B. Saunders.

Miller, M. A., and Rahe, R. H. (1997). Life changes scaling for the 1990s. *Journal of Psychosomatic Research,* 43(3):279–292.

O'Neill, D., and Kenny, E. (1998). Spirituality and chronic illness. *Image Journal Nursing School,* 30(3):275.

Rahe, R. H. (1995). Stress and psychiatry. In H. I. Kaplan and B. J. Sadock (Eds.), *Comprehensive textbook of psychiatry* (6th ed.) (Vol. 2, pp. 1545–1559). Baltimore: Williams & Wilkins.

Salmon, P. (2001). Effects of physical exercise on anxiety, depression, and sensitivity to stress: A unifying theory. *Clinical Psychological Review,* 21(1):33–61.

Selye, H. (1974). *Stress without distress.* Philadelphia: J. B. Lippincott.

Selye, H. (1993). History of the stress concept. In L. Goldberger and S. Breznitz (Eds.), *Handbook of stress: Theoretical and clinical aspects* (2nd ed.) (pp. 7–17). New York: Free Press.

Stoyva, J. M., and Carlson, J. G. (1993). A coping/rest model of relaxation and stress management. In L. Goldberger and S. Breznitz (Eds.), *Handbook of stress: Theoretical and clinical aspects* (2nd ed.) (pp. 724–756). New York: Free Press.

Trauger-Querry, B., and Haghighi, K. R. (1999). Balancing the focus: Art and music therapy for pain control and symptom management in hospice care. *Hospice Journal,* 14(1):25–38.

Varcarolis, E. M. (1996) Relaxation. In S. Lego (Ed.), *Psychiatric nursing: A comprehensive reference* (pp. 143–153). Philadelphia: J. B. Lippincott.

Warda, M. R. (1999). Cultural diversity in health care delivery. In Shea, C. A., Pelletier, L. R., Poster, E. C., Stuart, G. W., and Verhey, M. P. (Eds), *Advanced Practice Nursing in Psychiatric Mental Health Care.* St. Louis: Mosby.

Warner, C. D., et al. (1992). The effectiveness of teaching relaxation techniques to patients undergoing elective cardiac catheterization. *Journal of Cardiovascular Nursing,* 6(2):66.

Weinberger, R. (1991). Teaching the elderly stress reduction. *Journal of Gerontological Nursing,* 17(10):23.

Wickramasekera, I. (1999). How does biofeedback reduce clinical symptoms and do memories and beliefs have biological consequences? Toward a model of mind-body healing. *Applied Psychophysiological Biofeedback,* 24(2):91–105.

Visit the **Evolve** website at
http://evolve.elsevier.com/Varcarolis
for a pre-test on the content in this chapter.

Outline

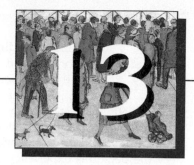

13

Understanding Anxiety and Anxiety Defenses

ELIZABETH M. VARCAROLIS

Key Terms and Concepts

The key terms and concepts listed here also appear in color where they are defined or first discussed in this chapter.

acting out behaviors

acute (state) anxiety

altruism

anxiety

chronic (trait) anxiety

denial

devaluation

displacement

dissociation

fear

humor

idealization

mild anxiety

moderate anxiety

panic levels of anxiety

passive aggression

projection

psychotic denial

rationalization

reaction-formation

repression

severe anxiety

somatization

splitting

sublimation

suppression

undoing

Objectives

After studying this chapter, the reader will be able to

1. Explore the difference between normal anxiety, acute anxiety, and chronic anxiety.

2. Contrast and compare the four levels of anxiety in relation to perceptual field, ability to learn, and physical and other defining characteristics.

3. Summarize five properties of the defense mechanisms.

4. Define and give a clinical example of each of the defense mechanisms identified by Vaillant under the following categories: mature, neurotic, immature, psychotic.

*A*n understanding of anxiety and anxiety defense mechanisms is basic to the practice of psychiatric nursing. One of Hildegarde Peplau's (1909–1999) greatest legacies to nursing is operationally defining the four levels of anxiety and suggesting interventions appropriate to the level of anxiety the person is experiencing.

ABOUT ANXIETY

Stress is a state produced by a change in the environment that is perceived as challenging, threatening, or damaging to a person's well-being. Stress can lead to a variety of psychological responses, the most common of which is anxiety.

Anxiety is a universal human experience that is a stranger to no one. It is the most basic of emotions. Dysfunctional behavior is often a defense against anxiety. When behavior is recognized as dysfunctional, interventions to reduce anxiety can be initiated by the nurse. As anxiety decreases, dysfunctional behavior will frequently decrease, and vice versa.

Anxiety is experienced on four levels: mild, moderate, severe, and panic anxiety. It can be broken down into three categories—normal, acute, and chronic—and it can be operationally defined.

Hildegard Peplau, a nurse theorist who had profound impact on shaping the psychiatric mental health nursing profession, identifies anxiety as one of the most important concepts in psychiatric nursing. Nurses can use the concept of anxiety to explain many clinical observations. Peplau (1968) conceptualized an anxiety model useful to the practice of nursing. Conceptualizing anxiety using Peplau's model has led to principles that serve as guides in nursing intervention. This conceptual basis of anxiety can be used by nurses as a framework to guide therapeutic approaches to clients in any setting.

Anxiety can be defined as a feeling of apprehension, uneasiness, uncertainty, or dread resulting from a real or a perceived threat whose actual source is unknown or unrecognized.

Fear is a reaction to a specific danger, whereas anxiety is a vague sense of dread relating to an unspecified danger. However, the body reacts in similar ways physiologically to both anxiety and fear.

An important distinction between anxiety and fear is that anxiety attacks us at a deeper level than does fear. Anxiety invades the central core of the personality. It erodes the individual feelings of self-esteem and personal worth that contribute to a sense of being fully human.

Normal anxiety is a healthy life force that is necessary for survival. It provides the energy needed to carry out the tasks involved in living and striving toward goals. Anxiety motivates people to make and survive change. It prompts constructive behaviors, such as studying for an examination, being on time for job interviews, preparing for a presentation, and working toward a promotion.

Acute anxiety is also referred to as state anxiety. **Acute (state) anxiety** is precipitated by an imminent loss or change that threatens an individual's sense of security. It may be seen in performers before a concert. For example, Barbra Streisand admits to experiencing acute anxiety before live concerts. Patients preparing for surgery often experience acute anxiety. The death of a loved one can stimulate acute anxiety when there is great disruption in one's life. In general, crisis involves the experience of acute anxiety.

Trait anxiety is another name for chronic anxiety. **Chronic (trait) anxiety** is anxiety that the person has lived with for a time. Ego psychologists suggest that in a nurturing environment the developing personality incorporates the primary caregivers' positive attributes, thus allowing the child to tolerate anxiety. When conditions for personality growth are less than adequate, positive values may not be incorporated, and the child may become anxiety ridden, a state that often covers up overwhelming, angry, and hostile impulses (Sullivan 1953). A child may demonstrate chronic anxiety by a permanent attitude of apprehension or by overreaction to all unexpected environmental stimuli. In adults, chronic anxiety may take the form of chronic fatigue, insomnia, discomfort in daily activities, discomfort in personal relationships, and ineffective job performance. When the subjective feelings of anxiety become too overwhelming, anxiety is unconsciously placed out of awareness (repressed) and is expressed in behavioral characteristics or symptoms.

An understanding of the types, levels, and defensive patterns used in response to anxiety is basic to psychiatric nursing care. This understanding is essential for assessing and planning interventions to lower a client's level of anxiety, as well as one's own, effectively. With practice, one becomes more skilled both at identifying levels of anxiety and the defenses used to alleviate it, and at evaluating the possible stressors contributing to increases in a person's level of anxiety.

LEVELS OF ANXIETY

Levels of anxiety range from mild to moderate to severe to panic. Peplau's (1968) classic delineation of these four levels of anxiety is based on Sullivan's work (refer to Chapter 2 for more on Peplau and anxiety). Assessment of a client's level of anxiety is basic to therapeutic intervention in any setting—psychiatric, hospital, or community. Determination of specific levels of anxiety can be used as guidelines for intervention (Table 13–1). Anxiety is experienced on a continuum from mild to moderate to severe to panic, and overlapping can and does occur. Use Table 13–1 as a guide for making observations.

Mild Anxiety

Mild anxiety occurs in the normal experience of everyday living. The person's ability to perceive reality is brought into sharp focus. A person sees, hears, and grasps more information, and problem solving becomes more effective. A person may display physical symptoms such as slight discomfort, restlessness, irritability, or mild tension-relieving behaviors (e.g., nail biting, foot or finger tapping, fidgeting).

Moderate Anxiety

As anxiety escalates, the perceptual field narrows, and some details are excluded from observation. The person in moderate anxiety sees, hears, and grasps less information than someone not in that state. Individuals may experience **selective inattention**, in which only certain things in the environment are seen or heard unless they are brought to the person's attention. Although the ability to think clearly is hampered, learning and problem solving can still take place, though not at an optimal level. At the moderate level of anxiety, the person's ability to solve problems is greatly enhanced by the supportive presence of another. Physical symptoms include tension, pounding heart, increased pulse and respiration rate, perspiration, and mild somatic symptoms (gastric discomfort, headache, urinary urgency). Voice tremors and shaking may be noticed. Mild or moderate anxiety levels can be constructive, because anxiety can be viewed as a signal that something in the person's life needs attention.

Severe Anxiety

The perceptual field of a person experiencing severe anxiety is greatly reduced. A person in severe anxiety may focus on one particular detail or many scattered details. The person may have difficulty noticing what is going on in the environment, even when it is pointed out by another. Learning and problem solving are not possible at this level, and the person may be dazed and confused. Behavior is automatic and aimed at reducing or relieving anxiety. The person may complain of increased severity of somatic symptoms (headache, nausea, dizziness, insomnia), trembling, and pounding heart. The person may also experience hyperventilation and a sense of impending doom or dread.

Panic Level of Anxiety

The panic level of anxiety is the most extreme form and results in markedly disturbed behavior. The person is not able to process what is going on in the environment and may lose touch with reality. The behavior that results may be manifested by confusion, shouting, screaming, or withdrawal. Hallucinations, or false sensory perceptions such as seeing people or objects that are not there, may be experienced by people in panic levels of anxiety. Physical behavior may be erratic, uncoordinated, and impulsive. Automatic behaviors are used to reduce and relieve anxiety, although such efforts may be ineffective. Acute panic may lead to exhaustion. Review Table 13–1 to identify the levels of anxiety in relation to (1) perceptual field, (2) ability to learn, and (3) physical and other defining characteristics.

Mild to Moderate Anxiety

A person in mild to moderate levels of anxiety is still able to solve problems; however, the ability to concentrate decreases as anxiety increases. You can help the client focus and solve problems with the use of specific communication techniques, such as employing open-ended questions, giving broad openings, and exploring and seeking clarification. These techniques can be useful to a client experiencing mild to moderate anxiety. Closing off topics of communication and bringing up irrelevant topics can increase a person's anxiety and are tactics that usually make the *nurse* feel better, not the client.

Reducing the anxiety level and preventing escalation of anxiety to more distressing levels can be aided by a calm presence, recognition of the anxious person's distress, and willingness to listen. Evaluation of effective past coping mechanisms is useful. Often the nurse can help the client to consider alternatives to problem situations and offer activities that may temporarily relieve feelings of inner tension. Table 13–2 identifies counseling techniques useful in people in moderate levels of anxiety.

TABLE 13–1   *Anxiety Levels*

MILD	MODERATE	SEVERE	PANIC
Perceptual Field			
Perceptual field can be heightened	Perceptual field narrows. Person grasps less of what is going on	Perceptual field greatly reduced	Unable to focus on the environment
Is alert and can see, hear, and grasp what is happening in the environment	Can attend to more *if pointed out by another* (selective inattention)	Focus is on details or one specific detail Attention is scattered	Experiences the utmost state of terror and emotional paralysis. Feels he or she "ceases to exist."
Can identify things that are disturbing and are producing anxiety		Completely absorbed with self	In panic, hallucinations or delusions may take the place of reality
		May not be able to attend to events in the environment *even when pointed out by others*	
		In severe to panic levels of anxiety, the environment is blocked out. It is as if these events are not occurring.	
Ability to Learn			
Ability to effectively work toward a goal and examine alternatives	Able to solve problems but not at optimal ability	Unable to see connections between events or details	May be mute or have extreme psychomotor agitation leading to exhaustion
	Benefits from guidance of others	Distorted perceptions	Disorganized or irrational reasoning
Mild and moderate levels of anxiety can alert the person that something is wrong and can stimulate appropriate action		**Severe and panic levels prevent problem solving and finding effective solutions. Unproductive relief behaviors are called into play, thus perpetuating a vicious cycle**	
Physical or Other Characteristics			
Slight discomfort Attention-seeking behaviors Restlessness Irritability or impatience Mild tension-relieving behavior: foot or finger tapping, lip chewing, fidgeting	Voice tremors Change in voice pitch Difficulty concentrating Shakiness Repetitive questioning Somatic complaints, e.g., urinary frequency and urgency, headache, backache, insomnia Increased respiration rate Increased pulse rate Increased muscle tension More extreme tension-relieving behavior; pacing, banging hands on table	Feelings of dread Ineffective functioning Confusion Purposeless activity Sense of impending doom More intense somatic complaints, e.g., dizziness, nausea, headache, sleeplessness Hyperventilation Tachycardia Withdrawal Loud and rapid speech Threats and demands	Experience of terror Immobility or severe hyperactivity or flight Dilated pupils Unintelligible communication or inability to speak Severe shakiness Sleeplessness Severe withdrawal Hallucinations or delusion likely out of touch with reality

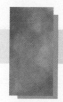

TABLE 13–2 *Interventions for Mild to Moderate Levels of Anxiety*

INTERVENTION	RATIONALE

Nursing Diagnosis: **Moderate anxiety related to situational event or psychological stress, as evidenced by increase in vital signs, moderate discomfort, narrowing of perceptual field, and selective inattention**

INTERVENTION	RATIONALE
1. Help the client identify anxiety. "Are you comfortable right now?"	1. Validate observations with the client, name the anxiety, and start to work with the client to lower anxiety.
2. Anticipate anxiety-provoking situations.	2. Escalation of anxiety to a more disorganizing level is prevented.
3. Use nonverbal language to demonstrate interest, e.g., lean forward, maintain eye contact, nod your head.	3. Verbal and nonverbal messages should be consistent. The presence of an interested person provides a stabilizing focus.
4. Encourage client to talk about his or her feelings and concerns.	4. When concerns are stated aloud, problems can be discussed and feelings of isolation decreased.
5. Avoid closing off avenues of communication that are important for the client. Focus on the client's concerns.	5. When staff anxiety increases, "changing the topic" or "offering advice" is common but leaves the person isolated.
6. Ask questions to clarify what is being said. "I'm not sure what you mean. Give me an example."	6. Increased anxiety results in scattering of thoughts. Clarifying helps the client identify thoughts and feelings.
7. Help the client identify thoughts or feelings before the onset of anxiety. "What were you thinking right before you started to feel anxious?"	7. Helps the client identify thoughts and feelings, facilitates problem solving.
8. Encourage problem solving with the client.*	8. Encouraging clients to explore alternatives increases sense of control and decreases anxiety.
9. Assist in developing alternative solutions to a problem through role play or modeling behaviors.	9. Encourage the client to try out alternative behaviors and solutions.
10. Explore behaviors that have worked to relieve anxiety in the past.	10. Encourage the mobilization of successful coping mechanisms and strengths.
11. Provide outlets for working off excess energy, e.g., walking, pingpong, dancing, exercises.	11. Physical activity can provide relief of built-up tension, increase muscle tone, and increase endorphins.

*Clients in mild to moderate anxiety levels can problem solve.

Severe to Panic Anxiety

A person in severe to panic levels of anxiety is unable to solve problems and may have a poor grasp of what is happening in the environment. Unproductive relief behaviors may take over and the person may not be in control of his or her actions. Extreme regression or running about aimlessly are behavioral manifestations of a person's intense psychic pain. The nurse is concerned with the client's safety and, at times, the safety of others. Physical needs (e.g., fluids and rest) have to be met to prevent exhaustion. Anxiety reduction measures may take the form of removing the person to a quiet environment where there is minimal stimulation and providing gross motor activities to drain off some of the tension. The use of medications may have to be considered, but both medications and restraints should be used only after other more personal and less restrictive interventions have failed to decrease anxiety to safer levels. Although communication may be scattered and disjointed, themes can often be heard, and the nurse can address these themes. The feeling that one is understood can decrease the sense of isolation and also reduce anxiety.

Because the person in severe to panic levels of anxiety is unable to solve problems, communication techniques suggested for the person in mild to moderate levels of anxiety are not always effective. Because clients in severe to panic anxiety levels are out of control, they need to know that they are safe from their own impulses. **Firm, short, and simple statements are useful.** Reinforcing commonalities in the environment and pointing out reality when there are distortions can also be useful interventions for the severely anxious person. Table 13–3 suggests basic nursing interventions for the client in severe to panic levels of anxiety.

Refer to the Case Study at the end of the chapter for a demonstration of how many of these techniques can be used with a person in severe anxiety. Chapter 12 offers many cognitive and behavioral

TABLE 13–3   *Interventions for Severe to Panic Levels of Anxiety*

INTERVENTION	RATIONALE

Nursing Diagnosis: Anxiety related to severe threat (biochemical, environmental, psychosocial), as evidenced by verbal or physical acting out, extreme immobility, sense of impending doom, inability to differentiate reality (possible hallucinations or delusions), and inability to problem solve

INTERVENTION	RATIONALE
1. Maintain a calm manner.	1. Anxiety is communicated interpersonally. The quiet calm of the nurse can serve to calm the client. The presence of anxiety can escalate anxiety in the client.
2. Always remain with the person in acute severe to panic levels of anxiety.	2. Alone with immense anxiety, a person feels abandoned. A caring face may be the only contact with reality when confusion becomes overwhelming.
3. Minimize environmental stimuli. Move to a quieter setting and stay with the client.	3. Further escalation of anxiety to self and to others in the setting is prevented.
4. Use clear and simple statements and repetition.	4. A person has difficulty concentrating and processing information with severe to panic levels of anxiety.
5. Use a low-pitched voice, speak slowly.	5. A high-pitched voice can convey anxiety. Low pitch can decrease anxiety.
6. Reinforce reality if distortions occur, e.g., seeing objects that are not there or hearing voices when no one is present.	6. Anxiety can be reduced by focusing on and validating what is going on in the environment.
7. Listen for themes in communication.	7. In severe to panic levels of anxiety, verbal communication themes may be the only indication of the client's thoughts or feelings.
8. Attend to physical and safety needs when necessary, e.g., warmth, fluids, elimination, pain relief, need for family contact.	8. High levels of anxiety may obscure the client's awareness of physical needs.
9. Because safety is an overall goal, physical limits may need to be set. Speak in a firm, authoritative voice: "You may not hit anyone here. If you can't control yourself, we will help you."	9. A person who is out of control is often terrorized. Staff must offer the client and others protection from destructive and self-destructive impulses.
10. Provide opportunities for exercise, e.g., pacing with nurse, punching bag, ping-pong.	10. Physical activity helps channel and dissipate tension and may temporarily lower anxiety.
11. When a person is constantly moving or pacing, offer high-caloric fluids.	11. Prevent dehydration and exhaustion.
12. Assess the person's need for medication or seclusion after other interventions have been tried and have not been successful.	12. Prevent exhaustion and physical harm to self and others.

strategies for decreasing stress and anxiety, and Chapter 14 identifies cognitive-behavioral techniques used in treating anxiety disorders.

DEFENSES AGAINST ANXIETY

Stress leads to increased anxiety, which then triggers some form of relief behavior. **Defense mechanisms**, or coping styles, are automatic psychological processes that protect the individual against anxiety and from the awareness of internal or external dangers or stressors (APA 2000). Defense mechanisms are relief behaviors used by everyone. They serve to lower anxiety, maintain ego function, and protect one's sense of self (Fig. 13–1).

High levels of anxiety can disturb problem solving and learning as well as perception and functioning. Unconscious defensive maneuvers are mobilized so that an individual can continue to meet personal and social goals in acceptable ways. All defense mechanisms are mobilized by the ego, with the exception of regression. In regression, the ego itself (personality) is relegated to a less mature, although more comfortable, mode of operation. Most defense mechanisms are mobilized on an unconscious level. A notable exception is suppression, which uses the conscious mind.

Adaptive use of defense mechanisms helps people lower anxiety to achieve goals in acceptable ways. Maladaptive use of defense mechanisms may lead to distortions in reality and self-deception that can interfere with individual growth and interpersonal sat-

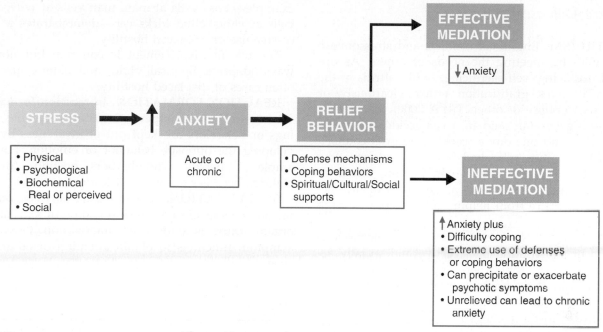

Figure 13–1 Anxiety, operationally defined.

isfaction. Determination of the effective use of defense mechanisms is based on frequency, intensity, and duration of use.

Sigmund Freud and his daughter Anna Freud outlined most of the defense mechanisms that we acknowledge today. The following summarizes five of their most important properties (Vaillant 1994):

1. Defenses are a major means of managing conflict and affect.
2. Defenses are relatively unconscious.
3. Defenses are discrete from one another.
4. Although often the hallmarks of major psychiatric syndromes, defenses are reversible.
5. Defenses are adaptive as well as pathological.

Over the years, researchers have hypothesized that defense mechanisms could be organized into a hierarchy of relative psychopathology. Devised by Vaillant (1994), Table 13–4 arranges specific defense mechanisms into four general classes of psychopathology. The ones identified as immature defenses are often associated with the personality disorders.

Definitions of many common mature, neurotic, and immature defenses follow. They are presented in the order of Vaillant's hierarchy. Actually, all defense mechanisms except sublimation and altruism can be used in both healthy and not-so-healthy ways. (Sublimation and altruism are always healthy coping mechanisms.) Most people use a variety of

defense mechanisms but not always on the same level. The adaptive or maladaptive use of defense mechanisms is determined for the most part by their frequency, intensity, and duration of use.

TABLE 13–4 *Ego Defenses Organized into Hierarchy of Psychopathology*

CATEGORY	DEFENSE
Mature defenses	Suppression
	Altruism
	Humor
	Sublimation
Neurotic (intermediate) defenses	Intellectualization, isolation
	Repression
	Reaction-formation
	Displacement, somatization
	Undoing, rationalization
Immature defenses	Passive aggression
	Acting out
	Dissociation
	Projection
Psychotic defenses	Denial (of external reality)
	Distortion (of external reality)

Adapted from Vaillant, G. (1994). Ego mechanisms of defense and personality psychopathology. *Journal of Abnormal Psychology,* 103 (1):44–50.

Mature Defenses

ALTRUISM. Emotional conflicts and stressors are dealt with by meeting the needs of others. As opposed to being self-sacrificing, with altruism the person receives gratification either vicariously or from the response of others (APA 2000). Six months after losing her husband in a car accident, Jeanette began to spend one day a week doing grief counseling with families who had lost a loved one. She found that she was effective in helping others in their grief, and she obtained a great deal of satisfaction and pleasure from helping others work through their pain.

SUBLIMATION. Sublimation is an unconscious process of substituting constructive and socially acceptable activity for strong impulses that are not acceptable in their original form. Often, these impulses are sexual or aggressive in nature. A man with strong hostile feelings may choose to become a butcher, or he may be involved with rough contact sports. A person who is unable to experience sexual activity may channel this energy into something creative, such as painting and gardening.

HUMOR. The individual deals with emotional conflicts or stressors by emphasizing the amusing or ironic aspects of the conflict or stressor through humor (APA 2000). A man goes to an interview that means a great deal to him. He is being interviewed by the top executives of the company. He has recently had foot surgery and, in entering the interview room, he stumbles and loses his balance. There is a stunned silence, and then the man states calmly, "I was hoping I could put my best foot forward." With everyone laughing, the interview continues in a relaxed manner.

SUPPRESSION. Suppression is the conscious denial of a disturbing situation or feeling. A student who has been studying for the state board examinations says, "I can't worry about paying my rent until after my exam tomorrow."

Neurotic (Intermediate) Defenses

REPRESSION. Repression is the exclusion of unpleasant or unwanted experiences, emotions, or ideas from conscious awareness. Forgetting the name of a former husband and forgetting an appointment to discuss poor grades are examples. Repression is considered the cornerstone of the defense mechanisms, and it is the first line of psychological defense against anxiety.

DISPLACEMENT. Transfer of emotions associated with a particular person, object, or situation to another person, object, or situation that is nonthreatening is called displacement. The frequently used example—boss yells at man, man yells at wife, wife yells at child, child kicks cat—demonstrates a successive use of displaced hostility.

The use of displacement is common but not always adaptive. Spousal, child, and elder abuse are often cases of displaced hostility.

REACTION-FORMATION. In reaction-formation (also termed **overcompensation**), unacceptable feelings or behaviors are kept out of awareness by developing the opposite behavior or emotion. For example, a person who harbors hostility toward children becomes a Boy Scout leader.

SOMATIZATION. Transforming anxiety on an unconscious level to a physical symptom that has no organic cause is a form of somatization. Often the symptom functions to obtain attention or as an excuse.

Vignette

■ A *professor develops laryngitis on the day he is scheduled to defend a research proposal to a group of peers. A woman who does not want to go out with her boss's brother calls to say "her back went out" and she cannot make the date (and, in fact, her back is sore).*

UNDOING. Undoing makes up for an act or communication (e.g., giving a gift to undo an argument). A common behavioral example of undoing is compulsive handwashing. This can be viewed as cleansing oneself of an act or thought perceived as unacceptable.

RATIONALIZATION. Rationalization consists of justifying illogical or unreasonable ideas, actions, or feelings by developing acceptable explanations that satisfy the teller as well as the listener. Common examples are "If I had Lynn's brains, I'd get good grades, too," or "Everybody cheats, so why shouldn't I?" Rationalization is a form of self-deception.

Immature Defenses (Personality Disorders)

PASSIVE AGGRESSION. A passive-aggressive individual deals with emotional conflict or stressors by indirectly and unassertively expressing aggression toward others. On the surface, there is an appearance of compliance that masks covert resistance, resentment, and hostility (APA 2000). With passive aggression, resistance is expressed through procrastination, inefficiency, and stubbornness, especially in response to assigned tasks or demands for independent action (Gunderson and Phillips 1995).

Vignette

■ *Sam promises his boss that he is working on the presentation for important clients, even though he constantly "forgets" to bring in samples of the presentation. The day of the presentation, Sam calls in sick with the flu.*

ACTING OUT BEHAVIORS. An individual deals with emotional conflicts or stressors by actions rather than reflections or feelings (APA 2000). For example, a person may lash out in anger verbally or physically to distract the self from threatening thoughts or feelings (e.g., powerlessness). The verbal or physical expression of anger can make a person feel temporarily less helpless or vulnerable (i.e., more powerful and more in control). By lashing out at others, an individual can transfer the focus from personal doubts and insecurities to some other person or object. **Acting out behaviors** demonstrate a destructive coping style.

Vignette

■ *When Harry was turned down a third time for a promotion, he went to his office and tore apart every client file in his file cabinet. His initial feeling of worthlessness and lowered self-esteem related to the situation was interpreted by Harry to mean "I am no good." This thinking resulted in Harry's quickly transforming these painful feelings into actions of anger and destruction. Temporarily, Harry felt more powerful and less vulnerable.*

DISSOCIATION. A disruption in the usually integrated functions of consciousness, memory, identity, or perception of the environment is known as **dissociation**.

Vignette

■ *A young mother who watched her son run over by a car was taken to a neighbor's house while the police dealt with the accident. Later she told the policeman "I really don't remember what happened. The last thing I remember was going out the door to check on Johnny."*

At that moment, to protect herself from an unbearable situation, she split off the threatening event from awareness until she could begin to deal with her feelings of devastation.

DEVALUATION. **Devaluation** occurs when emotional conflicts or stressors are dealt with by attributing negative qualities to self or others (APA 2000). When devaluing another, the individual then appears good by contrast.

Vignette

■ *A woman who is very jealous of a co-worker says, "Oh yes, she won the award. Those awards don't mean anything anyway, and I wonder what she had to do to be chosen." In this way she minimizes the other's accomplishments and keeps her own fragile self-esteem intact.*

IDEALIZATION. Emotional conflicts or stressors are dealt with by attributing exaggerated positive qualities to others (APA 2000). **Idealization** is an important aspect of the development of the self. Children who grow up with parents they can respect and idealize develop healthy standards of conduct and morality (Merikangas and Kupfer 1995).

When people idealize and overvalue a person in a new relationship, they are sure to be disappointed when the object of the idealization turns out to be human. This leads to a great deal of disappointment and painful lowering of self-esteem. Such individuals may then end up devaluing and rejecting the object of their affection to protect their own self-esteem. This pattern can be repeated over and over on a job, within friendships, and within marriages.

Vignette

■ *Mary met the most "wonderful and perfect" man. No one could tell Mary that Jim was nice but had some quirks, like everyone else. Mary wouldn't listen. When Jim failed to live up to Mary's expectations of giving her constant attention, adoration, and gifts, Mary was devastated. Shortly thereafter, she was saying that Jim was, like all men, a brute, and that she wanted no more to do with such an insensitive person.*

SPLITTING. **Splitting** is the inability to integrate the positive and negative qualities of oneself or others into a cohesive image. Aspects of the self and of others tend to alternate between opposite poles, for example, either good, loving, worthy, nurturing; or bad, hateful, destructive, rejecting, worthless (APA 2000). This is prevalent in personality disorders, especially the borderline ones.

Vignette

■ *Alice viewed her therapist as the most wonderful, loving, and insightful therapist she had ever had. When her therapist refused to write her a prescription for Valium, Alice shouted at her that she was the "stupidest, most uncaring, and thickheaded person" and she demanded another therapist "right away."*

PROJECTION. A person unconsciously rejects emotionally unacceptable personal features and attributes them to other people, objects, or situations through projection. This is the hallmark of blaming or scapegoating, which is the root of prejudice. People who always feel that others are out to deceive or cheat them may be projecting onto others those characteristics in themselves that they find distasteful and cannot consciously accept.

Projection of anxiety can often be seen in systems (family, hospital, school, business). In a family in which there are problems, the child is often scapegoated, and the pain and anxiety within the family are projected onto the child: "the problem is Tommy." In a larger system in which anxiety and conflict are present, the weakest members are scapegoated: "the problem is the nurses' aides, the students, the new salesman." When pain and anxiety exist within a system, projection can be an automatic relief behavior. Once the cause of the anxiety is identified, changes in relief behavior can ensue, and the system can become more functional and productive.

Psychotic (Severe) Defenses

DENIAL. Denial involves escaping unpleasant realities by ignoring their existence. For example, a man might believe physical limitations to be a negative reflection on one's manhood. Thus, he may deny chest pains, even though heart attacks run in his family, because of a threat to his self-image as a man. A woman whose health has deteriorated because of alcohol abuse denies she has a problem with alcohol by saying she can stop drinking whenever she wants.

The term psychotic denial is used when there is gross impairment in reality testing. A schizophrenic man who says he wants to stay out of the hospital tells the nurse it is his medication, not the cocaine, that makes him frankly psychotic and aggressive. Refer to Table 13–5 for examples of mild and severe (psychotic) defense mechanisms.

TABLE 13–5 *Defense Mechanisms*

MILD USE	EXTREME EXAMPLE
Repression	
Man forgets wife's birthday after a marital fight	Woman is unable to enjoy sex after having pushed out of awareness a traumatic sexual incident from childhood
Sublimation	
Woman who is angry with her boss writes a short story about a heroic woman. By definition, use of sublimation is always constructive	None
Regression	
Four-year-old boy with a new baby brother starts sucking his thumb and wanting a bottle	Man who loses a promotion starts complaining to others, hands in sloppy work, misses appointments, and comes in late for meetings
Displacement	
Patient criticizes a nurse after his family fails to visit	Child who is unable to acknowledge fear of his father becomes fearful of animals
Projection	
Man who is unconsciously attracted to other women teases his wife about flirting	Woman who has repressed an attraction toward other women refuses to socialize. She fears another woman will make homosexual advances toward her

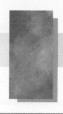

TABLE 13–5 *Defense Mechanisms (Continued)*

MILD USE	EXTREME EXAMPLE
Compensation	
Short man becomes assertively verbal and excels in business	Individual drinks alcohol when self-esteem is low to diffuse discomfort temporarily
Reaction-Formation	
Recovering alcoholic constantly preaches about the evils of drink	Mother who has an unconscious hostility toward her daughter is overprotective and hovers over her to protect her from harm, interfering with her normal growth and development
Denial	
Man reacts to news of the death of a loved one: "No, I don't believe you. The doctor said he was fine."	Woman whose husband died 3 years ago still keeps his clothes in the closet and talks about him in the present tense
Conversion	
Student is unable to take a final examination because of terrible headache	Man becomes blind after seeing his wife flirt with other men
Undoing	
After flirting with her male secretary, a woman brings her husband tickets to a show	Man with rigid and moralistic beliefs and repressed sexuality is driven to wash his hands when around attractive women to gain composure
Rationalization	
"I didn't get the raise because the boss doesn't like me."	Father who thinks his son was fathered by another man excuses his malicious treatment of the boy by saying "He is lazy and disobedient," when that is not the case
Identification	
Five-year-old girl dresses in her mother's shoes and dress and meets daddy at the door	Young boy thinks a neighborhood pimp with money and drugs is someone to look up to
Introjection	
After his wife's death, husband has transient complaints of chest pains and difficulty breathing—the symptoms his wife had before she died	Young child whose parents were overcritical and belittling grows up thinking that she is not any good. She has taken on her parent's evaluation of her as part of her self-image
Suppression	
Business man who is preparing to make an important speech that day is told by his wife that morning that she wants a divorce. Although visibly upset, he puts the incident aside until after his speech, when he can give the matter his total concentration	A woman who feels a lump in her breast shortly before leaving for a 3-week vacation puts the information in the back of her mind until after returning from her vacation

Visit the **Evolve** website at
http://evolve.elsevier.com/Varcarolis
for more Case Studies.

CASE STUDY 13–1   *A Person in Severe Levels of Anxiety*

The following case study describes a man in severe levels of acute anxiety. See if you can match his signs and symptoms with those in Table 13–1.

Tom Michaels, a 63-year-old man, came into the emergency department (ED) with his wife Anne, who had taken an overdose of sleeping pills and antidepressant medications. Ten years before, Anne's mother had died, and since that time Anne had suffered several episodes of severe depression with suicidal attempts. She had needed hospitalization during these episodes. Anne Michaels had been released 2 weeks earlier after treatment for depression and threatened suicide.

Tom had long established a routine of giving his wife her antidepressant medications in the morning and her sleeping medication at night and keeping the bottles hidden when he was not at home. Today, he had forgotten to hide the medications before he went

to work. His wife had taken the remaining pills from both bottles with large quantities of alcohol. When Tom returned home for lunch, Anne was comatose.

In the ED, Anne suffered a cardiac arrest and was taken to the intensive care unit (ICU).

Tom appeared very jittery. He moved about the room aimlessly. He dropped his hat, a medication card, and his keys. His hands were trembling, and he looked around the room, bewildered. He appeared unable to focus on any one thing. He said over and over, in a loud, high-pitched voice, "Why didn't I hide the bottles?" He was wringing his hands and began stamping his feet, saying "It's all my fault. Everything is falling apart."

Other people in the waiting room appeared distracted and alarmed by his behavior. Tom appeared to be oblivious to his surroundings.

ASSESSMENT

Russell Brown, the psychiatric nurse clinician working in the ED, came into the waiting room and assessed Tom's behavior as indicative of a severe anxiety level. After talking with Tom briefly, Mr. Brown believed nursing intervention was indicated.

Mr. Brown based his conclusion on the following assessment of the client.

Objective Data

■ Unable to focus on anything
■ Purposeless activity (walking around aimlessly)
■ Oblivious to his surroundings
■ Confused and bewildered
■ Unproductive relief behavior (stomping, wringing hands, dropping things)

Subjective Data

■ "Everything is falling apart."
■ "Why didn't I hide the bottles?"
■ "It's all my fault."

NURSING DIAGNOSIS

Mr. Brown formulated the following nursing diagnosis:

Anxiety (severe) related to the client's perception of responsibility for his wife's coma and possible death, as evidenced by inability to focus, confusion, and the feeling that "everything is falling apart."

OUTCOME CRITERIA

Client will use effective coping strategies.

PLANNING

Mr. Brown thought that if he could lower Tom's anxiety to a moderate level, he could work with Tom to get a clear picture of his situation and place the events in a more realistic perspective. He also thought that Tom needed to talk to someone and share some of his pain and confusion in order to sort out his feelings. Mr. Brown identified two short-term goals (outcomes):

1. Client's anxiety will decrease to moderate levels by 4 PM.
2. Client will talk about his feelings and plans by 4 PM.

CASE STUDY 13–1   A Person in Severe Levels of Anxiety (Continued)

INTERVENTION

Mr. Brown took Tom to a quiet room in the back of the ED. He introduced himself to Tom and said he noticed that Tom was upset. He said "I will stay with you." At first, Tom found it difficult to sit down and continued pacing around the room. Mr. Brown sat quietly and calmly, listening to Tom' self-recriminations. He listened carefully to what Tom was saying and what he was not saying, to identify themes.

After a while, Tom became calmer and was able to sit next to Mr. Brown. Mr. Brown offered him orange juice, which he accepted and held tightly.

Mr. Brown spoke calmly, using simple, clear statements. He used communication tools that were helpful to Tom in sorting out his feelings and naming them.

DIALOGUE		THERAPEUTIC TOOL/COMMENT
Tom:	Yes . . . yes . . . I forgot to hide the bottles. She usually tells me when she feels bad. Why didn't she tell me?	
Nurse:	You think that if she had told you she wanted to kill herself you would have hidden the pills?	The nurse asks for clarification on Tom's thinking.
Tom:	Yes, if I had only known, this wouldn't have happened.	
Nurse:	It sounds as if you believe you should have known what your wife was thinking without her telling you.	Here the nurse clarifies Tom's expectations that he should be able to read his wife's mind.
Tom:	Well . . . yes . . . when you put it that way . . . I just don't know what I'll do if she dies.	

When Mr. Brown thought that Tom had discussed his feelings of guilt sufficiently, he asked Tom to clarify his thinking about his wife's behavior. Tom was able to place his feelings of guilt in a more realistic perspective. Next, Mr. Brown brought up another issue—the question of whether Tom's wife would live or die.

DIALOGUE		THERAPEUTIC TOOL/COMMENT
Nurse:	You stated that if you wife dies, you don't know what you will do.	Reflecting.
Tom:	Oh God (he begins to cry), I can't live without her . . . she's all I have in the world.	
Silence.		
Nurse:	She means a great deal to you.	The nurse reflects Tom's feelings back to him.
Tom:	Everything. Since her mother died, we are each other's only family.	
Nurse:	What would it mean to you if your wife died?	The nurse asks Tom to evaluate his feelings about his wife.
Tom:	I couldn't live by myself, alone. I couldn't stand it. (Starts to cry again.)	

Case Study continued on following page

CASE STUDY 13–1   *A Person in Severe Levels of Anxiety* (Continued)

Nurse:	It sounds as if being alone is very frightening to you.	The nurse restates in clear tones Tom's experience.
Tom:	Yes . . . I don't know how I'd manage by myself.	
Nurse:	A change like that could take time adjusting to.	The nurse validates that if Tom's wife died it would be very painful. At the same time, he implies hope that Tom could work through the death in time.
Tom:	Yes . . . it would be very hard.	

Again, Mr. Brown gave Tom a chance to sort out his feelings and fears. Mr. Brown helped him focus on the reality that his wife might die and encouraged him to express fears related to her possible death. After a while, Mr. Brown offered to go up to the ICU with Tom to see how his wife was doing. On arrival at the ICU, Anne, although still comatose, was stabilized and breathing on her own.

After arrival at the ICU, Tom started to worry about whether he had locked the door at home. Mr. Brown encouraged him to call neighbors and ask them to check the door. At this time, Tom was able to focus on everyday things. Mr. Brown made arrangements to see Tom the next day when he came in to visit his wife.

The next day, Mrs. Michaels regained consciousness, and she was discharged 1 week later. At the time of discharge, Tom and Anne Michaels were considering family therapy with the psychiatric nurse clinician once a week in the outpatient department.

EVALUATION

The first goal was to lower anxiety from severe to moderate within a given time. Mr. Brown could see that Tom had become more visibly calm: his trembling, wringing of hands, and stomping of feet had ceased, and he was able to focus on his thoughts and feelings with the aid of Mr. Brown.

The second short-term goal set for Tom was that he would talk about his feelings and plans within a given time. Tom was able to identify and discuss with the nurse feelings of guilt and fear of being left alone in the world if his wife should die. Both these feelings were overwhelming him. He was also able to make tentative plans with Mr. Brown for the future.

SUMMARY

Stress is a state produced by change in the environment that is perceived as challenging, threatening, or damaging to a person's well-being. Stress can lead to a variety of psychological and psychobiological responses, the most common of which is anxiety.

The basic emotion of anxiety is differentiated from fear in that the source of anxiety is unknown or unrecognized, while that of fear is a reaction to a specific threat. Anxiety can be normal, acute, or chronic in nature. Peplau opera-tionally defined four levels of anxiety. The client's perceptual field, ability to learn, and physical and other characteristics (see Table 13–1) are experienced differently at each level.

Effective psychosocial interventions are different for a person in mild to moderate levels of anxiety from those needed by a person in severe to panic levels of anxiety. Effective psychosocial nursing approaches are suggested in Tables 13–2 and 13–3. The Case Study at the end of the chapter gives good examples of how these interventions can be incorporated when working with a person in severe to panic levels of anxiety.

Ego defenses against anxiety can be adaptive or maladaptive. Vaillant has organized ego defenses into a hierarchy from mature, neurotic, immature, and psychotic defenses. Each of these levels on the hierarchy has been identified and the defenses under each level defined. Table 13–5 illustrates examples of adaptive and maladaptive use of many of the more commonly used defense mechanisms.

Visit the **Evolve** website at
http://evolve.elsevier.com/Varcarolis
for a post-test on the content in this chapter.

Visit the **Evolve** website at
http://evolve.elsevier.com/Varcarolis
for additional self-study exercises.

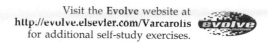

Critical Thinking and Chapter Review

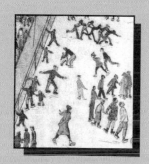

Critical Thinking

1. Tom La Rue is a senior at college and is taking his final exams for an engineering course. He is caught looking on and copying from his willing partner, June's, exam paper. Tom's paper is taken away, and he is asked to see the professor after the exams are all in. His heart starts to pound, his pulse and respiration rates increase, and he has to wipe perspiration from his hand and face several times. He feels as if he has to vomit and has a throbbing in his head. When speaking to the professor after the exams, he initially has difficulty focusing, and when he starts to speak his voice has tremors. Tom says that June convinced him that cheating was done all of the time and, in fact, it was her idea. Tom goes on to say that this "silly little exam" doesn't mean anything anyway, that he already passed the important courses. He tells the professor, "I thought you were the greatest, and now I see that you are a fool." When the professor remains calm, and explains that no matter Tom's thoughts on this matter, Tom was caught cheating, that he would have to take responsibility for his actions, and that the choice to cheat was his. He would have Tom go before the disciplinary board, which was the well-known procedure when one was caught cheating. When Tom realized this incident could affect his graduating on time, he began to yell at the professor and call him unflattering names. Another professor who had come in to take the exams to the grading machine witnessed this encounter.

   ■ Identify what level of anxiety Tom was in once caught cheating, and identify all of the signs and symptoms that helped you determine the correct level.
   ■ Identify and define five defense mechanisms that Tom used to lessen his anxiety.
   ■ Given the circumstances, once caught, how could Tom have reacted in a manner that would reflect more self-responsibility using more mature defenses?
   ■ If Tom at a later date used the defense mechanism altruism, in light of this situation, what are some of the ways he could do this?

Chapter Review

1. Shortly after being told that he has 90% blockage of three major coronary arteries and needs emergency coronary artery bypass surgery, Paul is noted by the nurse to appear dazed. His thoughts are scattered, as evidenced by his conversation jumping from topic to topic. He is unable to give direction to his wife when she asks him whom he wants her to notify. His pulse rate rises 15 points. The nurse can assess the type of anxiety Paul is experiencing as

   1. Normal anxiety.
   2. Sublimated anxiety.
   3. Acute (state) anxiety.
   4. Chronic (trait) anxiety.

2. Shortly after being told that he has 90% blockage of 3 major coronary arteries and needs emergency CABG surgery Paul is noted by the nurse to appear dazed. His thoughts are scattered as evidenced by his conversation jumping from topic to topic. He frequently states, "I'm overwhelmed. I don't know what to do." He is unable to give direction to his wife when she asks him whom he wants her to notify. His pulse rate rises 15 points. The nurse can assess Paul's level of anxiety as

   1. Mild.
   2. Moderate.
   3. Severe.
   4. Panic.

3. Nursing interventions that are helpful in lowering a client's level of anxiety from severe to moderate include

   1. Speak rapidly in a high-pitched voice.
   2. Permit existence of reality distortions.
   3. Validate themes client expresses.
   4. Provide solitude for client.

4. Defense mechanisms are

   1. A means of managing conflict.
   2. Predominantly conscious.
   3. Entirely pathological.
   4. Irreversible.

5. Which characteristic is true of mature ego defenses that is not true of ego defenses at the other levels? Mature defenses

   1. Arise from experiencing panic level anxiety.
   2. Do not distort reality to a significant degree.
   3. Disguise reality to make it less threatening.
   4. Are exclusively maladaptive.

REFERENCES

American Psychiatric Association (2000). *Diagnostic and statistical manual of mental disorders* (4th ed. Revised). Washington, D.C.: Author.

Gunderson, J. G., and Phillips, K. A. (1995). Personality disorders. In H. I. Kaplan and B. J. Sadock (Eds.), *Comprehensive textbook of psychiatry* (6th ed.) (Vol. 2, pp. 1425–1462). Baltimore: Williams & Wilkins.

Merikangas, K. R., and Kupfer, D. J. (1995). Mood disorders: Genetic aspects. In H. I. Kaplan and B. J. Sadock (Eds.), *Comprehensive textbook of psychiatry* (6th ed.) (Vol. 1, pp. 1102–1115). Baltimore: Williams & Wilkins.

Peplau, H. E. (1968). A working definition of anxiety. In S. F. Burd and M. A. Marshall (Eds.), *Some clinical approaches to psychiatric nursing.* New York: Macmillan.

Sullivan, H. S. (1953). *The interpersonal theory of psychiatry.* New York: W. W. Norton.

Vaillant, G. E. (1994). Ego mechanisms of defense and personality psychopathology. *Journal of Abnormal Psychology*, 103(1):44.

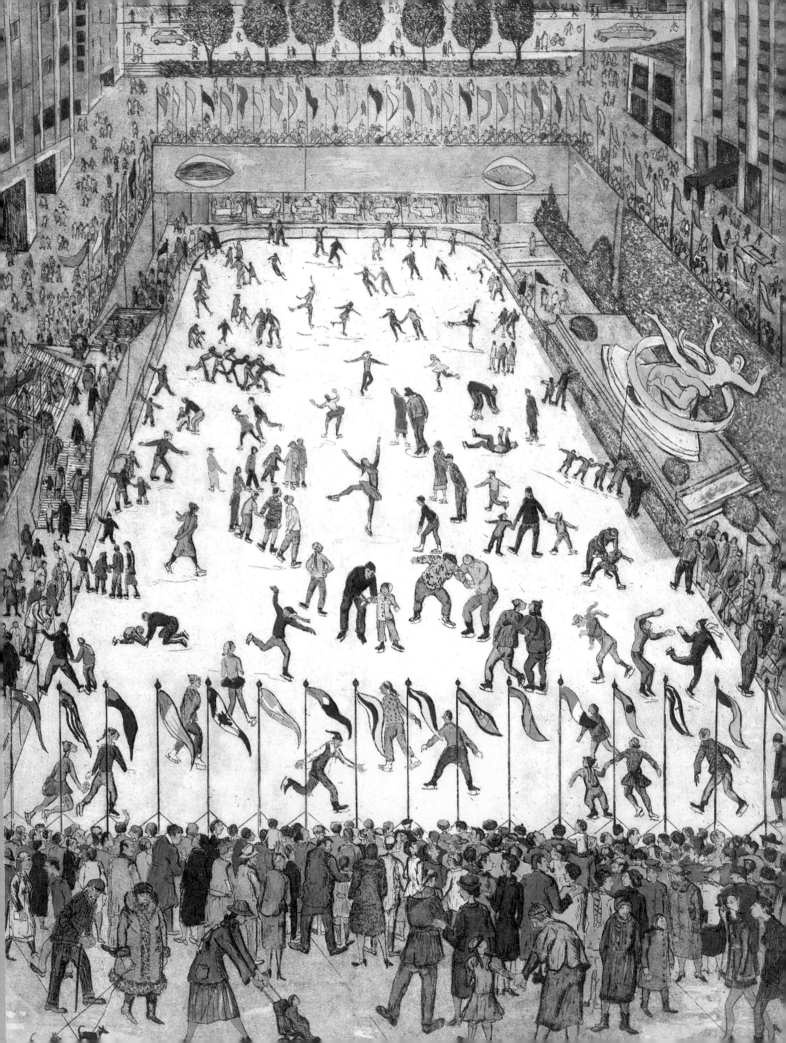

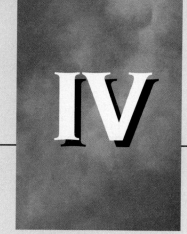
Psychobiological Disorders: Moderate to Severe

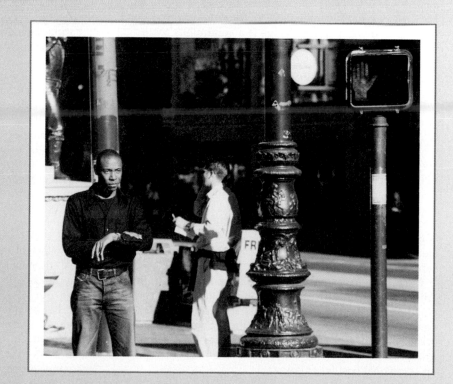

One of the symptoms of a nervous breakdown is the belief that one's work is terribly important.

BERTRAND RUSSELL
(1872–1970)

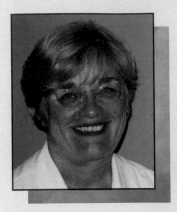

SHARON SHISLER

One of the values many nurses have in common is that of wanting to make a positive difference. One of my challenges during the last four years as a seasoned psychiatric clinical nurse specialist in a psychiatric treatment center of a general hospital has been conducting groups for clients with severe and chronic mental illness.

Making a difference with these clients is difficult for many reasons. For clients with chronic mental illness, change comes very slowly. Their imperceptible moves toward change are very difficult to identify and measure. There are no quick leaps into health as might be seen in a crisis. Patterns are relentlessly repeated. Cryptic reporting of subtle shifts in mood or behavior could mean a small step towards recovery or imminent danger with an acute break. Long-term compliance is seldom achieved, and short-term ownership for change is a continuous challenge for the client and the leader.

The group ranges in age from 34 to 72 years old. Most do not work, are on entitlements, and live in apartments or group residences with supervised, intensive outreach services. Their religious background is Catholic, Protestant, or Jewish. Few are married or have been married.

All show evidence of varying levels of cognitive and emotional functioning in their everyday life and relationships. Their diagnostic labels are depression, schizophrenia, dissociative identity disorder, schizo-affective disorder, borderline personality disorder, addictive disorders, mental retardation, early dementia, and brain damage related to seizures. These psychiatric conditions are further complicated by many chronic physical conditions such as sleep apnea, obesity, diabetes mellitus, emphysema, and cancer.

Most have had one or more psychiatric hospitalizations. All have a psychiatrist and an individual therapist. Most clients have attempted suicide, and for many, suicide is a consistent companion and ready option. Some participants actively hallucinate or experience other states during group sessions. Violence has been a rare event, except for an occasional hostile remark.

Before entering the group, each client goes through an assessment interview. Each participant describes their past experiences with groups and their perceptions of the strengths and weakness of any previous group experience. They also develop their individual goals for group therapy experience. These goals can relate to their emotional well-being, physical wellness, relationships, daily activities, losses, medications, and life stresses. They learn that the group has open membership with participants entering and leaving and meets twice per week for 1½ hours with a 15-minute break. Their length of stay may range from 3 months to 4 years. They also agree to interdisciplinary communications so that I can discuss events, mood, or changes with their psychiatrists and therapists and vice versa.

Various activities are incorporated into the process of the group, such as poetry, drawings, humor, relaxation techniques, meditation, visualizations, self-talk, positive affirmations, newspaper articles, television programs, previous group experiences, AA meetings, and emergent thoughts that occur at the time of the discussion. Since all of these clients experience multiple cognitive distortions, many strategies are used to increase retention and the likelihood of using group suggestions through the use of handouts, writing things down on flip charts or note books, anagrams, repetition, calendars, schedules, and role playing.

Topics for the groups include, but are not limited to, communication, triangles, empathetic confrontation, saying no and sticking to it, appropriate distancing vs. isolation, anger management, money management, nutrition, health issues, friendships, stigma and shame, active listening, connections, and how to get and keep support. Topics evolve out of the initial discussion for that week and could be the theme for one and up to four sessions, with introduction of a particular theme at later times.

The group members and leader mutually and spontaneously evolved a number of shortcuts, catchy phrases, or anagrams to repeat or emphasize specific premises and beliefs about the work of the group. Many of these shorthand expressions will be highlighted by the group's interactions with one of the participants, Arlene.

Arlene is a 32-year-old single woman with depression, alcohol addiction, obesity, diabetes, and an IQ of 80. She lives alone in an apartment with her cat, after taking more than 1 year to leave her mother's house. She has few friends, but is very close to another woman she met in an addiction recovery program.

She repetitively talked about her apparent lack of control with her mother, whom she described as demanding and domineering. She would attempt not seeing her every day and not running frequent errands for her. The group listened, made suggestions for more assertive actions, took the role of her mother and herself in role play situations, and verbalized her poor self-esteem, which she validated, all to no apparent success.

The group next tried a technique used with another member, called the *"Chain of Events"* exercise, and found that when Arlene attempted to assert herself, her mother rejected her. She then felt lonely, guilty, isolated, agitated, and sad. She found these separations intolerable and would be very vulnerable to manipulation by others, who would use her for her money. To gain "friends," she would give them money. On a few occasions, she stole money to be included in their drinking. She would become drunk and engage in dangerous activities, such as unprotected sex and walking on busy roads with no street lights or sidewalks. Her mother would then begin seeing her again and berate her for her behaviors, repeating the cycle again. This allowed the group to empathize with her loneliness and isolation and Arlene to begin to verbalize the dynamic process between her mother and herself.

The group then conducted a *"Cost-Benefit Analysis,"* or the positives and negatives of her relationship with her mother, and discovered many surprises. Although Arlene complained bitterly about the domination, blaming, and shaming by her mother (the minuses), she experienced many plusses by interacting with her mother: free lunch, interest and concern, and an imposed structure for her day that prevented her from feeling lonely. She also discovered that she used her separations as excuses for her impulsive behaviors of drinking and unsafe behaviors with a group of peers (a desired but destructive and dangerous end).

Once the group recognized the ambivalent nature of Arlene's relationship with her mother, they and the leader validated the positive side of her relationship with her mother and decreased their pressure for Arlene's complete separation from her mother. Arlene was acknowledged, recognized, and validated as being a very powerful person, who was able to refuse the group's suggestions and efforts to change according to their ideas.

After using various exercises and techniques, the group's awareness of Arlene's needs shifted and Arlene gradually was able to secure a doctor of her choice, get enrolled in a healthy living exercise and nutrition program, seek out more appropriate friends, and spend shorter periods of time with her mother, negotiating which errands she would do.

Listening with compassion and courage to the feelings, thoughts, and behaviors of the members of this group brought me to feel motivated and to creatively mobilize their inner and sometimes hidden strengths. The group's development of anagrams and other exercises serves many functions. They facilitate memory and actions, draw together a group of individuals with many heterogeneous issues but similar needs, and develop a culture of acceptance to help with the isolation of a mental illness and the stresses of life. This mutual process of creating exercises and anagrams from the "stuff" of their lives allows me to feel like I am making a difference in their lives and that they certainly are making a difference in the way my therapy has evolved. This in turn has helped to revitalize my work and prevent burnout.

Outline

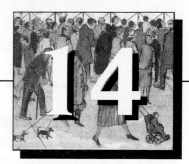

Anxiety Disorders

ELIZABETH M. VARCAROLIS

Key Terms and Concepts

The key terms and concepts listed here also appear in color where they are defined or first discussed in this chapter.

agoraphobia

anxiolytic drugs
(antianxiety drugs)

cognitive restructuring

compulsions

flashbacks

flooding

generalized anxiety
disorder

graduated exposure

modeling

obsessions

panic disorder

phobia

posttraumatic stress
disorder

response prevention

social phobias

specific phobias

systematic desensitization

Objectives

After studying this chapter, the reader will be able to

1. Identify various theories of the causes of anxiety disorders.

2. Describe clinical manifestations of each anxiety disorder.

3. Formulate appropriate nursing diagnoses that can be used with a person with an anxiety disorder.

4. Propose realistic outcome criteria for a client with (a) generalized anxiety disorder, (b) phobia, (c) posttraumatic stress disorder, (d) obsessive compulsive disorder.

5. Identify two nursing interventions appropriate for each of the following disorders: (a) generalized anxiety disorder, (b) phobia, (c) posttraumatic stress disorder, (d) obsessive-compulsive disorder.

6. Evaluate the effectiveness of care based on established outcome criteria.

7. Identify treatment modalities useful for each anxiety disorder.

8. Write a medication teaching plan for an individual on a benzodiazepine.

9. Recognize feelings that are commonly experienced by nurses caring for clients with anxiety disorders.

MENTAL HEALTH CONTINUUM FOR ANXIETY DISORDERS

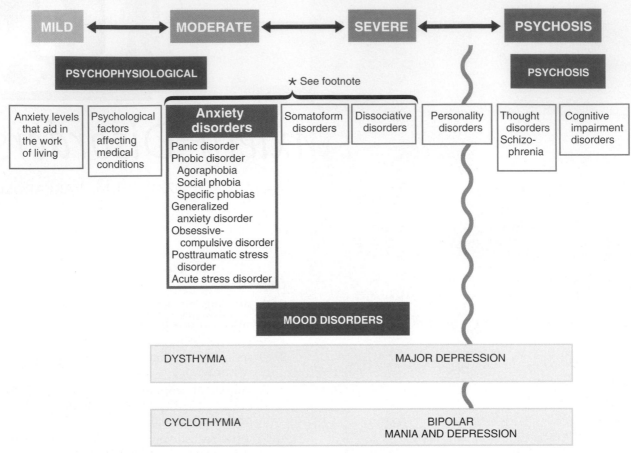

* These disorders are currently classified by presenting clinical symptoms. Previously they were called "neurotic" disorders.

Figure 14–1 The mental health continuum for anxiety disorders.

nxiety is a normal response to threatening situations. Anxiety becomes a problem when it interferes with adaptive behavior, causes physical symptoms, or exceeds a tolerable level.

Individuals with anxiety disorders use rigid, repetitive, and ineffective behaviors to try to control anxiety. The common element of these disorders is that individuals experience a degree of anxiety that is so high that it interferes with personal, occupational, or social functioning. Recent studies also suggest that chronic anxiety disorders may increase the rate of cardiovascular-related deaths. Anxiety disorders tend to be persistent and often disabling. Placement of these disorders on the mental health continuum can be seen in Figure 14–1.

PREVALENCE

Anxiety disorders are the most common of all psychiatric disorders and result in considerable distress and functional impairment among those who experience one or more of them (Hollander 1999). Refer to

Table 14–1 for prevalence rates for the individual anxiety disorders in the United States. People often have more than one anxiety disorder. **A note of caution:** differences in culture may affect the manifestation of anxiety disorders.

COMORBIDITY

Clinicians and researchers now recognize that anxiety disorders and depression occur together frequently. When they do, the illness is usually more severe and carries a poorer prognosis than either disorder alone (Gorman 1999). The *Diagnostic and Statistical Manual of Mental Disorders, Fourth Edition, Text Revised* (DSM-IV-TR) criteria (APA 2000) for mixed anxiety–depressive disorder is still being researched. The criteria are

A. Persistent or recurrent dysphoric mood lasting at least 1 month

The Editor would like to thank Helene S. Charron for her contribution to this chapter in the Third Edition of *Foundations of Psychiatric Mental Health Nursing.*

TABLE 14-1 *Prevalence Rates and Comorbidity of Anxiety Disorders*

DISORDER	PREVALENCE IN POPULATION	AGE OF ONSET	COMORBIDITY
Panic disorder (PD)	1–3.5%	Early 20s—60% Older than 30—40%	Agoraphobia (30%–40%) Major depression
Generalized anxiety disorder (GAD)	4–5%	Early 20s—chronic disorder	Agoraphobia Panic disorder Major depression Somatoform disorder
Phobias Agoraphobia (SPD)	2.8–5.3%—without PD	Between 20 and 40	Major depression (21.3%) Anxiety disorder
Social phobia	7.9–13%	Midteens to early 20s	Alcohol or other substance abuse
Obsessive-compulsive disorder (OCD)	2–2.5%	Mid 20s to early 30s	Major depression Panic disorder Phobia (simple/social) Alcohol dependence Tourette's syndrome
Posttraumatic stress disorder (PTSD)	1% in general population 20% in people exposed to traumatic life events, e.g., war, rape, catastrophe	After a traumatic life event	Panic attacks Substance abuse Depression Somatization diagnosis

Data from Welkowitz, L. A., Strvening, E. L., Pittman, J., Guardino, M., and Welkowitz, J. (2000). Obsessive-compulsive disorder and comorbid anxiety problems in a national anxiety screening sample. *Journal of Anxiety Disorders,* 14(5):471–482; and Horwath, E., and Weissman, N. M. (2000). The epidemiology and cross-national presentation of obsessive-compulsive disorder. *Psychiatric Clinics of North America,* 23(3):493–507.

B. The dysphoric mood is accompanied by at least 1 month of four (or more) of the following symptoms:
  1. Difficulty concentrating or mind going blank
  2. Sleep disturbance (difficulty falling or staying asleep or restless, unsatisfied sleep)
  3. Fatigue or low energy
  4. Irritability
  5. Worry
  6. Being easily moved to tears
  7. Hypervigilance
  8. Anticipating the worst
  9. Hopelessness (pervasive pessimism about the future)
  10. Low self-esteem; worthlessness

Other frequent comorbid disorders include substance abuse, somatization, and, as mentioned, other anther anxiety disorders. Table 14–1 identifies other common comorbid conditions for each of the other anxiety disorders.

THEORY

There is no longer any doubt that biological correlates predispose some individuals to pathological anxiety states (e.g., phobias, panic attacks). By the same token, traumatic life events, psychosocial factors, and sociocultural factors are also etiologically significant.

Genetic Correlates

Numerous studies substantiate that anxiety disorders tend to cluster in families. Nearly half of all clients with panic disorder have a relative with the disorder. Twin studies indicate a genetic component to both panic disorder and obsessive-compulsive disorder (OCD) (APA 2000). First-degree biological relatives of persons with OCD and persons with phobias have a higher frequency of these disorders than exists in the general population (APA 2000). An interesting set of findings concerns the possible relationship between a subset of OCDs and Tourette's disorder. Since there is considerable evidence for a genetic contribution to Tourette's disorder, there seems to be a genetic role in certain cases of OCDs (Fryer 1999).

Twin studies determined that phobias were mostly accounted for by genetic factors: heredity was 30% to 40%, depending on specific phobias

(Kendler et al. 1992). Social phobia also occurs more frequently among first-degree biological relatives of those with the disorder compared to the general population (APA 2000). First-degree biological relatives of people with panic disorder are up to eight times more likely to develop panic attacks (APA 2000). Even with posttraumatic stress disorder (PTSD), there is evidence of a heritable component (APA 2000).

For generalized anxiety disorder (GAD), there is a 19.5% morbidity risk among relatives of GAD clients compared with 3.5% risks in normal control relatives (Noyes et al. 1987).

Overall there is evidence of specific genetic contributions that increase a person's susceptibility to specific anxiety disorders. However, what has emerged is that genetics have something to do with anxiety disorders, but no anxiety disorder is likely to be the result of a specific gene (Gorman 1999). The actual genetics of anxiety disorders may be much more complicated than previous genetic theories supposed (Fryer 1999).

Biological Findings

Generalized Anxiety and Panic Disorders

Certain anatomic pathways (the limbic system) provide the structure for electrical impulses that either receive or send anxiety-related responses. Neurons release chemicals (neurotransmitters) that convey these messages. The neurochemicals that regulate anxiety in clients include epinephrine, norepinephrine, dopamine, serotonin, and γ-aminobutyric acid (GABA).

One theory, among many, is the GABA benzodiazepine theory. Recently discovered benzodiazepine receptors are linked to a receptor for inhibiting the neurotransmitter GABA. Binding of the benzodiazepines to the benzodiazepine receptor facilitates the action of GABA, which in turn slows neural transmission, giving a calming effect. This theory proposes that either the aberrant production of a substance that interferes with the binding of the benzodiazepine receptors or altered receptor sensitivity that interferes with proper benzodiazepine receptor function is involved with the unregulated anxiety levels (Hollander et al. 1999).

Numerous studies have linked sodium lactate infusions and CO_2 inhalation with the precipitation of panic attacks. Still other studies have shown an abnormal regulation of brainstem respiratory control centers and nonadrenergic and serotoninergic nuclei, and of their connections with key subcortical sites (Roy-Byrne and Cowley 1999).

A number of biological theories of both panic and GAD are prominent. Findings from numerous studies argue strongly against the notion that panic is a reaction to nonspecific stressors but rather point to a biological basis (Hollander 1999).

Phobias

Social phobias are accompanied by a surge of plasma epinephrine. People with social phobias exhibit a blunted growth hormone response to clonidine challenges, suggesting an underlying noradrenergic dysfunction similar to that seen in clients with panic disorder.

Obsessive-Compulsive Disorder

Neuroimaging techniques point to orbitofrontal-limbic-basal ganglia circuit dysfunction. For example, obsessions may be related to a defect in neural inhibition of dominant frontal systems, leading to the inability to inhibit unwanted verbal ideation, mental representations, and their corresponding motor sequences (Hollander 1999).

Neurochemistry of OCD points to serotonin (5-hydroxytryptamine), which normally is a mediator of impulsivity, suicidality, aggression, anxiety, social dominance, and learning. "Dysregulation of this behaviorally inhibitory neurotransmitter may possibly contribute to the repetitive obsessions and ritualistic behaviors seen in OCD clients" (Hollander 1999, p. 605).

Posttraumatic Stress Disorder

There are a number of biological theories associated with PTSD. Some investigators suggest that extreme stress in the form of physical, sexual, or psychological abuse is associated with damaging effects to the brain. Other studies support the hypothesis that abuse affects brain structure by reduction in the hippocampal size in clients with PTSD (Bremner et al. 1997).

Psychological Factors

Early theories about the development of anxiety disorders center around the idea that unconscious childhood conflicts are the basis for symptom development. **Freud** taught that anxiety resulted from the threatened breakthrough of repressed ideas or emotions from the unconscious into consciousness. Freud also suggested that ego defense mechanisms are used by the individual to keep anxiety at manageable levels. Later in this chapter, Table 14–9 defines and gives examples of defense mechanisms commonly used by individuals with anxiety disorders. The use of defense mechanisms results in behavior that is not wholly adaptive because of its rigidity and repetitive nature. Chapters 2 and 13 provide the reader with more depth on the dynamics of defense mechanisms.

Harry Stack Sullivan placed anxiety in an interpersonal context. He believed that all anxiety is linked either to the emotional distress caused when early needs go unmet or to the anxiety transmitted to the infant from the caregiver through the process of empathy. Thus, the anxiety experienced early in life becomes the prototype for that experienced when unpleasant events occur later in life.

Learning theories provide another view. Behavioral psychologists conceptualize anxiety as a learned response that can be unlearned. Some individuals may learn to be anxious from the modeling provided by parents or peers. For example, a mother who is fearful of thunder and lightning and who hides in closets during storms may transmit her anxiety to her children, who continue to adopt her behavior even into adult life. Such individuals can unlearn behaviors by observing others who react normally to a storm.

Cognitive theorists take the position that anxiety disorders are caused by distortions in an individual's thinking and perceiving. Ellis (1978) suggested that socially anxious people believe they must be approved of by everyone at all times. Because such individuals believe that any mistake they make will have catastrophic results, they experience acute anxiety.

Cultural Considerations

Reliable data on the incidence of anxiety disorders and ritualistic behaviors in this and other cultures are sparse. Leff (1988) suggested that traditional or culture-bound illnesses must be differentiated from anxiety disorders. Hispanic Americans may suffer a traditional illness called *susto* (fright). Susto is believed to cause a part of the self (the spirit) to separate from the body. As the spirit leaves, cold air rushes in. The victim experiences anxiety, fear, weakness, malaise, and anorexia. A traditional illness identified among African Americans is the *nervous breakdown*, characterized by increased anxiety, tension, altered self-care activities, and (in some instances) sadness and the hearing of voices. In some cultures, panic attacks may involve intense fear of witchcraft or magic (APA 2000).

Values conflicts created by immigration and assimilation into a new culture may be responsible for increased anxiety. For example, young adult émigrés of certain cultures (e.g., Asian Americans, Puerto Rican Americans, Vietnamese Americans) often experience increased anxiety when they challenge the traditional belief that the father is the authoritarian head of the family. Sociocultural variation in symptoms of anxiety disorders has also been noted. The way in which anxiety is manifested differs from culture to culture. Individuals of some cultures express anxiety through somatic symptoms, while in other cultures, cognitive symptoms of anxiety predominate. In some cultures, panic attacks involve fear of magic or witchcraft. Panic attacks experienced by Latin Americans and Northern Europeans often involve sensations of choking, smothering, numbness, or tingling, as well as fear of dying. Because fear of magic or spirits is considered normal in some cultures, it cannot be diagnosed as phobic unless the fear is excessive **in the context of the culture.** Social phobias manifested by individuals from the Japanese and Korean cultures may involve extreme anxiety centered on a belief that the individual's blushing, eye contact, or body odor is offensive to others (APA 2000). Similarly, one must be aware of the cultural norm before labeling ritualistic behavior as obsessive-compulsive. Nurses must be particularly alert for symptoms of PTSD in individuals who have recently emigrated from areas of social and civil unrest (APA 2000).

THE CLINICAL PICTURE

Anxiety disorders refer to a number of disorders, including the following:

■ Panic disorders
■ Phobias
■ OCDs
■ GAD
■ Stress response
■ Anxiety due to medical conditions
■ Anxiety due to substance use

DSM-IV-TR lists 11 anxiety disorders, each of which is explored in this section. Figure 14–2 presents the DSM-IV-TR criteria for various anxiety disorders.

Panic Disorder

The panic attack is the key feature of panic disorder, which is characterized by a pattern of recurring panic attacks. See the following Vignette for signs and symptoms of panic attacks. Panic disorder without agoraphobia is characterized by recurrent unexpected panic attacks, about which the individual is persistently concerned (APA 2000).

A **panic attack** involves the sudden onset of extreme apprehension or fear, usually associated with feelings of impending doom. The feelings of terror present during a panic attack are so severe that normal function is suspended, the perceptual field is severely limited, and misinterpretation of reality may occur. Severe personality disorganization is evident. Persons experiencing a panic attack may believe that they are losing their mind or are having a heart attack. The attacks are often accompanied by highly uncomfortable physical symptoms, such as palpitations, chest pain, breathing difficulties, nausea, feelings of choking, chills, and hot flashes. Typically, panic attacks come "out of the blue" (i.e., suddenly and not necessarily provoked by stress), are extremely intense, last a matter of minutes, and then subside.

Vignette

■ *Dora, a 30-year-old pharmacist, lives at home and cares for her mother. After her mother's death from heart disease, Dora begins to experience tension, irritability, and sleep disturbance. On several occasions, Dora awakens gasping for breath. Her heart pounds, and she feels a tight sensation, like a band around her chest. Her pulse typi-*

DSM-IV-TR CRITERIA FOR ANXIETY DISORDERS

ANXIETY DISORDERS

Panic Disorder

1. Both A and B
   A. Recurrent episodes of panic attacks.
   B. At least one of the attacks has been followed by one month (or more) of the following:
      1. Persistent concern about having additional attacks
      2. Worry about consequences ("going crazy," having a heart attack, losing control)
      3. Significant change in behavior

2. A. Absence of agoraphobia = **Panic disorder without agoraphobia.**
   B. Presence of agoraphobia = **Panic disorder with agoraphobia.**

Phobias

1. Irrational fear of an object or situation that persists although the person may recognize it as unreasonable.

2. Types include:
   • **Agoraphobia**: Fear of being alone in open or public places where escape might be difficult. May not leave home.
   • **Social phobia**: Fear of situations where one might be seen and embarrassed or criticized; speaking to authority figures, public speaking, or performing.
   • **Specific phobia**: Fear of a single object, activity, or situation (e.g., snakes, closed spaces, flying).

3. Anxiety is severe if the object, situation, or activity cannot be avoided.

Obsessive-Compulsive Disorder (OCD)

1. Either obsessions or compulsions
   A. Preoccupation with persistent intrusive thoughts, impulses, or images (obsession), or
   B. Repetitive behaviors or mental acts that the person feels driven to perform in order to reduce distress or prevent a dreaded event or situation (compulsion).

2. Person knows the obsessions/compulsions are excessive and unreasonable.

3. The obsession/compulsion can cause increased distress and is time-consuming.

Generalized Anxiety Disorder (GAD)

1. A. Excessive anxiety or worry more days than not over 6 months.
   B. Cannot control the worrying.

2. Anxiety and worry associated with 3 or more of the following symptoms:
   A. Restless, keyed-up
   B. Easily fatigued
   C. Difficulty concentrating, mind goes blank
   D. Irritability
   E. Muscle tension
   F. Sleep disturbance

3. Anxiety or worry or physical symptoms cause significant impairment in social, occupational, or other areas of important functioning.

Figure 14–2 DSM-IV-TR diagnostic criteria for anxiety disorders. (Adapted from American Psychiatric Association. [2000]. *Diagnostic and statistical manual of mental disorders* [4th ed., text revised]. Washington, D.C.: Author. Copyright 2000, American Psychiatric Association.)

cally increases to more than 110 beats per minute, and she experiences dizziness. She fears that she is going to die. On these occasions, Dora telephones a friend. The friend finds her wringing her hands, moaning, and appearing totally disorganized. In each instance, the friend takes Dora to the emergency department, where she remains overnight for observation and tests. All diagnostic test results are normal. The physician suggests that because no apparent organic basis exists for the episodes, they likely are panic attacks.

Beck (1996) emphasized that nurses can best help their clients if they learn to view panic as a separate concept from anxiety, especially in the clinical setting. Panic is not, according to Beck, a continuation of anxiety from moderate to severe; panic itself has an all-or-nothing quality, noted by its sudden and unexpected onset. Table 14–2 is a generic care plan for panic disorder.

Panic Disorder with Agoraphobia

Panic disorder with agoraphobia is characterized by recurrent panic attacks combined with agoraphobia. Agoraphobia involves intense, excessive anxiety or fear about being in places or situations from which escape might be difficult or embarrassing, or in which help might not be available if a panic attack occurred (APA 2000). The feared places are avoided by the individual in an effort to control anxiety. Examples of places or situations that are commonly avoided by clients with agoraphobia include being alone outside; being alone at home; traveling in a car, bus, or airplane; being on a bridge; and riding in an elevator. Avoidance behaviors can be debilitating and life constricting. Consider the effect on a father whose avoidance renders him unable to leave home and who thus cannot see his child's high school graduation, or the businesswoman whose avoidance of flying prevents her from attending distant business conferences, or the individual who avoids elevators and has no way to get to the 27th floor for an appointment. Refer to Figure 14–2 for the DSM-IV-TR criteria for panic disorders.

Vignette

■ *Jim is a 28-year-old man who suffers from panic attacks with agoraphobia. He once lived a very active life, often participating in thrill-seeking activities, like bungee jumping*

and skydiving. Jim's father, who had severe cardiovascular disease, died 2 years ago on his way to work. Since that time, Jim has become increasingly fearful of the outdoors. He gradually stopped leaving the family home because he experienced panic attacks; he feared that he would die if he left home.

Simple Agoraphobia

Agoraphobia without a history of panic disorder (i.e., unaccompanied by panic attacks) occurs only rarely, and it occurs early in the client's history. Over time, agoraphobia with panic attacks usually develops (Pine 1999).

Phobias

A phobia is a persistent, irrational fear of a specific object, activity, or situation that leads to a desire for avoidance, or actual avoidance, of the object, activity, or situation (APA 2000).

SPECIFIC PHOBIAS. Specific phobias are characterized by the experience of high levels of anxiety or fear provoked by a specific object or situation, such as dogs, spiders, heights, storms, water, sight of blood, closed spaces, tunnels, and bridges (APA 2000). Specific phobias are common and usually do not cause much difficulty because people can contrive to avoid the feared object. Clinical names for common phobias are given in Table 14–3.

Vignette

■ *Tran, who lives and works in Philadelphia, developed a morbid fear of closed spaces, such as elevators, after he read about the bombing of the World Trade Center in New York, even though he was not involved in the bombing. As his fear and anxiety intensified, it became necessary for him to use only stairs or escalators. Tran even became anxious if he had to enter closets or small storage rooms. Claustrophobia (fear of closed spaces) had developed.*

SOCIAL PHOBIAS. Social phobias are characterized by severe anxiety or fear provoked by exposure to a social situation or a performance situation (e.g., saying something that sounds foolish in public, not being able to answer questions in a classroom, eating in public, and performing on stage). Fear of public speaking is the most common social phobia.

TABLE 14–2 Interventions for Panic Disorder

NURSING DIAGNOSIS

Anxiety evidenced by sudden onset of fear of impending doom/dying; increased pulse, respirations, shortness of breath, possible chest pain, dizziness, abdominal distress, panic attacks.

Outcome criteria: Panic attacks will become less intense and time between episodes will lengthen so that clients can function comfortably at their usual level.

SHORT-TERM OUTCOMES	INTERVENTION	RATIONALE
1. Client's anxiety will decrease to moderate by (date).	1a. If hypercapnia occurs, instruct client to take slow, deep breaths. Breathe with client to obtain cooperation.	1a. Shifts focus from distressing symptoms.
	1b. Keep expectations minimal and simple.	1b. Anxiety limits ability to attend to complex tasks.
2. Client will gain mastery over panic episodes by (date).	2a. Help client connect feelings before attack with onset of attack: ■ "What were you thinking about just before the attack?" ■ "Can you identify what you were feeling just before the attack?"	2a. Physiological symptoms of anxiety usually appear first as the result of a stressor. They are immediately followed by automatic thoughts, such as "I'm dying" or "I'm going crazy," which are distorted assessments.
	2b. Help client recognize symptoms as resulting from anxiety, not from a catastrophic physical problem, for example. ■ Explain physical symptoms of anxiety. ■ Discuss the fact that anxiety causes sensations similar to physical events, such as a heart attack.	2b. Factual information and alternative interpretations can help client recognize distortions in thought.
	2c. Identify for client effective therapies for panic episodes.	2c. Cognitive-behavioral treatment is highly effective. Antipanic medication is highly appropriate.
	2d. Teach client abdominal breathing, to be used immediately when anxiety is detected.	2d. Breaks cycle of escalating symptoms of anxiety.
	2e. Teach client to use positive self-talk, such as "I can control my anxiety."	2e. Cognitive restructuring is an effective way to replace negative self-talk.
	2f. Teach client and family about any medication ordered for client's panic attacks (e.g., alprazolam, SSRIs).	2f. Client and family need to know what the medication can do, side effects, toxic effects, and who to call if untoward reactions occur.

SSRI, selective serotonin reuptake inhibitor.

Characteristically, phobic individuals experience overwhelming and crippling anxiety when they are faced with the object of the phobia. Phobic people go to great lengths to avoid the feared object or situation. A phobic person may not be able to think about or visualize the object or situation without becoming severely anxious. The life of a phobic person becomes more restricted as activities are given up so that the phobic object is avoided. All too frequently, complications ensue when people try to decrease anxiety through self-medication with alcohol or drugs. Identify on Figure 14–2 the DSM-IV-TR criteria for phobias, and see Table 14–4, which is a generic care plan for phobia.

Vignette

■ *Tim, a 22-year-old music theater major, develops a fear of performing on stage. He suffers severe anxiety attacks whenever he is scheduled to appear in a student production. Recently, he has become severely anxious when he is faced with classroom readings or singing solo in music class. He is thinking about changing his major.*

TABLE 14–3   Clinical Names for Common Phobias

CLINICAL NAME	FEARED OBJECT OR SITUATION
Acrophobia	Heights
Agoraphobia	Open spaces
Astraphobia	Electrical storms
Claustrophobia	Closed spaces
Glossophobia	Talking
Hematophobia	Blood
Hydrophobia	Water
Monophobia	Being alone
Mysophobia	Germs or dirt
Nyctophobia	Darkness
Pyrophobia	Fire
Xenophobia	Strangers
Zoophobia	Animals

Obsessive-Compulsive Disorder

Obsessions are defined as thoughts, impulses, or images that persist and recur, so that they cannot be dismissed from the mind. Obsessions often seem senseless to the individual who experiences them (ego-dystonic), while still causing the individual to experience severe anxiety.

Compulsions are ritualistic behaviors that an individual feels driven to perform in an attempt to reduce anxiety. The compulsive act temporarily reduces high levels of anxiety. Primary gain is achieved by compulsive rituals, but because the relief is only temporary, the compulsive act must be repeated again and again.

Although obsessions and compulsions can exist independently of each other, they most often occur together. Examples of common obsessions and compulsions are given in Table 14–5. Obsessive-compulsive disorder (OCD) behavior exists along a continuum. "Normal" individuals may experience mildly obsessive-compulsive behavior. Nearly everyone has had the experience of having a persistent tune run through the mind, despite attempts to push it away. Many people have had nagging doubts as to whether a door is locked or the stove is turned off. These doubts require the person to go back to check the door or stove. Minor compulsions, such as touching a lucky charm, knocking on wood, and making the sign of the cross on hearing disturbing news, are not harmful to the individual. Mild compulsions about timeliness, orderliness, and reliability are valued traits in U.S. society.

At the pathological end of the continuum are obsessive-compulsive symptoms that typically involve

TABLE 14–4   Interventions for Phobia

NURSING DIAGNOSIS
Fear related to a specific object or situation (social or specific)

CLIENT OUTCOMES	INTERVENTION	RATIONALE
1. Client will use adaptive coping strategies instead of avoidance.	1a. Determine type of phobia and when it first appeared.	1a. Determines whether phobia developed as a result of trauma, childhood experiences, or adult experiences.
	1b. Have client list consequences of contacting feared object.	1b. Isolates a specific fear associated with the object, e.g., a specific fear of flying may be a fear of getting hurt in a plane crash. These data can aid the therapist using cognitive therapy.
	1c. Identify for client which therapies have been highly effective with individuals who have the same disorder.	1c. Cognitive-behavioral techniques and treatment of panic attacks (if present) are highly successful.
	1d. Teach client relaxation techniques (deep breathing exercises, meditating, progressive muscle relaxation).	1d. Enhances client control over feelings and over level of anxiety.
	1e. Model unafraid behavior in phobic situation and discuss with client.	1e. Role modeling provides an opportunity to see healthy response to the phobic object or situation.

TABLE 14–5   *Common Obsessions and Compulsions*

TYPE OF OBSESSION	EXAMPLE	ACCOMPANYING COMPULSION
Doubt/need to check	"Did I turn off the stove?" repeatedly intrudes on the thinking of a woman who has recently gone from being a housewife to holding a secretarial position.	Checks to see if appliance is turned off, returning home several times each workday.
Sexual imagery or ideation	Young woman has recurrent thought when in presence of a man, "Pat his buttocks."	Avoids the presence of men if possible; if with men, excuses self to wash hands every 10–15 minutes.
Need for order	"Everything must be in its place" is the recurrent thought.	Arranges and rearranges items.
Violence	Man repeatedly has the thought "I should kill her" when he sees blonde women.	Abruptly turns head away from women and squints eyes to try to avoid seeing blondes.
Germs or dirt	Woman ruminates, "Everything is contaminated."	Avoids touching all objects. Scrubs hands if she is forced to touch any object.
Illness or death	Adolescent boy repeatedly thinks, "My teeth are decaying."	Repeats ritual of brushing and flossing up to a dozen times an hour.
Counting	Man counts aloud each step he takes.	Counting prevents mistakes and often serves to keep troublesome thought out of awareness.
Touching	Anorexic girl touches each doorknob she sees.	"Touch the knob or be a blob."
Washing or cleaning	Young woman repeatedly washes hands.	"Wash away my sins." Thought appeared after sexual encounter with a married man.
Avoidance	Man uses paper towel to touch objects touched by others.	"Maybe somebody with AIDS touched it."
Doing or undoing	Woman walks forward, then backward, sits in chair, then gets up and sits down again.	"Whatever I do has to be perfect or my husband won't love me."
Symmetry	Secretary lines up objects in rows on her desk, then realigns them repeatedly during the day.	"Secretaries who practice neatness never get fired."

AIDS, acquired immune deficiency syndrome.

issues of sexuality, violence, contamination, illness, or death. These obsessions or compulsions cause marked distress to the individual. People often feel humiliation and shame regarding these behaviors. The rituals are time consuming and interfere with normal routine, social activities, and relationships with others. Severe OCD consumes so much of the individual's mental processes that the performance of cognitive tasks may be impaired. Figure 14–3 shows positron-emission tomographic scans of OCD before and after successful pharmacological and behavioral treatment. Identify in Figure 14–2 the DSM-IV-TR criteria for OCD.

The Case Study at the end of the chapter gives an example of a young woman with OCD.

Generalized Anxiety Disorder

Generalized anxiety disorder (GAD) is characterized by excessive anxiety or worrying about numerous things that lasts for 6 months or longer (APA 2000). The individual with GAD also displays many of the following symptoms:

■ Restlessness
■ Fatigue
■ Poor concentration
■ Irritability
■ Tension
■ Sleep disturbance

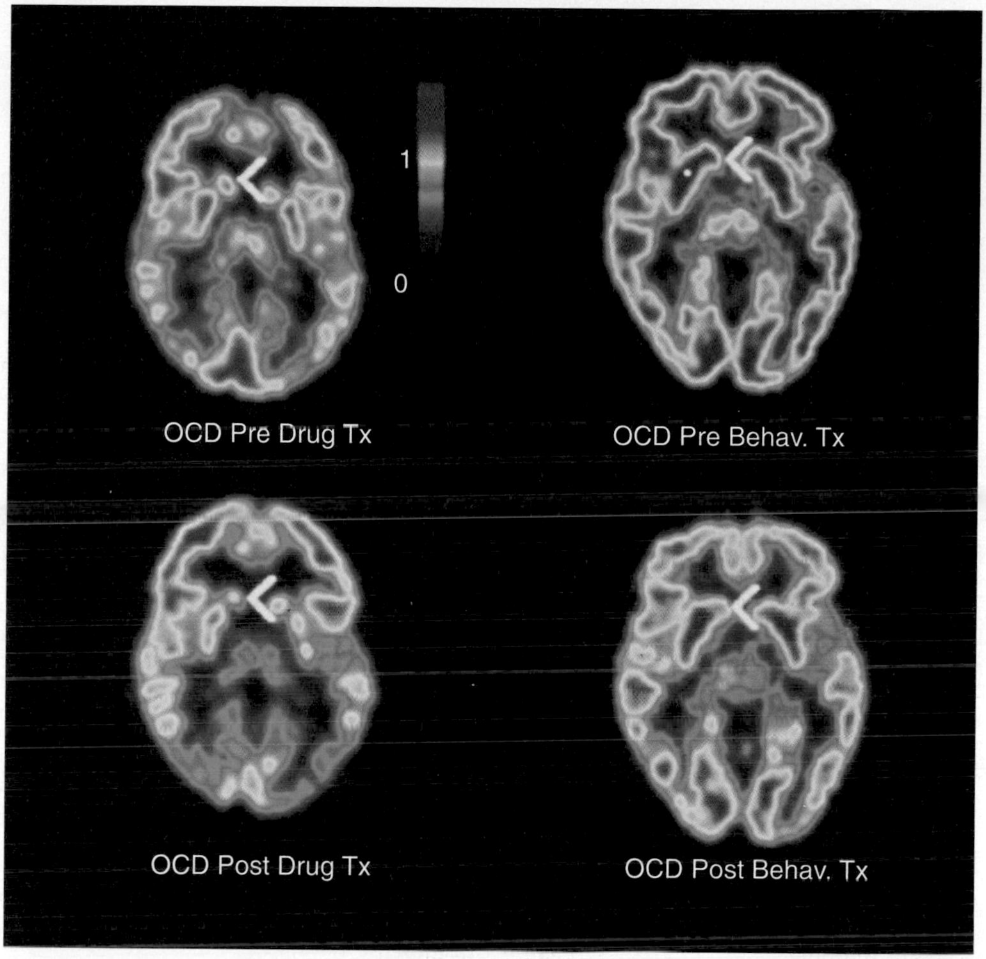

Figure 14-3 Positron-emission tomography scans of obsessive-compulsive disorder (OCD) clients show that the same reductions in brain caudate nucleus activity (center of brain) that occur after successful drug treatment (Tx) with clomipramine are also produced by successful behavior therapy. The scans provide tangible evidence that OCD involves a brain dysfunction that can be corrected by treatment—behavioral or pharmacological. (From Lewis Baxter, MD, University of Alabama. Courtesy of the National Institutes of Mental Health.)

The individual's worry is out of proportion to the true impact of the event or situation about which the individual is worried. Examples of worries typical in GAD are inadequacy in interpersonal relationships, job responsibilities, finances, health of family members, household chores, and lateness for appointments. Sleep disturbance is common because the individual worries about the day's events and real or imagined mistakes, reviews past problems, and anticipates future difficulties. Decision making is difficult, owing to poor concentration and dread of making a mistake. Check Figure 14–2 for the DSM-IV-TR criteria for GAD, and see Table 14–6 for a generic care plan for GAD.

Vignette

■ June is a 49-year-old legal secretary. She comes to the clinic complaining of feeling "so anxious I could jump out of my skin." She is shaky and diaphoretic; she has dilated pupils, an elevated pulse, and a quivering voice. She tells the nurse, "It was probably foolish to come here. Nobody understands me." June's only daughter is expecting her first child. Although the pregnancy is going well, June worries that something is wrong with the baby. "What if it's premature?" "What if it's deformed?"

June describes herself as tense and irritable. She has difficulty initiating sleep and cannot concentrate at work. She worries about making mistakes at work, about being fired from her position, and about the financial problems that could result. She often says "I just can't cope." Her daughter has begun calling several times a day to reassure her that all is well with the pregnancy and to try to decrease June's worry over other matters. The daughter has also begun shopping and housecleaning for June "to help her get some rest."

Anxiety Due to Medical Conditions

In anxiety due to medical conditions, the individual's symptoms of anxiety (panic attack, GAD, obsessive or compulsive) are a direct physiological result of a medical condition, such as pheochromocytoma, hyperthyroidism, pulmonary embolism, car-

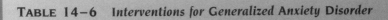

TABLE 14–6 *Interventions for Generalized Anxiety Disorder*

NURSING DIAGNOSIS
Ineffective coping: Related to persistent anxiety, fatigue, difficulty concentrating.
Outcome criteria: Client will maintain role performance.

SHORT-TERM GOALS	INTERVENTION	RATIONALE
1. Client will state that immediate distress is relieved by end of the session.	1a. Stay with client.	1a. Conveys acceptance and ability to give help.
	1b. Speak slowly and calmly.	1b. Conveys calm and promotes security.
	1c. Use short, simple sentences.	1c. Promotes comprehension.
	1d. Assure client that you are in control and can assist him or her.	1d. Severe anxiety gives feeling of loss of control.
	1e. Give brief directions.	1e. Reduces indecision. Conveys belief that client can respond in healthy manner.
	1f. Decrease excessive stimuli; provide quiet environment.	1f. Reduces need to focus on diverse stimuli. Promotes ability to concentrate.
	1g. After assessing level of anxiety, administer appropriate dose of anxiolytic agent, if warranted.	1g. Reduction of anxiety allows client to use coping skills.
	1h. Monitor and control own feelings.	1h. Anxiety is transmissible. Displays of negative emotion can cause client anxiety.
2. Client will be able to identify sources of anxiety by (date).	2a. Encourage client to discuss preceding events.	2a. Identification of stressors promotes future change.
	2b. Link client's behavior to feelings.	2b. Promotes self-awareness.
	2c. Teach cognitive therapy principles: ■ Anxiety is the result of a dysfunctional appraisal of a situation. ■ Anxiety is the result of automatic thinking.	2c. Provides a basis for behavioral change.
	2d. Ask questions that clarify and dispute illogical thinking: "What evidence do you have?" "Explain the logic in that." "Are you basing that conclusion on fact or feeling?" "What's the worst thing that could happen?"	2d. Helps promote accurate cognition.
	2e. Have client give alternative interpretation.	2e. Broadens perspective. Helps client think in a new way about problem or symptom.
3. Client will identify strengths and coping skills by (date).	3a. Identify what has provided relief in the past.	3a. Provides awareness of self as individual with some ability to cope.
	3b. Have client write assessment of strengths.	3b. Increases self-acceptance.
	3c. Reframe situation in ways that are positive.	3c. Provides a new perspective and converts distorted thinking.

diac dysrhythmias, and chronic obstructive pulmonary disease (APA 2000). To determine whether the anxiety symptoms are due to a medical condition, a careful and comprehensive assessment of multiple factors is necessary (APA 2000). Evidence needs to be present from the history, physical examination, or laboratory findings that the disturbance is the direct result of a general medical condition (APA 2000). Refer to Table 14–7 for a list of medical disorders that may contribute to anxiety symptoms.

Vignette

■ *Edmund is a 67-year-old man who has poorly controlled atrial fibrillation. His chief complaint is that he feels anxious most of the time. Edmund often experiences a feeling of impending doom and describes himself as "worrying a lot about my heart."*

Substance-Induced Anxiety Disorder

Substance-induced anxiety disorder is characterized by symptoms of anxiety, panic attacks, obsessions,

TABLE 14–7 *Medical Causes of Anxiety*

SYSTEM	DISORDERS
Respiratory	Chronic obstructive pulmonary disease
	Pulmonary embolism
	Asthma
	Hypoxia
	Pulmonary edema
Cardiovascular	Angina pectoris
	Arrhythmias
	Congestive heart failure
	Hypertension
	Hypotension
	Mitral valve prolapse
Endocrine	Hyperthyroidism
	Hypoglycemia
	Pheochromocytoma
	Carcinoid syndrome
	Hypercortisolemia
Neurological	Delirium
	Essential tremor
	Complex partial seizures
	Parkinson's disease
	Akathisia
	Otoneurological disorders
	Postconcussion syndrome
Metabolic	Hypercalcemia
	Hyperkalemia
	Hyponatremia
	Porphyria

and compulsions that developed with the use of the substance or within a month of stopping use of the substance (APA 2000). Once again, evidence needs to be established through the history, physical examination, or laboratory findings that either substance use, intoxication, or withdrawal from a substance is occurring (e.g., alcohol, amphetamine-like substance, inhalant, hallucinogenic, rave drugs, and others) (APA 2000).

Vignette

■ *Juana is a 46-year-old advertising executive whose physician had prescribed diazepam (Valium) "for nerves" for 2 years. When Juana changes physicians, she stops using diazepam. Three weeks after stopping the benzodiazepine, Juana begins to experience symptoms of severe anxiety and contacts her physician, who makes the diagnosis of substance-induced anxiety disorder arising as a result of diazepam withdrawal.*

Anxiety disorder not otherwise specified, including mixed anxiety-depressive disorder, is a diagnostic category used for the coding of disorders in which anxiety or phobic avoidance predominates and that do not meet other diagnostic criteria.

Posttraumatic Stress Disorder

Posttraumatic stress disorder (PTSD) (APA 2000) is characterized by repeated re-experiencing of a highly traumatic event that involved actual or threatened death or serious injury to self or others, to which the individual responded with intense fear, helplessness, or horror. PTSD may occur after any traumatic event that is outside the range of usual experience; examples are military combat; experience as a prisoner of war; natural disasters, such as floods, tornadoes, and earthquakes; human disasters, such as plane and train accidents; crime-related events, such as bombings, assaults, muggings, rapes, and hostage taking; or a diagnosis of a life-threatening illness. PTSD symptoms often begin within 3 months after the trauma, but a delay of months or years is not uncommon (Fig. 14–4). The major features of PTSD are

■ Persistent re-experiencing of the trauma through recurrent intrusive recollections of the event, through dreams, and through flashbacks. (Flashbacks are dissociative experiences during which the event is relived and the person behaves as though he or she is experiencing the event at that time.)
■ Persistent avoidance of stimuli associated with the trauma that results in the individual's avoiding

DSM-IV-TR CRITERIA FOR ANXIETY DISORDERS-STRESS RESPONSE

ANXIETY DISORDERS: STRESS RESPONSE

POSTTRAUMATIC STRESS DISORDER

1. The person experienced, witnessed, or was confronted with an event that involved actual, threatened death to self or others, responding in fear, helplessness, or horror.

2. The event is persistently reexperienced by:
   (a) Recurrent and intrusive recollections of the event, including images, thoughts, or perceptions
   (b) Distressing dreams or images
   (c) Reliving the event through flashbacks, illusions, hallucinations

3. Persistent avoidance of stimuli associated with trauma:
   (a) Avoidance of thoughts, feelings, conversations
   (b) Avoidance of people, places, activities
   (c) Inability to recall aspects of trauma
   (d) Decreased interest in usual activities
   (e) Feelings of detachment, estrangement from others
   (f) Restriction in feelings (love, enthusiasm, joy)
   (g) Sense of shortened feelings

4. Persistent symptoms of increased arousal (two or more):
   (a) Difficulty falling/staying asleep
   (b) Irritability/outbursts of anger
   (c) Difficulty concentrating

5. **Duration more than 1 month:**
   • Acute: Duration less than 3 months
   • Chronic: Duration 3 months or more
   • Delayed: If onset of symptoms is at least 6 months after stress

ACUTE STRESS RESPONSE

1. The person experienced, witnessed, or was confronted with an event that involved actual, threatened death to self or others, responding in fear, helplessness, or horror.

2. Three or more of the following dissociative symptoms:
   (a) Sense of numbing, detachment, or absence of emotional response
   (b) Reduced awareness of surroundings (e.g., "in a daze")
   (c) Derealization
   (d) Depersonalization
   (e) Amnesia for an important aspect of the trauma

3. The event is persistently reexperienced by:
   (a) Distressing dreams or images
   (b) Reliving the event through flashbacks, illusions, hallucinations
   (c) Distress on exposure to reminders of the traumatic event

4. Marked avoidance of stimuli that arouse memory of trauma (thoughts, feelings, people, places, activities, conversations).

5. Marked symptoms of anxiety:
   (a) Difficulty falling/staying asleep
   (b) Irritability/outbursts of anger
   (c) Difficulty concentrating

6. Causes impairment in social, occupational, and other functioning, or impairs ability to complete some memory tasks.

7. **Not due to drug of abuse/medications or medical condition.**

8. **Lasts from 2 days to 4 weeks, and occurs within 4 weeks of the traumatic event.**

Figure 14–4 DSM-IV-TR diagnostic criteria for acute stress disorder. (Adapted from American Psychiatric Association. [2000]. *Diagnostic and statistical manual of mental disorders* [4th ed., text revised]. Washington, D.C.: Author. Copyright 2000, American Psychiatric Association.)

talking about the event or avoiding activities, people, or places that arouse memories of the trauma
■ After the trauma, experiencing of persistent numbing of general responsiveness, as evidenced by feeling detached or estranged from others, feeling empty inside, feeling turned off to others
■ After the trauma, experiencing of persistent symptoms of increased arousal, as evidenced by irritability, difficulty sleeping, difficulty concentrating, hypervigilance, or exaggerated startle response

Difficulty with interpersonal, social, or occupational relationships nearly always accompanies PTSD, and trust is a common issue of concern. Child and spousal abuse may accompany hypervigilance and irritability. Chemical abuse may begin as an attempt to self-medicate to relieve anxiety. Table 14–8 is a generic care plan for PTSD.

Vignette

■ *While visiting in Mexico, Julio experienced a severe earthquake. He was unhurt except for cuts and bruises, but he was trapped for 2 days in a collapsed building. Six months later, back in the United States, Julio says of himself, "I'm a mess! I can't relate to my friends the way I used to. I feel numb inside, and I can't concentrate on what anyone is saying to me." He re-experiences hearing and seeing the building collapse around him and feels the sense of fear he experienced when he thought that he might not be found in the rubble (flashback). He startles at any crackling, creaking, or rumbling noise. He is awakened at night by nightmares in which he is trapped.*

It is important for health care workers to realize that exposure to stimuli that are reminiscent of the original trauma may cause an exacerbation of the trauma. For example, Noyes (1996) concluded that the infamous bombing of Oklahoma City caused an exacerbation of symptoms in veterans from World War II, the Korean war, and the Vietnamese conflict.

Acute Stress Disorder

Acute stress disorder occurs within 1 month after exposure to a highly traumatic event, such as those listed in the section on PTSD. To be diagnosed with acute stress disorder, the individual must display at least three dissociative symptoms either during or after the traumatic event: a subjective sense of numbing, detachment, or absence of emotional responsiveness from the emotional experience; a reduction in awareness of surroundings; derealization (a sense of unreality related to the environment);

TABLE 14–8 Interventions for Posttraumatic Stress Disorder

NURSING DIAGNOSIS
Posttraumatic stress response: precipitated by a specific overwhelming and devastating event(s).

CLIENT OUTCOMES	INTERVENTION	RATIONALE
1. Client will cope effectively with thoughts and feelings associated with traumatic events.	1a. Be honest, nonjudgmental, and empathetic.	1a. Builds trust.
	1b. Assess the type of trauma, e.g., natural or human induced.	1b. Victims of natural disasters experience less guilt. Victims of human disasters experience more humiliation and guilt.
	1c. Assess immediate posttraumatic reaction and later coping.	1c. Numbing and denial are common. Knowing the range of behavior can help assess impact and meaning of trauma.
	1d. Assess functioning before event, including drug and alcohol use.	1d. Knowing premorbid function may suggest additional diagnoses.
	1e. Assess drug and alcohol use since the event.	1e. Attempts to self-medicate are common to reduce anxiety or induce sleep.
	1f. Explore shattered assumptions, e.g., "I'm a good person; why did this happen to me?" "This is a safe world."	1f. Victims need to find meaning in the event. Helplessness and anxiety result from lost feelings of safety.
	1g. Promote discussion of possible meanings of event. Compare this situation with others that are worse.	1g. Helps clients see themselves as less victimized and the world as more understandable.
	1h. Suggest that client was not responsible for traumatic event but is responsible for learning to cope.	1h. Reduces powerlessness.
	1i. Identify social support for client in community and encourage participation.	1i. Can decrease feelings of loneliness and alienation.
	1j. Encourage attendance at support group.	1j. Share experiences, feel understood, start to heal.
	1k. Encourage client to keep a journal focusing writing about the trauma.	1k. Writing about a trauma can lessen the intensity and preoccupation with the event over time.

depersonalization (experiencing a sense of unreality or self-estrangement); or dissociative amnesia (loss of memory) (APA 2000).

Vignette

■ *Barbara, a 22-year-old college student, is sexually assaulted by a family friend. In the emergency department, she describes feeling detached from her body and being unaware of her surroundings during the assault, "as though it took place in a vacuum." She displays virtually no affect (i.e., she does not cry or appear anxious, angry, or sad). Barbara finds it difficult to concentrate on the examiner's questions. Three days later, Barbara still feels as though her mind is detached from her body; she reports having difficulty sleeping, poor concentration, and startling whenever anyone touches her. When she sees the nurse 4 weeks after the event, Barbara expresses feelings of anger and sadness over the assault, displays the ability to concentrate, and states that she no longer feels as though her mind and body were detached. She describes being able to "sleep better" and "not being so jittery and easily startled."*

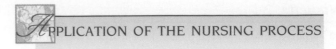

APPLICATION OF THE NURSING PROCESS

ASSESSMENT

Overall Symptoms of Anxiety

People with anxiety disorders rarely need hospitalization unless they are suicidal or have injuring compulsions (cutting self, banging a body part). Therefore, most clients prone to anxiety are encountered in a variety of community settings. A common example is an individual who is taken to an emergency department to rule out a heart attack when, in fact, the individual is experiencing a panic attack. Therefore, one of the first things that may need to be determined is if the anxiety is from a secondary source (medical or chemical condition, disease conditions, and substances) or from a primary source, as in an anxiety disorder. Refer to Table 14–7 for a list of medical disorders that might masquerade as anxiety symptoms.

TABLE 14–9   *Defenses Used in Anxiety Disorders*

PHENOMENON	DEFENSE	PURPOSE	EXAMPLE
Phobia	Displacement	In phobias, anxiety is reduced when strong feelings about the original object are directed at a less threatening object and that object is avoided.	Client has abnormal fear of cats. In therapy, it is discovered that the client unconsciously links cats to a feared and cruel mother.
Compulsion	Undoing	Performing a symbolic act cancels out an unacceptable act or idea.	Symbolic rituals, e.g., handwashing, cleaning, and checking. Handwashing removes guilt. Cleaning removes dirty thoughts. Checking protects against hostile thoughts.
Obsession	Reaction-formation	Anxiety-producing unacceptable thoughts or feelings are kept out of awareness by the opposite feeling or idea.	Client with strong aggressive feelings toward husband repeatedly thinks the opposite ("I love him with all my heart") to keep hostile feelings out of awareness.
	Intellectualization	Excessive use of reasoning, logic, or words is used to prevent the person from experiencing associated feelings.	Person talks in detail about parents' funeral but is unable to feel the associated pain of loss.
Posttraumatic stress disorder	Isolation	Facts associated with an anxiety-laden event remain conscious, but associated painful feelings are separated from the experience.	Client describes feeling "numb and empty inside."
	Repression		Client is unable to trust authority figures at work after taking orders from commanding officer to kill civilians while in combat.

Some preliminary symptoms of anxiety are when clients as discussed in Chapter 13 include the following reports:

■ Feel like they are going to die or have a sense of impending doom
■ Have narrowing perceptions and difficulty concentrating and problem solving
■ Have increased vital signs (blood pressure, pulse, and respiration), increased muscle tension, sweat glands activated, and dilated pupils
■ Complain of palpitations, urinary urgency and/or frequency, nausea, tightening throat, or unsteady voice
■ Complain of fatigue, difficulty sleeping, irritability, and disorganization

SYMPTOMS OF ANXIETY DISORDERS

Some symptoms of anxiety disorders are

■ **Panic attacks:** symptoms of severe anxiety that involves unpleasant physical, psychological, and cognitive symptoms (e.g., palpitations, feelings of impending death, inability to concentrate)
■ **Phobias:** excessive, irrational fears that cause the individual to avoid the feared object or situation in an attempt to control anxiety
■ **Obsessions:** persistent, recurrent, and intrusive thoughts, impulses, or images that cannot be dismissed from the mind
■ **Compulsions:** ritualistic behaviors that an individual feels driven to perform repetitively in an attempt to reduce anxiety, even against his or her own will

DEFENSES USED IN ANXIETY DISORDERS

People use a variety of ego defenses and behaviors to lessen the uncomfortable levels of anxiety. From a psychodynamic point of view, theorists believe that people who suffer from anxiety disorders employ specific defenses (Table 14–9). There is a simple preliminary screening test for anxiety disorders (Box 14–1). For a more comprehensive and sophisticated assessment tool, the Hamilton Rating Scale for Anxiety is a popular tool (Table 14–10). See how you rate on either or both these tools. **A word of caution:** This rating scale highlights important areas in the assessment of anxiety. Since many answers are subjective in nature, experienced clinicians use this tool as a guide when planning care in addition to their knowledge of their clients.

Self-Assessment

When working with an individual with an anxiety disorder, nurses may experience uncomfortable personal reactions. Often, anxiety originating in the cli-

BOX 14–1 *Preliminary Screening for Assessing Anxiety Symptoms*

1. Do you ever experience a sudden unexplained attack of intense fear, anxiety, or panic for no apparent reason?
2. Have you been afraid of not being able to get help or not being able to escape in certain situations, like being on a bridge, in a crowded store, or in a similar situation?
3. Do you find it difficult to control your worrying?
4. Do you spend more time than is necessary doing things over and over again, such as washing your hands, checking things, or counting items?
5. Do you either avoid or feel very uncomfortable in situations involving people, such as parties, weddings, dating, dances, or other social events?
6. Have you ever had an extremely frightening, traumatic, or horrible experience such as being a victim of a crime, seriously injured in a car accident, sexually assaulted, or seeing someone injured or killed?

From National Mental Illness Screening Project. (1999). National Anxiety Disorders Screening Day page: Sample test for anxiety disorder screening. *http://www.nmisp.org*; reprinted with permission. © 1999.

ent is experienced by the nurse empathetically. The nurse may experience feelings of frustration or anger while working with the anxiety-disordered client. The rituals of the client with OCD may frustrate the nurse's need to accomplish certain tasks within a given time. Communication with the client with OCD can also be frustrating. These clients correct and clarify repeatedly, as though they cannot let go of any topic. If the nurse uses therapeutic communication techniques, such as reflecting and paraphrasing, the client takes this opportunity to review material again and again, often angrily implying that the nurse has not understood. The client may introduce detail after detail, although the conversation becomes less and less clear. Communication requires much patience and the ability to provide clear structure.

In caring for the phobic client, the nurse may become frustrated after realizing that both client and nurse regard the fear as exaggerated and unrealistic, but the client is still unable to overcome the avoidant behavior. Behavioral change is often accomplished slowly. The process of recovery is different from that seen in a client with an infection, who is given antibiotics and demonstrates improvement within 24 hours. Nurses tend to become impatient

TABLE 14–10   *Hamilton Rating Scale for Anxiety*

Max Hamilton designed this scale to help clinicians gather information about anxiety states. The symptom inventory provides scaled information that classifies anxiety behaviors and assists the clinician in targeting behaviors and achieving outcome measures. Provide a rating for each indicator based on the following scale: 0 = None; 1 = Mild; 2 = Moderate; 3 = Disabling; 4 = Severe, Grossly Disabling.

ITEM	SYMPTOMS	RATING
1. Anxious mood	Worries, anticipation of the worst, fearful anticipation, irritability	_____
2. Tension	Feelings of tension, fatigability, startle response, moved to tears easily, trembling, feelings of restlessness, inability to relax	_____
3. Fear	Of dark, strangers, being left alone, animals, traffic, crowds	_____
4. Insomnia	Difficulty in falling asleep, broken sleep, unsatisfying sleep and fatigue on waking, dreams, nightmares, night terrors	_____
5. Intellectual (cognitive)	Difficulty in concentration, poor memory	_____
6. Depressed mood	Loss of interest, lack of pleasure in hobbies, depression, early waking, diurnal swings	_____
7. Somatic (sensory)	Tinnitus, blurring of vision, hot and cold flushes, feelings of weakness, picking sensation	_____
8. Somatic (muscular)	Pains and aches, twitchings, stiffness, myoclonic jerks, grinding of teeth, unsteady voice, increased muscular tone	_____
9. Cardiovascular symptoms	Tachycardia, palpitations, pain in chest, throbbing of vessels, fainting feelings, missing beat	_____
10. Respiratory symptoms	Pressure of constriction in chest, choking feelings, sighing, dyspnea	_____
11. Gastrointestinal symptoms	Difficulty in swallowing, wind, abdominal pain, burning sensations, abdominal fullness, nausea, vomiting, borborygmi, looseness of bowels, loss of weight, constipation	_____
12. Genitourinary symptoms	Frequency of micturition, urgency of micturition, amenorrhea, menorrhagic, development of frigidity, premature ejaculation, loss of libido, impotence	_____
13. Autonomic symptoms	Dry mouth, flushing, pallor, tendency to sweat, giddiness, tension headache, raising of hair	_____
14. Behavior at interview	Fidgeting, restlessness or pacing, tremor of hands, furrowed brow, strained face, sighing or rapid respiration, facial pallor, swallowing, belching, brisk tendon jerks, dilated pupils, exophthalmos	_____

Adapted from Hamilton, M. (1959). The assessment of anxiety states by rating. *British Journal of Medical Psychology, 32*:50–55.

with the anxious client and may feel angry when the client does not make rapid progress. Negative feelings are easily transmitted to the client, who then feels increasingly anxious.

The nurse who feels anger or frustration may withdraw from the client both emotionally and physically. This results in the client's feeling increasingly anxious and also withdrawing. Staging outcomes in small attainable steps can help prevent the nurse from feeling overwhelmed by the client's slow progress and can help the client gain a sense of control.

At the very least, the nurse often experiences increased tension and fatigue from mental strain when working with anxious clients. Unlike the client whose dressing needs to be changed several times a week, the client with anxiety requires emotional bandaging many times a week.

By having a clear understanding of the emotional pitfalls of working with clients who have anxiety disorders, the nurse is more prepared to minimize and avoid guilt associated with strong negative feelings. By examining personal feelings, the nurse is better able to understand their origin and to act objectively and constructively.

Assessment Guidelines

ASSESSMENT GUIDELINES: ANXIETY DISORDERS

1. A sound physical and neurological examination helps determine if the anxiety is primary or secondary to another psychiatric disorder, medical condition, or substance.
2. Assess for potential for self-harm, because it is known that people suffering from high levels of intractable anxiety may become desperate and attempt suicide.

3. Do a psychosocial assessment. Always ask the person: "Why do you think you are so anxious?" The client may identify a problem that should be addressed by counseling (stressful marriage, recent loss, stressful job or school situation).
4. Check for suicidal ideations (e.g., 20% of clients with panic disorder attempt suicide).
5. **Note:** Differences in culture can affect how anxiety is manifested.

NURSING DIAGNOSIS

Several nursing diagnoses should be considered for clients experiencing anxiety and anxiety disorders. The "related-to" component will vary with individual clients. Table 14–11 identifies potential nursing diagnoses for the anxious or client with acute anxiety disorder. Included are the signs and symptoms that might be found on assessment that support the diagnoses.

OUTCOME CRITERIA

The Nursing Outcomes Classification (NOC) (Johnson et al. 2000) has identified desired outcomes for clients with anxiety or anxiety-related disorders. The defining data for a nursing diagnosis correspond to the chosen hoped-for outcome, for example, for posttraumatic stress response related to a specific event as evidenced by flashbacks, nightmares, difficulty coping, the possible outcomes include

■ Reports decreased duration of episodes
■ Reports increased time between episodes

TABLE 14–11 *Potential Nursing Diagnosis for The Anxious Client*

SIGNS AND SYMPTOMS	NURSING DIAGNOSES
■ Concern that a panic attack will occur ■ Exposure to phobic object or situation ■ Presence of obsessive thoughts ■ Recurrent memories of traumatic event ■ Fear of panic attacks	Anxiety (moderate, severe, panic) Fear
■ High levels of anxiety interfere with the ability to work, disrupt relationships, and change ability to interact with others ■ Avoidance behaviors (phobia, agoraphobia) ■ Hypervigilance after a traumatic event ■ Inordinate time taken for obsession and compulsions	Ineffective coping Deficient diversional activity Social isolation Ineffective role performance
■ Difficulty with concentration ■ Preoccupation with obsessive thoughts ■ Disorganization associated with exposure to phobic object ■ Intrusive thoughts and memories of traumatic event ■ Excessive use of reason and logic associated with overcautiousness and fear of making a mistake	Disturbed thought processes Post-trauma syndrome
■ Unable to go to sleep related to intrusive thoughts, worrying, replaying a traumatic event, hypervigilance, fear	Disturbed sleep pattern Sleep deprivation Fatigue Hopelessness Chronic low self-esteem Spiritual distress
■ Feelings of hopelessness, inability to control one's life, low self-esteem related to inability to have some control in one's life	
■ Inability to perform self-care related to rituals	Self-care deficit
■ Skin excoriation related to rituals of excessive washing or excessive picking at the skin	Impaired skin integrity
■ Inability to eat because of constant ritual performance ■ Feeling of anxiety or excessive worrying overrides appetite and need to eat ■ Excessive overeating to appease intense worrying or high anxiety levels	Imbalanced nutrition (less or more than body requirements)

■ Uses effective coping strategies
■ Maintains social support
■ Reports adaptive steps
■ Maintains role expectation

The outcomes describe the client's state or situation that are expected to be influenced by nursing interventions (Johnson et al. 2000).

Suggestions for NOC outcome criteria for a per-

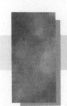

TABLE 14–12 *Nursing Outcomes: Anxiety Control*

Definition: Personal actions to eliminate or reduce feelings of apprehension and tension from an unidentifiable source

ANXIETY CONTROL INDICATORS	NEVER DEMON- STRATED 1	RARELY DEMON- STRATED 2	SOMETIMES DEMON- STRATED 3	OFTEN DEMON- STRATED 4	CONSISTENTLY DEMON- STRATED 5
1. Monitors intensity of anxiety	1	2	3	4	5
2. Eliminates precursors of anxiety	1	2	3	4	5
3. Decreases environmental stimuli when anxious	1	2	3	4	5
4. Seeks information to reduce anxiety					
5. Plans coping strategies for stressful situations	1	2	3	4	5
6. Uses effective coping strategies	1	2	3	4	5
7. Uses relaxation techniques to reduce anxiety	1	2	3	4	5
8. Reports decreased duration of episodes	1	2	3	4	5
9. Reports increased length of time between episodes	1	2	3	4	5
10. Maintains role performance	1	2	3	4	5
11. Maintains social relationships	1	2	3	4	5
12. Maintains concentration	1	2	3	4	5
13. Reports absence of sensory perceptual distortions	1	2	3	4	5
14. Reports adequate sleep	1	2	3	4	5
15. Reports absence of physical manifestations of anxiety	1	2	3	4	5
16. Behavioral manifestations of anxiety absent	1	2	3	4	5
17. Controls anxiety response	1	2	3	4	5
18. Other _____ (specify)	1	2	3	4	5

From Johnson, M., Mass, M., and Moorehead, S. (2000). *Nursing outcomes classification* (2nd ed.) (p. 116). St. Louis: Mosby.

son with an anxiety disorder are seen in Table 14–12. Suggestions for short-term and intermediate goals for specific anxiety disorders are in Table 14–13.

TABLE 14–13 *Suggested Short-Term and Intermediate Goals for Specific Anxiety Disorders*

ANXIETY DISORDER	SHORT-TERM OR INTERMEDIATE GOALS
Phobia	Clients will ■ Develop skills at reframing anxiety-provoking situation (date) ■ Work with nurse to desensitize self to feared object or situation (date) ■ Demonstrate one new relaxation skill that works well for them (date)
Generalized anxiety disorder	Clients will ■ State increased ability to make decisions and problem solve ■ Demonstrate ability to perform usual tasks even though still moderately anxious by (date) ■ Demonstrate one cognitive or behavioral coping skill that helps reduce anxious feelings by (date)
Obsessive-compulsive disorder	Clients will ■ Demonstrate techniques that can distract and distance self from thoughts that are anxiety producing by (date) ■ Decrease time spent in ritualistic behaviors ■ Demonstrate increased amount of time spent with family, friends and on pleasurable activities ■ State they have more control over intrusive thoughts and rituals by (date)
Posttraumatic stress disorder	Clients will ■ Attend support group at least once a week by (date) ■ Increase social support by one each month with aid of nurse/counselor ■ Report increase in restful sleep periods ■ Report decrease in nightmares or flashbacks ■ Demonstrate two new anxiety-reduction techniques (cognitive or behavioral) that work well for them

PLANNING

Anxiety disorders are encountered in numerous settings. Nurses encounter people with anxiety disorders in medical-surgical units while the people are undergoing treatment for physical illness in settings such as outpatient medical or psychiatric clinics, their homes, schools, day hospitals, and nursing homes. Cost-containment measures generally preclude admitting clients with anxiety disorders to inpatient psychiatric units. Therefore, planning for care usually involves selecting interventions that can be implemented in a community setting.

Whenever possible, the client should be encouraged to participate actively in planning. By sharing decision making with the client, the nurse increases the likelihood that positive outcomes will be attained. Shared planning is especially appropriate with a client with mild or moderate anxiety. When the client is experiencing severe levels of anxiety, the client may be unable to participate in planning, requiring the nurse to take a more directive role.

Most facilities have generic care plans or care maps for clients with specific anxiety disorders. On the previous pages you were given examples of useful strategies for clients with a number of common anxiety disorders.

INTERVENTIONS

The nurse uses the *Scope and Standards of Psychiatric–Mental Health Nursing Practice* when intervening with clients. Overall guidelines for nursing intervention include the following:

1. Identify community resources that can offer the client the development of skills that have been proven to be highly effective for people with a variety of anxiety disorders:

   ■ Cognitive restructuring
   ■ Relaxation training
   ■ Modeling techniques
   ■ Systematic desensitization/graduated exposure
   ■ Flooding (implosion therapy)
   ■ Behavior therapy

2. Identify community support groups for people with specific anxiety disorders.
3. Assess the need for interventions for families and significant others (support groups, family therapy, and help with issues that may be leading to relationship stress and turmoil).
4. When medications are used in conjunction with therapy, clients and their significant others will

need thorough teaching. Written information and instructions are given to the client/family/partner.

Counseling

Psychiatric mental health nurses use counseling to assist clients to improve or regain coping abilities, to foster mental health, and to prevent mental illness and disability. Treatment approaches that produce positive outcomes for clients with anxiety disorders include cognitive restructuring; relaxation training; and the behavioral techniques of modeling, graduated exposure (systematic desensitization therapy), flooding, and response prevention. Research has shown that combinations of these therapies may be more effective than single therapies (Gorman 1999). Advanced practice psychiatric mental health nurses may prescribe and conduct the therapies described in this section. While nurse generalists do not prescribe therapy, they are often the health professionals who implement the prescribed counseling; thus, nurse generalists must have a clear understanding of the various therapies.

COGNITIVE THERAPY

COGNITIVE RESTRUCTURING. Cognitive therapy, which was introduced in Chapter 2, assumes that cognitive errors made by the client produce mistaken negative beliefs that persist, despite evidence to the contrary. These distortions in thinking result in negative self-talk.

Counseling to promote cognitive restructuring calls for the nurse to assist the client to identify automatic negative anxiety-arousing thoughts and negative self-talk, to help the client discover the basis for these thoughts, and to assist the client to appraise the situation realistically and to replace the negative self-talk with supportive and calming self-talk.

Vignette

■ *Initially, June is assisted to identify several possible outcomes of making a mistake at work. The next step is to help her test the faulty thinking that making a mistake would automatically result in her being fired. June is able to see that being fired for making a mistake is highly unlikely. The same process is used to help June restructure her thinking about her daughter's pregnancy. In addition to working with June, the nurse gets in touch with June's daughter. Often, clients with anxiety disorders have "trained" significant others to act in ways that support their symptoms; this allows the client to receive secondary gains. June's daughter has taken over shopping and housecleaning for her mother. The nurse counsels June's daughter to allow her mother to gradually resume these activities.*

Cognitive restructuring was used to help June, a client with generalized anxiety disorder. Cognitive restructuring was also helpful to Jim.

Vignette

■ *Jim is required to monitor and record his automatic thoughts and phobic avoidance behaviors. Whenever Jim is faced with the need to leave his home, automatic thinking takes place: "When my father left home to go to work, he died. I'll die if I leave home to go to work." The nurse helps Jim to explore his father's health status in comparison with his own. This understanding helps Jim make a more rational appraisal of the possibility of his death.*

COGNITIVE-BEHAVIORAL THERAPY (CBT). CBT is a highly effective treatment modality for the anxiety disorders. CBT included a variety of approaches: psychoeducational, continuous panic monitoring, breathing retraining, development of anxiety management skill, cognitive restructuring, and in vivo (live) exposure to the feared object or situation.

Chapter 12 on stress reduction identifies a number of behavioral techniques used by many nurses that help reduce their and their client's anxiety and stress.

BEHAVIORAL THERAPY

RELAXATION TRAINING. Muscle groups cannot be both tense and relaxed at the same time; therefore, teaching a client how to relax the body results in tension reduction. Relaxation produces physiological effects that are opposite to those produced by anxiety (e.g., slowed heart rate, neuromuscular relaxation, calm state of mind). Anxious clients should be counseled that learning an effective relaxation method can be beneficial. Various relaxation techniques are described in Chapter 12.

MODELING. This technique, explained in Chapter 2, permits a client to see how an individual copes effectively with an object or a situation. In modeling, the client is expected to imitate the healthy coping behavior. The nurse often serves as a model of healthy behavior for clients, but family members and friends may also assume the role. Modeling was used by the nurse who, while working with Tran, did not show anxiety as she used elevators and obtained materials from storage.

SYSTEMATIC DESENSITIZATION THROUGH GRADUATED EXPOSURE. The technique of systematic desensitization through graduated exposure involves gradually introducing the client to a phobic object or situation in a predetermined sequence of least to most frightening. The following strategy might be used for an agoraphobic client like Jim.

At the direction of the therapist, the client may be asked to visualize being in a public place. When anxiety becomes severe, the client may be instructed to use a relaxation technique. When the imagined encounters become tolerable for the client, he or she goes on to work through a hierarchy of in vivo exposures, for example:

1. Opening the door and leaving the house
2. Walking down a street within a block from home
3. Riding in a car with a trusted person more than a block from home
4. Entering a small shop to purchase one item
5. Going to a supermarket to purchase a small list of items
6. Attending a movie or a play

Often, the activity is first undertaken with a trusted supportive person present, then it is undertaken alone. A psychiatrist, psychologist, or nurse therapist is usually responsible for setting up the hierarchy and for conducting the graduated exposure. However, the nurse generalist is often responsible for reinforcing gains made by the client by providing support as various objects on the continuum are revisited. At the Institute of Psychiatry in London, Marks (1995) reported that self-exposure treatment is being used more often to avoid frequent therapy sessions and to contain costs. The clinician's role is to teach the client how to perform the self-exposure.

FLOODING (IMPLOSION THERAPY). The purpose of flooding is to extinguish anxiety as a conditioned response. Flooding involves exposing an individual to large amounts of a stimulus that he or she finds undesirable. This technique may require the client to touch an object that is feared or found revolting or severely anxiety producing. For example, Sam, a client so obsessed with the idea of avoiding contamination that he used a paper towel to touch things, was required to touch objects in the room with his bare hand for an hour. Gradually, the client demonstrated less anxiety over having to touch "dirty" objects.

RESPONSE PREVENTION. Response prevention therapy is performed by a nurse practitioner or a clinical nurse specialist only on physician's orders. When compulsive individuals feel anxiety, they respond by performing a ritualized behavior with the hope of reducing anxiety; not permitting the individual to perform the compulsive behavior is termed **response prevention**. From response prevention, a form of behavior therapy, the client learns that anxiety can be managed if the compulsion is not carried out. Arlene, a client who engaged in handscrubbing after touching any object or person, was helped gradually to lengthen the time before scrubbing and to shorten the time of scrubbing. Eventually, the urges subsided. Such therapy not only changes behavior but also can change the brain's chemistry (Schwartz et al. 1996). At the beginning of the session, Arlene's anxiety was severe, but by the end, with support from the nurse, her anxiety had decreased to the point that she was able to touch a "clean" object without experiencing the urge to scrub.

THOUGHT STOPPING. Thought-stopping techniques have proved helpful to some clients with OCD. One technique calls for the client to shout "Stop!" when the obsession comes to mind. Eventually, the client learns to give the command silently. Another technique is to place a rubber band on the client's wrist with instructions to snap it whenever the obsession comes into awareness. Both techniques serve the purpose of helping the client dismiss the obsessive thought.

Milieu Therapy

As mentioned earlier, most clients who demonstrate anxiety disorders can be treated successfully as outpatients. Hospital admission is necessary only if prolonged severe anxiety is present, if symptoms that interfere with the individual's health are present, or if the individual is suicidal. When hospitalization is necessary, the following features of the therapeutic milieu can be especially helpful to the client:

- Structuring the daily routine to offer physical safety and predictability, thus reducing anxiety over the unknown
- Providing daily activities to prevent constant focus on anxiety or symptoms
- Providing therapeutic interactions
- Evaluating and communicating the effects of the environment on the client to facilitate nursing care planning

Self-Care Activities

Clients with anxiety disorders are usually able to meet their own basic physical needs. Self-care activities that are most likely to be affected are discussed in the following sections.

NUTRITION AND FLUID INTAKE

Clients who use ritualistic behaviors may be too involved with their rituals to take time to eat and drink; some phobic clients may be so afraid of germs that they cannot eat. In general, nutritious diets with snacks should be provided. Adequate intake should be firmly encouraged, but without entering into a power struggle. Weighing clients frequently (e.g., three times a week) is useful in assessing nutrition.

PERSONAL HYGIENE AND GROOMING

Some clients, especially those with OCD and phobias, may be excessively neat and may engage in time-consuming rituals associated with bathing and dressing. Hygiene, dressing, and grooming may take many hours. Maintenance of skin integrity may become a problem when the rituals involve excessive washing and the skin becomes excoriated and infected.

Some clients are indecisive about bathing or about what clothing should be worn. For the latter, limiting choices to two outfits is helpful. In the event of severe indecisiveness, simply presenting the client with the clothing to be worn may be necessary. The nurse may also need to remain with the client to give simple directions: "Put on your shirt . . . now, put on your slacks." Matter-of-fact support is effective in assisting the client to perform as much of the task as possible. The client should be encouraged to express thoughts and feelings about self-care. This communication can provide a basis for later health teaching or for ongoing dialogue about the client's abilities.

ELIMINATION

Clients with OCD may be so involved with the performance of rituals that they may suppress the urge to void and defecate. Constipation and urinary tract infections may result. Interventions may include creating a regular schedule for taking the client to the bathroom.

SLEEP

Anxious clients frequently have difficulty sleeping. Ritualistic clients may perform their rituals to the exclusion of resting and sleeping. Physical exhaustion may occur in highly ritualistic clients. Clients with GAD, PTSD, and acute stress disorder often experience sleep disturbance from nightmares. Monitoring sleep and keeping a sleep record may be useful in establishing the diagnosis of **sleep pattern disturbance** and evaluating progress.

Psychopharmacology

The evidence is not yet available to know for sure whether anxiety disorders are caused by an underlying neurochemical imbalance or psychological (cognitive, behavioral, or psychodynamic) problems. However, medication management of most anxiety disorders, with or without psychotherapy, is one of the most successful treatments in medicine today (Papp 1999). Four classes of medications have been found to be effective in the treatment of anxiety disorders:

1. Anxiolytics
2. Antidepressants
3. Beta blockers
4. Antihistamines

Selective serotonin reuptake inhibitors (SSRIs) and monoamine oxidase inhibitors (MAOIs) are more effective in **social phobia** than tricyclic antidepressants (TCAs) or beta blockers. SSRIs are more effective with OCD than are nonadrenergic antidepressants. SSRIs are more effective in panic disorders than TCAs or benzodiazepines (Sheehan, 1999). Table 14–14 presents the actions, indications for use, and daily doses of drugs commonly used in the treatment of anxiety disorders.

ANXIOLYTICS

Anxiolytic (antianxiety) drugs are often used to treat the somatic and psychological symptoms of anxiety disorders. When moderate to severe anxiety is reduced, clients are better able to participate in treatments directed at their underlying problems.

Symptoms of severe anxiety, such as that seen in panic disorder, can be treated with alprazolam (Xanax) and other short-acting benzodiazepines. Benzodiazepines (e.g., diazepam, alprazolam, lorazepam) should be used only on a short-term basis because dependence and addiction can develop quickly. However, Blair and associates (1996) cautioned against fear of addiction and undertreatment of anxiety disorders that could result from withholding a client's prn antianxiety dose.

Benzodiazepines have many side effects, making it necessary for the nurse to take care in assessing clients' reactions to the drugs. The more common side effects of the benzodiazepines are sedation (10%), dizziness, and ataxia (especially the elderly). Accumulation of active metabolites can lead to

■ Increased sedation
■ Decreased cognitive function
■ Ataxia

The **benzodiazepines** should not be given during pregnancy or when the client is breast feeding. See Box 14–2 for important information regarding client teaching.

Buspirone is a **nonbenzodiazepine anxiolytic** and does not cause dependence. Unlike the benzodiazepines and diphenylmethane antihistamines, buspirone does not produce an immediate calming effect. Thus, it cannot be given as a prn medication. Initial effects are experienced in 2 to 3 weeks, and full effects may take 4 to 6 weeks or even longer. Buspirone is particularly useful for the treatment of GAD, which tends to be a long-term disorder. Clients tak-

TABLE 14-14 *Medications for Anxiety Disorders*

GENERIC NAME	TRADE NAME	USUAL DAILY DOSE (MG/DAY)	ACTION AND INDICATION
Benzodiazepines			
Alprazolam	Xanax	0.75–4	Increase GABA release and receptor binding at synapses. Show preferential effect on limbic system. Useful for short-term treatment of anxiety; dependence and tolerance can develop
Clonazepam	Klonopin	1.5–20	
Diazepam	Valium	4–40	
Lorazepam	Ativan	0.5–6	
Oxazepam	Serax	30–120	
Chlordiazepoxide	Librium	15–100	
Prazepam	Centrax	20–60	
Halazepam	Paxipam	20–160	
Antihistamines			
Hydroxyzine hydrochloride	Atarax	100–300	Depress subcortical centers. Produce **no dependence, tolerance, or intoxication.** Can be used for anxiety relief for indefinite periods
Hydroxyzine pamoate	Vistaril	100–300	
Nonbenzodiazepine antianxiety agents			
Buspirone hydrochloride	BuSpar	15–40	Alleviates anxiety. Less sedating than the benzodiazepines. **Does not appear to produce physical or psychological dependence.** Requires 3 weeks or more to be effective
Beta Blockers			
Propranolol	Inderal	15–40	Used to relieve physical symptoms of anxiety, as in stage fright. Acts by attaching to sensors that detect arousal messages
Tricyclics			
Clomipramine	Anafranil	50–125	Used to prevent panic attacks, phobias, and PTSD. Act by regulating brain's reactions to serotonin. Clomipramine helpful for some in lowering obsessions in OCD
Imipramine	Tofranil	150–500	
Nortriptyline	Aventyl, Pamelor	75–125	
Desipramine	Norpramin	150–200	
MAOIs			
Phenelzine	Nardil	30–90	Used to treat panic disorders, phobias, and PTSD. Acts by blocking reuptake of norepinephrine and serotonin in central nervous system
SSRIs			
Sertraline	Zoloft	50–200	Used to treat OCD, panic, agoraphobia, generalized anxiety disorder. **Effective with mixed anxiety and depression**
Fluoxetine	Prozac	20–80	
Paroxetine	Paxil	20–60	
Fluvoxamine	Luvox	100–150	
Citalopram	Celexa	20–40	

GABA, γ-aminobutyric acid; MAOI, monoamine oxidase inhibitor; OCD, obsessive-compulsive disorder; PTSD, posttraumatic stress disorder; SSRI, selective serotonin reuptake inhibitor.

Box 14–2 *Client and Family Medication Teaching: Anxiety Disorders*

1. Caution the client

   ■ Not to increase dose or frequency of ingestion without prior approval of therapist.
   ■ That these medications reduce ability to handle mechanical equipment, e.g., cars, saws, and machinery.
   ■ Not to drink alcoholic beverages or take other antianxiety drugs because depressant effects of both would be potentiated.
   ■ To avoid drinking beverages containing caffeine because they decrease the desired effects of the drug.

2. Recommend that the client avoid becoming pregnant because taking benzodiazepines increases the risk of congenital anomalies.
3. Advise the client not to breast-feed because the drug is excreted in the milk and would have adverse effects on the infant.
4. Teach clients who are taking monoamine oxidase inhibitors about the details of tyramine-restricted diet (see Chapter 18).
5. Teach the client that

   ■ Stoppage of benzodiazepines after 3 to 4 months of daily use may cause withdrawal symptoms, e.g., insomnia, irritability, nervousness, dry mouth, tremors, convulsions, and confusion.
   ■ Medications should be taken with, or shortly after, meals or snacks to reduce gastrointestinal discomfort.
   ■ Drug interactions can occur: Antacids may delay absorption; cimetidine interferes with metabolism of benzodiazepines, causing increased sedation; central nervous system depressants, e.g., alcohol and barbiturates, cause increased sedation; serum phenytoin concentration may build up because of decreased metabolism.

6. Lower doses should be considered for elderly clients.

ing this drug should be counseled to take the drug regularly for maximal effectiveness. Two to 3 weeks or longer may be required before the full antianxiety effect of this drug is achieved.

ANTIDEPRESSANTS

Antidepressants also have a place in the treatment of anxiety disorders. TCAs, such as imipramine (Tofranil), desipramine (Norpramine), and clomipramine (Anafranil), are used to reduce the frequency and intensity of panic attacks with or without agoraphobia. Clomipramine is the TCA of choice for the treatment of OCD. PTSD is effectively treated with imipramine and amitriptyline (Elavil) (Sutherland and Davidson 1994). TCAs have anticholinergic side effects that may be annoying enough to cause people to discontinue their use. Clients should be counseled that these side effects often disappear with time. Clients should also be counseled that TCAs may require 2 to 4 weeks to take effect.

MAOIs, such as phenelzine (Nardil) and tranylcypromine (Parnate), have also been found to be effective in the treatment of panic attacks and social phobias. An important nursing consideration is that clients taking MAOIs must adhere to a tyramine-free diet or risk life-threatening hypertensive crisis (see Chapter 18).

SSRIs, such as fluoxetine (Prozac), sertraline (Zoloft), paroxetine (Paxil), and fluvoxamine (Luvox), are used to treat panic disorder, agoraphobia, OCD (DeVeaugh-Geiss 1994), and GAD. SSRIs are less likely than TCAs to produce anticholinergic side effects but may cause agitation, headaches, gastrointestinal disturbances, or sexual dysfunction. The SSRIs are commonly used in clients with a comorbid anxiety and depression.

BETA BLOCKERS

Beta blockers, such as propranolol (Inderal) and atenolol (Tenormin), can be helpful with anxiety disorders that are characterized by marked physical symptoms of anxiety, such as social phobia. Beta blockers are often given in a single dose to relieve severe physical symptoms of anxiety before a theatrical or concert performance, a public speaking engagement, or a job interview.

Box 14–2 summarizes the nursing implications and important client teaching as they relate to antianxiety drug therapy.

ANTIHISTAMINES

By contrast, diphenylmethane antihistamines, such as hydroxyzine hydrochloride (Atarax) and hydroxyzine pamoate (Vistaril), relieve symptoms of anxiety but produce no dependence, tolerance, or intoxication. This group of drugs can be used for anxiety relief over an indefinite period. The nurse generalist is responsible for administering medications; evaluating client response; educating clients and families about the medications, their side effects, and ways to diminish them; and educating about when to call the physician.

The advanced practice psychiatric mental health nurse may have prescriptive privileges to treat anxiety disorders with pharmacological agents, in addition to determining other aspects of the treatment plan. Table 14–15 summarizes accepted pharmaco-

TABLE 14–15 *Selected Treatment for Anxiety Disorders*

DISORDER	PHARMACOTHERAPY	THERAPEUTIC MODALITY	COMMENTS
Panic disorder	**Antidepressants** a. TCAs (imipramine) b. SSRIs c. MAOIs (second-line therapy because of dietary restrictions **Benzodiazepines** a. Alprazolam (Xanax) Lorazepam (Ativan) Clonazepam (Klonopin)	Cognitive-behavioral therapy (CBT) Behavioral therapy Relaxation techniques Breathing techniques	Current CBT emphasizes a. Information on anxiety and the panic cycle b. Symptom management (relaxation breathing) c. Cognitive restructuring d. Systematic desensitization e. In vivo exposure aimed at elementary avoidance behavior
Agoraphobia	a. Treatment of panic attacks (above) if present b. Phenelzine (Nardil), an MAOI, may have antiagoraphobic effects	Behavioral Cognitive therapy Insight-oriented psychotherapy	Systematic desensitization Deep muscle relaxation Rebreathing techniques Self-hypnosis Biofeedback Recognition of irrational beliefs Stopping of irrational thoughts Replacing of irrational thoughts with new thoughts or activities Especially for agoraphobia without history of panic disorder
Generalized anxiety disorder	a. Benzodiazepines b. Buspirone c. TCAs, especially imipramine	Cognitive therapy Behavioral therapy	
Posttraumatic stress disorder	a. MAOIs (especially phenelzine) may diminish nightmares and flashbacks b. TCAs (imipramine and amitriptyline) and SSRIs for depressive symptoms	Psychotherapy Family therapy Vocational rehabilitation Group therapy Relaxation techniques	**More than one treatment modality should be used.** a. Establish support b. Focus on abreaction, survivor guilt or shame, anger and helplessness
Obsessive-compulsive disorder	a. SSRIs (fluvoxamine [Luvox] and fluoxetine [Prozac]) b. Clomipramine (Anafranil) (TCA)	Behavioral therapy	Effective and necessary in addition to serotonergic medications Exposure in vivo plus response prevention are the crucial essential factors

TCA, tricyclic antidepressant; MAOI, monoamine oxidase inhibitor; SSRI, selective serotonin reuptake inhibitor.

logical therapy and effective therapeutic modalities for selected anxiety disorders.

Alternative and Complementary Therapies

Chapter 12 identified a number of complementary practices that are being widely used today to help people cope with their stressful lives. As mentioned in Chapter 36, consumers are using a wide number of herbs and dietary supplements, and many of these have demonstrable effects on mood, memory, and insomnia (Fugh-Berman and Cott 1999). However, herbs and dietary supplements are not subject to the rigorous testing that prescription medications need to undergo for approval in the U.S. market. Also, herbs and dietary supplements are not required to be uniform, and there is no guarantee of bioequivalence of the active compound across preparations (McEnany 2000). Problems that can occur with the use of psychotropic herbs include overuse or abuse, side effects, and herb-drug interactions (Tinsley 1999). It is important for nurses and other health care providers to improve their knowledge of these products so that they can discuss and provide their clients with reliable information.

Kava is one herb that has promise in the treatment of anxiety. Kava is an herb that has long been used by natives of the Pacific Islands and after the 18th century by Europeans. Kava is known for its antianxiety effects and its use in treating anxiety. Along with its antianxiety properties, kava is also used to reduce pain and relax muscles, and it has anticonvulsant effects. It may also help with insomnia, low energy, and muscle tension (Fontaine 2000).

Clinical trials demonstrate kava to be superior to placebo in seven double-blind, randomized, placebo-controlled trials (Pittler and Ernst 2000). Clinical trials also found kava to be roughly equivalent to the benzodiazepines oxazepam (15 mg/day) or bromazepam (9 mg/day) in its ability to decrease anxiety (Cauffield and Forbes 1999).

Desirable attributes of kava include the improved side effect profile over the benzodiazepines. For example, kava does not impair motor function or mental function when used in normal doses (50 to 75 mg three times per day) (Limon 2000) and seems to have a low potential for tolerance or dependence (McEnany 2000). Adverse effects can include gastrointestinal complaints, headache, dizziness, and allergic skin reactions (Limon 2000). Kava should not be taken together with substances that also act on the

---

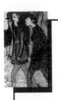

RESEARCH FINDINGS

Kava-Kava Used to Treat Postmenopausal Anxiety

Objective

To evaluate the effectiveness of the use of kava-kava extracts combined with hormone replacement therapy (HRT) compared with HRT used alone to treat postmenopausal anxiety.

Methods

Forty women who had been in menopause (either physiologic, i.e., natural, or brought about through surgery) for the past 1 to 12 years participated. Women in physiologic menopause were randomly assigned to one of the following protocols:

■ HRT (50 micrograms/day of natural estrogens with progestin) + 100 mg of kava-kava
■ HRT (50 micrograms/day of estrogen with progestin) + a placebo

Women in surgical menopause were randomly assigned to one of the following protocols:

■ Estrogen replacement therapy, or ERT (50 micrograms/day of natural estrogens) + 100 mg of kava-kava

■ ERT (50 micrograms/day of natural estrogens) + a placebo

Each treatment cycle lasted for 6 months.

Results

There was a significant reduction in the Hamilton Rating Scale for Anxiety (HAMA) score after 3 and 6 months of treatment in all four groups of women studied. The groups treated with HRT plus kava-kava and ERT plus kava-kava showed a greater reduction in the HAMA score compared with women in those groups that were treated with hormones alone.

Conclusions

The association of HRT/ERT and kava-kava extract may be an excellent therapy for the treatment of women in stabilized menopause, in particular those suffering from anxiety and depression, since kava-kava speeds up the resolution of the psychological symptoms without diminishing the therapeutic action of the estrogens on disorders such as osteoporosis and cardiovascular disease.

Source: De Leo, V., et al. (2000). Assessment of the association of kava-kava extract and hormone replacement therapy in the treatment of postmenopause anxiety. *Minerva Ginecol*, 52(6): 263–267.

central nervous system, such as alcohol, barbiturates, antidepressants, and antipsychotic drugs (Herbal Medicine 2000).

Initial studies on the effectiveness and use of kava for anxiety are encouraging, but as McEnany (2000) suggests, the reader should exercise caution in drawing conclusions. Kava seems as if it may be a potential option in the treatment of anxiety. (Go to www.holisticonline.com/herbal-med/_Herbs/h24.htm for more information on kava.)

Refer to the Research Findings box for an initial study of how kava can help ameliorate anxiety in postmenopausal women.

EVALUATION

Identified outcomes serve as the basis for evaluation. In general, evaluation of outcomes for clients with anxiety disorders deals with questions such as the following:

- Is the client experiencing a reduced level of anxiety?
- Does the client recognize symptoms as anxiety related?
- Does the client continue to display obsessions, compulsions, phobias, worry, or other symptoms of anxiety disorders? If still present, are they more or less frequent? More or less intense?
- Is the client able to use newly learned behaviors to manage anxiety?
- Can the client adequately perform self-care activities?
- Can the client maintain satisfying interpersonal relations?
- Can the client assume usual roles?

Visit the **Evolve** website at
http://evolve.elsevier.com/Varcarolis
for more Case Studies.

CASE STUDY 14–1 *Obsessive-Compulsive Disorder*

Tina, a 32-year-old single parent, seeks treatment for OCD. Tina was born 12 years after her older sister to parents who were aloof, perfectionistic, and morally strict. She often felt she was an unwanted child. Tina, like her sister, majored in business administration in college. During her senior year, she became pregnant. She did not seek an abortion because she believed it would be morally wrong. The father of the baby became so anxious that he moved away from the area. Tina, too embarrassed to return home, quit school to support herself and the child. She worked as a secretary, took courses at night, and presently holds a job in a prominent law firm. The only change in her life occurred several weeks ago, when a new secretary was hired for the office.

Recently, Tina started to have intrusive thoughts that some harm would come to her daughter. Even though she knows these thoughts are irrational, the thought **(obsession)** persists. The only way Tina can reduce her anxiety is to check on her daughter's safety **(compulsion)**. She calls the school hourly. She does not allow her daughter to play sports, screens her daughter's friends, monitors her daughter's activities, and gener-

ally tries to control her daughter's every move. Her daughter feels embarrassed by her mother's behavior of checking up on her.

Tina gets to the point where she hardly eats. She sleeps very little at night because of the need to go to her daughter's room to "check that she is safe." She states that she thinks she is stupid for not being able to manage her life as well as her sister and for not being able to get rid of her senseless worries. Her physician sets up an appointment for her at a nearby mental health clinic.

The nurse clinician avoids the use of psychoanalytic techniques. Although they may promote an intellectual understanding of the illness, they will not help the person attain appropriate emotions or change behavior. Instead, the clinician stays active and energetic, intervening whenever Tina's conversation becomes rambling. Tina is able to identify a precipitating stressor—the hiring of a new secretary, who symbolizes the sister with whom she competed. Tina was also started on fluvoxamine (Luvox), an SSRI effective with OCD.

The nurse weighs the options of using response prevention or of gradually reducing Tina's ritualization.

Case Study continued on following page

CASE STUDY 14–1   *Obsessive-Compulsive Disorder* (Continued)

Response prevention involves asking the client to refrain from the compulsive behaviors altogether. The therapist opts for gradual reduction.

The therapist tries to help Tina accomplish the following:

1. Discriminate between thoughts and actions
2. Accept "forbidden" desires and "bad" thoughts as common to most people
3. Discriminate between real and imagined danger and

act accordingly, especially as they relate to her daughter's activities
4. Achieve thought stopping by snapping a rubber band worn on her wrist whenever the obsessive thoughts begin

After 3 months of SSRI medication and behavioral therapy, Tina is doing remarkably well. She will continue the medication and reduce sessions to twice a month. She is sleeping 6 hours a night and is slowly gaining weight.

Visit the **Evolve** website at
http://evolve.elsevier.com/Varcarolis
for the other Nursing Care Plan diagnoses and for
more Nursing Care Plans.

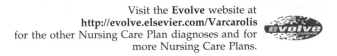

NURSING CARE PLAN 14–1   *A Person with Obsessive-Compulsive Disorder*

NURSING DIAGNOSIS
Ineffective coping: Related to time consumed with obsessions and compulsions

Supporting Data

■ Reported obsessive thoughts that daughter will be harmed
■ Compulsive checking designed to ensure daughter's safety

CLIENT OUTCOMES	INTERVENTION	RATIONALE	EVALUATION
1. By (date) client will experience a decrease in incidence of obsessive thinking and compulsive behavior, as evidenced by ■ Normal food and fluid intake ■ Six hours of sleep per night ■ No calls to school	1a. Anticipate needs, e.g., need for information. 1b. Focus on client rather than on symptoms. 1c. Permit client to call school six times per day for 2 days, then four times per day for 4 days, twice daily for 2 days, and no calls thereafter.	1a. Increases feelings of security. 1b. Reinforces self-worth. 1c. Allowing performance of ritual prevents panic. Reduction in frequency of rituals leads to extinction.	*GOAL MET* Client states that she likes the idea that the nurse explains things to her; she states that she worries less. Client is able to adhere to a schedule. Client has been able to call school according to schedule and not exceed moderate-level anxiety.

NURSING CARE PLAN 14–1 **A *Person with Obsessive-Compulsive Disorder*** *(Continued)*

CLIENT OUTCOMES	INTERVENTION	RATIONALE	EVALUATION
	1d. Firmly encourage client to attend and eat meals. Encourage nutritious snacks between meals.	1d. Limits must be placed on behaviors that threaten health.	Client is able to sit through meals without checking on daughter. Two-pound weight gain in past week. Client initiates sleep within 45 minutes but awakens several times nightly. Refuses sedation because she has daytime grogginess.
	1e. Advise client to take sedation if client has not initiated sleep by midnight.	1e. Promotes relaxation and sleep.	
	1f. Avoid hurrying client.	1f. Hurrying client increases anxiety and performance of rituals.	
	1g. Stay on fluvoxamine (Luvox) 100 mg per day.	1g. A highly effective medication for clients with obsessive-compulsive disorder.	
2. By (date) client will state that she is able to dismiss obsessive thoughts and will acknowledge that compulsion is not carried out.	2a. Teach to interrupt obsessive thoughts by snapping on wrist rubber band.	2a,b. Gives control over obsessive thinking and compulsive rituals. Positive reinforcement promotes repetition of adaptive behavior.	*GOAL MET* By the sixth day, client states, "It's getting easier to ignore my obsessive thoughts."
	2b. Give positive reinforcement for non-ritualistic behavior.		

SUMMARY

Individuals with anxiety disorders experience high levels of anxiety or use ritualistic behaviors. Clients who have panic and generalized anxiety disorders experience diffuse symptoms of anxiety.

Clients with phobias experience extreme fear of certain objects or situations and go to great lengths to avoid the feared object or situation.

Clients who have obsessions and compulsions experience the presence of repetitive, intrusive thoughts and the repetitive need to perform ritualized actions designed to relieve anxiety. Clients with acute and posttraumatic stress disorders experience the symptoms of acute anxiety, in addition to re-experiencing the traumatic event via nightmares, flashbacks, and illusions.

There is a great deal of evidence that anxiety disorders have biochemical and genetic correlates, although no one gene or biochemical dysfunction can be singled out. Stress, early childhood trauma, and environment all can play a part.

Clients with anxiety disorders have the ability to stay in touch with reality while not being in touch with their true feelings. Individuals with anxiety disorders expend great amounts of psychological energy and use multiple ego defenses to cope with anxiety, only to find that the defenses are inadequate for long-term anxiety reduction. These individuals recognize that the symptoms being experienced are odd or strange (ego-dystonic).

Issues of primary and secondary gain are present with anxiety disorders. Primary gain relieves discomfort, while secondary gain reinforces the sick role. Individuals with anxiety disorders share the common experience of low self-esteem associated with powerlessness to control ego-dystonic symptoms.

The presence of negative self-talk is nearly universal among clients with anxiety disorder; in clients who use it, cognitive restructuring may be helpful. Research has demonstrated positive responses to combined therapies involving cognitive, behavioral, educative, and psychobiological approaches.

Clients with anxiety disorders seem to have the ability to incite predictable negative feelings in health care workers, making it necessary for nurses to practice self-assessment and use supervision to resolve uncomfortable reactions. Clients with anxiety disorders usually have positive responses to staff who demonstrate a nonjudgmental, calm demeanor.

Nurses are challenged to use the nursing process to provide effective treatment for clients with anxiety disorders. Nurses are called on to educate both clients and significant others regarding the need for active participation in the treatment process to produce desired outcomes.

Visit the **Evolve** website at
http://evolve.elsevier.com/Varcarolis
for a post-test on the content in this chapter.

Visit the **Evolve** website at
http://evolve.elsevier.com/Varcarolis
for additional self-study exercises.

Critical Thinking and Chapter Review

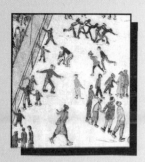

Critical Thinking

1. Ms. Smith, a client with obsessive-compulsive disorder, washes her hands until they are cracked and bleeding. Your nursing goal is to promote healing of her hands. What interventions will you plan?

2. This is Mr. Olivetti's third emergency department visit in a week. He is experiencing severe anxiety accompanied by many physical symptoms. He clings to you, desperately crying, "Help me! Help me! Don't let me die!" Diagnostic tests have ruled out a physical disorder. The client outcome has been identified as "Client anxiety level will be reduced to moderate/mild within 1 hour." What interventions should you use?

   Mr. Olivetti is given an appointment at the anxiety disorders clinic. How will you explain the importance of keeping the clinic appointment?

   At the clinic, Mr. Olivetti is assigned a case manager. If you were the case manager, what outcomes would you identify? What interventions would you plan?

3. Mr. Zeamans is a client with posttraumatic stress disorder. He has a history of substance abuse and is now a recovering alcoholic. During a clinic visit, he tells you he plans to ask his psychiatrist to prescribe diazepam (Valium) to use when he's feeling anxious. He asks whether you think this is a good idea. How would you respond? What action could you take?

4. You are to perform a nursing assessment for Ms. Lee, a Chinese American client with generalized anxiety disorder. What cultural considerations might play a role in conducting the assessment?

Chapter Review

Choose the most appropriate answer.

1. Interventions that would be helpful in caring for clients with anxiety disorders include

   1. Help client link feelings and behaviors.
   2. Leave anxious clients alone as much as possible.
   3. Advise client to minimize daily exercise to conserve endorphins.
   4. Teach clients the importance of maintaining caffeine intake at 750 mg or more daily.

2. One possible cause of obsessive-compulsive disorder is

   1. Faulty learning.
   2. Dopamine deficiency.
   3. Serotonin dysregulation.
   4. Clomipramine excess.

3. Mrs. T. is preoccupied with persistent intrusive thoughts and impulses and performs ritualistic acts repetitively. She expresses distress that her attention is

so consumed that she cannot accomplish her usual daily activities. These symptoms are most consistent with the DSM-IV-TR 2000 diagnosis of

1. Panic disorder.
2. Social phobia.
3. Generalized anxiety disorder.
4. Obsessive-compulsive disorder.

4. In addition to prescribing SSRIs to treat Mr. G's panic disorder, the nurse psychotherapist is likely to recommend

1. Family therapy.
2. Psychoanalysis.
3. Vocational rehabilitation.
4. Cognitive behavioral therapy.

5. A strategy nurses can employ to help clients with anxiety disorders replace negative self-talk is

1. Systematic desensitization/graduated exposure.
2. Counseling to promote cognitive restructuring.
3. Relaxation training.
4. Implosion therapy.

NURSE, CLIENT, AND FAMILY RESOURCES

ABIL (Agoraphobics Building Independent Lives), Inc.

3805 Cutshaw Avenue, Suite 415
Richmond, VA 23230
1-804-353-3964
mail to: abil1996@aol.com

Agoraphobics in Motion (AIM)

1719 Crooks
Royal Oak, MI 48067-1306
1-248-547-0400

Anxiety Disorder Association of America

11900 Parklawn Drive, Suite 100
Rockville, MD 20852
1-301-231-9350
http://www.adaa.org/

Obsessive-Compulsive Foundation, Inc.

P.O. Box 70
Milford, CT 06460-0070
1-203-878-5669
http://www.ocfoundation.org

Recovery, Inc.

802 N. Dearborn Street
Chicago, IL 60610
1-312-337-5661
http://www.recovery-inc.com
e-mail: spot@recovery-inc.com

REFERENCES

American Psychiatric Association. (2000). *Diagnostic and statistical manual of mental disorders* (4th ed., TR). Washington, D.C.: Author.

Beck, C. T. (1996). A concept analysis of panic. *Archives of Psychiatric Nursing,* 10(5):165.

Blair, B., et al. (1996). The undertreatment of anxiety: Overcoming the confusion and stigma. *Journal of Psychosocial Nursing and Mental Health Services,* 24(6):9.

Bremner, J. D., et al. (1997). Magnetic resonance imaging–based measurement of hippocampal volume in posttraumatic stress disorder related to childhood sexual abuse—a preliminary report. *Biological Psychiatry,* 41(1):23–32.

Cauffield, J. S., and Forbes, H. J. (1999). Dietary supplements used in the treatment of depression, anxiety, and sleep disorders. *Lippincott's Primary Care Practitioner,* 3(3):290–304.

DeVeaugh-Geiss, J. (1994). Pharmacological therapy of obsessive compulsive disorders. *Advances in Pharmacology,* 30:35.

Ellis, A. (1978). Rational emotive therapy. In R. Corsini (ed.), *Current psychotherapies* (2nd ed.). Itasca, Il: F. E. Peacock.

Fontaine, K. L. (2000). *Healing Practices: Alternative therapies for nursing.* Upper Saddle River, N.J.: Prentice Hall.

Fryer, A. J. (1999). Anxiety disorders: Genetics. In B. J. Sadock and V. A. Sadock (Eds.), *Kaplan and Sadock's comprehensive textbook of psychiatry* (7th ed.) (vol. 3, pp. 1457–1463). Philadelphia: Lippincott Williams & Wilkins.

Fugh-Berman, A., and Cott, J. M. (1999). Dietary supplements and natural produces as psychotherapeutic agents. *Psychosomatic Medicine,* 61(5):712–728.

Gorman, J. M. (1999). Anxiety disorders: Introduction and overview. In B. J. Sadock and V. A. Sadock (Eds.), *Kaplan and Sadock's comprehensive textbook of psychiatry,* (7th ed.) (Vol. 2, pp. 1441–1444). Philadelphia: Lippincott Williams & Wilkins.

Herbal Medicine. (2000). Medicine-herb/food interactions: Herbs and foods may lead to complication if you take them with drugs. *www.holisticonline.com/Herbal-Med/hol__herb__med__reac.htm*

Hollander, E. (1999). Anxiety disturbances. In R. E. Hales, S. C. Yudofsky, and J. A. Talbott (Eds.), *The American Psychiatric Press textbook of psychiatry* (3rd ed.) (pp. 567–634). Washington, D.C.: American Psychiatric Press.

Horwath, E. and Weissman, N. M. (2000). The epidemiology and cross-national presentation of obsessive-compulsive disorder. *Psychiatric Clinics of North America* 23(3): 493–507.

Johnson, M., Mass, M., and Moorehead, S. (2000). *Nursing outcomes classification* (2nd ed.). St. Louis: Mosby.

Kendler, K. S., Neale, M. C., Kessler, R. C., et al. (1992). The genetic epidemiology of phobias in women: The interrelationships of agoraphobia, social phobia, situational phobia, and simple phobia. *Archives of General Psychiatry*, 49:273–281.

Leff, J. (1988). *Psychiatry around the globe: A transcultural view* (2nd ed.). London: Royal College of Psychiatrists.

Limon, L. (2000, March 10–14). *Use of alternative medicine in women's health*. Presented at the annual meeting of the American Pharmaceutical Association, Washington, D.C.

Marks, I. (1995). Advances in behavioral-cognitive therapy of social phobia. *Journal of Clinical Psychiatry*, 56(Suppl. 5):25.

McEnany, G. (2000). Herbal psychotropics: III. Focus on kava, valerian, and melatonin. *Journal of the American Psychiatric Nurses Association*, 6(4):126–132.

Noyes, F. (1996). Oklahoma city bombing: Evaluation of symptoms in veterans with PTSD. *Archives of Psychiatric Nursing*, 10(1):55.

Noyes, R., and Holt, C. (1994). Anxiety disorders. In G. Winokur and P. Clayton (Eds.), *The medical book of psychiatry* (pp. 139–160). Philadelphia: W. B. Saunders.

Noyes, R., Clarkson, C., Crow, R. R., et al. (1987). A family study of generalized anxiety disorder. *American Journal of Psychiatry*, 144:1019–1024.

Papp, L. A. (1999). Anxiety disorders: Somatic treatment. In B. J. Sadock and V. A. Sadock (Eds.), *Kaplan and Sadock's comprehensive textbook of psychiatry* (7th ed.) (pp. 1490–1497). Philadelphia: Lippincott Williams & Wilkins.

Pine, D. S. (1999). Anxiety disorders: Clinical features. In B. J. Sadock and V. A. Sadock (Eds.), *Kaplan and Sadock's comprehensive textbook of psychiatry* (7th ed.) (pp. 1476–1489). Philadelphia: Lippincott Williams & Wilkins.

Pittler, M. H., and Ernst, E. (2000). Efficacy of kava extract for treating anxiety: Systematic review and meta-analysis. *Journal of Clinical Psychopharmacology*, 20(1):84–89.

Roy-Byrne, P. P., and Cowley, D. S. (1999). Assessment and treatment of panic disorder. In D. C. Duncan (Ed.), *Current psychiatric therapy*. Philadelphia: W. B. Saunders.

Schwartz, J. M., et al. (1996). Systematic changes in cerebral glucose metabolic rate after successful behavior modification treatments of obsessive-compulsive disorder. *Archives of General Psychiatry*, 53(2):109.

Sheehan, D. V. (1999). Current concepts in the treatment of panic disorder. *Journal of Clinical Psychiatry*, 60(18):16–21.

Sullivan, G. M., and Coplan, J. D. (1999). Anxiety disorders: Biochemical aspects. In B. J. Sadock and V. A. Sadock (Eds.), *Kaplan and Sadock's comprehensive textbook of psychiatry* (7th ed.) (pp. 1450–1456). Philadelphia: Lippincott Williams & Wilkins.

Sutherland, S., and Davidson, J. R. (1994). Pharmacotherapy for posttraumatic stress disorder. *Psychiatric Clinics of North America*, 17(2):409.

Tinsley, J. A. (1999). The hazards of psychotropic herbs. *Minnesota Medicine*, 88(5):20–31.

Welkowitz, L. A., Struening, E. L., Pittman, J., Guardino, M., and Welkowitz, J. (2000) Obsessive-compulsive Disorder and comorbid anxiety problems in a national anxiety screening sample. *Journal of Anxiety Disorders*, 14(5):471–482.

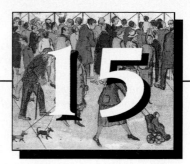

15

Somatoform and Dissociative Disorders

ELIZABETH M. VARCAROLIS

Key Terms and Concepts

The key terms and concepts listed here also appear in color where they are defined or first discussed in this chapter.

alternate personality (alter) or subpersonality

body dysmorphic disorder

conversion disorder

depersonalization disorder

dissociative amnesia

dissociative disorders

dissociative fugue

dissociative identity disorder

factitious disorder

hypnotherapy

hypochondriasis

la belle indifférence

malingering

pain disorder

secondary gains

somatization

somatization disorder

Objectives

After studying this chapter, the reader will be able to

1. Compare and contrast essential differences between the somatoform and the dissociative disorders.

2. Differentiate symptoms of somatoform disorder (a) from those of psychosomatic-psychophysiological disorder; (b) from those of malingering; and (c) from those of factitious disorder.

3. Give a clinical example of what you would find in each of the somatoform disorders.

4. Do a psychosocial assessment on a client using the psychosocial assessment tool included in this chapter (see Box 15–1). Describe how it is particularly useful in dealing with a client with a somatoform disorder.

5. Implement at least five psychosocial interventions that would be appropriate for a client with somatic complaints.

6. Plan interventions for a somatizing client (e.g., conversion disorder) who is receiving a great deal of secondary gain from his or her "blindness." Include self-care, referrals, family teaching.

7. Explain the concept of dissociation and the steps in dissociation in relation to early childhood trauma and/or sexual or physical abuse.

8. Compare and contrast the differences between amnesia and fugue and give a brief clinical example of each.

9. Write at least eight questions that are useful in assessing a client with a dissociative identity disorder.

10. Identify the most important outcome criteria for a client with dissociative identity disorder and the reason why. Describe other outcome criteria that are important for the client and family's quality of life.

11. Analyze some of the inherent factors in a person with dissociative identity disorder that makes therapy complex and challenging. Include cognitive factors, comorbid conditions, family reactions, and responses of health care professionals.

*A*nxiety exerts a powerful influence on the lives of individuals. People vary a great deal in their ability to cope with anxiety successfully. The ways in which anxiety is manifested dysfunctionally also differ considerably. In this chapter, the nurse will learn about the nursing care of clients who experience somatoform disorders and clients with dissociative disorders. The placement of these disorders on the mental health continuum can be seen in Figure 15–1.

Somatoform Disorders

PREVALENCE

The *Diagnostic and Statistical Manual of Mental Disorders*, 4th Edition, Text Revision (DSM-IV-TR) (APA 2000) defined the somatoform disorders as a group of disorders in which

■ Physical symptoms suggest a physical disorder for which there is no demonstrable base.
■ There is a strong presumption that the symptoms are linked to psychobiological factors.

Somatoform as a concept was first described in the DSM-III in 1980. Somatoform disorders should not be confused with the concept of **psychosomatic**. In somatoform disorders, physical changes are not evident. The "classic" **psychosomatic illness** (psychophysiological) described by Alexander in 1950 includes bronchial asthma, ulcerative colitis, thyrotoxicosis, essential hypertension, rheumatoid arthritis, neurodermatitis, and peptic ulcer (Martin and Yutzy 1999). All these entities are illnesses considered as general medical conditions that may be affected by stress or other psychobiological factors.

The current DSM-IV-TR somatoform disorders include

■ Somatization disorder
■ Undifferentiated somatoform disorder
■ Conversion disorder
■ Pain disorder
■ Hypochondriasis
■ Body dysmorphic disorder
■ Somatoform disorder not otherwise specified

See Table 15–1 for a brief description of each of the disorders; the prevalence of the disorder, if known; whether they interfere with the person's ability to function (yes or no); and a brief description of the course of the disorder.

COMORBIDITY

Studies have demonstrated that 50% to 70% of people with a mental disorder initially present with a somatic symptom, such as backache, fatigue, and headache (Katon 1997). Also, a high rate of misdiagnosis primarily occurs in clients who have somatic symptoms as an expression of psychosocial distress (Katon 1997). Somatoform disorders, therefore, exemplify the mind-body interaction (stress acted out through physical symptoms that are real to the individual). The brain, in ways still not understood, sends signals to the body indicating a serious problem in the body, when, in fact, there is no serious, demonstrable, peripheral organic disorder (Guggenheim 1999).

Although there may be comorbid substance abuse in somatoform pain disorder, most efforts by medical personnel rule out organic causes of somatoform disorders (Guggenheim 1999). Some of the disorders that are commonly confused with somatoform disorders and may need to be ruled out include

■ Multiple sclerosis
■ Brain tumor
■ Hyperparathyroidism
■ Lupus erythematosus
■ Myasthenia gravis
■ Hyperthyroidism

The author would like to thank Helene (Kay) Charron for her contributions from the third edition of this book.

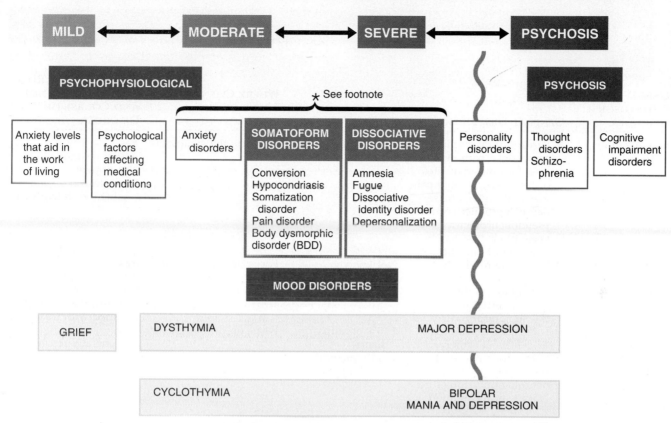

MENTAL HEALTH CONTINUUM FOR SOMATOFORM AND DISSOCIATIVE DISORDERS

* *These disorders are currently classified by presenting clinical symptoms. Previously they were called "neurotic" disorders.*

Figure 15–1 Mental health continuum for somatoform and dissociative disorders.

THEORY

Soma is the Greek word for body. Somatization can be defined as the expression of psychological stress through physical symptoms. Somatoform disorders are a group of conditions in which somatization is present. They are characterized by the following elements:

■ Complaints of physical symptoms that cannot be explained by physiological tests
■ Psychological factors and conflicts seem important in initiating, exacerbating, and maintaining the disturbance
■ Client's inability to control the symptom voluntarily
■ Symptoms not intentionally produced, as in malingering (making a conscious attempt to deceive others by pretending to have a false or exaggerated symptom, usually for financial gain) or factitious disorder (Munchausen's syndrome, in which physical signs of illness are produced through voluntary physiological tampering)

Biological Factors

Studies reported by Guggenheim (1999) provide information about the possible neurophysiological basis for somatoform disorders. Research suggests that the physical symptoms that are unexplained by medical disease can arise from faulty perceptions and incorrect assessments of body sensations associated with attention deficits and cognitive impairments (e.g., increased distractibility, impressionistic tendencies, partial and circumstantial associations). Symptoms seen in somatization disorder (a condition in which an individual experiences numerous unexplainable physical symptoms) and hypochondriasis (an intense preoccupation with fear of disease) may develop this way.

Somatoform disorders may involve a considerable variety of neuronal pathways—from brain–brain signals and perceptual pathways, in addition to efferent signals to motor apparatus and blood vessels (Guggenheim 1999).

Clients who experience somatoform pain disorder (pain unrelated to a medical disease) may be predis-

TABLE 15–1 *Somatoform Disorders*

DSM-IV-TR SOMATOFORM DISORDER	GENERAL DESCRIPTION	PREVALENCE	WHERE CLIENT PUTS FOCUS OF THE CONFLICT	IMPAIRMENT IN ROLE FUNCTION (YES/NO) AND COURSE OF DISORDER
Somatization disorder	■ History of many physical complaints: pain in at least four different sites or functions, two nonpain gastrointestinal, one sexual or reproductive, one pseudoneurologica (conversion) or dissociative ■ Most tend to be chronic	0.2–2% women Less than 0.2% men	Focus on the symptoms	**Yes** **Acute:** responds to brief treatment **Chronic:** can be contained with treatment
Undifferentiated somatoform disorder	■ One or more physical complaints ■ Much more common ■ Often referred to as **partial somatoform disorder**	Not known	Focus on the symptoms	**Yes** **Acute:** responds to brief treatment **Chronic:** can be contained with treatment
Conversion disorder	■ Unexplained symptoms or deficits affecting voluntary motor or sensory function suggesting a neurological or other general medical condition	1–3% of outpatients 1–14% medical-surgical inpatients	Focus on the symptoms	**Yes** ■ Generally resolve over time ■ May continue with chronic symptoms ■ Recurrence is common
Pain disorder	■ Pain as predominant focus of clinical presentation, of sufficient severity to warrant clinical attention.	10–15% of adults in United States with back pain alone 9–40% of clients with pain disorder reported disability in the past 6 months	Focus on the symptoms	**No if acute** pain resolves in short period **Yes if chronic**
Hypochondriasis	■ Preoccupation with fears of having, or the idea that one has, a serious disease based on the misinterpretation of bodily symptoms. Persists despite appropriate medical evaluation and reassurance	1–5% general population 2–7% in outpatient population	Preoccupation with interpretation and possible implication of bodily symptoms	**No** if part of other primary disorder (e.g., depression) **Yes,** tends to be chronic with some remissions and exacerbation Stress related
Body dysmorphic disorder	■ Preoccupation (may be of delusional intensity) with imagined defect in appearance or markedly excessive concern with slight physical anomaly	■ Unknown—general ■ With anxiety or depression, 5–40% In cosmetic surgery, 6–15%	Focus on imagined or exaggerated defect in appearance	Can interfere Symptoms wax and wane over time Usually continues over time
Somatoform disorder not otherwise specified	■ Disorders with specified somatoform symptoms. Examples: pseudocyesis; disorders of less than 6 months' duration with fatigue or body weakness, nonpsychotic hypochondriacal symptoms, or other physical complaints	No data		

posed to the experience of severe pain because of abnormalities in brain chemical balance or because of structural abnormalities of the sensory or limbic systems. Serotonin and endorphin deficiency in an individual may cause the individual to perceive incoming pain stimuli as being more intense than would others. Serotonin deficiency is also being considered as a causal factor in the development of misperceptions about one's body (body dysmorphic disorder).

Biological factors related to central nervous system arousal disturbances are implicated in the development of pseudoneurological symptoms, such as loss of sensory abilities and loss of voluntary motor function (conversion disorder). Abnormal regulation of the cytokine system is also being considered to result in some somatoform disorder symptoms, such as fatigue and anorexia. Cytokines are the messenger molecules the immune system uses to communicate among its parts and with the brain and nervous system.

Genetic Factors

Studies show that somatoform disorders may have a genetic component. Somatization disorder tends to run in families, occurring in 10% to 20% of first-degree female relatives of clients with somatization disorder (DSM-IV-TR). One study reported a concordance rate for somatization disorder of 29% in monozygotic twins and 10% in dizygotic twins. Other researchers showed an increased likelihood (7.7%) that first-degree relatives of individuals with hypochondriasis disorder would be diagnosed with the disorder (Noyes et al. 1999), and twin studies have shown an increased prevalence of somatization among identical twins (Kendler et al. 1995).

Cultural Factors

The DSM-IV-TR provides information about the role of culture in somatoform disorders and states that the type and the frequency of somatic symptoms vary across cultures. Burning hands and feet or the experience of worms in the head or ants under the skin is more common in Africa and southern Asia than in North America. Alteration of consciousness with falling is a symptom commonly associated with culture-specific religious and healing rituals. Somatization disorder, which is rarely seen in men in the United States, is more often reported in Greek and Puerto Rican men, suggesting that cultural mores may permit these men to use somatization as an acceptable approach to dealing with life stress.

Symptoms related to male reproductive function are more prevalent in Eastern cultures. For example, Leff, in his work *Psychiatry Around the Globe* (1988), discussed syndromes or illnesses that are confined to a particular culture, including *koro*, which is an illness seen in Chinese men. The affected individual becomes convinced that his genitals are withdrawing into his abdomen and that when the last of the genitals disappears, he will die. Panic-level anxiety ensues.

Conversion disorder is reported to be more common in individuals in low socioeconomic groups, those in rural settings, and those with little education. The incidence is higher in developing regions (Steinhausen et al. 1989).

In some cultures, certain physical symptoms are believed to result from spells having been cast on the individual. Spellbound individuals often seek the help of traditional healers in addition to modern medical help. The modern medical diagnostician may point to the presence of a non–life-threatening somatoform disorder, while the traditional healer may offer an entirely different explanation and prognosis. The individual may not show improvement until the traditional healer removes the spell.

Psychosocial Factors

Psychoanalytical Theory

Psychoanalytical theorists believe that psychogenic complaints of pain, illness, or loss of physical function are related to repression of a conflict (usually of an aggressive or sexual nature), and transformation of anxiety into a physical symptom that is symbolically related to the conflict. In conversion disorder, the ego defense mechanisms involved are repression and conversion. According to Freudian theory, conversion symptoms allow a forbidden wish or urge to be partly expressed but sufficiently disguised so that the individual does not have to face the unacceptable wish. Therefore, the symptom is said to be symbolic of the conflict.

Freudian theory suggests that conversion symptoms also permit the individual to communicate a need for special treatment or consideration from others. The following vignette is an example of how a symptom can be both symbolic of, and a solution to, a conflict.

Vignette

■ *Anita, aged 18 years, lives with her mother and stepfather. The stepfather has been physically abusive to Anita for many years. Anita hates him but is dependent on him for financial support. One day, as the family steps off the curb to cross a busy street, the stepfather is hit by a speeding automobile. Anita attempts to shout at her stepfather to warn him, but no sound comes out. She suffers aphonia (loss of voice) that lasts until psychotherapy helps her regain her ability to speak. It is obvious that the conflict was whether to warn her physically abusive and hated stepfather. The loss of her voice solved the problem and made it impossible to save him.*

Hypochondriasis is considered by many clinicians to have psychodynamic origins. These clinicians suggest that anger, aggression, or hostility that had its origins in past losses or disappointments is expressed as a need for help and concern from others. Other clinicians suggest that hypochondriasis is a defense against guilt or low self-esteem. In this hypothesis, the somatic symptoms that the individual has are experienced as deserved punishment. In

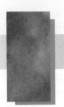

TABLE 15–2 *Somatoform Disorders: Defense and Examples*

DEFENSE MECHANISMS	EXAMPLE*
Conversion Disorder	
Conversion	Jan, a 28-year-old former secretary, awakens one morning to find that she has a tingling in both hands and cannot move her fingers. Two days earlier, her husband had told her that he wanted a separation and that she would have to go back to work to support herself. The conversion of anxiety relates the separation and increase in dependency needs to "paralysis of her fingers" so that she is unable to work.
Pain Disorder	
Displacement	Henry, 47, a laborer, "pulled a muscle" in his back a year ago. Two weeks before this, his wife, a waitress, told him that she wanted to go back to school to get her bachelor's degree. He suffers severe, constant pain, despite negative results from myelography, computed tomography, magnetic resonance imaging, and neurological examinations. He watches television all day and collects disability. His wife, unable now to go back to school, waits on him and has assumed his home responsibilities. Henry displaces his anxiety over the threat to his own self-esteem by his wife's potential change of status onto "pain in his back." The focus of his anxiety is now on his back and not on his threatened self-esteem.
Body Dysmorphic Disorder	
Symbolism and projection	Michele, a young, attractive woman, is preoccupied that her nose is too long and "ugly." She is preoccupied and distressed over her perception. Two plastic surgeons she consulted are hesitant to reshape her nose but have not altered her thinking that her nose makes her ugly.
Somatization Disorder	
Somatization	Deanna, 27, presents at the physician's office with excessive, heavy menstruation. She tells the nurse that recently she experienced pain "first in my back and then going to every part of my body." She states that she is often bothered with constipation and frequent vomiting when she "eats the wrong food." She states she was "unwell" and had suffered from seizures and still has them occasionally. The nurse becomes confused, not knowing what symptoms she wants the physician to evaluate. Deanna tells the nurse that she lives at home with her parents because her poor health makes it hard for her to hold a job.
Hypochondriasis	
Denial and somatization	Julio, 52, lost his wife to colon cancer 5 months ago, which he "took very well." Recently, he saw the sixth physician with the same complaint. He believes that he has liver cancer, despite repeated and extensive diagnostic tests, which are all negative. He has ceased seeing his friends, has dropped his hobbies, and spends much of his time checking his sclera and "resting his liver." His son finally demands that he see a doctor.

* All entail somatization.

pain disorder, the individual's pain may serve an unconscious function, such as atonement, a way to obtain the love and concern of others, and punishment for real or imagined wrongdoing. The defense mechanisms responsible are repression and displacement.

In cases of body dysmorphic disorder, some theorists believe that the individual invests a part of the body with special meaning that may be traceable to some event occurring at an earlier stage of psychosexual development. The original event is repressed, and the attachment of special meaning to a part of the body comes about through symbolization. Projection is used when the individual makes statements such as "It makes everyone look at me with horror" and "I know my husband hates it." Table 15–2 provides clinical examples of each of the somatoform disorders and their defenses.

Behavioral Theory

Behaviorists suggest that somatoform symptoms are learned ways of communicating helplessness and that they allow the individual to manipulate others. The symptoms become more intense when they are reinforced by attention from others. In the United States, most individuals are concerned about others who have pain, and physicians and nurses are taught to be attentive and responsive to a client's reports of pain. Other reinforcers include avoiding activities that the individual considers distasteful, obtaining financial gain from the pain, and gaining some advantage in interpersonal relationships as a result of the pain.

Cognitive Theory

Cognitive theorists believe that the client with hypochondriasis focuses on body sensations, misinterprets their meaning, and then becomes excessively alarmed by them.

DSM-IV-TR CRITERIA AND THE CLINICAL PICTURE OF SOMATOFORM DISORDERS

DSM-IV-TR listed five somatoform disorders that are reviewed in this section. Clinical vignettes accompany the criteria for each disorder.

Somatization Disorder

The diagnosis of somatization disorder requires that the client have a history of many physical complaints, beginning before the age of 30 years, that occur over a period of years and result in treatment being sought or in significant impairment in social, occupational, or other areas of functioning. The symptoms are displayed in Figure 15–1. In addition, the symptoms experienced by the client cannot be explained by a medical condition, or if they are explained by a medical condition, the complaints or social and occupational impairment that result are in excess of what would be expected.

Vignette

■ *Susanne, a 26-year-old beautician, is admitted to the hospital after an overdose of sedatives. She states that she is sick of not being able to get help from anyone. In describing herself, she mentions being unwell since the age of 14, shortly after her father died of valvular heart disease. She describes having seizures, fainting spells, and occasional weakness of the left leg. One year ago, she began having abdominal pain, nausea, and diarrhea. Exploratory surgery revealed no pathology. The symptoms still recur "sometimes." She mentions experiencing painful menstruation and excessive bleeding over a period of several years. Recently, she has experienced palpitations and tightness of her chest after emotionally trying events.*

Susanne lived at home with her mother until 6 months ago, when she married a man 15 years her senior. She says that she is "turned off by sex," and she reveals that her husband is upset by her constant illness. He is considering divorce. She has attempted suicide, and a brief admission is advised.

Hypochondriasis

Nondelusional preoccupation with having a serious disease or the fear of having a serious disease marks hypochondriasis. The preoccupation or fear is based on the client's misinterpretation of bodily symptoms, despite medical evaluation and reassurance, and has lasted more than 6 months, causing the client significant distress or impaired social or occupational function (see Fig. 15–2).

Vignette

■ *Anthony, aged 54 years, is referred to the mental health center outpatient clinic from the sexually transmitted disease (STD) clinic. Anthony has visited the clinic almost weekly for 2 years, asking for diagnostic tests for various STDs. He is always told that the test results are negative and that he has no illness. Most recently, his preoccupation has centered on acquired immunodeficiency syndrome (AIDS).*

DSM-IV-TR CRITERIA FOR SOMATOFORM DISORDERS

SOMATOFORM DISORDERS*

SOMATIZATION DISORDER

1. History of many physical complaints beginning before 30 years of age, occurring over a period of years and resulting in impairment in social, occupational, or other important areas of functioning.

2. Complaints must include all of the following:
   - History of pain in at least **four** different sites or functions
   - History of at least **two** gastrointestinal symptoms other than pain
   - History of at least **one** sexual or reproduction symptom
   - History of at least **one** symptom defined as or suggesting a neurological disorder

CONVERSION DISORDER

1. Development of one or more symptoms or deficit suggesting a neurologic disorder (blindness, deafness, loss of touch) or general medical condition.

2. Psychological factors are associated with the symptom or deficit because the symptom is initiated or exacerbated by psychological stressors.

3. Not due to malingering or factitious disorder and not culturally sanctioned.

4. Cannot be explained by general medical condition or effects of a substance.

5. Causes impairment in social or occupational functioning, causes marked distress, or requires medical attention.

HYPOCHONDRIASIS

For at least 6 months:

1. Preoccupation with fears of having, or the idea that one has, a serious disease.

2. Preoccupation persists despite appropriate medical tests and reassurances.

3. Other disorders are ruled out (e.g., somatic delusional disorders).

4. Preoccupation causes significant impairment in social or occupational functioning or causes marked distress.

PAIN DISORDER

1. Pain in one or more anatomical sites is a major part of the clinical picture.

2. Causes significant impairment in occupational or social functioning or causes marked distress.

3. Psychological factors thought to cause onset, severity, or exacerbation. **Pain associated with psychological factors.**

4. Symptoms not intentionally produced or feigned. If medical condition present, it plays minor role in accounting for pain.

5. **Pain may be associated with a psychological and/or medical condition.** Both factors are judged to be important in onset, severity, exacerbation, and maintenance of pain.

BODY DYSMORPHIC DISORDER (BDD)

1. Preoccupation with some imagined defect in appearance. If the defect is present, concern is excessive.

2. Preoccupation causes significant impairment in social or occupational functioning or causes marked distress.

3. Preoccupation not better accounted for by another mental disorder.

* The symptoms cannot be explained by a known medical condition or substance (drug/medication) or other mental disorder.

Figure 15–2 DSM-IV-TR criteria for somatoform disorders.

Anthony, a widower (his wife died of uterine cancer 3 years ago), is a self-employed plumber. Since the onset of his wife's illness and his own preoccupation with illness, his two daughters have visited at least weekly. He has no other social contacts, having given up attendance at an ethnic social club he once enjoyed.

The client was brought up in a strict religious environment, joined the Navy at age 17, and married shortly after discharge. Anthony reveals that despite his religious upbringing, he had several encounters with prostitutes while he was in the Navy. When his wife's illness was diagnosed, he began to wonder if he had acquired a "disease" and passed it on to her. He appears worried as he discusses with the nurse therapist his concern about having an STD and shares the story of his unsuccessful search for accurate diagnosis and treatment.

Pain Disorder

Diagnostic criteria for pain disorder cite pain in one or more anatomical sites as the predominant feature of this disorder. The pain must be of sufficient severity to cause significant distress, deserve clinical attention, and cause impaired social or occupational functioning. Psychological factors must be judged to play an important role in the onset, severity, exacerbation, or maintenance of the pain (see Fig. 15–2).

Vignette

■ Robert, aged 36 years, is referred to the outpatient mental health clinic by his private physician. He has suffered from chronic back pain for 2 years, during which he has been unable to work as a longshoreman. He leans heavily on a cane and moves slowly and deliberately when he walks. Robert states that he has had myelography, computed tomography (CT), and magnetic resonance imaging (MRI) that have shown no cause for his pain. He has used diazepam (Valium) and a variety of analgesics that afford him little relief. He states that he is never free of severe pain.

His back pain began after he played baseball at a picnic celebrating his wife's graduation from a community college nursing program. She had returned to school against his wishes when their youngest child entered high school. When his wife completed the program, he grudgingly agreed to her acceptance of a part-time position, but she instead chose a full-time position. He now states, "It's a good thing she went against me, because she's the breadwinner and has to take care of me, now that I can't work."

Body Dysmorphic Disorder

Body dysmorphic disorder involves preoccupation with an imagined defect in appearance that causes significant distress or impairment in social or occupational functioning (see Fig. 15–2).

Vignette

■ Anna, a 32-year-old office worker, is referred to the mental health center clinic by a plastic surgeon. She has been preoccupied with the size of her breasts for several years. Initially, she sought breast augmentation from the referring surgeon. After augmentation surgery, she reported seeing another plastic surgeon in hopes of having her breast size increased still further. Two years later, she returned to the first surgeon, seeking breast reduction. She was persuaded not to have surgery at that time. Two months ago, she again returned to the surgeon, expressing dissatisfaction with the size and shape of her breasts.

Conversion Disorder

Conversion disorder is characterized by the presence of one or more symptoms that suggest the presence of a neurological disorder that cannot be explained by a known neurological or medical disorder or a culturally bound symptom. Psychological factors, such as stress and conflicts, are present that are associated with the onset or exacerbation of the symptom (see Fig. 15–2).

Vignette

■ Pat, a fashion model, is admitted to the neurological unit on the eve of her 30th birthday, after the sudden onset of convulsions during a modeling assignment. She is an attractive woman whose manner with female nursing staff is indifferent and with male nursing staff and physicians is coy and flirtatious.

The first seizure recorded after hospitalization happens during morning rounds. As staff enter her room, Pat arches her back and begins pelvic thrusting motions while thrashing her arms and legs about on the bed. No loss of consciousness occurs. She is not incontinent, nor does she bite her tongue. Afterward, she is alert and oriented. The second seizure episode occurs in the afternoon during a visit from her mother and father and lasts 5 minutes. It begins with an outcry that brings nurses running. This time, Pat exhibits a period of generalized muscular rigidity, followed by pelvic thrusting and thrashing of her limbs. Again, no biting of the tongue or incontinence occurs during the sei-

tinue to be able to read, write, and perform skills such as driving a car. This use of automatic behaviors is similar to what goes on in our everyday lives when we say we have been operating on automatic pilot, performing an act or skill without concentrating on it.

PREVALENCE

There are no known data regarding actual prevalence of somatoform disorders.

DISSOCIATIVE AMNESIA. Although frequency of occurrence has not been adequately researched, it is believed that dissociative amnesia is more common than previously believed. People are often amnesic for traumatic events, and research investigations have found that 59% and 64% of study samples were amnesic for having been sexually abused prior to the age of 18 (Steinberg 1999).

DISSOCIATIVE FUGUE. Because of its rarity, little is known about the prevalence of fugues. Fugues are known to increase in prevalence in times of stress, such as war or natural disasters (Coons 1999).

DISSOCIATIVE IDENTITY DISORDER. Available epidemiological data is insufficient to state prevalence. It is believed that women have a higher incidence of DID, in a 5:1 to 9:1 women-to-men ratio (Putnam and Lowenstein 1999). Untreated, it is a chronic and recurring disorder (Spiegel and Maldonado 1999).

COMORBIDITY

DISSOCIATIVE AMNESIA. Clients may report depressive symptoms, anxiety, depersonalization, trance states, and spontaneous age regression, according to the DSM-IV-TR. Individuals with dissociative amnesia may also meet criteria for conversion disorder, a mood disorder, a substance-related disorder, or a personality disorder.

DISSOCIATIVE FUGUE. After returning to the individual's prefugue state, depression, dysphoria, anxiety, grief, shame, guilt, or suicidal or aggressive impulses may be present. Individuals with dissociative fugue may have a mood disorder, posttraumatic stress disorder, or a substance-related disorder (DSM-IV-TR).

DISSOCIATIVE IDENTITY DISORDER. North (1997) emphasized that the comorbid disorders that are always present and that are critical to the treatment plan include somatization disorder, borderline personality disorder, antisocial personality disorder, and substance abuse. Other phenomena that may

also be present include self-mutilative behavior, suicidal behavior, or impulsivity (DSM-IV-TR).

THEORY

The actual cause of dissociative disorders is unknown. However, childhood sexual abuse has been associated with adult dissociation symptomatology. DID is closely linked to severe experiences of childhood trauma (rates reported from 85% to 97% [Steinberg 1999]). Several theories are reviewed in the following sections.

Biological Factors

Current research suggests that the limbic system may be involved in the development of dissociative disorders. Traumatic memories are processed in the limbic system, and the hippocampus stores this information. Animal studies show that early prolonged detachment from the caretaker negatively affects the development of the limbic system. If this is true in humans, early trauma could remain detached from memory, and stress could precipitate dissociation. Significant early trauma and lack of attachment have also been demonstrated to have effects on neurotransmitters (specifically, serotonin).

Depersonalization disorder has a possible neurological link. The perception of change in one's own reality has been associated with neurological diseases, such as epilepsy and brain tumors, and psychiatric disorders, such as schizophrenia. Depersonalization is also experienced by individuals under the influence of certain drugs (e.g., alcohol, barbiturates, benzodiazepines, hallucinogens, and beta-adrenergic antagonists).

Genetic Factors

Several studies suggest that DID is more common among first-degree biological relatives of individuals with the disorder than in the population at large.

Cultural Factors

Certain culturally bound disorders exist in which there is a high level of activity, a trancelike state, and running or fleeing, followed by exhaustion, sleep, and amnesia regarding the episode. These syndromes include *piblokto*, seen in native people of the Arctic, Navajo *frenzy* witchcraft, and *amok* in Western Pacific natives. These syndromes, if seen in individuals native to these geographical areas, must be differentiated from dissociative disorders.

DSM-IV-TR lists dissociative trance disorder, which may involve a possession state, among diagnoses in need of further study. Possession is a concept that is often culturally determined. In the possession state, the individual believes the self to be controlled by a force, demon, deity, or other person. Clients and families profess little faith in conventional psychiatric treatment and instead seek rituals of atonement and exorcism.

Psychosocial Factors

Learning theory suggests that dissociative disorders can be explained as learned methods for avoiding stress and anxiety. The pattern of avoidance occurs when an individual deals with an unpleasant event by consciously deciding not to think about it or suppressing it (i.e., tuning out). The more anxiety-provoking the event, the greater the need not to think about it. Some individuals practice tuning out and become good at it, as evidenced by students tuning out what goes on in lectures or marriage partners seeming oblivious to the nagging of a spouse. It seems that the more dissociation is used, the more likely it is to become automatic. When stress is intolerable and ego disintegration becomes a possibility, the individual may unconsciously use dissociation to force the offending memory out of awareness.

All dissociative disorders are believed to be linked with traumatic life events, such as childhood abuse, kidnapping, incest, rape, postwartime combat, other threats of death or physical violence, or even being a witness to violence (Steinberg 1999). Abused individuals may learn to use dissociation to defend against feeling pain and to avoid remembering.

DSM-IV-TR AND THE CLINICAL PICTURE OF DISSOCIATIVE DISORDERS

DSM-IV-TR lists four major dissociative disorders: (1) depersonalization disorder, (2) dissociative amnesia, (3) dissociative fugue, and (4) DID.

Depersonalization Disorder

DSM-IV-TR describes depersonalization disorder as a persistent or recurrent alteration in the perception of the self to the extent that the sense of one's own reality is temporarily lost while reality testing ability remains intact. The person experiencing depersonalization may feel mechanical, dreamy, or detached from the body. These experiences of feeling a sense of deadness of the body, of seeing self from a distance, or of perceiving the limbs to be larger or smaller than normal are described by clients as being very disturbing (ego dystonic) (Fig. 15–3).

Vignette

■ Margaret describes becoming very distressed at perceiving changes in her appearance when she looks in a mirror. She thinks that her image looks wavy and indistinct. Soon after, she describes feeling as though she is floating in a fog with her feet not actually touching the ground. Questioning reveals that Margaret's son has recently revealed to her that he is HIV positive.

Dissociative Amnesia

Dissociative amnesia is marked by an inability to recall important personal information, often of a traumatic or stressful nature, that is too pervasive to be explained by ordinary forgetfulness (see Fig. 15–3). Clients with generalized amnesia are unable to recall information about their entire lifetime.

Vignette

■ A young woman, found wandering in a Florida park, is partly dressed and poorly nourished. She has no knowledge of who she is. Her parents identify her 2 weeks later when she appears in an interview on a national television show. She had just broken up with her boyfriend of 3 years.

The client with localized amnesia is unable to remember all events of a circumscribed period, from a few hours to a few days (e.g., the hours following the death of a loved one).

Vignette

■ Ann, a college student, is found walking along a major highway by a police road patrol. She can give her name and address but is not able to account for how she came to be walking along the highway. She is able to remember going to a party off-campus but has no recall of the party or events after. Hospital examination reveals the probability of recent rape.

Selective amnesia involves the ability to remember some events, but not others, during a short period (e.g., remembering an automobile accident but not remembering the death of someone involved in the accident).

DSM–IV–TR CRITERIA FOR DISSOCIATIVE DISORDERS

DISSOCIATIVE DISORDERS

DISSOCIATIVE AMNESIA*	DISSOCIATIVE FUGUE*	DISSOCIATIVE IDENTITY DISORDER* (DID)	DEPERSONALIZATION DISORDER*
1. One or more episodes of inability to recall important information — usually of a traumatic or stressful nature. 2. Causes significant distress or impairment in social, occupational, or other important areas of functioning.	1. Sudden, unexpected travel away from home or one's place of work with inability to remember past. 2. Confusion about personal identity or assumption of new identity. 3. Symptoms cause significant distress or impairment in social, occupational, or other important areas of functioning.	1. Existence of two or more distinct subpersonalities, each with its own patterns of relating, perceiving, and thinking. 2. At least two of these subpersonalities take control of the person's behavior. 3. Inability to recall important information too extensive to be explained by ordinary forgetfulness.	1. Persistent or recurrent experience of feeling detached from and outside of one's mental processes or body. 2. Reality testing remains intact. 3. The experience causes significant impairment in social or occupational functioning or causes marked distress.
*Not due to substance, medical, neurological, or other psychiatric disorder.	*Not due to substance, medical, neurological, or other psychiatric disorder.	*Not due to substance, medical, neurological, or other psychiatric disorder.	*Not due to substance, medical, neurological, or other psychiatric disorder.

Figure 15–3 DSM-IV-TR criteria for dissociative disorders.

Dissociative Fugue

Dissociative fugue is characterized by sudden, unexpected travel away from the customary locale and inability to recall identity and information about some or all of the past; in rare cases, a fugue has involved the assumption of a new identity. If a new identity is assumed, the new personality may be somewhat more outgoing. During a fugue state, individuals tend to lead rather simple lives, rarely calling attention to themselves. After a few weeks to a few months, they may remember their former identities and become amnesic for the time spent in the fugue (see Fig. 15–3 for DSM-IV-TR criteria).

Vignette

■ A *middle-aged woman awakens one morning and notices snow outside the window, swirling around unfamiliar buildings and streets. The radio tells her it is December. She is perplexed to find herself in a residential hotel in Chicago with no idea of how she got there. She feels confused and shaken. As she leaves the hotel, she is surprised to have strangers recognize her and say "Good morning, Sally." The name Sally does not seem right, but she cannot remember her true identity. She finds her way to a hospi-tal, where she is evaluated and referred to the psychiatric nurse in the emergency department. A day later, "Sally" is able to remember her true identity, Mary Hunt. She tells the nurse tearfully that she can now recall that her husband came home one day and "out of the blue" told her he wanted a divorce to marry a younger woman. Mary calls her sister in New York, who comes to Chicago to take her home.*

Most theorists agree that spontaneous loss of memory, as in amnesia and fugue, will have been preceded by a severely traumatic event. Amnesia or fugue is most likely to occur during a time of great disorganization, such as a war or a disaster in which the threat of physical injury or death exists. Other stressors severe enough to produce psychogenic amnesia or fugue include the loss of a loved one and the stress of having to face the unacceptability of certain impulses or acts, such as an extramarital affair.

Dissociative Identity Disorder

The essential feature of dissociative identity disorder (DID) is the presence of two or more distinct alternate personality (alter) or subpersonality states that recurrently take control of behavior. Each alter, or subpersonality, has its own pattern of perceiving, relating to, and thinking about the self and the environment. It is believed that severe sexual, physical, or psychological trauma in childhood predisposes an individual to the development of DID. The steps in the development of dissociated personalities identified by Greenberg (1982) are as follows:

1. A young child is confronted with an intolerable terror-producing event at a time when defenses are inadequate to handle the intense anxiety.
2. The child dissociates the event and the feelings associated with the event. The dissociated processes are split off from the memory of the primary personality.
3. The dissociated part of the personality takes on an existence of its own, becoming a subpersonality.
4. The subpersonality learns to deal with feelings and emotions that could overwhelm the primary personality.

This process may occur several times, creating one or several subpersonalities. When the individual is faced with an anxiety-producing situation, one of the subpersonalities takes over to protect the primary personality from disorganization and disintegration.

Each alternate personality or subpersonality is a complex unit with its own memories, behavior patterns, and social relationships that dictate how the person acts when that personality is dominant. Often, the original or primary personality is religious and moralistic, and the subpersonalities are quite different: aggressive, pleasure seeking, nonconforming, or sexually promiscuous. They may think of themselves as being a different sex, race, religion, or sexual orientation. Sometimes, the dominant hand is different, and the voice may sound different; intelligence and electroencephalographic findings may also be different. Alternate or subpersonalities may exhibit signs of emotional disturbance. A common alternate personality is a fearful, insecure child. Some subpersonalities have names for themselves. Some may be identified by roles they play: *host*, who provides the social front for interacting with the world; *protector*, who defends against harm; and *persecutor*, who attempts to harm other personalities.

Typical cognitive distortions include the insistence that alternative personalities inhabit separate bodies and are unaffected by the actions of one another. The primary personality is usually not aware of the alternate or subpersonalities but may be aware of, and perplexed by, lost time and unexplained events. Experiences such as finding unfamiliar clothing in the closet, being called a different name by a stranger, waking up or coming out of a blank spell in strange surroundings, or not having childhood memories are characteristic of DID. Subpersonalities are often aware of the existence of each other to some degree. Some may even interact with each other. Occasionally, one alternate personality may attempt to harm another. Alternate personalities may listen in on whatever personality is dominant at the time. Transition from one personality to another often occurs during times of stress and may range from a dramatic to a barely noticeable event. Some clients experience the transition when awakening. Shifts from personality to personality last from minutes to months, although shorter periods are more common.

Vignette

■ **Andrea**, *a conservative, 28-year-old electrical engineer, is the primary personality. Three alternate personalities coexist and vie for supremacy.*

*   **Michele** is a 5-year-old who is sometimes playful and sometimes angry. She speaks with a slight lisp and with the facial expressions, voice inflections, and vocabulary of a precocious child. She likes to play on swings, draw with a crayon, and eat ice cream. She likes to cuddle a teddy bear and occasionally sucks her thumb. Her favorite outfit is jeans and a Mickey Mouse sweatshirt.*

*   **Ann** is an accomplished ballet dancer. She is shy but firm about needing time to practice. When she is dominant, she likes to wear white and fixes her hair in a severe, pulled-back style. She does little but dance when she is in control.*

*   **Bridget** is near Andrea's age; although she says a lady never tells her age. She dresses seductively in bright colors, wears her hair tousled, and likes to frequent bars and stay out late. She often drinks to excess and has several male admirers. Bridget has many moods. She states that she would like to get rid of Ann and Andrea because they're such "goody-goodies."*

*   Andrea does not drink, hates ice cream, and sees herself as somewhat awkward. She does not dance. Instead, she is a paid soloist in a church choir. Andrea takes public transportation, but Ann and Bridget have driver's licenses. Andrea goes to bed and arises early, but Bridget and Michele like to stay up late.*

*   Andrea seeks treatment when she finds herself behind the wheel of a moving car and realizes that she does not know how to drive. She has been concerned for some time because she has found strange clothes in her closet. She has also received phone calls from men who insist that she has flirted with them in bars. She sometimes misses appointments and cannot account for periods of time. Al-*

though she goes to bed early, she is often unaccountably tired in the morning.

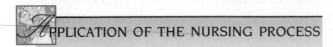

APPLICATION OF THE NURSING PROCESS

ASSESSMENT

For a diagnosis of dissociative disorder to be made, medical and neurological status, substance use, and coexistence of other psychiatric disorders need to be ruled out. Therefore, medical personnel collect objective data from physical examination, electroencephalography, CT, or MRI to rule out organic or other medical or psychiatric disorders. Most of the time the DID client will be treated in the community. However, a client with DID is admitted to a psychiatric unit when suicidal or in need of crisis stabilization. At that time, nursing assessment takes place through observation over a period as the nurse gathers information about identity, memory, consciousness, life events, mood, suicide risk, and impact of the disorder on the client and the family.

The student is urged to see the film "Sybil" (1976) which is a movie of an actual case study of a person with multiple personalities (DID). An older movie, "The Three Faces of Eve" (1957), also depicts a story of a person being treated for multiple personalities.

Overall Assessment

IDENTITY AND MEMORY

Assessing clients' ability to identify themselves requires more than asking clients to state their name. In addition, inability to identify self, or changes in client behavior, voice, and dress, might signal the presence of an alternate personality. Referring to self by another name or in the third person, using the word "we" instead of "I," are indications that the client may have assumed a new identity, as occurs in some fugue states. The nurse should consider the following when assessing memory:

- Can the client remember recent and past events?
- Is the client's memory clear and complete or partial and fuzzy?
- Is the client aware of gaps in memory, such as lack of memory for events such as a graduation or a wedding?
- Do the client's memories place the self with a family, in schools, in an occupation?

Clients with amnesia and fugue may be disoriented for time and place as well as person. Relevant assessment questions include the following:

- Do you ever lose time or have blackouts?
- Do you find yourself in places with no idea how you got there?

CLIENT HISTORY

The nurse must gather information about events in the person's life. Has the client sustained a recent injury, such as a concussion? Does the client have a history of epilepsy, especially temporal lobe epilepsy? Does the client have a history of early trauma, such as physical, mental, and sexual abuse? If DID is suspected, pertinent questions include the following:

- Have you ever found yourself wearing clothes you don't remember?
- Have you ever found strange clothing in your closet?
- Have you ever found among your belongings new items that you can't remember buying?
- Have you ever had strange people greet and talk to you as though they were old friends?
- Have you ever found writing or drawing that you can't remember doing?
- Does your ability to do things such as athletics, artistic activities, or mechanical tasks seem to change?
- Do you have differing sets of memories about childhood? (This is often an indicator of DID.)

MOOD

Is the individual depressed, anxious, or unconcerned? Many clients with DID seek help when the primary personality is depressed. The nurse also observes for mood shifts. When subpersonalities of DID take control, their predominant moods may be different from that of the principal personality. If the subpersonalities shift frequently, marked mood swings may be noted. Clients with DID or fugue may seem indifferent and unconcerned or may be uneasy or perplexed. A client with DID is likely to exhibit moderate to severe anxiety. This client often seeks help because of fear of "going crazy."

USE OF ALCOHOL AND OTHER DRUGS

Specific questions should be asked to identify drug or alcohol use or abuse. Dissociative episodes may be associated with recent alcohol use. Marijuana is known to produce symptoms of depersonalization. Some clients with dissociative disorders turn to alcohol in an attempt to cope with the disorder itself.

IMPACT ON CLIENT AND FAMILY

Has the client's ability to function been impaired? Have disruptions in family functioning occurred? Is secondary gain evident? In fugue states, individuals often function adequately in their new identities by choosing simple, undemanding occupations and having few intimate social interactions. The families of clients in fugue states report being highly distressed over the client's disappearance. Clients with amnesia may be more dysfunctional. Their perplexity often renders them unable to work, and their memory loss impairs normal family relationships. Families often direct considerable attention and solicitude toward the client but may exhibit concern over having to assume roles that were once assigned to the client. Clients with DID often have both family and work problems. Families find it difficult to accept the seemingly erratic behaviors of the client. Employers dislike the lost time that may accompany subpersonalities' being in control. Clients with depersonalization disorder are often fearful that others may perceive their appearance as distorted and may avoid being seen in public. If they exhibit high anxiety, the family is likely to find it difficult to keep relationships stable.

SUICIDE RISK

Whenever a client's life has been substantially disrupted, the client may have thoughts of suicide. The nurse gathering data should be alert for expressions of hopelessness, helplessness, or worthlessness and for verbalization or other behavior of a subpersonality that indicates the intent to engage in self-destructive or self-mutilating behaviors.

Self-Assessment

Nurses may experience feelings of skepticism while caring for clients with dissociative disorders. They may find it difficult to believe in the authenticity of the symptoms the client is displaying.

Feeling confused and bewildered by the presence of multiple identities is not unusual. Anger is commonly experienced as a reaction toward a subpersonality of a client with DID, if one personality is perceived as immature, challenging, or unpleasant. Some nurses experience feelings of fascination and are caught up in the intrigue of caring for a client with multiple identities. A sense of inadequacy may accompany the need to be ready to interact in a therapeutic way with whatever personality is in control at the moment.

Similarly, the nurse may feel inadequate when establishment of a trusting relationship occurs slowly. It is important for the nurse to remember that the client with a dissociative disorder has often experienced relationships in which trust was betrayed. When subpersonalities vie for control and attempt to embarrass or harm each other, crises are common. The nurse must be alert and ready to intervene and must always be prepared for the unexpected, including the possibility of a client's suicide attempt. Continuing hypervigilence by staff can eventually lead to feelings of fatigue. Anxiety may also be experienced by the nurse caring for a client with dissociative disorder in any of the following situations:

■ When a client who has regained memory develops panic-level anxiety related to guilt feelings
■ When a client becomes assaultive because of extreme confusion or panic-level anxiety
■ When a client attempts self-harm by acting out against the primary personality or other personalities
■ When a client develops panic-level anxiety during a depersonalization experience

If the client manifesting symptoms of a dissociative disorder has been involved in the commission of a crime, the nurse may experience concern over the fact that the medical record is likely to be a court exhibit. Nurses may feel anger in this situation if they believe that the client is faking illness to avoid being found guilty of the crime.

Supervision should always be available for staff and clinicians caring for a client with a dissociative disorder in all settings. By discussing feelings as well as the plan for care with a competent peer or peers, the nurse can better ensure objective and appropriate care for the client.

Hospitalization of clients with dissociative disorders is brief and crisis centered, if it is required at all. Most therapy is conducted at the outpatient level. Planning should involve the client. Opportunities to participate in the care of the self combat feelings of helplessness and powerlessness.

NURSING DIAGNOSIS

Nursing diagnoses for clients with dissociative disorders include those discussed in this section. For example, the nurse needs to remember that nursing diagnoses may be required for subpersonalities as well as for the primary personality (Table 15–5).

TABLE 15–5 *Potential Nursing Diagnosis for Dissociative Disorders*	
SIGNS AND SYMPTOMS	**NURSING DIAGNOSIS**
■ Amnesia or fugue related to a traumatic event	**Disturbed personal identity**
■ Symptoms of depersonalization; feelings of unreality and/or body image distortions	**Disturbed body image**
■ Alterations in consciousness, memory, or identity	**Ineffective coping**
■ Abuse of substances related to dissociation	**Ineffective role performance**
■ Disorganization or dysfunction in usual patterns of behavior (absence from work, withdrawal from relationships, changes role function)	
■ Disturbances in memory and identity	**Interrupted family processes**
■ Interrupted family processes related to amnesia or erratic and changing behavior	**Impaired parenting**
■ Feeling out of control of memory, behaviors, and awareness	**Anxiety** **Spiritual distress** **Risk for other-directed violence**
■ Unable to explain actions or behaviors when in altered state	**Risk for self-directed violence**

OUTCOME CRITERIA

Outcomes must be established for each nursing diagnosis. Because each client presents an individual set of circumstances, outcomes must be highly individualized and consistent with each client's assessment. Some potential outcome criteria for a client with a dissociative disorder (amnesia, fugue, depersonalization, DID) might be that the client will

■ Demonstrate ability to integrate identity and memory
■ Demonstrate a reduction in anxiety and/or depression
■ Resume pre-illness roles (occupational, family, friend)
■ Interact appropriately on a social level with family and peers

■ Refrain from attempts at self-harm or violent aggressive outbursts

Another outcome criteria would be that the family will demonstrate interactions that promote optimal functioning of client and family.

PLANNING

Planning nursing care for the client with a dissociative disorder relies heavily on the assessment and the priority of care needed. For example, is the client in crisis (suicidal or homicidal)? Is the client able to function in his or her primary role (family member, employee, student)? Is the client suffering from overwhelming degrees of anxiety or depression that might benefit from treatment? Do any of the subpersonalities require specialized medical treatment? Could the client benefit from specific social skills training? Is family therapy or couples therapy indicated? Is there support for the family or significant others? A good rule of thumb in planning care for any client, especially one which may have as many complex needs as a client with DID is always "safety first." Longer-term goals need to be realistic since clients with DID may require long-term skilled psychotherapy, perhaps with crisis intervention at various intervals.

INTERVENTION

Because nurses see relatively few clients with dissociative disorders, they are often anxious and unsure about the clinical decisions they are called on to make.

Psychosocial Interventions

Basic psychosocial interventions are aimed at offering emotional presence during the recalling of painful experiences, to provide a sense of safety, and to encourage an optimal level of functioning (Table 15–6).

Psychotherapy

Individual counseling for clients with amnesia, fugue, and depersonalization disorder focuses on creating a therapeutic alliance in which the client trusts the therapist and feels safe and relaxed. Feelings, conflicts, and situations that the client experienced before the onset of the dissociative disorder can then be explored. It is important to identify, as early as possible, triggers in the environment that lead to dissociation.

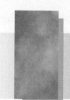

TABLE 15–6 *Psychosocial Interventions and Rationales: Dissociative Disorders*

INTERVENTION	RATIONALE
1. Ensure client safety by providing safe, protected environment and frequent observation.	1. Sense of bewilderment may lead to inattention to safety needs; some subpersonalities may be thrill seeking, violent, or careless
2. Provide nondemanding, simple routine.	2. Reduces anxiety
3. Confirm identity of client and orientation to time and place.	3. Supports reality and promotes ego integrity
4. Encourage clients to do things for themselves and make decisions about routine tasks.	4. Enhances self-esteem by reducing sense of powerlessness, and reduces secondary gain associated with dependence
5. Assist with other decision making until memory returns.	5. Lowers stress and prevents client from having to live with the consequences of unwise decisions
6. Support client during exploration of feelings surrounding the stressful event.	6. Helps lower the defense of dissociation used by the client to block awareness of the stressful event
7. Do not flood the client with data regarding past events.	7. Memory loss serves the purpose of preventing severe to panic levels of anxiety to overtake and disorganize the individual
8. Allow client to progress at own pace as memory is recovered.	8. Prevents undue anxiety and resistance
9. Provide support during disclosure of painful experiences.	9. Can be healing while minimizing feelings of isolation
10. Help client see consequences of using dissociation to cope with stress.	10. Increases insight and helps client understand own role in choosing behaviors
11. Accept client's expression of negative feelings.	11. Conveys permission to have negative or unacceptable feelings
12. Teach stress reduction methods.	12. Provides alternatives for anxiety relief
13. If client does not remember significant others, work with involved parties to re-establish relationships.	13. Helps client experience satisfaction and relieves sense of isolation

Psychotherapy for clients with DID have included psychoanalytic psychotherapy, cognitive-behavioral therapy, and hypnotherapy predominantly (Putnam and Lowenstein 1999). Therapy with DID clients is complex and requires the therapist to provide continuity, stability, and respectful impartiality toward the different alter (sub) personalities.

The ultimate goal for psychotherapy for DID clients is the integration of the disparate states of unconscious entities. Therapists often use the *rule of thirds* in therapy sessions to integrate all the subpersonalities into the main personality (Kluft 1991a, 1991b):

1. **First Third**: Assess individual's mental state and life problem areas that might benefit from retrieval into conscious memory and working through.
2. **Second Third**: Assess and work through the memory.
3. **Final Third**: Help client assimilate the information and regulate and modulate the emotional responses.

Hypnotherapy can be helpful in therapy as well as in diagnosis (Spiegel and Maldonado 1999). Hypnotherapy allows the client's conscious control to relax so the therapist and the client can access material from the unconscious or make contact with subpersonalities. Counseling for clients with DID is of much longer duration and moves through several phases.

Family counseling may assist in exploring and reducing role strain and family dysfunction. Often, the family member who has been physically absent because of fugue, mentally absent because of amnesia, or socially absent because of self-imposed isolation associated with depersonalization episodes must be reassimilated into the family. Families with members who are being treated for multiple identities need support to cope with the chaotic behaviors and to accept the integrated personality at the conclusion of therapy.

Milieu Therapy

When the client is in a crisis that requires hospitalization for stabilization, or if the client is suicidal, providing a safe environment is fundamental. Other desirable characteristics of the environment are that it is quiet, simple, structured, and supportive. Confusion and noise increase anxiety and the potential for depersonalization, delayed memory return, or shifts among subpersonalities. Group therapy has not proved to be helpful, but task-oriented groups, such as occupational and art therapy, give an opportunity for self-expression. Attendance at community or unit milieu meetings relieves feelings of isolation.

Teaching Coping Skills

Preventing dissociative episodes is a skill the nurse can help the client learn. It involves becoming aware of triggers to dissociation and developing a plan to interrupt the dissociative episode. Clients are encouraged to play an instrument or sing, engage in a specific physical activity, or interact with another person. Staff and significant others are made aware of the plan to foster their cooperation.

Clients should also be taught to write a daily journal. The journal puts the client in touch with feelings and provides concrete examples of overcoming triggers to dissociation. The journal should be shared with the nurse therapist on a periodic basis. If a client has never written a journal, the nurse should suggest beginning with a 5- to 10-minute daily writing exercise.

Case Management

Clients with dissociative disorders may require long-term case management. It may be necessary for the case manager to interact with numerous health professionals and health care agencies to facilitate the client's access to services and to maintain psychosocial functioning.

Psychopharmacology

There is no evidence that medication of any type has been therapeutic with the dissociative experience (Spiegel and Maldonado 1999). Antidepressants are the most useful class of psychotropics for use with DID. Many clients with DID have dysthymia disorder, or major depression, and can be suicidal at times (Spiegel and Maldonado 1999).

EVALUATION

Treatment is considered successful when outcomes are met. In the final analysis, the evaluation is positive when

- Client safety has been maintained
- Anxiety has been alleviated and the client has returned to a state of comfort
- Conflicts have been explored
- New coping strategies have permitted the client to function at his or her optimal level
- Stress is handled adaptively, without the use of dissociation

Visit the **Evolve** website at
http://evolve.elsevier.com/Varcarolis
for the other Nursing Care Plan diagnoses and for
more Nursing Care Plans.

NURSING CARE PLAN 15-1   A *Person with Conversion Disorder*: Pat

NURSING DIAGNOSIS

Ineffective Coping: use of conversion symptoms [seizures] related to low self-esteem and unmet needs for recognition and attention

Supporting Data

- No incontinence. No injury. Seizures vary and occur only in the presence of others
- Relates with seductive behavior toward men
- Relates with superiority and contempt toward friends
- Bland affect regarding personal problems (la belle indifférence)

Outcome Criteria: Client will cope effectively with life stress without using conversion

SHORT-TERM GOAL	INTERVENTION	RATIONALE	EVALUATION
1. Client will adjust to unit routine by (date).	1. Explain routine. Establish expectations regarding unit routines, e.g., do not allow special privileges. Expect client to eat in dining room, perform activities of daily living (ADLs), attend activities.	1. Reduces anxiety. Reduces secondary gain and manipulation.	*OUTCOME MET* Client initially refuses to leave room for meals. Misses one meal. Goes to dining room thereafter. Performs all ADLs, with special attention to applying make-up.
2. Client will remain free of injury.	2. Provide safety measures during seizures but limit attention and discussion about seizures afterward. Monitor physical condition unobtrusively.	2. Prevents harm. Reduces secondary gain. Minimizes secondary gain while condition is assessed.	Client does not sustain injury during seizures. States, "I guess my seizures don't interest staff. No one will talk to me about them." Client has no seizures after day 3 on psychiatric unit.
3. Client will identify one or two stressors by (date).	3. Encourage client to discuss life, work, significant others, and goals.	3. Uncovers stress, conflict, and strengths.	Client repeatedly mentions that 30th birthday means she is over the hill as a model.
4. Client will express at least feelings about the stressors by (date).	4. Encourage exploration of feelings.	4. Conveys interest.	Client states she is scared of losing her glamorous appearance and her job. Demonstrates appropriate affect.

Nursing Care Plan continued on following page

NURSING CARE PLAN 15-1   *A Person with Conversion Disorder:* **Pat** *(Continued)*

SHORT-TERM GOAL	INTERVENTION	RATIONALE	EVALUATION
5. Client will problem solve possible solutions to the problem by (date).	5. Focus on alternatives available to her to earn a living when modeling is no longer an option.	5. Encourages problem solving.	Client shows fashion sketches to nurse and reveals that she had once thought that she might be a good designer. With encouragement, decides to explore evening classes in illustration and design to prepare for second career.
6. Client will name three alternative ways to cope with stress by (date).	6. Encourage use of alternative anxiety reduction techniques. Encourage client to select and learn such a method.	6. Develops skill in use of a healthy technique.	Client chooses to use jogging and progressive muscle relaxation and attends teaching sessions after discharge.

SUMMARY

Somatoform disorders involve client complaints of physical symptoms that closely resemble actual medical conditions. Physical examination and diagnostic testing reveal no organic basis for the symptoms. Dissociative disorders make up a group of relatively rare conditions involving alteration in consciousness, memory, or identity. The cause of somatoform and dissociative disorders is assumed to be psychological (i.e., the appearance of symptoms provides relief of anxiety associated with a conflict or a traumatic event). Secondary gain is often present and must be minimized if treatment is to be successful.

Common nursing diagnoses are

■ Anxiety
■ Ineffective coping
■ Impaired social interaction
■ Compromised family coping
■ Chronic low self-esteem
■ Self-care deficit

Discussions of planning and intervention for clients with these disorders include the need to provide for client safety, to reduce secondary gain, to encourage performance of self-care activities, to promote effective communication, and to provide a therapeutic milieu.

Psychotherapy is the treatment of choice for clients with somatoform and dissociative disorders. The nurse's roles include providing counseling, developing and implementing plans for behavioral change, assisting with cognitive restructuring, teaching anxiety-reducing strategies, and engaging in health promotion and maintenance activities.

Visit the **Evolve** website at
http://evolve.elsevier.com/Varcarolis
for a post-test on the content in this chapter.

Visit the **Evolve** website at
http://evolve.elsevier.com/Varcarolis
for additional self-study exercises.

Critical Thinking and Chapter Review

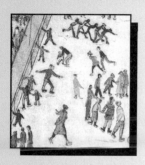

Critical Thinking

1. A client with suspected somatization disorder has been admitted to the medical-surgical unit after an episode of chest pain with possible electrocardiographic changes. While on the unit, she frequently complains of palpitations, asks the nurse to check her vital signs, and begs staff to stay with her. Some nurses take her pulse and blood pressure when she requests it. Others evade her requests. Most staff try to avoid spending time with her. Consider why staff wish to avoid her. Design interventions to cope with the client's behaviors. Give rationales for your interventions.

2. A client with body dysmorphic disorder talks incessantly about how big her nose is, the way those around her are offended by her appearance, and how her appearance has negatively affected her employment and her social life. What interventions could you take to promote cognitive restructuring?

3. A client with dissociative identity disorder has been admitted to the crisis unit for a short-term stay after a suicide threat. On the unit, the client has repeated the statement that she will kill herself to get rid of "all the others," meaning her subpersonalities. The client refuses to sign a "no harm" contract. Design a care plan to meet her safety and security needs.

Chapter Review

Choose the most appropriate answer.

1. Nurses working with clients with somatization and dissociative disorders can expect that these clients will fit on the continuum of psychobiological disorders at the

   1. Mild level.
   2. Moderate-severe level.
   3. Severe-psychotic level.
   4. They do not belong on the continuum, as anxiety has been reduced by ego defense mechanisms.

2. Mr. R. presents with a history of having assumed a new identity in a distant locale and of having no recollection of his former identity. Which DSM-IV-TR diagnosis can the nurse expect the psychiatrist to make?

   1. Hypochondriasis.
   2. Conversion disorder.
   3. Dissociative fugue.
   4. Depersonalization disorder.

3. The data that are least relevant when assessing a client with a suspected somatoform disorder are

   1. Whether the symptom is under voluntary control.
   2. Results of diagnostic work-ups.
   3. Limitations in activities of daily living.
   4. Potential for violence.

4. A suitable outcome criterion for the nursing diagnosis *Ineffective coping* related to dependence on pain relievers to treat chronic pain of psychological origin would be: client will

   1. Resume pre-illness roles.
   2. Cope adaptively as evidenced by use of alternative coping strategies.
   3. Demonstrate improved self-esteem as evidenced by focusing less on weaknesses.
   4. Replace demanding, manipulative behaviors with more socially acceptable behavior.

5. Which nursing diagnosis would be LEAST likely to be used for a client with hypochondriasis?

   1. Self-care deficit.
   2. Ineffective denial.
   3. Deficient diversional activity.
   4. Interrupted family processes.

REFERENCES

American Psychiatric Association. (1994). *Diagnostic and statistical manual of mental disorders* (4th ed.). Washington, D.C.

American Psychiatric Association. (2000). *Diagnostic and statistical manual of mental disorders* (4th ed., text revision). Washington, D.C.

Castle, D. J., and Morkell, D. (2000). "Imagined ugliness," a symptom which can become a disorder. *Medical Journal of Australia*, 173(4):205–207.

Coons, P. M. (1999). Dissociative fugue. In B. J. Sadock and V. A. Sadock (Eds.), *Kaplan and Sadock's comprehensive textbook of psychiatry* (7th ed., Vol. 1.) (pp. 1549–1551). Philadelphia: Lippincott Williams & Wilkins.

Greenberg, W. C. (1982). The multiple personality. *Perspectives in Psychiatric Care*, 20(3):100.

Grinspoon, I. (Ed.). (1992). Dissociation and dissociative disorders: I. *Harvard Mental Health Letter*, 8(9):1.

Guggenheim, F. G. (1999). Somatoform disorders. In B. J. Sadock and V. A. Sadock (Eds.), *Kaplan and Sadock's comprehensive textbook of psychiatry* (7th ed., Vol. 1.). Philadelphia: Lippincott Williams & Wilkins.

Hollander, E., et al. (1999). Clomipramine vs. desipramine crossover trial in body dysmorphic disorder: Selective efficacy of a serotonin reuptake inhibitor in imagined ugliness. *Archives of General Psychiatry*, 56(11):1033–1039.

Kaplan, H., et al. (1994). *Kaplan and Sadock's synopsis of psychiatry.* Baltimore: Williams & Wilkins.

Katon, W. (1997). Somatization disorder, hypochondriasis, and conversion disorder. In D. Dunner (Ed.), *Current psychiatric therapy II* (pp. 346–352). Philadelphia: W. B. Saunders.

Kendler, K. S., et al. (1995). A twin-family study of self-report symptoms of panic-phobia and somatization. *Behavioral Genetics*, 25(6):499–515.

Kluft, R. P. (1991a). Hospital treatment of multiple personality disorder. *Psychiatric Clinics of North America*, 14(3): 695–719.

Kluft, R. P. (1991b). Clinical presentation of multiple personality disorder. *Psychiatric Clinics of North America* 14(3): 605–629.

Kopelman, J. D. (1987). Amnesia: Organic and psychogenic. *British Journal of Psychiatry*, 144:293.

Leff, J. (1988). *Psychiatry around the globe: A transcultural view* (2nd ed.). London: Royal College of Physicians.

Martin, R. L., and Yutzy, S. H. (1999). Somatoform disorders. In R. Hales, S. C. Yudofsky, and J. A. Talbott (Eds.), *The American Psychiatric Press textbook of psychiatry* (3rd ed.) (pp. 663–694). Washington, D.C.: American Psychiatric Press.

North, C. S. (1997). Multiple personality disorders, fugue states, and amnesic disorders. In D. Dunner (Ed.), *Current psychiatric therapy II* (pp. 358–363). Philadelphia: W. B. Saunders.

Noyes, R., Jr., Happel, R. L., and Yagla, S. J. (1999). Correlates of hypochondriasis in a nonclinical population. *Psychosomatics*, 40(6):461–469.

Perkins, R. J. (1999). SSRI antidepressants are effective for treating delusional hypochondriasis [letter]. *Medical Journal of Australia*, 170(3):140–141.

Putnam, F. W., and Lowenstein, R. J. (1999). Dissociative identify disorder. In B. J. Sadock and V. A. Sadock (Eds.), *Kaplan and Sadock's comprehensive textbook of psychiatry* (7th ed., Vol. 1.) (pp. 1552–1563). Philadelphia: Lippincott Williams & Wilkins.

Spiegel, D., and Maldonado, J. R. (1999). Dissociative disorders. In R. Hales, S. C. Yudofsky, and J. A. Talbott (Eds.), *The American Psychiatric Press textbook of psychiatry* (3rd ed.) (pp. 711–738). Washington, D.C.: American Psychiatric Press.

Steinberg, M. (1999). Depersonalization disorder. In B. J. Sadock and V. A. Sadock (Eds.), *Kaplan and Sadock's comprehensive textbook of psychiatry* (7th ed., Vol. 1.) (pp. 1564–1569). Philadelphia: Lippincott Williams & Wilkins.

Steinberg, M. (1999). Dissociate amnesia. In B. J. Sadock and V. A. Sadock (Eds.), *Kaplan and Sadock's comprehensive textbook of psychiatry* (7th ed., Vol. 1.) (pp. 1544–1548). Philadelphia: Lippincott Williams & Wilkins.

Steinhausen, H. C., von Aster, M., Pfeiffer, E., and Gobel, D. (1989). Comparative studies of conversion disorders in childhood and adolescence. *Journal of Child Psychological Psychiatry*, 30(4):615–621.

Zlotnick, C., et al. (1994). The relationship between characteristics of sexual abuse and dissociative experiences. *Comprehensive Psychiatry*, 35(6):465.

Outline

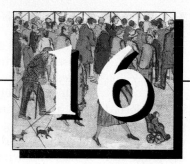

Personality Disorders

ELIZABETH M. VARCAROLIS

Key Terms and Concepts

The key terms and concepts listed here also appear in color where they are first defined or discussed in this chapter.

antisocial personality disorder

borderline personality disorder

devaluation

histrionics

idealization

limit setting

manipulation

narcissism

personality disorder

personality traits

self-mutilation

splitting

Objectives

After studying this chapter, the reader will be able to

1. Analyze the interrelatedness of biological determinants, chronic trauma, and psychodynamic issues in the cause of personality disorders.

2. Compare and contrast the main characteristics of each of the three clusters of personality disorders.

3. Describe the *Diagnostic and Statistical Manual of Mental Disorders*, fourth edition, text revision (2000) characteristics as seen on assessment of one personality disorder from each cluster and give a clinical example.

4. Formulate two nursing diagnoses that are characteristic of each personality disorder.

5. Discuss the nature and the importance of crisis intervention for people with personality disorders.

6. Become aware of the feelings that are experienced by nurses/others when working with people with a personality disorder.

7. Explain the importance of keeping clear boundaries when working with a person with a personality disorder.

8. Plan basic interventions for an impulsive, aggressive, or manipulative client.

*A*n individual's personality encompasses enduring and consistent attitudes, beliefs, desires, values and patterns of behavior. Personality has been referred to as an evolving pattern of thinking, perceiving, and experiencing. Personality patterns determine whether an individual is liked, how others judge him or her, and what his or her goals and accomplishments are in life. To a certain extent, these patterns are acquired in early childhood and become lifelong patterns of behavior (Gunderson and Phillips 1995).

The American Psychiatric Association (APA) states that "only when personality traits are inflexible and maladaptive and cause significant functional impairment or subjective distress, do they constitute a personality disorder" (APA 2000). The ability to achieve developmental tasks such as trust, autonomy, independence, and meaningful relationships is limited for individuals diagnosed with personality disorders.

Their long-term nature and repetitive maladaptive and often self-defeating behaviors characterize **personality disorders** (PDs). These behaviors are not experienced as uncomfortable or disorganized by the individual, as are the symptoms experienced by a client with anxiety disorders, mood disorders, schizophrenia, or other mental disorders. It is important to note that with PDs, other areas of personal functioning may be very adequate. The predominant maladaptive behaviors may affect only one aspect of the person's life. Therefore, many individuals with PDs do not seek treatment unless a severe crisis or trauma precipitates other symptoms.

All of the PDs have four characteristics in common: (1) inflexible and maladaptive response to stress; (2) disability in working and loving; (3) ability to evoke interpersonal conflict; and (4) capacity to "get under the skin" of others.

1. **Inflexible and maladaptive response to stress.** Personality patterns are deeply ingrained in the personality structure and persist, unmodified, over long periods of time. At times, these **personality** patterns and **traits** may be compatible with and acceptable within societal norms and are valued by the culture or occupation. For instance, an engineer or administrator needs to possess some compulsive traits, such as the ability to organize complex details and meet deadlines. At other times, these same compulsive traits, when too rigid and limited, may interfere with personal, occupational, or social functioning.

2. **Disability in working and loving, which is generally more serious and pervasive than the similar disability found in other disorders.** Certain characteristics, e.g., withdrawal, grandiosity, and extreme suspiciousness, observed in people with PDs are similar to those seen in people with mood disorders and schizophrenic disorders. The difference is that, for the most part, individuals with PDs have normal ego functioning and reality testing. There are, however, great disturbances in their ability to find intimate and satisfactory interpersonal relationships or to function at their optimum creative level.

3. **Ability to evoke interpersonal conflict.** In individuals with PDs, intense upheavals and hostility within a precarious interpersonal context mark interpersonal relationships. People with PDs lack the ability to see themselves objectively. Therefore, the need or desire to alter aspects of their behavior to enrich or maintain important interpersonal relationships is lacking. Thus, annoying and distancing behaviors continue and are usually met with strong negative reactions from others.

4. **Capacity to "get under the skin" of others.** Getting under the skin of others refers to the uncanny ability of people with PDs to merge personal boundaries with others. This merging is manifested by the intense effect they have on others. The process is often unconscious and the result undesirable.

Judgments about an individual's personality functioning must take into account the person's ethnic, cultural, and social background. Since PDs are often overdiagnosed in clients who are ethnically and culturally different from the health care provider, it is important for the clinician to obtain additional information from others from the individual's cultural background (APA 2000). Therefore, the client's national, cultural, and ethnic background should be reflected in the assessment. Box 16–1 identifies the *Diagnostic and Statistical Manual*, 4th edition–text revision (DSM-IV-TR), criteria for PDs.

Cloninger and Svrakic (1999) point out that besides individuals with a PD having chronic impairments in their ability to work and love, they tend to be less educated, single, drug addicts and sex offenders, and to have marital difficulties and be unemployed. They are often perpetrators of violent and nonviolent crimes. People with PDs are often

The editor would like to thank Francesca Profiri for her contribution to this chapter in the third edition of *Foundations of Psychiatric Mental Health Nursing*, 1998. The case study of the Borderline Personality Disorder is from Dr. Suzy Lego from the second edition of *Foundations of Psychiatric Mental Health Nursing*, 1994. Acknowledgment is also given to Dr. Kem Louie for her contribution of the Nursing Assessment and the therapeutic dialogue with the antisocial client from her contribution in the second edition of *Foundations of Psychiatric Mental Health Nursing*, 1994.

perceived as aggravating and demanding, or they may be seductive and dependent and elicit inappropriate responses from the health care providers, such as sexual interest or the urge to rescue (Cloninger and Svrakic 1999). Therefore, the potential for value judgments and preconceived ideas on the part of health care providers may negatively affect the care given to an individual with a PD. Nehls (1999), in speaking to nurses regarding clients with borderline PDs, suggests that mental health personnel confront prejudice, understand self-harm, and safeguard opportunity for dialogue. The caution regarding confronting personal prejudice is particularly sound when working with any individual with a PD.

Often people with PDs seek help from primary care physicians for physical complaints, rather than seeking help in the mental health arena. Under stress, some people with PD may become psychotic;

therefore, the diagnosis of PD borders on the severe and psychosis on the mental health continuum (Fig. 16–1).

PREVALENCE

Prevalence for PDs ranges from 11% to 23%, depending on severity (Cloninger and Svrakic 1999). Prevalence appears higher in medical and psychiatric populations (one third in general hospital psychiatry; one half with alcohol and substance abusing individuals) (Goldberg 1998). The appearance of PDs is exacerbated by significant stress or loss (Goldberg 1998).

COMORBIDITY

PDs are predisposing factors for many other psychiatric disorders. Both major depression and panic disorders have an estimated 25% to 50% comorbidity rate (Goldberg 1995). PDs also appear to co-exist in a host of other Axis I disorders, e.g., substance use disorders, eating disorders, anxiety disorders, posttraumatic stress disorder, and somatization and impulse control disorders. Recurrent suicide attempts and chronic pain may also compound the picture (Cloninger and Svrakic 1999). An individual with one PD may also have other PDs as well, e.g., paranoid PD with narcissistic PD.

THEORY

The answer to what causes PDs is that there is unlikely to be any single cause for a discrete PD. There are environmental influences (e.g., child abuse) and biological influences (e.g., genetic) as well as psychological (developmental or environmental factors) that all seem to come into play. An increasing number of studies of environmental factors of PDs (e.g., family environment and sexual and physical abuse) show that these factors are likely to be predominant in the lives of people with specific PDs (e.g., borderline PD) (Phillips and Gunderson 1999). On the other hand, family, twin, and adoption studies provide evidence that antisocial PD and schizotypal PDs have a substantial degree of hereditability (Phillips and Gunderson 1999). Valliant (1994) stresses the role defense mechanisms play in the expression of PDs, which are characterized by the less mature defense mechanisms such as projecting, acting out, and splitting (refer to Chapter 13).

Box 16–1 DSM-IV-TR Criteria for a Personality Disorder

1. An enduring pattern of inner experience and behavior that deviates markedly from the expectations of the individual's culture. This pattern is manifested in two (or more) of the following areas:

   ■ Cognition (i.e., ways of perceiving and interpreting self, other people, and events)
   ■ Affect (i.e., range, intensity, lability, and appropriateness of emotional response)
   ■ Interpersonal functioning
   ■ Impulse control

2. The enduring pattern is inflexible and pervasive across a broad range of personal and social situations.
3. The enduring pattern leads to clinically significant distress or impairment in social, occupational, or other important areas of functioning.
4. The pattern is stable and of long duration, and its onset can be traced back at least to adolescence or early adulthood.
5. The enduring pattern is not better accounted for as a manifestation or consequence of another mental disorder.
6. The enduring pattern is not due to the direct physiological effects of a substance (e.g., a drug of abuse, a medication) or a general medical condition (e.g., head trauma).

Adapted from American Psychiatric Association (2000). *Diagnostic and statistical manual of mental disorders* (4th ed.) Washington, DC: American Psychiatric Association. Reprinted with permission. Copyright 2000 American Psychiatric Association.

ances; second, a healing relationship can intervene to reconstruct the personality chemically, cognitively, and experientially.

Tables 16–1, 16–2, and 16–3 summarize findings and theories from various etiologic studies as compiled by Phillips and Gunderson (1999) and Cloninger and Svrakic (1999) and give the prevalence and prognoses for each of the PDs.

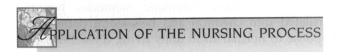

APPLICATION OF THE NURSING PROCESS

ASSESSMENT

Overall Assessment

ASSESSMENT TOOLS

The Minnesota Multiphasic Personality Inventory (MMPI) is the best-known standardized test for evaluating personality. There are many others in use.

ASSESSING PAST HISTORY

Taking a full medical history can help determine if this is a psychiatric problem, a medical problem, or both. Medical illness should never be ruled out as the cause until the data support this conclusion. Questions regarding a history of suicidal or homicidal ideation, intent, gestures, or attempts and current use of medicines, illegal substances, food, and money elicit information about the client's current level of crisis as well as dysfunctional coping styles. These are important data regarding clients who have PDs.

Important areas to explore are elicited through questions that detail involvement with the courts; current or past physical, sexual, or emotional abuse; and level of current endangerment from self or others. At times, immediate interventions may be needed to ensure the client's or others' safety. Information regarding prior use of any medication, including psychopharmacological agents, is important. This information gives evidence of other contacts the client has made for help and indicates how the health care provider found the client at that time.

PSYCHOSOCIAL NURSING ASSESSMENT

See Box 16–2, a tool for assessing people with PDs.

Self-Assessment

Finding an approach for helping clients with PDs who have overwhelming needs can be overwhelming for caregivers as well. These individuals can evoke intense feelings in the nurse (often the same feelings being experienced by the client). Being in the role of caregiver can result in feeling chronically confused, helpless, angry, and frustrated; these clients tell the nurse that the nurse is inadequate, incompetent, and abusive of authority. Clients with PD can be manipulative and may disparage the nurse to peers in such a way that the peers begin to believe the client; usually, this is the peers' attempt to defend against their own feelings of frustration and powerlessness, but the result is that substantial conflict can ensue in the workplace, with teams splitting or factions forming. Therefore, the interventions discussed next can be used on behalf of both clients and staff. O'Brian (1998) stresses that nurses working with individuals with borderline PDs should have adequate education, support, and su-

	TABLE 16–1 *Etiologies of Cluster A Disorders (Odd or Eccentric)*		
PERSONALITY DISORDER	**ETIOLOGICAL COMPONENTS**	**PREVALENCE IN GENERAL POPULATION**	**PROGNOSIS**
Schizotypal	■ Heredity and genetically linked to schizophrenia ■ Increased ventricular-brain ratio on computed tomographic (CT) scan, and other characteristics similar to schizophrenia	3%	Up to 25% go on to schizophrenia
Paranoid	■ Studies indicate that both biogenetic contributors and environmental factors play a role	0.5–2.5%	Fair to poor
Schizoid	■ Often history of cold, neglectful early childhood experiences ■ Shyness—introversion appears highly heritable	up to 7.5%	Fair to poor

TABLE 16–2   Etiology of Cluster B Disorders (Dramatic, Emotional, Erratic)

PERSONALITY DISORDER	ETIOLOGICAL COMPONENTS	PREVALENCE IN GENERAL POPULATION	PROGNOSIS
Borderline	■ Documented high frequency of early traumatic abandonment, physical abuse, and sexual abuse; child develops an enduring rage and self-hatred ■ Some evidence for genetic component as well	2%, more common in females	Chronic instability—in 4th or 5th decade relationships and functioning may improve
Antisocial	■ Early family life often poses severe environmental handicaps (abusive/inconsistent/neglectful parents) ■ Twin/adoption studies show genetic component ■ Impulsive and aggressive behavior may be mediated by abnormal serotonin transport in the brain	3% males 1% females	After 30 years old, flagrant antisocial behavior tends to decrease
Histrionic	■ Runs in families ■ Recent research suggests that qualities such as emotional expressiveness and attention seeking may be biologically determined temperament ■ Psychoanalytic theory proposes origins in oedipal phase of development	2–3%, more frequent in women	Some remission with age
Narcissistic	■ Little evidence available ■ Reconstruction and observation in psychoanalytic treatment pose a childhood of criticism, disdain, or neglect; protect selves as self-sufficient and invulnerable to protect self-esteem	1%	Chronic course of narcissism may decrease after 40 when pessimism increases

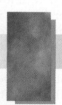

TABLE 16–3   Etiology of Cluster C Disorders (Anxious or Fearful)

PERSONALITY DISORDER	ETIOLOGICAL COMPONENTS	PREVALENCE IN GENERAL POPULATION	PROGNOSIS
Dependent	■ Genetic or constitutional factors may account for submissiveness ■ Culture and social roles may play a part for some	Most frequent personality disorder	Modified with medication
Avoidant	■ Some research implicates biological inborn impairment ■ Psychodynamic theory holds that early life experiences lead to exaggerated need for acceptance and intolerance for criticism	0.5–1%	Begins in childhood Modification good with medication
Obsessive-Compulsive	■ Excessive parental continual criticism and shaming; has rigid rules to prevent punishment and condemnation	1% Twice as common in males as in females	Modification good with medication

BOX 16-2 *Nursing Assessment Guide for People with Personality Disorders*

■ What is the presenting problem according to the client? What is it according to others (e.g., family, employer, police)?
■ Who has identified and defined the problem?
■ What is the client's emotional state? Is the client:
  ■ Suspicious
  ■ Anxious
  ■ Experiencing helplessness
  ■ Expressing boredom
  ■ Unconcerned
  ■ Lacking in empathy
  ■ Lacking remorse for hurting others
  ■ Suffering from low self-esteem
■ What particular circumstances or stress precipitated the behavior?
■ How is the client handling the problem? How has the client handled problems in the past?
■ Is the client suicidal? Self-mutilating?
■ How would the client like to see the problem resolved?
■ Does the client have any meaningful or lasting relationships? Friends, lovers, family?
■ What is the client's developmental history?
■ Is the client employed? What is the pattern of employment?
■ How does the behavior affect the job or role functioning?
■ What is the client's physical condition and status?
■ What behaviors or defenses does the client exhibit?
  ■ Manipulation
  ■ Splitting
  ■ Projection
  ■ Withdrawal
  ■ Angry, hostile, violent
  ■ Paranoia
  ■ Demanding
■ What substances (i.e., drugs and alcohol) are abused? How much is taken? When was the last time it was taken?
■ Has the client ever been arrested or convicted of a crime?

Adapted from Louie, K. B. (1994). Personality disorders: Antisocial, paranoid, and borderline. In E. M. Varcarolis (Ed.), *Foundations of psychiatric mental health nursing* (2nd ed.). Philadelphia: W. B. Saunders.

Assessment Guidelines

ASSESSMENT GUIDELINES: PERSONALITY DISORDERS

1. Does client have a medical disorder or another psychiatric disorder that may be responsible for symptoms?
2. Assess for suicidal or homicidal thoughts—if yes, will need immediate attention.
3. Assessment about personality functioning needs to be viewed within the person's ethnic, cultural, and social background.
4. Personality disorders are often exacerbated following the loss of significant supporting people or in a disruptive social situation.
5. A change in personality in middle adulthood or later signals the need for a thorough medical work-up or assessment for unrecognized substance abuse disorder.

Clinical Picture of Cluster A Disorders (Odd, Eccentric)

Figure 16–2 shows the DSM-IV-TR criteria for cluster A disorders.

PARANOID PERSONALITY DISORDER

Individuals with paranoid PD greatly fear that others will exploit, harm, or deceive them, to the point of endangering their lives. Even when no evidence exists, clients with paranoid PD interpret all experience from the perspective that they have been done irreversible damage by others; therefore, people with paranoid PD are extremely reluctant to share information about themselves. Compliments or loyalty is misread as manipulation or attempts to disempower them. These individuals are hypervigilant, anticipate hostility, and can actually create hostile responses by *initiating* a "counterattack." Jealousy, controlling behaviors, avoidance of others, and unwillingness to forgive all are characteristics of paranoid PD. Because of their excessive suspiciousness and fear of attack, people with paranoid PD are usually argumentative, sarcastic, and complaining, or they are quietly hostile and aloof (Gunderson and Phillips 1995). The best approach with paranoid individuals is neutral, matter of fact, and respectful. A warm, enthusiastic approach is perceived as being intrusive, insincere, and threatening.

Psychotic episodes can occur with these individuals, especially during times of stress (e.g., mourning, illness, change). Experiences that overwhelm them with frustration and anger aggravate their preexisting high level of fear, increase their need for solitude, and exacerbate their poor peer relationships and social anxiety. As people with paranoid PD age, their

pervision to avoid significant occupational stress arising from the population. This would be apt advice for working with other clients with PDs as well, e.g., antisocial PD, paranoid PD, narcissistic PD, and others.

DSM-IV-TR CRITERIA FOR CLUSTER A PERSONALITY DISORDERS

CLUSTER A (Odd or Eccentric)

PARANOID PERSONALITY DISORDER

A. A pervasive distrust and suspiciousness of others such that their motives are interpreted as malevolent, beginning by early adulthood and present in a variety of contexts, as indicated by four (or more) of the following:

(1) Suspects, without sufficient basis, that others are exploiting, harming, or deceiving self
(2) Is preoccupied with unjustified doubts about the loyalty or trustworthiness of friends or associates
(3) Is reluctant to confide in others because of unwarranted fear that the information will be used maliciously against self
(4) Reads hidden demeaning or threatening meanings into benign remarks or events
(5) Persistently bears grudges (i.e., is unforgiving of insults, injuries, or slights)
(6) Perceives attacks on his or her character or reputation that are not apparent to others and is quick to react angrily or to counterattack
(7) Has recurrent suspicions, without justification, regarding fidelity of spouse or sexual partner

8) HAS Comorbid cmrbm
9) Guarded
defensefuch
projection
intellectuali
Rationalizaton

SCHIZOID PERSONALITY DISORDER

A. A pervasive pattern of detachment from social relationships and a restricted range of expression in interpersonal settings, beginning by early adulthood and present in a variety of contexts, as indicated by four (or more) of the following:

(1) Neither desires nor enjoys close relationships, including being part of a family
(2) Almost always chooses solitary activities
(3) Has little, if any, interest in having sexual experiences with another person
(4) Takes pleasure in few, if any, activities
(5) Lacks close friends or confidants other than first-degree relatives
(6) Appears indifferent to the praise or criticism of others
(7) Shows emotional coldness, detachment, or flattened affect

- Precursor to Schizophrenie
- Lacking personal Skills
- Blunt Affect
- mou males

SCHIZOTYPAL PERSONALITY DISORDER

A. A pervasive pattern of social and interpersonal deficits marked by acute discomfort with, and reduced capacity for, close relationships as well as by cognitive or perceptual distortions and eccentricities of behavior, beginning by early adulthood and present in a variety of contexts, as indicated by five (or more) of the following:

(1) Ideas of reference (excluding delusions of reference)
(2) Odd beliefs or magical thinking that influence behavior and are inconsistent with subcultural norms (e.g., superstitiousness, belief in clairvoyance, telepathy, or "sixth sense"; in children or adolescents, bizarre fantasies or preoccupations)
(3) Unusual perceptual experiences, including bodily illusions
(4) Odd thinking and speech (e.g., vague, circumstantial, metaphorical, overelaborate, or stereotyped)
(5) Suspiciousness or paranoid ideation
(6) Inappropriate or constricted affect
(7) Behavior or appearance that is odd, eccentric, or peculiar
(8) Lack of close friends or confidants other than first-degree relatives
(9) Excessive social anxiety that does not diminish with familiarity and tends to be associated with paranoid fears rather than negative judgments about self

more males

Know
More Bizarre

enjoyable Activities
Social Skills trg
consistency
self directed
wrk c one Person
remove stress
Support
Independence

Figure 16–2 DSM-IV-TR criteria for cluster A personality disorders. (Adapted from American Psychiatric Association. [2000]. *Diagnostic and statistical manual of mental disorders* [4th ed.-TR]. Washington, DC: Copyright 2000, American Psychiatric Association.)

isolation, underachievement, and hypersensitivity give them a more idiosyncratic and eccentric presentation. They may even develop peculiar habits in dress, language, and thoughts that further set them apart.

Individuals with paranoid PD rarely initiate contact with a medical system and are usually in contact with health care professionals against the cli-

ent's will or in an emergency situation in which they have no choice. Once in the system, people with paranoid PD may suddenly flee or sign out against medical advice because of suspicion and fear (Goldberg 1998).

To counteract fear, straightforward explanations of tests, history taking, and procedures are helpful. The person with paranoid PD should be warned about the side effects of drugs, any changes in the treatment plan, and the possibility of further procedures.

Paranoid PD is most commonly diagnosed in males and is more prevalent in families with a history of schizophrenia. However, paranoid ideation is common. Paranoid ideation is expected when found in populations where harm, betrayal, and isolation have occurred, e.g., refugees, prisoners of war, the elderly, or the hearing-impaired (Gunderson and Phillips 1995). Cocaine-related disorders can look similar to paranoid PD (APA 2000).

An example of a client with paranoid PD follows.

Vignette

■ *Mr. Cortez, a 50-year-old employed factory worker, is seen in the emergency department after complaining of heart palpitations and chest pain. He refuses to have his blood drawn, to have lab tests done, or to answer questions. He also refuses to give his address and telephone number, stating that there are no relatives he wishes to have contacted, and begins a long and complicated diatribe against the medical system. The nurse explains calmly, and in reassuring detail, why all these questions need to be answered and the tests need to be done (Profiri 1998).*

Obtaining Mr. Cortez's permission to complete each task would facilitate his cooperation and compliance. Increasing his sense of power over what is happening to him by giving him control and information can measurably decrease his paranoia.

SCHIZOID PERSONALITY DISORDER

The client with schizoid PD has difficulty expressing any emotion, whether it be anger at being abused or joy in a fine meal. Usually, people with schizoid PD are seen as drifters on the periphery of society, avoiding relationships of even the most superficial type. Their lack of desire for companionship or sexual relationships produces social isolation. People who have schizoid PD infrequently marry, but when they do, the marriage is impaired by their lack of affect and flat experience of emotions. Occupational functioning is poor, especially if they must relate interpersonally, but they tend to do well if they can be the lone wolf. In response to stress, they may become delusional. People with this disorder appear cold and aloof, indifferent to the approval or criticism of others. However, in rare instances, people with schizoid PD reveal having painful feelings, especially related to social interaction (APA 2000).

Schizoid PD can be a precursor to schizophrenia or delusional disorder; the prevalence is increased if a family history of schizophrenia or schizotypal PD exists. If persistent psychotic symptoms (e.g., delusions, hallucinations) exist, schizoid disorder is ruled out. Sometimes, it is difficult to differentiate schizoid PD from autistic disorder, especially in the presence of long-term substance abuse.

Onset begins in early adulthood and is wide reaching in its effects on the client's life and family. Because schizoid individuals lack social awareness and insight into other people's behaviors, their relationship skills become rigid, maladaptive, and distressing to themselves; hence, they increasingly avoid others. This fear of others is fed by the confusion in other people's responses to them. In dealing with others, the schizoid client's most common experience is failure.

It is dangerous to assume that street people, hermits, and shut-ins may be diagnosed with schizoid PD, as other medical and psychiatric problems have a schizoid appearance. For example, speaking only a foreign language, being a new immigrant to this country, or being extremely agoraphobic or obsessive-compulsive can all present a picture similar to that of schizoid PD (APA 2000).

The following is an example of a person with schizoid PD.

Vignette

■ *Mr. Wong, a 28-year-old homeless man, is admitted to the hospital after a physical assault. Although compliant with his treatment, he spends most of his time in the smoking area of the hospital, sitting cross-legged and staring at the floor. He does not respond verbally when spoken to. He avoids eye contact and remains a passive recipient in his treatment and discharge planning. At night, Mr. Wong is often found in the darkest and most secluded area of the unit, sleeping on the floor in a fetal position with all his possessions around him. When spoken to, he gets up and walks away. All nursing interventions for socialization are rejected, although he continues to be outwardly compliant (Profiri 1998).*

Mr. Wong is likely to be most responsive when the nurse tells him what he can expect, and what is expected from him, on a task-by-task basis. Simplification and clarity can decrease his anxiety.

SCHIZOTYPAL PERSONALITY DISORDER

The history of a client with schizotypal PD shows eccentricity from early childhood, with strong although uncommon beliefs that display perceptual and cognitive distortions. Many cultures have beliefs that may appear eccentric outside of that culture but within it are adaptive and enhancing. This is not the case with clients with schizotypal PD. Their behavior, which is far outside cultural norms, is maladaptive. Such clients broadcast their beliefs, calling attention to themselves even though they do not seek attention. Their eccentric ideas stem from incorrect interpretations of internal and external events; the clients then spiritualize or concretize these distortions, convinced of their reality, and present them with significant conviction (which seems superstitious, magical, or grandiose to other members of the culture).

Clients with schizotypal PD may have magical rituals or a belief that they can control the actions of others; perceptually, they may hear murmuring voices or the presence of another person when no one is there. Their speech is idiosyncratic in phrasing and syntax. Their conversation is loose, in that they easily digress, are vague, or may become incoherent. They can be concrete and abstract, sometimes on the same topic; while it all makes sense to them, to others it may appear illogical. As a consequence, these clients become suspicious of others who do not share their reality. They may perceive others as dense or crazy, and as likely to undermine them.

Because people with schizotypal PD cannot pick up on interpersonal cues, they relate stiffly, apprehensively, and inappropriately. Their range of affect can be constricted, even though their beliefs may be fantastical. Their eccentric and unkempt behaviors and inattention to social conventions make it impossible for them to have a give-and-take conversation. Consequently, they can be frightened and paranoid in social situations.

Unlike those with schizoid PD, whose behavior suggests that they want diminished social contact, people with schizotypal PD are unhappy about having no functional relationships. Their social anxiety does not abate over time, and tension and unhappiness increase; their life is plagued by social and interpersonal deficits. This disorder is most prevalent in first-degree relatives of schizophrenics.

Vignette

■ *Ms. Carol, a 36-year-old unemployed woman receiving permanent psychiatric disability, enters day treatment after her fifth psychiatric hospitalization. She is appropriately dressed except for opera-length gloves and a lace scarf that is wrapped as a turban around her head. She is quiet and sits separately in a corner of the community room during most of her time there, appearing to be deep in thought and occasionally talking to herself. However, during group meetings, she suddenly begins to speak very loudly (but with flat affect) about how she is going to become an independent movie producer, director, and writer, to prove once and for all that the unidentified foreign objects visiting us are really angels from heaven and that 21st-century space ships have taken the place of 14th-century wings (Profiri, 1998).*

The nursing strategy is to calm Ms. Carol's apparent anxiety about being in a group setting by introducing her to each individual in day treatment and identifying their reason for being there. For example, Ms. Carol is told that the case manager will be helpful with housing and disability, and the nurse with therapy and medications. Other clients are introduced by their goals: "Mr. Tom wants to learn how to stay out of the hospital."

Clinical Picture of Cluster B Disorders (Dramatic, Emotional, Erratic)

The cluster B PDs include antisocial, borderline, histrionic, and narcissistic PDs. Individuals in cluster B often appear dramatic, emotional, or erratic. Figure 16–3 presents the DSM-IV criteria for cluster B disorders.

ANTISOCIAL PERSONALITY DISORDER

In the past, this PD has been called psychopathy, sociopathy, or dyssocial PD because it is characterized by deceit, manipulation, revenge, and harm to others with an absence of guilt or anxiety. People with antisocial PD have a sense of entitlement (i.e., they believe they have the right to hurt others). This disorder may be underdiagnosed in females and overdiagnosed in clients in lower socioeconomic areas of cities. Currently, 3% of males and 1% of females in the population are diagnosed as having antisocial PD. These traits may become less evident as the client ages, especially in the early forties or fifties, when antisocial criminal behavior—and, often, associated substance abuse—tends to decline.

Usually, first contact with this client occurs because of court-ordered treatment; the norm is a long history of illegal activity. The presentation of clients with antisocial PD is one of intent to deceive, along with impulsivity in action, so that the combination of reckless disregard for others and themselves is evident. They neglect responsibilities to others, lie, and repeatedly perform destructive acts—which may include vandalism, unsafe sex, driving under the influence, and assault—without developing any insight as to the predictable consequences. It is difficult for them to hold a job, to parent or relate to others, or to pay their bills because of their consistently defaulting on responsibility. Indifference to their own pain or the pain they inflict on others is defended by clients with antisocial PD by their presumed right to hold themselves above others; their assumption is that if they do not do these things to others first, then others will do these things to them. They accept no traditional value or moral as a boundary for their actions.

This lack of empathy combines with a contemptuous attitude toward others and an arrogant or gran-

DSM-IV-TR CRITERIA FOR CLUSTER B PERSONALITY DISORDERS

CLUSTER B (Dramatic, Emotional, or Erratic)

ANTISOCIAL PERSONALITY DISORDER

A. A pervasive pattern of disregard for and violation of the rights of others occurring since age 15, as indicated by three (or more) of the following:

(1) Failure to conform to social norms with respect to lawful behaviors as indicated by repeatedly performing acts that are grounds for arrest
(2) Deceitfulness, as indicated by repeatedly lying, use of aliases, or conning others for personal profit or pleasure
(3) Impulsivity or failure to plan ahead
(4) Irritability and aggressiveness, as indicated by repeated physical fights or assaults
(5) Reckless disregard for safety of self or others
(6) Consistent irresponsibility, as indicated by repeated failure to sustain consistent work behavior or honor financial obligations
(7) Lack of remorse, as indicated by being indifferent to, or rationalizing, having hurt, mistreated, or stolen from another

B. The individual is at least 18 years of age.

C. There is evidence of conduct disorder with onset before age 15 years.

(handwritten: "or oppositional")

BORDERLINE PERSONALITY DISORDER

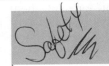 *(handwritten: "Safety")* *(handwritten: "they split staff")*

A. A pervasive pattern of instability of interpersonal relationships, self-image, and affects, and marked impulsivity beginning in early adulthood and present in a variety of contexts, as indicated by five (or more) of the following:

(1) Frantic efforts to avoid real or imagined abandonment. *Note:* Do not include suicidal or self-mutilating behavior covered in criterion 5.
(2) A pattern of unstable and intense interpersonal relationships characterized by alternating between extremes of idealization and devaluation *(handwritten: "re: stopping friend")*
(3) Identity disturbance: markedly and persistently unstable self-image or sense of self
(4) Impulsivity in at least two areas that are potentially self-damaging (e.g., spending, sex, substance abuse, reckless driving, binge eating). *Note:* Do not include suicidal or self-mutilating behavior covered in criterion 5.
(5) Recurrent suicidal behavior, gestures, or threats, or self-mutilating behavior
(6) Affective instability due to a marked reactivity of mood (e.g., intense episodic dysphoria, irritability, or anxiety, usually lasting a few hours and rarely more than a few days)
(7) Chronic feelings of emptiness
(8) Inappropriate intense anger or difficulty controlling anger (e.g., frequent displays of temper, constant anger, recurrent physical fights) *(handwritten: "self mutilate")*
(9) Transient, stress-related paranoid ideation or severe dissociative symptoms

NARCISSISTIC PERSONALITY DISORDER

A. A pervasive pattern of grandiosity (in fantasy and behavior), need for admiration, and lack of empathy, beginning in early adulthood and present in a variety of contexts, as indicated by five (or more) of the following:

(1) Has a grandiose sense of self-importance (e.g., exaggerates achievements and talents, expects to be recognized as superior without commensurate achievements)
(2) Is preoccupied with fantasies of unlimited success, power, brilliance, beauty, or ideal love
(3) Believes that he or she is "special" and unique and can only be understood by, or should associate with, other special or high-status people (or institutions)
(4) Requires excessive admiration
(5) Has sense of entitlement (i.e., unreasonable expectations of especially favorable treatment or automatic compliance with personal expectations)
(6) Is interpersonally exploitative (i.e., takes advantage of others to achieve personal ends)
(7) Lacks empathy: is unwilling to recognize or identify with the feelings and needs of others
(8) Is often envious of others or believes that others are envious of self
(9) Shows arrogant, haughty behaviors or attitudes

HISTRIONIC PERSONALITY DISORDER

A. A pervasive pattern of excessive emotionality and attention seeking, beginning in early adulthood and present in a variety of contexts, as indicated by five (or more) of the following:

(1) Is uncomfortable in situations in which self is not the center of attention
(2) Interaction with others is often characterized by inappropriate sexually seductive or provocative behavior
(3) Displays rapidly shifting and shallow expression of emotions
(4) Consistently uses physical appearance to draw attention to self
(5) Has a style of speech that is excessively impressionistic and lacking in detail
(6) Shows self-dramatization, theatricality, and exaggerated expression of emotion
(7) Is suggestible (i.e., easily influenced by others or circumstances)
(8) Considers relationships to be more intimate than they actually are

Figure 16-3 DSM-IV-TR criteria for cluster B personality disorders. (Adapted from American Psychiatric Association. [2000]. *Diagnostic and statistical manual of mental disorders.* [4th ed.-TR]. Washington, DC: Copyright 2000, American Psychiatric Association.)

diose opinion of self. Verbally, these clients can be adept, charming, and self-assured. This superficial charm engages others in their web of intrigue, which is designed for exploitation. They have difficulty tolerating boredom, seek out high stimulation to avoid depression, and can become tense if they do not feel in control of others. Frustration is familiar to them, as is compulsive behavior regarding food, alcohol, sex, and gambling.

Research among non–blood-related families (e.g., in cases of adoption) indicates that both genetic and environmental factors contribute to the risk of developing antisocial PD. Adopted children resemble their biological parents more than their adoptive ones, but the environment of the adoptive family highly influences the risk of this pathology (APA 2000). These clients rarely seek help but may be hospitalized when they are remanded by the courts or found to be a danger to others or even to themselves. Antisocial PD clients are extremely **manipulative** and often **aggressive**.

Vignette

■ *Mr. James, a 23-year-old unemployed truck driver, is admitted to the unit after an episode of drunken driving. He is on bed rest and traction, owing to a broken pelvis. In his admission work-up, he denies any active drug or alcohol use. When bathed by the nursing staff, he requests sexual contact. He complains loudly and angrily that his pain medication regimen is not adequate. When his requests are not met immediately, he begins to scream and throw objects around the room. His constant demanding behavior overwhelms the staff. His call light is always on, and the nursing staff begin to avoid answering it. On his third day of hospitalization, his temperature and blood pressure begin to rise, and he begins pharmacological treatment for drug and alcohol withdrawal (Profiri 1998).*

To promote optimal client care and avoid staff burnout, the staff formulate a written plan of care that is posted in his room detailing Mr. James' daily regimen: when his bath is to be given, what his meds are and when they are to be given, when he is to receive his meals, when the doctor can be expected to visit, when as-needed nursing contacts are to be made, and so on. Clarification of boundaries and consistent adherence to the routine in the nursing care plan are designed to minimize Mr. James' acting out behaviors, especially when his opportunities for manipulation are drastically reduced.

BORDERLINE PERSONALITY DISORDER

People with borderline PD experience overwhelming needs, both internal and external, which they seek to have met in relationships. A major defense of the client with borderline PD is splitting, or alternating between idealizing and devaluation. Splitting is a failure to integrate the positive and negative qualities of self or others (Kernberg 1985). For example, on first meeting, they idealize others (lovers, health care providers), imagining in that idealization that at last they have found someone to give them what they need. But, at the first disappointment, frustration, or denied request, they dramatically shift to devaluation and despising the other person. They threaten abandonment and may actually abandon the other person, but internally they are frantically searching to reattach; alternately, they try to find someone new to attach to as quickly and as intensely as before. Splitting is a primitive defense in which people see themselves or others as either all good or all bad and are unable to integrate the positive and negative qualities of the self or others into an integrated whole (Lego 1994). The person may alternately idealize and devalue the same person (APA 2000). This behavior results in unstable and difficult interpersonal relationships; this situation, in turn, diminishes self-esteem.

People with borderline PD have little tolerance for being alone. Internally, the client exists in a state of intense fear of abandonment. Just as they experience others as either perfect or worthless, they experience themselves in similarly dramatic terms. A continuous cycle of failure with themselves and others produces great internal despair. A repetitive pattern of despair leads to feelings of deadness, panic, and fury. Self-mutilation and suicide-prone behaviors are responses to their sensitivity to present or anticipated stress and loss. Self-mutilation is the "deliberate alteration or destruction of body tissue without conscious suicidal intent" (Favazza and Rosenthal 1993). Self-mutilation is usually not meant to be lethal. It generally occurs sporadically or repetitively. Examples include skin cutting, head banging, scratching, burning, eyeball pressing, and self-punching (Bonnivier 1996).

Completed suicide occurs in 8% to 10% of people with borderline PD (APA 2000). Self-mutilation is more common and usually occurs during a dissociative period. Paradoxically, self-mutilation may be used as a self-soothing behavior, which can become a ritualized part of the attempt to gain boundaries and clarity. People who have borderline PD also display impulsive self-destructive behaviors. For example, they may spend money irresponsibly, gamble, abuse substances, engage in unsafe sex, drive recklessly, or binge eat. These self-destructive acts are usually precipitated by threats of separation or rejection or by expectations that they assume increased responsibility (APA 2000). Without adequate nurturing, support, and provision of clarity and boundaries, people with borderline PD can lose the feeling of existing at all. Frantically, they act as victim, then rescuer, then perpetrator, trying to fill their inner emptiness.

Dysphoria, irritability, or anxiety can be intense, although short-lived. **Chronic depression** is common. Clients with borderline PD rarely experience feelings of satisfaction or well-being. Rather, they are extremely angry, and intervention needs to target their anger. Anger management is difficult but crucial in helping the client with borderline PD to regulate emotions. These clients often direct extreme sarcasm, enduring bitterness, or angry outbursts toward others. Their aggression and the need to destroy is an expression of intense and primitive rage, and it can undermine any treatment, especially if the destructive impulse is experienced by the client as filling a need. Treatment is often complicated by the client's self-destructive tendencies and instability. Goldberg (1998) states that when behavioral problems emerge, the therapeutic goals and boundaries must be calmly reviewed. Limit setting is defi-

nitely necessary but in the short run may lead to hostility, noncompliance, termination of treatment, or suicide attempt.

Sadly, people with borderline PD may have a history of leaving functional relationships, quitting jobs that are going well, or leaving school just before graduating. It may be no surprise, in light of this, that the occurrence of physical or sexual abuse, neglect, hostile conflict, and early parental loss or separation is common in clients' early childhood (see the Research Findings box).

About 2% of the population is estimated to have borderline PD. Borderline PD is thought to occur in 30% to 60% of all of the clinical populations with PD and accounts for about 20% of the inpatient population. Common co-occurring disorders include mood disorder (depression), substance abuse, eating disorders (bulimia), and posttraumatic stress disorder; it may also occur with other PDs (APA 2000). People with borderline PD are high users of all health and mental health resources, chronically traveling from one crisis to another and from one care-

---

RESEARCH FINDINGS

The Role of Biparental Abuse and Neglect in the Development of Borderline Personality Disorder

Objective

To assess the role of biparental abuse and neglect in the development of Borderline Personality Disorders (BPD).

Methods

A semistructured research interview was used to do a blind assessment of childhood experiences of biparental abuse and neglect reported by 358 hospitalized clients with BPD and 109 Axis II (personality disorders) as controls.

Results

Eighty-four % of BPD clients reported biparental abuse or neglect before age 18; 55% reported a childhood history of biparental abuse; 77% reported a history of biparental neglect. Among the Axis II controls, 61% reported biparental abuse or

neglect; 31% reported biparental abuse; 55% reported biparental neglect. Clients with BPD were significantly more likely than the Axis II controls to report having been verbally, emotionally, and physically but not sexually abused by caretakers of both sexes. They were also significantly more likely to report that both male and female caretakers denied the validity of their thoughts and feelings, failed to protect them; neglected their physical care; withdrew from them emotionally; and treated them inconsistently. Finally, female clients with BPD who reported a previous history of neglect by a female caretaker and abuse by a male caretaker were at significantly higher risk for having been sexually abused by a noncaretaker.

Conclusions

These results suggest that biparental failure (abuse and neglect, lack of validation for thoughts and feelings, inconsistency, and emotional withdrawal) may be a significant factor in the cause of BPD. The results also indicate that biparental failure may significantly increase a pre-BPD girl's risk of being sexually abused by someone other than her parents.

Source: Zanarini, M. C., Frankenburg, F. R., Reich, D. B. et al. (2000). Biparental failure in the childhood experiences of borderline patients. *Journal of Personality Disorders* 14(3):264–273.

taker to another. Females are about 75% more likely than males to be diagnosed with borderline PD; males are more likely to be diagnosed with a psychosis-related disorder.

Vignette

■ *Mrs. Suez, a 35-year-old mother of two with a history of psychiatric hospitalizations, has come for her usual clinic appointment. Her hand bears razor marks spelling "adios," her most recent self-mutilation. This is her last session before her nurse therapist leaves for a 2-week vacation. Mrs. Suez begins the session by saying that she wants to terminate therapy. She tells her nurse therapist: "I know you don't like me and I hope you have a really wonderful vacation with that sexy boyfriend of yours. Don't worry about me. No one else does . . . " (Profiri 1998).*

The nurse therapist helps Mrs. Suez understand that she is angry at her for going on vacation. She asks Mrs. Suez if she is thinking about or planning suicide. The nurse therapist again clarifies the resources available to Mrs. Suez during the vacation (e.g., who will be seeing her while the nurse therapist is gone, exactly when she will return) and reassures her that no matter what happens during the vacation, the two of them will continue to meet and work together on Mrs. Suez's problems afterward.

HISTRIONIC PERSONALITY DISORDER

Histrionics is a dramatic presentation of oneself with pervasive and excessive emotionality in order to seek attention, love, and admiration. People with histrionic PD may appear flamboyant, seductive, charming, and confident. They need to be the center of attention, the "life of the party," and when they are not, they often do something dramatic to regain attention.

Clients with histrionic PD are overly concerned with impressing others and are preoccupied with their appearance. Their dramatic and intense emotional expressions are frequently shallow, with rapid shifts from person to person or idea to idea. These people seductively draw others to them in relationships or work projects, but the attraction is usually short lived. Soon, they begin to embarrass these new friends and co-workers through their theatrical and exaggerated expression of emotion. They also begin to get caught in stories they have made up to aggrandize themselves. Thus, others experience their intense and short-term ardor as shallow, with no enduring substance.

Clients with histrionic PD effusively embrace their new health care practitioner, endowing instantaneous trust, and assume that the caregiver experiences the same intimacy. They have elaborate fantasies about those whom they instantly idealize, especially those in authority over them, imagining that they are involved in a great meeting of mind and heart with their caregiver. When they are disappointed, these clients plummet from exaggerated loyalty to suspected betrayal; their need to control, manipulate, and idolize is an attempt to prevent this fall from grace.

Understandably, others experience people with histrionic PD as smothering, destructive, and unable to understand anyone else's experience. Highly impaired relationships result. Without the instant gratification from others' admiration, clients with histrionic PD can experience significant to major depression. During this time, they are most likely to be seen in a health care setting. All suicidal ideation and gestures must be taken seriously by the health care practitioner, but doing so is difficult with this type of client.

The behavior of the client with histrionic PD can be interpreted as coercive and attention seeking. However, underresponding in such situations may put the caregiver in the role of enabling a potential suicide. When clients with histrionic PD receive the appropriate responsiveness, they are likely to be on to the next novelty—all life being a stage, with them as the playwright, director, and star. Although they initiate activities with great enthusiasm, when real obstacles and limitations set in, they lose interest and search anew for something that will be more immediately gratifying (APA 2000).

Vignette

■ *Mrs. Mahoney, a 51-year-old widow, initiates psychotherapy after the death of her husband. Unaccustomed to being alone and no longer having her mate to take care of her, she seeks out a nurse therapist, whom she immediately views as nurturing and caring. Mrs. Mahoney describes herself in grandiose terms as she outlines her ideas for success now that she is "free."*

However, she has a history of never completing her schooling, a job, or any of her many other projects. She indicates that she richly deserved the adoration of her late husband and implies that the nurse therapist is not giving her enough "praise and celebration" for doing as well as she is doing—that is, writing checks for the first time in her life.

Mrs. Mahoney makes frequent phone calls to the nurse, soliciting help with everyday tasks, such as balancing her check book and knowing when to schedule her car for a tune-up. When it becomes clear that the nurse therapist will not respond to her demands for adoration and enabling caretaking, Mrs. Mahoney becomes insulting to her therapist. She devalues and berates her, while dramatizing her own suffering, finally threatening to kill herself if her therapist is not more accommodating (Profiri, 1998).

The nurse therapist initially assesses Mrs. Mahoney's degree of lethality and offers support in the form of clear parameters of psychotherapy. She encourages Mrs. Mahoney to discuss her everyday problems in the session, where new skills can be taught. Approaching the client's dependence as a strength and refusing to identify with the client's devaluation are essential to working with clients with histrionic PD.

NARCISSISTIC PERSONALITY DISORDER

The primary feature in narcissistic PD is a pervasive pattern of grandiosity, a need for admiration, and a lack of empathy for others (APA 2000). Clients who have narcissistic PD exploit others to meet their own needs and desires; when they are successful, they experience a sense of superiority and omnipotence. Often, they are admired and envied by others for what appears to be a rich and talented life. Eventually, they require this admiration in greater and greater quantity because they believe that if they are not admired, they are "bad." Conversely, they may begrudge others their success or possessions, feeling that they deserve the admiration and privileges more (APA 2000).

A sense of shame compels clients with narcissistic PD never to make a mistake and never to tolerate the mistakes of others. This shame defends against the fear that if they are "bad," they will be abandoned or annihilated. Internally, a great pendulum exists, swinging from a grandiose position to one of intense feelings of inferiority, danger, and shame. During the grandiose cycle, clients with narcissistic PD feel invulnerable and perfect; during the shame cycle, their fear causes them intense anxiety, and they frantically search for what they have done wrong and exhaust themselves correcting others' opinions of them. They fear that if they do not carry out these acts, great harm will come to them. Having human limitations and disappointing or frustrating others can feel like a life-or-death situation. Conversely, disappointment or frustration regarding others' limitations can also feel like life or death, and they are as intolerant of that in others as they are in themselves (APA 2000).

Internally, therefore, clients with narcissistic PD do not have the ability to recognize realistic limitations. Frequently, they feel that others do not give them the rewards they deserve. In overestimating themselves and underestimating others, they find that what others give them never seems enough, and they frequently have fantasies of unlimited success, power, brilliance, and beauty.

When seen in a health care setting, these clients can demand "the best of everything," including practitioners. They measure their self-worth by surrounding themselves with what they project as being the "crème de la crème" (APA 2000). This feeling of entitlement has significant impact. Clients with narcissistic PD, who demonstrate lack of sensitivity, envy, demands, and disparagement of others, are seen as arrogant, highly critical, patronizing, and rude. However, this constant need for admiration, overevaluation of their own ability, and devaluation of others covers a fragile sense of self (APA 2000).

When these clients are corrected, when their boundaries are defined, or when limits are set on their behavior, they are left feeling humiliated, degraded, and empty. To reestablish internal balance, they may launch a counterattack. Sometimes, vocational endeavors are minimal, reflecting an attempt to avoid injury in competitive or risky situations. Social withdrawal, depression, and mood disorders may result.

Narcissism is essentially a maladaptive social response characterized by egocentric attitude, fragile self-esteem, constant seeking of praise or admiration, and envy. At about 4 years of age, narcissism is normal. During adolescence, many narcissistic traits are seen as being culturally normal, and, after a period of adjustment, this narcissism usually evolves into a greater scope of understanding of self and others. In the mental health care setting, those diagnosed with narcissistic PD are predominantly male (APA 2000).

Vignette

■ *Mr. Varick is a 43-year-old gay man who has lived with his partner for 15 years. He thinks of himself as a successful salesman, going into debt to drive a sports car and live on the "right" street. In his belief, being seen with the "right" people is more important than liking them. As his partner has grown older, Mr. Varick's sexual attention has focused outside their relationship on handsome younger men. These encounters help Mr. Varick believe that he himself is still young and handsome. However, Mr. Varick's sexual encounters are usually in the bushes of a park or in public bathrooms, and he has twice been arrested for indecent exposure, which has led to his initiating psychotherapy.*

Once in therapy, he regales his nurse therapist with stories that he hopes will amuse and impress her, but her response is a neutral one, listening but not displaying the hoped-for responses. Mr. Varick escalates his attempts to amuse and impress, until he finally expresses anger at his therapist for not being worldly enough to appreciate him. He wonders aloud whether another therapist might be better for him (Profiri 1998).

The nurse therapist compassionately identifies his attempts to seek and become perfect, his grandiosity, and his sense of entitlement. The therapist shows how this thinking ends up hurting his partner, in addition to placing both of them at great risk through his sexual acting out. Because his actions are making him feel more inadequate rather than fulfilled, he despairs that he is beyond help; his shaming of his nurse therapist expresses the fear that she cannot help him either.

Over time, clients with narcissistic PD can use such confrontation to begin to have compassion for themselves and, eventually, others.

Clinical Picture of Cluster C Disorders (Anxious, Fearful)

Cluster C includes the avoidant, dependent, and obsessive-compulsive PDs. Individuals with cluster C PDs often appear anxious or fearful. Figure 16–4

DSM-IV-TR CRITERIA FOR CLUSTER C PERSONALITY DISORDERS

CLUSTER C (Anxious or Fearful)

DEPENDENT PERSONALITY DISORDER	OBSESSIVE-COMPULSIVE PERSONALITY DISORDER	AVOIDANT PERSONALITY DISORDER
A. A pervasive and excessive need to be taken care of that leads to submissive and clinging behavior and fear of separation, beginning by early adulthood and present in a variety of contexts, as indicated by five (or more) of the following: (1) Has difficulty making everyday decisions without an excessive amount of advice and reassurance from others (2) Needs others to assume responsibility for most major areas of life (3) Has difficulty expressing disagreement with others because of fear of loss of support or approval. *Note:* Does not include realistic fears of retribution. (4) Has difficulty initiating projects or doing things on own (because of a lack of self-confidence in judgment or abilities rather than a lack of motivation or energy) (5) Goes to excessive lengths to obtain nurturance and support from others, to the point of volunteering to do things that are unpleasant (6) Feels uncomfortable or helpless when alone because of exaggerated fears of being unable to care for self (7) Urgently seeks another relationship as a source of care and support when a close relationship ends (8) Is unrealistically preoccupied with fears of being left to take care of self	A. A pervasive pattern of preoccupation with orderliness, perfectionism, and mental and interpersonal control, at the expense of flexibility, openness, and efficiency, beginning by early adulthood and present in a variety of contexts, as indicated by four (or more) of the following: (1) Is preoccupied with details, rules, lists, order, organization or schedules to the extent that the major point of the activity is lost (2) Shows perfectionism that interferes with task completion (e.g., is unable to complete a project because overly strict personal standards are not met) (3) Is excessively devoted to work and productivity to the exclusion of leisure activities and friendships (not accounted for by obvious economic necessity) (4) Is overconscientious scrupulous, and inflexible about matters of morality, ethics, or values (not accounted for by cultural or religious identification) (5) Is unable to discard worn-out or worthless objects even when they have no sentimental value (6) Is reluctant to delegate tasks or to work with others unless they submit exactly to own way of doing things (7) Adopts a miserly spending style toward both self and others; money is viewed as something to be hoarded for future catastrophes (8) Shows rigidity and stubbornness	A. A pervasive pattern of social inhibition, feelings of inadequacy, and hypersensitivity to negative evaluation, beginning by early adulthood and present in a variety of contexts, as indicated by four (or more) of the following: (1) Avoids occupational activities that involve significant interpersonal contact, because of fears of criticism, disapproval, or rejection (2) Is unwilling to get involved with people unless certain of being liked (3) Shows restraint within intimate relationships because of fear of being shamed or ridiculed (4) Is preoccupied with being criticized or rejected in social situations (5) Is inhibited in new interpersonal situations because of feelings of inadequacy (6) Views self as socially inept, personally unappealing, or inferior to others (7) Is unusually reluctant to take personal risks or to engage in any new activities because they may prove embarrassing

Figure 16–4 DSM-IV-TR criteria for cluster C personality disorders. (Adapted from American Psychiatric Association. [2000]. *Diagnostic and statistical manual of mental disorders* [4th ed.-TR]. Washington, DC: Copyright 2000, American Psychiatric Association.)

presents the DSM-IV-TR criteria for the cluster C disorders.

AVOIDANT PERSONALITY DISORDER

Shyness and avoidance of conflict, risk, and new situations are common in early childhood and are expected to diminish by the end of adolescence. Attainment and mastery of psychomotor skills, as well as skill development that becomes transferable to new situations, ordinarily make avoidance behaviors diminish with age. When avoidance instead grows into a pervasive pattern of social inhibition, with accompanying feelings of inadequacy and hypersensitivity to criticism, then avoidant PD is a possible diagnosis. Preoccupation with fear of rejection and criticism is the hallmark of this disorder.

Clients with avoidant PD have little tolerance for normal group process and perceive that they are receiving the rejection they most fear. Because their social presentation appears shy, timid, and socially inept, with low self-esteem and poor self-care, they can become objects of derision in any group. Although they can emphasize only the negative perceptions they receive, clients with avoidant PD often exaggerate the dangers of these experiences. Internally, they are fearful that the self-doubts they have of themselves will be seen by others, and they attempt to hide from others, which leaves them emotionally and physically isolated.

Restricted interpersonal contacts diminish the likelihood that they will learn how to interact with others and reinforces shame over such things as blushing or crying in the presence of others. Their low self-esteem and hypersensitivity increase as support networks decrease. Demands in the workplace and in normal adult daily living can begin to overwhelm them, and they may retreat to an inner world of fantasy where their desires for ideal love and acceptance can be met.

Clients with avoidant PD may long to feel part of a group or family, but hypersensitivity to the slightest hint of disapproval prevents them from joining in, even if they are given repeated reassurances and generous offers of support and nurturance. Building a therapeutic relationship with these clients is difficult. They enter the relationship with the projection that their caregiver will harm them through disapproval, and they perceive rejection where it does not exist. They have great difficulty trusting a correction of their interpretations, and they are unwilling to trust unless they are certain they will be liked. Because they have so often experienced shame and ridicule in social situations, even when trust is built, they restrain themselves from

the intimacy that they desire in order to avoid the anticipated pain of rejection. These inhibitions, their conviction that they are inferior and unable to learn how to be with people, and their reluctance to take risks hinder the caregiver at every turn.

Vignette

■ Ms. Knight is a 48-year-old single woman who is retired from a career in the army and now works for an electronics firm. She has never been involved in an intimate relationship with another adult but was able to make superficial contacts while in the military because of the clear social structure. Since she moved 3 years ago, Ms. Knight has met many people but has not made friends. She rarely speaks with her co-workers and faithfully returns to her mobile home each evening after work. Her sense of loneliness has become unbearable, and she finally seeks psychotherapy because she does not know where else to turn (Profiri, 1998).

The nurse-therapist's strategy is to teach and facilitate Ms. Knight's socialization skills, while providing positive feedback from which Ms. Knight can build her self-esteem.

DEPENDENT PERSONALITY DISORDER

Self-sacrifice, or toleration of physical, sexual, or emotional abuse when alternatives for self-care and escape exist, is the most startling aspect of dependent PD. The person with dependent PD has a poignant sense of being incapable of survival if left alone; this may be expressed in lack of ability even to pick out the day's wardrobe without considerable reassurance and guidance. Clients with dependent PD experience a deep foreboding about personal incompetence; consequently, they solicit caretaking by clinging and being pervasively and excessively submissive. By early adulthood, these people perceive themselves as being unable to separate from others and to work independently. They believe that it is necessary to be dependent on others in order to function at all. They are passive and follow other people's preferences or advice, even when they know it to be inaccurate and potentially harmful to themselves or others. If others do not initiate or take responsibility for them, then their needs remain neglected.

In clients with dependent PD, anger and assertiveness are suppressed by a passivity that masks a fear of others' retaliation or alienation. When they are able to maintain a dependent position in a stable relationship, they can function adequately; however, they may still fear appearing too competent, which could lead to abandonment. Thus, they often avoid skill-enhancing learning, instead mastering dependency-perpetuating behaviors.

Submissive behaviors intended to strengthen attachment to their partner, spouse, or family often result in unbalanced and distorted relationships. When a close relationship ends—whether because of children leaving home, death, or divorce—clients with dependent PD may become anxious, and this is the time they are most likely to seek a health care practitioner. They become intensely and prematurely attached to another person without pausing to evaluate the consequences. This inability to discriminate and discern stems from the fearfully held certainty that they will not survive on their own. These clients see themselves as so dependent that even the thought of loss is anxiety provoking. Their fears are excessive, extreme, persistent, and not amenable to logic.

The pessimism of clients with dependent PD pervades any logical cognitive intervention. Their self-doubt is projected onto others, and they devalue others' helpfulness unless it is the idealized, self-sacrificial caretaking they perceive as being "just good enough." Any setting of realistic expectations can deflate their self-esteem, and they then devalue themselves. This perpetual cycle of losing faith in themselves reinforces their belief in the necessity of self-sacrifice, making them willing to endure anything to remain attached. This can appear as **masochism** (soliciting dominance from others), but they feel it is what they must do to get the protection they need from others.

When a decision is left up to them, clients who have dependent PD experience painful levels of anxiety that derive from the belief that they will make a horrible mistake, and then not only will they suffer the sadism of others but they will also be abandoned in their misery. They can obsessively ruminate and fantasize about abandonment, even when it is not threatened.

The client with dependent PD is at greater risk for anxiety and mood disorders, and dependent PD can occur with borderline, avoidant, and histrionic PDs. This disorder commonly occurs in individuals who have a general medical condition or a disability that requires them to be dependent on others. Long-term inability to care independently for the self erodes confidence, autonomy, and personal integrity. Fear of losing support can be life threatening for this population (APA 2000). More insightful clients often benefit from psychodynamic psychotherapy that targets the client's low self-esteem, fears regarding autonomy, and relationship with the therapist. Others may benefit from supportive group therapy and/or assertiveness training.

Vignette

■ *Mrs. Patterson, a 70-year-old widow of an abusive spouse, is seen for the first time at a mental health clinic. She presents with suicidal ideation arising from intractable pain of osteoarthritis. She has been a widow for 15 years, but her most recent loss is that of her 50-year-old son, who is leaving his childhood home after returning to it periodically during his adulthood, never having fully emancipated himself from his family. This last extended return was of 3 years' duration. Mrs. Patterson says she could not live without her son to take care of her (Profiri, 1998).*

Nursing strategies include finding solutions to Mrs. Patterson's chronic pain. She is given antidepressants to quell her anxiety, and workers are assigned to assist her with adult daily living chores that will increase her sense of adequacy. Supportive therapy is encouraged in order to teach her new skills of problem solving, and it has the desired outcome of increasing her self-confidence.

OBSESSIVE-COMPULSIVE PERSONALITY DISORDER

Pack-rat behaviors, endlessly repeating tasks until perfection is achieved, rigid and literal enforcement of rules or laws designed to avoid disorder—all are essential features of obsessive-compulsive PD. On presentation, clients with obsessive-compulsive PD stubbornly insist that their way of doing things is the only right way. Gathering a history can be inordinately time consuming as the client offers endless irrelevant details.

Although excessive in verbosity, these clients are miserly with material goods, emotions, and behaviors. Their rationale is that catastrophe is imminent and that they must prepare by hoarding and protecting their resources. "You never know when you'll need it" is a frequently heard refrain from the individual with obsessive-compulsive PD about the tidy stacks of old newspapers, magazines, and appliances that cause havoc for families or roommates. Their resistance to help arises partly from this fear of catastrophe and partly from the belief that no one can perform these acts better. They tend to take firm control of everything in their lives and refuse to delegate tasks, even when they are unable to keep deadlines that could endanger their work life.

Although they may appear devoted to their work or occupation, in reality, the work behaviors of individuals with obsessive-compulsive PD cause much friction with others. If they do turn over some task, it is with high expectations, along with minutely detailed instructions, and they are angry if any deviation from their directions occurs. Highly critical of others, they hold themselves to a scrupulous moral code that allows little room for the ambiguities of normal adult life. Thus, they are also merciless with themselves when they make a mistake, and they almost never forgive what they see as a wrong; for them, the world is black and white.

In relationships, individuals with obsessive-compulsive PD can be taskmasters, turning even the most leisurely activity into a lesson or an opportunity to perfect oneself. They often believe that they cannot afford to rest, take time off, or go on vacation. There may be such a great emphasis on cleanliness, making lists, and refining that attempted projects never reach a stage of completion, causing considerable stress for themselves and those around them. Insight regarding the impact that their actions have on others is slight, if present at all.

Individuals with obsessive-compulsive PD experience a loss of control when they are called on to make decisions, prioritize, or streamline; they find these processes time consuming, difficult, and painful. When such activities are called for, the person with obsessive-compulsive PD is likely to respond defensively (although not with anger). Although they ruminate endlessly about what has displeased them, this activity serves only to make them more anxious about what is the right thing to do.

Intimacy in relationships is superficial and rigidly controlled, even though clients with obsessive-compulsive PD may feel deep and genuine affection for friends and family. Their everyday interactions have a formal and serious quality. Internally, they rehearse over and over again how they will react or what they will say in social situations. Emotional displays by others seem childish to them, and they have great difficulty trying to convey tender feelings of their own. When confronted with situations that demand flexibility or compromise, they are unable to compromise and often lose many opportunities in relationships and in the workplace (APA 2000).

Vignette

■ *Mr. Lopez, a 48-year-old married man who is a middle manager for a microchip company, keeps canceling the appointment for his yearly health check-up by the company nurse. His reason is that he has to do so much of his unit's job himself because his staff is incompetent. When he finally keeps an appointment, he is 30 minutes late and begins to give directions to the nurse: she should take his blood pressure on his right arm instead of his left, her name tag is on crooked, and the scale is 2¾ pounds off his scale at home.*

Mr. Lopez's blood pressure is high, and he complains of not sleeping well and of trouble at home with his teenaged children about their curfew. He also complains of severe heartburn and an 80-hour work week. He has been passed over for promotion for the past 5 years and has received poor job reviews for high employee turnover in his work unit (Profiri, 1998).

The nurse refers Mr. Lopez to a primary care provider for a cardiac and gastrointestinal work-up. She asks him if he feels he would like some help from someone who specializes in teaching relaxation techniques and problem-solving skills. Mr. Lopez declines these, saying that he does not have time, and besides, he knows all he needs to know about such things.

NURSING DIAGNOSIS

People with PDs are usually admitted to psychiatric institutions for reasons other than their disorder (e.g., for substance abuse, suicide attempts, or self-mutilation, or by court order). PDs seen most often in the health care system are borderline PD and antisocial PD. Because the behaviors central to these disorders often cause upheaval and disruption on psychiatric units, as well as on medical-surgical wards and clinics, nursing diagnoses and interventions for these two disorders are emphasized. Emotions such as anxiety, rage, and depression and behaviors such as withdrawal, paranoia, and manipulation are among the most frequent areas that health care workers need to address. See Box 16–3 for common potential nursing diagnoses.

OUTCOME CRITERIA

Realistic goal setting with individuals with PDs comes from the perspective that personality change happens one behavioral solution and one learned skill at a time. This can be expected to take much time and repetition. No matter how intelligent they may appear or how insightful they can be about themselves and others, these clients find that change is slow and occurs via trial and error, with the support of affect management and much interpersonal reinforcement. No shortcuts occur with the client with a PD; in permanent change, the learning can literally be integrated at the cellular level. In practical terms, this means that by the time they come for help, these clients may have already seen several caregivers and are likely to take whatever the nurse/counselor can give and then move on to the next caregiver. Theirs is a long and circuitous road, and the nurse is their most recent attempt to find healing (Profiri 1998).

Since larger steps are not realistic with PD clients, realistic outcomes need to be very modest and obtainable. For some individuals, overall outcome criteria might include

BOX 16-3 *Potential Nursing Diagnoses for Personality Disorder*

SYMPTOM	NURSING DIAGNOSIS
Crisis, high levels of anxiety	Ineffective Coping Anxiety Self-Mutilation
Anger and aggression; child, elder or spouse abuse	Risk for Other-Directed Violence Ineffective Coping Impaired Parenting Disabled Family Coping
Withdrawal	Social Isolation
Paranoia	Fear Disturbed Sensory Perception Disturbed Thought Process Defensive Coping
Depression	Hopelessness Helplessness Risk for Suicide Self-Mutilation Chronic Low Self-Esteem Spiritual Distress
Difficulty in relationships, manipulation	Ineffective Coping Impaired Social Interaction Defensive Coping Interrupted Family Processes Risk for Loneliness
Not keeping medical appointments, late for appointments, not following prescribed medical procedure/medication	Ineffective Therapeutic Regimen Management Noncompliance

■ Minimizing self-destructive or aggressive behavior
■ Reducing the effect of manipulative behaviors
■ Linking consequences to both functional and dysfunctional behaviors
■ Learning and mastering skills that facilitate functional behaviors
■ Practicing the substitution of functional alternatives during crisis
■ Initiating functional alternatives to prevent a crisis
■ Ongoing management of anger, anxiety, shame, and happiness
■ Creating a life style that prevents regressing

PLANNING

Basically, clients with PDs do not come voluntarily for treatment. People with antisocial PD and borderline PD are, however, frequently seen in health care settings for other reasons, and manifestations of both these disorders can cause a disruption for the nurse, staff, or system where they are seen.

People with borderline PD are impulsive (e.g., suicidal, self-mutilating), aggressive, manipulative, and even psychotic under periods of stress. People with antisocial PD most often are seen in the health care system through court order. They are also manipulative, aggressive, and impulsive. Generic care plans for manipulation (Table 16–4), aggressive behavior (Table 16–5), and impulsive behaviors (Table 16–6) are presented here.

Intervention for suicide and anger management are covered in Chapter 23 and Chapter 24, respectively. A more thorough discussion of interventions for manipulation is covered in Chapter 19.

INTERVENTION

It is often difficult to create a therapeutic relationship with clients with PD. Because most have expe-

TABLE 16–4   *Interventions for Manipulation*

Nursing Diagnosis: *Impaired Social Interaction:* related to need for immediate gratification and disregard for the rights of others, as evidenced by manipulation of others.
Outcome Criteria: Demonstrate limit setting on own manipulative behaviors.

GOAL	INTERVENTION
Client will demonstrate limit setting for manipulative behavior by (date)	1. Identify manipulative behaviors by client. 2. Set clear, consistent, enforceable limits on manipulative behaviors by communicating expected behaviors. 3. Convey to the team consistency of approach in setting limits. 4. Be realistic as to which behaviors can be limited. 5. Be clear with client about the consequences of exceeding limits. 6. Follow through with consequences in a nonpunitive manner. 7. Assist client in developing means of setting limits on own behavior. 8. Assess degree of insight into manipulative behavior and motivation to change. 9. Avoid getting into power struggles by accusing and arguing with client.
Client will develop two alternative nonmanipulative behaviors by (date).	1. Discuss client's behaviors in nonjudgmental and nonthreatening manner. 2. Assist client in identifying personal strengths and effective communication skills. 3. Assist client in testing out alternative behaviors for obtaining needs or fulfilling expectations. 4. Support client and provide feedback in trying new behaviors.

Data from Chitty, K. K., and Maynard, C. K. (1986). Managing manipulation. *J Psychosocial Nurs and Mental Health Services*, 24(6):9; Varcarolis, E. (2000). *Psychiatric nursing clinical guide*. Philadelphia: W. B. Saunders; Louie, K. B. (1994). Personality disorders: Antisocial, paranoid, and borderline. In E. M. Varcarolis (Ed.), *Foundations of psychiatric mental health nursing* (2nd ed.). Philadelphia: W. B. Saunders.

TABLE 16–5   *Interventions for Aggressive Behavior*

Nursing Diagnosis: *Other-Directed Violence:* related to rage reaction as evidenced by aggression (verbal/physical) toward others.
Outcome Criteria: Refrain from aggressive behaviors.

INTERMEDIATE GOAL	INTERVENTION
1. Client will demonstrate control and responsibility in two situations in which he or she previously used aggressive action by (date).	1a. Encourage client to spend time talking out instead of acting out intense feelings of frustration. 1b. Communicate positive expectations to the client. 1c. Assist client in developing concrete external controls. 1d. Assist client in problem-solving techniques to cope with frustration or tension. 1e. Provide feedback on results 1f. Limit choices to those that are safe and appropriate. 1g. Identify medications if appropriate for rage reaction.
2. Client will cope with stress and aggression in a nonviolent manner most of the time by (date).	2a. Assist client in identifying feelings of anxiety, expectations, anger, frustration, disappointment, or perceived threats. 2b. Assist client in verbalizing these feelings. 2c. Assist client in describing precipitating events or situations leading to aggressive behavior. 2d. Assist client in exploring present situation by discussing situations in the past that have aroused similar feelings. 2e. Assist client in identifying previous coping behaviors. 2f. Assist client in exploring consequences of behavior on self and others. 2g. Assist client in developing more effective coping behaviors and interpersonal skills. 2h. Teach client about anger reducing medications he/she is on—monitor for side effects.

Adapted from Louie, K. B. (1994). Personality disorders: Antisocial, paranoid, and borderline. In E. M. Varcarolis (Ed.), *Foundations of psychiatric mental health nursing* (2nd ed.). Philadelphia: W. B. Saunders.

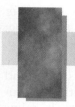

TABLE 16-6 *Interventions for Impulsive Behavior*

Nursing Diagnosis: *Ineffective Coping:* related to loss of impulse control as evidenced by impulsive behavior (self-mutilation, aggression)
Outcome Criteria: Demonstrate success in refraining from impulsive acts.

GOAL	INTERVENTION
1. Client will identify impulsive acts and give examples of situations in which they occur by (date).	1a. Identify the needs and feelings preceding the impulsive acts. 1b. Discuss current and previous impulsive acts. 1c. Explore impact of such acts on self and others. 1d. Recognize cues of impulsive behaviors that may injure others.
2. Client will role play alternatives to take when urges to act impulsively arise by (date).	2a. Teach or refer client to appropriate place to learn needed coping skills (anger management, assertive skills). 2b. Identify situations that trigger impulsivity and discuss alternative behavior. 2c. Role play one new skill/behavior at a time.

Adapted from Louie, K. B. (1994). Personality disorders: Antisocial, paranoid, and borderline. In E. Varcarolis (Ed.), *Foundations of psychiatric mental health nursing* (2nd ed.). Philadelphia: W. B. Saunders.

rienced a series of interrupted therapeutic alliances, their suspiciousness, aloofness, and hostility can be a set-up for failure. The guarded and secretive style of these clients tends to produce an atmosphere of combativeness. When clients blame and attack others, the nurse needs to understand the context of their complaints; these attacks spring from feeling threatened, and the more intense the complaints, the greater the fear of potential harm or loss.

Lacking the ability to trust, clients with PD require a sense of control over what is happening to them. Giving them choices—whether to come to a clinic appointment in the morning or afternoon, for example—may enhance compliance with treatment. Because clients with PD are hypersensitive to criticism yet have no strong sense of autonomy, the most effective teaching of new behaviors builds on their own existing skills.

When people with PDs exhibit fantasies that attribute malevolent intentions to the nurse or others, it is important to orient them to reality. They need to know that even though they have insulted or threatened their caregiver, they will still be helped and protected from being hurt. When they are hurt by others, as naturally happens in everyday life, the nurse takes time to dissect the situation with them, asking when, where, and how it happened, and honestly maps out for them how people, systems, families, and relationships work. It is important to be honest about their limitations and assets. The client with a PD may already be aware of them, but acknowledging them demonstrates trustworthiness. Tables 16–7, 16–8, and 16–9 identify

- nursing guidelines
- useful therapies
- effective psychopharmacology

for each of the PDs.

Communication Guidelines

Everyone has his or her own communication style. This style not only conveys what people have to say but also represents who people see themselves to be. Nurses greatly enhance their ability to be therapeutic when they combine limit setting, trustworthiness, dealing with manipulations, and authenticity with their own natural style. Many nurse clinicians work with clients who have PDs as therapists in clinics, health care centers, private practice, and institutes. These nurses are prepared at the advanced practice level and have had special training in conducting therapy.

Box 16–4 is an example of a nurse-client interaction: Donald, a client with antisocial PD, has instigated a fight with another client on a psychiatric unit (Louie 1994).

Milieu Therapy

Individuals with PD may, at times, be treated within a therapeutic milieu: inpatient, partial hospital, or day treatment settings. The primary therapeutic goal of milieu therapy is affect management in a group context. Community meetings, problem-solving groups, coping skills groups, and socializing groups are all areas in which clients can interact with peers, discuss relationship problems, delegate and take responsibility for certain tasks, discuss goals, collectively deal with problems that arise in the milieu, and learn problem-solving skills. Through desensitization via social group experience, overwhelming and painful internal states can be felt and endured, even while the task of the group is accomplished. Viewing acting out as unconscious communication that needs to be made conscious and verbal, so that it is possible to understand the need that it communicates, enables the group and the individual to decide how to meet that need.

Psychopharmacology

Clients with PD may be supported by a broad array of psychotropics, all geared toward maintaining cognitive function and managing affect. However, with clients who have PD, it is important to remember that medications are both a curse and a blessing; they can be simultaneously intrusive, untrustworthy, and soothing. Enhancing medication compliance with these clients requires that they understand their experiences consciously. Clients with PD usually do not like taking medicine unless it calms them down. They worry if they do not have an adequate supply but have difficulty organizing themselves to fill the prescription. Sometimes, they panic, somatocize about side effects, and stop taking the medication, while still demanding more tranquilizing drugs. As these complaints demonstrate, clients with PD are fearful about taking something over which they have no control.

Despite these cautions about prescribing drugs, antipsychotics may be useful for brief periods to control agitation, rage, and brief psychotic episodes.

TABLE 16-7 *Nursing and Therapy Guidelines for Cluster A Disorders (Odd or Eccentric)*

PERSONALITY DISORDER	CHARACTERISTICS	NURSING GUIDELINES	SUGGESTED THERAPIES
Schizotypal	■ Ideas of reference ■ Cognitive/perceptual distortions ■ Socially inept ■ Anxious	1. Respect the client's need for social isolation. 2. Be aware of client's suspiciousness and employ appropriate interventions. 3. As with the schizoid client, careful diagnostic assessment may be needed to uncover any other medical or psychological symptoms that may need intervention (e.g., suicidal thoughts).	1. Skills-oriented psychotherapy 2. Cognitive and behavioral measures 3. **Low-dose antipsychotics**
Paranoid (PPD)	■ Projects blame ■ Suspicious ■ Hostile/violent ■ Cognitive/perceptual distortions	1. Avoid being too "nice" or "friendly." 2. Give clear and straightforward explanations of tests and procedures beforehand. 3. Use simple clear language, avoid ambiguity. 4. Project a neutral but kind affect. 5. Warn about any changes, side effects of medications, and reasons for delay. Such interventions may help allay anxiety and minimize suspiciousness. 6. A written plan may help encourage cooperation.	1. Client distrusts therapist's motives. 2. Supportive psychotherapy, later cognitive-behavioral techniques 3. **Low dose of antipsychotics** if cognitive/perceptual problems chronic
Schizoid	■ Reclusive ■ Avoidant ■ Uncooperative	1. Avoid being too "nice" or "friendly." 2. Do not try to re-socialize these clients (Goldberg 1995). 3. A thorough diagnostic assessment may be needed to identify symptoms or disorders that the client is reluctant to discuss.	1. Supportive psychotherapy 2. Group therapy 3. **Antipsychotic, antidepressant, anxiolytics often short term**

Data from American Psychiatric Association (2000). *Diagnostic and statistical manual of mental disorders* (4th ed.-TR). Washington, DC: American Psychiatric Association; Varcarolis, E. M. (2000). *Psychiatric nursing clinical guide: Assessment tools and diagnosis.* Philadelphia: W. B. Saunders; Cloninger, C. R., and Svrakic, D. M. (1999). Personality disorders. In B. J. Sadock and V. A. Sadock (Eds.), *Comprehensive textbook of psychiatry-VII* (7th ed.). Philadelphia: Lippincott Williams & Wilkins; and Gunderson, J. G., and Phillips, K. A. (1995). Personality disorders. In H. I. Kaplan and B. J. Sadock (Eds.), *Comprehensive textbook of psychiatry-VI* (6th ed., Vol. 2, pp 1425–1462). Baltimore: Williams & Wilkins.

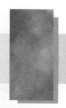

TABLE 16–8 *Nursing and Therapy Guidelines for Cluster B Disorders (Dramatic, Emotional, Erratic)*

PERSONALITY DISORDER	CHARACTERISTICS	NURSING GUIDELINES	SUGGESTED THERAPIES
Borderline (BPD)	■ Separation anxiety ■ Ideas of reference ■ Impulsive acts (suicide, self-mutilation) ■ Splitting (adoring/devaluing persons)	1. Set realistic goals, use clear action words. 2. Be aware of manipulative behaviors (flattery, seductiveness, guilt instilling) 3. Provide clear and consistent boundaries and limits. 4. Use clear and straightforward communication. 5. When behavioral problems emerge, calmly review the therapeutic goals and boundaries of treatment. 6. Avoid rejecting or rescuing. 7. Assess for suicidal and self-mutilating behaviors, especially during times of stress.	1. Dialectical (behaviorally based therapy, DBT) 2. **SSRIs for anger and depression** 3. **Carbamazepine (anticonvulsant for dyscontrol and self-harm)** 4. Low-dose antipsychotics for cognitive disturbance (paranoia, magical thinking, illusions)

Antisocial (ASPD)	■ Manipulative
	■ Exploits others
	■ Aggressive
	■ Callous towards others
		1. Try to prevent or reduce untoward effects of manipulation (flattery, seductiveness, instilling guilt):
		  ■ Set clear and realistic limits on specific behavior
		  ■ All limits should be adhered to by all staff involved
		  ■ Carefully document objective physical signs of manipulation or aggression when managing clinical problems
		  ■ Document behaviors objectively (give times, dates, circumstances)
		  ■ Provide clear boundaries and consequences
		2. Be aware that antisocial clients can instill guilt when they are not getting what they want. Guard against being manipulated through feeling guilty.
		3. Treatment of substance abuse is best handled through a well-organized treatment program *before* counseling and other forms of therapy are started.
			1. No treatment of choice—don't seek treatment
			2. Therapeutic community/token economics for some
			3. **Pharmacology for aggression (lithium, anticonvulsants, SSRIs)**

Narcissistic (NPD)	■ Exploitive ■ Grandiose ■ Disparaging ■ Rageful ■ Increased sensitivity to rejection, criticism	1. Remain neutral, avoid power struggles or becoming defensive in response to the client's disparaging remarks, no matter how provocative the situation may be. 2. Convey unassuming self-confidence.	1. No known effective treatment 2. Don't seek treatment 3. Treat comorbid Axis I disorder
Histrionic (HPD)	■ Seductive ■ Flamboyant ■ Seeks attention ■ Shallowness ■ Depression/suicidal when admiration withdrawn	1. Understand seductive behavior as a response to distress. 2. Keep communication and interactions professional, despite temptation to collude with the client in a flirtatious and misleading manner. 3. Encourage and model the use of concrete and descriptive language rather than vague and impressionistic. 4. Teach and role model assertiveness.	1. No known effective therapy: research lacking 2. Treat comorbid PDs (BPD common) 3. MAOIs may help with atypical depression

BPD, bipolar disorder; MAOIs, monoamine oxidase inhibitors; SSRIs, selective serotonin reuptake inhibitors.
Data from American Psychiatric Association (2000). *Diagnostic and statistical manual of mental disorders* (4th ed.-TR). Washington, DC: American Psychiatric Association; Varcarolis, E. M. (2000). *Psychiatric nursing clinical guide: Assessment tools and diagnosis.* Philadelphia: W. B. Saunders; Cloninger, C. R., and Svrakic, D. M. (1999). Personality disorders. In B. J. Sadock and V. A. Sadock (Eds.), *Comprehensive textbook of psychiatry-VII* (7th ed.). Philadelphia: Lippincott Williams & Wilkins, and Philips, K. A., and Gunderson, J. G. (1999). Personality disorders. In R. E. Hales, S. C. Yudofsky, and J. A. Talbott (Eds.), *The American psychiatric textbook of psychiatry* (3rd ed.). Washington, DC: The American Psychiatric Press.

TABLE 16-9 *Nursing and Therapy Guidelines for Cluster C Disorders (Anxious or Fearful)*

PERSONALITY DISORDER	CHARACTERISTICS	NURSING GUIDELINES	SUGGESTED THERAPIES
Dependent (DPD)	■ Excessive clinging ■ Self-sacrificing, submissive ■ Needy, gets others to care for him/her	1. Identify and help address current stresses. 2. Try to satisfy client's needs at the same time as you set up limits in such a manner that the client does not feel punished and withdraw. 3. Strong countertransference often develops in clinicians because of the client's excessive clinging (demands of extra time, nighttime calls, crisis before vacations); therefore, supervision is well advised. 4. Teach and role model assertiveness.	1. Combination of psychotherapy, supportive therapy, cognitive behavioral therapy may be the most advantageous.
Obsessive-Compulsive (OCD)	■ Perfectionistic ■ Need for control ■ Inflexible/rigid ■ Preoccupation with details ■ Highly critical of self and others	1. Guard against engaging in power struggles with an OCD client. Need for control is very high for these clients. 2. Intellectualization, rationalization, and reaction formation are the most common defense mechanisms with which clients with OCD use.	1. Supportive or insightful psychotherapy—also cognitive-behavioral therapy, depending on goals 2. **Clomipramine (tricyclic antidepressant) and SSRIs helpful for obsessional thinking and depression.**
Avoidant (APD)	■ Excessive anxiety in social situation ■ Hypersensitive to negative evaluuation	1. A friendly, gentle, reassuring approach is the best way to treat clients with APD. 2. Being pushed into social situations can cause extreme and severe anxiety for APD clients.	1. Social phobia treated with desensitization, social skills training—other cognitive-behavior therapies. 2. **MAOIs may help social anxieties.** 3. Benzodiazepines may help panic episodes.

MAOIs, monoamine oxidase inhibitors; SSRIs, selective serotonin re-uptake inhibitors.
Data from American Psychiatric Association. (2000). *Diagnostic and statistical manual of mental disorders* (4th ed.-TR). Washington, DC: American Psychiatric Association; Varcarolis, E. M. (2000). *Psychiatric nursing clinical guide: Assessment tools and diagnosis.* Philadelphia: W. B. Saunders; Cloninger, C. R., and Svrakic, D. M. (1999). Personality disorders. In B. J. Sadock and V. A. Sadock (Eds.), *Comprehensive textbook of psychiatry-VII* (7th ed.). Philadelphia: Lippincott Williams & Wilkins; and Philips, K. A., and Gunderson, J. G. (1999). Personality disorders. In R. E. Hales, S. C. Yudofsky, and J. A. Talbott (Eds.), *The American psychiatric textbook of psychiatry* (3rd ed.). Washington, DC: The American Psychiatric Press.

Pimozide (Orap) has been helpful in reducing paranoid ideation in some clients, and antidepressants may be useful at times, particularly for clients with borderline PD. Refer to Tables 16–7, 16–8, and 16–9 for effective pharmacology for individuals with PDs.

CASE MANAGEMENT

Case management is usually required for clients with PD who are persistently and severely impaired, have been hospitalized previously, have been unable to maintain work or personal relationships, and are relatively alone in their attempts to care for themselves. Most clients with PD are high functioning, but a significant number still need assistance in order to stay out of the hospital. Case management of a client, therefore, is geared toward reducing the necessity for hospitalization by creating a homeostasis that is based on the client's highest functioning level. Very little change is expected with most clients who have PD, and the primary focus is on health promotion and maintenance through stress reduction and crisis intervention.

BOX 16–4   *Dialogue with a Client with Manipulative, Aggressive, and Impulsive Traits*

DIALOGUE	THERAPEUTIC TOOL/COMMENT
Nurse: Donald, I would like to talk with you about what happened this morning.	Be clear as to purpose of interview.
Mr. Mann: OK, shoot.	
Nurse: Tell me what started the incident.	Use open-ended statements. Maintain a nonjudgmental attitude.
Mr. Mann: Well, as I told you before, I always had to fight to get what I wanted in life. My father and mother abandoned me emotionally when I was a child.	
Nurse: Yes, but tell me about this morning.	Redirect client to present problem or situation.
Mr. Mann: OK. I disliked Richard from the first. He has it in for me, I just know it. He doesn't get along with anyone here. Just 2 days ago, he almost had a fight.	
Nurse: Donald, what do you mean, Richard has it in for you?	Explore situation.
Mr. Mann: When I'm talking to one of the nurses, he stares and makes comments under his breath.	
Nurse: What does he say?	Encourage description.
Mr. Mann: How I'm "in" with the nurses. I'm just trying to do what is expected of me here.	
Nurse: You mean that Richard is envious of your relationship with the nurses?	Validate client's meaning.
Mr. Mann: Right. He really doesn't want to be here. He doesn't care about all that therapeutic junk.	
Nurse: You seem to know a lot about how Richard thinks, I wonder how that is?	Assist client to make association to present situation.
Mr. Mann: He reminds me of someone I knew when I was young. His name was Joe. We called him "Bones."	
Nurse: Tell me more about Bones.	Explore situation further.
Mr. Mann: We called him Bones because he was skinny. He was into drugs and never ate. He was also called Bones because he was selfish. He never shared anything. He never even had a girl that I knew about.	
Nurse: So Richard reminds you of someone who is selfish and lonely?	Make interpretation of information. Note increasing anxiety.
Mr. Mann: That's right. I've had three marriages and girlfriends on the side. No one can take them away from me. *(angrily)* Just let them try!	
Nurse: What makes you so angry now?	Identify feelings and explore threat or anxiety.
Mr. Mann: Richard! I know he wants to be like me, but he can't. I'll hurt him if he makes any more comments about me.	
Nurse: Donald, you will *not* hurt anyone here on the unit.	Set limits on, and expectations of, client's behavior.
Mr. Mann: I'm sorry, I didn't mean that.	
Nurse: It's important that we examine your part in the incident this morning and how to cope without threats or violence.	Focus on client's responsibility and suggest alternative methods of coping with situation.

Box continued on following page

Box 16–4 *Dialogue with a Client with Manipulative, Aggressive, and Impulsive Traits*
(Continued)

DIALOGUE	THERAPEUTIC TOOL/COMMENT
Mr. Mann: Listen, I know I've gotten into trouble because I can't control my temper, but that's because I won't get any respect until I can show them I don't fear them.	Exhibits rationalization.
Nurse: Who are "they"?	Clarify pronoun.
Mr. Mann: People like Richard.	
Nurse: You've told me that fighting was a way of survival as a child, but as an adult, there are other ways of handling situations that make you angry.	Shows understanding and suggests other means of coping.
Mr. Mann: You're right. I've thought about this. Do you think it would help if you give me some meds to control my anger?	Exhibits superficial and concrete thinking—possible manipulation.
Nurse: I wasn't thinking of medications but of a plan for being aware of your anger and talking it out instead of fighting it out.	Clarifying meaning toward behavioral change. Starts to explore alternatives Donald can use when angry instead of fighting.
Mr. Mann: I told you before, I have to fight.	
Nurse: Have you thought about the consequences of your fighting?	Identify results of impulsive behavior.
Mr. Mann: I feel bad afterwards. Sometimes I wish it hadn't happened.	Continues to explore.

EVALUATION

Evaluating effectiveness with this population is difficult. Nurse clinicians may never know the real measure of their interventions. Clients with PD generally find a long-term relationship too intimate an experience to remain long enough for useful evaluation; if they do, they probably no longer have PD. In these circumstances, self-care for the nurse clinician becomes important. Perhaps effectiveness can be measured by how successfully the nurse was able to be genuine with the client, to maintain a helpful posture, to offer substantial instruction, and to still care for himself or herself. The mixed therapeutic picture of effectiveness and lack of effectiveness with clients is a given. This means that it is important that the caregiver not measure personal effectiveness on the basis of the client's ability to change. Learning to find meaning and peace in the process, rather than proof of personal effectiveness, is the reward that is possible with these clients.

Visit the **Evolve** website at
http://evolve.elsevier.com/Varcarolis
for more Case Studies.

CASE STUDY 16–1   *Borderline Personality Disorder*

Mary Drake was a 24-year-old single secretary who lived alone. She had been seen in the emergency room several times for superficial suicide attempts. She was admitted because she had cut her wrists, ankles, and vagina with glass and had lost a lot of blood. This event was precipitated by her graduation from a community college.

Upon admission she was sweet, serene, and grateful to all the nurses, calling them "angels of mercy." Within one week she was angry at half of the nurses, demanding a new primary nurse, saying that the one she had (to whom she had grown attached) hated her. She has a history of heavy drinking and had managed to sneak alcohol onto the unit. She was found in bed with a young male client. She continually broke unit rules and then pleaded to have this behavior forgiven and forgotten. When angry, she threatened to cut herself again. When asked why she cut herself, Ms. Drake stated, "I was tired." She appeared restless and tense and frequently asked for antianxiety medication. When asked what she was anxious about, she said "Uh . . . I don't know . . . I feel so empty inside." Ms. Drake frequently paced up and down the halls looking both angry and bored.

DSM-IV Diagnosis

Axis I—Substance Abuse (alcohol)
Axis II—Borderline PD
Axis III—None
Axis IV—None
Axis V—GAF 65

ASSESSMENT

Ms. McCarthy, a recent graduate and Ms. Drake's primary nurse, organized the data into subjective and objective components.

Objective Data

1. Makes frequent, superficial suicide attempts
2. Requests antianxiety medication frequently
3. Paces up and down the hall much of the day
4. Threatens self-mutilation when anxious
5. Brings alcohol onto the unit after pass
6. Is found in bed with male client

Subjective Data

1. Initially "loved" her primary nurse, now "hates" her and wants another nurse
2. States she is restless and tense
3. Complains of feeling empty inside
4. Describes self as angry and bored much of the time

SELF-ASSESSMENT

Ms. McCarthy talked to Ms. Drake's therapist twice a week in staff meetings. The therapist impressed upon Ms. McCarthy the difficulty health care workers have in dealing effectively with people with borderline PDs. These clients constantly act out their feelings in self-destructive and maladaptive ways. They usually are not aware of their feelings or what triggered their actions.

The most difficult area for many health care workers is dealing with the intense feelings and reactions these clients can instill and provoke in others. Ms. McCarthy set a time twice a week for supervision with Ms. Drake's therapist. At the next meeting, common goals and intervention strategies were discussed.

Case Study continued on following page

CASE STUDY 16–1   *Borderline Personality Disorder (Continued)*

NURSING DIAGNOSIS

Ms. McCarthy formulated three initial nursing diagnoses that had the highest priority during this time.

1. *Anxiety* related to change in and loss of self-concept, as evidenced by inability to relax

   - States she feels "empty"
   - Is restless and tense
   - Requests antianxiety medication frequently

2. *Ineffective Coping* related to inadequate psychological resources, as evidenced by self-destructive behaviors

   - After stating that she feels frustrated, client goes on pass and comes back with alcohol

   - After stating that she loves her therapist, client is found in bed with a male client
   - After stating that she hates her primary nurse, client demands a new primary nurse

3. *Self-Mutilation* related to anxiety and emptiness, as evidenced by suicidal gestures and poor impulse control

   - Is admitted following self-mutilation
   - Threatens self-mutilation when anxious
   - Threatens self-mutilation on the unit

OUTCOME CRITERIA

Learning coping skills to deal with anxiety

PLANNING

The nurse decided on the following goals:

NURSING DIAGNOSIS	LONG-TERM GOALS	SHORT-TERM GOALS
1. *Anxiety* related to change in and loss of self-concept, as evidenced by inability to relax	1. Client will state that she feels relaxed more than she feels tense by discharge.	1. By (date) client will state she is relaxed in a situation that usually produces anxiety, e.g., after visiting hours.
2. *Ineffective Coping* related to inadequate psychological resources, as evidenced by self-destructive behaviors	2. Client will solve problems in a manner that injures neither self nor others by (date).	2. By (date) client will discuss feelings of frustration and deal with them appropriately rather than acting them out.
3. *Self-Mutilation* related to anxiety and emptiness, as evidenced by suicidal gestures and poor impulse control	3. Client will state that she will use an alternative coping device when thoughts of self-mutilation occur.	3. By (date) client will discuss desire to mutilate self rather than doing so.

INTERVENTION

Working with Ms. Drake, the nurse found, was not easy. Many times the nurse felt angry and frustrated with Ms. Drake when acting out behaviors occurred. With supervision, Ms. McCarthy was better able to deal with her feelings. The nurse became better able to focus on Ms. Drake's actions and work with her to figure out what feelings and events triggered the actions. See Ms. Drake's nursing care plan, including interventions and rationales (Nursing Care Plan 16–1).

CASE STUDY 16-1   *Borderline Personality Disorder* (Continued)

EVALUATION

Ms. Drake appeared to come a long way. Her acting out behaviors decreased. She had not threatened or attempted to mutilate herself since admission. Although her sessions with her therapist were often stormy, there was more discussion of feelings. Her pacing of the halls had decreased, and she appeared less tense most of the time. She still continued to ask for her antianxiety medication at frequent intervals but was willing to talk about what she thought the anxiety was about with both her primary nurse and the therapist. She agreed to continue therapy with her therapist on a biweekly basis after discharge.

Adapted from Lego, S. (1994). Personality disorders: Antisocial, paranoid and borderline. In E. M. Varcarolis (Ed.), *Foundations in Psychiatric Mental Health Nursing* (2nd Ed., pp. 403–406). Philadelphia: W. B. Saunders.

Visit the **Evolve** website at
http://evolve.elsevier.com/Varcarolis
for the other Nursing Care Plan diagnoses and for
more Nursing Care Plans.

NURSING CARE PLAN 16-1   *Borderline Personality Disorder*

NURSING DIAGNOSIS
Anxiety related to change in and loss of self-concept, as evidenced by inability to relax

Supporting Data

- States that she feels "empty"
- Is restless and tense
- Requests antianxiety medication frequently

Long-Term Goal: Ms. Drake will state that she feels relaxed more than she feels tense by discharge.

SHORT-TERM GOAL	INTERVENTION	RATIONALE	EVALUATION
1. By (date) Ms. Drake will state she is relaxed in a situation that usually produces anxiety (e.g., after visiting hours).	1a. Talk to client prior to event to help her observe and describe what she is expecting from the event.	1a. Understanding expectations that may or may not be met helps to identify source of anxiety and opens the way to more effective problem solving for unmet needs.	*GOAL MET* Client was able to discuss situation that was potentially anxiety provoking and appeared relaxed after discussion.
	1b. Engage client in physical activity, such as jogging or aerobics class.	1b. Exercise reduces physical tension and can increase endorphins, thereby increasing feelings of well-being.	Instead of pacing the halls today, she talked pleasantly with other clients after exercise class.

Nursing Care Plan continued on following page

NURSING CARE PLAN 16–1   *Borderline Personality Disorder* (Continued)

NURSING DIAGNOSIS

Ineffective Coping related to inadequate psychological resources, as evidenced by self-destructive behaviors

■ After stating that she feels "frustrated," client goes on pass and returns with alcohol.
■ After stating that she loves her therapist, client is found in bed with another client.
■ After stating that she hates her primary nurse, client demands a new primary nurse.

Long-Term Goal: Ms. Drake will solve problems in a manner that injures neither herself nor others by (date).

SHORT-TERM GOAL	INTERVENTION	RATIONALE	EVALUATION
1. By (date) Ms. Drake will discuss feelings of frustration and deal with them appropriately rather than acting them out.	1. Talk with client when she is frustrated regarding her goal, the block to the goal, and ways to either change the goal or reach it in an appropriate way. 2. Talk with client when she is experiencing strong positive or negative transference feelings, helping her to understand and experience all her feelings without acting them out.	1. Discussing and understanding the dynamics of frustration help to reduce the frustration by helping the client take positive action. 2. Discussing and understanding the meaning of transference feelings and splitting help to reduce the potential for acting out.	*GOAL MET* Ms. Drake was able to experience problems and deal with them appropriately. Acting out was minimal or absent. For example, client had an appointment for a job interview. She wanted to stay in bed and avoid the interview. Instead, she talked with her nurse about the fear of "growing up" and was able to get up and go to the interview.

NURSING DIAGNOSIS

Self-Mutilation related to anxiety and emptiness, as evidenced by suicidal gestures and poor impulse control

■ Is admitted following self-mutilation
■ Threatens self-mutilation when anxious
■ Attempts self-mutilation on the unit

NURSING CARE PLAN 16-1   *Borderline Personality Disorder (Continued)*

Long-Term Goal: Ms. Drake will state that she no longer has the desire to mutilate herself.

SHORT-TERM GOAL	INTERVENTION	RATIONALE	EVALUATION
1. By (date) Ms. Drake will discuss desire to mutilate herself rather than doing so.	1a. Assist client in observing potential situations for self-mutilation.	1a. Observing, describing and analyzing thoughts and feelings reduce the potential for acting them out destructively.	*GOAL MET* Ms. Drake was able to experience troubling thoughts and feelings without self-mutilation. Stated, "I was mad at my therapist today and decided to cut my arms after the session. Instead, I told her I was angry, and together we figured out why."
	1b. Encourage more appropriate ways to deal with these feelings.	1b. Offers alternative behaviors that can be more satisfying and growth promoting.	
	1c. Take care to safeguard environment at times when staff is busy and client's anxiety is acute.	1c. Times of increased anxiety, frustration, or anger without external controls could increase probability of client self-mutilating behaviors.	

Adapted from Lego, S. (1994). Personality disorders: Antisocial, paranoid, and borderline. In E. M. Varcarolis (Ed.), *Foundations in Psychiatric Mental Health Nursing* (2nd ed., pp. 403–406). Philadelphia: W. B. Saunders.

SUMMARY

The special needs of the client with PD project from an inner core of terror, rage, and confusion, around which neurochemical pathways have formed to create thoughts, feelings, and actions that are rigid and maladaptive. The role of the nurse with such clients is to understand the theoretical underpinnings of their disorder, along with its many diagnostic expressions, and to be able to intervene to change the crisis-oriented client into the client who is consciously aware of the consequences of his or her behavior and can soothe inner painful states while still accomplishing the tasks of adult daily living.

Visit the **Evolve** website at
http://evolve.elsevier.com/Varcarolis
for a post-test on the content in this chapter.

Visit the **Evolve** website at
http://evolve.elsevier.com/Varcarolis
for additional self-study exercises.

Critical Thinking and Chapter Review

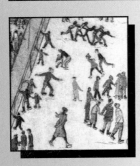

Critical Thinking

1. Mr. Rogers is undergoing surgery for a broken leg. He is very suspicious of the staff and believes that everyone is trying to harm him and to "do him in." He scans his environment constantly for danger (hypervigilant) and speaks very little to the nurses or the other clients. He has a paranoid personality disorder.

   ■ Why would being friendly and outgoing be threatening to Mr. Rogers?
   ■ Explain how being matter of fact and neutral, and sticking to the facts would be the most useful to Mr. Rogers.
   ■ What would be some ways to give Mr. Rogers some control over his situation in a hospital setting?
   ■ How would you best handle his sarcasm and hostility so that both you and he would feel most comfortable?

2. Mr. Stowe is a 29-year-old man who has been in and out of jail several times for stealing and selling drugs. He is HIV positive and often works as a prostitute to get money, never using a condom. He states: "Let them get what I have. Why should I be the only one?" When he wants something, he can be very charming and tells people anything to get what he wants from them. He has an antisocial personality disorder.

   ■ What other behaviors would you assess for in a person with an antisocial personality disorder? (Does he feel remorse? care for others' feelings? take drugs or engage in thrill-seeking behaviors? plan for his future? What other characteristics are commonly observed?)
   ■ When he is caught for selling drugs to minors, he tells his lawyer that the police planted the drugs on him, and told the police that all lawyers are corrupt. This is an example of what type of behavior?
   ■ How would you best respond to him when he tries to convince you that the police planted the drugs on him? What principle would that relate to?
   ■ How could you best deal with your thoughts and emotions about his not using a condom with others when he is HIV positive?

3. Ms. Pemrose is brought into the emergency department (ED) after slashing her wrist with a razor. She has previously been in the ED for drug overdose and has a history of addictions. The ED staff avoids her because they find her behavior trying and exhausting. Ms. Pemrose can be sarcastic, belittling, and aggressive to those who try to care for her. She has a history of difficulty with interpersonal relationships at her job. When a new advanced practice nurse comes in to examine her, she is at first adoring and compliant, telling him, "You are the best therapist I have ever seen, and I truly want to change." When he refuses to support her request for diazepam (Valium) and meperidine (Demerol) for "pain," she yells at him, "You are a stupid excuse for a therapist. I want a real doctor immediately." Ms. Pemrose has a borderline personality disorder.

■ What defense mechanisms is Ms. Pemrose using?
■ How could the advanced practice nurse therapist best handle this situation in keeping with setting limits and offering concern and useful interventions?

Chapter Review

Choose the most appropriate answer.

1. Which of the following best describes people with personality disorders?

   1. Readily assume the roles of compromiser and harmonizer
   2. Often seek help to change maladaptive behaviors
   3. Have the ability to tolerate high levels of anxiety
   4. Have difficulty working and loving

2. With which client is the nurse most likely to need to plan interventions to minimize overtly manipulative behavior?

   1. Mr. A, who has been diagnosed with obsessive-compulsive personality disorder
   2. Miss B, who has been diagnosed with borderline personality disorder
   3. Mr. C, who has been diagnosed with paranoid personality disorder
   4. Mrs. D, who has been diagnosed with schizoid personality disorder

3. A priority nursing intervention undertaken by the nurse dealing with clients with personality disorder is

   1. Offering advice
   2. Probing for etiological factors
   3. Encouraging diversional activity
   4. Combining limit-setting, trustworthiness, dealing with manipulations, and authenticity

4. Which statement will provide a foundation for understanding clients with personality disorders?

   1. The backgrounds of clients with personality disorder are usually trouble free.
   2. The tendency to develop personality disorders may have biological determinants.
   3. Clients with personality disorders are best treated in the inpatient setting.
   4. Personality disorders are more amenable to treatment than anxiety disorders.

5. Of the emotional states listed below, the nurse caring for a client with a personality disorder is most likely to experience

   1. Anger
   2. Depression
   3. Pleasure
   4. Spiritual distress

NURSE, CLIENT, AND FAMILY RESOURCES

Association

National Alliance for the Mentally Ill (NAMI)
200 North Glebe Road, Suite 1015
Arlington, VA 22203-3754
1-800-950-6264

Internet Sites

Online Screening for Personality Disorders
http://www.med.nyu.edu/psych/screens/pds.html

StrongeR—Destroying the Myth of Self-Harm
Recovery information for those who self-mutilate
http://www.geocities.com/SoHo/Study/8174/
frontpage.html

Borderline Personality Disorder Page
Recovery information for people with borderline PD
http://www.navicom.com/~patty/
http://mentalhelp.net/disorders

Self-Injury Page
Self-mutilation
http://www.palace.net/~llama/psych/injury.html

BPD Central
Borderline PD web site
http://www.bpdcentral/index.html
http://www.bpdcentral.com

Internet Mental Health
For a good overview of all the personality disorders
http://www.mentalhealth.com

Avoidant Personality Disorder Home Page
http://www.geocities.com/hotsprings/3764

Cognitive Therapy for Personality Disorders
http://www.mhsource.com/pt/p960241.html

REFERENCES

American Psychiatric Association (2000). *Diagnostic and statistical manual of mental disorders* (4th ed.-TR). Washington, DC: American Psychiatric Association.

Baker, L. A., and Daniels, D. (1990). Nonshared environmental influences and personality differences in adult twins. *Journal of Personality and Social Psychology*, 58:103–110.

Bonnivier, J. F. (1996). Management of self-destructive behaviors in an open inpatient setting. *Journal of Psychosocial Nursing and Mental Health Services*, 34(2):38–42.

Chitty K. K., and Maynard, C. K. (1986). Managing manipulation. *Journal of Psychosocial Nursing and Mental Health Services*, 24(6):9.

Cloninger, C. R., and Svrakic, D. M. (1999). Personality disorders. In B. J. Sadock and V. A. Sadock (Eds.), *Comprehensive textbook of psychiatry-VII* (7th ed.). Philadelphia: Lippincott Williams & Wilkins.

Cloninger, C. R., Svrakic, D. M., and Przybeck, T. R. (1993). A psychobiological model of temperament and character. *Archives of General Psychiatry*, 50:975–990.

Dawson, G., and Fischer, K. W. (Eds.). (1994). *Human behavior and the developing brain*. New York: Guilford Press.

Dunn, J., and McGuire, S. (1993). Young children's non-shared experiences: A summary of studies in Cambridge and Colorado. In E. M. Hetherington, D. Reiss, and R. Plomin (Eds.), *Nonshared environments* (pp 111–128). Hillsdale, NJ: Lawrence Eribaum.

Favazza, A. R., and Rosenthal, R. J. (1993). Diagnostic issues in self-mutilation. *Hospital and Community Psychiatry*, 44:134–140.

Goldberg, R. J. (1998). *Practical guide to the care of the psychiatric patient* (2nd ed.). St. Louis: C. V. Mosby.

Gunderson, J. G., and Phillips, K. A. (1995). Personality disorders. In H. I. Kaplan and B. J. Sadock (Eds.), *Comprehensive textbook of psychiatry-VI* (6th ed., Vol. 2, pp 1425–1462). Baltimore: Williams & Wilkins.

Horowitz, M. J. (1992). *Stress response syndromes*. Northvale, NJ: Jason-Aronson.

Kaplan, H. I., and Sadock, B. J. (1991). *Synopsis of psychiatry*. Baltimore: Williams & Wilkins.

Kernberg, O. (1985). *Internal world and external reality*. London: Aronson.

Kohut, H. (1984). *How does analysis cure?* Chicago: University of Chicago Press.

Lego, S. (1994). Personality disorders: Antisocial, paranoid, and borderline. In E. M. Varcarolis (Ed.), *Foundations of psychiatric mental health nursing* (2nd ed.). Philadelphia: W. B. Saunders.

Lewis-Herman, J. (1992). *Trauma and recovery*. New York: HarperCollins.

Louie, K. B. (1994). Personality disorders: Antisocial, paranoid, and borderline. In E. M. Varcarolis (Ed.), *Foundations of Psychiatric Mental Health Nursing* (2nd ed.). Philadelphia: W. B. Saunders.

Lyons, M. J., et al. (1995). Differential heritability of adult and juvenile antisocial traits. *Archives of General Psychiatry*, 52(11):906–915.

Maier, W., Lichtermann, D., Minges, J., and Heun, R. (1994). Personality disorders among the relatives of schizophrenia patients. *Schizophrenia Bulletin*, 20(3):481–493.

Maxmen, J. S., and Ward, N. G. (1995). *Psychotropic drugs fast facts* (2nd ed.). New York: W. W. Norton.

Maxmen, J. S., and Ward, N. G. (1996). *Essential psychopathology and its treatment* (2nd ed.). New York: W. W. Norton.

McGee, D. E., and Linehan, M. M. (1997). Cluster B personality disorders. In D. L. Dunner (Ed.), *Current psychiatric therapy* (2nd ed.). Philadelphia: W. B. Saunders.

Nehls, N. (1999). Borderline personality disorder: The voice of patients. *Residential Nursing and Health*, 22(4):285–293.

O'Brian, L. (1998). Inpatient nursing care of patients with borderline personality disorder: A review of the literature. *Australian and New Zealand Journal of Mental Health Nursing*, 7(4):172–183.

Oldham, J. M., et al. (1995). Comorbidity of axis I and axis II disorders. *American Journal of Psychiatry*, 152(4):571–578.

Philips, K. A., and Gunderson, J. G. (1999). Personality disorders. In R. E. Hales, S. C. Yudofsky, and J. A. Talbott (Eds.), *The American psychiatric textbook of psychiatry* (3rd ed.). Washington, D.C.: The American Psychiatric Press.

Post, R. M. (1992). Transduction of psychosocial stress into the neurobiology of recurrent affective disorder. *American Journal of Psychiatry*, 149:999–1007.

Profiri, F. (1998). Personality disorders. In E. M. Varcarolis (Ed.), *Foundations of psychiatric mental health nursing* (3rd ed.). Philadelphia: W. B. Saunders.

Store, M. H. (1997). Cluster C personality disorders. In D. L. Dunner (Ed.), *Current psychiatric therapy* (2nd ed.). Philadelphia: W. B. Saunders.

Valliant, G. E. (1994). Ego mechanisms of defense and personality psychopathology. *Journal of Abnormal Psychology*, 103:44–50.

Varcarolis, E. M. (2000). *Psychiatric nursing clinical guide: Assessment tools and diagnosis*. Philadelphia: W. B. Saunders.

Zale, C. F., O'Brien, M. M., Trestman, R. L., and Siever, L. J. (1997). Cluster A personality disorders. In D. L. Dunner (Ed.), *Current psychiatric therapy* (2nd ed.). Philadelphia: W. B. Saunders.

Outline

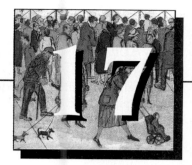

Eating Disorders

KATHLEEN IBRAHIM

Key Terms and Concepts

The key terms and concepts listed here also appear in color where they are defined or first discussed in this chapter.

anorexia nervosa

binge eating disorder

binge/purge cycle

bulimia nervosa

cognitive distortions

ideal body weight

Objectives

After studying this chapter, the reader will be able to

1. Differentiate between the four theories of eating disorders discussed in this chapter.
2. Compare and contrast the signs and symptoms (clinical picture) of anorexia nervosa with those of bulimia nervosa.
3. Identify three life-threatening conditions stated in terms of nursing diagnoses for a client with an eating disorder.
4. Develop three realistic outcome criteria for (a) a client with anorexia and (b) a client with bulimia nervosa.
5. Recognize which therapeutic interventions are appropriate for the acute phase of anorexia and which are appropriate for the long-term phase of treatment.
6. Explain the basic premise of cognitive-behavioral therapy in the treatment of anorexia nervosa and bulimia nervosa.
7. After reading the chapter, try to empathize with, and describe in your own words the possible thoughts and feelings of, a young anorectic girl during the acute phase of her illness.
8. Distinguish between the needs and treatment(s) for an acute bulimic client with bulimic individuals in long-term therapy.
9. Differentiate between the long-term prognosis of anorexia, bulimia nervosa, and binge eating disorder.

411

PREVALENCE

Individuals with eating disorders are often in severe psychic pain. The physical result of starvation, bingeing-purging, suicide, or self-mutilation may require immediate hospitalization or death may ensue. These are serious long-term illnesses that can manifest themselves in different ways at different points during the course of their illness (APA 2000b).

The estimated lifetime prevalence of anorexia nervosa among women ranges from 0.5% for narrowly defined criteria to 3.7% for more broadly defined anorexia nervosa (APA 2000a). The lifetime prevalence among women for bulimia nervosa ranges from 1.1% to 4.2% depending on the criteria applied. Some studies suggest that the incidence of bulimia nervosa in the United States may have decreased slightly (APA 2000a). The disorder is more common in females, and estimates of male/female ratios range from 1:6 to 1:10. Within the younger population, however, 19% to 30% are males (APA 2000b). A review of twin studies by Bulik and colleagues (2000) reveals a strong genetic liability for bulimia nervosa but the inheritability of anorexia nervosa appears less conclusive. Strober and colleagues (2000) interviewed first-degree relatives of individuals with anorexia nervosa and bulimia nervosa and found evidence of familial transmission of both disorders compared to first-degree relatives of never-ill individuals.

African American women were found overall to have the same incidence of eating disordered behavior as white women (Striegel-Moore et al. 2000c). The pattern of weight control was more likely as a result of fasting or abusing diuretics or laxatives rather than vomiting in the African-American group.

There is an overall increase worldwide in eating disorders, appearing now in cultures in which the disorder was previously rarely seen (APA 2000b). Becker (2000) reported on a survey in 1998 in Fiji done after 3 years of Western influence that showed a marked increase in eating disorder symptoms compared to a survey in 1995. Chinese women in Hong Kong and Australia are showing increased rates of eating disordered behaviors (Lake et al. 2000), as are adolescents in Iran (Nobakht and Dezhkam 2000).

Female athletes, especially those in sports that emphasize thinness, i.e., gymnastics, ballet dancing, figure skating, and distance running, have demonstrated an increase in eating disorders (Powers and Johnson 1999). Pope and associates (1993) found a high rate of anorexia nervosa (2.8%) among the male bodybuilders in his study compared to the 0.02% incidence found among the general American male population.

COMORBIDITY

The incidence of comorbid psychiatric illness is high in eating disorder patients who seek treatment. Major depressive disorder or dysthymia is diagnosed in 50% to 75% of patients with anorexia nervosa and bulimia nervosa (APA 2000a). Dysthymia in adolescents was predictive of eating disorder symptoms in a study by Zaider and colleagues (2000). Bipolar disorder is found in 4% to 6%, but some report a rate as high as 13%. The incidence of obsessive-compulsive disorder has been reported as high as 25% and is common among patients with bulimia nervosa. Anxiety disorders, particularly social phobia, are common. Substance abuse has been found in as many as 30% to 37% of those with bulimia nervosa and 12% to 18% of those with anorexia nervosa occurring primarily with binge/purge subtype (APA 2000b).

The pattern of comorbidity for psychiatric illness, including personality disorders, was noted to be the same in men as in women. Homosexuality/bisexuality was also noted as a specific risk factor for males, particularly those diagnosed with bulimia nervosa (Carlat et al. 1997). Male veterans with eating disorders were found to have a high rate of comorbid substance use and mood disorders, including those with anorexia nervosa who were at high risk for schizophrenia or another psychotic disorder. Males with bulimia nervosa were at risk for comorbid organic mental disorder, schizophrenia, and psychotic disorders (Striegel-Moore et al. 1999).

Comorbid personality disorder estimates range from 42% to 75%. There is a noted association between bulimia nervosa and cluster B and C personality disorders, especially borderline personality disorder and avoidant personality disorder, and between anorexia nervosa and cluster C—avoidant personality disorder and obsessive compulsive personality disorder (APA 2000b). Obsessive-compulsive personality disorder predicted eating disorder symptoms in adolescents in a community sample (Zaider et al. 2000). Obsessive-compulsive features are often prominent, both food-related and food-not-related (APA 2000b). Personality disorders are more common among individuals with binge/purge subtype of anorexia nervosa than the restricting type or normal weight clients with bulimia nervosa (APA 2000a).

Sexual abuse has been reported in 20% to 50% of people with bulimia nervosa (Bulik et al. 1989) and those with anorexia nervosa (Schmidt et al. 1993; Vize et al. 1995) although it is more common in clients with bulimia nervosa than with the restricting subtype of anorexia nervosa. A sexual abuse history is more common in eating disorders than in the general population. Women with a history of eating disorders and sexual abuse have a higher rate of other comorbid psychiatric illness than other women diagnosed solely with eating disorders (Pope and Hudson 1992).

Anorexia nervosa carries a significant risk of death and suicide. The features associated with a fatal outcome are longer duration of illness, bingeing and purging, comorbid substance abuse, and affective disorders (Herzog et al. 2000).

THEORY

The eating disorders—anorexia nervosa, bulimia nervosa, and binge eating not otherwise specified (NOS)—are actually entities or syndromes and are not specific diseases with a common cause, common pathology, or common treatment (Halmi 1999). It is more appropriate to conceptualize them as syndromes on the basis of the cluster of symptoms they present (Halmi 1999).

Neurobiological/Neuroendocrine Interactions

Several conceptual models of eating disorders exist. The coexistence (comorbidity) of eating disorders and depression has received considerable focus in the literature. The symptoms of undereating and overeating in eating disorders parallel the primary symptoms of melancholic and atypical depression. Devlin and Walsh (1989) proposed hypothetical relationships: The eating disorder either causes a depression or is a variant of a depressive disorder. Another relationship they hypothesized is one of common biopsychosocial vulnerabilities that lead to depression and/or eating disorders. Further, these authors noted the increased frequency of depression in biological relatives of clients with eating disorders. In some cases, major depressive disorder predated the eating disorder; in other cases, it developed after treatment of the eating disorder. In depression, as in eating disorders, complex interrelationships of altered neurotransmitters exist as well as aberrant patterns involving multiple systems and pathways. However, Devlin and Walsh (1989) also cautioned against assuming similar pathological features in eating disorders and depression based on the treatment response to antidepressant medication in the two groups.

Similar neuroendocrine abnormalities have been noted in both diagnostic entities, and neuroendocrine abnormalities have been much researched and documented in eating disorders (Hsu 1990). Irwin

1993). Whether the relationships are causal or result from starvation or abnormal eating behaviors is not clear. Cholecystokinin, an intestinal hormone, is present at low levels in bulimic persons; endogenous opioids, gastrointestinal hormones, and vasopressin have received attention, but the findings are not clear. The aforementioned findings represent the biological abnormalities observed in people with eating disorders and may help to explain the drive toward dieting, hunger, preoccupation with food, and tendency toward binge eating (Devlin et al. 1990).

Psychological Interactions

Anorexia nervosa results in amenorrhea and physiological changes, which interfere with the development of an age-appropriate sexual role. Psychoanalytical theorists long believed that conflict over one's sexual role was primary for anorectic persons (Bruch 1985). Bruch's work with anorectic women failed to prove these theoretical assumptions but postulated developmental factors that led to anorexia nervosa.

According to Bruch, girls who go on to have anorexia experience themselves as ineffectual, passive, and unable to assert their will. Misguided efforts to separate and establish an autonomous adult existence lead to self-starvation and a distorted sense of being special and powerful. People with anorexia are anxious about losing control over their eating and do not accurately experience hunger or satiety. These sensations result in a feeling of powerlessness and in a lack of ability to identify what they need. Defiance regarding eating occurs in an effort to define oneself, but it represents a futile endeavor to establish independence. The inauthentic identity has a veneer of competence, while underneath the individual has panic about losing control and feeling ineffectual.

Hsu (1990) stated that "affective overcontrol and intolerance, lack of self-direction, and personal effectiveness" are maladaptive responses to the developmental tasks of adolescence. Bruch (1985) described anorectic females who feel powerless and attempt to regulate their anxiety and feelings of effectiveness by controlling their eating, and, in so doing, achieve a societal ideal. Some individuals learn to control their feelings of depression (dysphoria) by binge eating and to numb their negative feelings by eating. These behaviors contribute to the avoidance of experiencing underlying negative emotions, which become replaced by the distress over binge eating and purging (Hsu 1990). Affective instability and poor impulse control are consistently associated with bulimia. Current research studies of mothers and daughters (Pike 1991) suggest a possible connection. Mothers of daughters with eating disorders had a longer dieting history and had a higher incidence of eating disorders compared with mothers of daughters who were not eating disordered.

It is a popular notion that sexual abuse is causal in the development of eating disorders, and frequently clinicians expect to uncover a history of such abuse. Welch and Fairburn (1994) noted that sexual abuse is a risk factor for the development of a psychiatric disorder, including bulimia nervosa, but it is not specific to bulimia. Pope and Hudson (1992) reviewed controlled retrospective studies of sexual abuse in individuals with eating disorders, uncontrolled studies, and studies of sexual abuse in the general population. They determined that sexual abuse does not constitute a specific risk factor for bulimia nervosa.

Sociocultural Models

The far greater incidence of eating disorders in westernized countries compared to developing countries is evidenced by the role of the perpetuating cultural pressure to be thin (Becker and Hamburg 1996). The media promotes the body as a commodity, and bodily preoccupation has become an acceptable form of self-promotion. Although the numbers of individuals who are overweight continue to increase, individuals with eating disorders have internalized the societal ideal to be thin as a compelling force. The feminist perspective is to assist women to resist a pathogenic culture (Wooley 1995).

The western ideal for women who are at risk is to be competent in traditional and nontraditional ways. For these women, being a mother and homemaker as well as a career woman may be experienced as a conflict. Bemporad (1996) noted that eating disorders do not flourish in male-dominated societies, where women are forced into a stereotypical nurturing role; rather, the incidence of eating disorders has risen in a society in which women have a choice in social roles. The increase in eating disorders in non-Western women assimilating into a Western society may be due either to the conflict of acculturation or due to identification with the new culture and its emphasis on a thin ideal female body (Lake et al. 2000).

Hsu (1990) noted that the characteristics of men with eating disorders are similar to those of women with eating disorders. In a study of college men, Olivardia and colleagues (1995) noted that men with eating disorders had characteristics similar to those of women with eating disorders but were different from men without eating disorders. Joiner and colleagues (2000) compared the bulimic symptoms of males and females and found males reported more perfectionism and distrust while females reported more drive for thinness. Males were more likely to have a later onset of their eating disorder and to be involved in a sport or occupation in which weight control was associated with performance according to Braun and others (1999), but the core pathology and comorbid illness remain very similar.

Biopsychosocial Models

Numerous hypotheses and studies are providing new data on eating disorders. Currently, an integrated biopsychosocial model is applied to the understanding and treatment of eating disorders. One study that looked for genetic factors found a 56% concordance rate in monozygotic twins for anorexia nervosa (Holland et al. 1984). The genetic vulnerability that might be responsible for the development of anorexia nervosa might lead to poor affect, poor impulse control, or an underlying neurotransmitter dysfunction. A family history of affective disorder and alcohol abuse was found to be common in monozygotic sets of twin pairs, in which one of the pair was diagnosed with bulimia nervosa. Kendler and colleagues (1991) found a 22.9% concordance rate for bulimia in monozygotic twins and an 8.7% rate in dizygotic twins. Hsu (1990) suggested that "significant psychiatric symptoms, such as depression, social anxiety and phobia, and obsessive-compulsive features" may contribute along with the dieting to the development of an eating disorder. Fairburn and colleagues (1999) question the findings of twin studies and view their results as inconsistent, favoring an etiological view that includes environmental mechanisms and gene-environment interactions.

Thiel and associates (1995) found a significant incidence of obsessive-compulsive disorder in a sample of anorectic clients and bulimic clients, who had obsessions and compulsions that were unrelated to eating behaviors.

According to Hsu (1990), "dieting provides the entree into an eating disorder" in the context of adolescent turmoil. Brewerton and colleagues (2000) confirmed that dieting is more likely to precede binge eating. However, this is not the only trigger; other mediating factors are subsumed into a biopsychosocial model. Obviously, eating disorders do not develop in all dieters, but certain risk factors increase the potential for such development. All of the previously cited theories postulate factors that could contribute to the risk of developing an eating disorder.

Excessive exercise has long been seen as a risk factor for the development of eating disorders, especially anorexia nervosa. The constellation of symptoms, e.g., disturbed eating behavior, amenorrhea, and osteoporosis has resulted in such terms as the "female athlete triad" and "anorexia athletica" (Powers and Johnson 1999). Athletes who participate in sports that emphasize a thin body are particularly at risk. Smolak and colleagues (2000) looked at athletic participation and eating problems and noted a significant risk, particularly in those sports emphasizing thinness, but also found athletic participation could be protective in certain situations, i.e., non-elite and non-lean sports. Pope and colleagues (1993) found a high rate of anorexia nervosa among the male bodybuilders in their study. They also describe a condition called "reverse anorexia" in which subjects developed a disordered body image in which they thought they were small and weak despite the opposite physical condition. The development of this reverse syndrome may precipitate or lead to continued use of anabolic steroids in some athletes.

Crisp (1995) has long maintained that the development of anorexia nervosa results in the desired avoidance of the sexual role. Hsu (1990) postulates that females in Western countries experienced adolescent turmoil as unhappiness significantly more than their male counterparts. This same finding was true of Japanese females, who expressed lower self-esteem than males (Lerner et al. 1980).

Physical attractiveness and its importance to the female have been demonstrated in many studies to be correlated with self-esteem. Davis and colleagues (2000) in their study of young women examined objective ratings of physical attractiveness and found physical beauty a risk for eating disorders. The impact of drive for thinness resulted in bulimia, depression, and body dissatisfaction in the study by Wiederman and Pryor (2000). Depression was also correlated with estimation of body size; those of normal weight who overestimated their size were more depressed than those who did not perceive themselves as fat (Kandel and Davies 1982).

Several researchers (Bruch 1985; Crisp 1995) have highlighted the conflict the female faces in establishing an identity. The adolescent female is expected to be both nurturing and competitive and to combine these extremes into a consistent female identity. No clear guidelines exist for the adolescent female, and the expectations may seem conflicting.

A comprehensive, biopsychosocial theory would subsume all of the aforementioned contributing factors, with specific risk factors playing more of a role in the development of an eating disorder in certain individuals.

All important, however, is the experienced event of dieting. The perception of being overweight is the most immediate cause for dieting that predisposes an individual to an eating disorder. Hsu (1990) postulated that once aberrant eating behaviors are established, they are reinforced through positive and negative factors, and the eating disorder becomes self-perpetuating. According to Fairburn and Cooper (1989), most of the problematic behaviors of anorexia nervosa and bulimia nervosa occur as a result of the overvalued ideas regarding weight, shape, and body image.

FUNDAMENTAL ASSESSMENT OF EATING DISORDERS

Anorexia and bulimia nervosa are two separate syndromes and, as such, present two clinical pictures on assessment. Table 17–1 identifies the clinical fea-

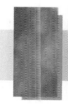

TABLE 17–1 *Possible Signs and Symptoms of Anorexia and Bulimia*

Phenomena Associated with Anorexia Nervosa

- Terrified of gaining weight
- Preoccupied with thoughts of food
- See themselves as fat even when emaciated
- Peculiar handling of food
  Cutting food into small bits
  Pushing pieces of food around plate
- May develop rigorous exercise regimens
- Self-induced vomiting, laxatives, and diuretics may be used
- Cognition so disturbed that they judge their self-worth by their weight

CLINICAL PRESENTATION	CAUSAL RELATIONSHIPS
■ Low weight	Caloric restriction, excessive exercising
■ Amenorrhea	Low weight
■ Yellow skin	Hypercarotenemia
■ Lanugo	Starvation
■ Cold extremities	Starvation
■ Peripheral edema	Hypoalbuminemia and on refeeding
■ Muscle weakening	Starvation, electrolyte imbalance
■ Constipation	Starvation

Table continued on following page

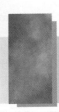

TABLE 17–1 *Possible Signs and Symptoms of Anorexia and Bulimia*
(Continued)

CLINICAL PRESENTATION	CAUSAL RELATIONSHIPS
■ **Abnormal lab values**	
Low T3, T4 levels	Starvation
■ CT scans, EEG changes	Starvation
■ Cardiovascular abnormalities	Starvation, dehydration
■ Hypotension	Electrolyte imbalance
■ Bradycardia	
■ Heart failure	
■ Impaired renal function, dehydration	
■ Hypokalemia (low K)	
■ Anemic pancytopenia	Starvation
■ Decreased bone density	Estrogen deficiency, low calcium intake

Phenomena Associated with Bulimia Nervosa

- Binge eating behaviors
- Often followed by self-induced vomiting (or laxative/diuretic use)
- 1/4 to 1/3 may have history of anorexia nervosa
- Have depressive signs and symptoms
- Have problem with
    Interpersonal relationships
    Self-concept
    Impulsive behaviors
- Experience increased levels of anxiety and compulsivity
- Chemical dependency may be common
- Impulsive stealing may occur

CLINICAL PRESENTATION	CAUSAL RELATIONSHIPS
■ Normal to slightly low weight	Excessive caloric intake with purging, excessive exercising
■ Dental caries, erosion	Vomiting (HCl reflux over enamel)
■ Parotid swelling	Increased serum amylase levels
■ Gastric dilation, rupture	Binge eating
■ Calluses, scars on hand	Self-induced vomiting, called **Russell's sign**
■ Peripheral edema	Rebound fluid especially if diuretic
■ Muscle weakening	Electrolyte imbalance
■ Abnormal lab values	
Electrolyte imbalance Hypokalemia Hyponatremia	Purging: vomiting, laxative, diuretic use
■ Cardiovascular abnormalities Cardiomyopathy ECG changes	Electrolyte imbalance—**can lead to death**
■ Cardiac failure (cardiomyopathy)	Ipecac intoxication

---

tures, potential lab results, and possible behaviors found on assessment.

Eating disorders are serious and in extreme cases can lead to death. Box 17–1 identifies a number of

BOX 17–1 *Some Medical Complications of Eating Disorders*

COMPLICATION	LABORATORY RESULTS
Cardiovascular	Electrocardiographic abnormalities
Bradycardia	
Postural hypotension	
Dysrhythmias	
Metabolic	
Acidosis (laxatives)	↓ K$^+$
Alkalosis (vomiting)	↑ Cholesterol
Hypokalemia	↑ Liver function tests
Hypocalcemia	↓ Mg2$^+$
Hypomagnesemia	↓ Na$^+$
Osteoporosis	↓ CA2$^+$
Dehydration	↓ Bone density
Renal	
Hematuria	↑ Blood urea nitrogen
Proteinuria	
Gastrointestinal	
Hyperamylasemia	↑ Serum amylase
Parotid swelling—hypertrophy	
Dental erosion (vomiting HCl)	
Esophagitis, esophageal tears (vomiting)	
Pancreatitis	
Diarrhea (laxative abuse)	
Gastric dilation–bingeing	
Hematological	
	Leukopenia
	↑ Erythrocyte sedimentation rate
	Abnormal complete blood count
Anemias (iron and vitamin B$_{12}$ deficiency)	Lymphocytosis
Endocrine	
Amenorrhea	↓ Follicle-stimulating hormone, luteinizing hormone, estradiol levels
	Urinary and plasma gonadotropins
Hypercortisolism	↑ Corticotropin-releasing hormone
Abnormal thyroid function test	↓ Tri-iodothyronine

Box 17-2   *Criteria for Hospital Admission for Clients with an Eating Disorder*

PHYSICAL CRITERIA

- Weight loss over 30% over 6 months
- Rapid decline in weight
- Severe hypothermia due to loss of subcutaneous tissue, or dehydration (T <36°C or 96.8°F)
- Inability to gain weight with outpatient treatment
- Heart rate less than 40 beats/min
- Systolic blood pressure less than 70 mm Hg.
- Hypokalemia—under 3 meq/L—or other electrolyte disturbances not corrected by oral supplementation.
- ECG changes (especially arrhythmias)
- Inability to gain weight repeatedly with outpatient treatment

PSYCHIATRIC CRITERIA

- Suicidal or severely out-of-control, self-mutilating behaviors
- Out-of-control use of laxatives, emetics, diuretics, or street drugs
- Failure to comply with treatment contract
- Severe depression
- Psychosis
- Family crisis/dysfunction

complications that can occur and the lab findings that may result in individuals with eating disorders. Because the eating behaviors in these conditions are so extreme, Box 17–2 identifies when an individual should be hospitalized; often hospitalization is via the emergency room. Table 17–2 provides the reader with a clinical tool and identifies some of the behaviors that when in extreme intensity or duration may signal the need for health intervention.

It needs to be emphasized that fundamental to all care for individuals with eating disorders is the establishment of a caring and trusting relationship. This will take time as well as diplomacy on the part

TABLE 17-2   *The Body Shape Questionnaire*

We would like to know how you have been feeling about your appearance over the PAST FOUR WEEKS. Please read the questions and circle the appropriate number to the right. Please answer all the questions.

OVER THE PAST FOUR WEEKS:	NEVER	RARELY	SOMETIMES	OFTEN	VERY OFTEN	ALWAYS
1. Has feeling bored made you brood about your shape?	1	2	3	4	5	6
2. Have you ever been so worried about your shape that you have been feeling you ought to diet?	1	2	3	4	5	6
3. Have you ever thought that your thighs, hips, or bottom is too large for the rest of you?	1	2	3	4	5	6
4. Have you ever been afraid that you might become fat (or fatter)?	1	2	3	4	5	6
5. Have you ever worried about your flesh not being firm enough?	1	2	3	4	5	6
6. Has feeling full (e.g., after eating a large meal) made you feel fat?	1	2	3	4	5	6
7. Have you ever felt so bad about your shape that you have cried?	1	2	3	4	5	6
8. Have you avoided running because your flesh might wobble?	1	2	3	4	5	6
9. Has being with thin women made you feel self-conscious about your shape?	1	2	3	4	5	6

Table continued on following page

TABLE 17–2 *The Body Shape Questionnaire (Continued)*

We would like to know how you have been feeling about your appearance over the PAST FOUR WEEKS. Please read the questions and circle the appropriate number to the right. Please answer all the questions.

OVER THE PAST FOUR WEEKS:	NEVER	RARELY	SOMETIMES	OFTEN	VERY OFTEN	ALWAYS
10. Have you worried about thighs spreading out when sitting down?	1	2	3	4	5	6
11. Has eating even a small amount of food made you feel fat?	1	2	3	4	5	6
12. Have you noticed the shape of other women and felt that your own shape compared unfavorably?	1	2	3	4	5	6
13. Has thinking about your shape interfered with your ability to concentrate (e.g., while watching TV, reading, listening to conversation)?	1	2	3	4	5	6
14. Has being naked, such as when taking a bath, made you feel fat?	1	2	3	4	5	6
15. Have you avoided wearing clothes which make you particularly aware of the shape of your body?	1	2	3	4	5	6
16. Have you ever imagined cutting off fleshy areas of your body?	1	2	3	4	5	6
17. Has eating sweets, cakes, or other high-calorie food made you feel fat?	1	2	3	4	5	6
18. Have you not gone out to social occasions (e.g., parties) because you have felt bad about your shape?	1	2	3	4	5	6
19. Have you felt excessively large and rounded?	1	2	3	4	5	6
20. Have you felt ashamed of your body?	1	2	3	4	5	6
21. Has worry about your shape made you diet?	1	2	3	4	5	6
22. Have you felt the happiest about your shape when your stomach has been empty?	1	2	3	4	5	6
23. Have you thought that you are the shape you are because of lack of self-control?	1	2	3	4	5	6
24. Have you worried about other people seeing rolls of flesh around your waist and stomach?	1	2	3	4	5	6
25. Have you felt that it is not fair that other women are thinner than you?	1	2	3	4	5	6
26. Have you vomited in order to feel thinner?	1	2	3	4	5	6
27. When in company, have you worried about taking up too much room (e.g., sitting on a sofa or a bus seat)?	1	2	3	4	5	6
28. Have you worried about your flesh being dumpy?	1	2	3	4	5	6
29. Has seeing your reflection (e.g., in a mirror or shop window) made you feel bad about your shape?	1	2	3	4	5	6
30. Have you pinched areas of your body to see how much fat there is?	1	2	3	4	5	6
31. Have you avoided situations where people could see your body (e.g., communal changing rooms or swimming baths)?	1	2	3	4	5	6
32. Have you taken laxatives to feel thinner?	1	2	3	4	5	6
33. Have you been particularly self-conscious about your shape when in the company of other people?	1	2	3	4	5	6
34. Has worry about your shape made you feel you ought to exercise?	1	2	3	4	5	6

From Cooper, P. J., Cooper, Z., Fairburn, C. G., and Taylor, M. J. (1987). The Development and Validation of the Body Shape Questionnaire. *International Journal of Eating Disorders,* 6(4):485–494. Copyright © 1987 John Wiley & Sons. Reprinted with permission of John Wiley & Sons, Inc.

of the nurse. Establishing and maintaining a therapeutic alliance are the bases for ongoing treatment.

In clients who have been sexually abused or who have otherwise been the victim of boundary violations, it is critical that the nurse and other health care workers maintain and respect clear boundaries (APA 2000b).

Figure 17–1 identifies the DSM-IV-TR criteria for anorexia nervosa, bulimia nervosa, and eating disorders not otherwise specified (NOS).

DSM-IV-TR CRITERIA FOR EATING DISORDERS

ANOREXIA NERVOSA

A. Refusal to maintain body weight at or above a minimally normal weight for age and height, e.g., weight loss leading to maintenance of body weight less than 85% of that expected, or failure to make expected weight gain during period of growth, leading to body weight less than 85% of that expected.

B. Intense fear of gaining weight or becoming fat, even though underweight.

C. Disturbance in the way in which one's body weight or shape is experienced, undue influence of body weight or shape on self-evaluation, or denial of the seriousness of the current low body weight.

D. In females, postmenarcheal amenorrhea, i.e., the absence of at least three consecutive menstrual cycles. (A woman is considered to have amenorrhea if her periods occur only after hormone, e.g., estrogen administration.)

Specify type:

Binge eating/purging type: During the episode of anorexia nervosa, the person engages in recurrent episodes of binge eating or purging behaviors.

Restricting type: During the episode of anorexia nervosa, the person does *not* engage in recurrent episodes of binge eating or purging behaviors.

BULIMIA NERVOSA

A. Recurrent episodes of binge eating. An episode of binge eating is characterized by both of the following:

(1) Eating in a discrete period (e.g., within any 2-hour period) an amount of food that is definitely larger than most people would eat during a similar period and under similar circumstances.
(2) A sense of lack of control over eating during the episode (e.g., a feeling that one cannot stop eating or control what or how much one is eating).

B. Recurrent inappropriate compensatory behavior to prevent weight gain such as self-induced vomiting; misuse of laxatives, diuretics, enemas, or other medications; fasting; or excessive exercise.

C. The binge eating and inappropriate compensatory behavior both occur on average at least twice a week for 3 months.

D. Self-evaluation is unduly influenced by body shape and weight.

E. The disturbance does not occur exclusively during episodes of anorexia nervosa.

Specify type:

Purging type: During the current episode of bulimia nervosa, the person has regularly engaged in self-induced vomiting or the misuse of laxatives, diuretics, or enemas.

Nonpurging type: During the current episode of bulimia nervosa, the person has used other inappropriate compensatory behaviors such as fasting or excessive exercise, but has not regularly engaged in self-induced vomiting or the misuse of laxatives, diuretics, or enemas.

EATING DISORDER NOT OTHERWISE SPECIFIED (NOS)

The eating disorder not otherwise specified category is for disorders of eating that do not meet the criteria for any specific eating disorder. Examples include:

1. For females, all the criteria for anorexia nervosa are met except that the individual has regular menses.

2. All the criteria for anorexia nervosa are met except that despite significant weight loss, the individual's current weight is in the normal range.

3. All the criteria for bulimia nervosa are met except that the binge eating and inappropriate compensatory mechanisms occur at a frequency of less than twice a week or a duration of less than 3 months.

4. The regular use of inappropriate compensatory behavior by an individual of normal body weight after eating small amounts of food (i.e., self-induced vomiting after the consumption of two cookies).

5. Repeatedly chewing and spitting out, but not swallowing, large amounts of food.

6. Binge eating disorder: recurrent episodes of binge eating in the absence of the regular use of inappropriate compensatory behaviors characteristic of bulimia nervosa.

Figure 17–1 DSM-IV-TR criteria for eating disorders. (Adapted from American Psychiatric Association [2000] *Diagnostic and statistical manual of mental disorders* (4th ed, text revision), (DSM-IV-TR). Washington, DC: American Psychiatric Association. Copyright 2000, American Psychiatric Association.)

Anorexia Nervosa

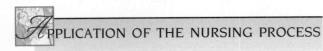

APPLICATION OF THE NURSING PROCESS

ASSESSMENT

Overall Assessment

Anorectic individuals often enter the health care system by being admitted to an intensive care unit with electrolyte imbalance. This condition may be due to the fact that the restrictive anorectic subtype is receding in incidence, and the purging subtype is becoming more common.

The nurse assessing the anorectic client observes a severely underweight male or female who may have fine, downy hair growth on the face and back (lanugo) with mottled, cool skin of the extremities, and low blood pressure, pulse, and temperature readings, consistent with a malnourished, dehydrated state. Refer to Table 17–1 for the signs and symptoms of anorexia and bulimia.

Vignette

■ *On admission to an eating disorder unit for inpatient treatment of anorexia nervosa, Tina, a 16-year-old young woman at 60% of ideal body weight, appears cachectic. She presents with a fine lanugo over most of her body and prominent parotid glands. She is further assessed to be hypotensive (86/50 mm Hg) and dehydrated. Additionally, she has a low serum potassium level and dysrhythmias that appear on an electrocardiogram. A decision is made to transfer her to the intensive care unit until she is medically stabilized. As an intravenous catheter is inserted, her severe weight phobia and fear of fat are underscored when she cries, "There's not going to be sugar in the IV?" The nurse responds, "I hear how frightened you are. We need to do what's necessary to get you past this crisis."*

As with any comprehensive psychiatric nursing assessment, a complete evaluation of biopsychosocial function is mandatory. The areas to be covered include the client's perception of the problem, the eating habits and history of dieting, the methods used to achieve control (restricting, purging, exercising), the value attached to a specific shape and weight, the client's interpersonal and social functioning, and an assessment of mental status with psychological and physiological parameters (Fairburn and Cooper 1989).

Self-Assessment

The nurse caring for the anorectic client may find it difficult to appreciate the compelling force of the illness, regarding it as trivial especially as compared to a diagnosis of schizophrenia. Because the client "chooses" to engage in behaviors that put her health at risk, nurses may find themselves blaming the client for bringing on her problems, especially as the client attempts to control the treatment. In an effort to motivate the client and take advantage of the decision to seek help and be healthier, the nurse may find encouragement is crossing the line towards authoritarianism and a parental role. As the nurse struggles to build a therapeutic alliance and be empathic, the client's terror at gaining weight and resistance to nursing interventions may engender significant frustration. Nurses must guard against any tendency to be coercive in their approach and be aware that one of the primary goals of treatment—weight gain—is the very thing the client fears. Frequent acknowledgement of how difficult it is for the client and of the constant struggle that so characterizes the treatment will help during times of extreme resistance.

Assessment Guidelines

ASSESSMENT GUIDELINES: ANOREXIA NERVOSA

Determine if:
1. The client has a medical or psychiatric situation that warrants hospitalization (see Box 17–1).
2. The family has information about the disease and knows where to get support.
3. The client is amenable to attending, or compliant with appropriate therapeutic modalities.
4. Family counseling has been offered to the family or individual family members for support, or to target a family or individual family member's problem.
5. A thorough physical examination with appropriate blood work has been done.
6. Other medical conditions have been ruled out.
7. The family and client need further teaching or information regarding client's treatment plan (e.g., psychopharmacological interventions, behavioral therapy, cognitive therapy, family therapy, individual psychotherapy). If the client is a candidate for partial hospitalization, can the family/client discuss those functions?
8. The client and family desire a support group; if yes, provide referrals.

NURSING DIAGNOSIS

Imbalanced nutrition: less than body requirements is usually the most compelling nursing diagnosis initially for individuals with anorexia. Altered nutrition: less than body requirements generates further nursing diagnoses, for example, **Decreased cardiac output, Risk for injury (electrolyte imbalance)**, and **Risk for imbalanced fluid volume**, which would have first priority when problems are addressed. Other nursing diagnoses include **Disturbed body image, Anxiety, Chronic low self-esteem, Deficient knowledge, Ineffective coping, Powerlessness**, and **Hopelessness**.

OUTCOME CRITERIA

In order to evaluate the effectiveness of treatment, outcome criteria are established to measure treatment results. The objectives that guide the treatment plan lead to the expected outcomes. Some common outcome criteria for clients with anorexia nervosa follow.

The individual will

- Normalize eating patterns, as evidenced by eating 75% of three meals/day plus two snacks
- Achieve 85% to 90% of ideal body weight
- Be free of physical complications
- Demonstrate healthy eating habits
- Demonstrate improved self-acceptance, as evidenced by both verbal and behavioral data
- Address maladaptive beliefs, thoughts, and activities related to the eating disorder
- Participate in treatment of associated psychiatric symptoms (defects in mood, self-esteem)
- Demonstrate behaviors and interests that are appropriate to age
- Participate in long-term treatment to prevent relapse

PLANNING

The focus of the therapeutic interventions is guided by the intensity of the disordered eating and the impact on the life of the anorectic person. Although a range of treatment modalities from psychoanalysis to nutrition counseling has been applied to anorexia nervosa, cognitive therapy has shown improved outcomes (Fairburn and Cooper 1989).

The type of treatment for anorexia nervosa is partly determined by the severity of the weight loss. Anorectic individuals whose weight is below 75% of ideal body weight are considered to be medically unstable (Hsu 1990). Admission to an inpatient unit may be necessary to reverse the downward spiral of dietary restriction and weight loss. Indeed, anorexia nervosa is a chronic illness requiring both inpatient and outpatient management, with therapeutic interventions that include individual, group, and family therapy and psychopharmacological therapy during different phases of the illness. The nature of the treatment is determined both by the intensity of the symptoms, which may vary over time, and the experienced disruption of one's life. The mainstay of treatment, however, is outpatient therapy.

In the current health care climate, reimbursement for inpatient treatment is limited. Brief hospitalization can address only acute complications, such as electrolyte imbalance, dysrhythmias, limited weight restoration, and acute psychiatric symptoms.

A potentially catastrophic treatment complication is the **refeeding syndrome**, in which the demands that a replenished circulatory system places on a nutritionally depleted cardiac mass result in cardiovascular collapse (Mehler 1996). Another acute symptom targeted on the acute inpatient unit is depression. The more persistent symptoms that attend undernutrition and fear of weight gain with distorted body image are more likely to be addressed on an outpatient basis.

General inpatient psychiatric units, although providing excellent care for most psychiatric disorders, are not structured to address the requirements of acute treatment of anorectic clients in the weight-restoration phase. Ideally, before the client is discharged from an acute care setting, a comprehensive outpatient treatment plan is arranged.

INTERVENTION

Acute Interventions

Typically, when the client with an eating disorder is admitted to the inpatient psychiatric facility, it is due to a crisis state. The nurse has a challenging task to establish trust and monitor the eating pattern, which is the client's coping strategy for deep-seated feelings. This is especially true when the client's hospital stay is usually of short duration (O'Meara 2000).

MILIEU THERAPY

Clients who are admitted to an inpatient unit designed to treat eating disorders participate in a treatment program that consists of an interdisciplinary team and a combination of therapeutic modalities. These modalities are designed to normalize eating patterns and to begin to address the issues raised by the illness. The milieu of an eating disorder unit is purposefully organized to assist the client to establish more adaptive behavioral patterns, including normalization of eating. The highly structured milieu includes precise meal times, adherence to the selected menu, observation during and after meals, and regularly scheduled weighings. Close monitoring of clients includes all trips to the bathroom after eating to ensure there is no self-induced vomiting. The client may also need monitoring on bathroom trips after visitors and any hospital pass. The latter is to ensure that the client has not had access to, and ingested, any laxatives or diuretics (O'Meara 2000). Groups are led by nurses and other interdisciplinary team members and are tailored to issues of clients with eating disorders. Client privileges are correlated with weight gain and treatment plan compliance.

In the current climate of health care reform, with managed care and critical pathways that define treatment options, acute treatment of anorexia nervosa now occurs increasingly in an outpatient setting. As stated earlier, anorexia nervosa requires both inpatient and outpatient management composed of various therapeutic interventions, including individual, group, and family therapy and psychopharmacological therapy at different phases of the illness. The mainstay of treatment, however, has been outpatient therapy.

COMMUNICATION GUIDELINES

The nurse on an inpatient unit may have multiple roles: primary nurse, group leader, and psychotherapist (advanced practice). Interventions include teaching, counseling, and psychotherapeutic functions. The initial focus depends on the results of a comprehensive assessment. Any acute psychiatric symptoms, such as suicidal ideation, must be immediately addressed. At the same time, the anorectic client begins a weight-restoration program that allows for incremental weight gain. Based on height, a treatment goal is set at 90% of ideal body weight, the weight at which most women are able to menstruate.

Establishing a therapeutic alliance with the anorectic client is difficult because the compelling force of the illness runs counter to therapeutic interventions. As clients begin to refeed, they ideally begin to participate in the milieu therapy, attending individual psychotherapy and group therapy sessions as well as nutritional counseling. The cognitive distortions perpetuate the illness and must be confronted consistently by all members of the interdisciplinary team. While the eating behavior is targeted, the underlying emotions of anxiety, dysphoria, and low self-esteem and the feelings of lack of control are also addressed.

Vignette

■ In a multifamily group on an inpatient unit, Mrs. Demi (who last saw her anorectic daughter before she had gained 40 pounds) is asked by the group leader how she regards her daughter Lila. Mrs. Demi replies, "She looks healthy." Her daughter responds with an angry, sullen look. She ultimately verbalizes that comments about her "healthy" appearance are experienced as "You look fat." The group leader points out that it is interesting that Lila equates "health" with "fat." In the multifamily group, there is a commonly expressed view that the illness "is not about weight," but that thinness conferred a feeling of being special, and being at a normal weight (healthy) meant that special status was lost.

HEALTH TEACHING

Self-care activities are an important part of the treatment plan. These activities include learning more constructive coping skills, improving social skills, and developing problem-solving and decision-making skills. The skills become the focus of both therapy sessions and supervised food shopping trips. As the client approaches the goal weight, he or she is encouraged to expand the repertoire to include eating out in a restaurant, preparing a meal, and eating forbidden foods. The following vignette exemplifies some of the issues that may complicate discharge.

Vignette

■ Alice, a 35-year-old woman with a long history of refractoriness to treatment for anorexia, wants to leave the hospital on reaching 75% of her ideal body weight (regarded as the minimum weight at which an individual may be considered medically stable). Discharge is feasible for this client only if her mother agrees to take Alice home. Initially, the mother allied herself with the treatment team and refused to go along with Alice's decision to leave at this low weight. The mother relents when Alice becomes threatening and angry, saying, "I won't love you anymore." Although the mother fears for Alice's life, the perceived emotional abandonment and separation from her seems more real and threatening.

The hastily arranged discharge plan for outpatient follow-up includes a counseling referral for this mother. Discharge planning is a critical component in treatment and, as the aforementioned example demonstrates, can be complex. Often, family members benefit from counseling. The discharge planning process must address living arrangements, school, and work, as well as feasibility of an independent financial status, applications for state/federal program assistance (if needed), and follow-up outpatient treatment.

PSYCHOTHERAPY

Whether in a partial hospitalization program, community mental health center, psychiatric home care program, or the more traditional outpatient treatment consisting of individual, group, or family therapy, the goals of treatment remain the same: weight restoration with normalization of eating habits and beginning treatment of psychological, interpersonal, and social issues that are integral to the experience of the client. In the acute, weight-restoration phase, the focus of the therapeutic interventions is almost wholly determined by the client's medically unstable weight. Attention to the underlying psychodynamic conflict is not feasible at this stage; a cognitive-behavioral approach to treatment is required at this time. Box 17–3 identifies some common types of cognitive distortions held by people with eating disorders.

Like the general psychiatric inpatient units, many existing day programs and partial hospitalization programs are not set up to care for the anorectic client in the weight-restoration phase. However, outpatient partial hospitalization programs designed to treat eating disorders are structured to achieve outcomes comparable with those of inpatient eating disorder units. Formerly, many therapists contracted with anorectic clients regarding the terms of treatment; outpatient treatment could continue only if the client maintained an agreed-on weight. If weight loss below the goal occurred, other treatment arrangements had to be made until the client returned to the goal weight. The highly structured approach to clients whose weight is below 75% of ideal body weight is necessary, even for therapists who are psychodynamically oriented. Techniques such as assisting the client with a daily meal plan, reviewing a journal of meals and dietary intake maintained by the client, and providing for weighing weekly (ideally 2 to 3 times a week) are essential if the client is to reach a medically stable weight.

One alternative to the traditional acute treatment of anorexia nervosa is being developed. The alternative is a psychiatric home care program for clients who meet the criteria for inpatient admission (with the exception of acute suicidal risk). Critical pathways for clients with eating disorders are being developed with outcomes that compare with those of a 3-month hospitalization. A comprehensive, multidisciplinary treatment approach includes a complete biopsychosocial assessment with laboratory and diagnostic tests. The psychiatric home care nurse/clinical specialist both coordinates and provides care. This is a unique role for the psychiatric nurse that allows for a wide range of interventions. Behavioral

Box 17–3 *Cognitive Distortions*

Overgeneralization: A single event affects unrelated situations.

■ "He didn't ask me out. It must be because I'm fat."
■ "I was happy when I wore a size 6. I must get back to that weight."

All-or-nothing thinking: Absolute, extreme reasoning in mutually exclusive terms of black or white, good or bad.

■ "If I have one popsicle, I must eat five."
■ "If I allow myself to gain weight, I'll blow up like a balloon."

Catastrophizing: Magnifying the consequences of an event.

■ "If I gain weight, my weekend will be ruined."
■ "When people say I look better, I know they think I'm fat."

Personalization: Overinterpretation of events as having personal significance.

■ "I know everybody is watching me eat."
■ "I think people won't like me unless I'm thin."

Emotional reasoning: Subjective emotions determine reality.

■ "I know I'm fat because I feel fat."
■ "When I'm thin, I feel powerful."

Adapted from Garner, D., and Bemis, K. (1982). A cognitive-behavioral approach to anorexia nervosa. *Cognitive Therapy and Research, 6*:123–150.

strategies include psychoeducation about the eating disorder, meal planning, relaxation techniques, and cognitive-behavioral therapy to address the distorted perceptions and values regarding eating, body shape, and weight. The psychiatric home care nurse plans the frequency and duration of the home visits, with the expected objectives to be accomplished by the client at predicted intervals. Issues of food preparation, including shopping for food, may be arranged for by a family member or a home health attendant. The psychiatric home care nurse must be innovative in the approach to the client with an eating disorder. Such nontraditional nursing interventions as eating a meal and shopping for food with the client are crucial (Rosedale 1996).

Long-Term Treatment

THERAPY

Clients with a diagnosis of anorexia nervosa are at various stages of recovery according to the percentage of ideal body weight that has been achieved, the extent to which self-worth is defined by shape and weight, and the amount of disruption of their personal life. Clinical specialists and nurse practitioners in an advanced-practice model are providers of long-term follow-up treatment of anorectic clients, often in collaboration with other mental health professionals. Long-term treatment includes a variety of modalities to ensure a successful outcome (e.g., individual therapy, family therapy, couples therapy, and psychopharmacological treatment) (APA 2000b).

Anorexia nervosa is a disease with deep psychopathological features and individuals require support throughout recovery. Therefore, psychotherapeutic interventions require from one year to 5 or 6 years (Strober et al. 1997).

In long-term treatment, the underlying issues affecting the client's illness and personal goals can be addressed. In addition to weight maintenance, the overriding goal for the client is to achieve a sense of self-worth and self-acceptance that is not exclusively based on appearance. Clients need assistance to find satisfaction in other areas of their lives (e.g., interpersonal, social, vocational). The combination of individual, group, and family therapy (especially for the younger client) provides the anorectic client with the greatest chance for a successful outcome.

Clients with anorexia nervosa have failed to achieve a sense of independence. Some clients report that the disordered eating behavior is a way to obtain nurturance and to cope with loneliness. They may even admit that these behaviors were unsuccessful in meeting those needs. Families often report feeling powerless in the face of behavior that is mystifying. Clients are often unable to experience compliments as supportive and therefore are unable to internalize the support. They often seek attention from others but feel scrutinized when they receive it. Clients want their families to care for and about them, but are afraid that they do not care. Reasonable expressions of caring are not experienced as such. When others do respond in an attempt to show love and support, it is not internalized as a good feeling. The following three vignettes demonstrate this phenomenon.

Vignette

■ In a family session, a grandmother says to Gina (her 18-year-old anorectic granddaughter), "Gina, you're young, you're smart, you're beautiful. You can do anything." When the client does not react to the statement by feeling praised, the grandmother looks bewildered. After exploring what Gina is feeling, it becomes clear that such statements result in her feeling guilty and more ineffectual since she does not perceive herself as either beautiful or smart but feels that she should be acting both smart and beautiful.

Vignette

■ In a multifamily group setting, Terri's mother tells a poignant story of concern for her anorectic daughter. She describes lying awake at night, afraid that in the morning she would find her daughter dead. Although it seems to the group that this expressed sentiment is genuine, the daughter appears to be unmoved. It is later pointed out by the group and the group leader that although Terri often verbalizes that her mother does not care, she is actually unable to receive expressions of concern for her health as caring.

Often, families and significant others are seeking a way to communicate with the anorectic client. Much miscommunication occurs between the client and others. This confusion of thoughts and feelings leads to the client's inability to validate perceptions. Consequently, families experience the tension of saying or doing the wrong thing and then feeling responsible if a setback occurs. Psychiatric nurse clinicians have an important role in assisting families and significant others to develop strategies for improved communication and to search for ways to be comfortably supportive to the client.

The following vignette demonstrates a young anorectic client's awareness of how she has been communicating and a breakthrough in her treatment.

Vignette

■ Harriet, an anorectic client, has made significant strides in her treatment and comes to recognize that her emotions are being expressed through her eating behaviors. In the presence of her family, she says, "It's up to me. Only I can do it." This is said with fierce pride. The issue of control, which is commonly expressed in clients with eating disorders, is highlighted in this exchange. Harriet and other clients like her frequently find it difficult to ask for appropriate help.

PSYCHOPHARMACOLOGY

As with most other psychiatric diagnoses, psychopharmacological treatment has become a common component of the successful treatment of eating disorders. The selective serotonin reuptake inhibitors (SSRIs), such as fluoxetine (Prozac), are promising pharmacological agents that have been shown to improve the rate of weight gain and reduce the occurrence of relapse in anorexia nervosa (Walsh and Devlin 1995; Peterson and Mitchell 1999). However, Ferguson and colleagues (1999) found that fluoxetine had no effect on the symptomatology of underweight anorectic clients. Olanzapine (Zyprexa) has been reported to decrease agitation and resistance to treatment along with improving weight gain (La Via et al. 2000).

EVALUATION

The process of evaluation is ongoing, and short-term and intermediate goals are revised as necessary to achieve the treatment outcomes established. These goals are the daily guides to reaching successful outcomes and must be continually re-evaluated for their appropriateness.

The long-term outcome of anorexia nervosa is protracted in terms of symptom recovery with a less favorable outcome compared to bulimia nervosa or binge eating disorder (Fichter and Quadflieg 1999).

Essentially, the outcomes are:
Has the client:

- Regained a healthy weight?
- Remained free of physical complications?
- Substituted healthy eating habits?
- Described a more realistic perception of body size and shape in relation to height and body type?
- Demonstrated commitment to long-term treatment to prevent relapses?
- Refrained from the excessive use of exercise for the sole purpose of losing weight?

See Case Study 17–1 and Nursing Care Plan 17–1 later in chapter.

Bulimia Nervosa

Bulimia as a diagnosis first entered the DSM-III in 1980, but without purging or inappropriate compensatory behaviors as a criterion. The diagnosis became bulimia nervosa with the addition of the preceding criterion in 1987. Currently, in DSM-IV-TR (APA 2000a), it is further subtyped as purging or nonpurging type (see Fig. 17–1).

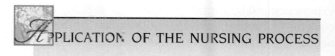

APPLICATION OF THE NURSING PROCESS

ASSESSMENT

Overall Assessment

Clients with bulimia nervosa may not initially appear to be physically or emotionally ill. They are often at or slightly above or below ideal body weight. However, as the assessment continues and the nurse makes further observations, the physical and emotional problems of the client become apparent. On inspection, the client demonstrates enlargement of the parotid glands with dental erosion and caries if the client has been inducing vomiting. The history disclosed may be one of difficulties with impulse control. Family relationships may be chaotic and reflect a lack of nurturing (Halmi 1999). Their lives may reflect chaotic and troublesome interpersonal relationships as well. Behaviors are often marked by impulsivity and compulsivity. Impulsive stealing is not uncommon (e.g., food, clothing, jewelry) (Halmi 1999). Refer back to Table 17–1 for a comparison of the characteristics of bulimia with anorexia nervosa.

Vignette

- *Jenny is being admitted to an inpatient eating disorder unit. During the initial assessment, the nurse wonders if Jenny is actually in need of hospitalization. The nurse is struck by how well the client presents, appearing healthy looking, well dressed, and articulate. As Jenny continues to relate her history, she tells of restricting her intake all day until early evening, when she buys her food and begins to binge as she is shopping. She arrives home and immediately induces vomiting. For the remainder of the evening and into the early morning hours, she "zones out" while watching television and binge eating. Periodically, she goes to the bathroom to vomit. She does this about 15 times during the evening. The nurse admitting Jenny to the unit reminds her of the goals of the hospitalization, including interrupting the binge/purge cycle and normalizing eating. The nurse further explains to Jenny that she has the support of the eating disorder treatment team and the milieu of the unit to assist her toward recovery.*

Self-Assessment

In working with the bulimic client, the nurse needs to be aware that the client is very sensitive to others' perceptions of her illness. The client may be experiencing significant shame and feeling out of control. In building a therapeutic alliance, the nurse needs to empathize with the bulimic's feelings of low self-esteem, unworthiness, and dysphoria. The nurse may feel the client is not being honest when she does not report actively bingeing or purging or that the client is being manipulative. An accepting, nonjudgmental approach along with a comprehensive understanding of the bulimic's subjective experience will help to build trust.

Assessment Guidelines

> ### ASSESSMENT GUIDELINES: BULIMIA NERVOSA
>
> 1. Medical stabilization is the first priority. Problems resulting from purging are disruptions in electrolyte and fluid balance and cardiac function. Therefore, a thorough medical examination is vital.
> 2. Medical evaluation usually includes a thorough physical, as well as pertinent lab values:
>
>   - Electrolytes
>   - Glucose
>   - Thyroid function tests
>   - Neuroimaging of pituitary
>   - Complete blood count
>   - ECG
>
> 3. Psychiatric evaluation is advised because treatment of psychiatric comorbidity is important to outcome.

NURSING DIAGNOSIS

The assessment of the client with bulimia nervosa yields nursing diagnoses that result from the disordered eating and weight control behaviors. Problems resulting from purging are a first priority because electrolyte and fluid balance and cardiac function are affected. Common nursing diagnoses include **Decreased cardiac output, Risk for injury (electrolyte imbalance), Disturbed body image, Powerlessness, Chronic low self-esteem, Anxiety,** and **Ineffective coping (substance abuse, impulsive responses to problems).**

OUTCOME CRITERIA

The effectiveness of treatment interventions is evaluated against established outcome criteria. Some common outcomes for clients with bulimia follow:
The client will:

- Refrain from binge-purge behaviors
- Demonstrate new skills for managing stress/anxiety/shame (triggers to binge-purge behaviors)
- Obtain and maintain normal electrolyte imbalance
- Be free of self-directed harm
- Express feelings in a non–food-related way
- Verbalize desire to participate in ongoing treatment
- State she feels good about herself and about who she is as a person

PLANNING

The criteria for inpatient admission of a client with bulimia nervosa are included in the criteria for inpatient admission of a client with an eating disorder (see Box 17–2). Like the client with anorexia nervosa, the client with bulimia may be treated for life-threatening complications (i.e., gastric rupture [rare], electrolyte imbalance, cardiac dysrhythmias) in an acute care unit of a hospital. If the client is admitted to a general inpatient psychiatric unit for acute suicidal risk, again only the acute psychiatric manifestations are addressed short term.

Vignette

- *Iris weighs 85% of her ideal body weight. She has a history of diuretic abuse, and she became very edematous when she stopped their use and entered treatment. Iris could not tolerate the weight gain and the accompanying edema, despite education about the edema's being related to the use of diuretics and thus transient, and that it would resolve after normalization of eating habits and discontinuation of the diuretics. She restarted the diuretics, perpetuating the cycle of fluid retention and the risk of kidney damage. The nurse empathizes with her inability to tolerate the feelings of anxiety and dread that the client experiences because of her markedly swollen extremities.*

When planning care, the nurse is aware that, ideally, clients who are this severely ill are referred to an inpatient eating disorder unit for comprehensive treatment of their illness. The cognitive-behavioral model of treatment has been shown to be highly effective and can serve as the cornerstone of the therapeutic approach to the client. Inpatient units designed to treat eating disorders are especially structured to interrupt the cycle of binge eating and purging and to normalize eating habits. Therapy is begun to examine the underlying conflicts and the distorted perceptions of shape and weight that sustain the illness. Evaluation for treatment of comorbid disorders, such as major depression and sub-

RESEARCH FINDINGS

Bulimia and Abnormalities in Brain Serotonin

Objective

To determine the association between bulimia, impulsive, and depressive syndromes with abnormalities in brain serotonin mechanisms.

Method

Twenty-six bulimic women and 22 normal-eater women reported impulsive, affective, self-destructive, and bulimic symptoms, then give serial blood samples to measure (3H)-paroxetine binding in platelets and prolactin (PRL) responses following oral administration of meta-chlorophenyl-piperazine (m-CPP).

Results

Bulimia was associated with markedly reduced density of paroxetine-binding sites, modest blunt-ing of m-CPP stimulated PRL response, and greater nausea following administration of m-CPP. Biological variables did not co-vary with most psychopathological or eating-symptom indices. However, there were inverse associations (in bulimic women only) between scores indicating impulsivity and density of platelet 5-HT uptake sites.

Conclusion

There is a link between bulimia nervosa and altered 5-HT (serotonin) functioning and there may be a relatively symptom-specific association between impulsivity and reduced 5-HT reuptake.

Source: Steiger, H., Young, S. N., Kin, N. M., et al. (2001). Implications of impulsive and affective symptoms for serotonin function in bulimia nervosa. *Psychological Medicine*, 31(1): 85–95.

stance abuse, is also addressed (See Research Findings Box). In most cases of substance dependence, the treatment of the eating disorder must occur after the substance dependence is treated.

INTERVENTION

Acute Interventions

MILIEU THERAPY

The highly structured milieu of an inpatient eating disorder unit has as its primary goals the interruption of the binge/purge cycle and the prevention of the disordered eating behaviors. Interventions such as observation during and after meals to prevent purging, normalization of eating patterns, and appropriate exercise are integral elements of such a unit. The interdisciplinary team of the unit uses a comprehensive treatment approach to address the emotional and behavioral problems that arise when the client is no longer binge eating or purging. The underlying feelings have been masked by the disor-dered eating behaviors, and the interruption of the binge/purge pattern brings these psychodynamic issues to the fore.

PSYCHOTHERAPY

Central to the treatment approach of bulimia nervosa is the emphasis on educating clients and helping them avoid dieting and restricting of caloric intake, particularly for many hours, which sets up the response to binge eat and then compensate by purging or excessively exercising. While the client is attending individual, group, and family therapy sessions, it is hoped that the binge/purge cycle will be interrupted and the normalization of eating and meal planning can begin.

HEALTH TEACHING

The client is now ready to enter the second phase of treatment, in which there are carefully planned challenges to the client's newly developed skills. For instance, the client is expected to have a meal while "on pass" outside the hospital or to plan an overnight pass with meals at home. On return to the unit, the client shares the experience.

On discharge from the hospital, the client is referred for long-term care to solidify the goals that have been achieved and to treat both the attitudes and the perceptions that maintain the eating disorder and the psychodynamic issues that attend the illness.

Long-Term Treatment

THERAPY

Cognitive behavior therapy has been established as the most effective treatment for bulimia nervosa. Agras and colleagues (2000) developed outcome predictors for those best suited for cognitive behavior treatment. Reduction in purging by the sixth session predicted a successful outcome. Clients with bulimia nervosa, because of possible coexisting depression, substance abuse, and personality disorders, are often in various therapies. Although the specific eating-disordered behaviors may not be targeted specifically in some therapies, it is those very behaviors that are responsible for much of the client's emotional distress. It is imperative that irrational attitudes and perceptions of weight and shape be addressed. Therefore, restructuring faulty perceptions and helping individuals develop accepting attitudes towards themselves and their body is a primary focus of therapy. When the client does not indulge in these bulimic behaviors, issues of self-worth and interpersonal functioning become more prominent. The psychodynamic issues can be addressed by numerous psychotherapeutic approaches, but cognitive-behavioral therapy is most effective in the acute phase of bulimic behaviors. Compared with the food-restricting anorectic client, the client with bulimia nervosa often more readily establishes a therapeutic alliance with the advanced practice nurse because the eating-disordered behaviors are so ego-dystonic.

Vignette

■ *Patty, a 23-year-old client with a 6-year history of bulimia nervosa, struggles with issues of self-esteem. She expresses much guilt about "letting her father down" in the past by engaging in drinking alcohol excessively and binge eating and purging. She is determined that this time she is not going to fail at treatment. After her initial success in stopping the aforementioned behaviors, she says defiantly, "I'm doing this for me." Patty experiences her behavior as either pleasing or disappointing to others. She begins to realize that her feeling of self-worth is very much dependent on how others see her and that she needs to develop a better sense of herself.*

PSYCHOPHARMACOLOGY

tidepressant medication along with psychotherapy has been shown to bring about improvement in bulimic symptoms (Peterson and Mitchell 1999). The use of fluoxetine added to the cognitive-behavioral treatment added modestly to the treatment benefit (Walsh et al. 1997). According to a study by Goldstein and associates (1999), fluoxetine treatment reduced the number of binge eating and vomiting episodes in patients with and without comorbid depression.

EVALUATION

Evaluation of treatment effectiveness is ongoing, and goals are revised as necessary to reach the desired outcomes. See Case Study 17–2 and Nursing Care Plan 17–2 later in chapter.

Binge Eating Disorder (Obesity)

Binge eating disorder as a variant of compulsive overeating is presented here. Although considerable controversy exists over whether this proposed diagnosis constitutes a separate eating disorder, 20% to 30% of obese individuals seeking treatment report binge eating as a pattern of overeating (Marcus 1995). In the DSM-IV-TR appendix, research criteria are listed for further study of binge eating disorder (Fig. 17–2). Because there are no compensatory behaviors (purging, exercise) to attempt to control weight in this disorder, it is currently diagnosed as *eating disorder* not otherwise specified *(NOS)*. Wilfely and colleagues (2000) compared binge eating disorder to anorexia nervosa and bulimia nervosa, noting that patients with binge eating disorder had lower levels of self-restraint, had eating concerns similar to those anorectic clients but not as much as bulimic patients. Weight and shape concerns were similar to bulimic individuals and greater than anorectic clients. In a study comparing subthreshold binge eating disorder with binge eating disorder in a community sample, Striegel-Moore and colleagues (2000b) found no significant differences in the two eating disorder groups on measures of eating disorder psychopathology when adjusting for significant differences in weight.

Obese individuals in general are heavily stigmatized in our society and the myth is that all obesity

DSM-IV-TR CRITERIA FOR BINGE EATING DISORDER

Binge Eating Disorder (Compulsive Overeating)

A. Recurrent episodes of binge eating. An episode of binge eating is characterized by both of the following:
1. Eating, in a discrete period (e.g., within any 2-hour period), an amount of food that is definitely larger than most people would eat in a similar period under similar circumstances.
2. A sense of lack of control over eating during the episode (e.g., a feeling that one cannot stop eating or control what or how much one is eating).

B. The binge-eating episodes are associated with three (or more) of the following:
1. Eating much more rapidly than normal
2. Eating until feeling uncomfortably full
3. Eating large amounts of food when not feeling physically hungry
4. Eating alone because of being embarrassed by how much one is eating
5. Feeling disgusted with oneself, depressed, or very guilty after overeating

C. Marked distress regarding binge eating is present.

D. The binge eating occurs, on average, at least 2 days a week for 6 months.

Note: the method of determining frequency differs from that used for bulimia nervosa; future research should address whether the preferred method of setting a frequency threshold is counting the number of days on which binges occur or counting the number of episodes of binge eating.

E. The binge eating is not associated with the regular use of inappropriate compensatory behaviors (e.g., purging, fasting, excessive exercise) and does not occur exclusively during the course of anorexia nervosa or bulimia nervosa.

Figure 17–2 DSM-IV-TR criteria for binge eating disorder. (Adapted from American Psychiatric Association [2000]. *Diagnostic and statistical manual of mental disorders* (4th ed.), TR. Washington, DC: American Psychiatric Association. Copyright 2000 American Psychiatric Association.)

is a result of binge eating and gluttony of the individual. Research under way in obesity has implicated several metabolic and endocrine problems rather than binge eating and excessive nutritional intake as the cause of the problem (O'Meara 2000).

THERAPY

Cognitive-behavioral therapy (CBT) programs are at present the most effective and the most promising for individuals with binge eating disorders (Ricca et al. 2000).

The use of SSRIs in treating binge eating disorder has been studied. McElroy and associates (2000) found that sertraline reduced the frequency of binges and the overall severity of the illness. Devlin and colleagues (2000) added phentermine and fluoxetine to cognitive-behavioral therapy; however, patients regained significant weight after discontinuance of medication and found no advantage to the addition of medication.

In the United States, approximately 25% of the population is considered to be overweight (Williamson 1993), despite the national trend of attempting to live a healthier life style. The reasons for obesity are varied. The most appropriate treatment decisions consider the degree of overweight, associated illness, duration of being overweight, and heredity factors. The greater the above mentioned factors, the greater the need for professional intervention (Brownell and Wadden 1991). See Table 17–3 for matching classification of obesity with treatment.

In the World Health Organization's *ICD-10 Classification Of Mental And Behavioral Disorders*, overeating associated with other psychological disturbances, including obesity due to overeating as a reaction to a distressing event, is classified as an atypical eating disorder (World Health Organization 1992). However, obesity due to eating disturbances secondary to medical and psychiatric conditions is not classified as an eating disorder according to DSM-IV-TR criteria.

Overeating is frequently noted as a symptom of an affective disorder (i.e., atypical depression). Higher rates of affective and personality disorders were found among binge eaters (Marcus 1990). Binge eaters reported a history of major depression significantly more than non-binge eaters. They further reported that disordered eating occurred during negative mood states and that they experienced binge eating as soothing or serving the function of mood regulation. Although dieting is almost always an antecedent of binge eating in bulimia nervosa, in approximately 50% of a sample of obese binge eaters, no attempt to restrict dietary intake occurred (Marcus 1992).

An effective program for obese binge eaters must integrate modification of the disordered eating and the depressive symptoms with the ultimate goal of a more appropriate weight for the individual. Fairburn and associates (2000) found the course of binge eating disorder to be different from bulimia nervosa and with a better outcome. The overwhelming majority of women with binge eating disorder recover. Peterson and colleagues (2000) in their study found that the frequency of binge eating episodes prior to intervention was predictive of treatment outcome. See Case Study 17–3 and Nursing Care Plan 17–3 later in chapter

TABLE 17-3 *Conceptual Scheme for Selecting Treatment for Overweight Individuals*

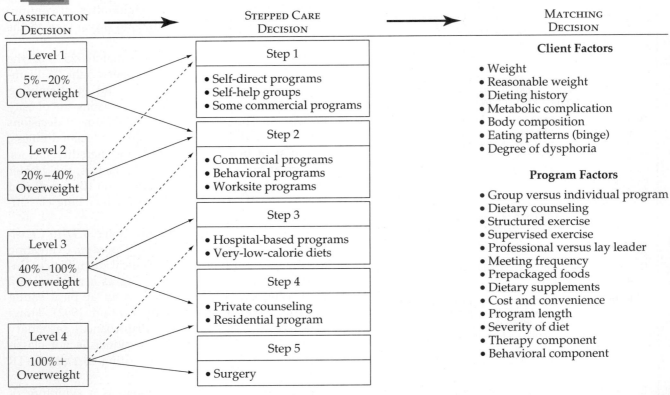

CLASSIFICATION DECISION	STEPPED CARE DECISION	MATCHING DECISION

CLASSIFICATION DECISION

Level 1 — 5%–20% Overweight

Level 2 — 20%–40% Overweight

Level 3 — 40%–100% Overweight

Level 4 — 100%+ Overweight

STEPPED CARE DECISION

Step 1
- Self-direct programs
- Self-help groups
- Some commercial programs

Step 2
- Commercial programs
- Behavioral programs
- Worksite programs

Step 3
- Hospital-based programs
- Very-low-calorie diets

Step 4
- Private counseling
- Residential program

Step 5
- Surgery

MATCHING DECISION

Client Factors
- Weight
- Reasonable weight
- Dieting history
- Metabolic complication
- Body composition
- Eating patterns (binge)
- Degree of dysphoria

Program Factors
- Group versus individual program
- Dietary counseling
- Structured exercise
- Supervised exercise
- Professional versus lay leader
- Meeting frequency
- Prepackaged foods
- Dietary supplements
- Cost and convenience
- Program length
- Severity of diet
- Therapy component
- Behavioral component

Adapted from Brownell, K. D., and Wadden, D. A. (1991). The heterogeneity of obesity. Fitting treatments to individuals. *Behavior Therapy*, 22:163–177. © 1991 by Association of Behavior Therapy. Reprinted by permission of the publisher.

Visit the **Evolve** website at
http://evolve.elsevier.com/Varcarolis
for more Case Studies.

CASE STUDY 17-1   A Client with Anorexia Nervosa

Cindy is a 20-year-old woman who is brought to the inpatient eating disorder unit of a psychiatric research hospital by two older brothers, who support her on either side. She is profoundly weak, holding her head up with her hands.

ASSESSMENT

Cindy gives a history of being a good student in elementary and high school. She delayed plans to attend college to care for her mother, who was very ill. The family further reports that Cindy began to attend exclusively to her mother and the household, totally neglecting herself and becoming extremely perfectionistic about her responsibilities. Although she had always been of normal weight with no prior eating problems, she began to restrict her food intake while spending an inordinate amount of time planning and preparing meals for others in the household. She rarely ate meals with the family and became increasingly socially isolated as she grew thinner.

On admission to the unit, her height and weight are taken: At 62 inches (5′2″) and 58 pounds, her weight is 50% of her

CASE STUDY 17-1   A Client with Anorexia Nervosa *(Continued)*

ideal body weight. A complete physical examination reveals her to be extremely hypotensive (74/50 mm Hg), bradycardic (54 beats/min), and anemic (hemoglobin, 9 g/dL). Other laboratory test results are abnormal as well, reflecting her extreme malnutrition. She is immediately placed on therapeutic bed rest to conserve energy and calories, and an intravenous line is started to increase her hydration.

Cindy presents her problem as being one of extreme fatigue and needing to have more energy. She does not acknowledge that her extreme fasting has created the illness. When informed that the treatment would commence with prescription of a dietary supplement to provide nutrition, she does not object.

As Cindy slowly begins to furnish a history of her eating pattern, she states that more recently she would begin the day with some water and half a piece of toast. During the day, she might have a piece of fruit. Her only "meal" is dinner, which consists of a very small quantity of turkey breast and carrots. She is ultimately unable to eat with others and avoids mealtimes. She eats in isolation. Her thoughts throughout the day are preoccupied with food. She maintains her extremely low weight both by exercising and restricting food intake. Ultimately, she is too lethargic to exercise and maintains her extremely low weight entirely by restricting her food intake. She denies

having a history of binge eating or purging. Cindy does not acknowledge that she is too thin, insisting instead that she is too fatigued. She speaks about examining her body daily for evidence of fat. When she sits down, she does not like her thighs to touch. Cindy's affect is constricted, and she reports that her mood is depressed. She denies having suicidal thoughts. She is oriented in all spheres, with good attention and memory. Her thinking is concrete when explaining a proverb.

This is Cindy's first hospitalization and her first treatment for anorexia nervosa. She denies having a history of substance abuse or depression before her weight loss. She reports having no history of physical or sexual abuse.

Cindy is the youngest of 12 children, with a 10-year difference between her and her next oldest sibling. Cindy's father died 2 years ago. Around that time, her 68-year-old mother became very ill. Cindy considers herself an only child because of the difference in ages between her and her siblings and because she lives alone with her mother at a great distance from the rest of the family. Since she began taking care of her mother, she has become socially isolated, which is further complicated by the development of anorexia. She has not maintained contact with high school friends in the past year. Currently, she says, "I do not know what I want to be when I grow up."

NURSING DIAGNOSES

The first two nursing diagnoses formulated for Cindy are **Imbalanced nutrition** and **Disturbed body image.** The first nursing diagnosis with interventions is developed here in the text. Please refer to the SIMON website for the goals and interventions for **Body image disturbance.**

PLANNING AND INTERVENTION

Initial measures are taken in order to address Cindy's unstable physiological state (e.g., restoring fluid and electrolyte balance, increasing red blood cell count, preventing hypothermia, and stabilizing vital signs). As Cindy begins the weight-restoration phase of treatment, she is placed on an 1800-calorie diet but is unable to eat and spends most of the mealtime poking at her food. A liquid supplement is prescribed, which is the exclusive source of her nutritional intake for several weeks, after which she slowly begins to eat solid food. As she gains weight, she can frequently be found doing jumping jacks in her room or speed walking down the corridors of the unit. Nursing Care Plan 17-1 provides an intervention for a client with anorexia nervosa.

CASE STUDY 17–2   A Client with Bulimia Nervosa

Sally is a 30-year-old college graduate who is an aspiring actress. She is currently working typing manuscripts as a "temp" for a publishing house. She is being admitted to a partial hospitalization program designed for clients with eating disorders. Partial hospitalization programs are designed to serve an alternative level of care (subacute care, transition from hospital to community) and to accommodate different levels of client functioning (working clients, clients requiring more structure and support than traditional outpatient therapy provides). Services vary from 2 to 5 days a week for several hours a day. Some programs have evening hours to further address the needs of working clients.

ASSESSMENT

Sally states that on returning home after her first semester at college, her mother met her at the airport and greeted her with, "You better go on a diet." Sally began to diet, fasting for most of the day and then beginning to eat in the evening. She quickly developed a pattern of fasting and binge eating at dinner, followed by vomiting. Her unstructured, chaotic life style contributed to her impulsivity and bulimic behaviors.

Sally's weight is approximately normal; at 65 inches (5'5") and 127 pounds, her weight is at 95% of ideal body weight. Physical examination reveals a blood pressure of 120/80 mm Hg sitting and 90/60 mm Hg standing; her pulse is 70 sitting and 96 standing. Her parotid glands are enlarged. There is considerable dental erosion present. Laboratory tests reveal a potassium level of 2.7 mmol/L (normal range, 3.3–5.5 mmol/L). Her electrocardiogram is abnormal, consistent with hypokalemia.

Sally has a dread of being fat, and the thought of not being slim makes her very anxious. She states that she cannot stop the cycle of binge eating and purging that causes her to feel guilty and ashamed. Sally fasts for most of the day, and then, once she begins to eat, she feels compelled to binge and then vomit. She finds this pattern to be particularly true if she eats certain foods, such as French fries. The cycle of binge eating and vomiting occurs at least 5 times a day. Sally works odd hours, doing her manuscript typing mostly at night. Because she works alone and can avoid being observed, she binge eats while doing her work and ultimately purges by inducing vomiting. Sally maintains her weight through vomiting and exercising for several hours daily at a gym. She reports that she has used laxatives and over-the-counter diuretics only a couple of times in the past. Sally thinks that her current weight, which is 96% of her ideal body weight, is "OK. If I gain an ounce, I'll be fat." She regards her slim figure as crucial to her success. Sally's affect is appropriate to her mood, which is anxious. She denies having suicidal ideation currently, although she has recently felt passively suicidal. The remainder of the mental status examination is normal.

Sally gives a history of being hospitalized for depression for 4 weeks at the age of 19. At that time, she was treated with an antidepressant and continued in outpatient treatment for about 6 months. She reports that her eating disorder was never diagnosed at that time. She also gives a history of intermittent marijuana and alcohol abuse but is not currently using substances. She stated her mother is in therapy for depression and is being treated with Prozac.

Sally was raised in an upper-middle-class family with highly successful parents and siblings who are all 3000 miles away. Of the five children in her family, she is the only one who does not have a career or an intimate relationship, both of which she very much wants. Sally states that her mother frequently uses her as a confidante in inappropriate ways. For instance, she shares with Sally that she is having an affair with her business partner. Sally regards her father as unapproachable and distant but feels guilty about not telling him about her mother's affair. Sally graduated from college but has never had a job that is appropriate to her education, settling for temporary work. She maintains that she needs the kind of job that is flexible and at off hours so that she can be available to attend acting and dance classes and auditions.

It is not clear how assiduously Sally pursues acting. She reports that she has never actually had an acting job. It becomes apparent that the aspiring actress is mostly a fantasy, with no real substance. In reality, her unstructured life style contributes to her impulsivity and her bulimic behaviors.

| NURSING DIAGNOSES | **Risk for injury** related to electrolyte imbalance and **Powerlessness**. Nursing Care Plan 17-2 provides interventions for a client with bulimia. The first nursing | diagnosis with intervention is developed here in the text. The diagnosis **Powerlessness**, including outcomes and interventions, is provided on the website. |

CASE STUDY 17-3   An Individual with an Eating Disorder (NOS) (Obesity)

Phyllis is a 25-year-old schoolteacher who gives a history of overeating since the age of 10 years. She seeks treatment at a community mental health center because she has recently felt more depressed.

| ASSESSMENT | Phyllis gives a history of being overweight since the age of 6 years. At the age of 10, she began to overeat in a more serious fashion. She reports that her overeating was related to her dysphoric mood, which is frequently associated with a perceived rejection. While attending a prestigious university, she began to binge eat several times a week but did not attempt to compensate by exercising or purging. Phyllis became very depressed in her third year of college and made a suicide attempt with 20 extra-strength acetaminophen tablets. She subsequently went into treatment with a psychiatrist, who diagnosed depression and prescribed fluoxetine, 60 mg daily. She subsequently stopped treatment because she continued to binge eat compulsively, although her mood was less dysphoric while she was taking fluoxetine.

Phyllis's weight is 200 pounds at a height of 61 inches (5'1"), placing her at 180% of ideal body weight. Her physical examination is otherwise unremarkable.

One of the reasons Phyllis gives for the increase in her depressive symptoms is her upcoming position as a first-grade teacher at an exclusive private school, a school she attended as a child. She speaks of the promise she once displayed as a child and of the low opinion she | currently has of herself and her accomplishments. She expresses having a lot of conflict about teaching students whom she calls "rich brats." She further states that the youngsters represent a promise for the future of which she is envious. "I once displayed that promise and look at me now."

Phyllis describes her appetite as voracious: "I'll eat anything in sight." She describes her eating pattern as constant if food is available. She states that she feels herself to be out of control in the presence of food. She reports eating a variety of foods, including nutritious ones, but in excess. Her attempts to restrict her intake have always been unsuccessful. She reports that Weight Watchers, Overeaters Anonymous, and dieting on her own have never had even minimal success. She denies using laxatives, diuretics, or self-induced vomiting. Phyllis feels guilty about being overweight and describes the envy and hostility she feels toward women who are slender. She is dressed neatly in loose, baggy clothing. Her affect is agitated with a depressed mood. She maintains good eye contact during the interview. She denies having an active suicidal plan but does admit to wishing that she would not wake up in the morning. |

Case Study continued on following page

CASE STUDY 17–3 *An Individual with an Eating Disorder* (NOS) (Obesity) *(Continued)*

Phyllis gives a history of depression with a serious suicide attempt. Treatment with fluoxetine improves her mood only slightly. She denies having a history of substance abuse. She reports no physical or sexual abuse. She states that her father has a drinking problem.

Phyllis is an only child of highly successful parents. She describes parents who are achievement oriented and who have high expectations for Phyllis. "My parents seem confident that I can do anything, but I'm not so sure. I feel I never measure up." She is currently living with her parents, a temporary arrangement until she begins teaching in 2 months. She has few close friends and tends to isolate herself. She states that she is interested in music, art, and reading but frequently is inactive and uninvolved.

NURSING DIAGNOSIS	**Altered nutrition: more than body requirements** and **Low self-esteem.** Nursing Care Plan 17–3 provides outcome criteria, interventions, and evaluation for Phyllis's care. The length of long-term follow-up, along with the effectiveness of the interventions for Phyllis, must be measured against the outcome criteria for	normalizing eating patterns, acceptable weight loss, and mood stabilization. The first nursing diagnosis provides outcomes and interventions for an obese individual with compulsive eating behavior. The nursing diagnosis **Low self-esteem** is developed with clear interventions on the website.

Visit the **Evolve** website at
http://evolve.elsevier.com/Varcarolis
for the other Nursing Care Plan diagnoses and for
more Nursing Care Plans.

NURSING CARE PLAN 17–1 *Interventions for a Client with Anorexia Nervosa*

NURSING DIAGNOSIS

Imbalanced Nutrition: Less Than Body Requirements related to restricting caloric intake, secondary to extreme fear of weight gain

Supporting Data
- 58 lb (50% of ideal body weight)
- Cachectic appearance, pale with fine lanugo; BP, 74/50 mm Hg; pulse, 54, barely palpable
- Depressed mood
- Denies being underweight: "I need treatment because I get fatigued so easily."
- Anemia (HGB = 9 g/dL)

Outcome Criteria: Client will reach 75% of ideal body weight—92 lb—by discharge.

NURSING CARE PLAN 17–1   *Interventions for a Client with Anorexia Nervosa (Continued)*

SHORT-TERM GOAL	INTERVENTION	RATIONALE	EVALUATION
1. Client will gain a minimum of 1/2 lb at each weigh-in (Mon-Wed-Fri).	1a. Acknowledge the emotional and physical difficulty the client is experiencing. Use client's extreme fatigue to engage her cooperation in the treatment plan.	1a. A first priority is to establish a therapeutic alliance.	*WEEK 1:* Client increases caloric intake with liquid supplement only. Client unable to eat solid food. Client does not gain weight. Client remains hypotensive, bradycardic, anemic (HGB = 9 g/dL).
	1b. Weigh the client daily for the first week; then three times a week. Client should be weighed in bra and panties only. There should be no oral intake, including a drink of water, before the early AM weigh-in. Do not negotiate the weight with the client nor reweigh the client. Client may choose not to look at the scale or request she not be told the weight.	1b. These measures ensure weight is accurate.	*WEEK 2:* Client gains 2 lb drinking liquid supplement—minimal solid food. Client remains hypotensive, bradycardic (HGB = 10 g/dL). *WEEK 3:* Client gains 3 lb drinking liquid supplement. Client selects meal plan but is unable to eat most of solid food. Client's BP = 84/60 mm Hg, pulse = 68, regular; HGB = 11 g/dL.
	1c. Vital signs TID until stable, then daily. Repeat ECG and laboratory tests until stable.	1c. As client begins to increase in weight, cardiovascular status improves to within normal range and monitoring is less frequent.	*WEEKS 4–6:* Client gains an average of 2 1/2 lb/week. Client samples more of solid food selected from meal plan. Client's BP = 90/60 mm Hg; pulse = 68, regular; HGB = 11.5 g/dL.
	1d. Provide a pleasant, calm atmosphere at mealtimes. Clients should be told the specific times and duration (usually a half hour) of meals.	1d. Mealtimes become episodes of high anxiety, and knowledge of regulations decreases tension in the milieu, particularly when the client has given up so much control by entering treatment.	

Nursing Care Plan continued on following page

NURSING CARE PLAN 17–1 *Interventions for a Client with Anorexia Nervosa (Continued)*

SHORT-TERM GOAL	INTERVENTION	RATIONALE	EVALUATION
	1e. Administer liquid supplement as ordered. 1f. Observe client during meals to prevent hiding or throwing away of food for at least 1 hour after meals and snacks to prevent purging. 1g. Encourage client to try to eat some solid food. Preparation of client's meals should be guided by likes and dislikes list, as client is unable to make own selections to complete menu. Morning weigh-in procedure is a high-anxiety time. Knowledge of the weight increasing induces feelings of being out of control, especially during initial phase of refeeding	1e. Client may be unable to eat solid food at first. 1f,g. The compelling force of the illness is such that these behaviors are difficult to stop. A power struggle between staff and client may emerge in which the client appears to comply but defies the rules (appearing to eat but throwing away food).	*WEEK 7:* Client weighs 71 lb (almost 60% of ideal body weight); calories are mostly from liquid supplement. Client selects balanced meals, eating more varied, solid food: turkey, carrots, lettuce, fruit. Client's HGB = 12.5 g/dL, maintains normal range of BP and pulse. Client continues to increase participation in social aspects of eating.
	1h. Be empathetic with client's struggle to give up control of her eating and her weight as she is expected to make minimum weight gain on a regular basis. Permit client to verbalize feelings at these times.	1h. The client is expected to gain at least three quarters of a pound on a specific schedule, usually three times a week (Mon-Wed-Fri).	*WEEKS 8–12:* Client gains an average of 2 1/2 lb/week and weighs 82 lb (approx. 68% of ideal body weight). Client is eating more varied solid food, but most caloric intake is still from liquid supplement. Client maintains normal vital signs and hemoglobin levels. Client maintains social interaction during mealtimes and snacks.

NURSING CARE PLAN 17–1   *Interventions for a Client with Anorexia Nervosa* (Continued)

SHORT-TERM GOAL	INTERVENTION	RATIONALE	EVALUATION
	1i. Monitor client's weight gain. A weight gain of 3 to 5 lb/week is medically acceptable.	1i. Weight gain of more than 5 lb in a week may result in pulmonary edema.	*WEEK 13:* Client has reached medically stable weight at the end of 16th week—92 lb (75% of ideal body weight).
	1j. Provide teaching regarding healthy eating as the basis of a healthy life style.	1j. Reinforces healthy aspects of eating, e.g. increased energy, rather than gaining weight.	Client continues to eat more solid food with relatively less liquid supplement.
	1k. Continue to provide a supportive, empathetic approach as client continues in weight restoration.	1k. Eating regularly for the anorectic client, even within the framework of restoring health, is extremely difficult.	Client is not able to participate in planned exercise program until client reaches 85% of ideal body weight.
	1l. Use a cognitive-behavioral approach to client's expressed fears regarding weight gain. Identify and examine dysfunctional thoughts, identify and examine values and beliefs that sustain these thoughts.	1l. Confronting irrational thoughts and beliefs is crucial to changing eating behaviors.	
	1m. As client approaches her target weight, there should be encouragement to make her own choices for menu selection.	1m. The client can assume more control of her meals, which is empowering for the anorectic client.	
	1n. Emphasize social nature of eating. Encourage conversation that does not have the theme of food during mealtimes.	1n. Eating as a social activity, shared with others and participating in conversation, serves as both a distraction from obsessional preoccupations and a pleasurable event.	

Nursing Care Plan continued on following page

NURSING CARE PLAN 17–1 *Interventions for a Client with Anorexia Nervosa* (Continued)

SHORT-TERM GOAL	INTERVENTION	RATIONALE	EVALUATION
	1o. The weight maintenance phase of treatment challenges the client. This is the ideal time to address more of the issues underlying the client's attitude toward weight and shape.	1o. At a healthier weight, the client is cognitively better prepared to examine emotional conflicts and themes.	
	1p. Focus on the client's strengths, including her good work in normalizing her weight and eating habits.	1p. The client who is beginning to normalize weight and eating behaviors has achieved a major accomplishment, of which she should be proud. Explores noneating activities as a source of gratification.	
	1q. Provide for a planned exercise program when the client reaches target weight.	1q. The client experiences a strong drive to exercise; this measure accommodates this drive by planning a reasonable amount.	
	1r. Encourage the client to apply all the knowledge, skills, and gains made from the various individual, family, and group therapy sessions.	1r. The client has been receiving intensive therapy and education, which have provided tools and techniques that are useful in maintaining healthy behaviors.	

NURSING CARE PLAN 17-2 *Interventions for a Client with Bulimia*

NURSING DIAGNOSIS

Risk for Injury: related to low potassium and other physical changes secondary to binge eating and purging.

Supporting Data

- Potassium level of 2.7 mmol/L
- Abnormal electrocardiogram
- Enlarged parotid glands
- Dental tooth enamel erosion, caries
- History of binge eating/purging

Outcome criteria: Client will demonstrate ability to regulate eating patterns in the absence of untoward signs and symptoms.

SHORT-TERM GOAL	INTERVENTION	RATIONALE	EVALUATION
1. Client will identify signs and symptoms of low potassium (K^+) level and K^+ level will remain within the normal limits throughout hospitalization.	1a. Educate the client regarding the ill effects of self-induced vomiting, low K^+ level, dental erosion.	1a. Health teaching is crucial to treatment. The client needs to be reminded of the benefits of normalization of eating behavior.	*WEEK 1:* Client begins to select balanced meals. Client demonstrates knowledge of untoward effects of vomiting and of K^+ deficiency.
	1b. Educate the client about binge/purge cycle and its self-perpetuating nature.	1b,c. The compulsive nature of the binge/purge cycle is maintained by the cycle of restricting, hunger, bingeing, purging accompanied by feelings of guilt, and then repeating the cycle over and over.	Client begins to demonstrate understanding of repetitive nature of binge/purge cycle.
	1c. Teach the client that fasting sets one up to binge eat.		
	1d. Explore ideas about trigger foods.	1d. Trigger foods are foods that provide the stimulus for a binge: french fries, donuts.	*WEEK 2:* Client begins to challenge irrational thoughts and beliefs. Client continues to plan nutritionally balanced meals, including dinner at home. Client begins to sample "forbidden foods" and discuss thoughts and attitudes about same.

Nursing Care Plan continued on following page

NURSING CARE PLAN 17–2   *Interventions for a Client with Bulimia* (Continued)

SHORT-TERM GOAL	INTERVENTION	RATIONALE	EVALUATION
	1e. Challenge irrational thoughts and beliefs about "forbidden" foods.	1e. The client also has a list of "forbidden foods," which cause excessive weight gain or cannot be eaten in normal amounts, e.g., ice cream, cake.	*WEEK 3:* Client discusses triggers to binge and resultant behavior. Client continues to challenge irrational thoughts and beliefs in individual and group sessions. Client plans meals, including "forbidden foods."
	1f. Teach the client to plan and eat regularly scheduled, balanced meals.	1f. Planning and structuring meals helps to ensure success in maintaining abstinence from binge/purge activity.	*WEEK 4:* Client reports no binge/purge behaviors at day program or outside. Client demonstrates understanding of repetitive nature of binge/purge cycle. Client continues to challenge irrational thoughts and beliefs.

NURSING CARE PLAN 17–3   *Interventions for a Client Who Is Obese*

NURSING DIAGNOSIS

Imbalanced Nutrition; More Than Body Requirements—180% of ideal body weight related to compulsive overeating, including episodes of bingeing

Supporting Data
- 200 lb (180% of ideal body weight)
- Uncontrollable eating pattern
- "I'll eat anything in sight."

Outcome Criteria: Client will normalize eating pattern and achieve a specific target date according to a predetermined plan.

NURSING CARE PLAN 17–3 *Interventions for a Client Who Is Obese (Continued)*

SHORT-TERM GOAL	INTERVENTION	RATIONALE	EVALUATION
1. Client will learn coping strategies that result in adhering to a structured meal schedule.	1a. The clinical nurse specialist can use many techniques of cognitive behavioral therapy in addressing the issues of overweight and disordered eating. The client should begin a journal.	1a. Cognitive-behavioral techniques can be useful in addressing automatic behaviors. Recording what and where one eats begins to identify patterns that can be modified.	*WEEK 1:* Client selects a meal plan with structured times and places; begins journal and maintains it consistently. Client begins to relate feelings around eating.
	1b. Teach the client to structure and plan ahead for times and places where she will have her meals and snacks for the day.	1b. Organization and structure can allow for a different choice.	*WEEK 2:* Client is able to adhere to structured meal schedule approximately 25%. Client expresses the struggle and feelings of tension around implementing structured meal schedule—some modifications are made to allow the client to be more successful. Client shares contents of journal, which she consistently maintains. Client reports weight is unchanged; client was unable to change pattern of exercise.
	1c. Teach the client not to abstain from eating for longer periods of time than planned in order to avoid rebound binge eating.	1c,d. Extended periods of abstinence, restrictive dietary intake, or very-low-calorie diet can result in rebound overeating.	*WEEK 3:* Client is adhering to schedule 50% of the time. Client shares journal entries and relates thoughts and feelings concerning eating. Client reports 1/2-lb weight loss. Client is beginning to walk for a half an hour as part of her daily routine.
	1d. Review the nutritional content of dietary intake to ensure a balanced diet.		
	1e. Review the journal with the client to identify areas for improvement in adhering to the treatment plan.	1e. The journal is an important tool in modifying eating behaviors.	*WEEK 4:* Client continues to adhere to structured schedule approximately 75% of the time.

Nursing Care Plan continued on following page

NURSING CARE PLAN 17–3 *Interventions for a Client Who Is Obese* (Continued)

SHORT-TERM GOAL	INTERVENTION	RATIONALE	EVALUATION
	1f. Explore with the client the thoughts and feelings she is experiencing about this new regimen. 1g. Identify thoughts and beliefs and underlying assumptions that reinforce disordered eating patterns.	1f,g. The nurse must be empathetic and supportive of the client's experience, which is one of struggle accompanied by feelings of tension. The nurse should explore the thoughts and beliefs accompanying the eating behavior.	Client walks regularly, experiencing a better sense of well-being. Client thinks she is up to the challenge of continuing the plan to normalize her eating pattern and increase her energy expenditure. Client's weight is 196 lb (− 4 lb); she acknowledges that progress has and will continue to be slow.
	1h. Establish a once-a-week schedule of weighing.	1h. There may be minimal or no weight reduction, leading to discouragement.	

SUMMARY

Many theoretical models help explain, at least in part, the origins of eating disorders. For example, neurobiological theories identify an association between eating disorders and depression and neuroendocrine abnormalities. Psychological theories explore issues of control in anorexia and affective instability and poor impulse control in bulimia. Sociocultural models look at both our present societal ideal of being thin and the ideal feminine role model in general. Interestingly, males with eating disorders share many of the characteristics of women with eating disorders. In those populations where eating disorders had been rare and are now appearing, the dynamics—the stress of acculturation versus identification with the new culture—are being examined. Biopsychosocial theories explore genetic vulnerabilities that may predispose people toward eating disorders and increasingly twin studies confirm genetic liability, perhaps interacting with environmental mechanisms. Anorexia nervosa can be a life-threatening eating disorder in young women and, less frequently, in men. Findings include severe underweight; low blood pressure, pulse, and temperature; and dehydration. Critical symptoms may include low serum potassium level and dysrhythmias. Altered nutrition: less than body requirements is a primary nursing diagnosis, and Decreased cardiac output, Risk for injury, Body image disturbance, and Powerlessness are other important considerations. Having the client achieve 85% to 90% of ideal body weight and normalizing eating patterns are among some of the main targeted outcome criteria. Initially, anorexia may be treated in an *inpatient treatment setting*, where milieu therapy, psychotherapy (cognitive), self-care skills, and psychobiological interventions can be implemented. Because of managed care and shorter length of hospital stays, *acute care: outpatient treatment* is needed, where psychotherapy and psychopharmacology continue. Long-term treatment aims to help clients maintain healthy weight and includes treatment modalities such as individual therapy, family therapy, group therapy, psychopharmacology, and nutrition counseling.

Bulimia nervosa clients are typically within normal weight range but some may be slightly below or above ideal body weight. On assessment, the client may have clear physical and emotional problems. For example, the client may have enlargement of the parotid glands and dental erosion and caries if she has induced vomiting. Nursing diagnoses can include Decreased cardiac output, Risk for injury, Disturbed body image, and Powerlessness. Among the outcome criteria for these clients is helping the client refrain from binge eating and purging and remain safe. Acute care may be necessary when life-threatening complications are present, such as gastric rupture (rare), electrolyte imbalance, and cardiac dysrhythmias. Within the highly structured milieu of the inpatient eating disorder unit, the goal of interventions is to interrupt the binge/purge cycle. Psychotherapy as well as self-care skill training are included. *Long-term treatment* focuses on therapy aimed at intervening with any coexisting depression, substance abuse, and/or personality disorders that are causing the client distress and interfering with the client's quality of life. Self-worth and interpersonal functioning eventually become issues that are useful for the client to target.

Eating disorders NOS include a variety of patterns, and in this chapter, obesity due to binge eating disorder was examined. Approximately 25% of Americans are overweight, despite the emphasis in the media on leading healthier lives. It is also true that binge eaters report a history of major depression significantly more often than non-binge eaters. An effective program for obese binge eaters must integrate modification of the disordered eating and the depressive symptoms with the ultimate goal of a more appropriate weight for the individual.

Family support and family psychotherapy are useful in helping individuals deal with family relationship problems that may contribute to maintaining the disorder (APA 2000b). Clients and their families are increasingly using on-line websites, news groups, and chat rooms as resources. Clinicians should inquire about these and other complementary approaches clients or their families may be using (APA 2000b).

Visit the **Evolve** website at
http://evolve.elsevier.com/Varcarolis
for a post-test on the content in this chapter.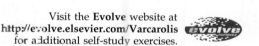

Visit the **Evolve** website at
http://evolve.elsevier.com/Varcarolis
for additional self-study exercises.

Critical Thinking and Chapter Review

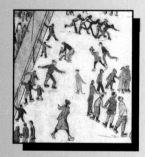

Critical Thinking

1. Tom Shift, a 19-year-old male model, has had a rapid decrease in weight over the last four months, after his agent told him he would have to lose more weight or lose a coveted account. Tom is 6'2", and is presently 132 pounds, down from his usual 176. He is brought to the emergency room with a pulse of 40, and severe arrhythmias. His laboratory work-up reveals severe hypokalemia. He has become extremely depressed, saying, "I am too fat . . . I won't take anything to eat . . . , if I gain weight my life will be ruined. There is nothing to live for if I can't model." Tom's parents are startled and confused, and his best friend, Dick Lamb, is worried and feels helpless to help Tom. "I tell Tom he needs to eat or he will die . . . I tell him he is a skeleton, but he refuses to listen to me. I don't know what to do."

   ■ Which physical and psychiatric criteria suggest that Tom should be immediately hospitalized? What other physical signs and symptoms may be found upon assessment?
   ■ What are some of the questions you would eventually ask Tom when evaluating his biopsychosocial functioning?

- ■ What are your feelings toward someone with anorexia? Can you make a distinction between your thoughts and feelings toward women with anorexia as compared to a man with anorexia?
- ■ What are some things you could do for Tom's parents and Tom's friend Dick in terms of offering them information, support and referrals? Identify specific referrals.
- ■ Explain the kinds of interventions or restrictions Tom may receive while hospitalized (e.g., weighing, observations after eating or visits, exercise, therapy, self-care).
- ■ How would you describe partial hospitalization programs or psychiatric home care programs when asked if Tom would have to be hospitalized for a long time?
- ■ What are some of Tom's cognitive distortions that would be a target for therapy?
- ■ Identify at least five criteria that would indicate that Tom was improving.

2. You and your close friend Mary Alice have been together since nursing school and you are now working on the same surgical unit. Mary Alice told you that in the past she has made several suicide attempts. Today you accidentally come upon her bingeing off unit, and she looks embarrassed and uncomfortable when she sees you. Several times you notice that she spends time in the bathroom and you hear sounds of retching. In response to your concern, she admits that she has been binge-purging for several years, but now she is getting out of control and feeling profoundly depressed.

   - ■ Although Mary Alice doesn't show any physical signs of bulimia nervosa, what would you look for when assessing an individual with bulimia?
   - ■ What kinds of emergencies could result from bingeing and purging?
   - ■ What would be the most useful type of psychotherapy for Mary Alice initially and what issues would need to be addressed?
   - ■ What kinds of new skills does a person with bulimia need to learn to lessen the compulsion to binge and purge?
   - ■ What would be some signs that Mary Alice is recovering?

Chapter Review

Choose the most appropriate answer.

1. The most pervasive cognitive distortion nurses will identify among clients with eating disorders is

   1. Thinness equates with self worth.
   2. I'm unpopular because I'm fat.
   3. Being thin is being powerful.
   4. Being fat is more harmful than being thin.

2. During the weight-restoration phase, a client with anorexia nervosa may have edema of the lower extremities related to

   1. Liver dysfunction
   2. Endocrine imbalance
   3. Poor cardiac function
   4. Compromised kidney function

3. Which client with an eating disorder would be at greatest risk for hypokalemia?

   1. An anorectic who loses weight by restricting food intake
   2. An anorectic who purges to promote weight loss
   3. A nonpurging bulimic

4. Eating disorder clients who are at risk for hyponatremia rather than hypokalemia

4. Which medication is likely to be used in treatment of clients with eating disorders?

1. An SSRI such as fluoxetine
2. A neuroleptic such as respirdone
3. An anxiolytic such as alprazolam
4. An anticonvulsant such as carbamazepine

5. Which risk factor for eating disorder is most commonly identified in the histories of adolescents with eating disorders?

1. Dieting
2. Purging
3. Overeating
4. Excessive exercise

NURSE, CLIENT, AND FAMILY TEACHING FOR EATING DISORDERS

Self-Help Groups

American Anorexia/Bulimia Association
293 Central Park West, #R
New York, NY 10024
1-212-891-8686
(for people with eating disorders)

National Association of Anorexia Nervosa and Associated Disorders (ANAD)
P.O. Box 7
Highland Park, IL 60035
1-847-831-3438
(for people with eating disorders)

National Eating Disorders Organization
6655 South Yale Avenue
Tulsa, OK 74136
1-918-481-4044
(for people with eating disorders, their families, and friends)

Eating Disorders Awareness and Prevention
603 Stewart Street, Suite 803
Seattle, WA 98101
1-206-382-3587

Internet Sites

Mirror Mirror Eating Disorders Home Page
http://www.mirror-mirror.org/eatdis.htm

The Center for Eating Disorders
http://www.eatingdisorder.org

Anorexia Nervosa and Related Eating Disorders, Inc.
http://www.anred.com

Academy for Eating Disorders
http://www.acadeatdis.org

Healthtouch Online
http://www.healthtouch.com

REFERENCES

Agras, W. S., et al. (2000). Outcome predictors for the cognitive behavior treatment of bulimia nervosa: Data from a multisite study. *The American Journal of Psychiatry,* 157(8):1302–1308.

American Psychiatric Association. (1980). *Diagnostic and statistical manual of mental disorders* (3rd ed.). Washington, DC: American Psychiatric Association.

American Psychiatric Association. (1987). *Diagnostic and statistical manual of mental disorders* (3rd ed., revised). Washington, DC: American Psychiatric Association.

American Psychiatric Association. (2000a). *Diagnostic and statistical manual of mental disorders* (4th ed.), TR. Washington, DC: American Psychiatric Association.

American Psychiatric Association. (2000b). *Practice guidelines for the treatment of psychiatric disorders: Compendium 2000.* Washington, DC: American Psychiatric Association.

Beck, A., Rush, A., Shaw, B., and Emery, G. (1979). *Cognitive therapy of depression.* New York: Guilford Press.

Becker, A. E. (2000). Presentation at American Psychiatric Association meeting in Washington, DC, May, 2000.

Becker, A. E., and Hamburg, P. (1996). Culture, the media, and eating disorders. *Harvard Review of Psychiatry,* 4:163–167.

Bemporad, J. (1995). Self-starvation through the ages: Reflections on the pre-history of anorexia nervosa. *International Journal of Eating Disorders,* 19(3):217–237.

Braun, D. L., Sunday, S. R., Huang, A., and Halmi, K. A. (1999). More males seek treatment for eating disorders. *International Journal of Eating Disorders,* 25(4):415–424.

Brewerton, T. D., Dansky, B. S., Kilpatrick, D. G., and O'Neil, P. M. (2000). Which comes first in the pathogenesis of bulimia nervosa: Dieting or bingeing? *International Journal of Eating Disorders,* 28(3):259–264.

Brownell, K. D., and Wadden, T. A. (1991). The heterogeneity of obesity: Fitting treatments to individuals. *Behavior Therapy,* 22(2):153–177.

Bruch, H. (1973). *Eating disorders: Obesity, anorexia, and the person within.* New York: Basic Books.

Bruch, H. (1985). Four decades of eating disorders. In D. M. Garner and P. E. Garfinkel (Eds.), *Handbook of psychotherapy for anorexia nervosa and bulimia* (pp 7–18). New York: Guilford Press.

Bulik, C. M., Sullivan, P. F., and Rorty, M. (1989). Childhood sexual abuse in women with bulimia. *Journal of Clinical Psychiatry,* 50:460–464.

Carlat, D. J., Camargo, C. A., Jr., and Herzog, D. B. (1997). Eating disorders in males: A report on 135 patients. *The American Journal of Psychiatry,* 154(8):1127–1132.

Chamorro, R., and Flores-Ortiz, Y. (2000). Acculturation and disordered eating patterns among Mexican-American women. *International Journal of Eating Disorders,* 28(1):125–129.

Crisp, A. H. (1995). *Anorexia nervosa: Let me be.* Hove, England: Erlbaum.

Davis, C., Claridge, G., and Fox, J. (2000). Not just a pretty face: Physical attractiveness and perfectionism in the risk for eating disorders. *International Journal of Eating Disorders,* 27:67–73.

Devlin, M. J., Goldfein, J. A., Carino, J. S., and Wolk, S. L. (2000). Open treatment of overweight binge eaters with phentermine and fluoxetine as an adjunct to cognitive-behavioral therapy. *International Journal of Eating Disorders,* 28(3):325–332.

Devlin, M. J., and Walsh, B. T. (1989). Eating disorders and depression. *Psychiatric Annals,* 19(9):473–476.

Devlin, M. J., et al. (1990). Metabolic abnormalities in bulimia nervosa. *Archives of General Psychiatry,* 47(2):144–148.

Fairburn, C. G., Cooper, Z., Doll, H. A., Norman, P., and O'Connor, M. (2000). The natural course of bulimia nervosa and binge eating disorder in young women. *Archives of General Psychiatry,* 57:659–665.

Fairburn, C. G., Cowen, P. J., and Harrison, P. J. (1999). Twin studies and the etiology of eating disorders. *International Journal of Eating Disorders,* 26(4):349–358.

Fairburn, C. G., and Cooper, P. J. (1989). Eating disorders. In K. Hawton, P. M. Salkovskis, J. Kirk, and D. M. Clark (Eds.), *Cognitive behaviour therapy for psychiatric problems* (pp. 277–314). New York: Oxford University Press.

Ferguson, C. P., La Via, M. C., Crossan, P. J., and Kaye, W. H. (1999). Are serotonin selective reuptake inhibitors effective in underweight anorexia nervosa? *International Journal of Eating Disorders,* 25(1):11–17.

Fichter, M. M., and Quadflieg, N. (1999). Six-year course and outcome of anorexia nervosa. *International Journal of Eating Disorders,* 26(4):359–385.

Garner, D. M., and Bemis, K. (1982). A cognitive-behavioral approach to anorexia nervosa. *Cognitive Therapy and Research,* 6: 123–150.

Garner, D. M., Olmsted, M. P., Bohr, Y., and Garfinkel, P. E. (1982). The Eating Attitudes Test: Psychometric features and clinical correlates. *Psychological Medicine,* 12:871–878.

Goldstein, D. J., Wilson, M. G., Ascroft, R. C., and Al-Banna, M. (1999). Effectiveness of fluoxetine therapy in bulimia nervosa regardless of comorbid depression. *International Journal of Eating Disorders,* 25(1):19–27.

Halmi, K. A. (1999). Eating disorders. In B. J. Sadock and V. A. Sadock (Eds.), *Kaplan & Sadock's comprehensive textbook of psychiatry* (7th ed.). Philadelphia: Lippincott Williams & Wilkins.

Herpetz, S., et al. (2000). Relationship of weight and eating disorders in type 2 diabetic patients: A multicenter study. *International Journal of Eating Disorders,* 28(1):68–77.

Herzog, D. B., et al. (2000). Mortality in eating disorders: A descriptive study. *International Journal of Eating Disorders,* 28:20–26.

Holland, A. J., et al. (1984). Anorexia nervosa: A study of 34 twin pairs and one set of triplets. *British Journal of Psychiatry,* 145: 414–418.

Hsu, L. K. G. (1990). *Eating disorders.* New York: Guilford Press.

Ibrahim, K., and Rosedale, M. (1994). Perspectives in multiple family group therapy with eating disordered patients. Paper presented at the meeting of the Society for Education and Research in Psychiatric Nursing, Rockville, MD, November 1994.

Irwin, E. G. (1993). A focused overview of anorexia nervosa and bulimia: I. Etiological issues. *Archives of Psychiatric Nursing,* 7(6): 342–346.

Joiner, T. E., Katz, J., and Heatherton, T. F. (2000). Personality features differentiate late adolescent females and males with chronic bulimic symptoms. *International Journal of Eating Disorders,* 27(2):191–197.

Kandel, D. B., and Davies, M. (1982). Epidemiology of depressive mood in adolescents. *Archives of General Psychiatry,* 39:1205–1212.

Keel, P. K., and Mitchell, J. E. (1997). Outcome in bulimia nervosa. *The American Journal of Psychiatry,* 154(3):313–321.

Kendler, K. S., et al. (1991). The genetic epidemiology of bulimia nervosa. *American Journal of Psychiatry,* 148(12):1627–1637.

Lake, A. J., Staiger, P. K., and Glowinski, H. (2000). Effect of western culture on women's attitudes to eating and perceptions of body shape. *International Journal of Eating Disorders,* 27:83–89.

La Via, M. C., Gray, N., and Kaye, W. (2000). Case reports of olanzapine treatment of anorexia nervosa. *International Journal of Eating Disorders,* 27(3):363–366.

Lehoux, P. M., Steiger, H., and Jabalpurlawa, S. (2000). State/trait distinctions in bulimic syndromes. *International Journal of Eating Disorders,* 27(1):36–42.

Lerner, R. M., et al. (1980). Self-concept, self-esteem, and body attitudes among Japanese male and female adolescents. *Child Development,* 51:847–855.

Marcus, M. D. (1997). Adapting treatment for patients with binge-eating disorder. In D. M. Garner and P. E. Garfinkel (Eds.), *Handbook of treatment for eating disorders* (2nd ed., pp 485–499). New York: Guilford Press.

Marcus, M. D. (1995). Binge eating and obesity. In K. D. Brownell and C. G. Fairburn (Eds.), *Eating disorders and obesity: A comprehensive handbook* (pp 441–444). New York: Guilford Press.

Marcus, M. D., Smith, D., Santelli, R., and Kaye, W. (1992). Characterization of eating disordered behavior in obese binge eaters. *International Journal of Eating Disorders,* 12(3):249–255.

Marcus, M. D., et al. (1990). Psychiatric disorders among obese binge eaters. *International Journal of Eating Disorders,* 9(1):69–77.

McElroy, S. L., et al. (2000). Placebo-controlled trial of sertraline in the treatment of binge eating disorder. *The American Journal of Psychiatry,* 157(6):1004–1006.

Mehler, P. S. (1996). Eating disorders: 1. Anorexia nervosa. *Hospital Practice (Office Edition),* 31(1):109–113, 117.

Metropolitan Life Insurance Company (1983). 1983 Height and weight tables. *Statistical Bulletin,* 64(1):3–9.

Minuchin, S. (1974). *Families and family therapy.* Cambridge, MA: Harvard University Press.

Nobakht, M., and Dezhkam, M. (2000). An epidemiological study of eating disorders in Iran. *International Journal of Eating Disorders,* 28(3):265–271.

Olivardia, R., Pope, G., Mangweth, B., and Hudson, J. (1995). Eating disorders in college men. *American Journal of Psychiatry,* 152(9):1279–1285.

O'Meara, N. (2000). Houston, Texas, Reviewer for Chapter 17.

Peterson, C. B., et al. (2000). Predictors of treatment outcome for binge eating disorder. *International Journal of Eating Disorders,* 28(2):131–138.

Peterson, C. B., and Mitchell, J. E. (2000). Psychosocial and pharmacological treatment of eating disorders: A review of research findings. *Journal of Clinical Psychology,* 55(6):685–697.

Pike, K. (1991). Mothers, daughters, and disordered eating. *Journal of Abnormal Psychology,* 1200(2):198–204

Pope, H. G., Katz, D. L., and Hudson, J. L. (1993). Anorexia nervosa and "reverse anorexia" among 108 male bodybuilders. *Comprehensive Psychiatry,* 34(6):406–409.

Pope, H. G., and Hudson, J. L. (1992). Is childhood sexual abuse a risk factor for bulimia nervosa? *American Journal of Psychiatry,* 149(4):455–463.

Powers, P. S., and Johnson, C. L. (1999). Small victories: Prevention of eating disorders among elite athletes. In N. Piran, M. P. Levine, and C. Steiner-Adair (Eds.), *Preventing eating disorders: A handbook of interventions and special challenges* (pp. 241–255). Philadelphia: Brunner/Mazel.

Ricca, V., Mannucci, E., Zucchi, T., Rotella, C. M., and Faravelli, C. (2000). Cognitive-behavioral therapy for bulimia nervosa and binge eating disorder. A review. *Psychotherapy and Psychosomatics*, 69(6): 287–295

Rosedale, M. (1996). *Eating disorders critical pathway*. New York: US Home Care.

Russell, G. (1979). Bulimia nervosa: An ominous variant of anorexia nervosa. *Psychological Medicine*, 9:429–448.

Russell, G. (1985). The changing nature of anorexia nervosa. *Journal of Psychiatric Research*, 19:101–109.

Rydall, A., Rodin, G., Olmsted, M., Devenyi, M., and Daneman, D. (1997). Disordered eating behavior and microvascular complications in young women with insulin-dependent diabetes mellitus. *New England Journal of Medicine*, 336(26):1849–1854.

Schmidt, U., Tiller, J., and Treasure, J. (1993). Self-treatment of bulimia nervosa: a pilot study. *International Journal of Eating Disorders*, 13:273–277.

Smolak, L., Murnen, S. K., Ruble, A. E. (2000). Female athletes and eating problems: A meta-analysis. *International Journal of Eating Disorders*, 27(4):371–380.

Striegel-Moore, R. H., et al. (2000a). One-year use and cost of inpatient and outpatient services among female and male patients with an eating disorder: Evidence from a national database of health insurance claims. *International Journal of Eating Disorders*, 27(4):381–389

Striegel-Moore, R. H., et al. (2000b). Subthreshold binge eating disorder. *International Journal of Eating Disorders*, 27(3):270–278.

Striegel-Moore, R., Wilfley, D. E., Pike, K. M., Dohm, F. A., and Fairburn, C. G. (2000c). Recurrent binge eating in black women. *Archives of Family Medicine*, 9(1):83–87.

Striegel-Moore, R. H., Garvin, V., Dohm, F., and Rosenheck, R. A. (1999). Psychiatric comorbidity of eating disorders in men: A national study of hospitalized veterans. *International Journal of Eating Disorders*, 25(4):399–404.

Strober, M., Freeman, R., Lampert, C., Diamond, J., and Kaye, W. (2000). Controlled family study of anorexia nervosa and bulimia nervosa: Evidence of shared liability and transmission of partial syndromes. *The American Journal of Psychiatry*, 157(3): 393–401.

Strober, M., Freeman, R., Morrell, W. (1997). The long-term course of severe anorexia nervosa in adolescents: Survival analysis of recovery, relapse, and outcome predictors over 10–15 years in a prospective study. *International Journal of Eating Disorders*, 22: 339–360.

Stunkard, A. (1993). A history of binge eating. In C. G. Fairburn and G. T. Wilson (Eds), *Binge eating: Nature, assessment, and treatment* (pp 15–34). New York: Guilford Press.

Thiel, A., et al. (1995). Obsessive-compulsive disorder among patients with anorexia nervosa and bulimia nervosa. *American Journal of Psychiatry*, 152(1):72–75.

Verrotti, A., Catino, M., DeLuca, F. A., Morgese, G., and Chiarelli, F. (1999). Eating disorders in adolescents with type I diabetes mellitus. *Acta Diabetologica*, 36(1/2):21–25.

Vize, C. M., and Cooper, P. J. (1995). Sexual abuse in patients with eating disorder, patients with depression, and normal controls: A comparative study. *British Journal of Psychiatry*, 167:80–85.

Walsh, B. T., and Devlin, M. (1995). Eating disorders. *Child and Adolescent Psychiatric Clinics of North America*, 4(2):343–357.

Walsh, B. T., and Garner, D. M. (1997). Diagnostic issues. In D. M. Garner and P. E. Garfinkel (Eds.), *Handbook of treatment for eating disorders* (2nd ed., pp 25–33). New York: Guilford Press.

Walsh, B. T., et al. (1997). Medication and psychotherapy in the treatment of bulimia nervosa. *The American Journal of Psychiatry*, 154:523–531.

Welch, S. L., and Fairburn, C. G. (1994). Sexual abuse and bulimia nervosa: Three integrated case control comparisons. *American Journal of Psychiatry*, 151(3):402–407.

Wiederman, M. W., and Pryor, T. L. (2000). Body dissatisfaction, bulimia, and depression among women: The mediating role of drive for thinness. *International Journal of Eating Disorders*, 27: 90–95

Wilfley, D. E., Schwartz, M. B., Spurrell, E. B., and Fairburn, C. G. (2000) Using the eating disorder examination to identify the specific psychopathology of binge eating disorder. *International Journal of Eating Disorders*, 27(3):259–269.

Williamson, D. F. (1993). Descriptive epidemiology of body weight and weight change in U.S. adults. *Annals of Internal Medicine*, 19(7):646–649.

Wooley, S. C. (1995). Feminist influences on the treatment of eating disorders. In K. D. Brownell and C. G. Fairburn (Eds.), *Eating disorders and obesity: A comprehensive handbook* (pp 294–298). New York: Guilford Press.

World Health Organization (1992). *ICD-10 Classification of mental and behavioral disorders: Clinical descriptions and diagnostic guidelines* (pp 176–181). Geneva: World Health Organization.

Zaider, T. I., Johnson, J. G., and Cockell, S. J. (2000). Psychiatric comorbidity associated with eating disorder symptomatology among adolescents in the community. *International Journal of Eating Disorders* 28(1):58–67.

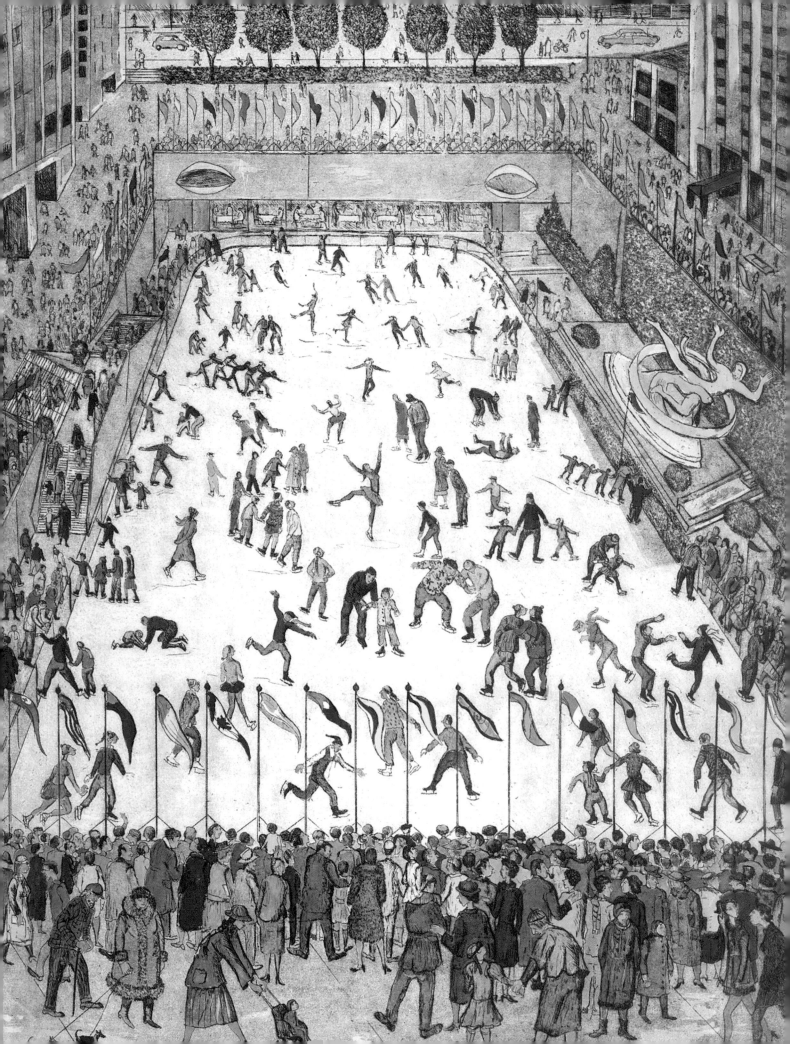

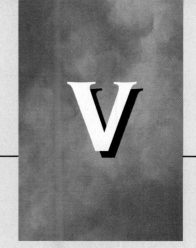
Psychobiological Disorders: Severe to Psychotic

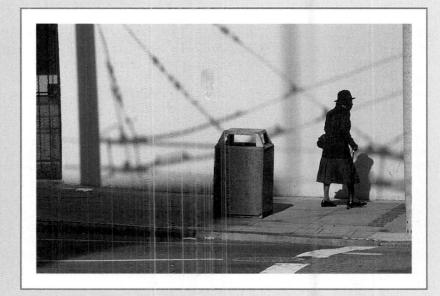

The worst solitude is to be destitute of sincere friendship.

FRANCIS BACON
(1561–1626)

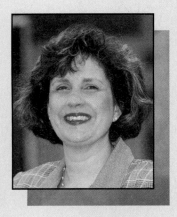

MARY LESNIAK

As a psychiatric nurse for more than twenty years I have held many positions from staff nurse to my present role of Director of Behavioral Health Services. During that time I encountered numerous problems but none so unsettling as the issue of **floating.**

To remedy fluctuations in census and staffing many hospitals use staffing techniques such as floating, which may have legal and ethical ramifications as well as quality-of-care issues. This technique requires staff from a low census unit to float to a high census or inadequately staffed area where they may lack the skills and knowledge to properly care for the clients. The practice of floating, although not new, had become more prevalent in recent years due to managed care, hospital downsizing, and a nursing shortage, and it is important for those entering the nursing profession to recognize the possibility of being mandated to float.

This practice affected the nurses I supervise when the client census took a drastic downward trend. The nurses were required to work in unfamiliar areas with little or no orientation and were very intimidated and frustrated with these assignments. They were also faced with a legal and ethical issue. Should they risk disciplinary action if they refused to float or risk the loss of their license if a client was harmed due to their lack of competence? As a nurse director, a nursing shift supervisor, and a former staff nurse, I recognized that this is a serious problem plaguing hospitals and health systems. I could empathize with the fears and frustrations of nurses who are requested to perform in an area where they have no recent experience. I can empathize with nursing supervisors who are responsible to provide adequate staffing in each nursing unit, and as a nurse director I recognize the need for quality and safety as well as cost-effective care. Subsequently, I reviewed the literature related to this issue to determine if floating strategies were available that would provide a safe environment for the client, the nurse, and the organization.

Since regulatory agencies do not mandate staffing patterns, it is the responsibility of hospital administration to provide appropriate client-staff ratios. With declining hospital profit margins, administrators are required to do more with less in terms of staffing and since there is a tendency for hospital administrators to believe that all nurse are generalists and are prepared to work in any nursing area, floating seems like a logical and responsible solution. Floating to unfamiliar areas, however, is a major source of stress for nurses who believe that each area of nursing is a specialty area and requires special knowledge and training. Nurses are very fearful that they will make an error that will be detrimental to the client and possibly result in a legal issue. A study of ICU nurses revealed "that only death outranks floating as a source of stress" (Davidhizar, Dowd, Brownson, 1998, p. 33). New graduate nurses are taught to assess all systems, but as a nurse specializes, client assessments take on a narrower focus with a better understanding of the specialty. A psychiatric nurse, for example, is trained to focus on the mental status examination of a client and over time may feel that he/she has become less proficient at assessing and managing medical problems (Krch-Cole, Lynch, Hughes and Naganiski, 1997).

Nurse practice acts do not specify whether floating is acceptable, and some professional nursing organizations believe a nurse should have the right to refuse to float (Davidhizar et al, 1998). However, if a hospital has a policy on floating, a nurse can be subject to disciplinary action for refusing the assignment.

Standards of nursing care defined in nurse practice acts are standards all nurses should follow to care safely for a client. If a nurse deviates from a standard and causes harm to the client, the nurse can be found guilty of negligence. If a nurse manager assigned a nurse to care for a client knowing she did not have the skills and competence to care for that client, this would be a deviation from the standard of care, and if the client was harmed because of this deviation from the standard, the nurse manager could be considered negligent (Showers, 1999).

There have been hospitals and health systems which have used float nurses to safely provide adequate staffing,

450

but measures must be taken to ensure success. The NIH Medical Center Nursing Department has developed guidelines for floating which include the following responsibilities for management and nursing staff:

- Orientation to the unit must be provided. Nurses must be shown the physical layout of the unit, the location of procedure manuals, and information regarding safety issues and unit rules.
- The nurse should be introduced to the other staff members and assigned a partner who will be a resource person and can assume the job responsibilities which the float nurse is not competent to do.
- Client assignments must be given according to the nurse's level of competence including generic nursing duties as well as documented clinical competence.
- The charge nurse should check on the float nurse regularly through the shift to provide support or assistance.
- The nurse manager/supervisor should complete an evaluation regarding the floating experience and provide feedback to the float nurse.
- The float nurse should communicate his/her level of competence to the charge nurse.
- The float nurse should work with the partner and express concerns or problems that assure support and direction.
- The float nurse should complete an evaluation form and obtain feedback from the nurse manager/supervisor (*http://www.cc.nih.gov/nursmg/allocnres.html*).

The Florida State Nurses Association has also developed guidelines for floating for the staff nurse. Before accepting the assignment, the Association recommends that the nurse consider the following:

- *Clarification.* Communicate with the charge person to be sure you understand the assignment. You need to know the acuity levels, the client workload, and what assistance will be available.
- *Assessment.* Examine your skill levels, knowledge, and experience to determine if this assignment will result in unsafe client care.

- *Option Identification.* If you feel you are capable of providing competent care, you should accept the assignment. If you feel you cannot safely provide care to the assigned clients, you should communicate this to the nurse manager/supervisor and request that other arrangements be made. It may be possible to accept part of the assignment or switch assignments with someone so all clients can be provided safe care (Kelter, 1994).

Reviewing the literature was an enlightening experience. I discovered that since most hospitals are faced with the problem of fluctuation in census and staffing, the issue of floating as a solution to this problem is a hot topic across the nation. The majority of nurses expressed similar fears of providing inadequate care and the majority of hospitals are in a quandary attempting to balance safety and quality with cost effectiveness. Floating can be successful but requires careful deliberation. Staff nurses, supervisors, and administrators need to recognize their responsibilities regarding this practice and need to be sensitive to each other's concerns. If these issues are addressed and policies are developed that are consistent with guidelines recommended by professional medical organizations, floating as a scheduling technique can be accomplished in a way that is both safe and beneficial to the client, the nurse, and the organization.

REFERENCES

Davidhizar, R., Dowd, I. B., and Brownson, K. (1998). An equitable nursing assignment structure. *Nurse Management*, 29(4):33–35.

Kelter, I. (1994). The ethical and legal implications of restructuring . . . floating without being properly trained. *American Nurse* 26(7):23.

Krch-Cole, E., Lynch, P., Hughes, J., and Naganiski, D.A. (1997). Bridging the chasm: Incorporating the medically compromised patient into psychiatric practice. *Psychosocial Nursing and Mental Health Services*, 36(3)28–32.

Showers, J. L. (1999). Protection from negligence lawsuits. *Nursing Management*, 30(9):23–26.

Outline

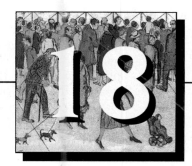

Mood Disorders: Depression

Elizabeth M. Varcarolis

Objectives

After studying this chapter, the reader will be able to

1. Compare and contrast major depression and dysthymia.

2. Discuss the links between the stress model of depression and the biological model of depression.

3. Assess behaviors for each of the following areas: (a) affect, (b) thought processes, (c) feelings, (d) physical behavior, (e) communication in a depressed individual at your clinical site.

4. Formulate five nursing diagnoses for a client who is depressed, and include outcome criteria.

5. Name unrealistic expectations that a nurse may have while working with a depressed person and compare them with your personal reactions.

6. Role-play six principles of communication that are useful with depressed clients.

7. Evaluate the advantages of using the selective serotonin reuptake inhibitors (SSRIs) rather than the tricyclic antidepressants.

8. Explain the uniqueness of two of the novel antidepressants in specific circumstances.

9. Develop a medication teaching plan for clients on the tricyclic antidepressants, including (a) common side effects, (b) adverse side effects, and (c) drugs that can trigger an adverse reaction.

10. Discuss two common side effects of the monoamine oxidase inhibitors, and state one serious adverse reaction identifying the appropriate medical intervention.

11. Write a medication teaching plan for a client on a monoamine oxidase inhibitor, including foods and drugs that are contraindicated with the use of that type of agent.

12. Recognize in what kinds of depressions electroconvulsive therapy is most helpful.

*N*o one is immune from brief depressive reactions. The term *depression* can mean many different things—from a major depressive episode, to bereavement, to loss of motivation secondary to brain disease (dementia). All races, all ages, males, females are susceptible to depressive episodes, although some are more susceptible than others.

PREVALENCE

Community prevalence of major depression in the USA is 3% to 5%, and the lifetime risk for depression is 5% to 12% for men and 10% and 25% for women, according to the *Diagnostic and Statistical Manual of Mental Disorders*, 4th edition, text revision (DSM-IV-TR) (APA 2000). Note that most studies do find that unipolar depression is twice as common in women as in men (Dubovsky and Buzan 1999). The prevalence rates for major depressive disorder appear unrelated to ethnicity, education, income or marital status (APA 2000). **Postpartum depression** occurs in about 10% of mothers. Children as young as 3 years of age have been diagnosed with depression. Major depressive disorder is said to occur in as many as 18% of preadolescents, perhaps a low estimate since depression in this age group is often underdiagnosed (Dubovsky and Buzan 1999). Children and adolescents between 9 and 17 years of age have a 6% prevalence of depression, with 4.9% having a major depression (NIMH 1999). Children whose families are depressed seem to become depressed earlier (ages 12 to 13 years) than children from families that are not depressed (16 to 17 years old) (Dubovsky and Buzan 1999). Major depression among adolescents is often associated with substance abuse and antisocial behavior, both of which can obscure accurate diagnosis (Kashani and Nair 1995).

Among the elderly, depression ranges from 3.5% in the community to 16% of those medically hospi-

talized, while nursing home prevalence is 15% to 20% (Dubovsky and Buzan 1999; Goldberg 1998). Depression can be as high as 40% in some older adult populations (Fuller and Sajalovic 2000).

Mixed anxiety-depression is perhaps one of the most common psychiatric presentations. Symptoms of anxiety occur in an average of 70% of cases of major depression. The prevalence of anxiety-depression is at least 5% of the population (Goldberg 1998).

COMORBIDITY

A depressive syndrome frequently accompanies other psychiatric disorders such as schizophrenia, substance abuse, eating disorders, and schizoaffective disorder. People with anxiety disorders often present with depression (as mentioned earlier) as well as people with personality disorders (PDs) (particularly borderline PD), adjustment disorder, and brief depressive reactions.

The problem of major depression greatly increases among people with a medical disorder. Chronic medical problems and a history of early abuse or trauma are considered relevant risk factors. Depression can also be secondary to a medical condition, mood disorders due to a general medical condition (Table 18–1), substance-induced mood disorder (from substances such as alcohol, cocaine, marijuana, heroin, and anxiolytics), and even prescription medication (Table 18–2). Depression is frequently an expected sequela of bereavement and grief. See Chapter 30 for end-of-life issues and bereavement.

DEPRESSIVE DISORDERS AND CLINICAL PRESENTATIONS

Figure 18–1 presents the two DSM-IV-TR depressive disorders (major depression and dysthymia), possible presenting symptoms and other clinical phenomena. Also see Table 18–3.

Major Depressive Disorder

Clients with a major depressive disorder experience substantial pain and suffering, as well as psychological, social, and occupational disability, during the depression. A client with a major depressive disorder presents with a history of one or more major depressive episodes and no history of manic or hypomanic episodes. In a major depression, the symp-

TABLE 18-1 *Medical Disorders Associated with Depressive Syndromes*	
SYNDROME	**DISORDERS**
Neurologic	Dementias, hydrocephalus, Huntington's chorea, infectious (including HIV, neurosyphilis), migraines, multiple sclerosis, myasthenia gravis, Parkinson's disease, seizure disorders, stroke, trauma, tumors, vasculitis, Wilson's disease
Endocrine	Addison's disease, Cushing's syndrome, diabetes mellitus, hyperparathyroidism, hyperthyroidism, hypoparathyroidism, hypothyroidism, menses-related depression, postpartum depression
Metabolic/nutritional	Folate deficiency, hypercalcemia, hypocalcemia, hyponatremia, pellagra, porphyria, uremia, vitamin B_{12} deficiency
Infectious/inflammatory	Influenza, hepatitis, mononucleosis, pneumonia, rheumatoid arthritis, Sjögren's disease, systemic lupus erythematosus, tuberculosis
Other	Anemias, cardiopulmonary disease, neoplasms (including gastrointestinal, lung, pancreatic), sleep apnea

Data from Mulner, K. K., Florence, T., and Glick, R. L. (1999). Mood and anxiety syndromes in emergency psychiatry. *Psychiatric Clinics of North America,* 22(4):761.

toms often interfere with the person's social or occupational functioning and in some cases may include psychotic features. Delusional or psychotic major depression is a severe form of mood disorder that is characterized by delusions or hallucinations. For example, clients might have delusional thoughts that interfere with their nutritional status (e.g., "God put snakes in my stomach and told me not to eat").

The emotional, cognitive, physical, and behavioral symptoms an individual exhibits during a major depressive episode represent a change in the person's usual functioning. See Figure 18-1 for DSM-IV-TR criteria for major depressive disorder and dysthymic disorder.

The course of major depressive disorder is variable. At least 60% of people can expect to have a second episode. Individuals who have experienced two episodes of major depression are 70% as likely to have a third. Those who have had three episodes have a 90% chance of future episodes (APA 2000).

Dysthymia

Dysthymia often has an early and insidious onset and is characterized by a chronic depressive syndrome that is usually present for most of the day, more days than not, for at least 2 years (APA 2000). The depressive mood disturbance, because of its chronic nature, cannot be distinguished from the person's usual pattern of functioning, such as "I've always been this way" (APA 2000). Because the individual has minimal social and occupational impairment, hospitalization is rarely necessary unless the person becomes suicidal. The age of onset is usually from early childhood-teenage years to early adulthood. Clients with dysthymia are at risk for developing major depressive episodes as well as other psychiatric disorders.

Differentiating a major depression from dysthymic disorder can be difficult because the disorders have similar symptoms. The main differences are in the duration and the severity of the symptoms (APA 2000).

TABLE 18-2 *Medications and Substances Associated with Depressive Syndromes*	
SYNDROME/ SUBSTANCES	**MEDICATIONS**
Neurologic/psychiatric	Amantadine, anticholinesterases, antipsychotics, baclofen, barbiturates, benzodiazepines, bromocriptine, carbamazepine, chloral hydrate, disulfiram, ethosuximide, levodopa, phenytoin
Antibacterial/antifungal	Ampicillin, griseofulvin, metronidazole, nalidixic acid, trimethoprim
Anti-inflammatory/analgesic	Corticosteroids, indomethacin, opiates, sulindac
Antineoplastic	Asparaginase, azothioprine, bleomycin, hexamethylamine, vincristine, vinblastine
Cardiovascular	Clonidine, digitalis, guanethidine, methyldopa, propanolol, reserpine
Gastrointestinal	Cimetidine, ranitidine
Other	Alcohol, caffeine, oral contraceptives, stimulant withdrawal

Data from Mulner, K. K., Florence, T., and Glick, R. L. (1999). Mood and anxiety syndromes in emergency psychiatry. *Psychiatric Clinics of North America,* 22(4):761.

DSM-IV-TR CRITERIA FOR DEPRESSION

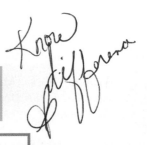

DEPRESSIVE DISORDERS

MAJOR DEPRESSION DISORDER

1. Represents a change in previous functions.

2. Symptoms cause clinically significant distress or impair social, occupational, or other important areas of functioning.

3. **Five or more** of the following occur nearly every day for most waking hours over the same 2-week period:
   • Depressed mood most of day, nearly every day
   • Anhedonia
   • Significant weight loss or gain (more than 5% of body weight in 1 month)
   • Insomnia or hypersomnia
   • Increased or decreased motor activity
   • Anergia (fatigue or loss of energy)
   • Feelings of worthlessness or inappropriate guilt (may be delusional)
   • Decreased concentration or indecisiveness
   • Recurrent thoughts of death or suicidal ideation (with or without plan)

DYSTHYMIA

1. Occurs over a 2-year period (1 year for children and adolescents), depressed mood.

2. Symptoms cause clinically significant distress in social, occupational, and other important areas of functioning.

3. Presence of **two or more** of the following:
   • Decreased or increased appetite
   • Insomnia or hypersomnia
   • Low energy or chronic fatigue
   • Decreased self-esteem
   • Poor concentration or difficulty making decisions
   • Feelings of hopelessness or despair

SPECIFIERS DESCRIBING MOST RECENT EPISODE

1. **Chronic.**

2. **Atypical features.**

3. **Catatonic features.**

4. **Melancholic features.**

5. **Postpartum onset.**

SPECIFY IF

1. Early onset (before 21 years old).

2. Late onset (21 years or older).

3. Atypical features.

Figure 18–1 DSM-IV-TR criteria for major depression and dysthymia. (Adapted from American Psychiatric Association. [2000]. *Diagnostic and statistical manual of mental disorders.* [4th ed., text revision]. Washington, D.C.: American Psychiatric Press).

Subtypes

The diagnosis of major depressions may include a specifier in clients with specific symptoms. Specifiers include

■ Psychotic features
■ Catatonic features
■ Melancholic features
■ Postpartum onset
■ Seasonal affective patterns (generally related to fall or winter and remitting in the spring) **(SAD)**
■ Atypical

THEORY

Although many theories attempt to explain the cause of depression, many psychological, biological, and cultural variables make identification of any one cause difficult. It is unlikely that there is a single cause for depression. It is becoming evident that depression is a heterogeneous systemic illness involving an array of different neurotransmitters, neurohormones, and neuronal pathways (Sadek and Nemeroff 2000). The idea that depression is the result of a simple hereditary process or traumatic life

TABLE 18–3 *Depressive Disorders: Specifiers and Clinical Phenomena*

DISORDER	DSM-IV-TR STATUS	SYMPTOMS AND COMMENTS
Major Depression (MDD)	Disorder	Specific DSM-IV-TR criteria outlined in Figure 18–1. Symptoms represent a change from usual functioning. Associated with high mortality rate. Increases in physical, social, and role functioning, as well as pain, and physical illness
with psychotic features	Specifier	Indicates the presence of delusions (guilt, being punished for sins), somatic (horrible disease or body rotting), poverty (going bankrupt), or hallucinations (usually auditory, voices berating person for sins or shortcomings)
with postpartum onset	Specifier	Occurs within 4 weeks after childbirth Can present with or without psychotic features. **Severe ruminations or delusional thoughts about infant signifies increase risk of harm to the infant**
with seasonal characteristics (SAD)	Specifier	Mostly, episodes begin in fall of winter and remit in spring. Characterized by anergia, hypersomnia, overeating, weight gain, and a craving for carbohydrates. Responds to light therapy
with chronic features	Specifier	MDD lasting 2 years or more
Dysthymia Disorder (DD)	Disorder	Specific DSM-IV-TR criteria presented in Figure 18–1. DD has an early and insidious onset (childhood to early adult). DD has a chronic course. 75% of people with DD go on to an MDD. When dysthymia is superimposed on a major depression it is called **double depression**
DD and MDD *with* Atypical Features	Specifier	Mood reactivity (can be cheered with positive events); rejection sensitivity (pathological sensitivity to perceived interpersonal rejection) presents through life and results in functional impairment. Also hypersomnia, hyperphagia (overeating), leaden paralysis (feeling weighed down in extremities), and so forth
Mixed anxiety-depression	RDC	Prevalence (5%). Significant functional disability. Criteria includes at least 1 month of persistent dysphoric mood, with possible hypervigilance, difficulty concentrating, fatigue, low self-esteem, irritability, and more, all causing **significant impairment/distress in functioning**
Recurrent brief depression	RDC	Meets criteria for depressive episode, but episodes last 1 day to 1 week. Depressive episode must recur at least once per month over 12 months or more. **Carries a high rate for suicide**
Premenstrual dysphoric disorder	RDC	More severe symptoms than premenstrual syndrome. Symptoms begin toward last week of luteal phase and are absent in the week following menses. Symptoms include depressed mood, anxiety, affective lability, or persistent and marked anger or irritability. Other symptoms include anergia, overeating, difficulty concentrating, feeling out of control/overwhelmed, and more
Minor depression	RDC	Sustained depressed mood without the full depressive syndrome. Pessimistic attitude and self-pity are required for the diagnosis (Dubovsky and Buzan 1999). Minor depressive disorder may be chronic and may be complicated by a superimposed major depressive episode

RDC, research diagnostic category; MDD, major depression disorder; SAD, seasonal affective disorder.

event that ultimately leads to a single neurotransmitter deficiency is simply unsubstantiated by the evidence (Sadek and Nemeroff 2000). Depression may result from a complex interaction between genetic predisposition to the illness and early untoward life events that ultimately lead to significant changes in the central nervous system (CNS). Four common theories of depression are discussed here: (1) biological, (2) psychodynamic influences and life events, (3) cognitive, and (4) learned helplessness.

Biological Theories

Genetic Theories

Twin studies consistently show that genetic factors play a role in the development of depressive disorders. Various studies reveal that the average concordance rate for mood disorders among monozygotic twins (twins sharing the same genetic structure) is 45% to 60%. The percentage for dizygotic twins (separate genetic structure) is 12%. Thus, identical twins (monozygotic) have a fivefold greater concordance rate than dizygotic twins (Merikangas and Kupfer 1995).

Thase (1999) pointed out that mood disorders are heritable for some people. Increased heritability is associated with an earlier age of onset, greater comorbidity, and increased risk of recurrent illness. However, any genetic factors that are present must interact with environmental factors for the development of depression (Dubovsky and Buzan 1999). Stressful life events, especially losses, seem to be a significant factor (Kendler et al 1993).

Biochemical Factors

The brain is a highly complex organ that contains billions of neurons. There is much evidence to support that depression is a biologically heterogeneous disorder; that is, many CNS neurotransmitter abnormalities can probably cause clinical depression. These neurotransmitter abnormalities may be the result of inherited or environmental factors, or even other medical conditions, such as cerebral infarction, hypothyroidism, acquired immunodeficiency syndrome (AIDS), and drug use. Therefore, specific neurotransmitters in the brain are believed to be related to altered mood states. Initially it was believed that the two main neurotransmitters were **serotonin** (5-hydroxytryptamine [5-HT]) and **norepinephrine.** Serotonin is an important regulator of sleep, appetite, and libido. A serotonin circuit dysfunction could result in poor impulse control, low sex drive, decreased appetite, and irritability (Sadek and Nemeroff 2000). Decreased levels of norepine-

phrine in the medical forebrain bundle may account for anergia, anhedonia, decreased concentration, and diminished libido in depression (Thase 1999). However, it is now considered unlikely that a catecholamine deficiency alone is the actual cause of depression.

Presently, however, it seems depression results from the dysregulation of a number of neurotransmitter systems in addition to serotonin and norepinephrine. The dopamine, acetylcholine, and gamma-aminobutyric acid systems are also believed to be involved in the pathophysiology of a major depressive episode (APA 2000).

Norepinephrine, serotonin, and acetylcholine also play a role in stress regulation. When these neurotransmitters become overtaxed through stressful events, neurotransmitter depletion may occur.

At this stage, no unitary mechanism of antidepressant action has been found. The relationships among the serotonin, norepinephrine, dopamine, acetylcholine, and gamma-aminobutyric acid systems are complex and need further assessment and research. However, treatment with medication has proved empirically successful for many clients. Figure 18–2 shows a positron-emission tomographic (PET) scan of the brain of a woman before and after taking medication. Refer to Chapter 3 (Fig. 3–6) for comparison of a PET scan of an individual when depressed and nondepressed.

Alterations in Hormonal Regulation

Although neuroendocrine findings are as yet inconclusive, the neuroendocrine symptom most widely studied in relation to depression has been hyperac-

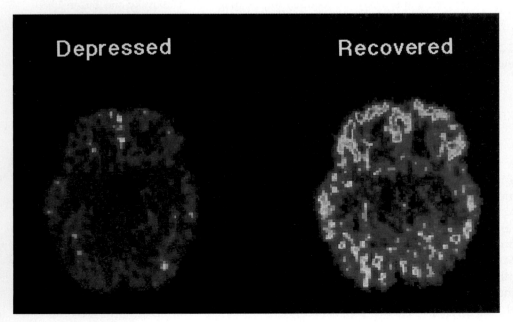

Figure 18–2 Positron-emission tomography (PET) scans of a 45-year-old woman with recurrent depression. The scan on the left was taken when she was on no medication and very depressed. The scan on the right was taken several months later when she was well, after she had been treated with medication for her depression. Note that her entire brain is more active when well, particularly the left prefrontal cortex. (From Mark George, MD, Biological Psychiatry Branch, National Institute of Mental Health.)

tivity of the cortical-hypothalamic-pituitary-adrenal axis. Evidence of increased cortisol secretion is apparent in 20% to 40% of depressed outpatients and 40% to 60% of depressed inpatients (Thase 1999). Dexamethasone, an exogenous steroid that suppresses cortisol, is used in the dexamethasone suppression test for depression. Results of the dexamethasone suppression test are abnormal in about 50% of depressed clients, indicating hyperactivity of the cortical-hypothalamic-pituitary-adrenal axis. However, the findings of this test may also be abnormal in people with obsessive-compulsive disorders and other medical conditions. Significantly, clients with psychotic major depression are among those with the highest rates of nonsuppression of cortisol on the dexamethasone suppression test.

Sleep Abnormalities

Sleep electroencephalogram abnormalities may be evident in 40% to 60% of outpatients and up to 90% of inpatients with a major depressive episode (APA 2000). People prone to depression tend to have a premature loss of deep, slow (delta) wave sleep and rapid eye movement (REM) latency. The phase of REM sleep associated with dreaming occurs earlier in two thirds of clients with bipolar and major depressive illnesses. This sign is referred to as **REM latency**, consistent with the expected behavior of an inherited trait. Reduced REM latency and deficits of slow wave sleep typically persist following recovery from a depressed episode (Thase 1999). Data also suggest that depressed clients without this sign are not likely to respond to tricyclic antidepressant (TCA) therapy, which suppresses early REM sleep. A study by Lauer and associates (1995) demonstrated that about 20% of nondepressed individuals who had at least one first-degree relative with a mood disorder had depression-like sleep patterns. Further follow-up studies may determine if specific sleep abnormalities do, indeed, represent a biological marker for vulnerability to depression.

Psychodynamic Influences and Life Events

The stress-diathesis model of depression in contemporary psychodynamic approaches to mood disorders takes into account the strong biological underpinnings of depression and bipolar disorder (Gabband 1999). What is almost certain is that psychosocial stressors and interpersonal events appear to trigger certain neurophysical and neurochemical changes in the brain (Gabband 1999). Early life trauma may result in long-term hyperactivity of the

CNS corticotropin-releasing factor (CRF) and norepinephrine systems with a consequent neurotoxic effect on the hippocampus that leads to neuronal loss. These changes could cause sensitization of the CRF circuits to even mild stress in adulthood, leading to an exaggerated stress response (Heim and Nemeroff 1999). With exposure to repeated stress in adulthood, these already stress-sensitive pathways become "markedly hyperactive leading to a persistent increase in CRF and cortisol secretion, which causes alterations in the glucocorticoid receptors and thus forms the basis for the development of mood and anxiety disorders" (Sadek and Nemeroff, 2000).

These stressors and life events may lead to a depressive syndrome in some individuals, particularly those who are biologically vulnerable to depression. Therefore, life events (psychosocial stressors and interpersonal events) may influence the development and recurrence of depression through the psychological and biological experience of stress in some people. Major depression following a stressful life event is no less likely to require or benefit from antidepressant medication than other depressive episodes. A relationship between a major life stressor (loss) and a major depressive disorder may be a good indicator for specific psychotherapy as well as psychopharmacology (APA 2000).

Cognitive Theory

Aaron T. Beck, one of the early proponents of cognitive therapy, applied the cognitive behavior theory to depression. Beck proposed that people acquire a psychological predisposition to depression through early life experiences. These experiences contribute to negative, illogical, and irrational thought processes that may remain dormant until they are activated during times of stress (Beck and Rush 1995). Beck found that depressed persons process information in negative ways, even in the midst of positive factors that affect the person's life. Beck believes three automatic negative thoughts are responsible for people becoming depressed. These three thoughts are called **Beck's cognitive triad.** They are

1. A negative, self-deprecating view of self
2. A pessimistic view of the world
3. The belief that negative reinforcement (or no validation for the self) will continue in the future

The phrase *automatic negative thoughts* refers to thoughts that are repetitive, unintended, and not readily controllable (Haaga and Beck 1992). This cognitive triad seems to be consistent in all depressions, regardless of clinical subtype.

The goal of cognitive behavior therapy is to change the way clients think and thus relieve the depressive syndrome. This is accomplished by assisting the client in the following:

1. Identifying and testing negative cognition
2. Developing alternative thinking patterns
3. Rehearsing new cognitive and behavioral responses

Cognitive therapy has been remarkably successful with acutely depressed individuals and is associated with a significantly lower rate of relapse (Hallon and Fawcett 1995).

Learned Helplessness

One of the most popular theories of the cause of depression is Martin Seligman's theory of learned helplessness. Seligman (1973) stated that although anxiety is the initial response to a stressful situation, anxiety is replaced by depression if the person feels that the self has no control over the outcome of a situation. A person who believes that an undesired event is his or her fault and that nothing can be done to change it is prone to depression. The theory of learned helplessness has been used to help explain the development of depression in certain social groups, such as the aged, people living in ghettos, and women.

A study by Gulesserian and Warren (1987) found data supporting the theory that "depression is linked with poor adaptational/coping abilities that may lead to learned helplessness, panic, and depression." The lack of the following specific coping skills appeared to increase the likelihood of depression: social supports, tension reduction skills, and effective problem-solving skills. The behavioral therapeutic approach helps individuals gain a sense of control and mastery of the environment by teaching depressed individuals new and more effective coping skills and ways to increase their self-confidence.

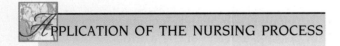

APPLICATION OF THE NURSING PROCESS

ASSESSMENT

Overall Assessment

Since depression can mean so many different things, Goldberg (1998) suggested an evaluation starting with depressive symptoms, then assessing possible cause and past episodes. Goldberg (1998) suggested

using the assessment tool in Figure 18–3 when assessing depressive symptoms.

ASSESSMENT TOOLS

There are numerous standardized screening instruments that help the clinician assess the type of depression a person may be experiencing. For example, the Beck Depression Inventory, the Hamilton Depression Scale, and the Geriatric Depression Scale all are valuable tools. The Zung Depression Scale is a short inventory that highlights predominant symptoms seen in depressed individuals and is presented here for its ease of use (Table 18–4).

The National Mental Health Association (NMHA) has launched **http://www.depression-screening.org,**

Initial Assessment Guide	
Depressive symptoms	**Duration**
Depressed mood	_____
Decreased energy	_____
Poor concentration	_____
Sleep change	_____
Appetite change	_____
Psychomotor change	_____
Guilt, poor self-esteem	_____
Anhedonia	_____
Suicidality	_____
Chronic pain	_____
Poor functional level	_____
Somatized symptoms	_____

Accompanying symptoms

Delusions	Panic attacks	Mania
Hallucinations	Generalized anxiety	

Possible precipitants

_____
_____
_____

Possible medical causes

_____
_____
_____

Past episodes

_____
_____
_____

From Goldberg, R. J. (1998). The care of the psychiatric patient. St. Louis: Mosby.

Figure 18–3 Initial assessment guide.

TABLE 18-4 *Nursing Assessment: Zung's Self-Rating Depression Scale**

	NONE OR LITTLE OF THE TIME	SOME OF THE TIME	A GOOD PART OF THE TIME	MOST OR ALL OF THE TIME
1. I feel down-hearted, blue, and sad.	1	2	3	4
2. Morning is when I feel the best.	4	3	2	1
3. I have crying spells or feel like it.	1	2	3	4
4. I have trouble sleeping through the night.	1	2	3	4
5. I eat as much as I used to.	4	3	2	1
6. I enjoy looking at, talking to, and being with attractive women/men.	4	3	2	1
7. I notice that I am losing weight.	1	2	3	4
8. I have trouble with constipation.	1	2	3	4
9. My heart beats faster than usual.	1	2	3	4
10. I get tired for no reason.	1	2	3	4
11. My mind is as clear as it used to be.	4	3	2	1
12. I find it easy to do the things I used to do.	4	3	2	1
13. I am restless and can't keep still.	1	2	3	4
14. I feel hopeful about the future.	4	3	2	1
15. I am more irritable than usual.	1	2	3	4
16. I find it easy to make decisions.	4	3	2	1
17. I feel that I am useful and needed.	4	3	2	1
18. My life is pretty full.	4	3	2	1
19. I feel that others would be better off if I were dead.	1	2	3	4
20. I still enjoy the things I used to do.	4	3	2	1

* A raw score of 50 or above is associated with depression requiring hospital treatment.
From Zung, W. K. (1965). A self-rating depression scale. *Archives of General Psychiatry*, 12:63. Copyright 1965, American Medical Association.

a new website enabling people to take a confidential screening test online for depression and find reliable information on the illness. The website's mission is threefold:

1. To educate people about depression
2. To offer a simple and confidential way for people to get screened for the illness
3. To guide people toward appropriate professional help when necessary

SAFETY FIRST

Evaluate for suicidal/homicidal ideation. About 10% to 15% of depressed people eventually commit suicide (Fuller and Sajatovic 2000). Initial suicide evaluation (Goldberg 1998) might include the following statements:

■ "You have said you are depressed. Tell me what that is like for you."
■ "When you feel depressed, what thoughts go through your mind?"
■ "Have you gone so far as to think about taking your own life?" "Do you have a plan?" "Do you have the means to carry out your plan?" "Is there

anything that would prevent you from carrying out your plan?"

Refer to Chapter 23 for suicide and strategies for suicide prevention. However, Box 18-1 gives the reader some critical risk factors and warning signs to assess in depressed individuals.

KEY FINDINGS

A depressed mood and anhedonia (an inability to find meaning or pleasure in existence) are the key symptoms in depression. Almost 97% of people with depression have anergia (reduction in or lack of energy). Anxiety, a common symptom in depression, is seen in about 60% of clients (Zajecka 1995).

When people are depressed, their thinking is slow, and their memory and concentration are usually affected. Depressed people dwell on and exaggerate their perceived faults and failures and are unable to focus on their strengths and successes. A person with major depression may experience delusions of being punished for doing bad deeds or being a terrible person. Feelings of worthlessness, guilt, anger, and helplessness are common. Psychomotor agitation may be evidenced by constant pac-

Box 18–1 *Risk Factors for Suicide Intent*

Risk factors for suicide include

- Previous suicide attempts
- Close family member who has committed suicide
- Past psychiatric hospitalization
- Recent losses—this may include the death of a relative, a family divorce, or a breakup with a girlfriend
- Social isolation—the individual does not have social alternatives or skills to find alternatives to suicide
- Drug or alcohol abuse—drugs decrease impulse control making impulsive suicide more likely. Additionally, some individuals try to self-medicate their depression with drugs or alcohol
- Exposure to violence in the home or the social environment—the individual sees violent behavior as a viable solution to life problems
- Handguns in the home, especially if loaded
- Age: teens, males older than 45 years of age, elderly

Warning signs include

- Suicidal talk
- Preoccupation with death and dying
- Signs of depression
- Behavioral changes
- Giving away special possessions and making arrangements to take care of unfinished business
- Difficulty with appetite and sleep
- Taking excessive risks
- Increased drug use
- Loss of interest in usual activities

From www.baltimorepsych.com/suicide.htm

ing and wringing of hands. The slowed movements of **psychomotor retardation**, however, are more common. Somatic complaints (headaches, malaise, backaches) are also common. **Vegetative signs of depression** (change in bowel movements and eating habits, sleep disturbances, and disinterest in sex) are usually present.

AREAS TO ASSESS

AFFECT. A person who is depressed sees the world through gray-colored glasses. Posture is poor, and clients may look older than their stated age. Facial expressions convey sadness and dejection, and the client may have frequent bouts of weeping. Con-

versely, the client may say that he or she is unable to cry. Feelings of hopelessness and despair are readily reflected in the person's affect. Often the individual will not make eye contact, speaks in a monotone, shows little or no expressions (flat affect), and may only make yes or no responses. Frequent sighing is common.

THOUGHT PROCESSES. Identifying the presence of suicidal thoughts and suicide potential has the highest priority in the initial assessment. Approximately two thirds of depressed people contemplate suicide, and up to 15% of untreated or inadequately treated clients give up hope and kill themselves (Akiskal 1995). Asking a depressed person openly "Have you thought about killing yourself?" can encourage the expression of painful, pent-up feelings (see Chapter 23). The risk of suicide is not necessarily correlated with the severity of the symptoms. Although depressed persons can attempt suicide at any time, the highest mortality exists within a year of discharge from a psychiatric hospital (Litman 1992).

During the time a person is depressed, the person's ability to solve problems and think clearly is negatively affected. Judgment is poor, and indecisiveness is common. People claim that their mind is slowing down. Memory and concentration are poor. Evidence of delusional thinking may be seen in a major depression. Common statements of delusional thinking are "I have committed unpardonable sins," "God wants me dead," or "I am wicked and should die."

FEELINGS. Feelings frequently reported by depressed people include anxiety, worthlessness, guilt, helplessness and hopelessness, and anger. As previously mentioned, **anxiety** is present in about 60% of depressed persons. Feelings of **worthlessness** range from feeling inadequate to having an unrealistic evaluation of self-worth. These feelings reflect the low self-esteem that is a painful partner to depression. Statements such as "I am no good; I'll never amount to anything" are common. Themes of one's inadequacy and incompetence are repeated relentlessly.

Guilt is a common accompaniment to depression. A person may ruminate over present or past failings. Extreme guilt can assume psychotic proportions: "I have committed terrible sins. God is punishing me for my evil ways."

Helplessness is evidenced by the inability to carry out the simplest tasks. Everything is too difficult to accomplish (e.g., grooming, doing housework, working, caring for children). With feelings of helplessness come feelings of **hopelessness**. Even though most depressive states are usually time limited, during a depressed period, people believe that things will never change. This feeling of utter hopelessness can lead people to look at suicide as a way out of constant mental pain. An analysis of the concept of hopelessness by Campbell (1987) cited findings in the literature that identified hopelessness as one of the core characteristics of depression and suicide, as well as a characteristic of schizophrenia, alcoholism, and physical illness. Campbell identified the common cognitive and emotional components of hopelessness as having the following attributes:

- Negative expectations for the future
- Loss of control over future outcomes
- Passive acceptance of the futility of planning to achieve goals
- Emotional negativism, as expressed in despair, despondency, or depression

Anger and **irritability** are natural outcomes of profound feelings of helplessness. Anger in depression is often expressed inappropriately. For example, anger may be expressed in destruction of property, hurtful verbal attacks, or physical aggression toward others. However, in people who are depressed, anger may be directed toward the self, resulting in feelings of low self-esteem and worthlessness. An extreme example of turning aggression against the self is suicide. One biological view links low levels of serotonin with an increase in suicidal behavior and violence.

PHYSICAL BEHAVIOR. Lethargy and fatigue can result in psychomotor retardation. Movements are extremely slow, facial expressions are decreased, and gaze is fixed. The continuum in psychomotor retardation may range from slowed and difficult movements to complete inactivity and incontinence. At other times, the nurse may note psychomotor agitation. For example, clients may constantly pace, bite their nails, smoke, tap their fingers, or engage in some other tension-relieving activity. At these times, clients commonly feel fidgety and unable to relax.

Grooming, dress, and personal hygiene are markedly neglected. People who usually take pride in their appearance and dress may be poorly groomed, allowing themselves to look shabby and unkempt.

Vegetative signs of depression are universal. Vegetative signs refer to alterations in those activities necessary to support physical life and growth (eating, sleeping, elimination, sex). For example, **changes in eating patterns** are common. About 60% to 70% of people who are depressed report having anorexia; overeating occurs more often in dysthymia.

Changes in sleep patterns are a cardinal sign of depression. Often, people have insomnia, waking at 3 or 4 AM and staying awake, or sleeping only for short periods. The light sleep of a depressed person tends to prolong the agony of depression over a 24-hour period. Deep stages of sleep (3 and 4) are usually decreased or totally absent (Akiskal 1999).

For some, sleep is increased (hypersomnia) and provides an escape from painful feelings. This is more common in young depressed individuals or those with bipolar tendencies (Akiskal 1999). In any event, sleep is rarely restful or refreshing.

Changes in bowel habits are common. Constipation is seen most frequently in clients with psychomotor retardation. Diarrhea occurs less frequently, often in conjunction with psychomotor agitation.

Interest in sex declines (loss of libido) during depression. Some men experience impotence, which can further complicate marital and social relationships.

COMMUNICATION. A person who is depressed may speak very slowly. Their comprehension is slow. The lack of an immediate response by the client to a remark does not mean that the client has not heard or chooses not to reply: the client just needs a little more time to compose a reply. In extreme depression, however, a person may be mute.

Self-Assessment

Depressed clients often reject the overtures of the nurse and others. When they are depressed, people do not appear to respond to nursing interventions and they seem resistant to change. When this occurs, nurses can experience feelings of frustration, hopelessness, and annoyance. Nurses can alter these problematic responses by

- Recognizing any unrealistic expectations they have of themselves or the client
- Identifying feelings they are experiencing that originate with the client
- Understanding the part that neurotransmitters play in the precipitation and maintenance of a depressed mood

UNREALISTIC EXPECTATIONS OF SELF

Health care workers new to working with depressed individuals may have expectations of themselves and their clients that are not realistic, and problems result when these expectations are not met. Unmet expectations usually result in the nurse feeling anxious, hurt, angry, helpless, or incompetent. Unrealistic expectations of oneself and others may be held even by experienced health care workers, and this phenomenon contributes to staff burnout. Many of the nurse's expectations may not be conscious. However, when these expectations are made conscious and worked through with peers and more experienced clinicians (supervisors), more realistic expectations can be formed and attainable goals can be set. Realistic expectations of oneself and the client can decrease feelings of helplessness and can increase the nurse's self-esteem and therapeutic potential.

Unrealistic expectations are common, especially for nursing students and nurses who are new to the psychiatric setting.

CLIENT FEELINGS EXPERIENCED BY THE NURSE

Intense feelings of anxiety, frustration, annoyance, and helplessness may be experienced by the nurse, although the feelings may originate in the client. These feelings can be important diagnostic clues to the client's experience. Often, the nurse senses what the client is feeling through empathy.

When the nurse's feelings of annoyance, hopelessness, and anxiety are the result of empathetic communications with the client, the nurse can discuss these feelings with peers and supervisors to separate personal feelings from those originating in the client. If personal feelings are not recognized, named, and examined, withdrawal by the nurse is likely to occur. People naturally stay away from situations and persons that arouse feelings of frustration, annoyance, or intimidation. If the nurse has unresolved feelings of anger and depression, the complexity of the situation is compounded. There is no substitute for competent and supportive supervision to facilitate growth, both professionally and personally. Supervision by a more experienced clinician and sharing with peers help minimize feelings of confusion, frustration, and isolation and can increase therapeutic potential and self-esteem in the nurse.

Assessment Guidelines

ASSESSMENT GUIDELINES: DEPRESSION

1. A thorough medical and neurological examination helps determine if the depression is primary or secondary to another disorder. Depression is a mood that can be secondary to a host of medical or other psychiatric disorders, as well as medications. Essentially, the nurse evaluates if

   ■ The client is psychotic
   ■ The client has taken drugs or alcohol
   ■ Medical conditions are present
   ■ The client has a history of comorbid psychiatric syndrome (eating disorders, borderline, anxiety disorders)

2. Always evaluate the client's risk of harm to self or others. Overt hostility is highly correlated with suicide (see Chapter 23 for assessment of and interventions for dealing with suicidal ideation and suicide attempts)

3. Assess past history of depression, what happened, what worked and did not work

4. Assess support systems, family and significant others, and need for information and referrals

NURSING DIAGNOSIS

During the initial assessment, a high priority for the nurse is identification of the presence of suicide potential. Therefore, the nursing diagnosis of **risk for self-directed violence** should always be considered. Table 18–5 identifies signs and symptoms commonly experienced in depression and offers potential nursing diagnoses.

OUTCOME CRITERIA

Outcome criteria and short-term goals are formulated for each nursing diagnosis. Each client is different, and goals are devised according to each person's individual needs. When possible, the nurse and client discuss desired outcomes of health care interventions. Outcome criteria are identified, and concrete, measurable steps are formulated as short-term goals. Depression is complex. Depressed individuals present with a variety of needs. Therefore, nursing diagnoses are many. Table 18–6 outlines outcome criteria from the Nursing Outcomes Classification (Johnson et al. 2000).

Outcome criteria for any of the vegetative or physical signs of depression should be formulated such that they show evidence of weight gain, return to normal bowel activity, duration of sleep of 6 to 8 hours per night, or return of sexual desire.

For an individual whose work and interpersonal relationships have been negatively affected during the depressive episode, the ability to use previous adaptive coping skills would be an important outcome criteria. For a family in which altered family processes have occurred, the outcome criteria would be resumption of previously satisfying and desired family coping behaviors.

PLANNING

Planning care for people with depression is geared toward the phase of depression the person is in and the particular symptoms the person is exhibiting. At all times, the nurse and all members of the health care team are cognizant of the potential for suicide, and assessment of self-harm (or harm to others) is ongoing during the care of the depressed person. We know that a combination of therapy (cognitive, interpersonal, and other) and psychopharmacology is an effective approach to the treatment of this disease—depression—that robs individuals of their quality of life. The nurse is aware that the vegetative signs of depression (changes in eating, sleeping, sexual satisfaction, etc.) often need targeting, as well as changes in concentration, activity level, social inter-

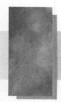

TABLE 18–5 *Potential Nursing Diagnosis for Depression*

SIGNS AND SYMPTOMS	POTENTIAL NURSING DIAGNOSES
Previous suicidal attempts, putting affairs in order, giving away prized possessions, suicidal ideation (has plan, ability to carry it out), makes overt or covert statements regarding killing self, feelings of worthlessness, hopelessness, helplessness	Risk for violence: self-directed Risk for self-mutilation
Lack of judgment, memory difficulty, concentration poor, inaccurate interpretation of environment, negative ruminations, cognitive distortions	Disturbed thought processes
Difficulty with simple tasks, inability to function at previous level, poor problem solving, poor cognitive functioning, verbalizations of inability to cope	Ineffective coping Interrupted family processes Risk for impaired parent/infant/child attachment Ineffective role performance Decisional conflict
Difficulty making decisions, poor concentration, inability to take action	
Feelings of helplessness, hopelessness, powerlessness	Hopelessness Powerlessness
Questions meaning of life, own existence, unable to participate in usual religious practices, conflict over spiritual beliefs, anger toward spiritual deity or religious representatives	Spiritual distress
Feelings of worthlessness, poor self-image, negative sense of self, self-negating verbalizations, feels like a failure, expressions of shame or guilt, hypersensitive to slights or criticism	Chronic low self-esteem Situational low self-esteem
Withdrawn, noncommunicative, speaks only in monosyllables, shies away from contact with others	Impaired social interaction Social isolation Risk for loneliness
Vegetative signs of depression: changes in sleeping, eating, grooming and hygiene, elimination, sexual patterns	Self-care deficit (bathing/hygiene, dressing/grooming) Imbalanced nutrition: less than body requirements Disturbed sleep pattern Constipation Sexual dysfunction

action, care for personal appearance, and so on. Therefore, planning care for a client who is depressed is based on the individual's symptoms and attempts to encompass a variety of areas in the person's life. Safety is always the highest priority.

INTERVENTION

Recovery from depression can be conceptualized as a process. Kupfer (1991) identified the following three phases in the treatment of and recovery from a major depression:

1. Acute (6 to 12 weeks)
2. Continuation (4 to 9 months)
3. Maintenance (1 or more years)

During the acute phase, hospitalization may be necessary. With the advent of managed care, lengthy hospital stays have been greatly decreased.

The **acute phase** includes psychiatric management (e.g., suicidal concerns) and participation in the initial treatment (pharmacology, psychotherapy, electroconvulsive therapy [ECT], light therapy).

The **continuation phase** is continuation of medication to prevent relapse. There is growing evidence to support the use of specific psychotherapy during the continuation phase (APA 2000).

The **maintenance phase** treatment includes a continuation of full-dose antidepressants used during the acute and intermediate phase to prevent relapse.

Counseling and Communication Strategies

Nurses often have great difficulty communicating with a client without talking. However, some depressed clients are so withdrawn that they are unwilling or unable to speak. Just sitting with a client in silence may seem like a waste of time to the nurse. Often, the nurse becomes uncomfortable not doing something, and, as anxiety increases, the nurse may start daydreaming, feel bored, remember something that "must be done now," and so on. It is important to be aware that this time spent together can be meaningful to the depressed person, especially if the nurse has a genuine interest in learning about the depressed individual.

Vignette

■ Doris, a senior nursing student, is working with a depressed, suicidal, withdrawn woman. The instructor notices in the second week that Doris spends a lot of time talking with other students and their clients and little time with her own client. In postconference, Doris acknowledges feeling threatened and useless and says that she wants a client

TABLE 18−6 *Depression Control*: Nursing Outcomes Classification*

DEPRESSIVE CONTROL INDICATORS	NEVER DEMON-STRATED 1	RARELY DEMON-STRATED 2	SOMETIMES DEMON-STRATED 3	OFTEN DEMON-STRATED 4	CONSISTENTLY DEMON-STRATED 5
1. Monitors ability to concentrate	1	2	3	4	5
2. Monitors intensity of depression	1	2	3	4	5
3. Identifies precursors of depression	1	2	3	4	5
4. Plans strategies to reduce effects of precursors	1	2	3	4	5
5. Behavioral manifestations of depression absent	1	2	3	4	5
6. Reports adequate sleep	1	2	3	4	5
7. Reports improved libido	1	2	3	4	5
8. Reports absence of physical manifestations of depression	1	2	3	4	5
9. Reports improved mood	1	2	3	4	5
10. Maintains stable weight	1	2	3	4	5
11. Follows treatment plan	1	2	3	4	5
12. Takes medication as prescribed	1	2	3	4	5
13. Follows exercise plan	1	2	3	4	5
14. Adheres to therapy schedule	1	2	3	4	5
15. Reports changes in symptoms	1	2	3	4	5
16. Decreases use of alcohol	1	2	3	4	5
17. Decreases use of non-prescribed drugs	1	2	3	4	5
18. Maintains personal hygiene and grooming	1	2	3	4	5
19. Other _____ (Specify)	1	2	3	4	5

Definition: Personal actions to minimize melancholy and maintain interest in life events.
From Johnson, H., Maas, M., Meriden, M., and Moorehead, S. (2000). *Nursing outcomes classification (NOC)*, (2nd ed.). St. Louis: Mosby.

who will interact with her. *After reviewing the symptoms of depression, its behavioral manifestations, and the needs of depressed persons, Doris turns her attention back to her client and spends time rethinking her plan of care. After 4 weeks of sharing her feelings in postconferences, working with her instructor, and trying a variety of approaches with her client, Doris is rewarded. On the day of discharge, the client tells Doris how important their time together was for her:* "I actually felt someone cared."

It is difficult to say when a withdrawn or depressed person will be able to respond. However, certain techniques are known to be useful in guiding effective nursing interventions. Some communication techniques are listed in Table 18−7 for a severely withdrawn client. Counseling guidelines for depressed persons are offered in Table 18−8.

Health Teaching

Health teaching is done with both clients and their families. It is important for both to understand that depression is a legitimate medical illness over which the client has no voluntary control. Depressed clients and their families need to learn about the biological symptoms of depression, as well as about the psychosocial and cognitive changes in depression. Review of the medications, side effects, and toxic effects helps families evaluate clinical change and stay alert for reactions that might affect client compliance. The section Psychobiological Interventions provides information on the side effects of antidepressants and specific areas to be covered in client and family teaching.

When a client has been hospitalized and is leaving the hospital, predischarge counseling should be performed with the client and the client's relatives. One

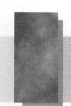

TABLE 18–7 *Communication Guidelines with Severely Depressed Persons*

INTERVENTION	RATIONALE
1. When a client is mute, use the technique *making observations:* "There are many new pictures on the wall" or "You are wearing your new shoes."	1. When a client is not ready to talk, direct questions can raise the client's anxiety level and frustrate the nurse. Pointing to commonalities in the environment draws the client into, and reinforces, reality.
2. Use simple, concrete words.	2. Slowed thinking and difficulty concentrating impair comprehension.
3. Allow time for the client to respond.	3. Slowed thinking necessitates time to formulate a response.
4. Listen for covert messages and ask about suicide plans.	4. People often experience relief and decrease in feelings of isolation when they share thoughts of suicide.
5. *Avoid platitudes,* such as "Things will look up" or "Everyone gets down once in a while."	5. Platitudes tend to minimize the client's feelings and can increase feelings of guilt and worthlessness because the client cannot "look up" or "snap out of it."

purpose of this counseling is to clarify the interpersonal stresses and discuss steps that can alleviate tension for the family system. Predischarge counseling can be performed by the psychiatrist, the psychiatric nurse clinician, or the psychiatric social worker. Including families in discharge planning can bring about the following results:

■ Increase the family's understanding and acceptance of the depressed family member during the aftercare period
■ Increase the client's use of aftercare facilities in the community
■ Contribute to higher overall adjustment in the client after discharge

Self-Care Activities

A depressed person may report having many physical complaints. Depressed clients suffer from intense feelings of hopelessness, despair, low self-worth, and fatigue. Therefore, the nurse and family often notice signs and symptoms of physical neglect.

Nursing measures for improving physical well-being and promoting adequate self-care are then initiated. Some effective interventions targeting the physical needs of the depressed client are listed in Table 18–9. Nurses in the community can work with family members to encourage a depressed family member to perform and maintain his or her health care needs.

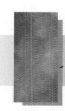

TABLE 18–8 *Counseling Guidelines for Depressed Persons*

INTERVENTION	RATIONALE
1. Help client question underlying assumptions and beliefs and consider alternate explanations to problems.	1. Reconstructing a healthier and more hopeful attitude about the future can alter depressed mood.
2. Work with the client to identify cognitive distortions that encourage negative self-appraisal. For example: a. Overgeneralizations b. Self-blame c. Mind reading d. Discounting positive attributes	2. Cognitive distortions reinforce negative, inaccurate perception of self and world. a. Taking one fact or event and making a general rule out of it ("He always"; "I never"). b. Consistent self-blame for everything perceived as negative. c. Assuming others don't like you, and so forth, without any real evidence that assumptions are correct. d. Focusing on negative.
3. Encourage activities that can raise self-esteem. Identify need for (a) problem-solving skills, (b) coping skills, and (c) assertiveness skills.	3. Many depressed people, especially women, are not taught with range of problem solving and coping skills. Increase social, family and job skills can change negative self-assessment.
4. Encourage exercise, running and/or weight lifting.	4. Can improve self-concept and potentially shift neurochemical balance.
5. Encourage forming of supportive relationships, such as support groups, therapy, and peer support.	5. Reduce social isolation, enable client to work on personal goals and relationship needs.
6. Provide information referrals, when needed, for religious or spiritual information (e.g. readings, programs, tapes, community resources).	6. Spiritual and existential issues may be heightened during depressive episodes—many people find strength and comfort.

TABLE 18–9 *Targeting the Vegetative Signs of Depression*

INTERVENTION	RATIONALE
Nutrition-Anorexia	
1. Offer small high-calorie and high-protein snacks frequently throughout the day and evening.	1. Low weight and poor nutrition render the client susceptible to illness. Small, frequent snacks are more easily tolerated than large plates of food when the client is anorexic.
2. Offer high-protein and high-calorie fluids frequently throughout the day and evening.	2. These fluids prevent dehydration and can minimize constipation.
3. When possible, encourage family or friends to remain with the client during meals.	3. This strategy reinforces the idea that someone cares, can raise the client's self-esteem, and can serve as an incentive to eat.
4. Ask the client which foods or drinks he or she likes. Offer choices. Involve the dietician.	4. The client is more likely to eat the foods provided.
5. Weigh the client weekly and observe the client's eating patterns.	5. Monitoring the client's status gives the information needed for revision of the intervention.
Sleep-Insomnia	
1. Provide periods of rest after activities.	1. Fatigue can intensify feelings of depression.
2. Encourage the client to get up and dress and to stay out of bed during the day.	2. Minimizing sleep during the day increases the likelihood of sleep at night.
3. Provide relaxation measures in the evening (e.g., back rub, tepid bath, or warm milk).	3. These measures induce relaxation and sleep.
4. Reduce environmental and physical stimulants in the evening—provide decaffeinated coffee, soft lights, soft music, and quiet activities.	4. Decreasing caffeine and epinephrine levels increases the possibility of sleep.
Self-Care Deficits	
1. Encourage the use of toothbrush, washcloth, soap, make-up, shaving equipment, and so forth.	1. Being clean and well groomed can temporarily increase self-esteem.
2. Give step-by-step reminders such as "Wash the right side of your face, now the left."	2. Slowed thinking and difficulty concentrating make organizing simple tasks difficult.
Elimination-Constipation	
1. Monitor intake and output, especially bowel movements.	1. Many depressed clients are constipated. If the condition is not checked, fecal impaction can occur.
2. Offer foods high in fiber and provide periods of exercise.	2. Roughage and exercise stimulate peristalsis and help evacuation of fecal material.
3. Encourage the intake of fluids.	3. Fluids help prevent constipation.
4. Evaluate the need for laxatives and enemas.	4. These measures prevent fecal impaction.

Milieu Therapy

When a person is acutely and severely depressed, hospitalization may be indicated. The depressed person needs protection from suicidal acts, a supervised environment for regulating antidepressant medications, and (when indicated) a course of ECT. Often, being removed from a stressful interpersonal situation in itself has therapeutic value. Hospitals have protocols regarding the care and protection of the suicidal client. Chapter 23 on suicide discusses the nurse's responsibility for providing a therapeutic environment that is structured to protect the client against self-inflicted harm.

During the continuation phase of depression (4 to 9 months) and maintenance phase (longer than 1 year), people find that various short-term therapies—individual and group—are useful for dealing with the presence and aftermath of a major depressive episode. Numerous support groups may also prove extremely valuable; these include groups sponsored by the National Alliance for the Mentally Ill or bipolar support groups.

Psychotherapy

Studies have demonstrated that traditional psychotherapies (e.g., psychoanalytic psychotherapy) are only slightly more effective than placebo in reducing depressive symptoms (Beck and Young 1985). Most recently, there has been an increased emphasis on short-term therapies. Therapies that have received the most attention in outcome research include behavioral therapy, interpersonal psychotherapy, brief psychodynamic therapy, and cognitive therapy.

Cognitive-behavioral therapy (CBT), interpersonal therapy (IPT), and time-limited focused psychotherapy all are especially effective in the treatment of depression (Agras and Berkowitz 1999). However, superior maintenance has been demonstrated with only CBT and IPT (Agras and Berkowitz 1999). CBT has been shown to be at least as effective as medications, with CBT showing a lower relapse rate (Beck and Young 1985). Many clinicians believe in both medication and therapy. See Box 18–2 for an overview of these psychotherapies in the treatment of depression.

A review of several studies (Haaga and Beck 1992) showed apparent prophylactic effects with cognitive therapy in depressed clients, especially those with unipolar depression; that is, people seem to learn something in cognitive therapy that is helpful after the acute phase of treatment, and this knowledge may help minimize a relapse.

Social skills training is also effective in the treatment of depression. Social skills such as assertiveness training and effective social and coping skills that help increase positive reinforcements from other people and the environment are most effective. CBT and social skills training are also effective in childhood depression. The goals are the same as for adults, that is, to decrease depressive thinking, enhance social skills, and increase pleasant activities (Agras and Berkowitz 1999).

Group treatment is a widespread modality for the treatment of depression. One advantage of group treatment is that it increases the number of people who can receive treatment at a decreased individual cost. A second advantage is that groups increase clients' socialization and offer people an opportunity to share common feelings and concerns, thereby decreasing feelings of isolation. Support from other group members can lessen feelings of hopelessness and helplessness. A widely used model for outpatient group treatment is fashioned after Beck's cognitive theory of depression (Luby and Yalom 1992).

Another popular group approach is **interactional group therapy**. In this type of therapy, groups consist of clients with different types of disorders. The therapist in this setting focuses on the here and now. Maladaptive behaviors displayed within the group are interpreted as the kinds of psychopathology the person displays in his or her outside relationships. Therefore, the target of treatment is not the depression itself but rather the interpersonal manifestations of the disorder (Luby and Yalom 1992).

Psychopharmacology

As mentioned elsewhere, the combination of specific psychotherapies (e.g., cognitive-behavioral) and antidepressants has been found to be superior to either psychotherapy or psychopharmacology alone (APA 2000, Keller et al. 2000).

WHAT ANTIDEPRESSANTS CAN DO

Antidepressant drugs can positively alter poor self-concept, degree of withdrawal, vegetative signs of depression, and activity level. Target symptoms include

1. Sleep disturbance
   - Early morning awakening
   - Frequent awakening
   - Hypersomnia (excessive sleeping)

Box 18–2 *Overview of Cognitive-Behavioral Therapies and Interpersonal Psychotherapy for Depression*

Cognitive-Behavioral Therapy

Problems; negative thoughts about

- Oneself—leads to lower self-esteem
- World—leads to increased caution/guardedness
- Future—leads to pessimism and hopelessness

Treatment techniques

- Identify negative automatic thoughts
- Question negative automatic thoughts
- Behavioral experiments

Interpersonal Therapy

Goals

- Reduce depressive symptoms
- Improve self-esteem
- Develop better social and interpersonal functioning

Target problems

- Grief
- Role changes
- Interpersonal disputes
- Deficits in interpersonal relationships

2. Appetite disturbance (decreased or increased)
3. Fatigue
4. Decreased sex drive
5. Psychomotor retardation or agitation
6. Diurnal variations in mood (often worse in the morning)
7. Impaired concentration or forgetfulness
8. Anhedonia

One drawback to the use of antidepressant medication is that the client may have to take antidepressant agents for 1 to 3 weeks before improvement is noticed. However, if a client is acutely suicidal, 2 to 3 weeks may be too long to wait. At these times, ECT may be the treatment of choice.

FACTORS USED IN CHOOSING A SPECIFIC ANTIDEPRESSANT

All antidepressants work equally as well. However, they have different side effects, costs, safety features, and maintenance considerations. Gitlin (1999) proposed the following primary and secondary considerations when choosing a specific antidepressant:

PRIMARY CONSIDERATIONS
■ Side effect profile
■ Ease of administration
■ History of past response
■ Safety and medical considerations
■ Specific subtype (if applicable)

SECONDARY CONSIDERATIONS
■ Neurotransmitter specificity
■ Family history of response
■ Blood level considerations
■ Cost

Table 18–10 highlights some drugs of choice for specific problems.

PSYCHOPHARMACOLOGICAL TREATMENT OPTIONS

Basic antidepressant classes (Gitlin 1999) include the following:

1. **First-line agents**

   ■ Selective serotonin reuptake inhibitors (SSRIs)
   ■ Novel new antidepressants: bupropion (Wellbutrin), venlafaxine (Effexor), nefazodone (Serzone), mirtazapine (Remeron)
   ■ Cyclic antidepressants: tricyclics (TCAs)

2. **Second-line agents**

   ■ Monoamine oxidase inhibitors (MAOIs)
   ■ ECT

SELECTIVE SEROTONIN REUPTAKE INHIBITORS. The selective serotonin reuptake inhibitors (SSRIs) represent an important advance in pharmacotherapy. They are neither TCAs nor MAOIs. Es-

TABLE 18–10 *Special Problems and Medications of Choice*

PROBLEM	DRUGS OF CHOICE
1. High suicide risk	1. Trazodone, fluoxetine, sertraline, paroxetine, bupropion, venlafaxine
2. Concurrent depression and panic attacks	2. Phenelzine, imipramine, fluoxetine, paroxetine
3. Chronic pain with or without depression	3. Amitriptyline, doxepin
4. Weight gain on other antidepressants	4. Fluoxetine, bupropion, sertraline, paroxetine
5. Sensitivity to anticholinergic side effects	5. Trazodone, fluoxetine, phenelzine, tranylcypromine, bupropion, sertraline, paroxetine
6. Orthostatic hypotension	6. Nortriptyline, bupropion, sertraline
7. Sexual dysfunction	7. Bupropion, nefazodone

Note: Most antidepressants are quite toxic when taken in an overdose. Extreme caution should be taken in prescribing to high-risk suicidal patients. Of the existing antidepressants, trazodone appears to have the lowest degree of cardiotoxicity.

From Preston, J., and Johnson, J. (1998). *Clinical psychopharmacology made ridiculously simple.* Miami: MedMaster.

sentially, the SSRIs selectively block the neuronal uptake of serotonin. Therefore, through blockade of the reuptake process, serotonergic neurotransmission is enhanced, thereby permitting serotonin to act for an extended period at the synaptic binding sites in the brain. Chapter 3 provides more information on how the SSRIs work.

SSRIs are recommended as first-line therapy in all depressions *except* psychotic depression (in which ECT may be the first choice), melancholic depression, or mild outpatient depression.

SSRI antidepressant drugs have a lower incidence of anticholinergic side effects (dry mouth, blurred vision, urinary retention), less cardiotoxicity, and faster onset of action than the TCAs. Clients are more likely to comply with the SSRIs than the TCAs, and compliance is a crucial step toward recovery or remission. The SSRIs seem to be effective in depressions with anxious features as well as in clients with psychomotor agitation.

Since SSRIs cause fewer side effects and, because of their low cardiotoxicity, they are less dangerous when they are taken in overdose. The SSRIs, selective serotonin/norepinephrine reuptake inhibitors, and atypical antidepressants have a low lethality risk for suicide attempts compared with the TCAs, which have a very high potential for lethality with overdose.

Types and Indications. The SSRIs have a broad

TABLE 18-11 *Selective Serotonin Reuptake Inhibitors (SSRIs)*

SSRIs	SEDATION	WEIGHT GAIN	SEXUAL DYSFUNCTION	OTHER KEY SIDE EFFECTS
	Minimal	Rare	Yes	Initial: nausea, loose bowel movements, headache, insomnia Toxic effects, rare serotonin syndrome

Generic Name	Trade Name	Initial Dose (mg/day)	Dose After 4–8 weeks (mg/day)	Maximum Dose
Citalopram	Celexa	10–20	20–60	—
Fluoxetine	Prozac	10–20	20–80	80
Fluvoxamine*	Luvox	50–100	100–200	300
Paroxetine	Paxil	10–20	20–50	50
Sertraline	Zoloft	50	50–200	200

*Clients with hepatic disease and elderly clients should start with 50% less than the standard doses listed in the table. This applies to clients with coexisting panic or anxiety symptoms.

base for clinical use. In addition to their use in depressive disorders, the SSRIs have been prescribed with success in some of the anxiety disorders, in particular, obsessive-compulsive disorder and panic disorder (see Chapter 14). SSRIs are effective in some women who suffer from late luteal phase dysphoric disorder (Marangell et al. 1999).

Common Side Effects. Agents that selectively enhance synaptic serotonin within the CNS may induce agitation, anxiety, sleep disturbance, tremor, sexual dysfunction (primarily anorgasmia), or tension headache. Autonomic reactions (e.g., dry mouth, sweating, weight change, mild nausea, and loose bowel movements) may also be experienced with the SSRIs. See Table 18–11 for general side effects profile of the SSRIs, specific SSRIs, and dosage.

Serious Side Effects. One rare and life-threatening event associated with the SSRIs is the **central serotonin syndrome**. This is thought to be related to overactivation of the central serotonin receptors, either from too high a dose or in combination with other drugs. Symptoms include abdominal pain, diarrhea, sweating, fever, tachycardia, elevated blood pressure, altered mental state (delirium), myoclonus, increased motor activity, irritability, hostility, and mood change. Severe manifestation can induce hyperpyrexia, cardiovascular shock, or death. The risk of this syndrome seems to be the greatest when an SSRI is administered temporally with a second serotonin-enhancing agent, such as an MAOI. For example, a person taking fluoxetine (Prozac) would have to be medication free for a full 5 weeks before being

switched to an MAOI (5 weeks is the half-life for fluoxetine). If clients are already taking an MAOI, they should wait at least 2 weeks before starting fluoxetine therapy. Other SSRIs have shorter lives; for example, sertraline and paroxetine have half-lives of 2 weeks, so there would need to be a 2-week gap between medications. Table 18–12 lists

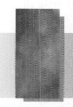

TABLE 18-12 *Symptoms and Interventions for Central Serotonin Syndrome*

SYMPTOMS	EMERGENCY MEASURES

1. Hyperactivity/restlessness
2. Tachycardia → cardiovascular shock
3. Fever → hyperpyrexia
4. Elevated blood pressure
5. Altered mental states (delirium)
6. Irrationality, mood swings, hostility
7. Seizures → status epilepticus
8. Myoclonus, incoordination, tonic rigidity
9. Abdominal pain, diarrhea, bloating
10. Apnea → death
	1. Remove offending agent(s)
	2. Symptomatic treatments
	  a. Block serotonin receptors: cyproheptadine, methysergide, propranolol
	  b. Hyperthermia: Cooling blankets, chlorpromazine
	  c. Muscle rigidity/rigors: dantrolene, diazepam
	  d. Anticonvulsants
	  e. Artificial ventilation
	  f. Paralysis

the signs and symptoms of central serotonin syndrome, and Box 18–1 offers emergency treatment guidelines. Box 18–3 is a useful tool for clients and family teaching about the SSRIs.

NOVEL ANTIDEPRESSANTS. Nefazodone, venlafaxine, bupropion, and mirtazapine all are effective novel antidepressants.

Nefazodone (Serzone). Nefazodone inhibits serotonin, is a potent antagonist of serotonin (5-HT2) receptors, and binds to the serotonin transmitter. Nefazodone also binds to the norepinephrine transporter. It is different from other antidepressants because of its two actions in the serotonin system: moderate serotonin selective reuptake blocking and direct 5-HT2 antagonisms that may be more anxiolytic than other antidepressants. It is also useful for depressed clients who have a coexisting sexual dysfunction. It appears to be a safe and well-tolerated drug after both short-term and long-term use.

The most common adverse effects of nefazodone are nausea, somnolence, dry mouth, dizziness, constipation, asthenia, lightheadedness, and blurred vision. Much to its credit, the drug causes a low incidence of sexual dysfunction, weight change, sleep dysfunction, and cardiotoxicity.

Venlafaxine (Effexor). Venlafaxine is a potent inhibitor of serotonin as well as norepinephrine in the CNS. This drug has demonstrated effective antidepressant properties with a good side effect profile. Preliminary data suggest that it may be useful in people with chronic pain and other disorders in which SSRIs are effective.

The main side effects are nausea, somnolence, dry mouth, dizziness, constipation, nervousness, sweating, asthenia, abnormal ejaculation and orgasm, and anorexia. A 33% to 40% response rate to venlafaxine has been reported in clients who have not improved with adequate trials of other treatments (Marangell et al. 1999; Post 1995). Modest dose-dependent increases in blood pressure may occur with venlafaxine treatment.

Wellbutrin (Bupropion Hydrochloride). Bupropion is effective in depressed clients, especially those who are refractory or intolerant to the TCAs. A significant advantage of bupropion is its relative lack of sexual side effects. It has had some success in individuals with rapid-cycling bipolar II disorder (see Chapter 19). It has been used successfully with children with attention-deficit hyperactivity disorder and in some clients with chronic fatigue syndrome (Golden et al. 1995). Bupropion is currently being marketed under the name **Zyban for smoking cessation.** Bupropion has a favorable side effect profile, although nausea can occur in some clients. Disadvantages include an increased risk of medication-induced seizures, and for this reason the drug is contraindicated in people with epilepsy, major head injury, bulimia, and anorexia nervosa. Refer to Table 18–13 for an overview of the side effects and dosage profile for these novel antidepressants.

Alprazolam. Alprazolam is a benzodiazepine anxiolytic (see Chapter 14). Although this is an effective drug for anxiety disorders (e.g., panic disorders, agoraphobia), it is also as effective as the TCAs for the treatment of mild to moderate depression with anxious features. Its side effect profile (sedation, minimal cardiovascular effects, lack of anticholinergic activity) can be advantageous for some individuals (Golden et al. 1995). The downside is that the benzodiazepines can cause potentially severe withdrawal reactions after abrupt discontinuation.

Box 18–3 *Client and Family Teaching for Use of Selective Serotonin Reuptake Inhibitors (SSRIs)*

- SSRIs may cause sexual dysfunction or lack of sex drive—inform nurse or physician
- SSRIs may cause insomnia, anxiety, and nervousness—inform nurse or physician
- SSRIs may interact with other medications—be sure physician knows other medications client is taking (digoxin, warfarin). SSRIs should not be taken within 14 days of the last dose of a monoamine oxidase inhibitor
- Do not take any over-the-counter drugs without first notifying the physician
- Common side effects include fatigue, nausea, diarrhea, dry mouth, dizziness, tremor, and sexual dysfunction or lack of sex drive
- Because of the potential for drowsiness and dizziness, client should not drive or operate machinery until these side effects are ruled out
- Avoid alcohol
- Client should have liver and renal function tests performed and blood counts checked periodically
- **Do not discontinue medication abruptly.** If side effects become bothersome, client should ask physician about changing to a different drug. Abrupt withdrawal can lead to serotonin withdrawal

Report any of the following symptoms to a physician immediately:

- Rash or hives
- Rapid heartbeat
- Sore throat
- Difficulty urinating
- Fever, malaise
- Anorexia and weight loss
- Unusual bleeding
- Initiation of hyperactive behavior
- Severe headache

TABLE 18–13 *Novel Antidepressants*

GENERIC NAME	TRADE NAME	INITIAL DOSE (MG/DAY)	DOSE AFTER 4–8 WEEKS (MG/DAY)	SIDE EFFECTS PROFILE
Bupropion	Wellbutrin	100–150	200–450	Initial: nausea, headache, insomnia, anxiety/agitation; seizure risk **Low: weight gain/sedation/sexual dysfunction**
Nefazodone	Serzone	100–200	300–500	Initial: nausea, dizziness, confusion, visual changes, rarely blurred vision **High: sedation** **Low: weight gain/sexual dysfunction**
Trazodone	Desyrel	50	150–400	Initial: sedation, **priaprism,** dizziness, orthostasis **Not recommended as first-line treatment** **High: sedation** **Low: weight gain/sexual dysfunction**
Venlafaxine	Effexor	50–75	75–375	Similar to SSRIs; dose-dependent hypertension **High: sexual dysfunction** **Minimal:** sedation Low: weight gain
Mirtazapine	Remeron	7.5–15	15–45	Anticholinergic*; may increase serum lipids; rare: orthostasis, hypertension, peripheral edema, agranulocytosis **High: sedation, weight gain** Low: sexual dysfunction

*Anticholinergic side effects: dry mouth, blurred vision, constipation, urinary retention, tachycardia, and possible confusion.
SSRIs, selective serotonin reuptake inhibitors.

TRICYCLIC ANTIDEPRESSANTS. The tricyclic antidepressants (TCAs) inhibit the reuptake of norepinephrine and serotonin by the presynaptic neurons in the CNS. Therefore, the amount of time that norepinephrine and serotonin are available to the postsynaptic receptors is increased. This increase in norepinephrine and serotonin in the brain is believed by many to be responsible for mood elevations when TCAs are given to depressed persons.

TCAs benefit about 65% to 80% of people with nondelusional depressive disorders but only about 33% of those with delusional depression (Maxmen and Ward 1995). Clients with delusional depression respond well to ECT (75% to 85%). Antipsychotic agents, given along with an antidepressant, are also effective for some depressed clients (65% to 70%) who have psychotic symptoms (Maxmen and Ward 1995).

Clients must take therapeutic doses of TCAs for 10 to 14 days or longer before these agents start to work. The full effects may take from 4 to 8 weeks to be seen. An effect on some symptoms of depression, such as insomnia and anorexia, may be noted earlier. Currently, a person who has had a positive response to TCA therapy would probably be maintained on that medication from 6 to 12 months to prevent an early relapse. Choice of TCA is based on

■ What has worked for the client or a family member in the past
■ The drug's side effects

For example, for a client who is lethargic and fatigued, a more stimulating TCA, such as desipramine (Norpramin) and protriptyline (Vivactil), may be best. If a more sedating effect is needed for agitation or restlessness, drugs such as amitriptyline (Elavil) and doxepin (Sinequan) may be more appropriate choices. **No matter which TCA is given, the dose should always be low initially and gradually increased.** Caution should be used, especially in elderly persons, in whom slow drug metabolism may be a problem. Trimipramine (Surmontil) is a good choice for the elderly because of its low side effect profile and its rapid effects on promoting sleep.

Common Side Effects. The chemical structure of the TCAs is similar to that of the antipsychotic medications. Therefore, the **anticholinergic** actions are similar (e.g., dry mouth, blurred vision, tachycardia, constipation, urinary retention, and esophageal reflux). These side effects are both more common and more severe in clients taking antidepressants. These side effects are usually not serious and are often transitory, but **urinary retention and severe constipation warrant immediate medical attention.**

The alpha-adrenergic blockade of the TCAs can produce postural-orthostatic hypotension and tachycardia as well. Postural hypotension can lead to dizziness and increase the risk of falls.

Administering the total daily dose of TCA at night is beneficial for two reasons. First, most TCAs have sedative effects, thereby aiding sleep. Second, the minor side effects occur during sleep, thereby increasing compliance with drug therapy. Table 18–14 reviews the common side effects, TCAs in common use, and dose range.

Serious Side Effects. The most serious side effects of the TCAs are cardiovascular: Dysrhythmias, tachycardia, myocardial infarction, and heart block have been reported. Because the cardiac side effects are so serious, the TCAs are considered a risk in clients with cardiac disease and in the elderly. Cli-

ents should have a thorough cardiac work-up before beginning TCA therapy.

Adverse Drug Interactions. Individuals taking TCAs can have adverse reactions to numerous other medications. For example, use of an MAOI along with a TCA is contraindicated. A few of the more common medications usually *not* given while the TCAs are being administered are listed in Box 18–4. Any client who is taking any of these medications along with the TCAs should have medical clearance because some of the reactions can be fatal.

Antidepressants may precipitate a psychotic episode in a person with schizophrenia. An antidepressant can precipitate a manic episode in a client with bipolar disorder. Depressed clients with bipolar disorder often receive lithium along with the antidepressant.

Contraindications. People who have recently had a myocardial infarction (or other cardiovascular problems), those with narrow-angle glaucoma or a history of seizures, and pregnant women should not be treated with TCAs, except with extreme caution and careful monitoring.

Client Teaching. Teaching clients and their family

TABLE 18–14 *Tricyclic Antidepressants (TCAs): Overall Side Effects and Dose Range*

TCAs	Sedation	Weight Gain	Sexual Dysfunction	Other Key Side Effects
	Most/Yes	Yes	Yes	■ Anticholinergic* ■ Orthostasis ■ CHF effects (tachycardia, arrhythmias, ECG changes, heart failure) ■ Lethal in overdose

Generic Name	Trade Name	Initial Dose (mg/day)	Therapeutic Dosage Range (mg/day)	Maximum Dose
Amitriptyline	Elavil, Endep	25–50	150–300	300
Amoxapine	Asendin	50–100	150–450	400
Desipramine	Norpramin, Pertofrane	25–50	75–200	300
Doxepin	Adapin, Sinequan	25–50	150–300	300
Imipramine	Tofranil	25–50	150–300	300
Nortriptyline	Aventyl, Pamelor	10–25	50–150	150
Protriptyline	Vivactil	10	15–45	60
Trimipramine	Surmontil	25–50	100–250	300
Maprotiline	Ludiomil	25–50	100–150	225

*Anticholinergic side effects: dry mouth, blurred vision, constipation, urinary retention, tachycardia, and possible confusion.
CHF, congestive heart failure; ECG, electrocardiograph.

Box 18–4 *Drugs Used with Caution in Clients Taking a Tricyclic Antidepressant*

■ Phenothiazines
■ Barbiturates
■ Monoamine oxidase inhibitors
■ Disulfiram (Antabuse)
■ Oral contraceptives (or other estrogen preparations)
■ Anticoagulants
■ Some antihypertensives (clonidine, guanethidine, reserpine)
■ Benzodiazepines
■ Alcohol
■ Nicotine

18–6 for foods and Box 18–7 for medications that are high in tyramine and that need to be avoided or curtailed.

Since people who are depressed are often lethargic, confused, and apathetic, adhering to strict dietary limitations may not be feasible. That is why MAOIs, although highly effective, are not often given as a first-line measure.

MAOIs are particularly effective for people with atypical depression (refer to Table 18–3) as well as other disorders (e.g., panic disorder, social phobia, generalized anxiety disorder, obsessive-compulsive disorder, posttraumatic stress disorder, bulimia). The common MAOIs presently used in the United States are phenelzine (Nardil) and tranylcypromine sulfate (Parnate).

Common Side Effects. Some common and trou-

members about medications is an expected nursing responsibility. Medication teaching should be started in the hospital when a client is hospitalized. The nurse or another qualified health care provider needs to review with the client and, whenever possible, one or more family members, the client's medications, expected side effects, and necessary client precautions. Areas for the nurse to discuss when teaching clients and their families about TCA therapy are presented in Box 18–5. Clients and family members need to have written information to refer to when at home. Written information should be provided for all medications people will be taking at home.

MONOAMINE OXIDASE INHIBITORS. The enzyme monoamine oxidase is responsible for inactivating certain brain amines such as norepinephrine, serotonin, dopamine, and tyramine. When a person ingests an MAOI, these amines do not get inactivated, or broken down, and there is an increase of these amines available for synaptic release in the brain. The increase in norepinephrine, serotonin, and dopamine are the hoped for effects since they can raise the mood of depressed persons. The increase in tyramine, on the other hand, poses a problem. When the amine tyramine increases and is not broken down by MAO, this increase can lead to high blood pressure, hypertensive crisis, and eventually to a cerebrovascular accident. Therefore, people taking these drugs have to reduce their intake of tyramine, so that tyramine does not rise to dangerous levels. For that reason, foods and drugs that are high in tyramine have to be curtailed, or the depressed individual can experience a hypertensive crisis. See Box

Box 18–5 *Teaching Clients and Their Families About Tricyclic Antidepressants*

■ Tell the client and the client's family that mood elevation may take from 7 to 28 days. It may take up to 6 to 8 weeks for the full effect to take place and for major depression symptoms to subside.
■ Have the family reinforce this frequently to the depressed family member because depressed people have trouble remembering and respond to ongoing reassurance.
■ Reassure the client that drowsiness, dizziness, and hypotension usually subside after the first few weeks.
■ When the client starts taking tricyclic antidepressants (TCAs), caution the client to be careful working around machines, driving cars, and crossing streets because of possible altered reflexes, drowsiness, or dizziness.
■ Alcohol can block the effects of antidepressants. Tell the client to refrain from drinking.
■ If possible, the client should take full dose at bedtime to reduce the experience of side effects during the day.
■ If the client forgets the bedtime dose (or the once-a-day dose), the client should take the dose within 3 hours; otherwise the client should wait for the next day. The client should *not* double the dose.
■ Suddenly stopping TCAs can cause nausea, altered heartbeat, nightmares, and cold sweats in 2 to 4 days. The client should call the physician or take one dose of TCA until the physician can be contacted.

BOX 18–6 *Foods That Can Interact with Monoamine Oxidase Inhibitors*

FOODS THAT CONTAIN TYRAMINE

CATEGORY	UNSAFE FOODS (HIGH TYRAMINE CONTENT)	SAFE FOODS (LITTLE OR NO TYRAMINE)
Vegetables	Avocados, especially if overripe; fermented bean curd; fermented soybean; soybean paste; sauerkraut	Most vegetables
Fruits	Figs, especially if overripe; bananas, in large amounts	Most fruits
Meats	Meats that are fermented, smoked, or otherwise aged; spoiled meats; liver, unless very fresh; beef and chicken liver	Meats that are known to be fresh (exercise caution in restaurants—meats may not be fresh)
Sausages	Fermented varieties; bologna, pepperoni, salami, others	Nonfermented varieties
Fish	Dried, pickled or cured fish; fish that is fermented, smoked, or otherwise aged; spoiled fish	Fish that is known to be fresh; vacuum-packed fish, if eaten promptly or refrigerated only briefly after opening
Milk, milk products	Practically all cheeses	Milk, yogurt, cottage cheese, cream cheese
Foods with yeast	Yeast extract (e.g., Marmite, Bovril)	Baked goods that contain yeast
Beer, wine	Some imported beers, Chianti	Major domestic brands of beer; most wines
Other foods	Protein dietary supplements; soups (may contain protein extract); shrimp paste; soy sauce	

FOODS THAT CONTAIN OTHER VASOPRESSORS

FOOD	COMMENTS
Chocolate	Contains phenylethylamine, a pressor agent; large amounts can cause a reaction
Fava beans	Contain dopamine, a pressor agent; reactions are most likely with overripe beans
Ginseng	Headache, tremulousness, and manic-like reactions have occurred
Caffeinated beverages	Caffeine is a weak pressor agent; large amounts may cause a reaction

From Lehne, R. A., et al. (1994). *Pharmacology for nursing* (2nd ed.). Philadelphia: W. B. Saunders.

---

blesome long-term side effects of the MAOIs are orthostatic hypotension, weight gain, edema, change in cardiac rate and rhythm, constipation, urinary hesitancy, sexual dysfunction, vertigo, overactivity, muscle twitching, hypomanic and manic behavior, insomnia, weakness, and fatigue.

Adverse Reactions. The most serious reactions to these agents involve an increase in blood pressure, with the possible development of intracranial hemorrhage, hyperpyrexia, convulsions, coma, and death. Therefore, routine monitoring of blood pressure, especially during the first 6 weeks of treatment, is necessary.

Because so many other drugs, foods, and beverages can have adverse interactions with the MAOIs, increase in blood pressure is a constant concern. The beginning of a hypertensive crisis usually occurs within a few hours of ingestion of the contraindicated substance. The crisis may begin with headaches; stiff or sore neck; palpitations; increase or decrease in heart rate, often associated with chest pain; nausea; vomiting; or increase in temperature (pyrexia). When a hypertensive crisis is suspected, immediate medical attention is crucial. Antihypertensive medications, such as phentolamine (Regitine), are slowly administered intravenously. Pyrexia is treated with hypothermia blankets or ice packs. Box 18–8 identified common side effects and toxic effects. Box 18–9 can be used as a teaching guide for clients on an MAOI and their families.

Contraindications. MAOIs may be contraindicated in

Box 18-7 *Drugs That Can Interact with Monoamine Oxidase Inhibitors*

Drug restrictions that apply to clients taking a monoamine oxidase inhibitor include the following:

- Over-the-counter medications for colds, allergies, or congestion (any product containing ephedrine, phenylephrine hydrochloride, or phenylpropanolamine)
- Tricyclic antidepressants (imipramine, amitriptyline)
- Narcotics
- Antihypertensives (methyldopa, guanethidine, reserpine)
- Amine precursors (levodopa, L-tryptophan)
- Sedatives (alcohol, barbiturates, benzodiazepines)
- General anesthetics
- Stimulants (amphetamines, cocaine)

- Cerebrovascular disease
- Hypertension and congestive heart failure
- Liver disease
- Foods containing tyramine, tryptophan, and dopamine (see Box 18-4)
- Medications (see Box 18-5)
- Recurrent or severe headaches
- People having surgery in 10 to 14 days
- Children younger than 16 years of age

See Table 18-15 for overview of side effects and MAOIs in current use and dose range.

Electroconvulsive Therapy

Electroconvulsive therapy (ECT) can achieve a higher than 90% remission rate in depressed clients within 1 to 2 weeks. Since 20% to 30% of depressed individuals do not respond to antidepressants, ECT remains an effective treatment for depression (Mendelowitz et al. 2000). According to Dubovsky and Buzan (1999), ECT is indicated when

- There is a need for a rapid, definitive response when a client is suicidal or homicidal.

Box 18-8 *Common Side Effects and Toxic Effects of Monoamine Oxidase Inhibitors*

SIDE EFFECTS	COMMENTS
■ Hypotension ■ Sedation, weakness, fatigue ■ Insomnia ■ Changes in cardiac rhythm ■ Muscle cramps ■ Anorgasmia or sexual impotence ■ Urinary hesitancy or constipation ■ Weight gain	Hypotension is the most critical side effect (10%); the elderly, especially, may sustain injuries from it.

TOXIC EFFECTS	COMMENTS

Hypertensive crisis*
 	
■ Severe headache
■ Stiff, sore neck
■ Flushing, cold, clammy skin
■ Tachycardia
■ Severe nosebleeds, dilated pupils
■ Chest pains, stroke, coma, death
■ Nausea and vomiting
	1. Client should go to local emergency department immediately—blood pressure should be checked.
	2. May receive one of the following to lower blood pressure
	
	  ■ 5 mg intravenous phentolamine (Regitine)
	      or
	  ■ Oral chlorpromazine
	      or
	  ■ Nifedipine (calcium channel blocker), 10 mg sublingually

*Related to interaction with foodstuffs and cold medication.

BOX 18–9 *Teaching Clients and Their Families About Monoamine Oxidase Inhibitors (MAOIs)*

■ Tell the client and the client's family to avoid certain foods and all medications (especially cold remedies) unless prescribed by and discussed with the client's physician (see Box 20–6 for specific food and drug restrictions).

■ Give the client a wallet card describing the MAOI regimen (Parke-Davis will supply them if contacted at 1-800-223-6432).

■ Instruct the client to avoid Chinese restaurants (sherry, brewer's yeast, and other products may be used).

■ Tell the client to go to the emergency department right away if he or she has a severe headache.

■ Ideally, blood pressure should be monitored during the first 6 weeks of treatment (for both hypotensive and hypertensive effects).

■ After stopping the MAOI, the client should maintain dietary and drug restrictions for 14 days.

■ A client is in extreme agitation or stupor.
■ The risks of other treatments outweigh the risks of ECT.
■ The client has a history of poor drug response, a history of good ECT response, or both.
■ The client prefers it.

ECT is useful in clients with major depressive and bipolar depressive disorders, especially when psychotic symptoms are present (delusions of guilt, somatic delusions, or delusions of infidelity). Clients who have depressions with marked psychomotor retardation and stupor also respond well.

ECT is also indicated in manic clients whose conditions are resistant to lithium and antipsychotic drugs and in clients who are **rapid cyclers.** A rapid cycler is a client with bipolar disorder who has many episodes of mood swings close together (four or more in 1 year). People with schizophrenia (especially catatonia), those with schizoaffective syndromes, psychotic clients who are pregnant, and clients with Parkinson's disease can also benefit from ECT.

However, ECT is not necessarily effective in clients with dysthymic depressions, those with atypical

TABLE 18–15 *Monamine Oxidase Inhibitors (MAOIs): Overview of Side Effects and Dose Range*

MAOIs	SEDATION	WEIGHT GAIN	SEXUAL DYSFUNCTION	OTHER KEY SIDE EFFECTS
	Rare	Yes	Yes	■ Orthostatic hypotension ■ Insomnia ■ Peripheral edema (avoid in patients with CHF) ■ Avoid phenelzine in patients with hepatitis ■ Potential life-threatening drug interactions ■ Strict dietary and medication restrictions (see Boxes 18–4, 18–5)

Generic Name	Trade Name	Initial Dose (mg/day)	Dose After 4–8 weeks (mg/day)	Maximum Dose
Phenelzine	Nardil	45–75	45–75	75
Tranylcypromine	Parnate	20–30	20–60	30
Reversible inhibitors of MAO not yet available in United States				
Moclobemide	Manerix Aurorix	300	300–600	900

depression and personality disorders, those with drug dependence, or those with depression secondary to situational or social difficulties.

A usual course of ECT for a depressed client is 6 to 12 treatments given two or three times per week. Although no absolute contraindications to ECT exist, according to Fink (1992), several conditions have special risks that demand special attention and skill; these include clients with recent myocardial infarction, cerebrovascular accident, and cerebrovascular malformation or intracranial mass lesion. Clients with these high-risk conditions are usually not treated with ECT unless the need is compelling (Fink 1992).

PROCEDURE. The procedure is explained to the client, and informed consent must be obtained when voluntary clients are being treated. For involuntary clients, when informed consent cannot be obtained, permission may be obtained from the next of kin, although in some states treatment must be court ordered.

Generalized anesthesia and muscle-paralyzing agents have revolutionized the comfort and safety of ECT (Mendelowitz et al. 2000).

POTENTIAL SIDE EFFECTS. The major side effects with bilateral treatments are confusion, disorientation, and short-term memory loss. On awakening, the client may be confused and disoriented. The nurse and family may need to orient the client frequently during the course of treatment. Many people state that they have memory deficits for the first few weeks before and after the course of treatment. Memory usually recovers, although not always. ECT is not a permanent cure for depression, and maintenance treatment with TCAs or lithium decreases the relapse rate. Maintenance ECT (once a week to once a month) may also help to decrease relapse rates for clients with recurrent depression.

Alternative and Complementary Therapies for Depression

Zahourek (2000) has highlighted an array of complementary, alternate, and integrative approaches in the treatment of depression that includes supplements, exercise, massage, light therapy, homeopathy, and rapid rate transcranial magnetic stimulation (TMS). Many products are on the market over the counter for the treatment of dysphoric mood. Herbal products and supplements for depression have become a multi-million dollar industry; however, the long-term effects of these products have not been studied nor are they presently known. Zahourek (2000) cautioned that since many of these methods are not supported by research, they should be used with caution. Psychiatric nurses do need to become knowledgeable about these alternatives and serve as a resource person to clients. The approaches briefly discussed here are light therapy, St. John's wort, exercise, and TMS. Refer to Chapter 36 for more discussion on alternative and complementary approaches.

LIGHT THERAPY

Light therapy has been successfully used for seasonal affective disorders (SAD) and has become first-line treatment for SAD (see Table 18–3). People with SAD often live in climates in which there are marked seasonal differences in the length of daylight. Dubovsky and Buzan (1999) noted that seasonal variations in mood disorders in the Southern Hemisphere are the reverse of those in the Northern Hemisphere. Light therapy may also be useful as an adjunct in chronic major depressive disorder or dysthymia with seasonal exacerbations (APA 2000).

Light therapy is thought to be effective because of the influence of light on melatonin. Melatonin is secreted by the pineal gland and is necessary in maintaining and shifting biological rhythms. Exposure to light suppresses the nocturnal secretion of melatonin that seems to have a therapeutic effect on people with SAD (Zahourek 2000). Treatments consist of light balanced to resemble sunlight, for example, a 10,000-lux light box slanted toward the client's face, in the amount of 30 minutes a day either once or in two divided doses (APA 2000). Light treatment has been found to be equally as effective in reducing depressive symptoms compared with medications in people with SAD (Zahourek 2000).

ST. JOHN'S WORT (HYPERICUM PERFORATUM)

St. John's wort is a whole plant product with antidepressant properties that is not regulated by the U.S. Food and Drug Administration. In a recent review of 14 short-term double-blind studies in people with mild to moderate depression, St. John's wort demonstrated a superior efficacy to placebo and was generally comparable to low-dose TCA treatment (APA 2000). The herb is not to be taken in certain situations (e.g. major depression, pregnancy, children younger than 2 years of age) (Fuller and Sajatovic 2000). Nor should St. John's wort be taken with certain substances, such as amphetamines or other stimulants, other antidepressants (MAOIs, SSRIs), levodopa, and 5-HT (Fuller and Sajalovic 2000). When taken with other antidepressant medications, there is a potential for additive effects and serotonin syndrome (Zahourek 2000). A person taking this herb should also avoid tyramine-containing foods (Box 18–10). Nangia and colleagues (2000) have stressed the need for dose standardization and adequate trial lengths before St. John's wort can be used as a first-line antidepressant.

Box 18–10 *Alternative and Complementary Therapies for Depression: St. John's Wort (Hypericum perforatum)*

USE

St. John's wort is an herb with antidepressant properties. It has been found effective in mild to moderate depression and has also been used traditionally for treatment of stress and insomnia. Fourteen double-blind studies have shown that St. John's wort is superior to placebo and comparable to low-dose tricyclic antidepressant treatment. The proportion experiencing side effects was lower among those taking St. John's wort.

DOSE (Based on *Hypericum* Content)

Oral: 300 mg three times daily (not to be used longer than 8 weeks)
Liquid extract: 2 to 4 mL three times daily
Tincture: 2 to 4 mL three times daily
Herb: 2 to 4 g three times daily

SIDE EFFECTS

Hypersensitivity to sunlight, skin rash, gastrointestinal upset

ADVERSE REACTIONS

The following have been reported: sinus tachycardia, photosensitivity, abdominal pain. Serotonin malignant syndrome is a dangerous possibility if taken with other antidepressants.

CONTRAINDICATIONS

People with endogenous depressions (severe psychomotor retardation, anorexia) and in pregnancy and children. See Drug Interactions.

DRUG INTERACTIONS

Avoid amphetamines or other stimulants; use with caution if taking a monoamine oxidase inhibitor, levodopa, avoid foods containing tyramine; avoid concurrent use with selective serotonin reuptake inhibitors or other antidepressants.

St. John's wort can interfere with indinavir (Crixivan) and human immunodeficiency syndrome protease inhibitor used to treat AIDS, and cyclosporine, which is used by heart transplant patients.

St. John's wort may also interact with birth control pills and possibly other medications (cardiac, seizure control, cold or flu over-the-counter preparations containing pseudoephedrine.)

BEWARE

Preparations lack standardization regarding their composition and potency. Differences in extract preparations make dose comparison difficult.

ADDITIONAL INFORMATION

The National Institute for Mental Health (NIMH) has launched a large-scale controlled study in the United States to determine if St. John's wort has a significant therapeutic effect in people with mild to moderate depression. Log onto the web (http://www.hypericum.rto.org).

APA (2000), Fuller and Sajatovic (2000), Tyler (2000), (ACS News Today, August 9, 2000).

EXERCISE

As discussed in Chapter 12, exercise can have a profound effect on stress reduction, and according to Andrew Weil (1995) can manage the transient syndrome of mild depression. Weil's prescription is for 30 minutes of aerobic exercise at least five times per week (Zahourek 2000).

Refer to the Research Findings box for a study of the benefits of exercise on depression.

TRANSCRANIAL MAGNETIC STIMULATION

Transcranial magnetic stimulation (TMS) is a new technology that hold great promise but is still being developed. TMS applies the principles of electromagnetism to deliver an electrical field to the cerebral cortices (Pridmore and Belmaker 1999). This technique in early studies seems to support further research for the treatment of serious, relapsing medication-resistant depression (Zahourek 2000). TMS, unlike ECT, does not involve seizure induction, as does ECT. This is a potential treatment for the future, but there is enough evidence for some that it will become an accepted treatment for depression (Pridmore and Belmaker 1999).

EVALUATION

Short-term goals and outcome criteria are frequently evaluated. For example, if the client comes into the

RESEARCH FINDINGS

Aerobic Exercise to Treat Depression

Objective

To evaluate the short-term effects of an aerobic exercise training program on clients with moderate to severe depression.

Method

Twelve clients participated (mean age 49 years): five men, seven women, all with a major depressive episode as defined by the DSM-IV criteria. The mean (SD) duration of the depressive episode was 35 (21) weeks (range 12–96). Aerobic exercise consisted of walking on a treadmill following interval training, for a total of 30 minutes per day for 10 days.

Results

At the end of the aerobic training program, there was a clinically relevant and statistically significant reduction in depression scores based on the Hamilton Rating Scale for Depression. Before, 19.5 (6.3); after 13 (5.5); $P = 0.002$. Self-assessed intensity of symptoms: before, 23.2 (7); after, 17.7 (8.1); $P = 0.006$. All values are mean (SD). Subjective and objective changes in depression scores correlated strongly ($r = 0.66$, $p = 0.01$).

Conclusion

Aerobic exercise can produce substantial improvement in mood in a short time in clients with major depressive disorders.

SD, standard deviation. r, correlation coefficient; P, level of significance.

Source: Dimec F.; Bauer, M; Varahram, I.; Proest, G.; Halter, U. (2001). Benefits from aerobic exercise in patients with major depression: A pilot study. *British Journal of Sports Medicine* 35 (2): 114–117.

unit with suicidal thoughts, the nurse evaluates whether suicidal thoughts are still present, whether the depressed person is able to state alternatives to suicidal impulses in the future, whether he or she is able to explore thoughts and feelings that precede suicidal impulses, and so forth. Outcomes relating to thought processes, self-esteem, and social interactions are frequently formulated because these areas are often problematic in people who are depressed. Physical needs warrant nursing or medical attention. If a person has lost weight because of anorexia, is the appetite returning? If a person was constipated, are the bowels now functioning normally? If the person was suffering from insomnia, is he or she now getting 6 to 8 hours of sleep per night?

If the goals have not been met, an analysis of the data, nursing diagnoses, goals, and planned nursing interventions is made. The care plan is reassessed and reformulated when necessary.

Visit the **Evolve** website at
http://evolve.elsevier.com/Varcarolis
for more Case Studies.

CASE STUDY 18–1 *Depression*

Mrs. Olston is a 35-year-old executive secretary. She has been divorced for 3 years and has two sons, 11 and 13 years of age. She is brought into the emergency department (ED) by her neighbor. She has some superficial slashes on her wrists and is bleeding. The neighbor states that both of Mrs. Olston's sons are visiting their father for the summer. Mrs. Olston has become more and more despondent after terminating a 2-year relationship with a married man 4 weeks ago. According to the neighbor, for 3 years after her divorce, Mrs. Olston talked constantly about not being pretty or good enough and doubted that anyone could really

Case Study continued on following page

love her. The neighbor states that Mrs. Olston has been withdrawn for at least 3 years. After the relationship with her boyfriend ended, she became even more withdrawn and sullen. Mrs. Olston is about 20 pounds overweight, and her neighbor states that Mrs. Olston often stays awake late into the night, drinking by herself and watching television. She sleeps through most of the day on the weekends.

After receiving treatment in the ED, Mrs. Olston is seen by a psychiatrist. The initial diagnosis is dysthymia with suicidal ideation. Although the physician does not think that Mrs. Olston is acutely suicidal at this time, a decision is made to hospitalize her briefly for suicide observation and evaluation for appropriate treatment.

The nurse, Ms. Weston, admits Mrs. Olston to the unit from the ED.

Nurse: Hello, Mrs. Olston, I'm Marcia Weston. I will be your primary nurse.

Mrs. Olston: Yeah . . . I don't need a nurse, a doctor, or anyone else. I just want to get away from this pain.

Nurse: You want to get away from your pain?

Mrs. Olston: I just said that, didn't I? Oh, what's the use. No one understands.

Nurse: I would like to understand, Mrs. Olston.

Mrs. Olston: Look at me. I'm fat . . . ugly . . . and no good to anyone. No one wants me.

Nurse: Who doesn't want you?

Mrs. Olston: My husband didn't want me . . . and now Jerry left me to go back to his wife.

Nurse: You think because Jerry went back to his wife that no one else could care for you?

Mrs. Olston: Well . . . he doesn't anyway.

Nurse: Because he doesn't care, you believe that no one else cares about you?

Mrs. Olston: Yes . . .

Nurse: Who do you care about?

Mrs. Olston: No one . . . except my sons . . . I do love my sons, even though I don't often show it.

Nurse: Tell me more about your sons.

Ms. Weston continues to speak with Mrs. Olston. Mrs. Olston talks about her sons with some affect and apparent affection; however, she continues to state that she does not think of herself as worthwhile.

ASSESSMENT

The nurse divides the data into objective and subjective components.

Objective Data

1. Slashed her wrists
2. Recently broke off with boyfriend
3. Has thought poorly of herself for 3 years, since divorce
4. Has two sons she cares about
5. Is 20 pounds overweight
6. Stays awake late at night, drinking by herself
7. Has been withdrawn since divorce

Subjective Data

1. "No one could ever love me."
2. "I'm not good enough."
3. "I just want to get rid of this pain."
4. "I'm fat and ugly . . . no good to anyone."
5. "I do love my sons, although I don't always show it."

CASE STUDY 18–1   Depression *(Continued)*

SELF-ASSESSMENT	Ms. Weston is aware that when clients are depressed, they can be negative, think life is hopeless, and be hostile toward those who want to help. When Ms. Weston was new to the unit, she withdrew from depressed clients and sought out clients who appeared more hopeful and appreciative of her efforts. The unit coordinator was very supportive of Ms. Weston when she was first on the unit. Ms. Weston, along with other staff, was sent to in-service education sessions on working with depressed clients and was encouraged to speak up in staff meetings about the feelings that many of these depressed clients evoked in her. As a primary nurse, she was now assigned a variety of clients. She found that as time went on, with the support of her peers and the opportunity to speak up at staff meetings, she was able to take what clients said less personally and not feel so responsible when clients did not respond as fast as she would like. After 2 years, she had had the experience of seeing many clients who seemed hopeless and despondent on admission respond well to nursing and medical interventions and go on to lead full and satisfying lives. This also made it easier for Ms. Weston to understand that even though the client may think that life is hopeless and may believe that there is nothing in life to live for, change is always possible.

NURSING DIAGNOSIS

The nurse evaluates Mrs. Olston's strengths and weaknesses and decides to concentrate on two initial nursing diagnoses that seem to have the highest priority.

1. **Risk for self-directed violence** related to separation from 2-year relationship, as evidenced by actual suicide attempt

   ■ Slashed her wrists
   ■ Recently broke off with boyfriend
   ■ Drinks at night by herself
   ■ Withdrawn for 3 years, since divorce

2. **Situational low self-esteem** related to divorce and recent termination of love relationship, as evidenced by derogatory statements about self

   ■ "I'm not good enough."
   ■ "No one could ever love me."
   ■ "I'm fat and ugly . . . no good to anyone."
   ■ "I do love my sons, although I don't always show it."

OUTCOME CRITERIA

Because Mrs. Olston is acutely suicidal, she is put on suicide precautions (see Chapter 24 for suicide precaution protocol). The nurse devises the following outcome criteria and short-term goals with some input from Mrs. Olston.

NURSING DIAGNOSIS	OUTCOME CRITERIA	SHORT-TERM GOALS
1. **Risk for self-directed violence** related to separation from 2-year relationship, as evidenced by actual suicide attempt	1. Client will remain safe.	1a. Client will state she has a reason to live by (date). 1b. Client will state two alternative actions she can take when feeling suicidal in the future.

Case Study continued on following page

CASE STUDY 18–1   *Depression* (Continued)

2. **Situational low self-esteem** related to divorce and recent termination of love relationship, as evidenced by derogatory statements about self

2. By discharge, client will identify a plan to deal with her poor self-esteem.

2. By (date), client will name two things she would like to change about herself.

PLANNING	Because Mrs. Olston was discharged after 48 hours, the *disturbance in self-esteem* issue is continued in her therapy after discharge. Ms. Weston later reviews the goals for her work with Mrs. Olston in the community. See Nursing Care Plan 18–1.
INTERVENTION	Mrs. Olston is put on 24-hour suicide precautions. She appears to respond positively to the attention from the nurses, as well as to that from some of the other clients on the unit. She tells the nurse that since her divorce she has become more withdrawn and has stopped socializing with others and participating in her usual outside activities. Her married boyfriend never took her out, and together they did not share any social activities. Just being around people who seemed interested in her made her feel better. After 2 days, Mrs. Olston says that she really did not want to kill herself. Mrs. Olston agrees that she will try therapy when she is discharged, because she wants her life to change. The following Monday, she starts therapy with Mr. Wiley, a nurse clinical specialist at the community health center near Mrs. Olston's home. During therapy sessions, Mr. Wiley uses various cognitive therapy approaches with Mrs. Olston. She is encouraged to look at her life and herself differently, to assess her strengths, and to identify those things she values. The therapist assists Mrs. Olston in questioning and changing inaccurate thoughts and beliefs she holds toward herself and her future. He first assists Mrs. Olston in learning new behaviors to cope with her loneliness, lack of motivation, and negative thinking. Mr. Wiley also works with Mrs. Olston to help her get her needs met through more assertive behavior. With the encouragement of Mr. Wiley, Mrs. Olston schedules activities throughout her day. A record of these activities will be kept by the client and discussed with Mr. Wiley at the following session. The nurse also role plays with Mrs. Olston some of the new behaviors she is learning in her therapy sessions (see Nursing Care Plan 18–1).
EVALUATION	During the course of her work with Mr. Wiley, Mrs. Olston decides to go to some meetings of Parents Without Partners. She states that she is looking forward to getting back to work and feels much more hopeful about her life. She has also lost 3 pounds while attending Weight Watchers. She states, "I need to get back into the world." Although Mrs. Olston still has negative thoughts about herself, she admits to feeling much better about herself, and she has learned important tools to deal with her negative cognitions.

Visit the **Evolve** website at
http://evolve.elsevier.com/Varcarolis
for the other Nursing Care Plan diagnoses and for
more Nursing Care Plans.

NURSING CARE PLAN 18-1   A *Person* With Depression

NURSING DIAGNOSIS (Hospital Focus)

Risk for self-directed violence: related to separation from two-year relationship, as evidenced by suicide attempt

Supporting Data

- Slashed her wrists
- Recently broke off with boyfriend
- Withdrawn for 3 years since divorce
- Drinks at night by herself
- "I just want to die."

Outcome Criteria: Client will remain safe while in the hospital

SHORT-TERM GOAL	INTERVENTION	RATIONALE	EVALUATION
1. Client will state she has a reason to live by (date).	1a. Observe the client every 15 minutes while she is suicidal. 1b. Remove all dangerous objects from the client. 1c. Spend regularly scheduled periods of time with the client throughout the day. 1d. Assist the client in evaluating the positive as well as the negative aspects of her life. 1e. Encourage the appropriate expression of angry feelings.	1a,b. Ensures client safety. Minimizes impulsive self-harmful behavior. 1c. Reinforces that she is worthwhile; builds up experience to begin to better relate to nurse on one-to-one basis. 1d. A depressed person is often unable to acknowledge any positive aspects of her life unless they are pointed out by others. 1e. Providing for expression of pent-up hostility in a safe environment can reinforce more adaptive methods of releasing tension and may minimize the need to act out self-directed anger.	*OUTCOME MET* By the end of the second day, Mrs. Olston states she really did not want to die, she just couldn't stand the loneliness in her life.

Nursing Care Plan continued on following page

NURSING CARE PLAN 18–1   A *Person With Depression* (Continued)

SHORT-TERM GOAL	INTERVENTION	RATIONALE	EVALUATION
	1f. Accept the client's negativism.	1f. Acceptance enhances feelings of self-worth.	
2. Client will state two alternative actions she can take when feeling suicidal in the future.	2a. Explore usual coping behaviors.	2a. Identifies behaviors that need reinforcing and new coping skills that need to be introduced.	*OUTCOME MET* By discharge, Mrs. Olston states that she is definitely going to try cognitive-behavior therapy. She also discusses joining a women's support group that meets once a week in a neighboring town.
	2b. Assist the client in identifying members of her support system.	2b. Evaluate strengths and weaknesses in the support available.	
	2c. Suggest a number of community-based support groups she might wish to discuss or visit (e.g., hotlines, support groups, women's groups).	2c. The client needs to be aware of community supports to use them.	
	2d. Assist the client in identifying realistic alternatives that she is willing to use.	2d. Unless the client is in agreement with any plan, she will be unable or unwilling to follow through in a crisis.	

SUMMARY

Depression is probably the most commonly seen mental syndrome in the health care system. There are a number of depressive subtypes and depressive clinical phenomena. The two primary depressive disorders are *major depressive disorder* and *dysthymia*. The symptoms in a major depression are usually severe enough to interfere with a person's social or occupational functioning. A person with major depressive disorder may or may not have psychotic symptoms, and the symptoms a person usually exhibits during a major depression are different from the characteristics of the normal premorbid personality.

In dysthymia, the symptoms are often chronic (lasting 2 years) and are considered mild to moderate. Usually, a person's social or occupational functioning is not greatly impaired. The symptoms in a dysthymic depression are often congruent with the person's usual pattern of functioning.

Many theories about the cause of depression exist. Four common theories are psychophysiological theory, cognitive theory, learned helplessness theory, and psychodynamic and life events issues.

Nursing assessment includes the assessment of affect, thought processes, feelings, physical behavior, and communication. The nurse also needs to be aware of the symptoms that mask depression.

Nursing diagnoses can be numerous. Depressed individuals are always evaluated for risk for self-directed violence. Some other common nursing diagnoses are altered thought processes, self-esteem disturbance, altered nutrition, bowel elimination, sleep pattern disturbance, ineffective individual coping, and ineffective family coping.

Working with people who are depressed can evoke intense feelings of hopelessness and frustration in health care workers. Initially, nurses need support and guidance to clarify realistic expectations of themselves and their clients and to sort out personal feelings from those communicated by the client via empathy. Peer supervision and individual supervision with an experienced nurse clinician or a psychiatric social worker or psychologist are useful in increasing therapeutic potential.

Interventions with clients who are depressed involve several approaches. The nurse intervenes therapeutically, using specific principles of communication, planning activities of daily living, administering or participating in somatic therapies, maintaining a therapeutic environment, and teaching clients about the biochemical aspects of depression.

Many short-term therapies have been found to be effective in the treatment of depression, including the following:

1. Interpersonal therapies
2. Cognitive-behavioral therapy
3. Skills training (assertiveness and social skills)
4. Some forms of group therapy

Evaluation is ongoing throughout the nursing process, and the client's outcomes are compared with the stated outcome criteria and short-term goals. The care plan is revised by use of the evaluation process when outcomes are not being met.

Visit the **Evolve** website at
http://evolve.elsevier.com/Varcarolis
for a post-test on the content in this chapter.

Visit the **Evolve** website at
http://evolve.elsevier.com/Varcarolis
for additional self-study exercises.

Critical Thinking and Chapter Review

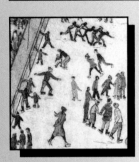

Critical Thinking

1. You are spending time with Mr. Plotsky, who is being worked up for depression. He hardly makes eye contact, he slouches in his seat, and his expression appears blank, although sad. Mr. Plotsky has had numerous bouts of major depression in the past, and says to you, "This will be my last depression. . . . I will never go through this again."

   A. If safety is first, what are the appropriate questions to ask Mr. Plotsky at this time?
   B. Give an example of the kinds of signs and symptoms you might find when you assess a client with depression in terms of behaviors, thought processes, activities of daily living, and ability to function at work and at home?
   C. Mr. Plotsky tells you that he has been on every medication there is but that none have worked. He asks you about the herb St. John's wort. What is some information he should have about its effectiveness for severe depression, its interactions with other antidepressants, and its regulatory status?
   D. What might be some somatic options for a person who is resistant to antidepressant medications?
   E. Mr. Plotsky asks what causes depression. In simple terms, how might you respond to his query?
   F. Mr. Plotsky tells you that he has never tried therapy because he thinks it is for babies. What information could you give him about various therapeutic modalities that have proven effective for some other depressed clients?

2. When you are teaching Mrs. Mac about her SSRI, sertraline (Zoloft), she asks you, "What makes this such a good drug?"

   A. What are some of the positive attributes of the SSRIs? What is one of the most serious, although rare, side effects of the SSRI?
   B. Devise a teaching plan for Mrs. Mac.

Chapter Review

Choose the most appropriate answer.

1. Which statement indicates that the nurse subscribes to the theory that learned helplessness is a major factor in the development of depression?

   1. TCAs, MAOIs, and SSRIs are the most useful tools to combat depression.
   2. Depression develops when a person believes he or she is powerless to effect change in a situation.
   3. Depressive symptoms result from experiencing significant loss and turning aggression against the self.

4. Psychosocial stressors and interpersonal events trigger neurophysical and neurochemical changes in the brain.

2. Which response by a nurse to a client experiencing depression would be helpful?

   1. "Don't worry, we all get down once in awhile."
   2. "Don't consider suicide. It's an unacceptable option."
   3. "Try to cheer up. Things always look darkest before the dawn."
   4. "I can see you're feeling down. I'll sit here with you for awhile."

3. Which symptom is considered a "vegetative" symptom of depression?

   1. Sleep disturbance.
   2. Trouble concentrating.
   3. Neglected grooming and hygiene.
   4. Negative expectations for the future.

4. Which is true of the cognition of a person with severe depression?

   1. Reality testing remains intact.
   2. Concentration is unimpaired.
   3. Repetitive negative thinking is noted.
   4. Ability to make decisions is improved.

5. When the nurse is caring for a depressed client, the problem that should receive the highest nursing priority is

   1. Powerlessness.
   2. Suicidal ideation.
   3. Inability to cope effectively.
   4. Anorexia and weight loss.

NURSE, CLIENT, AND FAMILY RESOURCES

Associations

National Alliance for the Mentally Ill (NAMI)
200 North Glebe Road, Suite 1015
Arlington, VA 22203-3754
1-800-950-NAMI

Depressed Anonymous: Recovery from Depression
DSS, Inc.
P.O. Box 17471
Louisville, KY 40217
502-569-1989

National Foundation for Depressive Illness
P.O. Box 2257
New York, NY 10016
1-800-248-4344

National Organization for Seasonal Affective Disorders (NOSAD)
P.O. Box 40133
Washington, DC 20016

National Depressive and Manic-Depressive Association
730 N. Franklin #501
Chicago, IL 60610
312-642-0049
http://www.ndmda.org

Internet Sites

Depression.com
Great general source
http://www.depression.com

NIMH—Depression/Awareness, Recognition, and Treatment
http://www.nimh.nih.gov/depression/index.html

Depression Resources List
http://www.execpc.com/~corbeau/

Internet Mental Health
Great resource for everything
http://www.mentalhealth.com

What You Should Know about Women and Depression
http://www.apa.org/pubinfo/depress.html

Pharmaceutical Information Network
Drug FAQs: Antidepressants
http://pharminfo.com/drugfaq/antidep_faq.html

Online Depression Screening Test
Short (10-question) assessment
http://www.med.nyu.edu/psych/screens/depres.html

REFERENCES

Agras, W. S., and Berkowitz, R. I. (1999). Behavior therapies. In R. E. Hales, S. C. Yudofsky, and J. A. Talbott (Eds.), *Textbook of psychiatry*. Washington, D.C.: American Psychiatric Press, Inc.

Akiskal, H. S. (1995). Mood disorders: Introduction and overview. In H. I. Kaplan and B. J. Sadock (Eds.), *Comprehensive textbook of psychiatry IV* (Vol. 1) (pp. 1067–1078). Baltimore: Williams & Wilkins.

American Psychiatric Association. (2000). *Diagnostic and statistical manual of mental disorders* (4th ed., Text Revision). Washington, D.C.: American Psychiatric Press.

American Psychiatric Association. (2000). *Practice guidelines for the treatment of psychiatric disorders*. Washington, D.C.: American Psychiatric Press.

Beck, A. T., and Rush, A. J. (1995). Cognitive therapy. In H. I. Kaplan and B. J. Sadock (Eds.), *Comprehensive textbook of psychiatry IV* (Vol. 2) (pp. 1847–1856). Baltimore: Williams & Wilkins.

Beck, A. T., and Young, J. E. (1985). Depression. In D. H. Barlow (Ed.), *Clinical handbook of psychological disorders*. New York: Guilford Press.

Burns, C. M., and Stuart, G. W. (1991). Nursing care in electroconvulsive therapy. *Psychiatric Clinics of North America*, 14(4):971.

Calarco, M. M., and Krone, K. P. (1991). An integrated nursing model of depressive behavior in adults: Theory and implementation. *Nursing Clinics of North America*, 26(3):573.

Campbell, L. (1987). Hopelessness. *Journal of Psychosocial Nursing*, 25(2):18.

Dubovsky, S. L., and Buzan, R. (1999). Mood disorders. In R. E. Hales, S. C. Yudofsky, and J. A. Talbott (Eds.), *Textbook of psychiatry* (pp 479–566). Washington, D.C.: American Psychiatric Press.

Fink, M. (1992). Electroconvulsive therapy. In E. S. Paykel (Ed.), *Handbook of affective disorders* (2nd ed.) (pp. 359–368). New York, Guilford Press.

Fuller, M. A., and Sajatovic, M. (2000). *Drug information handbook* (2nd ed.). Cleveland, Ohio: Lexi-Comp.

Gabband, G. O. (1999). Mood disorders: Psychodynamic aspects. In H. I. Kaplan and B. J. Sadock (Eds.), *Comprehensive textbook of psychiatry* (7th ed., Vol. 1). Philadelphia: Lippincott Williams & Wilkins.

Gitlin, M. (1999). *Psychopharmacology for psychotherapists*, parts 1–3. 12th Annual U.S. Psychiatric and Mental Health Congress, November 11–14.

Goldberg, R. J. (1998). *The care of the psychiatric patient*. St. Louis: Mosby.

Golden, R. N., et al. (1995). Trazodone and other antidepressants. In A. F. Schatzberg and C. B. Nemeroff (Eds.), *The American Psychiatric Press textbook of psychopharmacology* (pp. 195–214). Washington, D.C.: American Psychiatric Press.

Gulesserian, B., and Warren, C. J. (1987). Coping resources of depressed patients. *Archives of Psychiatric Nursing*, 1(6):392.

Haaga, D. F, and Beck, A. T. (1992). Cognitive therapy. In E. S. Paykel (Ed.), *Handbook of affective disorders* (2nd ed.) (pp. 511–524). New York: Guilford Press.

Hallon, S. D., and Fawcett, J. (1995). Combined medication and psychotherapy. In G. O. Gabbard (Ed.), *Treatment of psychiatric disorders* (2nd ed., Vol. 1) (pp. 1221–1263). Washington, D.C.: American Psychiatric Press.

Heim, C. and Nemeroff, C, B. (1999). The impact of early adverse experiences on brain systems involved in the pathophysiology of anxiety and affective disorders. *Social Biology Psychiatry*, 46:1–15.

Johnson, H., Maas, M., Meriden, M., and Moorehead, S. (2000). *Nursing outcomes classification* (2nd ed.). St. Louis: Mosby.

Kashani, J. H., and Nair, J. (1995). Affective/mood disorders. In J. M. Weiner (Ed.), *Diagnosis and psychopharmacology of childhood and adolescent disorders* (2nd ed.) (pp. 229–263). New York: Wiley.

Keller, M. B., et al. (2000). A comparison of natazedone, the cognitive-behavioral analysis system of psychotherapy, and their combination for treatment of chronic depression. *New England Journal of Medicine*, 342(20):1462–1470.

Keller, M. (1995). Depression in adults. Presented at the U. S. Psychiatric and Mental Health Congress, Marriott Marquis, New York, November 18, 1995.

Kendler, K. K., et al. (1993). The prediction of major depression in women: Toward an integrated etiologic model. *American Journal of Psychiatry*, 150:1139–1148.

Kramer, T. A. M. (2000). Transcranial magnetic stimulation and its effectiveness in affective disorders. 22nd Congress of the Collegium Internatinale Neuro-Psychophramacologieum, July 12, 2000, Brussels, Belgium.

Kupfer, D. J. (1991). Long-term treatment in depression. *Journal of Clinical Psychiatry*, 32(Suppl):28–34.

Lauer, C. J., et al. (1995). In the quest of identifying vulnerability markers for psychiatric disorders by all-night polysomnography. *Archives of General Psychiatry*, 52(2):145.

Litman, R. E. (1992). Predicting and preventing hospital suicides. In R. W. Maris, et al. (Eds.), *Assessment and prediction of suicide*. New York: Guilford Press.

Luby, J. L., and Yalom, I. D. (1992). Group therapy. In E. S. Paykel (Ed.), *Handbook of affective disorders* (2nd ed.) (pp. 475–486). New York: Guilford Press.

Marangell, L. B., Silver, J. M., and Yudofsky S. C. (1999). Psychopharmacology and electroconvulsive therapy. In R. E. Hales, S. C. Yudofsky, and J. A. Talbott (Eds.), *Textbook of psychiatry*. Washington, D.C.: American Psychiatric Press.

Maxmen, J. S., and Ward, N. G. (1995). *Psychotropic drugs: Fast facts* (2nd ed.). New York: W. W. Norton.

Mendelowitz, A. J., Dawkins, K., and Lieberman, J. A. (2000). Antidepressants. In J. A. Lieberman and A. Tasman (Eds.), *Psychiatric drugs*. Philadelphia: W. B. Saunders.

Merikangas, K. R., and Kupfer, D. J. (1995). Mood disorders: Genetic aspects. In H. I. Kaplan and B. J. Sadock (Eds.), *Comprehensive textbook of psychiatry IV* (Vol. 1) (pp. 1102–1116). Baltimore: Williams & Wilkins.

Nangia, M., Syed, W., and Doraiswamy, P. (2000). Efficacy and safety of St. John's wort for the treatment of major depression. *Public Health Nutrition*, 3(4A):487–494.

National Institute of Mental Health. (1999). *The invisible disease: Depression*. Washington, D.C.: Author. (www.nimh.nih.gov/publicat/invisiblecfm).

Post, R. (1995). Mood disorders: Somatic treatments. In H. I. Kaplan and B. J. Sadock (Eds.), *Comprehensive textbook of psychiatry* (4th ed., Vol. I) (pp. 1152–1172). Baltimore: Williams & Wilkins.

Pridmore, S., and Belmaker, R. (1999). Transcranial magnetic stimulation in the treatment of psychiatric disorders. *Psychiatry and Clinical Neuroscience*, 53(5):541–548.

Sadek, N., and Nemeroff, C. B. (2000). Update on the neurobiology of depression. www.medscape.com/Medscape/psychiatry/TreatmentUpdate/2000/tu03/public/toc-tu03.html.

Seligman, M. E. (1973). Fall into hopelessness. *Psychology Today*, 7: 43.

Thase, M. E. (1999). Mood disorders: Neurobiology. In H. I. Kaplan and B. J. Sadock (Eds.), *Comprehensive textbook of psychiatry* (7th ed., pp. 1318–1327, Vol. I). Philadelphia: Lippincott Williams & Wilkins.

Tyler, V. E. (2000). St. John's wort update. *Prevention*. I:117–120.

Weil, A. (1995). Dr. Andrew Weil's self-healing relieving depression simply. Watertown, Massachusetts: Thorne Communications.

Zahourek, R. (2000). Alternative, complementary, or integrative approaches to treating depression. *Journal of the American Psychiatric Nurses Association*, 6(3):77–86.

Zajecka, J (1995). *Treatment strategies for depression complicated by anxiety disorder.* Presented at the U. S. Psychiatric and Mental Health Congress. Marriott Marquis, New York, November 16, 1995.

Visit the **Evolve** website at
http://evolve.elsevier.com/Varcarolis
for a pre-test on the content in this chapter.

Outline

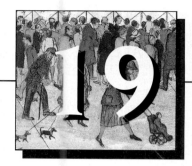

Chapter 19

Mood Disorders: Bipolar

ELIZABETH M. VARCAROLIS

Key Terms and Concepts

The key terms and concepts listed here also appear in bold where they are defined or discussed in this chapter.

acute phase of mania
antiepileptic drugs
bipolar I disorder
bipolar II disorder
clang associations
continuation phase
cyclothymia

electroconvulsive therapy
flight of ideas
hypomania
lithium carbonate
maintenance phase
mania
seclusion protocol

Objectives

After studying this chapter, the reader will be able to

1. Make an assessment of a manic client's (a) mood, (b) behavior, and (c) thought processes.
2. Formulate three nursing diagnoses appropriate for a manic client, including supporting data.
3. Explain the rationale for five principles of communication that may be used with a manic client.
4. Identify four expected side effects for a person on lithium therapy.
5. Distinguish between signs of early and severe lithium toxicity.
6. Write a medication care plan specifying five areas of client teaching regarding lithium carbonate.
7. Contrast and compare basic clinical conditions that may respond better to anticonvulsant therapy with those that may respond better with lithium therapy.
8. Evaluate specific indications for the use of seclusion with a manic client.
9. Defend the use of electroconvulsive therapy for a client in specific situations.
10. Review with a bipolar client at least three of the items stated in the teaching plan (Box 19–2).
11. Distinguish between the focus of treatment for a person in the acute manic phase and that of a person in the continuation or maintenance phase of a bipolar I disorder.
12. Access at least two websites using the Varcarolis SIMON site.

PREVALENCE

Bipolar disorder is a chronic mood syndrome that manifests as recurring mood episodes throughout a person's life. Alternating mood episodes include both period(s) of hypomania or mania, and depressive episodes. These mood episodes are characterized by mania, hypomania, depression, and concurrent mania and depression (mixed episodes—depressive symptoms during a manic attack). Periods of normal functioning may alternate with periods of illness (highs, lows, or mixed highs and lows). However, some 20% to 30% of bipolar individuals continue to display mood lability and other residual mood symptoms (DSM-IV-TR 2000). Up to 60% of bipolar I individuals may experience chronic interpersonal or occupational difficulties between acute episodes (DSM-IV-TR 2000).

Since there is no "cure," clients and families require support and education to reduce relapse and increase the quality of their lives.

Bipolar disorders currently include bipolar I, bipolar II, and cyclothymia.

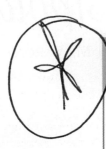

DSM-IV-TR CRITERIA FOR BIPOLAR DISORDER

1. A distinct period of abnormality and persistently elevated, expansive, or irritable mood for at least:
   - 4 days for hypomania
   - 1 week for mania

2. During the period of mood disturbance, **at least three (or more)** of the following symptoms have persisted (four if the mood is only irritable) and have been present to a significant degree:
   - Inflated self-esteem or grandiosity
   - Decreased need for sleep (e.g., the person feels rested after only 3 hours of sleep)
   - More talkative than usual or pressure to keep talking
   - Flight of ideas or subjective experience that thoughts are racing
   - Distractibility (i.e., the person's attention is too easily drawn to unimportant or irrelevant external stimuli)
   - Increase in goal-directed activity (either socially, at work or school, or sexually) or psychomotor agitation
   - Excessive involvement in pleasurable activities that have a high potential for painful consequences (e.g., the person engages in unrestrained buying sprees, sexual indiscretions, or foolish business investments)

HYPOMANIA

1. The episode is associated with an unequivocal change in functioning that is uncharacteristic of the person when not symptomatic.

2. The disturbance in mood and the change in functioning are observed by others.

3. Absence of marked impairment in social or occupational functioning.

4. Hospitalization is not indicated.

5. Symptoms are not due to direct physiological effects of substance (e.g., drug abuse, medication, or other medical conditions).

MANIA

1. Severe enough to cause marked impairment in occupational activities, usual social activities, or relationships.

   or

2. Necessitate hospitalization to prevent harm to self or others, or there are psychotic features.

3. Symptoms are not due to direct physiological effects of substance (drug abuse, medication) or general medical condition (e.g., hyperthyroidism).

Figure 19–1 Diagnostic criteria for bipolar disorder. From the Diagnostic and Statistical Manual of Mental Disorders, 4th edition, text revised (DSM-IV-TR). Washington, DC: American Psychiatric Association, copyright 2000.

Bipolar I Disorder: at least one episode of mania alternating with major depression

Bipolar II Disorder: hypomanic episode(s) alternating with major depression

Cyclothymia: hypomanic episodes alternating with minor depressive episodes (at least two years in duration).

The distinction between mania and hypomania for diagnostic purposes is made in the DSM-IV-TR and is shown in Figure 19–1.

Epidemiological surveys in general populations of different countries of the world found a lifetime prevalence rate for bipolar I disorders of about 0.8% to 1% of the general population over a lifetime. Bipolar I disorder seems to be somewhat more common among males than females (Wacker 2000). Bipolar II affects about .05% of the population over the course of a lifetime and is more common in women (APA 2000). Whereas, major depression usually starts between 25 and 30 years of age, bipolar disorders emerge between the ages of 18 and 30 (Wacker 2000). Mean age of the first episode of the disease appears younger for people with a familial history of the disease (Canceil 1999). A person 40 years or older who presents with a manic episode is more likely to have mania secondary to a general medical condition or substance abuse. The first episode in males is likely to be a manic episode, while in females the disease usually presents with a depressive episode. During the course of the illness, the episodes increase in number and severity as the person gets older.

Cyclothymia usually begins in adolescence or early adulthood. There is a 15% to 50% risk that an individual with cyclothymia will subsequently develop bipolar I or bipolar II disorder.

COMORBIDITY

Substance use disorders are exceptionally common in individuals with a bipolar disease, although the reasons for this are not clear (Strakowski and Del-Bello 2000). Substance abuse clients seem to have more rapid cycling and more mixed or dysphoric mania (Sonne et al. 1999). When this is the case, treatment for substance use and mood disorder should proceed at the same time whenever possible (APA 2000). Other associated disorders include personality disorders, anxiety disorders (panic disorder and social phobia), anorexia nervosa, bulimia nervosa, and attention deficit/hyperactivity disorder (DSM-IV-TR 2000). A study by Dunayevich and colleagues (2000) found that bipolar clients with co-occurring personality disorders had poorer outcomes

12 months after hospitalization for mania than those without personality disorders. A study by Colom and associates (2000) found this population had a greater tendency towards medication nonadherence.

Interestingly, a study by Johnson and associates (2000) found that another disorder may signal a future bipolar disorder. See Research Findings on Bipolar Disorder.

THEORY

Bipolar disorders (one or more episodes of both elated and depressed moods) are thought to be distinctly different, e.g., bipolar I vs. bipolar II vs. cyclothymia. Refer to Table 19–1 for differences between bipolar I and bipolar II disorders.

Individuals with bipolar I disorder have relatives with bipolar I illness, and the same is true for bipolar II disorder. Bipolar II clients are more likely to become depressed in winter than in summer (seasonal) and have more suicide attempts (Zerbe 1999).

Bipolar depression is also different from unipolar depression. Bipolar depression affects younger people, produces more episodes of illness, and requires more frequent hospitalization (Zerbe 1999). Table 19–2 clarifies the difference between bipolar and unipolar (major) depressions. Some theoretical data pertaining specifically to the cause of the bipolar disorders are genetic, neurobiological, social, and psychosocial.

TABLE 19–1 *Manifestations of Bipolar I and Bipolar II Disorder*

BIPOLAR I DISORDER	BIPOLAR II DISORDER
Psychosis	Personality disturbance or disorder of temperament (borderline-like)
Paranoia	
Rapid mood cycling	
Recurrent schizophrenia-like symptoms	Seasonal depression
Recurrent depression	Alcohol and/or substance abuse
Mania	Rapid mood cycling
Bizarre behavior	Premenstrual dysphoria; premenstrual mood disturbance
Substance abuse and/or self-medication	Impulse difficulties
	Interpersonal sensitivity
	Recurrent depression
	Mood instability

From Zerbe, K. J. (1999). *Women's mental health in primary care.* p. 57. Philadelphia: W. B. Saunders.

RESEARCH FINDINGS

Bipolar Disorder

OBJECTIVE

To identify the association between bipolar disorder and other psychiatric disorders during adolescence and early adulthood.

METHODS

The study identified a cross-section of the population and was conducted over a period of time (longitudinal study). Psychiatric interviews were administered to a community sample of 717 youths and their mothers in 1983 (mean age = 14 years), again in 1985–1986, and in 1991–1993.

RESULTS

A wide range of psychiatric disorders co-occurred with bipolar disorder during adolescence and early adulthood. Adolescent anxiety disorders were uniquely associated with increased risk for early adulthood bipolar disorder.

Manic symptoms during adolescence were associated with increased risk for anxiety and depressive disorders during early adulthood.

CONCLUSIONS

Adolescents with anxiety disorders may be at increased risk for bipolar disorder or clinically significant manic symptoms during early adulthood. Adolescents with manic symptoms may be at increased risk for anxiety and depressive disorders during early adulthood.

Source: Johnson, J.G., Cohen, P., and Brook, J.S. (2000). Association between bipolar disorder and other psychiatric disorders during adolescence and early adulthood: A community-based longitudinal investigation. *American Journal of Psychiatry*, 157(10):1679–1681.

TABLE 19–2 *Characteristic Differences Between Bipolar and Unipolar Depressive Disorders*

VARIABLE	BIPOLAR DISORDER	UNIPOLAR DEPRESSIVE DISORDER
Age of onset	Earlier: 19–30 years (mean, 21 years).	Later: 40–44 years (mean, 40 years).
Sex	Equally frequent in men and women	Twice as frequent in women as in men.
Childhood experience	May come from families with low perceived prestige in their community.	Evidence that early parental death and disruptive childhood environment may play a role.
Family environment	Higher rate of divorce and marital conflict.	Divorce rate same as in general population.
Stressful life events	Contributory in the occurrence of both.	Contributory in the occurrence of both.
Personality traits	Dominance, exhibition, and autonomy needs higher in bipolar disorder. More hypomanic drive toward success and achievement.	Defense of status and guilt feeling higher in depressive disorder. Tendency toward a lack of autonomy.
Symptoms in a depressed phase	*More likely to show* ■ Psychomotor retardation. ■ Hypersomnia. ■ Fewer somatic complaints. ■ Less anxiety.	*More likely to show* ■ Increased motor activity. ■ Insomnia. ■ Somatic complaints. ■ Hypochondriasis.
Course and outcome	Higher frequency of relapse than in a major depressive disorder.	Lower frequency of relapse than in bipolar disorder.
Residence	Greater risk in suburbs than inner city.	Greater risk in urban areas than rural areas.

Genetic Causes

Significant evidence exists to support the theory that bipolar disorders are a result of genetic transmission. For example, the rate of bipolar disorder is higher in relatives of people with bipolar disorders than in the general population (Kelsoe 1999). A study at the National Institutes of Mental Health found that 25% of relatives of bipolar clients had a bipolar or a major depressive disorder. For clients with a depressive disorder, 20% of relatives had a bipolar or major depressive disorder, compared with 7% of relatives of control clients (Nurnberger and Gershon 1992). Twin studies bear out a genetic marker for both the bipolar disorders and the depressive disorders; however, the incidence of illness is significantly higher in the bipolar disorders (Kelsoe 1999). Identical twins are 78% to 80% more concordant than fraternal twins (14% to 19%) for bipolar disorder (Merikangas and Kupfer 1995; Nurnberger and Gershon 1992). Twin, family, and adoption studies provide evidence for a partial genetic cause, but the modes of inheritance have not been identified (Ginns et al. 1996).

Neurobiological Causes   Sodium + Kt

The neurotransmitters (norepinephrine, dopamine, and serotonin) have been studied since the 1960s as causal factors in mania and depression. For example, during a manic episode, clients with bipolar disorder demonstrate significantly higher norepinephrine and epinephrine plasma levels than they do when they are depressed or *euthymic* (have normal mood) (Nathan et al. 1995; Freedman et al. 1999). Post et al. (1989) found acutely manic clients had higher cerebrospinal fluid levels of norepinephrine than depressed or euthymic persons. Among the manic clients, norepinephrine correlated with the degree of dysphoria, anger, and anxiety. Other research has found that the interrelationships within the neurotransmitter system are complex.

More complex hypotheses have developed since the amine hypotheses were originally proposed. Mood disorders are most likely a result of complex interactions among various chemicals, including neurotransmitters and hormones. (a type)

The hypothalamic-pituitary-thyroid adrenal axis has been closely scrutinized in people with mood disorders. Hypothyroidism is known to be associated with depressed moods, and hypothyroidism is seen in some clients who are experiencing rapid cycling. Some clients with rapid cycling respond to thyroid hormone treatment (Nathan et al. 1995).

Interestingly, early studies using MRI scans are showing different neurobiological alterations be-

tween bipolar I and bipolar II clients. The difference is that there is an increase in the left ventrical of the brain in clients with bipolar I disorder.

Social Status

Some evidence suggests that the bipolar disorders may be more prevalent in the upper socioeconomic classes. The exact reason for this is unclear; however, people with bipolar disorders appear to achieve higher levels of education and occupational status than nonbipolar depressed individuals. However, no difference exists in education across various socioeconomic classes with the nonbipolar depressions. Also, a high proportion of bipolar clients has been found among creative writers, artists, highly educated men and women, and professional people.

Psychosocial Factors

Although there is increasing evidence for genetic and biological vulnerabilities in the cause of the mood disorders, psychological factors may play a role in the precipitation of manic episodes for many individuals. Two studies of family atmosphere suggest an association between high expressed emotion and relapse. However, the relationship between psychosocial stress and bipolar disorder requires further and more detailed research (Ranaka and Bebbington 1995).

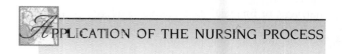

APPLICATION OF THE NURSING PROCESS

ASSESSMENT

Overall Assessment

RECOGNIZING MANIA

The three most common initial symptoms during the onset of mania are (1) elated mood, (2) increased activity, and (3) reduced sleep. Not all people in the manic state experience euphoria; some people become extremely irritable, especially when limits are set on their behavior. The nurse evaluates these characteristics when assessing a manic client's mood, behavior, and thought processes.

As many as 66% of treatable bipolar individuals never receive the care they need because the diagnosis is missed (Zerbe 1999). People with bipolar I disorder experience at least one bout of acute mania—possibly delirious mania. In bipolar II disorders, the highs are considered hypomania, and may

TABLE 19–3　*Mania on a Continuum*

HYPOMANIA	ACUTE MANIA	DELIRIOUS MANIA
Communication		
1. Talks and jokes incessantly, is the "life of the party," gets irritated when not center of attention.	1. May go suddenly from laughing to anger or depression. *Mood is labile.*	1. Totally out of touch with reality.
2. Treats everyone with familiarity and confidentiality; often borders on crude.	2. Becomes inappropriately demanding of people's attention, and intrusive nature repels others.	—
3. Talk is often sexual—can reach obscene, inappropriate propositions to total strangers.	3. Speech may be marked by profanities and crude sexual remarks to everyone (nursing staff in particular).	—
4. Talk is fresh; flits from one topic to the next. Marked by *pressure of speech.*	4. Speech marked by *flight of ideas*, in which thoughts race and fly from topic to topic. May have *clang associations.*	4. Most likely has *clang associations.*
Affect and Thinking		
1. Full of pep and good humor, feelings of euphoria and sociability; may show inappropriate intimacy with strangers.	1. Good humor gives way to increased irritability and hostility, short-lived period of rage, especially when not getting his or her way or controls are set on behavior. May have quick shifts of mood from hostility to docility.	1. May become destructive or aggressive—totally out of control.
2. Feels boundless self-confidence and enthusiasm. Has elaborate schemes for becoming rich and famous. Initially, schemes may seem plausible.	2. Grandiose plans are totally out of contact with reality. Thinks he or she is musician, prominent businessman, great politician, or religious figure, without any basis in fact.	2. May experience undefined hallucinations and delirium.
3. Judgment often poor. Gets involved with schemes in which job, marriage, or financial status may be destroyed.	3. Judgment is extremely poor.	—
4. May get involved with writing large quantities of letters to rich and famous people regarding schemes or may make numerous world-wide telephone calls.	—	—
5. Decreased attention span to both internal and external cues.	5. Decreased attention span and distractibility are intensified.	—
Physical Behavior		
1. Overactive, distractible, buoyant, and busily occupied with grandiose plans (not delusions); goes from one action to the next.	1. Extremely restless, disorganized, and chaotic. Physical behavior may be difficult to control. May have outbursts, e.g., throwing things or becoming briefly assaultive when crossed.	1. *Dangerous state.* Incoherent, extremely restless, disoriented, and agitated. Hyperactive. Motor activity is totally aimless (must have physical or chemical restraints to prevent exhaustion and death).
2. Increased sexual appetite; sexually irresponsible and indiscreet. Illegitimate pregnancies in hypomanic women and venereal disease in both men and women are common. Sex used for escape, not for relating to another human being.	2. Too busy—no time for sex. Poor concentration, distractibility, and restlessness are severe.	2. Same as in acute mania but in the extreme.

TABLE 19–3 *Mania on a Continuum (Continued)*

HYPOMANIA	ACUTE MANIA	DELIRIOUS MANIA
3. May have voracious appetite, eat on the run, or gobble food during brief periods.	3. No time to eat—too distracted and disorganized.	3. Same as acute mania but in the extreme.
4. May go without sleeping unaware of fatigue. However, may be able to take short naps.	4. No time for sleep—psychomotor activity too high; if unchecked, can lead to exhaustion and death.	—
5. Financially extravagant, goes on buying sprees, gives money and gifts away freely, can easily go into debt.	5. Same as in hypomania but in the extreme. Debt.	5. Too disorganized to do anything.

go unrecognized. People who have cyclothymia have mood swings ranging from hypomania on the one hand to dysthymia on the other. Table 19–3 identifies mania on a continuum from hypomanic-manic to delirious manic at the extreme. Please note the changes in communication, affect and thinking, and physical behavior as mania escalates.

ASSESSING CHARACTERISTICS OF MANIA

ASSESSING MOOD. The euphoric mood associated with a bipolar illness is unstable. During euphoria, clients may state that they are experiencing an intense feeling of well-being, are "cheerful in a beautiful world," or are becoming "one with God" (Silverstone and Hunt 1992). This mood may change to irritation and quick anger when the elated person is thwarted. The irritability and belligerence may be short-lived, or it may become the prominent feature of a person's manic illness. When elated, the person's overjoyous mood may seem out of proportion to what is going on, and a cheerful mood may be inappropriate to the circumstances.

The person in a manic state may laugh, joke, and talk in a continuous stream, with uninhibited familiarity. Manic people demonstrate boundless enthusiasm, treat everyone with confidential friendliness, and incorporate everyone into their plans and activities. They know no strangers. Energy and self-confidence seem boundless.

Elaborate schemes to get rich and famous and acquire unlimited power may be frantically pursued, despite objections and realistic constraints. Excessive phone calls and e-mails are made, often to famous and influential people all over the world. People in the manic phase are busy all hours of the day and night furthering their grandiose plans and wild schemes. To the manic person, no aspirations are too high and no distances are too far. No boundaries exist in reality to curtail the elaborate schemes.

In the manic state, a person often gives away money, prized possessions, and expensive gifts. The manic person throws lavish parties, frequents expensive nightclubs and restaurants, and spends money freely on friends and strangers alike. This spending, excessive use of credit cards, and high living continue, even in the face of bankruptcy. Intervention is often needed to prevent financial ruin.

HYPOMANIA TO MANIA. As the clinical course progresses, sociability and euphoria are replaced by a stage of hostility, irritability, and paranoia. The following is a client description of the painful transition from hypomania to mania (Jamison 1995):

At first when I'm high, it's tremendous . . . ideas are fast . . . like shooting stars you follow until brighter ones appear . . . all shyness disappears, the right words and gestures are suddenly there . . . uninteresting people, things become intensely interesting. Sensuality is pervasive. the desire to seduce and be seduced is irresistible. Your marrow is infused with unbelievable feelings of ease, power, well-being, omnipotence. euphoria . . you can do anything . . . but somewhere this changes. . . .

The fast ideas become too fast and there are far too many . . . overwhelming confusion replaces clarity . . . you stop keeping up with it—memory goes. Infectious humor ceases to amuse—your friends become frightened . . . everything now is against the grain . . . you are irritable, angry, frightened, uncontrollable, and trapped in the blackest caves of the mind—caves you never knew were there. It will never end. Madness carves its own reality.

Refer to Table 19–3.

ASSESSING BEHAVIOR

During Mania. When in full-blown mania, a person constantly goes from one activity to another, one place to another, and one project to another. Many projects may be started, but few, if any, are completed. Inactivity is impossible, even for the shortest period of time. Hyperactivity may range from mild, constant motion to frenetic, wild activity. The writing of flowery and lengthy letters and the making of numerous and excessive long-distance telephone calls are accentuated. Individuals become involved in pleasurable activities that can have painful consequences. For example, spending large sums of money on frivolous items, giving money away indiscriminately, or making foolish business investments can leave a family penniless. Sexual indiscretion can dissolve relationships and marriages.

Bipolar individuals can be manipulative, profane, fault finding, and adept at exploiting others' vulnerabilities. They constantly push limits. These behaviors often alienate family, friends, employers, health care providers, and others.

When people are hypomanic, they have voracious appetites for food as well as for indiscriminate sex. Although the constant activity of the hypomanic prevents proper sleep, short periods of sleep are possible. However, a reduced need for sleep is experienced by all manic clients, and some clients may not sleep for several days in a row. The manic person is too busy to eat, sleep, or engage in sexual activity. **This nonstop physical activity and the lack of sleep and food can lead to physical exhaustion and even death if not treated.**

Modes of dress often reflect the person's grandiose yet tenuous grasp on reality. Dress may be described as outlandish, bizarre, colorful, and noticeably inappropriate. Make-up may be garish or overdone. Manic people are highly distractible. Concentration is poor, and manic individuals go from one activity to another without completing anything. Judgment is poor. Impulsive marriages and divorces take place.

After Mania. People often emerge from a manic state startled and confused by the shambles of their lives. The following description conveys one client's experience (Jamison 1995):

> Now there are only others' recollections of your behavior—your bizarre, frenetic, aimless behavior—at least mania has the grace to dim memories of itself . . . now it's over, but is it? . . . Incredible feelings to sort through . . . Who is being too polite? Who knows what? What did I do? Why? And most hauntingly, will it, when will it, happen again? Medication to take, to resist, to resent, to forget . . . but always to take. Credit cards revoked . . . explanations at

work . . . bad checks and apologies overdue . . . memory flashes of vague men (what did I do?) . . . friendships gone, a marriage ruined.

ASSESSING THOUGHT PROCESSES. Flight of ideas is a nearly continuous flow of accelerated speech with abrupt changes from topic to topic that are usually based on understandable associations or plays on words. At times, the attentive listener can keep up with the changes, even though direction changes from moment to moment. Speech is rapid, verbose, and circumstantial (including minute and unnecessary details). When the condition is severe, speech may be disorganized and incoherent. The incessant talking often includes joking, puns, and teasing:

> How are you doing, kid, no kidding around, I'm going home . . . home sweet home . . . home is where the heart is, the heart of the matter is I want out and that ain't hay, . . . hey, Doc . . . get me out of this place . . .

The content of speech is often sexually explicit and ranges from grossly inappropriate to vulgar. Themes in the communication of the manic may revolve around extraordinary sexual prowess, brilliant business ability, or unparalleled artistic talents (e.g., writing, painting, and dancing). The person may actually have only average ability in these areas.

Speech is not only profuse, but also loud, bellowing, or even screaming. One can hear the force and energy behind the rapid words. As mania escalates, flight of ideas may give way to clang associations. Clang associations are the stringing together of words because of their rhyming sounds, without regard to their meaning (Schiller and Bennett 1994):

> Cinema I and II, last row. Row, row, row your boat. Don't be a cutthroat. Cut your throat. Get your goat. Go out and vote. And so I wrote . . .

Grandiosity (inflated self-regard) is apparent in either the ideas expressed or the person's behavior. Manic people may exaggerate their achievements or importance, state that they know famous people, or believe that they have great powers (Silverstone and Hunt 1992). The boast of exceptional powers and status can take delusional proportions in mania. Grandiose persecutory delusions are common. For example, manic people may think that God is speaking to them or that the Federal Bureau of Investigation is out to stop them from saving the world. Sensory perceptions may become altered as the mania escalates, and hallucinations may occur. However, in hypomania, no evidence of delusions or hallucinations is present.

Self Assessment

The manic client can elicit numerous intense emotions in the nurse. A manic client is out of control and resists being controlled. The client may use humor, manipulation, power struggles, or demanding behavior to prevent or minimize the staff's ability to set limits on and control dangerous behavior.

The behavior of a manic client is often aimed at decreasing the effectiveness of staff control. He or she might accomplish this by getting involved with power plays. For example, the client might taunt the staff by pointing out faults or oversights, drawing negative attention to one or more staff. Usually, this is done in a loud and disruptive manner, which serves to get staff defensive, thereby escalating the environmental tension and the client's degree of mania.

Another unconscious tactic is to divide staff as a ploy to keep the environment unsettled. The manic client is sensitive to the vulnerabilities and conflicts within a group. Often, a manic client manipulates staff by turning one group of staff against another in an unconscious attempt to discourage outside controls. For example, a client might tell the day shift, "You are the only nurse who listens. On evenings, they hardly look at you. You could drop dead, and the nurses wouldn't even know it." To the evening shift the client might say, "Thank God you're here. At last, someone who cares. All the day people do is push pills and drink coffee." This is a manipulative tactic called splitting, often seen with other clients as well (e.g., borderline and antisocial personality disorder, substance abusers).

The client can become aggressively demanding. This behavior often triggers frustration and exasperation in health care professionals. The manic is adept at distracting staff into defensive positions and setting up an environment that allows the manic defense to go unchecked. Setting limits is an important skill for staff to develop. Adequate administration of medications (anxiolytic, antipsychotic) is essential, particularly in the acute phase of mania.

When the staff start to feel confused and angry with each other, it is often an indication that a client is successfully splitting the staff. Frequent staff meetings dealing with the behaviors of the client and the nurses' responses to these behaviors can help minimize staff splitting and feelings of anger and isolation by the staff. The consistent setting of limits is the main theme for a person in mania.

Consistency among staff is imperative if the limits are to be carried out effectively.

ASSESSMENT GUIDELINES: BIPOLAR DISORDERS

1. Assess danger to self or others:
   - Manic clients can exhaust themselves to the point of death.
   - Client may not eat or sleep for days at a time.
   - Poor impulse control may result in harm to others or self.
   - Uncontrolled spending
2. Clients may give away all of their money or possessions, so they may need controls to protect them from bankruptcy.
3. Assess for need for hospitalization to safeguard and stabilize client.
4. Assess medical status. A thorough medical examination helps to determine if mania is primary (a mood disorder—bipolar/cyclothymia) or secondary to another condition. Mania can be:
   - Secondary to a general medical condition
   - Substance induced (use or abuse of drug, medication, or toxin exposure)
5. Assess for any co-existing medical or other conditions that warrant special intervention (e.g., substance abuse, anxiety disorder, legal or financial crises).
6. Assess the client's and family's understanding of bipolar disorder, knowledge of medications, support groups, and organizations that provide information on bipolar disorder.

NURSING DIAGNOSIS

Nursing diagnoses vary for the manic client. A primary consideration for a client in acute mania is the prevention of exhaustion and death from cardiac collapse. Because of the client's poor judgment, excessive and constant motor activity, probable dehydration, and difficulty evaluating reality, *risk for injury* is a likely and appropriate diagnosis if the client's activity level is dangerous to his or her health. Refer to Table 19–4 for a list of potential nursing diagnoses.

OUTCOME CRITERIA

Outcome criteria will be based on which phase of the illness the client is experiencing.

Phase I: Acute Phase (Acute Mania)

Outcomes will reflect safety issues:

- Be free of injury
  - Cardiac status stable

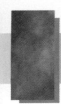

TABLE 19–4 *Potential Nursing Diagnosis*: Bipolar	
SIGNS AND SYMPTOMS	**NURSING DIAGNOSIS**
Excessive and constant motor activity Poor judgment Lack of rest and sleep Poor nutritional intake (excessive/relentless mix of above behaviors can lead to cardiac collapse)	**Risk for Injury**
Loud, profane, hostile, combative, aggressive, demanding Intrusive and taunting behaviors Inability to control behavior Rage reaction	**Risk for Other-Directed Violence/Self-Directed Violence** **Ineffective Coping**
Manipulative, angry, or hostile verbal and physical behaviors Impulsive speech and actions Can be destructive of property or lash out at others in a rage reaction	**Defensive Coping** **Ineffective Coping**
Racing thoughts, grandiosity, poor judgment	**Disturbed Thought Processes** **Ineffective Coping** **Interrupted Family Processes** **Caregiver Role Strain**
Gives away valuables, neglect of family, impulsive major life changes (divorce, career changes)	
Continuous pressured speech jumping from topic to topic (**flights of ideas**)	**Impaired Verbal Communication**
Constant motor activity, going from one person or event to another May annoy or taunt others; speech loud and crass Provocative behaviors	**Impaired Social Interaction**
Too distracted, agitated, and disorganized to eat, groom, bathe, dress self Too frantic and hyperactive to sleep: sleep deprivation can lead to exhaustion and death	**Imbalanced Nutrition, Less than Body Requirements** **Deficient Fluid Volume** **Self-Care Deficit: (Bathing/ Hygiene, Dressing/ Grooming)** **Disturbed Sleep Pattern**

- Well hydrated
- Remains free of abrasions

- Reports an absence of delusions, racing thoughts, and irresponsible behavior

- Obtains a balanced sleep and rest pattern with activity
- Demonstrates an absence of destructive behavior, including sexual activity

Phase II: Continuation of Treatment Phase

Continues for four to nine months: Goal is to prevent relapse:

- Demonstrates adherence to medication regime
- Client and family participate in psychoeducational classes, i.e.,

  - The nature of the disease
  - Medication classes
  - Community support and referrals
  - Effects of drugs and alcohol on precipitating future episodes
  - Clear understanding of early signs and symptoms of relapse

- Finds support in groups or therapy (cognitive-behavioral, interpersonal)
- Attends communication/problem-solving skills training

Phase III: Maintenance Treatment Phase

- Client and family/friends are aware of the prodromal signs of escalating mood or depression
- Adheres to follow-up appointments
- Family obtains support and counseling on ways to reduce daily stress and emotional reactivity
- Client participates in learning interpersonal strategies dealing with work, interpersonal, and family problems
- Client participates in psychotherapy, group, or other ongoing supportive therapy modality

PLANNING

Planning care for a bipolar individual usually is geared toward the particular phase of mania (acute, continuation, or maintenance) as well as any other co-occurring issues included on the assessment (e.g., risk of suicide, risk of violence to person or property, family crisis, legal crises, substance abuse, risk-taking behaviors).

Acute Phase

During the acute phase of mania, measures are taken to medically stabilize the client while maintaining client safety. When mania is acute, hospitalization is usually the safest place for a client. Nursing care is often geared toward lowering physical activity, increasing food and fluids, ensuring at least four to six hours of sleep per night, alleviating any bowel or bladder problems, and intervening with self-care needs. Provide a safe environment. Some clients may require seclusion or even electroconvulsive therapy, and certainly careful medication management.

Continuation Phase

During the continuation phase (lasts four to nine months), measures are taken to help maintain medication compliance and prevent relapse. Depending upon the assessment data regarding the client's interpersonal and stress reduction skills, cognitive functioning, employment status, substance-related problems, social support systems, and such, interventions are planned accordingly. During this time psychoeducational teaching is a must for client and family. Evaluation of the need for communication skills training and problem-solving skills training is an important consideration. The need for referrals to community programs, groups, support for any co-occurring disorders or problems (e.g., substance abuse, family problems, legal issues, and financial crises) is evaluated. People with bipolar disorders often have interpersonal problems that affect their work, family, and social life, as well as other emotional problems. Residual problems resulting from reckless, violent, withdrawn, or bizarre behavior that may have occurred during a manic episode often leave lives shattered and family and friends hurt and distant. For some clients, specific psychotherapy (in addition to medication management) is needed to address these issues, although the focus of psychotherapeutic treatment will vary over time for each individual (Hirschfeld et al. 2000).

Maintenance Phase

During the maintenance phase, the goals are to continue to prevent relapse and to limit the severity and duration of future episodes. Bipolar disorders are lifetime disorders and may require medications over long periods of time, if not a lifetime. Psychotherapy, groups, and periodic evaluations are all appropriate to help clients maintain their family and social life and continue employment, if they are employed.

INTERVENTION

Clients with bipolar disorders are often ambivalent about treatment. Clients may minimize the destructive consequences of their behaviors or deny the seriousness of the disease. Some clients are reluctant to give up the increased energy, euphoria, and heightened sense of self-esteem of hypomania, be-

fore the devastating features of full blown mania commence (Hirschfeld et al. 2000). Unfortunately, nonadherence with mood stabilizing medication is a major cause of relapse. Therefore, the establishment of a therapeutic alliance with the bipolar individual can be crucial.

Acute Phase

Hospitalization is the safest place for a client in acute mania (bipolar I) in order to provide external controls on destructive behaviors and to provide medical stabilization. Unfortunately, sufficient hospital time is not always possible under the present system of managed care. During the hospitalization period, unique approaches to clients are useful in communicating with a client in acute mania and maintaining client safety. Table 19–5 lists suggestions for communication and for providing physical and physiological safety. During this time, the staff will need to continuously set limits in a firm, nonthreatening, and neutral manner in order to prevent further escalation of mania and to provide safe boundaries for the client and others.

PSYCHOPHARMACOLOGY: MOOD STABILIZERS

LITHIUM CARBONATE. Lithium carbonate is effective in the acute treatment of mania and depressive episodes and the prevention of recurrent mania and depressive episodes. Once primary acute mania has been diagnosed, lithium is the first choice for treatment.

Lithium is most effective in up to 90% of clients with pure manic symptoms (elation and grandiosity); of that 90%, 70% experience a full initial response and 20% experience a partial initial response (Maxmen and Ward 1995). Lithium is less effective in people with mixed mania (elation and depression) or in those with rapid cycling (Bowden 1995).

Lithium is particularly effective (Maxmen and Ward 1995) in reducing

■ Elation, grandiosity, and expansiveness
■ Flights of ideas
■ Irritability and manipulativeness
■ Anxiety

To a lesser extent, lithium controls

■ Insomnia
■ Psychomotor agitation
■ Threatening or assaultive behavior
■ Distractibility

Initially, in the treatment of acute mania an antipsychotic drug is given. Antipsychotics act promptly to slow speech, inhibit aggression, and decrease psy-

TABLE 19–5 *Care of the Client in Acute Mania*

INTERVENTION	RATIONALE
Communication	
1. Use firm and calm approach: "John. Come with me. Eat this sandwich."	1. Provides structure and control for a client who is out of control. Can result in feelings of security: "Someone is in control."
2. Use short and concise explanations or statements.	2. Short attention span limits comprehension to small bits of information.
3. Remain neutral; avoid power struggles and value judgments.	3. Client can use inconsistencies and value judgments as justification for arguing and escalating mania.
4. Be consistent in approach and expectations.	4. Consistent limits and expectations minimize potential for client's manipulation of staff.
5. Have frequent staff meetings to plan consistent approaches and to set agreed-on limits.	5. Consistency of all staff is needed to maintain controls and minimize manipulation by client.
6. Staff decides on limits, tells client in simple, concrete terms with consequences, e.g., "John, do not yell at or hit Peter. If you cannot control yourself, we will help you," or "The seclusion room will help you feel less out of control and prevent harm to yourself and others."	6. Clear expectations help client experience outside controls as well as understand reasons for medication, seclusion, or restraints (if he or she is not able to control behaviors).
7. Legitimate complaints should be heard and acted on.	7. Reduces underlying feelings of helplessness and minimizes acting out behaviors.
8. Firmly redirect energy into more appropriate and constructive channels.	8. **Distractibility is the nurse's most effective tool with the manic client.**
Structure in a Safe Milieu	
1. Maintain low level of stimuli in client's environment (e.g., away from bright lights, loud noises, and people).	1. Helps decrease escalation of anxiety.
2. Provide structured solitary activities with nurse or aide.	2. Structure provides security and focus.
3. Provide frequent high-calorie fluids.	3. Prevents serious dehydration.
4. Provide frequent rest periods.	4. Prevents exhaustion.
5. Redirect violent behavior.	5. Physical exercise can decrease tension and provide focus.
6. Acute mania may warrant the use of phenothiazines and seclusion to minimize physical harm.	6. Exhaustion and death can result from dehydration, lack of sleep, and constant physical activity.
7. Observe for signs of lithium toxicity.	7. There is a small margin of safety between therapeutic and toxic doses.
8. Protect client from giving away money and possessions. Hold valuables in hospital safe until rational judgment returns.	8. Client's "generosity" is a manic defense that is consistent with irrational, grandiose thinking.
Physiological Safety: Self Care Needs **Nutrition**	
1. Monitor intake, output, and vital signs.	1. Ensures adequate fluid and caloric intake; minimizes dehydration and cardiac collapse.
2. Offer frequent high-calorie protein drinks and **finger foods** (e.g., sandwiches, fruit, milkshakes).	2. Constant fluid and calorie replacement are needed. Client may be too active to sit at meals. Finger foods allow "eating on the run."
3. Frequently remind client to eat. "Tom, finish your milkshake." "Sally, eat this banana."	3. The manic client is unaware of bodily needs and is easily distracted. Needs supervision to eat.
Sleep	
1. Encourage frequent rest periods during the day.	1. Lack of sleep can lead to exhaustion and death.
2. Keep client in areas of low stimulation.	2. Promotes relaxation and minimizes manic behavior.
3. At night, provide warm baths, soothing music, and medication when indicated. Avoid giving client caffeine.	3. Promotes relaxation, rest, and sleep.

TABLE 19–5 *Care of the Client in Acute Mania (Continued)*

INTERVENTION	RATIONALE
Hygiene	
1. Supervise choice of clothes, minimize flamboyant and bizarre dress, e.g., garish stripes, plaids, and loud, unmatching colors. 2. Give simple step-by-step reminders for hygiene and dress. "Here is your razor. Shave the left side . . . now the right side. Here is your toothbrush. Put the toothpaste on the brush."	1. Lessens the potential for ridicule, which lowers self-esteem and increases the need for manic defense. Assists client in maintaining dignity. 2. Distractibility and poor concentration are countered by simple, concrete instructions.
Elimination	
1. Monitor bowel habits; offer fluids and food that are high in fiber. Evaluate need for laxative. Encourage client to go to the bathroom.	1. Prevents fecal impaction resulting from dehydration and decreased peristalsis.

chomotor activity. The immediate action of the antipsychotic medication is to prevent exhaustion, coronary collapse, and death.

An adjunctive strategy is to initiate treatment of acutely manic clients with both lithium and benzodiazepines such as lorazepam or clonazepam. This strategy allows the clinician to immediately address the insomnia and hyperactivity without the potentially toxic effects of an antipsychotic (Schatzberg et al. 1997). In the case of psychotic features, an antipsychotic may be added as well.

Lithium must reach therapeutic levels in the client's blood to be effective. This usually takes from 7 to 14 days, or longer for some. As lithium levels become effective in reducing manic behavior, the antipsychotics are usually discontinued. Lithium is 70% to 90% effective in treating the manic phase of a bipolar disorder; however, it is not a cure. Many clients receive indefinite lithium maintenance and experience manic and depressive episodes if the drug is discontinued.

Trade names for lithium carbonate include Lithane, Eskalith, and Lithonate. During the *active phase*, 300 to 600 mg by mouth is given two to three times a day, to reach a clear therapeutic result or a lithium level of 0.8 to 1.4 mEq/L. **The actual maintenance blood levels should range between 0.4 and 1.3 mEq/L.** To avoid serious toxicity, lithium levels should *not* exceed 1.5 mEq/L (Hopkins and Gelenberg 2000). At serum levels above 1.5 mEq/L, early signs of toxicity can occur, at 1.5–2.0 advanced signs of toxicity, and at 2.0–2.5 mEq/L or above severe toxicity can occur, and emergency measures should be taken immediately.

In cases of severe lithium toxicity, 2.0 mEq/L or above, gastric lavage and treatment with urea, mannitol, and aminophylline can all hasten lithium excretion. Hemodialysis has also been used in extreme cases.

ADVERSE REACTIONS. A small range exists between the therapeutic dose and the toxic dose of lithium. Initially, blood levels are drawn weekly or biweekly until the therapeutic level has been reached. After therapeutic levels have been reached, blood levels are drawn every month. After 6 months to a year of stability, blood levels every 3 months may suffice (Schatzberg et al. 1997). Blood should be drawn 8 to 12 hours after the last dose of lithium is taken. Refer to Table 19–6 for side effects, signs of lithium toxicity, and interventions.

As mentioned, toxic effects are usually associated with lithium levels of 2.0 mEq/L or more, although they can occur at much lower levels (even within a therapeutic range).

Maintenance Therapy. According to Maxmen and Ward (1995), bipolar relapses occur within 2 years of onset in 20% to 40% of people taking lithium and in 65% to 90% of people not taking lithium. When clients stop taking lithium, relapse usually occurs within several weeks.

Some clinicians suggest that clients with bipolar disorder need to be given lithium for 9 to 12 months, and some clients may need lifelong lithium maintenance in order to prevent further relapses. Many clients respond well to lower doses during maintenance or prophylactic lithium therapy.

Lithium is unquestionably effective in preventing both manic and depressive episodes in clients with

TABLE 19-6   *Drug Information: Side Effects and Signs of Lithium Toxicity*

LEVEL	SIGNS*	INTERVENTIONS
Expected Side Effects		
<0.4–1.0 mEq/L **(therapeutic levels)**	Fine hand tremor, polyuria, and mild thirst.	Symptoms may persist throughout therapy.
	Mild nausea and general discomfort. Weight gain.	Symptoms often subside during treatment. Weight gain may be helped with diet, exercise, and nutritional management.
Early Signs of Toxicity		
<1.5 mEq/L	Nausea, vomiting, diarrhea, thirst, polyuria, slurred speech, muscle weakness.	Medication should be withheld, blood lithium levels drawn, and dose re-evaluated.
Advanced Signs of Toxicity		
1.5–2.0 mEq/L	Coarse hand tremor, persistent gastrointestinal upset, mental confusion, muscle hyperirritability, electroencephalographic changes, incoordination.	Use interventions outlined above or below, depending on severity of circumstances.
Severe Toxicity		
2.0–2.5 mEq/L	Ataxia, serious electroencephalographic changes, blurred vision, clonic movements, large output of dilute urine, seizures, stupor, severe hypotension, coma. Death is usually secondary to pulmonary complications.	There is no known antidote for lithium poisoning. The drug is stopped, and excretion is hastened. If client is alert, provide an emetic. Otherwise, gastric lavage and treatment with urea, mannitol, and aminophylline all hasten lithium excretion.
>2.5 mEq/L	Confusion, incontinence of urine or feces, coma, cardiac arrhythmia, peripheral circulatory collapse, abdominal pain, proteinuria, oliguria, and death.	Hemodialysis may also be used in severe cases.

Data from Scherer, J. C. (1985). *Nurse's drug manual* (pp. 631–632). Philadelphia: J. B. Lippincott; Lehne, R. A., et al. (1998). *Pharmacology for nursing care* (3rd ed., pp. 269–299). Philadelphia: W. B. Saunders; and Lieberman, J. A., and Tasman, A. (2000). *Psychiatric drugs*. Philadelphia: W. B. Saunders.

bipolar disorder. However, complete suppression may occur in only 50% of clients or fewer, even with compliance to maintenance therapy. Therefore, both the person with a bipolar disorder and his or her significant other need careful instructions about (1) the purpose and requirements of lithium therapy, (2) its side effects, (3) its toxic effects and complications, and (4) situations in which the physician should be contacted. Box 19–1 elaborates client and family teaching for a family member taking lithium.

Clients need to know that **two major long-term risks of lithium therapy are hyperthyroidism and impairment of the kidney's ability to concentrate urine.** Therefore, a person on lithium therapy needs to have periodic thyroid and renal follow-up. Health care providers need to stress to bipolar clients and

their families the importance of discontinuing maintenance therapy gradually.

Contraindications. Before the administration of lithium, a medical evaluation is performed to assess a client's ability to tolerate the drug. In particular, baseline physical and laboratory examinations should include renal function; thyroid status, including thyroxine and thyroid-stimulating hormone; and evaluation for dementia or neurological disorders, which signal a poor response to lithium.

Other clinical and laboratory assessments, including an electrocardiogram, are done as needed, depending on the individual's physical condition.

Lithium is generally contraindicated in persons with cardiovascular disease. Lithium may also harm the fetus and is not given to women who are preg-

Thyroid
CBC
24° Creat Cl
EKg Prior to
Lithium therapy

CHAPTER 19 ■ *Mood Disorders: Bipolar* **507**

Box 19–1   *Teaching Clients and Their Families About Lithium*

The client and the client's family should be instructed about the following, encouraged to ask questions, and given the material in written form as well.

1. Lithium can treat your current emotional problem and also helps prevent relapse. Therefore, it is important to continue taking the drug after the current episode is resolved.
2. Because therapeutic and toxic dosage ranges are so close, lithium blood levels must be monitored very closely, more frequently at first, then once every several months after that.
3. Lithium is not addictive.
4. A normal diet and normal salt and fluid intake (1500–3000 mL/day or six 12-ounce glasses) should be maintained. Lithium decreases sodium reabsorption by the renal tubules, which could cause sodium depletion. A low sodium intake causes a relative increase in lithium retention, which could lead to toxicity.
5. Stop taking drug if excessive diarrhea, vomiting, or diaphoresis occurs. Dehydration can raise lithium levels in the blood to toxic levels. **Inform your physician if you have any of these problems.**
6. Diuretics (water pills) are contraindicated with lithium.
7. Lithium is irritating to the gastric mucosa. Therefore, take lithium with meals.
8. **Periodic monitoring of renal functioning and thyroid function is indicated with long-term use.** Discuss follow-up with the doctor.
9. Avoid taking any over-the-counter medications without checking first with the doctor.
10. If weight gain is significant, client may need to see a physician or nutritionist.
11. Many self-help groups have been developed to provide support for people with bipolar disorder and their families. The local self-help group is (give name and telephone number).
12. You can find out more information by calling (give name and telephone number).
13. Keep side-effects/toxic effects on file handy with name and number of contact person (see Box 19–2).
14. **If lithium is to be discontinued, you will be tapered gradually to minimize risk of early relapse.**

---

nant whenever possible. Lithium is also contraindicated in people who have brain damage or renal or thyroid disease. Both the fear of and the wish to become pregnant are a major concern for many bi-

polar women taking lithium. Lithium is also contraindicated in mothers who are breast-feeding or persons who have myasthenia gravis and in children younger than 12 years of age.

ANTIEPILEPTIC DRUGS. As many as 40% of bipolar clients may not respond or respond sufficiently to lithium, or they may not tolerate it. Some subtypes of bipolar clients who may not respond well to lithium but might do well on antiepileptic drugs (AEDs) (Hopkins and Gelenberg 2000) are those with

■ Dysphoric mania (depressive thoughts and feelings during manic episodes)
■ Rapid cycling (four or more episodes a year)
■ EEG abnormalities
■ Substance abuse not associated with mood episodes
■ Progression in frequency and severity of symptoms
■ No family history of bipolar disorder among first-degree relations

The two most widely used AEDs useful in treating mood disorders are carbamazepine and valproic acid. Newer anticonvulsants seem to be effective in some cases of refractory bipolar disease (those cases not responding to traditional approaches). Antiepileptics have been found to:

■ Be superior for continuous cycling clients
■ Be more effective when there is a negative family history of bipolar disease
■ Dampen affective swings in schizoaffective clients
■ Diminish impulsive and aggressive behavior in some nonpsychotic clients
■ Facilitate alcohol and benzodiazepine withdrawal

Clinical benefits include the ability to control mania (within 2 weeks) and depression (within 3 weeks or more).

Carbamazepine (Tegretol). In 25% to 50% of clients with treatment-resistant bipolar disorder, carbamazepine has clear clinical benefits. Some treatment-resistant clients with bipolar disorder improve after taking carbamazepine and lithium or carbamazepine and an antipsychotic. Carbamazepine seems to work better in 60% of clients with rapid cycling and better in severely paranoid, angry, manic clients than in euphoric, overactive, overfriendly manic clients (Schatzberg et al. 1997). It is also thought to be more effective in dysphoric manic clients.

Blood levels of carbamazepine should be monitored at least weekly through the first 8 weeks of treatment because the drug can increase liver enzymes, which then speed its own metabolism (Schatzberg et al. 1997).

Valproic Acid (Depakene, Depakote). Valproic acid has been found helpful for lithium nonresponders in initial studies. It can be useful in treating lithium nonresponders who are in acute mania, who are in rapid cycles, who are in dysphoric mania, or who have not responded to carbamazepine. It has also been helpful in preventing future manic episodes. Numerous new antiepileptic drugs have been introduced.

Two of these newer antiepileptics being used in the treatment of refractory bipolar disorder are *lamotrigine* (Lamictal) and *gabapentin* (Neurontin). Presently there are just anecdotal reports that these agents have been successful in controlling rapid cycling and mixed states in people who have not been helped by other anti-manic agents (Hopkins and Gelenberg 2000). See Table 19–7 for anticonvulsant dose range and major concerns.

ANXIOLYTICS

Clonazepam and Lorazepam. Clonazepam (Klonopin) and lorazepam (Ativan) have been found to be useful in the treatment of acute mania in some treatment-resistant manic clients. These drugs are also effective in managing psychomotor agitation seen in mania. Further studies are needed to provide conclusive evidence for their universal use.

ELECTROCONVULSIVE THERAPY (ECT)

Electroconvulsive therapy (ECT) may also be used to subdue severe manic behavior, especially in treatment-resistant manic clients and clients with rapid cycling (i.e., those who suffer four or more episodes of illness a year). ECT has been found effective in bipolar clients with rapid cycling and those with paranoid-destructive features that often respond poorly to lithium therapy (Abou-Saleh 1992), or who are unable to safely tolerate one of the effective medications (Hirschfeld et al. 2000).

MILIEU THERAPY: SECLUSION

Within the confines of the managed care environment, people in the manic phase of a bipolar disorder have a shorter hospital stay than previously. Important aspects of clients' care are addressed in community-based health care centers at times when clients may still be having difficulty controlling their behavior and following medical guidelines. Therefore, the client must perform specific tasks, and sound discharge planning must be in place during the client's hospital stay. An important part of dis-

TABLE 19–7 *Anticonvulsants*

DRUG	DOSE RANGE	MAJOR CONCERN/SIDE EFFECT
Carbamazepine (Tegretol)	800–1200 mg/day	■ Agranulocytosis or aplastic anemia are most serious side effects. ■ Blood levels should be monitored through first eight weeks because drug induces liver enzymes that speed its own metabolism. Dose may need to be adjusted to maintain serum level of 6–8 mg/L. ■ Sedation is most common problem; tolerance usually develops. ■ Diplopia, incoordination, and sedation can signal excessive levels.
Valproate (Depakene)	750–1000 mg/day	■ Baseline liver function tests should be performed and monitored at regular intervals. Hepatitis, although rare, has been reported, with fatalities in children. ■ Signs and symptoms to watch for: fever, chills, right upper-quadrant pain, dark-colored urine, malaise, and jaundice. ■ Common side effects: tremors, gastrointestinal upset, weight gain, and rarely, alopecia. ■ Consider sedation/somnolence in the elderly.
Lamotrigine (Lamictal)	100–200 mg/day	**Life threatening rash reported in 1 in every 1000 adults; and 1:50–1:1000 in children.** ■ Use caution in renal, hepatic, or cardiac function impairment. ■ Dizziness, diplopia, headache, ataxia, somnolence among frequent side-effects.
Gabapentin (Neurontin)	900–1800 mg/day	■ Most serious side effects are difficulty in breathing, swelling of the lips, rash, slurred speech, drowsiness, and diarrhea. ■ Fatigue, somnolence, dizziness, ataxia, diplopia, hypertension are the more frequent signs and symptoms.

charge planning is finding support for clients' families and locating community resources.

Control during the acute phase of hyperactive behavior almost always includes immediate treatment with an antipsychotic, such as haloperidol (Haldol) or chlorpromazine (Thorazine). However, when a client is dangerously out of control, use of the seclusion room or restraints may also be indicated. The seclusion room can provide comfort and relief to many clients who can no longer control their own behavior.

Seclusion serves the following purposes:

■ Reduces overwhelming environmental stimuli
■ Protects a client from injuring self, others, or staff
■ Prevents destruction of personal property or property of others

Seclusion is warranted when documented data by the nursing and medical staff reflect the following points:

■ Substantial risk of harm to others or self is clear
■ Client is unable to control his or her actions
■ Behavior has been sustained (continues or escalates despite other measures)
■ Other measures have failed (e.g., setting limits or using chemical restraints)

The use of seclusion or restraints involves complex therapeutic, ethical, and legal issues. Most state laws prohibit the use of unnecessary physical restraint or isolation. Barring an emergency, the use of seclusion and restraints warrants the client's consent. Therefore, most hospitals have well-defined protocols for treatment with seclusion. **Seclusion protocols** include a proper reporting procedure through the chain of command when a client is to be secluded. For example, the use of seclusion and restraint is permitted only on the written order of a physician, which must be reviewed and rewritten every 24 hours. The order should also include the type of restraint to be used. As-necessary (prn) orders are updated.

Only in an emergency may the charge nurse place a client in seclusion or restraint; under these circumstances, a written physician's order needs to be obtained within a specified period of time (15 to 30 minutes).

Seclusion protocols also identify specific nursing responsibilities, such as how often the client's behavior is to be observed and documented (e.g., every 15 minutes), how often the client is to be offered food and fluids (e.g., every 30 to 60 minutes), and how often the client is to be toileted (e.g., every 1 to 2 hours). Because phenothiazines are of-

ten used with clients in seclusion, vital signs should be taken frequently (e.g., every 1 to 2 hours).

Careful and precise documentation is a legal necessity. The nurse documents

■ The behavior leading up to the seclusion/restraint
■ What actions were taken to provide the least restrictive alternative
■ The time the client was placed in seclusion
■ Every 15 minutes, the client's behavior, needs, nursing care, and vital signs
■ The time and type of medications given and their effects on the client

When a client does require seclusion to prevent harm to himself or herself or others, it is ideal to have one nurse on each shift work with the client on a continuous basis. Communication with a client in seclusion should be concrete and direct but should be kind and limited to brief instructions. Clients should be reassured that the seclusion is only a temporary measure, and that they will be returned to the unit when their behavior is safer and quieter.

Frequent staff meetings regarding personal feelings about seclusion are necessary to prevent possible dangers. Dangers include using seclusion as a form of punishment and leaving a client in seclusion for long periods of time without proper supervision. Restraints and seclusion should never be used as punishment or for the convenience of the staff. Chapter 4 discusses the legal implications of seclusion and restraints, and Chapter 24 provides more discussion and guidelines.

Continuation Phase

This phase is a crucial one for clients and families. The goal of this phase is to prevent relapse. This phase usually lasts 4 to 9 months. People with bipolar illness and their families can find support in most communities A client may attend a mental health center for medication follow-up. Other clients may attend day hospitals if they are not too excitable and are able to tolerate a certain amount of stimuli. Day hospitals can offer structure, encourage medication compliance, decrease social isolation, and help clients channel their time and energy. If clients are in a homebound status (medicine criteria), then home visits are appropriate for monitoring medications and side effects, supervising health care needs, and evaluating family needs. Community resources are chosen based on the needs of the client, the appropriateness of the referral, and the availability of community resources. Frequently, it is a case manager who evaluates appropriate follow-up care for clients and their families. Medication compliance during this phase is perhaps the most important goal of treatment. Clients and families need support and a place to go for health education when needed.

HEALTH TEACHING

Clients and families need information about bipolar illness, and the chronic and highly recurrent nature of the illness needs to be emphasized and reemphasized to both clients and families. Charts can be used to illustrate the high relapse rate and worsening course in untreated illness, as well as the dramatic effect of the mood stabilizers on the course of manic-depressive illness (Jamison 1995).

Clients and their families also need to be taught the symptoms of impending episodes. For example, changes in sleep patterns are particularly important, since they usually precede, accompany, or precipitate mania. Even a single night of unexplainable sleep loss can be taken for an early warning of impending mania. The regularization of sleep patterns, meals, exercise, and other activities should be stressed to clients (Jamison 1995). See Box 19–2 for guidelines for health teaching for clients with bipolar disease and their families.

Maintenance Phase

Maintenance therapy is aimed at preventing the recurrence of an episode of a bipolar illness. Along with some of the community resources cited earlier, clients and families often greatly benefit from mutual support and self-help groups mentioned later in this chapter.

PSYCHOTHERAPEUTIC APPROACHES

Pharmacology and psychiatric management are essential in the treatment of acute manic attacks. However, bipolar individuals suffer from the psychosocial consequences of their past episodes and their vulnerability to suffering future episodes. People who have bipolar disease also have to face the burden of long-term treatments that may involve some unpleasant side effects (APA 2000). During the course of their illness many clients have sustained strained interpersonal relationships, marriage and family problems, academic and occupational problems, and legal or other social difficulties. Psychotherapy can help people work through these difficulties and decrease some of the psychic distress and increase self-esteem. Psychotherapeutic treatments can also help clients improve their functioning between episodes and attempt to decrease the frequency of future episodes (APA 2000).

Actual research on specific psychosocial interventions for bipolar clients is sparse. Behavioral family management, family therapy, and psychoeducation seem to have helped families to stay together, to

Box 19–2 *Health Teaching: Bipolar Clients and Their Families*

1. Bipolar clients and their families need to know:
   a. About the chronic episodic nature of bipolar illness.
   b. That disease is long-term, therefore maintenance treatment will need to be long-term with a mood stabilizing agent(s).
   c. The expected side effects of medications, the toxic effects of medications, and who to call and where to go.
   d. The signs and symptoms of relapse that may "come out of the blue."
2. Beware of the use of alcohol, drugs of abuse, even small amounts of caffeine, and over-the-counter medications. Sometimes, even a little of these substances can exacerbate bipolar disorder.
3. Practice good sleep hygiene. The prodrome of a manic episode may be lack of sleep. In some cases, mania may be averted by the use of sleeping medications (e.g., temazepam).
4. Psychosocial strategies for dealing with work, interpersonal, and family problems help lower stress, increase sense of personal control, and increase functioning in the community.
5. Psychotherapies (group and/or individual) to gain skills to prevent relapse, gain insight, provide social support, and increase coping skills in interpersonal issues can improve medication compliance, reduce functional morbidity, and may cut down on the rate of hospitalizations.
6. Health care workers need to remember:
   a. Minimization and denial are common defenses that require gradual introduction of facts.
   b. Anger and abusive remarks, although aimed at the health care provider, are symptoms of the disease and are not personal.

Data from Zerbe, K.J. (1999). *Women's mental health in primary care.* Philadelphia: W.B. Saunders.

have lower rates of rehospitalization, and to have improved family functioning (APA 2000, Miklowitz et al. 2000). Cognitive behavioral treatments, which include teaching cognitive behavioral skills for coping with psychosocial stressors and attendant problems, facilitating compliance with treatment, and monitoring the occurrence and severity of symptoms have also been found effective (APA 2000). Currently a formalized psychotherapy called "interpersonal and social rhythm therapy" is being tested in combination with pharmacotherapy in randomized clinical trials for clients during the maintenance phase of bipolar illness (APA 2000).

Psychotherapy is particularly important in the treatment of bipolar illness in encouraging lithium compliance (Jamison 1995b). Often, the clients receiving medication and therapy place more value on psychotherapy than do clinicians. Moreover, clients treated with cognitive therapy more often took their medication as prescribed than did clients who were not in therapy (Jamison 1995).

A client describes her feelings about drug therapy and psychotherapy (Jamison 1995a):

> I cannot imagine leading a normal life without lithium. From startings and stoppings of it, I now know it is an essential part of my sanity. Lithium prevents my seductive but disastrous highs, diminishes my depressions, clears out the weaving of my disordered thinking, slows me, gentles me out, keeps me in my relationships, in my career, out of a hospital, and in psychotherapy. It keeps me alive, too. But psychotherapy heals, it makes some sense of the confusion, it reins in the terrifying thoughts and feelings, it brings back hope, and the possibility of learning from it all. Pills cannot, do not, ease one back into reality. They bring you back headlong, careening, and faster than can be endured at times. Psychotherapy is a sanctuary, it is a battleground, it is where I have come to believe that someday I may be able to contend with all of this. No pill can help me deal with the problem of not wanting to take pills, but no amount of therapy alone can prevent my manias and depressions. I need both.

The belief that bipolar clients are not suitable candidates for group therapy has become well accepted among therapists (Luby and Yalom 1992). Bipolar clients have generally been considered poor psychotherapeutic candidates because of their difficult defensive styles. However, two studies have demonstrated that a long-term homogeneous group of bipolar clients focusing on interpersonal issues can be successful for this population (Luby and Yalom 1992).

SUPPORT GROUPS

People with bipolar disorders who are receiving treatment benefit from forming mutual support groups, such as those sponsored by the National Depressive and Manic-Depressive Association (NDMDA), the National Alliance for the Mentally Ill (NAMI), the National Mental Health Association, and the Manic Depressive Association. Friends and families of people with bipolar disorders can also benefit from mutual support and self-help groups such as those sponsored by NDMDA and NAMI.

EVALUATION

The outcome criteria often dictate the frequency of evaluation of the short-term goals. For example, are the client's vital signs stable, and is he or she well hydrated? Is the client able to control his or her own behavior or respond to external controls? Is the client able to sleep for 4 or 5 hours per night or take frequent short rest periods during the day? Does the family have a clear understanding of the client's disease and need for medication? Do they know which the community agencies may be able to help them?

If goals are not met, the preventing factors are analyzed. Were the data incorrect or insufficient? Were nursing diagnoses inappropriate or goals unrealistic? Was the intervention poorly planned? After the goals and care plan are reassessed, the plan is revised, if indicated. Longer term outcomes include client medication compliance, level of functioning in the community, stability of family, work, and social relationships, stability of mood, and need for stress reduction or new coping skills.

Visit the **Evolve** website at
http://evolve.elsevier.com/Varcarolis
for more Case Studies.

CASE STUDY 19–1 *Mania*

Ms. Horowitz is brought into the emergency department after being found on the highway shortly after her car breaks down. When the police come to her aid, she tells them that she is "driving myself to fame and fortune." She appears overly cheerful, constantly talking, laughing, and making jokes. At the same time, she walks up and down beside the car, sometimes tweaking the cheek of one of the policemen. She is coy and flirtatious with the police officers, saying at one point, "Boys in blue are fun to do."

Case Study continued on following page

CASE STUDY 19–1 *Mania* (*Continued*)

She is dressed in a long red dress, a blue-and-orange scarf, many long chains, and a yellow-and-green turban. When she reaches into the car and starts drinking from an open bottle of bourbon, the police decide that her behavior and general condition might result in harm to herself or others. When they explain to Ms. Horowitz that they want to take her to the hospital for a general check-up, her jovial mood turns to anger and rage, yet 2 minutes after getting into the police car, she is singing "Carry Me Back to Old Virginny."

On admission to the emergency department, she is seen by a psychiatrist, and her sister is called. The sister states that Ms. Horowitz stopped taking her lith-ium about 5 weeks ago and is becoming more and more agitated and out of control. She states that Ms. Horowitz has not eaten in 2 days, has stayed up all night calling friends and strangers all over the country, and finally fled the house when the sister called an ambulance to take her to the hospital. The psychiatrist contacts Ms. Horowitz's physician, and previous history and medical management are discussed. It is decided to hospitalize her during the acute manic phase and restart her lithium therapy. It is hoped that medications and a controlled environment will prevent further escalation of the manic state and prevent possible exhaustion and cardiac collapse.

ASSESSMENT

On Ms. Horowitz's admission to the unit, Mr. Atkins is assigned as her primary nurse. Ms. Horowitz is unable to sit down. She strides ceaselessly up and down the halls, talking loudly, pointing to other clients, and making loud sexual or hostile comments. Some of the other clients laugh at her actions and her dress. Others become angry and defensive.

Mr. Atkins suggests that they go to a quieter part of the unit. Ms. Horowitz turns to him angrily and says, "Let me be . . . set me free, lover . . . I am untouchable . . . I'll get the FBI to set me free."

Mr. Atkins divides the data into subjective and objective components.

OBJECTIVE DATA

- Little if anything to eat for days
- Little if any sleep for days
- History of mania
- History of lithium maintenance
- Constant physical activity: unable to sit
- Very loud and distracting to others
- Anger when wishes are curtailed

- Flight of ideas
- Dress loud and inappropriate
- Remarks suggestive of sexual themes: calls nurse "lover"
- Some clients find her behavior amusing
- Remarks suggest grandiose thinking
- Poor judgment

SUBJECTIVE DATA

- "Driving myself to fame and fortune."
- "I'm untouchable . . . I'll get the FBI to set me free."
- "Let me be . . . set me free, lover."

SELF-ASSESSMENT

Mr. Atkins has worked on the psychiatric unit for 2 years. He has learned to deal with many of the challenging behaviors associated with the manic defense. For example, he no longer takes most of the verbal insults personally, although many of the remarks could be cutting and could hit "close to home." He is also better able to recognize and set limits on some of the tactics used by the manic client to split the staff. The staff on this unit work closely with each other, which makes the atmosphere positive and supportive; therefore, communication is good among staff. Frequent and effective communication is needed among those work-ing with clients who try to divide staff. Clear staff communication is vital to maximize external controls and maintain consistency in nursing care.

The only aspect of Ms. Horowitz's behavior that Mr. Atkins thought he might have some difficulty with is the sexual assaults and loud sexual comments she might make toward him. He knew that this could make him anxious, and his concern is that his anxiety might be picked up by the client.

When discussing this with the unit coordinator, they both decide that two nurses should provide care for Ms. Horowitz. A female nurse would spend time with her in her room, and Mr. Atkins would spend time with her in quiet areas on the unit. It is decided that neither Mr. Atkins nor any male staff member would be alone with Ms. Horowitz in her room at any time. Mr. Atkins should ask for relief if Ms. Horowitz's sexual remarks and acting-out behaviors make him anxious.

Mr. Atkins made the following Nursing Care Plan. See Nursing Care Plan 19-1.

NURSING DIAGNOSIS	Mr. Atkins discusses Ms. Horowitz's immediate needs with the admitting psychiatrist. The psychiatrist orders 5 mg of intramuscular haloperidol (Haldol), to be given immediately. Then, he prescribes 5 mg intramuscularly every 8 hours until she can take the medication by mouth. Thereafter, Ms. Horowitz is to receive an extra 5 mg every other day. If dystoria occurs, she is to be given an anticholinergic agent (benztropine [Cogentin], trihexyphenidyl [Artane]) (see Chapter 20). She is to be observed for behaviors that might indicate harm to herself or others. The medical staff state that if medication and nursing interventions do not reduce her activity level, the nurses should allow for possible periods of rest and ingestion of fluids. Failing that, the use of seclusion would have to be considered. It is agreed that her physical safety is greatly jeopardized. Mr. Atkins's initial diagnoses reflect the nursing and medical staffs' main concern: Ms. Horowitz's physical condition. Although she may present many possible nursing diagnoses and needs at the time, the following two nursing diagnoses are formulated because they focus on her physical safety. 1. **Risk for injury** related to dehydration and faulty judgment, as evidenced by inability to meet own physiological needs and set limits on own behavior ■ Has not slept for days ■ Has not consumed food or fluids for days ■ Constant physical activity; unable to sit 2. **Defensive coping** related to biochemical changes, as evidenced by change in usual communication patterns ■ Very loud and distracting to others ■ Remarks suggested sexual themes ■ Some clients found her behavior amusing ■ Remarks suggested grandiose thinking ■ Flight of ideas ■ Loud, hostile, and sexual remarks to other clients

OUTCOME CRITERIA	Mr. Atkins formulates the following goals:

NURSING DIAGNOSIS	LONG-TERM OUTCOME	SHORT-TERM GOALS
1. **Risk for injury** related to dehydration and faulty judgment, as evidenced by inability to meet own physiological needs and set limits on own behavior.	1. Client's cardiac status will remain stable during manic phase.	1a. Client will be well hydrated, as evidenced by good skin turgor and normal urinary output within 24 hours. 1b. Client will sleep or rest 3 hours during first night in hospital, with aid of medication and nursing intervention.

Case Study continued on following page

CASE STUDY 19–1 *Mania* (Continued)

OUTCOME CRITERIA	NURSING DIAGNOSIS	LONG-TERM OUTCOME	SHORT-TERM GOALS
			1c. Client's blood pressure and pulse will be within normal limits within 24 hours, with aid of medication and nursing measures.
	2. **Defensive coping** related to inadequate psychological resources, as evidenced by change in usual communication patterns.	2. Within 3 days, client will respond to verbal external controls when aggression escalates.	2. Client will engage in safe activities aimed at reducing aggressive energy within 24–48 hours.

INTERVENTION

Because the most immediate concerns for Ms. Horowitz on admission are those of physical safety, 5 mg of intramuscular haloperidol (Haldol) is given intramuscularly. Other clients are moved so that Ms. Horowitz can have a single room. She does not allow vital signs to be taken at first; however, vital signs are eventually taken and recorded at regular intervals. After the nurse spends 2 hours of pacing with Ms. Horowitz and coaxing her into less stimulating areas of the unit, Ms. Horowitz starts taking some fluids. Within 5 hours, she is drinking 8 ounces of high-caloric fluids per hour, after much reminding and encouragement.

By the next day, Ms. Horowitz's behaviors are much less hyperactive, and although her verbal sexual and aggressive assaults are less intense, she continues to provoke other clients. At this time, Mr. Atkins begins to assist her to channel some of her physical energy into less disruptive activities. He and Ms. Horowitz perform some slow exercises to relaxing music in a quiet part of the unit; he provides writing paper for her, and she spends 5 to 10 minutes writing furiously. She continues to pace and yell out to other clients, but with continued medication and nursing intervention, Mr. Atkins sees that this behavior is decreasing.

When Ms. Horowitz's sister comes to visit, she brings clothes, and Mr. Atkins spends some time with the sister finding out more about Ms. Horowitz. He learns that she is a schoolteacher, was depressed for 3 months before her first manic episode 2 years before, and is recently coming out of her second depressive episode. Although the second depressive episode is less severe than the first, the sister is concerned that Ms. Horowitz will "do something foolish," meaning suicide. Ms. Horowitz is separated from her husband and is having a difficult time adjusting to being back at work.

Mr. Atkins and the female nurse encourage Ms. Horowitz to dress and groom herself more appropriately because some of the other clients are beginning to laugh at her appearance. Mr. Atkins is aware that ridicule could further lower Ms. Horowitz's self-esteem, thus increasing her anxiety and need for the manic defense.

Ms. Horowitz's behavior is beginning to be controlled by the lithium about 10 days later, and she is being weaned off the haloperidol. At this time, she is able to talk to Mr. Atkins about how upset and depressed she is about her life (job and separation) and the fact that she must take medication for the "rest of my life." See Nursing Care Plan 19–1.

Mr. Atkins discusses with her some of the side effects of lithium that contributed to her noncompliance. He works with her to reduce and control some of her reactions to lithium. He then reviews other possible side effects and toxic effects of lithium and dietary and other

CASE STUDY 19–1 *Mania (Continued)*

precautions. At the end of her hospital stay, Ms. Horowitz states that she is resigned to continuing her lithium. After talking to Mr. Atkins, she decides to re-enter therapy to "help me get back into life."

EVALUATION

After 2 days, the medical staff think that Ms. Horowitz's cardiac status is stable. Her vital signs are within normal limits, she is consuming sufficient fluids, and her urinary output is normal. Although her hyperactivity persists, it does so to a lesser degree, and she is able to get periods of rest during the day and is sleeping 3 to 4 hours during the night.

Ms. Horowitz's hyperactivity continues to be a challenge to the nurses; however, she is able to attend to some activities that require gross motor movement. These activities are useful in channeling some of her aggressive energy. Shortly after her arrival on the unit, Ms. Horowitz starts a fight with another client, but

seclusion is avoided because she is able to refrain from further violent episodes as a result of medication and nursing interventions. She could be directed toward solitary activities, which channel some of her energies, at least for short periods.

As the effectiveness of the drugs progresses, Ms. Horowitz's activity level decreases, and by discharge, she is able to discuss issues of concern with the nurse and make some useful decisions about her future. She is to be followed up at the community center and agrees to join a family psychoeducational group with her sister and other families with a bipolar member.

Visit the **Evolve** website at
http://evolve.elsevier.com/Varcarolis
for the other Nursing Care Plan diagnoses and for
more Nursing Care Plans.

NURSING CARE PLAN 19–1 *Mania*

NURSING DIAGNOSIS

Risk for Injury: related to dehydration and faulty judgment, as evidenced by inability to meet own physiological needs and set limits on own behavior.

Supporting Data

- Has not slept for days.
- Has not taken in food or fluids for days.
- Constant physical activity—is unable to rest.

Outcome Criteria: Client's cardiac status will remain stable during manic phase.

Nursing Care Plan continued on following page

NURSING CARE PLAN 19–1 **Mania** *(Continued)*

SHORT-TERM GOAL	INTERVENTION	RATIONALE	EVALUATION
1. Client will be well hydrated, as evidenced by good skin turgor and normal urinary output and specific gravity within 24 hours.	1a. Give haloperidol intramuscularly immediately and as ordered.	1a. Continuous physical activity and lack of fluids can eventually lead to cardiac collapse and death.	*GOAL MET* After 3 hours, client takes small amounts of fluids (2–4 ounces per hour).
	1b. Check vital signs frequently (every 1–2 hours).	1b. Monitor cardiac status.	
	1c. Place client in private or quiet room (whenever possible).	1c. Reduce environmental stimuli—minimize escalation of mania and distractibility.	
	1d. Stay with client and divert client away from stimulating situations.	1d. Nurse's presence provides support. Ability to interact with others is temporarily impaired.	
	1e. Offer high-calorie, high-protein drink (8 ounces) every hour in quiet area.	1e. Proper hydration is mandatory for maintenance of cardiac status.	After 5 hours, client starts taking 8 ounces per hour with a lot of reminding and encouragement.
	1f. Frequently remind client to drink: "Take two more sips."	1f. Client's concentration is poor; she is easily distracted.	
	1g. Offer finger food frequently in quiet area.	1g. Client is unable to sit; snacks she can eat while pacing are more likely to be consumed.	
	1h. Maintain record of intake and output.	1h. Enables staff to make accurate nutritional assessment for client's safety.	
	1i. Weigh client daily.	1i. Monitoring nutritional status is necessary.	*GOAL MET* After 24 hours, specific gravity is within normal limits.

NURSING CARE PLAN 19–1 *Mania (Continued)*

SHORT-TERM GOAL	INTERVENTION	RATIONALE	EVALUATION
2. Client will sleep or rest 3 hours during the first night in the hospital with aid of medication and nursing interventions.	2a. Continue to direct client to areas of minimal activity. 2b. When possible, try to direct energy into productive and calming activities (e.g., pacing to slow, soft music; slow exercise; drawing alone; or writing in quiet area). 2c. Encourage short rest periods throughout the day (e.g., 3–5 minutes every hour) when possible. 2d. Client should drink decaffeinated drinks only—decaffeinated coffee, tea, or colas. 2e. Provide nursing measures at bedtime that promote sleep—warm milk, soft music.	2a. Lower levels of stimulation can decrease excitability. 2b. Directing client to paced, nonstimulating activities can help minimize excitability. 2c. Client may be unaware of feelings of fatigue. Can collapse from exhaustion if hyperactivity continues without periods of rest. 2d. Caffeine is a central nervous system stimulant that inhibits needed rest or sleep. 2e. Promotes nonstimulating and relaxing mood.	Client is awake most of the first night. Sleeps for 2 hours from 4 AM to 6 AM. Client is able to rest on the second day for short periods and engage in quiet activities for short periods (5–10 minutes).
3. Client's blood pressure (BP) and pulse (P) will be within normal limits within 24 hours with the aid of medication and nursing interventions.	3a. Continue to monitor blood pressure and pulse frequently throughout the day (every 30 minutes). 3b. Keep staff informed by verbal and written reports of baseline vital signs and client progress.	3a. Physical condition is presently a great strain on client's heart. 3b. Alerting all staff regarding client status can increase medical intervention if a change in status occurs.	Baseline measure on unit is not obtained because of hyperactive behavior. Information from family physician states BP 130/90 and P 88 baseline. BP at end of 24 hours is 130/70; P is 80.

SUMMARY

Genetic factors appear to play a role in the etiology of the bipolar disorder. In addition, little doubt exists that an excess of, and an imbalance in, neurotransmitters are also related to bipolar mood swings. The outward gaiety and expansive, self-confident facade of a manic client often mask feelings of depression. Mania can be observed on a continuum from hypomania to acute mania to delirious mania.

The three main features of mania are (1) euphoria, (2) hyperactivity, and (3) flight of ideas. The nurse assesses the client's mood, behavior, and thought processes to plan the appropriate nursing interventions.

The analysis of the data helps the nurse choose appropriate nursing diagnoses. Some of the nursing diagnoses appropriate for a client who is manic are risk for violence, defensive coping, ineffective coping, disturbed thought processes, and situational low self-esteem. During the acute phase of mania, physical needs often take priority and demand nursing interventions. Therefore, deficient fluid volume and imbalanced nutrition or elimination, as well as disturbed sleep pattern are usually part of the nursing plan. The diagnosis interrupted family processes is also an important consideration. Support groups, psychoeducation, and guidance for the family can greatly affect the client's participation in medication compliance.

Planning nursing care involves identifying the specific needs of the client and family during the three phases of mania. Can the client benefit from communication skills training, increased coping skills, legal or financial counseling, further psychoeducation teaching? What community resources best fit the client needs at this time?

Manic clients can be very demanding and manipulative. Setting limits in a firm, neutral manner as well as using specific communication interventions and interventions for client safety are necessary. Examples of manipulative behavior include pitting members of the staff against each other through manipulation, loudly and persistently pointing to faults and shortcomings in staff, constantly demanding attention and favors of the staff, and provoking clients as well as staff with profane and lewd remarks. The manic client constantly interrupts activities and distracts groups with his or her continuous physical motion and incessant joking and talking. The feelings aroused in such situations are often anger and frustration toward the client by health care workers, family, and friends. When these feelings are not examined and shared, the therapeutic potential of the staff is reduced, and feelings of confusion and helplessness remain.

Antimanic medications are available. Lithium has a narrow therapeutic index which necessitates thorough client and family teaching. Anticonvulsants such as carbamazepine and valproic acid are useful, especially in people refractory to lithium. Other medications may be used to augment the effectiveness of these drugs. At times, ECT may be the most appropriate medical treatment. Client and family teaching takes many forms and is most important in encouraging medication compliance and reducing the risk of relapse.

Evaluation includes examining the effectiveness of the nursing interventions, changing the goals as needed, and reassessing the nursing diagnoses. Evaluation is an ongoing process and is part of each of the other steps in the nursing process.

Visit the **Evolve** website at
http://evolve.elsevier.com/Varcarolis
for a post-test on the content in this chapter.

Visit the **Evolve** website at
http://evolve.elsevier.com/Varcarolis
for additional self-study exercises.

Critical Thinking and Chapter Review

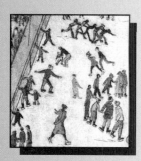

Critical Thinking

1. Donald has been taking lithium for 4 months. During his clinic visit, he tells you, his caseworker, that he does not think he will be taking his lithium anymore because he feels great and he is able to function well at his job and at home with his family. He tells you his wife agrees that "he has this thing licked."

   A. What are Donald's needs in terms of teaching?
   B. What are the needs of the family?
   C. Write out a teaching plan, or use an already constructed plan. Include these issues with sound rationales for the following teaching topics:

      ■ Use of alcohol, drugs, caffeine, over-the-counter medications
      ■ Need for sleep, hygiene
      ■ Types of community resources
      ■ Signs and symptoms of relapse

   D. Role play with a classmate how you could teach this family about bipolar illness and approach effective medication teaching, stressing the need for compliance and emphasizing those things that may threaten compliance.
   E. What referral information (websites, associations) could you give Donald and his family if they asked where they can access further information regarding this disease?

Chapter Review

Choose the most appropriate answer.

1. A major principle that should be observed when a nurse communicates with a client experiencing elated mood is

   1. use calm, firm approach
   2. give expanded explanations
   3. make use of abstract concepts
   4. encourage lightheartedness and joking

2. An outcome for a person in the continuation of treatment phase of bipolar disorder is

   1. client will avoid involvement in self-help groups
   2. client will adhere to medication regime
   3. client will demonstrate euphoric mood
   4. client will maintain normal weight

3. A medication teaching plan for a client receiving lithium should include

   1. rationale for lithium maintenance
   2. dietary teaching to restrict daily sodium intake
   3. importance of blood draws to monitor serum potassium level
   4. seeking medication change if side effects are troublesome

4. Which symptom related to communication is likely to be assessed in a manic client?

   1. mutism
   2. verbosity
   3. poverty of ideas
   4. confabulation

5. For assessment purposes the nurse should identify the body system most at risk for decompensation during a severe manic episode as

   1. renal
   2. cardiac
   3. endocrine
   4. pulmonary

NURSE, CLIENT, AND FAMILY RESOURCES

Associations

National Alliance for the Mentally Ill (NAMI)
200 North Glebe Road, Suite 1015
Arlington, VA 22203-3754
1-703-524-7600; 1-800-950-NAMI

Depressed Anonymous: Recovery from Depression
DSS, Inc.
P.O. Box 17471
Louisville, KY 40217
(502) 569-1989

National Foundation for Depressive Illness
P.O. Box 2257
New York, NY 10116
1-800-248-4344; 1-212-268-4260
http://www.depression.org

National Depressive and Manic-Depressive Association
730 N. Franklin #501
Chicago, IL 60610
1-800-82NDMDA
http://www.ndmda.org

Depression and Related Affective Disorders Association
Meyer #3-181
600 N. Wolfe St.
Baltimore, MD 21287-7381
1-410-955-4647
http://www.med.jhu.edu/drada/

For useful Internet websites, access the Varcarolis SIMON website.

REFERENCES

American Psychiatric Association (2000). *Diagnostic and statistical manual of mental disorders* (4th ed-TR.). Washington, DC: American Psychiatric Press.

American Psychiatric Association (2000). *Practice guidelines for the treatment of psychiatric disorders*. Washington, DC: American Psychiatric Press.

Akiskal, H.S., and Pinto, O. (1999). The evolving bipolar spectrum. *The Psychiatric Clinics of North America*, 22(3): 517–546.

Bowden, C. L. (1995). Treatment of bipolar disorder. In A. F. Schatzberg and C. B. Nemeroff (Eds.), *The American psychiatric press textbook of psychopharmacology* (pp. 603–614). Washington, DC: American Psychiatric Press.

Canceil, O., et al. (1999). First clinical episodes of bipolar disorder. *Encephale*, 25(6): 523–527.

Colom, F., et al. (2000). Clinical factors associated with treatment noncompliance in euthymic bipolar patients. *Journal of Clinical Psychiatry*, 61(8): 549–555.

Delgado, P. L., and Gelenberg, A. J. (1995). Antidepressant and antimanic medications. In G. O. Gabbard (Ed.), *Treatment of psychiatric disorders* (2nd ed., Vol. 1, pp. 1131–1168). Washington, DC: American Psychiatric Press.

Dunayevich, E., et. al. (2000) Twelve month outcome in bipolar patients with and without personality disorders. *Journal of Clinical Psychiatry*, 61(2): 134–139.

Freedman, M.P., and McElroy, S.L. (1999). Clinical picture and etiologic models of mixed states. *The Psychiatric Clinics of North America*, 22(3):535–546.

Gabbard, G. O. (1995). Mood disorders: Psychodynamic etiology. In H. I. Kaplan and B. J. Sadock (Eds.), *Comprehensive textbook of psychiatry IV* (Vol. 1, pp. 1116–1123). Baltimore: Williams & Wilkins.

Ginns, E. I., Ott, J., Egeland, J. M., Allen, C. R., et al. (1996). A genome-wide search for chromosomal loci linked to bipolar affective disorder in the Old Order Amish. *National Genetics*, 12(4):431.

Goldstein, M. J., Baker, B. L., and Jamison, K. R. (1980). *Abnormal psychology: Experiences, origins and interventions*. Boston: Little, Brown.

Hauser, P., Matochik, J., Altshuler, L.L., Denicoff, K.D., et al (2000). MRI-based measurements of temporal lobe and ventricular structures in patients with bipolar 1 and bipolar 11 disorders. *Journal of Affective Disorders*, 60(1): 25–32.

Hirschfeld, R.M.A., et. al. (2000). Practice guidelines for the treatment of patients with bipolar disorder. In *Practice guidelines for the treatment of psychotic disorders, compendium 2000*. Washington, DC: American Psychiatric Association.

Hopkins, H.S., and Gelenberg, A.J. (2000). Mood stabilizers. In J.A. Lieberman and A. Tasman (Eds.), *Psychiatric drugs*. Philadelphia: W.B. Saunders.

Jamison, K. R. (1995a). *An unquiet mind*. New York, A. A. Knopf.

Jamison, K. R. (1995b). Psychotherapy of bipolar patients. Presented at the U. S. Psychiatric and Mental Health Congress, Marriot Marquis, New York, November 18, 1995.

Kelsoe, J. R. (1999). Mood disorders: Genetics. In B. J. Sadock and V. A. Sadock (Eds.), *Kaplan and Sadock's Comprehensive Textbook of Psychiatry* (7th ed., Vol. 2), p. 1308–1317. Philadelphia: Lippincott Williams & Wilkins.

Klerman, G. L. (1978). Affective disorders. In A. M. Nicholi, Jr. (Ed.), *The Harvard guide to modern psychiatry*. Cambridge, MA: Belknap Press of Harvard University Press.

Lehne, R. A., et al. (1994). *Pharmacology of nursing* (2nd ed.). Philadelphia: W. B. Saunders.

Luby, J. L., and Yalom, I. D. (1992). Group therapy. In E. S. Paykel (Ed.), *Handbook of affective disorders* (2nd ed.), pp. 475–486. New York: Guilford Press.

Maxmen, J. S., and Ward, N. G. (1995). *Psychotropic drugs: Fast facts* (2nd ed.). New York: W. W. Norton.

Merikangas, K. R., and Kupfer, D. J. (1995) Mood disorders: Genetic aspects. In H. I. Kaplan and B. J. Sadock (Eds.), *Comprehensive textbook of psychiatry IV* (Vol. 1, pp. 1102–1115). Baltimore: Williams & Wilkins.

Miklowitz, D. J., Simoneau, T.L., George, E.L., Richards, J.A., et al (2000). Family-focused treatment of bipolar disorder: 1-year effects of a psychoeducational program in conjunction with pharmacotherapy. *Biological Psychiatry*, 48(6):582–592.

Moreno, F.A., et al. (1997). Maintenance treatment of bipolar disorder. In D.L. Dunner (Ed.), *Current psychiatric therapy* (2nd ed.), p. 277. Philadelphia: W.B. Saunders.

Nathan, K. I., et al. (1995). Biology of mood disorders. In A. F. Schatzberg and C. B. Nemeroff (Eds.), *The American psychiatric press textbook of psychopharmacology* (pp. 439–477). Washington, DC: American Psychiatric Press.

Nurnberger, J. I., Jr., and Gershon, E. S. (1992). Genetics. In E. S. Paykel (Ed.), *Handbook of affective disorders* (2nd ed.), pp. 131–148. New York: Guilford Press.

Perris, C. (1992). Bipolar-unipolar distinction. In E. S. Paykel (Ed.), *Handbook of affective disorders* (2nd ed.), pp. 57–76. New York: Guilford Press.

Post, R. M., Rubinow, D. R., and Uhde, T. W. (1989). Dysphoric mania: Clinical and biological correlates. *Archives of General Psychiatry*, 46:353–358.

Post, R. M. (1992). Anticonvulsants and novel drugs. In E. S. Paykel (Ed.), *Handbook of affective disorders* (2nd ed.), pp. 387–418. New York: Guilford Press.

Preston, J., and Johnson, J. (1995). *Clinical psychopharmacology made ridiculously simple*. Miami: MedMaster.

Ramana, R., and Bebbington, P. (1995). Social influences on bipolar affective disorders. *Social Psychiatry-Psychiatric Epidemiology*, 30(4):152.

Schatzberg, A. F., Cole, J. O., and Debattista, C. (1977). *Manual of clinical psychopharmacology*. (3rd ed.). Washington, DC: American Psychiatric Press.

Scherer, J. S. (1985). *Nurses' drug manual*. Philadelphia: J. B. Lippincott.

Schiller, L., and Bennett, A. (1994). *The quiet room*. New York: Warner Books.

Silverstone, T., and Hunt, N. (1992). Symptoms and assessment of mania. In E. S. Paykel (Ed.), *Handbook of affective disorders* (2nd ed.), pp. 15–24. New York: Guilford Press.

Sonne, S.C., and Brady, K.T. (1999). Substance abuse and bipolar comorbidity. *The Psychiatric Clinics of North America*, 22(3): 609–628.

Strakowski, S.M., and DelBello, M.P. (2000). The occurrence of bipolar and substance use disorders. *Clinical Psychology Review*, 20(2): 191–206.

Wacker, H.R. (2000). Epidemiology and comorbidity of depressive disorders. *Ther Umsch*, 57(2): 53–58.

Zerbe, K.J. (1999). *Women's mental health in primary care*. Philadelphia: W.B. Saunders.

effects and toxic effects, (d) needs for client and family teaching and follow-up, and (e) cost.

9. Analyze the effective strategies of individual, group, and family therapies that are most useful for schizophrenic clients and their families.
10. Differentiate among the three phases of schizophrenia as to symptoms, focus of care, and needs for intervention.
11. Apply the key elements of a teaching plan for a schizophrenic client and a family member to the nursing care of one client with schizophrenia.
12. Analyze the different approaches to care between a paranoid client and a disorganized client with schizophrenia.

EPIDEMIOLOGY

Schizophrenia is a devastating disease of the brain that affects a person's thinking, language, emotions, social behavior and ability to accurately perceive reality. Unfortunately, people with this disease are often misunderstood and stigmatized by even the medical community as well as the general population (Andreasen and Munich 1995). The lifetime prevalence of schizophrenia is 1% worldwide.

The most typical age for onset of schizophrenia is during the late teens and early 20s, although cases of onset at age 5 or 6 have been reported (DSM-IV-TR 2000). Men and women are equally represented in the population of individuals with this disease; however, there are some differences. Individuals with an early age of onset (18–25) are more often male and have poorer premorbid adjustments, more evidence of structural brain abnormalities, and more prominent negative symptoms (DSM-IV-TR 2000). Individuals with a later onset (25–35) are more likely to be female, have less evidence of structural brain abnormalities, and have better outcomes (DSM-IV-TR 2000).

Course

The course of the disease usually involves recurrent acute exacerbations of psychosis. Kissling (1991) stated that prevention of relapse is more important than risk of side effects from medications because most side effects are reversible, but the consequences of relapse may be irreversible. With each relapse of psychosis, there is an increase in residual dysfunction and deterioration. The phases in the course of the disease are:

1. Acute phase: periods of florid positive symptoms (e.g., hallucinations, delusions) as well as negative symptoms (e.g., apathy, withdrawal, no motivation).
2. Maintenance phase: period when acute symptoms decrease in severity. This phase can last up to 6 months or more after the acute phase.
3. Stable phase: period where symptoms are in remission.

COMORBIDITY

Substance abuse disorders occur in approximately 40% to 50% of individuals with schizophrenia (Blanchard et al. 2000), and the lifetime incidence is even higher at 60% (APA 2000). Substance abuse is associated with a variety of negative outcomes: incarceration, homelessness, violence, suicide, and HIV infection. Substance abuse in schizophrenia is also linked with male gender, more pronounced psychotic symptoms, nonadherence with medication, and poor prognosis (Soyka 2000).

Nicotine dependence is very common in schizophrenia and may be as high as 80% to 90% (DSM-IV-TR 2000). Nicotine addicted schizophrenic individuals have a high rate of emphysema and other pulmonary and cardiac problems (DSM-IV-TR 2000).

Depressive symptoms occur frequently in schizophrenia. Suicide is the leading cause of premature death in this population at 10% or perhaps higher (Andreasen 2000), with 20% to 40% making at least one attempt over the course of the illness. A significant percentage of suicides in schizophrenia occurs during periods of remission after 5 to 10 years of illness (APA 2000). Comorbid **anxiety disorders** are also found to be higher in individuals with schizophrenia than in the general population. **Psychosis-induced polydipsia** occurs in 6% to 20% of people with chronic mental illness. This phenomenon is the compulsive drinking of 4 to 10 liters of water a day.

THEORY

The causation of schizophrenia is clearly a complicated matter. What is known is that the brain chemistry and brain activity are different in a person suffering from schizophrenia compared with a person without schizophrenia (Andreasen 1999, Korn and Saito 2000, Schizophrenia 1999, Saito 2000).

Schizophrenia most likely occurs as a result of a combination of inherited genetic factors and extreme nongenetic factors (e.g., virus, birth injuries, nutritional factors), which can affect the genes governing the brain, or injure the brain directly (Andreasen 2000). These factors may alter the structures of the brain, affect the brain's neurotransmitter system, and disrupt the neural circuits, resulting in impairment in cognition.

The hypothesis shared by most investigators today is that schizophrenia is a disease of neural connectivity (communication within the brain) caused by multiple factors that affect brain development (Andreasen 2000, Andreasen 1999).

Research findings from numerous studies suggest

- A multifactorial cause is likely but unknown.
- Neurological, structural, and functional abnormalities have been identified.
- Neuropsychological evidence suggests a subcortical cognitive focus; the *N*-methyl-D-aspartate (NMDA) receptor complex has been implicated.
- No single region or transmitter abnormality explains the disease, although dopamine, serotonin, and glutamate all seem to play a part.
- A disease that arises from dysfunctional neural circuits may best explain schizophrenia.

Neurobiologic Findings

To make matters even more complex, schizophrenia is not a single disease, but a syndrome that involves neurobiochemical and neuroanatomic abnormalities with strong genetic links. Multiple nongenetic factors may also be present and may play a role in the development of schizophrenia.

Dopamine Hypotheses

For many years the most widely accepted explanation for the biochemical pathophysiology was the "dopamine hypothesis."

The dopamine theory of schizophrenia is derived from the study of the action of the antipsychotic drugs that have dopamine blocking agents (D2). These antipsychotics block some of the dopamine receptors in the brain (D2), which thereby limits the activity of dopamine and reduces some of the symptoms of schizophrenia. Amphetamines, cocaine, methylphenidate (Ritalin), and levodopa are drugs that increase the activity of dopamine in the brain. These drugs produce an excess of dopamine in the

brain and, in large doses, can exacerbate the symptoms of schizophrenia in psychotic clients. Amphetamines, cocaine, and other drugs can simulate symptoms of paranoid schizophrenia in a nonschizophrenic person.

Because the dopamine blocking agents do not ameliorate all the symptoms of schizophrenia, the "dopamine hypothesis" is no longer considered conclusive.

Alternative Biochemical Findings

More recent hypotheses include the role of other neurotransmitter systems (e.g., norepinephrine, serotonin, glutamate, γ-aminobutyric acid [GABA], neuropeptides, and neuromodulatory substances) in the pathophysiology of schizophrenia (Black and Andreasen 1999).

The development of the atypical antipsychotics that block serotonin as well as dopamine suggests that **serotonin** may play a role in the causation of the symptoms of schizophrenia. The understanding of how atypical antipsychotic drugs modulate the expression and targeting 5-hydroxytryptamine 2_A (5-HT_{2A}) may provide unique insight into schizophrenia (Yamada 2000).

It has long been noted that the phencyclidine piperidine (PCP) induces a state that closely resembles schizophrenia. This observation has resulted in a renewed interest in the NMDA receptor complex and the possible role of **glutamate** in the pathophysiology of schizophrenia (Wyall et al. 1999, Black and Andreasen 1999). Glutamate is a crucial neurotransmitter during periods of neural maturation, and abnormal maturation of the central nervous system (CNS) is considered to be a central factor in the development of schizophrenia (Korn and Saito 2000).

Genetic Findings

There is unquestionable evidence of a genetic contribution to some, and perhaps all, of the diseases classified as schizophrenic. It has long been observed that schizophrenia and schizophrenic-like symptoms occur at an increased rate in relatives with schizophrenia. For example (Black and Andreasen 1999, Carpenter and Buchanan 1995, Jones and Cannon 1998):

- If one parent has schizophrenia, about 12% of his or her children develop the disease.
- If both parents have schizophrenia, up to 46% of their children will get the disease.

- Among identical twins (from the same egg), 40% to 50% will both develop schizophrenia.
- Among fraternal twins (from two eggs), in 15% both twins will develop schizophrenia.
- Children of "normal" parents who are placed in foster homes in which a foster parent later had schizophrenia do not show an increased rate of schizophrenia.

Evidence suggests that several genes on different chromosomes interact with environmental factors to cause schizophrenia. In a study sponsored by the National Institutes of Mental Health, Brzustowicz and colleagues (2000) reported a strong statistical connection between a location on chromosome 1 and schizophrenia. Brzustowicz and her team (2000) also found evidence of a weaker linkage on chromosome 13.

Neuroanatomic Findings

Disruptions in the connecting and communication within neural circuitry (communication pathways) are thought to be severe in schizophrenia. Therefore, structural cerebral abnormalities could cause disruption to the entire circuit in the brain.

Brain-imaging techniques, such as computed tomography (CT), magnetic resonance imaging (MRI), and positron-emission tomography (PET), provide substantial evidence that some schizophrenic people have structural brain abnormalities. MRI and CT scans have found lower brain volume and more cerebral spinal fluid in people with schizophrenia than in those of healthy people (Kaplan and Sadock 1995).

Computed tomographic and magnetic resonance imaging studies provide evidence for structural cerebral abnormalities. Some findings include the following:

- Enlargement of the lateral cerebral ventricles
- Cortical atrophy
- Third ventricular dilation
- Ventricular asymmetry
- Cerebellar atrophy
- Atrophy of the frontal lobe

Some schizophrenic clients may also have changes in the cerebral cortex, the region of the brain that governs higher mental functions. During neurological testing, PET scans also show a low rate of blood flow and glucose metabolism in the frontal lobes of the cerebral cortex, which govern planning, abstract thinking, and social adjustment. Refer to Chapter 3 for a PET scan that demonstrates reduced brain activity in the frontal lobe of a person with schizophrenia.

Nongenetic Risk Factors

BIRTH AND PREGNANCY COMPLICATIONS. Theories in this area arise from the fact that infants born with a history of pregnancy or birth complications are at increased risk for developing schizophrenia as adults. Infections during pregnancy, poor nutrition during pregnancy, or exposure to toxins could all damage neurons or affect neurotransmitter systems in the fetus.

STRESS-RELATED THEORIES. Developmental and family stress and other social, physiological, or physical stress may play a significant role in the severity and course of the disease, as well as the person's quality of life. There is no evidence that stress causes schizophrenia, although it may precipitate it in a vulnerable individual.

Other risk factors include such things as birth during the winter, birth in urban areas, and low socioeconomic status.

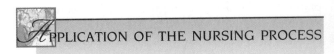

APPLICATION OF THE NURSING PROCESS

ASSESSMENT

DSM-IV-TR *Criteria for Schizophrenia*

In 1950, Eugen Bleuler, building on the observations of Emil Kraepelin, coined the term **schizophrenia.** Bleuler's fundamental signs of schizophrenia are referred to as the four As. The four As are

1. **Affect,** the outward manifestation of a person's feelings and emotions. In schizophrenia, one can observe flat, blunted, inappropriate, or bizarre affect.
2. **Associative looseness,** which refers to haphazard and confused thinking that is manifested in jumbled and illogical speech and reasoning. People also use the term *looseness of association.*
3. **Autism,** thinking that is not bound to reality but reflects the private perceptual world of the individual. Delusions, hallucinations, and neologisms are examples of autistic thinking in a person with schizophrenia.
4. **Ambivalence,** simultaneously holding two opposing emotions, attitudes, ideas, or wishes toward the same person, situation, or object. Ambivalence occurs normally in all relationships. Pathological ambivalence is paralyzing.

Vignette

■ *Sam, a 25-year-old man soon to be discharged from the hospital, constantly tells the social worker he wants his own apartment. When Sam is told that an apartment has been found for him, he states, "But who will take care of me?" Sam is acting out his ambivalence between his desire to be independent and his desire to be taken care of.*

In 1959, Kurt Schneider developed a system of diagnosing a person with schizophrenia by classifying ongoing symptoms as first rank and second rank. In 1975, the World Health Organization (WHO) identified a standard set of symptoms specific to the diagnosis of schizophrenia; this set is common to people in numerous countries. Today clinicians in the USA use the DSM-IV-TR (2000) criteria for the diagnosis of schizophrenia. Subtypes of schizophrenia include Paranoid, Catatonic, Disorganized, Undifferentiated, and Residual.

Symptoms in schizophrenia are many and not all people with schizophrenia have the same symptoms, even within a specific subtype. Figure 20–1 breaks down the signs and symptoms of schizophrenia into four main areas: positive symptoms, negative symptoms, cognitive symptoms and co-occurring problems.

Often before the acute onset of symptom identification, there are early (prodromal) signs of the disease that may puzzle and distress both client and family. The following narrative of early onset gives the reader an understanding of a young person's experience before the full-blown disease occurs. There is increased evidence that identifying and treating schizophrenia early on is associated with relatively favorable outcomes (Tsuang 2000).

OVERALL ASSESSMENT

Prodromal/Early Symptoms

Many people who have schizophrenia experience prodromal symptoms a month to a year before their first psychotic break. These symptoms represent a clear deterioration in previous functioning. Often, a person who has schizophrenia was withdrawn from others, lonely, and perhaps depressed as an adolescent. Plans for the future may appear vague or unrealistic to others.

In the early phase a person may complain about acute or chronic anxiety, phobias, obsessions, and

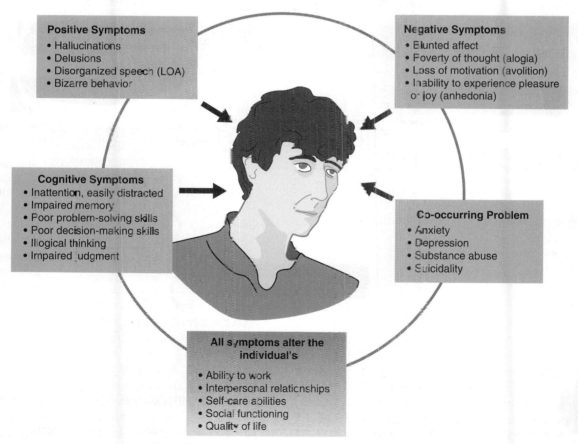

Figure 20–1 Signs and symptoms of schizophrenia.

compulsions, or he or she may have dissociative features. As anxiety mounts, indications of a thought disorder may be present. An adolescent may have difficulty with concentration and with the ability to complete school work or job-related work. Eventually, severe deterioration of work and deterioration of ability to cope with the environment occur. People report having "mind wandering," inability to concentrate, and a need to devote more time to maintaining one's thoughts. Finally, the ability to keep out unwanted intrusions into one's thoughts becomes impossible. Eventually, the person finds that his or her mind becomes so distracted that the ability to have ordinary conversations with others is lost (Kolb and Brodie 1982).

An individual may at first feel that something "strange" or "wrong" is going on. He or she misinterprets things going on in the environment and may give mystical or symbolic meanings to ordinary events. For example, they may think that certain colors hold special powers or that a thunderstorm is a message from God. Other people's actions or words may be mistaken for signs of hostility or evidence of harmful intent (Kolb and Brodie 1982).

As the disease develops, strong feelings of rejection, lack of self-respect, loneliness, and hopelessness begin to emerge. Emotional and physical withdrawal increase feelings of isolation, as does an inability to trust or relate to others. Difficulty in reality testing may become evident in hallucinations, delusions, and odd mannerisms. Some individuals think their thoughts are being controlled by others or that their thoughts are being broadcast to the world. Others may think that people are out to harm them or are spreading rumors about them. Voices are sometimes heard in the form of commands or derogatory statements about their character. The voices may seem to come from outside the room, from electrical appliances, or from other sources.

Early in the disease a person may be preoccupied with religion, matters of mysticism, or metaphysical causes of creation. Speech may be characterized by obscure symbolisms.

Later, words and phases may become indecipherable, and these can be understood only as part of the person's private world. Sometimes, he or she makes up words. People who have been ill with

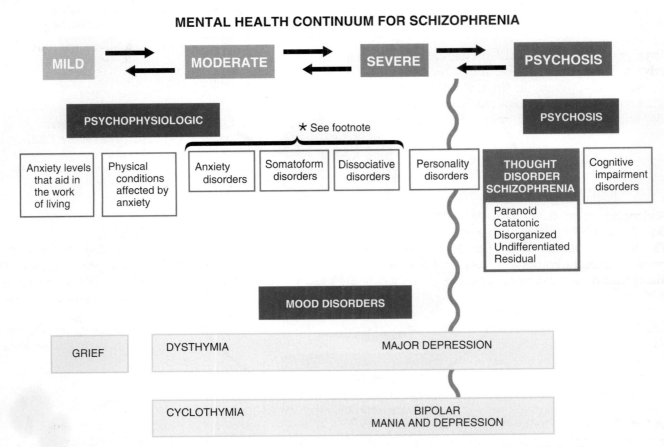

* These disorders are currently classified by presenting clinical symptoms. Previously they were called "neurotic" disorders.

Figure 20-2 Mental health continuum for schizophrenia.

schizophrenia for a long time often have speech patterns that are incoherent, rambling, and devoid of meaning to the casual observer.

Sexual activity is frequently altered in mental disorders. Preoccupation with homosexual themes may be associated with all psychoses but is most prominent in people with paranoid schizophrenia. Doubts regarding sexual identity, exaggerated sexual needs, altered sexual performance, and fears of intimacy are prominent in schizophrenia. The process of regression in schizophrenia is accompanied by increased self-preoccupation, isolation, and masturbatory behavior.

An abrupt onset with good premorbid functioning is usually a favorable prognostic sign. A slow, insidious onset over a period of 2 or 3 years is more ominous. Those whose prepsychotic personalities show good social, sexual, and occupational functioning have a greater chance for a good remission or a complete recovery. Childhood histories of withdrawn, seclusive, eccentric, and tense behavior are unfavorable diagnostic signs. The younger the client is at the onset of schizophrenia, the more discouraging the prognosis. Because schizophrenia is a psychotic disorder, it is placed on the high end of the mental illness continuum (Fig. 20–2).

Early psychiatric and medical treatment helps secure a more favorable eventual outcome. A delay of months or years allows the psychotic process to become more entrenched. No single symptom is always present in all cases of schizophrenia or occurs only in schizophrenia alone (refer back to Fig. 20–1). Figure 20–3 identifies the DSM-IV-TR criteria for schizophrenia. The various subtypes of schizophrenia, with symptoms, are outlined later in the chapter.

Assessing Symptoms

Schizophrenia is classified as a psychotic disorder. Box 20–1 briefly defines other psychotic disorders. The term **psychotic** here refers to "delusions, any prominent hallucinations, disorganized speech, or disorganized or catatonic behavior" (DSM-IV-TR 2000, p. 297).

The symptoms of schizophrenia can be classified into four overall groups of symptoms: Positive, Negative, Cognitive, and Disorganized.

The positive symptoms (e.g., hallucinations, delusions, bizarre behavior, and paranoia) are the attention-getting symptoms referred to as *florid psychotic symptoms*. Three decades of analysis of treatment and study findings indicate that perhaps these florid psychotic symptoms may not be the core deficiency after all. Actually, the crippling negative symptoms (e.g., apathy, lack of motivation, anhedonia, and

---

DSM-IV-TR Diagnostic Criteria for Schizophrenia

A. Characteristic Symptoms
Two or more of the following during a 1-month period (or less if successfully treated)
1. Delusions
2. Hallucinations
3. Disorganized speech (e.g., LOA)
4. Grossly disorganized or catatonic behavior
5. Negative symptoms (e.g., affective flattening, avolition, alogia)
If delusions bizarre or auditory hallucinations and
   a. voices keep a running commentary about person's thoughts/behaviors **or**
   b. two or more voices converse with each other
Then only one criterion is needed.

B Social/Occupational Dysfunction
If one or more major areas of the person's life are markedly below premorbid functioning (work, interpersonal relationships or self-care) **or**
If childhood or adolescence failure to achieve expected level of interpersonal, academic, or occupational achievement
Then meets criteria of **B**.

C. Duration
Continuous signs persist for at least 6 months with at least 1 month that meets criteria of **A** (Active Phase) and may include prodromal or residual symptoms.

D. 1. **All other mental diseases** (e.g., schizoaffective/ mood disorder) have been ruled out.
   2. **All other medical conditions** (substance use/ medications or general medical conditions) have been ruled out.
   3. **If history of pervasive developmental disorders**, then prominent hallucinations or delusions for 1 month are needed to make the diagnosis of schizophrenia.

Figure 20–3 Diagnostic criteria for schizophrenia. (Adapted from American Psychiatric Association [2000], *Diagnostic and statistical manual of mental disorders. Text Revision, 4th ed.* Washington, D.C.: American Psychiatric Association. Copyright 2000 American Psychiatric Association.)

---

poor thought processes) persist and seem the most destructive because they render the person inert and unmotivated (Black and Andreasen 1999). The positive-negative approach may correlate with prognosis as well as biological variables.

Positive symptoms, such as hallucinations, delusions, bizarre behavior, and paranoia, are associated with

- Acute onset
- Normal premorbid functioning
- Normal social functioning during remissions
- Normal computed tomographic findings
- Normal neuropsychological test results
- Favorable response to antipsychotic medication

BOX 20–1 *Other Psychotic Disorders*

SCHIZOPHRENIFORM DISORDER

The essential features of this disorder are exactly those of schizophrenia except that:

- The total duration of the illness is at least 1 month but less than 6 months.
- Impaired social or occupational functioning during some part of the illness is not apparent (although it may appear).

This disorder may or may not have a good prognosis.

BRIEF PSYCHOTIC DISORDER

This is a disorder in which there is a sudden onset of psychotic symptoms (delusions, hallucinations, disorganized speech) or grossly disorganized or catatonic behavior. The episode lasts at least 1 day but less than 1 month, and then the individual returns to his or her premorbid level of functioning. Brief psychotic disorders often follow extremely stressful life events.

SCHIZOAFFECTIVE DISORDER

This disorder is characterized by an uninterrupted period of illness during which time there is a major depressive, manic or mixed episode, concurrent with symptoms that meet the criteria for schizophrenia. The symptoms must not be due to any substance use or abuse or general medical condition.

DELUSIONAL DISORDER

This disorder involves nonbizarre delusions (situations that occur in real life such as being followed, infected, loved at a distance, or deceived by a spouse, or having a disease) of at least one month's duration. The person's ability to function is not markedly impaired nor is the person's behavior obviously odd or bizarre. Common types of delusions seen in this disorder are delusions of grandeur, persecution, jealousy, somatic, or mixed.

SHARED PSYCHOTIC DISORDER (FOLIE À DEUX)

A shared psychotic disorder is an occurrence in which one individual who is in a close relationship with another who has a psychotic disorder with a delusion, eventually comes to share the delusional beliefs either in total or in part. Apart from the shared delusion, the person who takes on the other's delusional behavior is not otherwise odd or unusual. Impairment of the person who shares the delusion is usually much less than the person who has the psychotic disorder with the delusion. The cult phenomenon is an example, as was demonstrated at Waco and Jonestown.

INDUCED OR SECONDARY PSYCHOSIS

Psychosis may be induced by substances (drugs of abuse, alcohol, medications or toxin exposure) or caused by the physiologic consequences of a general medical condition (delirium, neurological conditions, metabolic conditions, hepatic or renal diseases and many more). Medical conditions and substances of abuse must always be ruled out before a primary diagnosis of a schizophrenia or other psychotic disorder can be made.

Varcarolis, E. (2000). *Psychiatric nursing clinical guide*. Philadelphia: W.B. Saunders.

Negative symptoms, such as apathy, anhedonia, poor social functioning, and poverty of thought, are associated with

- Insidious onset
- Premorbid history of emotional problems
- Chronic deterioration
- Demonstration of atrophy on computed tomographic scans
- Abnormalities on neuropsychological testing
- Poor response to antipsychotic therapy

Cognitive symptoms represent the third group. Cognitive impairment affects at least 40% to 60% of people with schizophrenia and is now accepted as one of the major disabilities associated with schizophrenia (Andreasen et al 1998). Cognitive impairment involves difficulty with attention, memory, and executive functions (e.g., decision making and problem solving). Good verbal memory has been found to be the one indicator of eventual community functioning, since it helps with acquiring psychosocial skills, learning and retention skills. These are all necessary for eventual rehabilitation (Andreasen et al 1998).

The **disorganized** dimension describes the degree to which disorganized speech, disorganized behavior, or inappropriate affect is present (DSM-IV-TR 2000).

POSITIVE SYMPTOMS

The positive symptoms appear early in the first phase of the illness and often precipitate hospitalization. They are, however, the least important prognostically and usually respond to antipsychotic medication, both the standard and the newer atypical antipsychotics (AAPs). The positive symptoms are presented here in terms of alterations in thinking, and alterations in speech, perceiving, and behavior.

Alterations in Thinking

Delusions. Alterations in thinking can take many forms. Delusions are most often defined as false fixed beliefs that cannot be corrected by reasoning. They may be simple beliefs or part of a complex delusional system. In schizophrenia, delusions are often loosely organized and may be grotesque. Most commonly, delusional thinking involves the following themes:

- Ideas of reference
- Persecution
- Grandiosity
- Somatic
- Jealousy
- Control

Table 20–1 provides definitions and examples of delusions.

About 75% of schizophrenic people experience delusions at some time during their illness. In schizophrenia, persecutory and grandiose delusions are the most common, as are those involving religious or hypochondriacal ideas.

In the acute phase of schizophrenia, the person is overwhelmed by anxiety and is not able to distinguish what is inside (thoughts) from what is outside (reality). Therefore, a delusion may stimulate behavior for dealing with confusion and the resulting anxiety.

When delusional, a person truly believes what he or she thinks to be real is real. The person's thinking often reflects feelings of great fear and aloneness: "I know the doctor talks to the CIA about getting rid of me" or "Everyone wants me dead." Delusions may reflect the person's feelings of low self-worth through the use of reaction-formation (observed as grandiosity). "I'm the only one who can save the world, but they won't let me."

At times, delusions hold a kernel of truth. One client came into the hospital acutely psychotic. He kept saying that the Mafia was out to kill him. Later, the staff learned that he had been selling drugs, that he had not paid his contacts, and that gang members were out trying to find him and hurt him or even kill him.

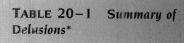

TABLE 20–1 Summary of Delusions*	
DEFINITION	**EXAMPLE**
Ideas of Reference	
Misconstruing trivial events and remarks and giving them personal significance	When Maria saw the doctor and nurse talking together, she believed they were talking against her. When she heard on the radio that a hurricane was coming, she believed this to be a message that harm was going to befall her.
Persecution	
The false belief that one is being singled out for harm by others; this belief often takes the form of a plot by people in power against the person	Sam believed that the Secret Service was planning to kill him. He became wary of the food he ate, since he believed that the Secret Service was poisoning his food.
Grandeur	
The false belief that one is a very powerful and important person	Sally believed that she was Mary Magdalene and that Jesus controlled her thoughts and was telling her how to save the world.
Somatic Delusions	
The false belief that the body is changing in an unusual way, e.g., rotting inside	David told the doctor that his brain was rotting away.
Jealousy	
The false belief that one's mate is unfaithful. May have so-called proof	Harry accused his girlfriend of going out with other men, even though this was not the case. His "proof" was that she came home from work late twice that week. He persisted in his belief, even when the girlfriend's boss explained that everyone had worked late.

*A false belief held and maintained as true, even with evidence to the contrary. This does not include unusual beliefs maintained by one's culture or subculture.

Other common delusions observed in schizophrenia are the following:

1. **Thought broadcasting,** the belief that one's thoughts can be heard by others (e.g., "My brain is connected to the world mind. I can control all heads of state through my thoughts.").
2. **Thought insertion,** the belief that thoughts of others are being inserted into one's mind (e.g., "They make me think bad thoughts.").
3. **Thought withdrawal,** the belief that thoughts have been removed from one's mind by an outside agency (e.g., "The devil takes my thoughts away and leaves me empty.").
4. **Delusions of being controlled,** beliefs that one's body or mind is controlled by an outside agency (e.g., "There is a man from darkness who controls my thoughts with electrical waves.").

Concrete Thinking. In psychiatry, the term concrete thinking usually implies overemphasis on specific details and an impairment in the ability to use abstract concepts. For example, during an assessment, the nurse might ask what brought the client to the hospital. The client might answer "a cab" rather than explaining the need for seeking medical or psychiatric aid. When asked to give the meaning of the proverb "people in glass houses shouldn't throw stones," the person might answer, "Don't throw stones or the windows will break." The answer is literal; the ability to use abstract reasoning is absent.

Alterations in Speech
Associative Looseness. Zelda Fitzgerald wrote her husband, the writer F. Scott Fitzgerald, an account of going mad:

> Then the world became embryonic in Africa—and there was no need for communication . . . I have been living in vaporous places peopled with one-dimensional figures and tremulous buildings until I can no longer tell an optical illusion from a reality . . . head and ears incessantly throb and roads disappear (Vidal 1982).

Associations are the threads that tie one thought to another and one concept to another. In schizophrenia, these threads are missing, and connections are interrupted. In looseness of association, thinking becomes haphazard, illogical, and confused:

Nurse: "Are you going to the picnic today?"
Client: "I'm not an elephant hunter, no tiger teeth for me."

At times, the nurse may be able to decipher, or decode, the client's messages and begin to understand the client's feelings and needs. Any exchange in which a person feels understood is useful. Therefore, the nurse might respond to the client in this way:

Nurse: "Are you saying, Tony, that you don't feel secure enough to go out with the others today?"
Client: "Yeah . . . no tiger getting me today."

Very often it is not possible to understand what the client may mean because the client's verbalizations are too fragmented. For example:

Client: I sang out for my mother . . . for this to hell I went. How long is road? This little said three hills, hop aboard, share the appetite of the Christmas mice spread . . . within three round moons the devil will be washed away.

If the nurse does not understand what the client is saying, it is important to let the client know this. Clear messages and complete honesty are an important part of working with schizophrenic persons. Letting the person know that the nurse does not understand but would like to understand or will try to understand is honest.

Neologisms. Neologisms are words a person makes up that have special meaning for the person. ("I was going to tell him the mannerologies of his hospitality won't do." "I want all the vetchkisses to leave the room and leave me be.")

Children and creative writers often make up their own words. Their creation of neologisms is imaginative, constructive, and adaptive. Neologisms in the schizophrenic reaction represent a disruption in thought processes.

Echolalia. Echolalia is the pathological repeating of another's word by imitation and is often seen in people with catatonia.

Nurse: Mary, come for your medication.
Mary: Mary, come for your medication.

Echolalia is the counterpart of echopraxia, mimicking the *movements* of another, and is also seen in catatonia.

Clang Associations. Clang association is the meaningless rhyming of words, often in a forceful manner, "On the track... have a Big Mac... or get the sack," in which the rhyming is often more important than the context of the word. This form of speech pattern may be seen in schizophrenia; however, it may also be seen in the manic phase of a bipolar disorder or in a person with a cognitive disorder, such as Alzheimer's disease or HIV-related dementia.

Word Salad. Word salad is a term used to identify a mixture of phrases that is meaningless to the listener and perhaps to the speaker as well. It may include a string of neologisms, as in the following example: "Birds and fishes... framewoes... mud and stars and thump-bump going."

Alterations in Perceiving

Hallucinations, especially auditory hallucinations, are the major example of alterations in perception in schizophrenia. The following alterations in perceptions are discussed in this section: hallucinations and loss of ego boundaries (depersonalization and derealization).

Hallucinations. Hallucinations can be defined as sensory perceptions for which no external stimulus exists. The most common types of hallucinations include

- Auditory—hearing voices or sounds.
- Visual—seeing persons or things.
- Olfactory—smelling odors.
- Gustatory—experiencing tastes.
- Tactile—feeling body sensations.

Table 20–2 provides examples of common hallucinations and also describes the difference between hallucinations and illusions.

It is estimated that 90% of people with schizophrenia experience hallucinations at some time during their illness. Although manifestations of hallucinations are varied, auditory hallucinations are most common in schizophrenia. Voices may seem to come from outside or inside the person's head. The voices may be familiar or strange, single or multiple. Voices speaking directly to the person or commenting on the person's behavior are most common in schizophrenia. A person may believe that the voices are from God, the devil, deceased relatives, or strangers. The auditory hallucinations may occasionally take the form of sounds rather than voices. **Command hallucinations** must be assessed carefully, because the voices may command the person to hurt himself or others. For example, a client might state that "the voices" are telling him to "jump out the window" or "take a knife and kill my child." Command hallucinations are often terrifying for the individual. Command hallucinations may signal a psychiatric emergency. Clients who can give an identity to the hallucinated voice are at somewhat greater risk of compliance with the hallucinated command than are those who can not (Junginger 1995).

Evidence of possible auditory hallucinatory behavior may be the turning or tilting of the head, as if the client is talking to someone, or frequent blinking of the eyes and grimacing. Sometimes, clients verbally respond to "unseen others."

Visual hallucinations are less often reported in schizophrenia (about 20%) and are more often noted in organic disorders. Olfactory, tactile, or gustatory

TABLE 20–2 Summary of Hallucinations*

DEFINITION	EXAMPLE
Auditory	
Hearing voices or sounds that do not exist in the environment but are projections of inner thoughts or feelings	Anna "hears" the voice of her dead mother call her a whore and a tramp.
Visual	
Seeing a person, object, or animal that does not exist in the environment	Charles, who is experiencing alcohol withdrawal delirium, "sees" hungry rats coming toward him.
Olfactory	
Smelling odors that are not present in the environment	Theresa "smells" her insides rotting.
Gustatory	
Tasting sensations that have no stimulus in reality	Sam will not eat his food because he "tastes" the poison the FBI† is putting in his food.
Tactile	
Feeling strange sensations where no external objects stimulate such feelings; common in delirium tremens	Jack, a paranoid schizophrenic, "feels" electrical impulses controlling his mind.

*A hallucination is a false sensory perception for which no external stimulus exists. They are different from **illusions** in that illusions are misperceptions or misinterpretations of a real experience. For example, a man saw his coat hanging on a coat rack and believed it to be a bear about to attack him. He did see something real but misinterpreted what it was.

†FBI, Federal Bureau of Investigation.

Common with DJT's (handwritten note)

hallucinations account for about 10% of hallucinations in people with schizophrenia (Moller 1989).

Personal boundary difficulties. People with schizophrenia often lack a sense of their body in relationship to the rest of the world—where they leave off and others begin. Clients might say that they are merging with others or are part of inanimate objects.

Depersonalization is a nonspecific feeling that a person has lost his or her identity, that the self is different or unreal. People may be concerned that body parts do not belong to them. People may have an acute sensation that their body has drastically changed. For example, a woman may see her fingers as snakes or her arms as rotting wood. A man may look in a mirror and state that his face is that of an animal.

Derealization is the false perception by a person that the environment has changed. For example, everything seems bigger or smaller, or familiar surroundings have become somehow strange and unfamiliar.

Both depersonalization and derealization can be interpreted as **loss of ego boundaries,** sometimes referred to as loose ego boundaries.

Alterations in Behavior

Bizarre and agitated behavior are associated with schizophrenia and may take a variety of forms.

Bizarre behavior. Bizarre behaviors may take the form of a stilted rigid demeanor, eccentric dress or grooming, and rituals. The following behaviors are often seen in catatonia:

■ **Extreme motor agitation.** Extreme motor agitation is agitated physical behavior, such as running about, in response to inner and outer stimuli. The person may become dangerous to others or may become exhausted or collapse and die if not stopped.
■ **Stereotyped behaviors.** Stereotyped behaviors are motor patterns that originally had meaning to the person (e.g., sweeping the floor, washing windows) but have become mechanical and lack purpose.
■ **Automatic obedience.** A catatonic client may perform, without hesitation, all simple commands in a robot-like fashion.
■ **Waxy flexibility.** Waxy flexibility consists of excessive maintenance of posture, evidenced when a person's arms or legs can be placed in any position and the position is held for long periods.
■ **Stupor.** The person who is in a stupor may sit motionless for long periods and may be motionless to the point of apparent coma.
■ **Negativism.** Negativism is equivalent to resistance. In *active negativism,* the people do the opposite of what they are told to do. When people do not do things they are expected to do (e.g., do not get out of bed, do not dress, do not eat), such behavior is termed *passive negativism.*

Slowness of movement, stupor, and negativism can be considered negative symptoms.

Agitated behavior. Clients with schizophrenia may have difficulty with impulse control when they are acutely ill. Because of cognitive deterioration, clients lack social sensitivity and may act out impulsively with others (e.g., grab another's cigarette, throw food on the floor, and get the television remote control and change channels abruptly).

NEGATIVE SYMPTOMS

The negative symptoms of schizophrenia develop over a long time. These are the symptoms that most interfere with the individual's adjustment and ability to survive. The presence of negative symptoms interferes with the person's ability to

■ Initiate and maintain relationships.
■ Initiate and maintain conversations.
■ Hold a job.
■ Make decisions.
■ Maintain adequate hygiene and grooming.

The presence of negative symptoms contributes to the person's poor social functioning and social withdrawal.

On assessment, specific phenomena are noted. During an acute psychotic episode, negative symptoms may be difficult to assess because the positive and more florid symptoms, such as delusions and hallucinations, may dominate. Some of the negative phenomena, which are outlined in Table 20–3, include poverty of speech content, poverty of speech, thought blocking, anergia, anhedonia, affective blunting, and lack of volition.

Affect is the observable behavior that expresses a person's emotions. The affect of a schizophrenic person can usually be categorized in three ways: flat or blunted, inappropriate, or bizarre.

A **flat** (immobile facial expressions or a blank look) or **blunted affect** (minimal emotional response) is commonly seen in schizophrenia. In schizophrenia, people's outward affect may not coincide with their inner emotions.

Inappropriate affect refers to an emotional response to a situation that is not congruent with the tone of the situation. For example, a young man, told that his father is ill, breaks into laughter.

Bizarre affect is especially prominent in the disorganized form of schizophrenia. Grimacing, giggling, and mumbling to oneself come under this heading. Bizarre affect is marked when the client is unable to relate logically to the environment. Review Table 20–4 for a comparison between positive and negative symptoms.

SELF-ASSESSMENT

Working with individuals diagnosed as schizophrenic will likely cause strong emotional reactions

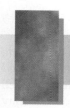

TABLE 20–3 *Negative Phenomena*

PHENOMENON	EXPLANATION
Affective blunting	In *affective blunting*, severe reduction in the expression and range and intensity of affect occurs; in *flat affect* no facial expression of emotion exists.
Anergia	Lack of energy: passivity, impersistence at work or school.
Anhedonia	Inability to experience any pleasure in activities that usually produce pleasurable feelings; result of profound emotional barrenness.
Avolition	Lack of motivation: unable to initiate tasks, e.g., social contacts, grooming, and other aspects of activities of daily living.
Poverty of content of speech	Speech that is adequate in amount but conveys little information because of vagueness, empty repetitions, or use of stereotypes or obscure phrases.
Poverty of speech	Restriction in the amount of speech—answers range from brief to monosyllabic one-word answers.
Thought blocking	A client may stop talking in the middle of a sentence and remain silent. After a client stops abruptly: Nurse: "What just happened now?" Client: "I forgot what I was saying. Something took my thoughts away."

from health care workers. The psychotic client is intensely anxious, lonely, dependent, and distrustful. The intensity of these emotions can evoke similarly intense, uncomfortable, and frightening emotions in all health care workers. Identification of one's feelings and responses is an important part of working with all clients.

If personal feelings and reactions are ignored by the health care worker, clinician, or nurse, feelings of helplessness may follow. Increased feelings of helplessness can increase anxiety. Without the support, opportunity, and willingness to explore these reactions with more experienced nursing staff, defensive behaviors emerge on the part of the health care professional. Defensive behaviors in the nurse (e.g., denial, withdrawal, avoidance) thwart the client's progress and undermine the nurse's self-esteem. These behaviors are associated with staff burnout. Statements such as "These clients are hopeless," "You can't understand these people," and "You waste your time with them" are examples of

unexamined or unrecognized emotional reactions to client's behaviors or feelings.

For nurses new to the psychiatric setting, especially for student nurses, the availability of supportive supervision is necessary if learning is to take place. The student's part in the supervisory process is a willingness to discuss and identify personal feelings and to identify problem behaviors. This can be, and often is, accomplished in group supervision. Experienced psychiatric nurses call this process **peer group supervision.**

Menninger (1934) discussed the extreme frustration that staff have with the slow progress of schizophrenic clients. This sense of frustration and feelings

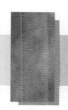

TABLE 20–4 *Negative and Positive Symptoms of Schizophrenia*

NEGATIVE SYMPTOMS	POSITIVE SYMPTOMS
Affective Flattening Unchanging facial expression Decreased spontaneous movements Paucity of expressive gestures Poor eye contact Inappropriate affect Lack of vocal inflections	**Hallucinations** Auditory Voices commenting Voices conversing Somatic-tactile Olfactory Visual
Alogia Poverty of speech Poverty of content of speech Blocking	**Delusions** Persecutory Jealous Grandiose Religious Somatic Delusions of reference Delusions of being controlled Delusions of mind reading Thought broadcasting Thought insertion Thought withdrawal
Avolition-apathy Impaired grooming and hygiene Lack of persistence at work or school Physical anergia	
Anhedonia-asociality Few recreational interests/activities Little sexual interest/activity Impaired intimacy/closeness Few relationships with friends/peers	**Bizarre behavior** Clothing, appearance Social, sexual behavior Aggressive-agitated Repetitive-stereotyped
Attention Social inattentiveness	**Positive formal thought disorder/speech patterns** Derailment Tangentiality Incoherence Illogicality Circumstantiality Pressure of speech Distractible speech Clanging

Adapted from Andreasen, N.C. (1987). The diagnosis of schizophrenia. *Schizophrenia Bulletin*, 13:9–22.

of helplessness can lead to burnout. Periodic reassessment of treatment goals and scaling down of expectations can benefit both the nurse and the client. Periodic review of frustrating clients can lead to a better understanding of the client's strengths and weaknesses. A team approach to reevaluating and establishing realistic, obtainable outcomes for clients can help energize staff, reduce helplessness, and benefit the client.

Clinical practice with adequate supervision can increase the nurse's skills, lower personal anxiety, increase confidence, and improve the quality of interpersonal relationships with clients, as well as relationships with others.

ASSESSMENT GUIDELINES

> **ASSESSMENT GUIDELINES FOR SCHIZOPHRENIA AND OTHER PSYCHOTIC DISORDERS**
>
> 1. Has the client had a medical work-up; has a medical or substance-induced psychosis been ruled out?
> 2. Assess for command hallucinations, e.g., voices telling the person to harm self or another. **If yes:**
>   - Do you plan to follow the command?
>   - Do you believe the voices are real?
> 3. Assess if the client has fragmented, poorly organized, well organized, systematized, or extensive system of beliefs that are not supported by reality (delusion). **If yes:**
>   - Assess if delusions have to do with someone trying to harm the client, and if the client is planning to retaliate against a person or organization.
>   - Assess if precautions need to be taken.
> 4. Assess for co-occurring disorders:
>   - Depression: Suicidality?
>   - Anxiety
>   - Substance abuse
>   - History of violence
> 5. Assess if client is on medications, what medications, and if he or she is treatment compliant.
> 6. How does the family respond to increased symptoms? Overprotective? Hostile? Suspicious?
> 7. How do family members and client relate?
> 8. Assess support system. Is family well informed about the disease (e.g., schizophrenia)? Does the family understand the need for medication adherence? Is family familiar with family support groups in the community, or where to go for respite and family support?
> 9. Assess client's global functioning (using the Global Assessment Scale—GAF—found in Chapter 1.

NURSING DIAGNOSIS

People with schizophrenia have multiple disturbing and disabling symptoms that invite a multifaceted approach to care and treatment of the client as well as the client's family. The positive symptoms may be ameliorated with medications. It is the negative symptoms that challenge health care personnel and are so destructive to the client and his family's quality of life. See Table 20–5 for potential nursing diagnoses for a person with schizophrenia.

OUTCOME CRITERIA

The desired outcome criteria may vary with the phase of the illness the client is experiencing.

Phase I—Acute Phase

The acute phase of the illness is essentially crisis intervention with client safety and medical stabilization as the overall goal. Therefore, if the client is at risk for violence to self or others, initial outcome criteria would address safety issues, e.g., "Client will remain safe while hospitalized." Other outcomes might include, "Client will adhere to the medication regime or refrain from acting upon delusions or hallucinations."

During the acute phase, the client's thought disorder will be most pronounced, therefore focus may be on outcomes that reflect improvement in the intensity and frequency of hallucinations and delusions, and increasing reality testing. Safety here is geared toward preventing the client from acting out self-damaging behaviors resulting from hallucinatory or delusional thinking. Table 20–6 identifies potential client outcomes for Thought Disorder.

Phase II (Maintenance) and Phase III (Stable)

Outcome criteria during these phases will focus on helping the client to adhere to medication regimes, understanding the nature of his or her illness, and the participation and availability of psychoeducational activities for both the client and his or her family.

Very important outcomes, during these phases, especially the later phase, ideally will focus on targeting the negative symptoms (those symptoms which rob the client of enjoyment and quality of life). Outcomes may include ability to perform special skills training (social, vocational, or self-care) and involvement in socializing groups at various levels. All people with schizophrenia are uniquely different and all have unique personal strengths and disease-associated deficits. Ideally, outcomes should reflect en-

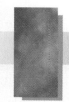

SYMPTOMS	NURSING DIAGNOSES	SYMPTOMS	NURSING DIAGNOSES
POSITIVE SYMPTOMS **Hallucinations:** ■ Hears voices (loud noises) that others do not hear. Hears voices telling them to hurt self or others (*command hallucinations*). **Distorted thinking not based on reality** For example: ■ **Persecution:** thinking that others are trying to harm them. ■ **Jealousy:** thinking that spouse or lover is being unfaithful, or thinking others are jealous of them when they are not. ■ **Grandeur:** thinking they have powers and talents that they do not possess, or they are someone powerful or famous. ■ Reference: believing all events within the environment are directed at or hold special meaning for them. ■ Loose association of ideas **(looseness of association).** ■ Uses words in a meaningless, disconnected manner **(word salad).** ■ Uses words that rhyme in a nonsensical fashion **(clang association).** ■ Repeats words that are heard (*echolalia*). ■ Does not speak **(mutism).** ■ The person delays getting to the point of communication because of unnecessary and tedious details **(circumstantiality).**	Disturbed Sensory Perception: Auditory/Visual Risk for Harm to Self and Others Disturbed Thought Processes Defensive Coping Impaired Verbal Communication Disturbed Thought Processes	■ Concrete thinking. The inability to abstract; uses literal translations concerning aspects of the environment. **NEGATIVE SYMPTOMS** Uncommunicative, withdrawn, no eye contact. Preoccupation with own thoughts. Expression of feelings of rejection or of aloneness (lies in bed all day . . . positions back to door). Talks about self as "bad" or "no good." Feels guilty because of "bad thoughts," extremely sensitive to real or perceived slights. Lack of energy (anergia) Lack of motivation (avolition), unable to initiate tasks (social contact, grooming, and other aspects of daily living) **Other** Families and significant others become confused, overwhelmed, lack knowledge of disease or treatment, feel powerless in coping with client at home Nonadherence to medications and treatment. Client stops taking medication (often from side effects), stops going to therapy groups, family and significant others not aware of need for medications and treatments.	Social Isolation Impaired Social Interaction Risk for Loneliness Chronic Low Self-Esteem Risk for Self-Directed Violence Ineffective Coping Self-Care Deficit (bathing, dressing, grooming and hygiene). Constipation Compromised Family Coping: Impaired Parenting Caregiver Role Strain Deficient Knowledge Noncompliance

Varcarolis, E. (2000). *Psychiatric Nursing Clinical Guide.* Philadelphia: W. B. Saunders, pp. 226–227.

hancing the person's strengths and minimizing the effects of the client's deficits.

PLANNING

Planning appropriate interventions is often guided by the phase of the illness.

Acute Phase

During this time, brief hospitalization may be indicated if the client is considered a danger to self or others, is refusing to eat or drink, or is too disorganized to care for him or her self. Other indications for hospitalization may be for specific observations, neurological work-up, or other medically related

TABLE 20–6   *Outcomes for Distorted Thought Control*

Definition: Self-restraint disruption in perception, thought processes, and thought content

DISTORTED THOUGHT CONTROL	NEVER DEMONSTRATED 1	RARELY DEMONSTRATED 2	SOMETIMES DEMONSTRATED 3	OFTEN DEMONSTRATED 4	CONSISTENTLY DEMONSTRATED 5
Indicators	1	2	3	4	5
1. Recognizes when hallucinations or delusions are occurring	1	2	3	4	5
2. Is able to refrain from attending to hallucinations or delusions	1	2	3	4	5
3. Refrains from responding to hallucinations or delusions	1	2	3	4	5
4. Verbalizes frequency of hallucinations or delusions	1	2	3	4	5
5. Describes content of hallucinations or delusions	1	2	3	4	5
6. Reports decrease in hallucinations or delusions	1	2	3	4	5
7. Asks for validation of reality	1	2	3	4	5
8. Affect appears consistent with mood	1	2	3	4	5
9. Interacts with others appropriately	1	2	3	4	5
10. Behaviors indicate accurate interpretation of environment	1	2	3	4	5
11. Exhibits logical thought flow patterns	1	2	3	4	5
12. Exhibits reality-based thinking	1	2	3	4	5
13. Exhibits appropriate thought content	1	2	3	4	5
14. Exhibits ability to grasp ideas of others	1	2	3	4	5
15. Other _____ (Specify)	1	2	3	4	5

From: Johnson, H., Maas, M., Meriden, M., and Moorehead, S. (2000). *Nursing Outcomes Classification (NOC), 2nd ed.,* St. Louis: Mosby.

tests or treatment. Planning care centers around client safety and acute symptom stability.

At this time the treatment team will identify long-term care needs and identify and provide appropriate referrals for client's and family's follow-up and supportive needs. Discharge planning needs to take into consideration the client's living arrangement, economic resources, social supports, family relationships, and vulnerability to stress. Relapse can be very devastating to a person's long-term functioning. Vigorous efforts should be made to refer clients to community agencies that can provide social supports and opportunities for helping clients learn about their illness, medications, and relapse prevention skills.

Maintenance and Stable Phases

During these phases the focus is geared toward client and family education and skills training. Relapse prevention skills are vital, as well as identifying the need for social skills, interpersonal skills, coping skills, or vocational skills. Planning is also focused on identifying appropriate social supports and community activities that can help maintain the optimum functioning of schizophrenic individuals.

INTERVENTION

As with outcome criteria and planning, interventions are geared toward the client's phase of schizophrenia. For example, during phase I, the acute phase, the clinical focus is on crisis intervention, acute symptom stabilization, and safety. Interventions are often hospital-based; however, more and more community-based settings and home care agencies are treating acute clients in the community.

A number of factors that affect the choice of treatment setting are based on the following (APA 2000):

■ Protection of the person from harm to self or others.
■ Client's needs for external structure and support.
■ Client's ability to cooperate with treatment.
■ Client's need for a particular treatment that may be available only in one setting.
■ Client's need for treatment of comorbid, general, medical, or psychiatric condition.
■ Availability of psychosocial support to facilitate receipt of treatment and give critical information to staff about clinical status and response to treatment.

Acute phase interventions include:

■ Acute psychopharmacological treatment.
■ Supportive and directive communications.
■ Limit setting.
■ Psychiatric, medical, and neurological evaluation.

Given the recent trend for decreasing lengths of hospital stays, alternatives such as partial hospitalization, halfway houses, and day treatment centers are being developed as cost-effective alternatives to hospitalization (Zerbe 1999).

When clients are hospitalized during the acute phase, the length of hospitalization is often short

(days). Once the acute symptoms are being treated, the client is discharged to the community, where appropriate treatment can be carried out during the maintenance phase (phase II) and the stable phase (phase III) of the disease. Effective long-term treatment of an individual with schizophrenia relies on a three-pronged approach: medications, nursing approaches, and community approaches. Family psychoeducation is a key component in effective treatment.

Phase II and III interventions include:

■ Client and family teaching about the disease.
■ Medication teaching and side-effect management.
■ Cognitive and social skills enhancement.
■ Identifying signs of relapse.
■ Attention to deficit in self-care, social, and work functioning.

Table 20–7 provides an overview of the clinical focus, intervention, and professional collaboration that are best suited to each phase.

Throughout the work with schizophrenic clients, the nurse and others attempt to minimize stress and anxiety levels. Lowered anxiety levels can decrease the intensity of schizophrenic symptoms and make the client more amenable to engaging in activities and relationships with others, improving family interactions, and becoming involved in nonthreatening activities.

Desired outcomes for a person with psychosis that may reduce his or her vulnerability to symptoms include (Mills 2000)

■ Maintain a regular sleep pattern.
■ Reduce alcohol, drug, and caffeine intake.
■ Keep in touch with supportive friends and family.
■ Keep active (exercise, hobbies, employment).
■ Have a routine daily and weekly schedule including enjoyable activities.
■ Take medication regularly.

When planning interventions, it is important that the nurse not overlook the adaptive skills of a psychotic client. **Attention should be given to the client's strengths and healthy functioning as well as to areas of deficiency.**

Milieu Therapy

ACTIVITIES

Effective hospital care involves more than protection of the client from a confusing family, social, or vocational environment. Slately (1994) reported finding that a structured milieu contributes to greater im-

TABLE 20−7 *Treatment Focus at Different Phases of Schizophrenia*

	PHASE I		PHASE II	PHASE III
	Acute: Onset, Exacerbation, or Relapse	Subacute and Convalescent	Maintenance Adaptive Plateau	Stable Plateau
Clinical focus	■ Crisis intervention ■ Safety ■ Acute symptom stabilization	■ Social supports ■ Stress and vulnerability assessment ■ Living arrangements ■ Daily activities ■ Economic resources	■ Understanding and acceptance of illness	■ Social, vocational, and self-care skills ■ Learning or relearning ■ Identifying realistic expectations ■ Adaptation to deficits

Intervention	■ Acute psychopharmacological treatment
	■ Limit setting
	■ Supportive and directive
	■ Psychiatric, medical, neurological evaluation
	■ Meet with family
		■ Psychosocial evaluation
		■ Linkage with
		  - Social services
		  - Human services
		  - Community treatment agencies
		■ Psychoeducational interventions with families
			■ Support and teaching
			■ Medication teaching and side effect management
			■ Direct assistance with situational problems
			■ Identification of prodromal and acute symptoms and signs of relapse
			■ Continued psychoeducational work with families as needed
				■ Attention to detail of self-care, social, and work functioning
				■ Direct intervention with family/employers
				■ Cognitive/social skills enhancement
				■ Medication maintenance
				■ Continued psychoeducational intervention with families as needed

Professional collaboration	■ Inpatient treatment team ■ Residential alternative to hospitalization ■ Community crisis intervention ■ Internist ■ Neurologist	■ Social work department ■ Health and human services ■ Day treatment or community support	■ Community support staff ■ Family support groups ■ Group therapies and self-help groups ■ Behavior therapies using educational models	■ Group therapists ■ Social, vocational, and self-care providers ■ Family, employer, community support staff

Adapted from Gabard GO (2001) *Treatment of Psychiatric Disorders*, 3/e. Washington, DC: American Psychiatric Publishing, Inc.

provement with schizophrenic clients in the acute phase than does an open unit where the clients have more freedom. Partial hospitalization, halfway houses, and day treatment centers are other treatment options that can provide a structured milieu. The milieu should also provide resources for resolving conflicts and opportunities for learning social and vocational skills.

Group work with schizophrenic clients is oriented toward providing support, an environment in which a client can develop social skills, and a format that allows friendships to begin (Black et al. 1988). Structured group therapy can target some of the negative symptoms of schizophrenia. For example, participation in activity groups, which is determined by the client's level of functioning, has been found to decrease withdrawal, promote motivation, modify unacceptable aggression, and increase social competence. People who respond to group therapy while hospitalized may benefit from group therapy on an outpatient basis, and group therapy would thus be an important part of the client's community milieu.

Group work with schizophrenic clients can result in increased self-concept scores. Such activities as drawing pictures, reading poetry, and listening to music can be used as a focus of conversation to reduce anxiety and promote socialization. Group functions, such as picnics, can result in growth in social concern for others and the ability to set limits for self and others. Nurses can use activity group therapy in many settings. Success at tasks and increased involvement with objects and individuals can lead to greater self-esteem in many settings.

In hospital and outpatient settings, the nurse may participate with other members of the health care team in providing appropriate, structured, and useful activities for the clients. Recreational, occupational, art, and dance therapists are available on many psychiatric units as well as in structured community settings (see Chapters 5 and 6).

SAFETY

A client, especially in the acute phase, may become physically violent, often in response to hallucinations or delusions. During this time, measures need to be taken to ensure the client's safety as well as the safety of others. After unsuccessful verbal de-escalation efforts, and if chemical restraints (antipsychotic medication) fail to lessen the person's aggression, measures such as physical restraints and seclusion may be indicated. (Refer to Chapters 8 and 19 for care of a client in seclusion or restraints.)

Communication Guidelines

Therapeutic strategies for working with schizophrenic clients often involve interventions that address specific behaviors. Interventions are aimed at lowering the client's anxiety, decreasing defensive patterns, encouraging participation in the milieu, and raising the level of self-worth. Refer to the appropriate sections for specific counseling techniques for schizophrenic clients with paranoid, withdrawn, excitable, and regressed behaviors.

All nurses should be familiar with the principles used in dealing with phenomena that are likely to arise with most schizophrenic clients: hallucinations, delusions, and looseness of association.

HALLUCINATIONS. As previously stated, voices are the most common hallucinatory experience reported by schizophrenic clients. It is important initially to understand what the voices are saying or telling the person to do. Suicidal or homicidal messages necessitate safety measures for all members of the health care team.

Hallucinations are real to the person who is experiencing them. A hallucinating client should be approached in a nonthreatening and nonjudgmental manner (Lipton and Cancro 1995). Moller (1989) emphasized that often when a person is hallucinating, the individual is experiencing anxiety, fear, loneliness, and low self-esteem, and the brain is not processing stimuli accurately.

During the acute phase of the illness, it is helpful to maintain eye contact, speak simply in a louder voice than usual, and call the person by name. Table 20–8 identifies basic communication strategies for a client who is hallucinating or delusional.

DELUSIONS. Delusions are a result of misperception of cognitive stimuli. It is best when the

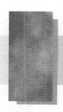

TABLE 20–8 *Communication Skills: Thought Disorders*	
IF THE CLIENT IS HALLUCINATING	**IF THE CLIENT IS EXPERIENCING DELUSIONS**
■ Ask patient directly about his or her hallucinations. For instance, you may say "Are you hearing voices? What are they saying to you?" ■ Watch patient for cues that he or she is hallucinating, such as eyes darting to one side, muttering, or watching a vacant area of the room. ■ Avoid reacting to hallucinations as if they are real. Do not argue back to the voices. ■ Do not negate patient's experience but offer your own perceptions. For instance, you may say "I don't see the devil standing over you, but I do understand how upsetting that must be for you." ■ Focus on reality-based diversions and topics such as conversations or simple projects. Tell patient, "Try not to listen to the voices right now. I have to talk with you." ■ Be alert to signs of anxiety in the patient, which may indicate hallucinations are increasing.	■ Be open, honest, and reliable in interactions to reduce suspiciousness. ■ Respond to suspicions in a matter-of-fact and calm manner. ■ Ask patient to describe the delusions, for instance, "Who is trying to hurt you?" ■ Avoid arguing about the content, but interject doubt where appropriate, for instance, "I don't think it would be possible for that petite girl to hurt you." ■ Focus on the feelings the delusions generate, such as "It must feel frightening to think there is a conspiracy against you." ■ Once a patient describes delusion, do not dwell on it. Rather, focus conversation on more reality-based topics. If patient obsesses on delusions, set firm limits on amount of time you will devote to talking about them. ■ Observe for events that trigger delusions. If possible, discuss these with patient. ■ Validate if part of the delusion is real, for instance, "Yes, there was a man at the nurse's station, but I did not hear him talk about you."

Data from Gorman, L. M., Sultan, D. F., and Raines, M. L. (1996). *Davis's manual of psychosocial nursing for general patient care.* Philadelphia: F. A. Davis Company.

nurse attempts to see the world as it appears through the eyes of the client. In that way, the nurse can better understand the client's delusional experience. For example:

> **Client**: You people are all alike . . . all in on the CIA plot to destroy me.
> **Nurse**: I don't want to hurt you, Tom. Thinking that people are out to destroy you must be very frightening.

First, the nurse clarifies the reality of the client's experience. Second, the nurse empathizes with the client's apparent experience, the feelings of fear. The nurse does not get drawn into the conversation regarding the content of the delusion (CIA and plot to destroy) but looks for the feelings that the person may be experiencing. Talking about the client's feelings can be helpful to the client; talking about delusional material is not.

It is *not* useful to argue with the client regarding the content of the delusion. Doing so can intensify the client's retention of irrational beliefs. Although the nurse does not argue with the client's delusions, clarifying misinterpretations of the environment is useful. For example:

> **Client**: I see the doctor is here, and he is out to get me and destroy me.
> **Nurse**: It is true the doctor wants to see you, but he wants to talk to you about your treatment. Would you feel more comfortable talking to him in the day room?

Interacting with the client on concrete realities in the environment can help minimize the client's time spent thinking delusional thoughts. Specific manual tasks within the scope of the client's abilities can often be useful as distractions from delusional thinking. The more time the client spends with reality-based activities or with people, the more opportunity the client has to become comfortable with reality.

There are a number of coping skills that may help some people minimize the disturbing effect of their voices and their "worrying" thoughts. Mills (2000) identifies some useful coping strategies. The counselor/nurse works with the client to find out which ones work and how best to use them. See Table 20–9 and the Research Findings Box.

LOOSENESS OF ASSOCIATION. Looseness of association often mirrors the client's autistic thoughts and reflects the person's poorly disorganized thinking. The client's autistic and disorganized ramblings may leave the nurse confused and frustrated. An increase in the client's autistic speech patterns can indicate increased anxiety on the part of the client and can reflect his or her difficulty in responding to internal and external stimuli.

TABLE 20–9   Ways of Coping With Voices and Worrying Thoughts

DISTRACTING	INTERACTING
Voices and strange, worrying thoughts: ■ Listening to music ■ Reading aloud ■ Counting backwards from 100 ■ Describing an object in detail ■ Watching TV	**Voices:** ■ Telling the voices to go away ■ Talking to the voices while pretending to use a mobile phone ■ Agreeing to listen to the voices at particular times

ACTIVITY	SOCIAL	PHYSICAL
Voices and strange, worrying thoughts: ■ Walking ■ Tidying the house ■ Having a relaxing bath ■ Playing the guitar ■ Singing ■ Going to the gym	**Voices and strange, worrying thoughts:** ■ Talking to a trusted friend or member of the family ■ Phoning a helpline ■ Avoiding people ■ Going to a drop-in center ■ Visiting a favorite place	**Voices and strange, worrying thoughts:** ■ Taking extra medication–**call your doctor** ■ Using ear plugs (voices) ■ Breathing exercises ■ Relaxation methods

From Mills, J. (2000). Dealing with voices and strange thoughts. In C. Gamble and G. Brennan (Eds.). *Working with serious mental illness: A manual for clinical practice.* London: Bailliere Tindall.

The following guidelines may be useful for spending time with a client whose speech is confused and disorganized.

1. Do not pretend that you understand the client's communications when you are confused by the client's words or meanings.
2. Tell the client that you are having difficulty understanding the communications.
3. Place the difficulty in understanding on yourself, *not* on the client. For example, say "I am having trouble following what you are saying," *not* "You are not making any sense."
4. Look for recurring topics and themes in the client's communications. For example, "You've mentioned trouble with your brother several times. I guess your relationship with your brother is on your mind."
5. Emphasize what is going on in the client's immediate environment (here and now) and involve the client in simple reality-based activities.

RESEARCH FINDINGS

The Use of Cognitive Therapy for Treating Delusions

Objective

To assess the effectiveness of cognitive therapy in modifying delusions in clients seen in routine clinical practice.

Methods

Eighteen clients with chronic delusions were treated using cognitive therapy, after the method of Chadwick and Lowe. A single-case multiple-baseline experimental design was used, including a control treatment. Each subject was used as his or her own control.

Results

Six clients showed a reduction in the conviction of their delusions during cognitive therapy but not during the control treatment. Seven clients did not show any change in the conviction of their delusions. Five clients showed a variable response. There was no decrease to zero in the degree of conviction for any of the clients. All of them reported that the therapy had helped them, while six said, without being asked, that they had experienced changes in psychotic thinking.

Conclusions

One third of the clients with chronic delusions who were treated in this study responded to delusion modification with a reduction in the degree of conviction in their delusions. Change within cognitive therapy sessions predicted outcome, as did change in the conviction in delusion during baseline. Finally, the goal of cognitive therapy to treat delusions should be to reduce stress as well as the degree of conviction in the delusions.

Source: Jakes, S., Rhodes, J., and Turner, T. (1999). Effectiveness of cognitive therapy for delusions in routine clinical practice. *British Journal of Psychiatry*, 175:331–335.

These measures can help the client better focus thoughts.

6. Tell the client what you do understand and reinforce clear communication and accurate expression of needs, feelings, and thoughts.

Client and Family Health Teaching

Teaching methods of health management to clients, families, and other caregivers is important in stabilizing the schizophrenic person's future adjustment. It is not just the level or source of stress in the client's environment that is crucial; also important are the manner in which people deal with the stress and how effectively stressful issues are resolved. Psychological strategies aimed at reducing exacerbation of the psychotic symptoms follow:

1. Educate the client and the client's family about the illness. Emphasize how stress and medication affect the illness. Such knowledge may increase medication adherence and motivate involvement in psychosocial activities.
2. Assist the client in improving his or her ability to solve problems related to environmental stress.
3. Teach the client coping strategies to deal with the source of symptoms of schizophrenia and the stressors in the social environment.
4. Assist family and client to identify sources for ongoing support in dealing with the illness.

Some of these steps may be implemented during the acute phase of the illness (e.g., educating family, identifying sources of support), while others may be implemented or continued once the client is discharged through community-based resources (see Table 20–8).

Studies have indicated the importance of the family environment for a schizophrenic client. When a schizophrenic client is returned to a family environment that consists of warmth, concern, and supportive behavior, a relapse is less likely to occur. An environment that is highly critical of the client's behavior or consists of intrusive involvement into the client's life has a higher correlation with recurrent episodes of schizophrenia.

Some of the judgmental attitudes toward people with schizophrenia result from a lack of understanding of the symptoms of schizophrenia, especially the negative symptoms. For example, the client's apathy and lack of drive and motivation may be wrongly interpreted as laziness. This erroneous assumption can foster hostility on the part of family members, caregivers, or people in the community. Thus, further teaching of the disease process of schizophrenia can reduce tensions in families and communities. Educating the client, families, and others is most effective when it is carried out over time. Table 20–10 can be used as a guide for client and family teaching. Later in this chapter, the pivotal role of family psychoeducation in enhancing a schizophrenic person's integration into society, decreasing relapse, and increasing the quality of life for schizophrenic persons and their families is discussed.

Case Management

Discharge planning is a vital part of managing schizophrenic clients. With the shifting of care for the seriously mentally ill from inpatient to community-based treatment centers, the need for transitional care is heightened. Case management by nurses and other health care professionals is one way that clients can be effectively monitored. Because of the limits on the length of hospital stays that have been established by third-party payers, clients are discharged to the community while they are still severely impaired and even frankly psychotic. Alternatives to hospitalization that work for many include partial hospitalization, halfway houses, and day treatment programs (Baldessarini 1996):

■ **Partial hospitalization:** Clients sleep at home and attend treatment sessions during the day or evening.
■ **Halfway houses:** Clients live in the community with a group of other clients, sharing expenses and responsibilities. Usually have staff who are present in the house 24 hours, 7 days a week.
■ **Day treatment programs:** Clients live in halfway house or on their own, sometimes with home visits, or in residential programs. Clients attend a structured program during the day.

Program may consist of

■ group therapy
■ supervised activities
■ individual counseling
■ specialized training and rehabilitation.

Nurses, physicians, and social workers need to be aware of the community resources for clients who

TABLE 20–10   *Client and Family Teaching Guidelines for Schizophrenia*

1. **Learn all you can about the illness:**
   ■ Attend psycho-educational groups
   ■ Attend support groups
   ■ Join NAMI (National Alliance for the Mentally Ill)
   ■ Contact the NIMH (National Institute for Mental Illness)
2. **Develop a relapse prevention plan**
   ■ Know the early warning signs of relapse of your loved one (e.g., social withdrawal, trouble sleeping, increased bizarre/magical thinking)
   ■ Know who to call and where to go when early signs of relapse appear
   ■ **Relapse is part of the illness, not a sign of failure**
3. **Take advantage of all psycho-educational tools**
   ■ Family, group, individual therapy
   ■ Learn new behaviors and cognitive coping skills to help handle interfamily stress, interpersonal, social, and vocational difficulties.
      1. Get information from health care workers (Nurse, Case Managers, Physician), NAMI, Community Mental Health Groups, Hospital
   ■ **Everyone needs a place to address their fears and losses, and to learn new ways of coping.**
4. **Comply with treatment**
   ■ Research has determined that people who do the best with the disease comply with treatment that works for them.
   ■ Tell your health care worker (nurse, caseworker, physician, social worker) about troubling side effects (e.g., sexual problems, gaining weight, "feeling funny").
   ■ Most side effects can be treated.
   ■ Keeping side effects a secret or stopping medication can prevent you from having the best quality of life. Share your concerns.
5. **Avoid alcohol and/or drugs. They can act on your brain and precipitate a relapse.**
6. **Keep in touch with supportive people**
7. **Keep healthy—Stay in balance**
   ■ Maintain a regular sleep pattern
   ■ Maintain self-care (e.g., diet and hygiene)
   ■ Keep active (hobbies, friends, groups, sports, job, special interests)
   ■ Learn ways to reduce stress

"I am always humbled by people's ability to bear the adversity associated with psychotic symptoms. Often people have adapted their lifestyle so much that the small sense of well-being they do have feels precariously balanced." (Jem Mills, 2000)

Data from Zerbe 1999, Mills 2000.

are to be discharged and their families. Some clients may feel more comfortable with self-help community groups, such as Recovery, Inc., and Schizophrenics Anonymous. Information on community resources should be made available to clients and families alike. Examples include community mental health services, home health services, work support programs, day hospitals, social skills/supportive groups, family educational skills groups, and respite care.

A major problem in some public programs is that there are not adequate treatment resources for optimal client care. Another occurs when case managers function independently and are not well integrated into the treatment team (DSM-IV-TR 2000).

Clients, families, or siblings should be given telephone numbers and addresses of local support groups that are affiliated with the National Alliance for the Mentally Ill (NAMI). (Information can be obtained at National Alliance for the Mentally Ill, 1901 North Fort Myers Drive, Suite 500, Arlington, VA 22209, (703) 525-7600. 1-800-950-NAMI can provide information regarding chapters nearest the reader.)

Psychotherapy

Medication maintenance has been shown to be the single most important factor in the prevention of relapse in a schizophrenic person. However, psychosocial interventions, in addition to drug therapy, result in an even lower rate of relapse than does drug therapy alone (Black and Andreasen 1999). Psychosocial therapies such as cognitive behavioral therapies (CBT), cognitive rehabilitation, and social skills training (SST) are particularly helpful with chronic schizophrenics with cognitive impairment (Hirayasu 2000).

Zahniser and colleagues (1991) identified relationship problems, family concerns, depression, losses, and medication as the most common concerns of schizophrenic clients in therapy. Hilde Bruch (1980) cited a study that identified the elements that contribute to successful therapeutic outcomes with schizophrenic clients, even though the therapists' disciplines were diverse:

> The highest improvement rate was associated with "active participation," with the therapist showing initiative in an empathetic inquiry, challenging the client's self-deprecatory attitude, and identifying realistic limits as to what is acceptable in the client's behavior.

INDIVIDUAL THERAPY

For people with schizophrenia, the most useful therapeutic modality is supportive therapy. Supportive therapy over long periods has great value and helps people make adjustments for more useful and satisfactory life. Two individual therapies that are especially effective in schizophrenia are social skills training and cognitive therapy techniques.

- **Skills training** can significantly enhance social functioning.
- **Cognitive rehabilitation** focuses on improving information processing skills such as memory, attention, and conceptual abilities.
- **Cognitive content (CBT)** aimed at changing abnormal thoughts or responses to hallucinations through coping strategies such as listening to music, etc. (Refer to Table 20–9.)

Beck and Rector (1998) have developed successful strategies for dealing with hallucinations, delusions, and some of the negative symptoms of schizophrenia. Beck and Rector (1998) cite a number of studies reporting promising results for schizophrenic individuals who had inadequate response to drug treatment. Many of the techniques in Table 20–10 are incorporated.

Individual therapy, ideally combined with group therapy, should be made available to the client and family on an outpatient basis as well as being part of inpatient treatment.

GROUP THERAPY

Group therapy is particularly useful for clients who have had one or more psychotic episodes. It has been shown that groups can help the client develop

- Interpersonal skills.
- Resolution of family problems.
- Effective use of community supports.

Groups provide opportunities for socialization in safe settings, for expression of tensions, and for sharing problems. The most useful types of groups for schizophrenic clients are those that help clients develop abilities to deal with such issues as solving day-to-day problems, sharing relevant experiences, learning to listen, asking questions, and keeping topics in focus. Groups available on a continuing outpatient basis allow individual growth in these areas.

Some hospitals and clinics offer medication groups for clients. Medication groups can help clients

- Deal more effectively with troubling side effects.
- Alert the nurse to potential adverse side effects or toxic effects.
- Minimize isolation among clients receiving antipsychotics.
- Increase medication adherence.

FAMILY THERAPY

Families with a schizophrenic member often endure considerable hardships while coping with the psychotic and residual symptoms of schizophrenia. Often, these families become isolated from their communities and relatives. To make matters worse, until recently, families were often blamed for causing or triggering episodes of schizophrenia in their schizophrenic member (Fenton and Cole 1995). The National Alliance for the Mentally Ill (NAMI) and the National Association for Research in Schizophrenia and Depression are actively involved in efforts to develop new and effective treatment strategies that involve families, making them partners in the treatment process (Fenton and Cole 1995).

Families are perhaps the most consistent factor in the client's life. Over 60% of clients discharged from a psychiatric facility return to their family of origin (Bustillo et al. 1999). Family education and family therapy are known to diminish the negative effects of family life on schizophrenic clients. It is well established that when family therapy is added to pharmacological therapy, the relapse rate is reduced to about half. The results of eight studies in the United States and England found that family intervention has reduced the average relapse rate from 44% to 12% (McFarlane 1995).

The following is an example of how a family came to distinguish between "Martha's problem" and "the problem caused by schizophrenia."

> It was a good idea, us all meeting in the comfort of our own home to discuss my sister's illness. We were all able to say how it felt and for the first time I realized that I knew very little about what she was suffering from or how much—the word schizophrenia meant nothing to me before but it's much clearer now. I used to think she was just being lazy until she told me in the meeting what it was really like. (Gamble and Brennan 2000, p. 192.)

Programs that provide support, education, coping skills training, and social network development are extremely effective. This approach is called **psychoeducational**, and it combines educational with behavioral approaches to family treatment. The psychoeducational approach assumes that families are not to be blamed for their schizophrenic member's illness but in fact are secondary victims of a biological illness (Hatfield 1990, McFarlane 1995). The challenge for the 21st century is for health care workers to move beyond the global concept of family and begin to address the great diversity among families with mental illness (Hatfield, 1997). In family therapy sessions, the family can identify fears, faulty communications, and distortions. Improved problem-solving skills can be taught, and healthier alternatives to situations of conflict can be explored. Family guilt and anxiety can be lessened, which facilitates change.

In a recent study, investigators concluded that families with schizophrenic members who have a high risk for relapse and who received psychoeducational treatment in multiple family groups did even better than those treated in single family groups. Over a two-year follow-up period, those treated in single family therapy had a 27% relapse rate, while those treated in multiple family therapy groups had only a 16% relapse (Gabbard and Callaway 1995). Both single and multiple family treatments are cost effective; multiple family groups are the more cost effective and the most advantageous to families and their schizophrenic member. Some factors that seem to be involved in improvement follow (Gabbard and Callaway 1995):

■ Expands the client's and their relatives' social network
■ Expands the problem-solving capacity available in groups
■ Lowers the emotional overinvolvement of families
■ Increases the overall positive tone that characterizes such groups

The family self-help movement has been an important development in the mental health field. Families of schizophrenic clients have formed local and national self-help and advocacy organizations.

Families with schizophrenic members have very real needs. They need to be part of the decision-making process, to have adequate and appropriate help in crises, and to have periodic respite from the hard work of coping with a schizophrenic member (Lamb et al. 1986). Families need help in

■ Understanding the disease and the role of medications.
■ Setting realistic goals for the schizophrenic person.
■ Developing problem-solving skills for handling tensions and misunderstandings within the family environment.
■ Identifying the early signs of relapse.

Whether this is in the form of family therapy, psychoeducational multiple family therapy, or educational counseling, the family unit needs to be included in the treatment plan and counseling made available if the schizophrenic member is to become stabilized.

Psychopharmacology

Until the 1960s, a client who had even one schizophrenic episode spent months to years in a state or private psychiatric hospital acting bizarrely and experiencing a great deal of emotional pain. Additionally, these episodes resulted in great emotional and financial burdens to the families. Refer to "A Nurse Speaks" at the beginning of Unit I. Only with the advent of antipsychotic drugs could symptoms be controlled and clients managed in the community. Although these drugs can alleviate many of the symptoms of schizophrenia, they cannot cure the underlying psychotic processes. Therefore, when clients stop taking their medications, psychotic symptoms usually return. Although each client is unique, a general rule exists regarding how long a client needs to take medication. A client who has experienced one psychotic break should take medications for at least 1 year. After two psychotic episodes, medications should be continued for at least 2 years. If a client has experienced three or more psychotic episodes, medications may have to be continued throughout the person's life (Slately 1994). A 1997 study by Meltzer and associates confirms previous data that indicated that people with an early onset of schizophrenia are often resistant to antipsychotic medication.

Drugs used to treat psychotic disorders are called antipsychotic medications. Two groups of antipsychotic drugs exist: **standard** (traditional dopamine antagonists [D_2]) and **atypical** (serotonin-dopamine antagonists [$5-HT_{2A}$]). In addition, some drugs are used to augment the antipsychotic agents for treatment-resistant clients; they are discussed later in this chapter.

The standard (traditional dopamine antagonists D_2) clinically active antipsychotic drugs are able to block postsynaptic dopamine receptors D_2 in the central nervous system and are effective in the treatment of schizophrenia. The choice of drug is often based on:

■ Desired side effects (e.g., an agitated client may be given a more sedating antipsychotic).
■ Avoiding adverse side effects (e.g., haloperidol [Haldol] may be used in a person with cardiac problems because of its reduced anticholinergic effects).
■ Client response (what drug worked well for a specific individual in the past).

The antipsychotic drugs are effective for most acute exacerbations of schizophrenia and for the prevention or mitigation of relapse. The standard typical (traditional) antipsychotics target the positive symptoms of schizophrenia (e.g., hallucinations, delusions, disordered thinking, and paranoia). The newer atypical (novel) antipsychotics (e.g., clozapine, risperidone, olanzapine, quetiapine and ziprasidone) can diminish the negative symptoms as well (deficits in social interaction, blunted or inappropriate emotional expression, and lack of motivation). Because

of the improvement in the negative symptoms as well as positive symptoms, and because of the more serious side effects of the standard antipsychotics, the atypical antipsychotics are often preferred as first-time agents (Marangell et al. 1999).

Antipsychotic drugs can cause

■ Reduction in disruptive and violent behavior.
■ Increase in activity, speech, and sociability in withdrawn or mute clients.
■ Improvement in self-care.
■ Improvement in sleep patterns.
■ Reduction in the disturbing quality of hallucinations and delusions.
■ Improvement in thought processes.
■ Decreased resistance to activity therapies and supportive psychotherapy.
■ Reduced rate of relapse (about 2.5 times less).
■ Decrease in the intensity of paranoid reactions.

Antipsychotic agents are usually effective 3 to 6 weeks after the regimen is started. Only about 10% of schizophrenic clients fail to respond to antipsychotic drug therapy. These clients should not continue to take medication that, for them, holds only risks and no benefit. Schizophrenia is the most common indication for antipsychotic medication. People in acute mania or psychotic depression may respond to a short course of antipsychotic drugs. These agents are also frequently effective in the treatment of the behavioral disorders associated with cognitive disorders such as dementia.

In order to understand why the newer atypical antipsychotics (AAPs) are so well received by clinicians as well as many clients, it is helpful to understand the more traditional (typical or standard) antipsychotics, which were the only medications available until the first atypical drugs were introduced in the early 1990s.

TYPICAL (TRADITIONAL) ANTIPSYCHOTICS

The properties and side effects of agents in the five classes are similar. The phenothiazines are usually considered the prototype for assessing the action and side effects of the traditional antipsychotics.

The choice of specific drugs is often made on the basis of major side effects, which include extrapyramidal side effects (EPSs), anticholinergic side effects, and sedation. Other side effects include orthostatic hypotension and lowered seizure threshold. For example, chlorpromazine (Thorazine) is the most sedating agent and has fewer EPSs than do other antipsychotic agents, but it causes hypotension in large doses. Haloperidol (Haldol) is the least sedating and is often used in large doses to reduce assaultive behavior but has a high incidence of EPS. The value of haloperidol for treating violent behav-

TABLE 20–11 *Typical (Traditional) Antipsychotics*

DRUG	ROUTES OF ADMINISTRATION	ACUTE (MG/DAY)*	MAINTENANCE (MG/DAY)*	SPECIAL CONSIDERATIONS
High Potency				
Haloperidol (Haldol)	PO, IM	5–50	2–20	Has low sedative properties; is used in large doses for assaultive patients, thus avoiding the severe side effect of hypotension. Appropriate for the elderly for the same reason as above; lessens the chance of falls from dizziness or hypotension. High incidence of extrapyramidal side effects.
Trifluoperazine (Stelazine)	PO, IM	10–60	5–30	Low sedation—good for withdrawn or paranoid symptoms. High incidence of extrapyramidal side effects. Neuroleptic malignant syndrome may occur.
Fluphenazine (Prolixin)	PO, IM, SC	2.5–20	2–20	Among the least sedative.
Thiothixene (Navane)	PO, IM	6–30	5–40	High incidence of akathisia.
Medium Potency				
Loxapine (Loxitane)	PO, IM	60–100	20–200	Possibly associated with weight reduction.
Molindone (Moban)	PO	50–100	20–200	Possibly associated with weight reduction.
Perphenazine (Trilafon)	PO, IM, IV	12–32	8–64	Can help control severe vomiting.
Low Potency				
Chlorpromazine (Thorazine)	PO, IM, R	200–1600	200–1000	Increases sensitivity to sun (as with other phenothiazines). Highest sedation and hypotension effects; least potent. May cause irreversible retinitis pigmentosis at 800 mg/day.
Chlorprothixene (Taractan)	PO, IM	50–600	75–600	Weight gain common.
Thioridazine (Mellaril)	PO	200–600	200–600	**Not recommended as first line antipsychotic.** Dose-related severe EKG changes, may cause sudden death (Kennedy 2000).
Mesoridazine (Serentil)	PO, IM	75–300	100–400	Among the most sedative; severe nausea and vomiting may occur in adults.
Decanoate: Long-Acting				
Haloperidol decanoate (Haldol)	IM	0	50–300	Given deep muscle Z-track IM **Given every 3–4 wk**
Fluphenazine decanoate (Prolixin)	IM	0	12.5–50	Given deep muscle Z-track IM **Effective every 2–4 wk**

*Dosages vary with individual responses to antipsychotic agent used.
IM, intramuscular; PO, oral; R, rectal; SC, subcutaneous; IV, intravenous.
Drug dosages from Tasman 2000, Kennedy 2000, Fuller and Sajatovic 2000.

iors is its effectiveness in controlling hallucinatory phenomena with a low incidence of hypotension. People who are functioning at work or at home may prefer less sedating drugs; clients who are agitated or excitable may do better with a more sedating medication.

The antipsychotics are often divided into low potency and high potency on the basis of their anticholinergic side effects (ACH), EPSs, and sedation:

■ Low Potency = High Sedation + High ACH + Low EPS
■ High Potency = Low Sedation + Low ACH + High EPS

However, all the standard antipsychotic drugs can cause tardive dyskinesia. The newer atypical antipsychotic drugs have dramatically fewer reports of tardive dyskinesia.

The phenothiazine-like drugs have some positive attributes. It is difficult to take a lethal overdose. Neither tolerance nor potential for abuse develops. Many of the side effects are minor or temporary, although a few can be very serious. These drugs are used with caution in people who have seizure disorders because they can lower the seizure threshold. Table 20–11 identifies which drugs are low, medium, and high potency, as well as doses for acute symptoms, usual maintenance doses, and other considerations.

Some of the more disturbing side effects caused by the dopamine blockade properties of the standard antipsychotics are the EPSs. Three of the more common EPSs are acute dystonia (muscle cramps of the head and neck), akathisia (internal and external restless pacing or fidgeting), and pseudoparkinsonism (stiffening of muscular activity in the face, body, arms, and legs). These side effects often appear early in therapy and can be minimized with treatment. Treatment usually consists of lowering the dosage or prescribing antiparkinsonian drugs, especially centrally acting anticholinergic drugs. Commonly used drugs include trihexyphenidyl (Artane), benztropine mesylate (Cogentin), diphenhydramine hydrochloride (Benadryl), and amantadine hydrochloride (Symmetrel). The first two in this list are antiparkinsonian drugs. Treatment with antiparkinsonian drugs is not completely benign, because the anticholinergic side effects of the antipsychotics may be intensified (e.g., urinary retention, constipation, failure of visual accommodation [blurred vision], cognitive impairment, and delirium) (Berkow et al. 1992).

Table 20–12 identifies common side effects and nursing and medical interventions for patients taking these antipsychotic medications.

Most clients develop tolerance to EPSs after a few months. Effective nursing and medical management is important during this time, to encourage compliance with the medications until the disturbing and frightening side effects have been properly managed. Table 20–13 identifies some of the more commonly used drugs for the treatment of EPS.

Perhaps the most troubling side effects for outpatients taking antipsychotics are weight gain, impotence, and tardive dyskinesia (TD). Weight gain is most frequently a problem with women and may result in as much as a 100-pound gain in some clients. Discontinuation of the antipsychotic medication may be necessary, along with the use of an alternative drug. Impotence is occasionally reported (but frequently experienced) by men and may also necessitate switching to alternative drugs. Sexual dysfunctions are perhaps the most common reasons for male noncompliance.

Tardive dyskinesia, an EPS that usually appears after prolonged treatment, is more serious and not always reversible. Tardive dyskinesia consists of involuntary tonic muscular spasms that typically involve the tongue, fingers, toes, neck, trunk, or pelvis. This potentially serious EPS most frequently affects women, older clients, and up to 50% of people receiving long-term large-dose therapy. Tardive dyskinesia varies from mild to moderate and can be disfiguring or incapacitating. Early symptoms of tardive dyskinesia are fasciculations of the tongue or constant smacking of the lips. These early oral movements can develop into uncontrollable biting, chewing, sucking motions, an open mouth, and lateral movements of the jaw. In many cases, the early symptoms of tardive dyskinesia disappear when the antipsychotic medication is discontinued. In other cases, however, early symptoms are not reversible and may progress. No proven cure for advanced tardive dyskinesia exists.

The National Institute of Mental Health has developed a brief test for the detection of tardive dyskinesia. The test is referred to as the Abnormal Involuntary Movement Scale (Box 20–2). (A copy of the Abnormal Involuntary Movement Scale is free to those who write to the National Institute of Mental Health, Schizophrenic Disorders Section, Somatic Treatments Branch, Rockville, MD 20857.) The three areas of examination are facial and oral movements, extremity movements, and trunk movement.

Nurses need to know about some rare—but serious and potentially fatal—toxic effects of these drugs. Toxic effects include neuroleptic malignant syndrome, agranulocytosis, and liver involvement.

Neuroleptic malignant syndrome (NMS) may occur in about 0.2% to 1% of clients who have taken antipsychotic agents. It is believed that the acute reduction in brain dopamine activity plays a role in the development of neuroleptic malignant syn-

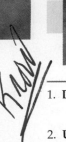

TABLE 20–12 *Nursing Measures for Side Effects of Antipsychotics*

SIDE EFFECTS	ONSET	NURSING MEASURES
Anticholinergic Symptoms (ACH)		
1. **Dry mouth**		1. Frequent sips of water and sugarless candy or gum. If severe, provide Xero-Lube, a saliva substitute.
2. **Urinary retention and hesitancy**		2. Check voiding; try warm towel on abdomen; consider catheterization if this doesn't work.
3. **Constipation**		3. Usually short term. May use stool softener. Assess for adequate water intake.
4. **Blurred vision**		4. Usually abates in 1 to 2 weeks. If patient is taking thioridazine, do not give it and check with physician.
5. **Photosensitivity**		5. Encourage client to wear sunglasses.
6. **Dry eyes**		6. Use artificial tears.
7. **Inhibition of ejaculation or impotence in men**		7. Alert physician; client may need alternative medication.
Extrapyramidal Side Effects		
1. **Pseudoparkinsonism:** masklike faces, stiff and stooped posture, shuffling gait, drooling, tremor, "pill-rolling" phenomena.	>5–30 days	1. Alert medical staff. An anticholinergic agent (e.g., trihexyphenidyl [Artane] or benztropine [Cogentin] may be used.
2. **Acute dystonic reactions:** acute contractions of tongue, face, neck, and back (tongue and jaw first) ■ **Opisthotonos:** tetanic heightening of entire body, head and belly up ■ **Oculogyric crisis:** eyes locked upward	1–5 days	2. **First choice:** Diphenhydramine hydrochloride (Benadryl) 25–50 mg IM/IV. Relief occurs in minutes. **Second choice:** Benztropine, 1–2 mg IM/IV. **Prevent further dystonias** with any anticholinergic agent (see Table 20–12). Experience is very frightening. Take patient to quiet area and stay with him or her until medicated.
3. **Akathisia:** motor inner-driven restlessness (e.g., tapping foot incessantly, rocking forward and backward in chair, shifting weight from side to side).	5–60 days	3. Physician may change antipsychotic agent or give antiparkinsonian agent. Tolerance does not develop to akathisia, but akathisia disappears when neuroleptic is discontinued. Propranolol (Inderal), lorazepam (Ativan), or diazepam (Valium) may be used.
4. **Tardive dyskinesia:** ■ **Facial:** Protruding and rolling tongue, blowing, smacking, licking, spastic facial distortion, smacking movements. ■ **Limbs:** **Choreic:** rapid, purposeless and irregular movements **Athetoid:** slow, complex and serpentine movements ■ **Trunk:** neck, shoulder, dramatic hip jerks and rocking, twisting pelvic thrusts.	6–24 mo to years	4. **No known treatment.** Discontinuing the drug does not always relieve symptoms. Possibly 20% of patients taking the drug for >2 years may develop tardive dyskinesia. Nurses and doctors should encourage patients to be screened for tardive dyskinesia at least every three months.

TABLE 20–12   *Nursing Measures for Side Effects of Antipsychotics* (Continued)

SIDE EFFECTS	ONSET	NURSING MEASURES
Cardiovascular Effects		
1. **Hypotension and postural hypotension**		1. Check blood pressure before giving; advise patient to dangle feet before getting out of bed to prevent dizziness and subsequent falls. A systolic pressure of 80 mm Hg when standing is indication to not give the current dose. This effect usually subsides when drug is stabilized in one to two weeks. Elastic bandages may prevent pooling. If condition is serious, physician orders volume expanders or pressure agents.
2. **Tachycardia**		2. Patients with existing cardiac problems should *always* be evaluated before the antipsychotic drugs are administered. Haloperidol is usually the preferred drug because of its low anticholinergic effects.
Rare and Toxic Effects		
1. **Agranulocytosis:** symptoms include sore throat, fever, malaise, and mouth sore. It is a rare occurrence, but one the nurse should be aware of; any flulike symptoms should be carefully evaluated.	Usually occurs suddenly and becomes evident in the first 12 weeks	1. Blood work usually done every week, then every two months. Physician may order blood work to determine presence of leukopenia or agranulocytosis. If test results are positive, the drug is discontinued, and reverse isolation may be initiated. Mortality is high if the drug is not ceased and if treatment is not initiated.
2. **Cholestatic jaundice:** Rare, reversible, and usually benign if caught in time; prodromal symptoms are fever, malaise, nausea, and abdominal pain; jaundice appears 1 week later		2. Drug is discontinued; bed rest and high-protein, high-carbohydrate diet is given. Liver function tests should be performed every six months.
3. **Neuroleptic malignant syndrome:** Somewhat rare, potentially fatal. ■ **Severe extrapyramidal:** e.g., severe muscle rigidity, oculogyric crisis, dysphasia, flexor-extensor posturing, cog wheeling. ■ **Hyperpyrexia** elevated temperature (≤103°F) ■ **Autonomic dysfunction:** e.g., hypertension, tachycardia, diaphoresis, incontinence.	Can occur in the first week of drug therapy but often occurs later. Rapidly progresses over 2 to 3 days after initial manifestation **RISK FACTORS:** ■ Using concomitant psychotropics ■ Being older ■ Being female (3:2) ■ Having a mood disorder (40%) ■ Undergoing rapid dose titration (Lieberman & Tasman 2000)	3. ■ Stop neuroleptic. ■ Transfer STAT to medical unit. ■ Bromocriptine can relieve muscle rigidity and reduce fever. ■ Dantrolene may reduce muscle spasms. ■ Cool body to reduce fever. ■ Maintain hydration with oral and IV fluids. ■ Correct electrolyte imbalance. ■ Arrhythmias should be treated. ■ Small doses of heparin may decrease possibility of pulmonary emboli. ■ Early detection increases client's chance of survival.

IM, intramuscular; IV, intravenous; STAT, immediately.

TABLE 20–13 *Treatment of Acute Extrapyramidal Side Effects*

DRUG	ORAL DOSE, MG	INTRAMUSCULAR OR INTRAVENOUS DOSE, MG	CHEMICAL GROUP
Trihexyphenidyl* (Artane)	2–5 tid	—	ACA
Benztropine mesylate* (Cogentin)	1–3 bid	1–2	ACA
Biperiden* (Akineton)	2 bid or qid	2	ACA
Diphenhydramine hydrochloride (Benadryl)	25–50 tid or qid	25–50	Antihistamine
Procyclidine hydrochloride (Kemadrin)	2.5–5 tid	—	ACA
Bromocriptine mesylate (Parlodel)		1.25–2.0	

* Antiparkinsonian drug.
ACA, anticholinergic agent (after one to six months of long-term maintenance antipsychotic therapy, most ACAs can be withdrawn); bid, twice a day; tid, three times a day; qid, four times a day.
From Maxmen, J. S., and Ward, N. G. (1995). *Psychotropic drugs: Fast facts* (2nd Ed.). New York: W. W. Norton.

drome. Neuroleptic malignant syndrome is fatal in about 10% of cases. It usually occurs early in the course of treatment but has been reported in people after 20 years of treatment.

Neuroleptic malignant syndrome is characterized by decreased level of consciousness, greatly increased muscle tone, and autonomic dysfunction, including hyperpyrexia, labile hypertension, tachycardia, tachypnea, diaphoresis, and drooling. Treatment consists of early detection, discontinuation of the antipsychotic agent, management of fluid balance, reduction of temperature, and monitoring for complications. Dopamine antagonists or dantrolene (Dantrium) and even electroconvulsive therapy are used in some cases (Caroff and Mann 1993).

Agranulocytosis is also a serious side effect and can be fatal. Liver involvement may occur. Nurses need to be aware of the prodromal signs and symptoms of these side effects and to teach them to their clients and clients' families. (Refer back to Table 20–12).

ATYPICAL ANTIPSYCHOTICS

These atypical antipsychotics (AAPs) are a new generation of antipsychotics, and first emerged in the early 1990s with clozapine (Clozaril). Clozapine, unfortunately, has a very real disadvantage. From 0.8% to 1% of people on this drug will develop agranulocytosis. However, the AAPs that eventually followed do not share this same disadvantage.

The important advantage to the AAPs is that they alleviate both the positive and the negative symptoms of schizophrenia. These newer atypical medications (Table 20–14) permit more than just control of the most alarming symptoms of this disease (e.g., hallucinations, delusions); they also allow for improvement in the quality of life for people with schizophrenia. **These drugs are often chosen as first line antipsychotics** because they:

■ Have few or no EPS or tardive dyskinesia (TD).
■ Treat both the distressing positive symptoms as well as the disabling negative symptoms of schizophrenia.
■ May improve the neurocognitive defects associated with schizophrenia.

The first of these newer drugs was clozapine, which caused dramatic changes in some clients resistant to the standard antipsychotics. Its major drawback is a high incidence of agranulocytosis and seizures, as mentioned previously. Those clients on clozapine have weekly white blood count monitoring for the first six months, then every other week thereafter. Next came risperidone, which has also had a beneficial effect on the functioning of people with schizophrenia and could be used as a first-line drug without the hematological concerns of clozapine. Newer atypical antipsychotics include olanzapine (Zyprexa), quetiapine (Seroquel), and ziprasidone (Geodon). None of the last four, however, causes agranulocytosis. They all make good choices for first line agents because of the lower side effects profile. One of the disadvantages of the AAPs is that all have a tendency (with the exception of ziprasidone) to cause weight gain in clients (Taylor and McAskill 2000). Consequences of weight gain for schizophrenic clients are (Keith 1999):

■ Increased risk of morbidity

　■ cardiovascular disease
　■ diabetes
　■ hypertension

Box 20-2 *Abnormal Involuntary Movement Scale*

DEPARTMENT OF HUMAN SERVICES PUBLIC HEALTH SERVICE Alcohol, Drug Abuse, and Mental Health Administration NIMH Treatment Strategies in Schizophrenia Study **ABNORMAL INVOLUNTARY MOVEMENT SCALE (AIMS)**	PATIENT NUMBER – – – –	DATA GROUP aims	EVALUATION DATE

PATIENT NUMBER – – – – DATA GROUP aims EVALUATION DATE _ _ _ _ _ M M D D Y Y

PATIENT NAME

RATER NAME

RATER NUMBER

– – –

EVALUATION TYPE (*Circle*)

1 Baseline	4 Start double-blind	7 Start open meds	10 Early termination
2 2-week minor	5 Major evaluation	8 During open meds	11 Study completion
3	6 Other	9 Stop open meds	

INSTRUCTIONS: Complete Examination Procedure (reverse side) before making ratings.
MOVEMENT RATINGS: Rate highest severity observed.

Code: 1 = None 3 = Mild
2 = Minimal, may be extreme normal 4 = Moderate 5 = Severe

		(Circle One)				
FACIAL AND ORAL MOVEMENTS:	**1. Muscles of facial expression** e.g., movements of forehead, eyebrows, periorbital area, cheeks; include frowning, blinking, smiling, grimacing	1	2	3	4	5
	2. Lips and perioral area e.g., puckering, pouting, smacking	1	2	3	4	5
	3. Jaw e.g., biting, clenching, chewing, mouth opening, lateral movement	1	2	3	4	5
	4. Tongue Rate only increase in movement both in and out of mouth, NOT inability to sustain movement	1	2	3	4	5
EXTREMITY MOVEMENTS:	**5. Upper** (*arms, wrists, hands, fingers*) Include choreic movements (i.e., rapid, objectively purposeless, irregular, spontaneous), athetoid movements (i.e., slow, irregular, complex, serpentine). Do NOT include tremor (i.e., repetitive, regular, rhythmic)	1	2	3	4	5
	6. Lower (*legs, knees, ankles, toes*) e.g., lateral knee movement, foot tapping, heel dropping, foot squirming, inversion and eversion of foot	1	2	3	4	5
TRUNK MOVEMENTS:	**7. Neck, shoulders, hips** e.g., rocking, twisting, squirming, pelvic gyrations	1	2	3	4	5
GLOBAL JUDGMENTS:	**8. Severity of abnormal movements**	None, minimal 1 Minimal 2 Mild 3 Moderate 4 Severe 5				

Box continued on following page

Box 20–2 *Abnormal Involuntary Movement Scale* (Continued)

GLOBAL JUDGMENTS: (CONT')	9. Incapacitation due to abnormal movements	None, minimal	1
		Minimal	2
		Mild	3
		Moderate	4
		Severe	5
	10. Patient's awareness of abnormal movements Rate only patient's report	No awareness	1
		Aware, no distress	2
		Aware, mild distress	3
		Aware, moderate distress	4
		Aware, severe distress	5
DENTAL STATUS:	11. Current problem with teeth and/or dentures?	No	1
		Yes	2
	12. Does patient usually wear dentures?	No	1
		Yes	2

EXAMINATION PROCEDURE

Either before or after completing the Examination Procedure observe the patient unobtrusively, at rest (e.g., in waiting room).

The chair to be used in this examination should be a hard, firm one without arms.

1. Ask patient to remove shoes and socks.
2. Ask patient whether there is anything in his/her mouth (i.e., gum, candy, etc.) and if there is, to remove it.
3. Ask patient about the *current* condition of his/her teeth. Ask patient if he/she wears dentures. Do teeth or dentures bother the patient *now?*
4. Ask patient whether he/she notices any movements in mouth, face, hands, or feet. If yes, ask to describe and to what extent they *currently* bother patient or interfere with his/her activities.
5. Have patient sit in chair with hands on knees, legs slightly apart, and feet flat on floor. (Look at entire body movements while in this position.)
6. Ask patient to sit with hands hanging unsupported: if male, between legs; if female and wearing a dress, hanging over knees. (Observe hands and other body areas.)
7. Ask patient to open mouth. (Observe tongue at rest within mouth.) Do this twice.
8. Ask patient to protrude tongue. (Observe abnormalities of tongue movement.) Do this twice.
9. Ask patient to tap thumb, with each finger, as rapidly as possible for 10 to 15 seconds: separately with right hand, then with left hand. (Observe each facial and leg movement.)
10. Flex and extend patient's left and right arms (one at a time). (Note any rigidity.)
11. Ask patient to stand up. (Observe in profile. Observe all body areas again, hips included.)
12. Ask patient to extend both arms outstretched in front with palms down. (Observe trunk, legs, and mouth.)
13. Have patient walk a few paces, turn, and walk back to chair. (Observe hands and gait.) Do this twice.

■ Diminished self-esteem
■ Causes problems with adherence to medication

Another disadvantage of the AAPs is that although they seem to target more symptoms, have fewer side effects, and improve the client's quality of life, they are more expensive than the traditional antipsychotics. Refer to Table 20–14 for the atypical antipsychotics, their dose range, some properties, and comments.

ADJUNCTS TO ANTIPSYCHOTIC DRUG THERAPY

Other drugs are often used in the treatment of drug-resistant schizophrenia.

ANTIDEPRESSANTS. Antidepressants are recommended along with antipsychotic agents for the

TABLE 20–14 Atypical Antipsychotic Agents

DRUG	DOSE RANGE, MG/DAY	EPS	ACH	OH	SED	COMMENTS
Clozapine (Clozaril)	25–600	No	High	High	High	■ Used in treatment refractory clients— **non–first-line** ■ 0.8%–0.1% incidence of agranulocytosis—weekly WBC ■ High seizure rate
Risperidone (Risperdal)	2–16	Mild	Very low	Mod	Mod	■ Weight gain significant ■ Doses >6 mg may see **TD**
Olanzapine (Zyprexal)	2.5–20	Mild	Mod	Mod	Mod	■ Weight gain significant ■ Once a day dose (long half-life) ■ Interaction with SSRIs may occur
Quetiapine (Seroquel)	150–750	Low	Mild	Mod	Mod	■ Risk of TD and NMS very low
Ziprasidone (Geodon)	40–200	Low	Mild	Mild	Low	■ ECG changes—QT prolongation. Not to be used with other drugs known to prolong QT interval. ■ Effective with the depressive symptoms of schizophrenia ■ Low propensity for weight gain

ACH, anticholinergic side effects (dry mouth, blurred vision, urinary retention, constipation, agitation); EPS, extrapyramidal side effects; NMS, neuroleptic malignant syndrome; OH, orthostatic hypotension; SED, sedation; TD, tardive dyskinesia.
Adapted from Fuller and Sajatovic 2000, Lieberman and Tasman 2000.

treatment of depression which is so common among these individuals. Refer to Chapter 18.

ANTIMANIC AGENTS. Lithium can be useful for suppressing episodic violence in schizophrenia as well as for targeting many of the more disturbing symptoms when the agent is used along with a more traditional antipsychotic. Grove et al (1979) found augmenting with lithium to improve the psychotic symptoms, especially the negative symptoms. It seems to also help alleviate comorbid depression in some clients (Learner et al 1988). Carbamazepine and valproic acid (Depakene) have also been found to alleviate symptoms in some drug-resistant clients who have schizophrenia when they are used along with a standard antipsychotic (see Chapter 19).

BENZODIAZEPINES. Benzodiazepines are also being studied as possible adjuncts in the treatment of selected clients with schizophrenia, especially in the acute phase. Several studies have demonstrated that benzodiazepines as adjuncts to antipsychotics can have positive effects on anxiety, agitation, psychosis or global impairment (DSM-IV-TR 2000).

WHEN TO CHANGE AN ANTIPSYCHOTIC REGIMEN

The following conditions suggest the need for a different antipsychotic agent:

■ Clear lack of efficacy of the current drug regimen
■ Need for supplemental medications (lithium, carbamazepine, valproate)
■ Occurrence of intolerable or persistent side effects

Electroconvulsive Therapy

In several studies of first-admission schizophrenic clients, electroconvulsive therapy (ECT) was found to be as effective as antipsychotic medication during the acute phase (APA 1997). It is not as effective with chronic schizophrenia (DSM-IV-TR 2000). Electroconvulsive therapy may be used for severely catatonic clients. It is also indicated when antipsychotic drug therapy fails or is contraindicated. Electroconvulsive therapy may be helpful for people who do not respond satisfactorily to drugs and are too old to be discharged—for example, for a client who appears to be tormented by hallucinations or delusional fears, or who has rapid or dramatic onset of psychosis, or who presents an ongoing or acute risk to his or her life (refusing food or fluids, maintaining active suicidal intent) (Johns 1996). A study in Nigeria, where ECT is widely used for schizophrenia, demonstrated that ECT facilitated recovery in drug treatment–resistant psychotic subjects (Ikeji and colleagues 1999).

However, ECT is mostly used in the United States for people with psychotic depression, or who are violent, suicidal, or participating in self-starvation.

NURSING INTERVENTIONS FOR SCHIZOPHRENIC SUBTYPES

The schizophrenias are a group of disorders. The DSM-IV-TR subtypes are found in Figure 20–4. In the following section you will be introduced to the

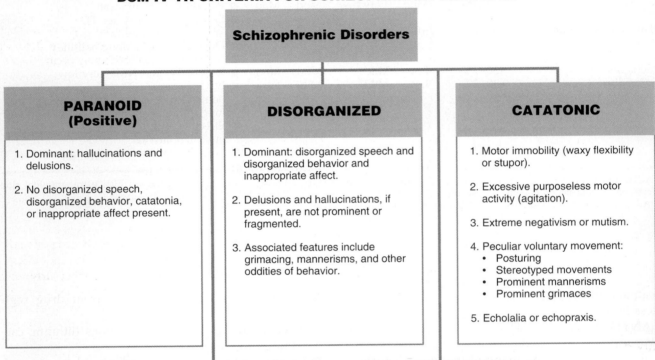

DSM-IV-TR CRITERIA FOR SCHIZOPHRENIA SUBTYPES

Schizophrenic Disorders

PARANOID (Positive)

1. Dominant: hallucinations and delusions.

2. No disorganized speech, disorganized behavior, catatonia, or inappropriate affect present.

DISORGANIZED

1. Dominant: disorganized speech and disorganized behavior and inappropriate affect.

2. Delusions and hallucinations, if present, are not prominent or fragmented.

3. Associated features include grimacing, mannerisms, and other oddities of behavior.

CATATONIC

1. Motor immobility (waxy flexibility or stupor).

2. Excessive purposeless motor activity (agitation).

3. Extreme negativism or mutism.

4. Peculiar voluntary movement:
   • Posturing
   • Stereotyped movements
   • Prominent mannerisms
   • Prominent grimaces

5. Echolalia or echopraxis.

RESIDUAL

1. No longer has active phase symptoms (e.g., delusions, hallucinations, or disorganized speech and behaviors).

2. However, persistence of some symptoms is noted, e.g.:
   • Marked social isolation or withdrawal
   • Marked impairment in role function (wage earner, student, or homemaker)
   • Markedly eccentric behavior or odd beliefs
   • Marked impairment in personal hygiene
   • Marked lack of initiative, interest, or energy
   • Blunted or inappropriate affect

UNDIFFERENTIATED (MIXED TYPE)

1. Has active phase symptoms (does have hallucinations, delusions, and bizarre behaviors).

2. No one clinical presentation dominates, e.g.:
   • Paranoid
   • Disorganized
   • Catatonic

Figure 20–4 DSM-IV-TR criteria for schizophrenia subtypes. (Adapted from American Psychiatric Association [2000], *Diagnostic and statistical manual of mental disorders, Text Revision, 4th ed.* Washington, D.C.: American Psychiatric Association. Copyright 2000 American Psychiatric Association.)

paranoid, catatonic (excited and withdrawn phase), and the disorganized person. Each one will identify guidelines for communication, self-care and milieu needs. A short case study will be given at the end of each section. The full nursing care plan for the paranoid client can be found at the end of this chapter. The full nursing care plans for the others are found on the SIMON website.

Paranoia

Any intense and strongly defended irrational suspicion can be regarded as paranoia. Paranoid ideas cannot be corrected by experiences and cannot be modified by facts or reality. **Projection** is the most common defense mechanism used by people who are paranoid. For example, when paranoid individuals feel self-critical, they experience others as being harshly critical toward them. When they feel anger, they experience others as being unjustly angry at them, as if to say "I'm not angry, you are!"

Paranoid states may occur in numerous mental or organic disorders. For example, a person experiencing a psychotic depression or manic episode may display paranoid thinking. Paranoid symptoms can be secondary to physical illness, organic brain disease, or drug intoxication.

Paranoid schizophrenia is one of the **primary** paranoid disorders (i.e., those in which the primary symptom is paranoid thinking). The others are paranoid delusional disorder and paranoid personality disorder. Chapter 16 addresses the paranoid personality disorder.

People with paranoid schizophrenia usually have a later age of onset (late twenties to thirties). Paranoid schizophrenia develops rapidly in individuals with good premorbid functioning and tends to be intermittent during the first 5 years of the illness. In some cases, paranoid schizophrenia is associated with a good outcome or with recovery (Fenton and McGlashan 1991). People with a paranoid disorder are usually frightened. Although not always consciously aware of their feelings, paranoid people have deep feelings of loneliness, despair, helplessness, and fear of abandonment. The paranoid facade is a defense against painful feelings. Useful nursing strategies are outlined in the following sections.

COMMUNICATION GUIDELINES

Because persons who are paranoid are unable to trust the actions of those around them, they are usually guarded, tense, and reserved. Although clients may keep themselves aloof from interpersonal contacts, impairment in actual functioning may be minimal. To ensure interpersonal distance, they may adopt a superior, hostile, and sarcastic attitude. A common defense used by paranoid individuals to maintain self-esteem is to disparage others and dwell on the shortcomings of others. The client frequently misinterprets the messages of others or gives private meaning to the communications of others (ideas of reference). For example, a client might see his primary nurse talking to the physician and believe that they are planning to harm him in some manner. Minor oversights are often interpreted as personal rejection.

During hospitalization, a paranoid client may make offensive yet accurate criticisms of staff and of ward policies. It is important that staff not react to these criticisms with anxiety or rejection of the client. Staff conferences, peer group supervision, and clinical supervision are effective ways of looking behind the behaviors to the motivations of the client. This provides the opportunity to reduce the client's anxiety and increase staff effectiveness. Refer to your communication card for guidelines to communication approaches for a paranoid person.

SELF-CARE NEEDS

People with paranoid schizophrenic disorder usually have stronger ego resources than do individuals with other schizophrenic disorders, particularly with regard to occupational functioning and capacity for independent living. Grooming, dress, and self-care may not be a problem. In fact, in some cases, grooming may be meticulous. Nutrition, however, may pose a problem. A common distortion or delusion is that the food is poisoned. In this case, special foods should be provided in enclosed containers to minimize the suspicion of tampering. If clients think that others will harm them when they are sleeping, they may be fearful of going to sleep. Therefore, adequate rest may become a problem that warrants nursing interventions.

MILIEU NEEDS

A paranoid person may become physically aggressive in response to hallucinations or delusions. Hostile drives are projected onto the environment and then acted on. Homosexual urges may be projected onto the environment as well, and fear of sexual advances from others may stimulate aggression or homosexual panic.

An environment that provides the client with a sense of security and safety should minimize anxiety and environmental distortions. Activities that distract the client from ruminating on hallucinations and delusions can also help decrease anxiety.

A vignette of a paranoid client follows.

Vignette

■ Tom is a 37-year-old man who is currently an inpatient at the Veterans Administration Hospital. He has been separated from his wife and four children for 6 years. His medical records state that because of his illness (which Tom describes as "hearing voices a lot"), he has been in and out of hospitals for 17 years. Tom is an ex-Marine who first "heard voices" at the age of 19, while he was stationed in Okinawa; he subsequently received a medical discharge.

The hospitalization was precipitated by an exacerbation of auditory hallucinations. "I thought people were following me. I hear voices, usually a woman's voice, and she's tormenting me. People say that it happens because I don't take my medications. The medications make me tired and I can't have sex." Tom also admits to using cocaine and marijuana. He is aware that marijuana and cocaine increase his paranoia and that taking drugs usually precedes hospitalization but says that "they make me feel good." Tom finished 11 years of school but did not graduate from high school. He says that he has no close friends. He was in prison for 5 years for manslaughter and told the nurse, "I was in prison because I did something bad." He was abusing alcohol and drugs at the time, and drug abuse has been related to each subsequent hospitalization.

Ms. Lally is Tom's primary nurse. When Tom meets the nurse, he is dressed in pajamas and bathrobe. His hygiene is good and he is well nourished. He tells the nurse that he does not sleep much because "the voices get worse at night." Ms. Lally notes in Tom's medical record that he has had two episodes of suicidal ideation. During those times, the voices were telling him to jump "off rooftops" and "in front of trains."

During the first interview, Tom only occasionally makes eye contact and speaks in a low monotone. At times, he glances about the room as if distracted, mumbles to himself, and appears upset.

Nurse: Tom, my name is Ms. Lally. I will be your nurse while you're in the hospital. We will meet every day for 30 minutes at 10 AM. During that time, we can discuss areas of concern to you.

Tom: Well . . . don't believe what they say about me. I want to start a new . . . Are you married?

Nurse: This time is for you to talk about *your* concerns.

Tom: Oh . . . *(Looks furtively around the room, then lowers his eyes.)* Someone is trying to kill me, I think . . .

Nurse: You appear to be focusing on something other than our conversation.

Tom: The voices tell me things . . . I can't say . . .

Nurse: I don't hear any voices except yours and mine. I am going to stay with you. Tell me what is happening and I will try to help you.

Tom: The voices tell me bad things.

Ms. Lally stays with Tom and encourages him to communicate with her. As Tom focuses more on the nurse, his anxiety appears to lessen. His thoughts become more connected, he is able to concentrate more on what the nurse is saying, and he mumbles less to himself.

The full nursing care plan for Tom is found at the end of this chapter.

Catatonia: Withdrawn Phase

The essential feature of catatonia is abnormal motor behavior. Two extreme motor behaviors are seen in clients with catatonia: extreme motor agitation and extreme psychomotor retardation (with mutism, even stupor). Other behaviors identified with catatonia include posturing, waxy flexibility, stereotyped behavior, extreme negativism or automatic obedience, echolalia, and echopraxia. The onset of catatonia is usually abrupt and the prognosis favorable. With chemotherapy and improved individual management, severe catatonic symptoms are rarely seen today. Useful nursing strategies are discussed in the following sections.

COMMUNICATION GUIDELINES

Clients in the withdrawn phase of catatonia can be so withdrawn that they appear comatose. They can be mute and may remain so for hours, days, or even weeks or months if they are not treated with antipsychotic medication. Although such clients may not appear to pay attention to events going on around them, the client is acutely aware of the environment and may remember events accurately at a later date. A withdrawn client has special needs, and the nurse can use the following guidelines. Developing skill and confidence in working with withdrawn clients takes practice. Refer to your communication card for guidelines on communicating with a withdrawn client.

SELF-CARE NEEDS

When a client is extremely withdrawn, physical needs take priority. A client may need to be hand fed or tube fed for adequate nutritional status to be maintained. Normal control over bladder and bowel functions can be interrupted. Assessment of urinary or bowel retention must be made and acted on when found. Incontinence of urine and feces may cause skin breakdown and infection. Because physical movements may be minimal or absent, range-of-motion exercises need to be carried out to prevent muscular atrophy, calcium depletion, and contractures. Dressing and grooming usually need direct nursing interventions.

The client with catatonic symptoms may trigger staff resistance to nursing interventions because the client may refuse to participate in activities or cooperate voluntarily.

MILIEU NEEDS

During the withdrawn state, the catatonic person may be on a continuum from decreased spontaneous movements to complete stupor. **Waxy flexibility,** or the ability to hold distorted postures for extensive periods, is often seen. The term *waxy* refers to the holding of any posture that the staff may place the person in. For example, if someone raises the client's arms over his head, the client may maintain that position for hours or longer. This phenomenon is often used as a diagnostic sign. When less withdrawn, a client may demonstrate stereotyped behavior, echopraxia, echolalia, or automatic obedience.

Caution is advised because even after holding a single posture for long periods, the client may suddenly and without provocation have brief outbursts of gross motor activity in response to inner hallucinations, delusions, and change in neurotransmitters. The following vignette is for a client who is withdrawn.

Vignette

■ Mrs. Chou is a 25-year-old woman. She left China for the United States 6 months ago to join her husband. Before she came to the United States, she lived with her parents and worked in a button factory. In China, Mrs. Chou had been educated to speak and understand English. She had always been shy and looked to her parents and now to her husband for guidance and support. Shortly after she arrived in the United States, her mother developed pneumonia and died, and Mrs. Chou was not able to go back to China for the funeral. Mr. Chou states that his wife thought that if she had stayed in China, her mother would not have become ill. She told him recently that evil would come to their one-year-old child because she was unable to take proper care of her mother. Three days before admission, Mrs. Chou became lethargic and spent most of the day staring into space and mumbling to herself. When Mr. Chou asked who she was talking to, she would answer, "My mother." She has not eaten for 2 days; at the time of admission, Mrs. Chou sits motionless and mute and appears stuporous.

The physician notices that when he takes Mrs. Chou's pulse, her arm remains in midair until he replaces it by her side. Mr. Chou says that once his wife became ex-

tremely agitated and started to scream and cry while tearing the curtains and knocking over objects. Shortly afterward, she returned to a withdrawn, mute state. Mr. Chou is extremely distraught and confused, and he fears for the safety of their child. Mr. Nolan is assigned to Mrs. Chou as her primary nurse.

Mrs. Chou is sloppily dressed, and her hair and nails are dirty. She is pale, and her skin turgor is poor. She sits motionless and appears to be unaware of anything going on around her. Mr. Nolan introduces himself and explains what he will be doing beforehand—for example, that he will be taking her blood pressure and pulse and offering her fluids.

While taking her vital signs, he tells Mrs. Chou the date, the time, and where she is. When he is finished taking her vital signs, he offers Mrs. Chou some fluids. She is able to take sips from a straw when the straw is placed in her mouth. Mrs. Chou's intake and output are monitored, and she is placed in a four-bed room next to the nurses' station.

Catatonia: Excited Phase

COMMUNICATION GUIDELINES

During the excited, or acute, stage, the person talks or shouts continually, and verbalizations may be incoherent. Communication is clear and directed, and concern is for the client's and others' safety.

SELF-CARE NEEDS

A person who is constantly and intensely hyperactive can become completely exhausted and can even die if medical attention is not available. Most often, a standard antipsychotic agent is administered intramuscularly. The client may continue to be agitated, but within limits that are not potentially harmful. During this time of heightened physical activity, the client's body has an increased need for fluids, calories, and rest. During the hyperactive state, a client may be destructive and aggressive to others in response to hallucinations or delusions. Many of these concerns and interventions are the same as for a bipolar client in a manic phase.

Disorganized Schizophrenia

The most regressed and socially impaired of all the schizophrenic disorders is the disorganized form. A person diagnosed with disorganized schizophrenia (formally hebephrenia) may have marked looseness of associations, grossly inappropriate affect, bizarre mannerisms, and incoherence of speech and may display extreme social withdrawal. Although delusions and hallucinations are present, they are fragmentary and not well organized. Behavior may be considered "odd," and giggling or grimacing in response to internal stimuli is common. Disorganized schizophrenia has an earlier age of onset (early to middle teens) and often develops insidiously. It is associated with poor premorbid functioning, a significant family history of psychopathologic disorders, and a poor prognosis. Often, these clients are in state hospitals and can live in the community safely only in a structured and well-supervised setting. Unfortunately, these clients now make up a good portion of the homeless population. Other clients may live at home, and their families have significant needs for community support, respite care, and day hospital affiliations.

COMMUNICATION GUIDELINES

People with disorganized schizophrenia experience persistent and severe perceptual problems. Verbal responses may be marked by looseness of associations or incoherence. Clang associations or word salad may be present. **Blocking,** a sudden cessation in the train of thought, is frequently observed.

SELF-CARE NEEDS

Grooming is neglected. Hair may be dirty and matted, and clothes may be inappropriate and stained. The client has no awareness of social expectations. The client may be too disorganized to carry out simple activities of daily living.

Basic goals for nursing intervention include encouraging optimal level of functioning, preventing further regression, and offering alternatives for inappropriate behaviors whenever possible.

MILIEU NEEDS

Behavior is often described as bizarre. A client may twirl around the room or make strange gestures with the hands and face. Social behavior is often primitive or regressed. For example, a client may eat with the hands, pick the nose, or masturbate in public. Typical behaviors include posturing, grimacing or giggling, and mirror gazing. A vignette of a person with disorganized schizophrenia follows.

Vignette

■ *Martin Taylor, a 36-year-old white, unemployed man, has been referred to the mental health center. He is accompanied by his mother and sister. He had been hospitalized for 3 years in a state hospital with the diagnosis of chronic schizophrenia and was doing well at home until 2 months ago. His only employment was for 5 months as a janitor after high school graduation. Other significant family his-*

tory includes a twin brother who died of a cerebral aneurysm in his teens. Martin tells the nurse he has used every street drug available, including LSD and intravenous heroin. His mother states that as a teenager, before his substance abuse, he was an excellent athlete who received average grades. At the age of 17, he had his first psychotic break when taking a variety of street drugs. His behavior became markedly bizarre (e.g., eating cat food, swallowing a rubber-soled heel that required an emergency laparotomy).

Ms. Lamb, a clinical nurse specialist, meets with Martin after speaking with his mother and sister. Martin is unshaven, and his appearance is disheveled. He is wearing a red headband in which he has placed popsicle sticks and scraps of paper. He chain smokes during the interview and frequently gets up and paces back and forth. He tells the nurse that he is Alice from Alice in the Underground and that people from space hurt him with needles. His speech pattern is marked by associative looseness and occasional blocking. For example, he often stops in the middle of a phrase and giggles to himself. At one point, when he starts to giggle, Ms. Lamb asks him what he was thinking about. He stated "You interrupted me." At that point, he began to shake his head while repeating in a sing-song voice "Shake them tigers . . . shake them tigers . . . shake them tigers." He denies suicidal or homicidal ideation. Ms. Lamb notes that Martin has a great deal of difficulty accurately perceiving what is going on around him. He has markedly regressed social behaviors. For example, he eats with his hands and picks his nose in public. He has no apparent insight into his problems; he tells Ms. Lamb that his biggest problem is the people in space.

Undifferentiated Schizophrenia

In the undifferentiated type of schizophrenia, *active signs of the disorder* (positive or negative symptoms) are present, but the individual does not meet the criteria for paranoia, catatonia, or disorganized type (APA 2000). Undifferentiated schizophrenia has an early and insidious onset (early to middle teens), like that of disorganized schizophrenia. However, the premorbid state is less predictable, and the disability remains fairly stable, although persistent, over time.

Residual Type of Schizophrenia

In the residual type of schizophrenia, active phase symptoms are no longer present, but evidence of two or more residual symptoms persists. Residual symptoms include

- Lack of initiative, interests, or energy.
- Marked social withdrawal.
- Impairment in role function (wage earner, student, homemaker).
- Marked speech deficits (circumstantial, vague, and poverty of speech or content of speech).
- Odd beliefs, magical thinking, and unusual perceptual experiences.

Principles of care similar to those applying to withdrawn, paranoid, and disorganized schizophrenia apply to undifferentiated and residual schizophrenia, as dictated by the client's behavior.

EVALUATION

Evaluation is always an important step in the planning of care. Evaluation is especially important with people who have chronic psychotic disorders. Modifications may have to be made in the goals set for specific clients. All goals need to be realistic and obtainable. Often, the goals set for people with chronic disorders are too ambitious. A former short-term goal often becomes a long-term goal. Change is a process that occurs over time; with a person diagnosed with schizophrenia, the time period may be pronounced. Therefore, for preventing both client frustration and staff burnout, short-term goals should be realistic and obtainable.

Another advantage of regularly scheduled evaluations with chronically ill clients is that they allow the health care personnel to consider new data and to reassess the client's problems. Is the client not progressing because a more important need is not being met? Is the staff using the client's strengths and interest to reach identified goals? Are more appropriate interventions available for this client to facilitate progress? If a newer antipsychotic agent is being tried, is there evidence of improvement or a lower level of functioning? Is the family involved, giving support, and do they understand the client's disease and treatment issues?

The active involvement of staff with the client's progress can help sustain interest and prevent feelings of helplessness and burnout. Input from the client can offer valuable data about why a certain desired behavior or situation has not occurred.

Visit the **Evolve** website at
http://evolve.elsevier.com/Varcarolis
for more Case Studies.

CASE STUDY 20–1	*Working With a Person Who Is Paranoid*

ASSESSMENT	This case study refers to Tom, the client in the first Vignette in this chapter. After the initial interview, Ms. Lally divides the data into objective and subjective components.

OBJECTIVE DATA

- Speaks in low monotone
- Poor eye contact
- Well nourished, adequate hygiene
- States that he has auditory hallucinations
- Has history of drug abuse—cocaine and marijuana

- Has no close friends
- Was first hospitalized at age 19 and has not worked since that time
- Has had suicidal impulses twice
- Imprisoned 5 years for violent acting out (manslaughter)
- Thoughts scattered when anxious

SUBJECTIVE DATA

- "Someone is trying to kill me . . . I think."
- "I don't take my medicine. It makes me tired and I can't have sex."
- "The voices get worse at night, and I can't sleep."
- Voices have told him to "jump off rooftops" and "in front of trains."

SELF-ASSESSMENT

On the first day of admission, Tom assaults another male client, stating that the other client accused him of being a homosexual and touched him on the buttocks. After assessing the incident, the staff agrees that Tom's provocation came more from his own projections (Tom's sexual attraction to the other client) than from anything the other client did or said.

Tom's difficulty with impulse control frightens Ms. Lally. She has concerns regarding Tom's impulse control and the possibility of Tom's striking out at her, especially when Tom is hallucinating and highly delusional. Ms. Lally mentions her concerns to the nursing coordinator, who suggests that Ms. Lally meet with Tom in the day room until he demonstrates more control and less suspicion of others. After 5 days, Tom is less excitable, and the sessions are held in a room set aside for client interviews. Ms. Lally also speaks with a senior staff nurse regarding her fear. By talking to the senior nurse and understanding more clearly her own fear, Ms. Lally is able to identify interventions to help Tom regain a better sense of control.

NURSING DIAGNOSIS

Ms. Lally formulates two nursing diagnoses on the basis of her assessment data.

1. **Disturbed thought processes** related to alteration in biochemical compounds, as evidenced by persecutory hallucinations and intense suspiciousness.

   - Voices have told him to "jump off rooftops" and "in front of trains."
   - "Someone is trying to kill me, I think."
   - Abuses cocaine and marijuana, although these increase paranoia, because "it makes me feel good."

CASE STUDY 20–1	*Working With a Person Who Is Paranoid (Continued)*

2. **Noncompliance** related to side effects of therapy, as evidenced by verbalization of noncompliance and persistence of symptoms.

- Does not take prescribed medication because "it makes me tired and I can't have sex."
- Chronic history of relapse of symptoms when client is out of hospital.

OUTCOME

Ms. Lally decides that initial concentration should be placed on establishing a relationship in which Tom can feel safe with the nurse and comfortable enough to discuss his voices and the events that precipitate them. The nurse is aware that if Tom's anxiety level can be lowered and his suspicions can be diminished, he will be able to participate more comfortably in reality-based activities and will have an increased ability to solve problems. Because noncompliance with his medications seems to be a major factor in the persistence of Tom's disturbing symptoms, this becomes an important focus for discussion. Ms. Lally plans to evaluate the medication and side effects with the physician and to work with Tom on alternatives to increase his medical compliance.

NURSING DIAGNOSIS	OUTCOME CRITERIA	SHORT-TERM GOALS
1. **Disturbed thought processes** related to alteration in biochemical compounds, as evidenced by persecutory hallucinations and intense suspiciousness.	1. Tom will refrain from acting upon his "voices" and suspicions, should they occur.	1a. By (date), Tom will state that he feels comfortable with the nurse. 1b. By (date), Tom will name two actions that precipitate voices and paranoia. 1c. By (date), Tom will name two actions he can take if the voices start to upset him.
2. **Noncompliance** related to side effects of medication, as evidenced by stating he is not taking medicine and persistence of symptoms.	2. Tom will adhere to medication regimen.	2a. By (date), Tom will name actions he can take to offset the side effects of medication. 2b. Tom will attend weekly support group for people with schizophrenia.

INTERVENTION

Ms. Lally makes out an initial nursing care plan (Nursing Care Plan 20–1). An important part of her plan consists of conferring with the physician about the legitimate concerns Tom had regarding his medication. The concerns Tom has regarding not being able to sustain an erection are legitimate, and the physician states that he

Case Study continued on following page

CASE STUDY 20–1 *Working With a Person Who Is Paranoid* (Continued)

will put Tom on one of the newer atypical antipsychotics, olanzapine (Zyprexa), which has little known sexual inhibitors. Ms. Lally works with Tom on continuing his participation in the support group. During team conference, the social worker suggests that if Tom becomes able to maintain contact with a support group, he might be a good candidate for a group home in the future.

Antipsychotic medications seem to greatly lower Tom's suspiciousness and his hallucinatory symptoms. This enables Tom to discuss with the nurse more reality-based concerns and to be more amenable to attending the weekly support group. After their fourth meeting, Tom seems to view the group more favorably and even speaks of making a friend in the group.

EVALUATION	When Tom is discharged home, he says he has a better understanding of his medications and what to do. He knows that marijuana and cocaine increase his symptoms, but he says that he sometimes got lonely and needed to "feel good." Tom continues with support group and outpatient counseling. The reason he gives for deciding to attend outpatient therapy is that he feels that Ms. Lally had really cared about him, and that made him feel good. He reports sleeping much better and says that he has more energy during the day.

Visit the **Evolve** website at
http://evolve.elsevier.com/Varcarolis
for the other Nursing Care Plan diagnoses and for
more Nursing Care Plans.

NURSING CARE PLAN 20–1   A *Person With Paranoia:* Tom

NURSING DIAGNOSIS

Disturbed thought processes: related to alteration in biochemical compounds, as evidenced by persecutory hallucinations and intense suspiciousness.

Supporting Data

■ Voices have told him to "jump off rooftops" and "in front of trains."
■ "Someone is trying to kill me, I think."
■ Abuses cocaine and marijuana although paranoia increases: "It makes me feel good."

Outcome Criteria: Tom will state that he is able to function without interference from his "voices" by discharge.

SHORT-TERM GOAL	INTERVENTION	RATIONALE	EVALUATION
By (date), Tom will state that he feels comfortable with the nurse.	1a. Meet with Tom each day for 30 minutes. 1b. Use clear, unambiguous statements. 1c. Provide activities that need concentration and are noncompetitive.	1a. Short, consistent meetings help establish contact and decrease anxiety 1b. Minimizes potential for misconstruing of messages. 1c. Increases time spent in reality-based activities and decreases preoccupation with delusional and hallucinatory experiences.	*GOAL MET* By the end of the first week, Tom says he looks forward to meeting with "my nurse."
By (date), Tom will name two actions that precipitate voices and paranoia.	2a. Investigate content of hallucinations with Tom. 2b. Explore those times that voices are the most threatening and disturbing.	2a. Identifies suicidal or aggressive themes. 2b. Identifies events that increase anxiety.	*GOAL MET* Tom is able to identify that the voices are worse at nighttime. He also states that after smoking marijuana and taking cocaine, he always thought people were trying to kill him.
Tom will name two actions that he can take if the voices start to upset him by (date).	3. Explore with Tim possible actions that can minimize anxiety.	3. Offers alternatives while anxiety level is relatively low.	*GOAL MET* Tom has the telephone number of a physician he can call when hallucinations start to escalate.

Nursing Care Plan continued on following page

NURSING CARE PLAN 20–1 **A *Person* With *Paranoia*: Tom** *(Continued)*

NURSING DIAGNOSIS

Noncompliance: related to side effects of therapy, as evidenced by verbalization of noncompliance and persistence of symptoms.

Supporting Data

■ Does not take prescribed medication: "It makes me tired and I can't have sex."
■ Chronic history of relapse symptoms when out of the hospital.

Outcome Criteria: Tom will adhere to medication regimen.

SHORT-TERM GOAL	INTERVENTION	RATIONALE	EVALUATION
By (date), Tom will name actions he can take to offset the side effects of medication.	1a. Evaluate medication response with physician in the hospital. 1b. Medication changed to olanzapine (Zyprexa) 1c. Educate Tom regarding side effects—how long they last and what actions can be taken.	1a. Identifies drugs and dosages that have increased therapeutic value and decreased side effects. 1b. Olanzapine (Zyprexa) causes no known sexual difficulties. 1c. Can give increased sense of control over symptoms.	*GOAL MET* Physician readjusts dose, with the large dose at bedtime to increase sleep and a small dose during the day to decrease fatigue. Tom states that he sleeps better at night but is still tired during the day.
Tom will attend weekly support group for people with schizophrenia by (date).	2. Encourage Tom to join support group for people with schizophrenia.	2. Mutual concerns and problems are discussed in an atmosphere of acceptance—concerns such as housing expenses, loneliness, and jobs. Group also provides peer support for drug therapy maintenance.	*GOAL MET* Week 1: Tom attends meeting. Week 2: Tom states that he has made a friend. He speaks in the group about "not feeling good" at times. Week 3: Tom says that he might go to group therapy after discharge from the hospital.

SUMMARY

Schizophrenia is a biologically based disease of the brain. Psychotic symptoms in schizophrenia are more pronounced and disruptive than are symptoms found in other disorders. The basic differences are in degree of severity, withdrawal, alteration in affect, impairment of intellect, and regression.

Neurochemical (catecholamines and serotonin), genetic, and neuroanatomic findings help explain the symptoms of schizophrenia. However, no one theory at present can account for all phenomena found in schizophrenic disorders.

During the nurse's work with schizophrenic clients, specific symptoms are evident. No one symptom is found in all cases. The positive and negative symptoms of schizophrenia are two of the major categories of symptoms. The **positive** symptoms are more florid (hallucinations, delusions, looseness of associations) and respond better to antipsychotic drug therapy. The **negative** symptoms of schizophrenia (poor social adjustment, lack of motivation, withdrawal) can be more debilitating and do not respond to antipsychotic therapy.

Some nursing diagnoses discussed include **Sensory-perceptual alterations, Altered thought process, Impaired verbal communications, Ineffective individual coping, Risk for violence directed at self or others,** and **Ineffective family coping: compromised or disabling.**

Planning outcomes involves setting short-term and long-term outcomes. An awareness of personal feelings and reactions to clients' feelings and behaviors is crucial.

Interventions for people with schizophrenia include special communication and counseling techniques, self-care strategies, and milieu intervention. Also necessary is an understanding of the properties, side effects, toxic effects, and doses of the traditional, atypical, and other medications used for schizophrenia.

Basic characteristics of paranoid, catatonic (withdrawn and excited), and disorganized schizophrenic are presented in this chapter. Specific nursing interventions are outlined in case studies.

Visit the **Evolve** website at
http://evolve.elsevier.com/Varcarolis
for a post-test on the content in this chapter.

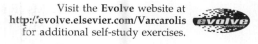

Visit the **Evolve** website at
http://evolve.elsevier.com/Varcarolis
for additional self-study exercises.

Critical Thinking and Chapter Review

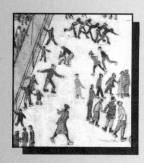

Critical Thinking

1. Using Table 20–8, teach a group (study group, co-workers) about the acute and long-term needs of people with schizophrenia. Identify the basic focus and interventions for the different phases.

2. Jamie, a 29-year-old woman, is being discharged in 2 days from the hospital after her first psychotic break (paranoid schizophrenia). Jamie is recently divorced and has been working as a legal secretary, although her work had become erratic, and her suspicious behavior was calling attention to herself at work. Jamie will be discharged in her mother's care until she is able to resume working. Jamie's mother is overwhelmed and asks the nurse how she is going to cope. "Jamie has become so distant, and she always takes things

the wrong way. I can hardly say anything to her without her misconstruing everything. She is very mad at me because I called 911 and had her admitted after she told me she was going to get justice back in the world by blowing up evil forces that have been haunting her life, and then proceeded to try to run over her ex-husband, thinking he was the devil. She told me there is nothing wrong with her and I am concerned she won't take her medications once she is discharged. What am I to do?"

Answer the following questions relating to the above case study. It is best if you can discuss and analyze responses to these situations with your classmates/instructor.

A. What are some of the priority concerns that the nurse could address in the hospital setting before Jamie's discharge?
B. How would you explain to Jamie's mother some of the symptoms that Jamie is experiencing? What suggestions could you give her to handle some of her immediate concerns?
C. What issues could you bring up to the staff about Jamie's medical compliance? What would be some ways to deal with this issue?
D. What are some of the community resources that the case manager could contact to help support this family and increase the chances of continuity of care? Identify some useful community referrals that would be supportive for Jamie and her mother. Name at least three and describe how they could be supportive to this family.
E. What do you think of Jamie's prognosis? Support your hypothesis with data on influences on the course of schizophrenia.

Chapter Review

Choose the most appropriate answer.

1. In which of the following situations can the nurse make the assessment that the client is experiencing auditory hallucinations?

   1. Mrs. D tells the nurse, "There are worms crawling on my arms and legs."
   2. Ms. E states, "I have seen the vorels who are planning to abduct me."
   3. Miss F mentions, "The food on my plate is poisoned. Take it away immediately."
   4. Mr. G who is seated by himself pleads, "I am a good person. Stop shouting those bad things about me."

2. To plan appropriate interventions the nurse must know that depersonalization and derealization are examples of

   1. delusions
   2. hallucinations
   3. automatic obedience
   4. personal boundary difficulties

3. Which symptoms of schizophrenia are most amenable to treatment with both low and high potency antipsychotic medications?

   1. hallucinations, delusions
   2. ambivalence, avolition
   3. inadequate hygiene, grooming
   4. poor social functioning, withdrawal

4. A nursing strategy that usually proves helpful when caring for a person with schizophrenia is

1. asking open-ended questions
2. focusing on what is happening in the here and now
3. limiting contact to one or two short interactions daily
4. assuming knowledge of what is meant when client talks about "they"

5. A nursing diagnosis that is universally applicable to clients with schizophrenia during the prodromal and acute phases is

1. noncompliance
2. body image disturbance
3. altered thought processes
4. risk for violence: other directed

NURSE, CLIENT AND FAMILY RESOURCES

Associations

National Alliance for the Mentally Ill (NAMI)
200 North Glebe Road, Suite 1015
Arlington, VA 22203-3754
1-800-950-NAMI
http://www.nami.org

Recovery, Inc.
802 North Dearborn Street
Chicago, IL 60610
1-312-337-5661

Internet Sites (For Nurses and Families)

Doctors' Guide to the Internet
Many articles; good site for schizophrenia information
http://www.pslgroup.com/schizophr.htm

Internet Mental Health
Vast amount of information/booklets/articles and general information
http://www.mentalhealth.com

National Alliance for Research on Schizophrenia and Depression
http://www.mhsource.com/narsad.html

Schizophrenia Home Page
http://www.schizophrenia.com/

REFERENCES

Addington, J., Addington, D., and Maticka-Tyndale, E. (1991). Cognitive functioning and positive and negative symptoms in schizophrenia. *Schizophrenia Research*, 5(2):123.

American Psychiatric Association (2000). *Diagnostic and statistical manual of mental disorders* TR (4th ed Text Revised). Washington, DC: American Psychiatric Association.

American Psychiatric Association (1997). Practice guidelines for the treatment of patients with schizophrenia. *American Journal of Psychiatry* (Suppl), 154(4):1.

American Psychiatric Association (APA) (2000). *Practice guidelines for the treatment of psychiatric disorders: Compendium 2000*. Washington, DC: American Psychiatric Association.

Andersson, C., Chakos, M., Mailman, R., and Lieberman, J. (1998). Emerging roles for novel antipsychotic medication in the treatment of schizophrenia. *Psychiatric Clinics of North America*, 21 (1):151–179.

Andreasen, N. C. (1987). The diagnosis of schizophrenia. *Schizophrenia Bulletin*, 13:9–22.

Andreasen, N., and Munich, R. L. (1995). Introduction. In G. O. Goddard (Ed.), *Treatment of psychiatric disorders* (2nd ed., Vol. 1, pp. 944–946). Washington, DC: American Psychiatric Press.

Andreasen, N. C.(1999). Understanding the causes of schizophrenia (editorial). *New England Journal of Medicine*, 340:645–647.

Andreasen, N. C. (2000). Schizophrenia: The fundamental question. *Brain Research Review*, 31(2–3):106–112.

Baldessarini, R. J. (1996). First episode psychosis: Effect of duration on hospital outcome. *Current Approaches to Psychosis*, 5(11):1, 4.

Beck, A. T., and Rector, N. A. (1998). Cognitive therapy for schizophrenic patients. *The Harvard Mental Health Letter*, 15(6):4–6.

Berkow, R., et al. (Eds.) (1992). *Merck manual* (16th ed.). Rahway, NJ: Merck Research Laboratories.

Black, D. W., Yates, W. R., and Andreasen, N. C. (1988). Schizophrenia, schizophreniform disorders and delusional paranoid disorders. In R. E. Hales, S. C. Yudofsky, J. A. Talbott (Eds.), *Textbook of psychiatry*. Washington, DC: American Psychiatric Press.

Black, D. W., and Andreasen, N. C. (1999). Schizophrenia, schizophreniform disorders, and delusional (paranoid) disorders. In R. E. Hales, S. C. Yudofsky, J. A. Talbott (Eds.). *Textbook of Psychiatry*. Washington, DC: American Psychiatric Press.

Blanchard, J. J., Brown, S. A., Horton, W. P., and Sherwood, A. R. (2000). Substance use disorders in schizophrenia: review, integration, and a proposed model. *Clinical Psychological Review*, 20(2):207–234.

Brekke, J. S., DeBonis, J. A., and Graham, J. W. (1994). The latent structure analysis of the positive and negative symptoms in schizophrenia. *Comprehensive Psychiatry*, 35(4):252.

Bruch, H. (1980). *Psychotherapy in schizophrenia: Historical considerations.* New York: Plenum.

Brzustowicz, L., Hodgkinson, K., Chow, E., Honer, W., Bassett, A. (2000). Location of major susceptibility locis for familial schizophrenia on chromosome 1q21–q22. *Science* (288):678–682.

Bugle, C., Andrew, S., Heath, J. (1992). Early detection of water intoxication. *Journal of Psychosocial Nursing*, 30(11):31.

Bustillo, J., Keith, S. J., and Lauriello, J. (1999) Schizophrenia: Psychosocial treatment. In B. J. Sadock and V. A. Kaplan (Eds.). *Kaplan and Sadock's comprehensive textbook of psychiatry, 7th ed.* Philadelphia: Lippincott Williams and Wilkins.

Caroff, S. N., and Mann, S. C. (1993). Neuroleptic malignant syndrome. *Medical Clinics of North America*, 77(1):185.

Carpenter, W., and Buchanan, R. W. (1995). Schizophrenia: Introduction and overview. In H. I. Kaplan and B. J. Sadock (Eds.), *Comprehensive textbook of psychiatry* (6th ed., Vol. 1, pp. 889–902). Baltimore: Williams & Wilkins.

Dowart, R. A., and Hoover, C. W. (1994). A national study of transitional hospital services in mental health. *American Journal of Public Health*, 84(8):1229.

Duke, P. J. (1994). South Westminster schizophrenic survey: Alcohol use and its relationship to symptoms, tardive dyskinesia and illness onset. *British Journal of Psychiatry*, 164(5):630.

Fenton, W. S., and Cole, S. A. (1995). Psychosocial therapies of schizophrenia: Individual, group, and family. In G. O. Goddard (Ed.), *Treatment of psychiatric disorders* (2nd ed., Vol. 1, pp.988–1018). Washington, DC: American Psychiatric Press.

Fenton, W. S., and McGlashan, T. H. (1991). Natural history of schizophrenic subtypes: I. Longitudinal study of paranoid, hebephrenic, and undifferentiated schizophrenia. *Archives of General Psychiatry*, 48(11):969.

Fuller, M. A., Sajatovic, M. (2000). *Drug information handbook for psychiatry.* Hudson, OH: Lexi-comp, Inc.

Gabbard, G. O., and Callaway, B. W. (1995). Multiple family groups reduce schizophrenia relapse. *The Menninger Letter*, 3(10):1.

Gamble, C., and Brennan, G. (2000) Working with families and informed careers. In C. Gamble and G. Brennan (Eds.). *Working with serious mental illness: A manual for clinical practice.* London: Bailliere Tindall.

Gordon, B. J., and Milke, D. J. (1995). Clozapine and recidivism. *Psychiatric Services*, 46(10):1079.

Gorman, L. M., Sultan, D. F., and Raines, M. L. (1996). *Davis's manual of psychosocial nursing for general patient care.* Philadelphia: F. A. Davis Company.

Grebb, J. A., and Cancro, R. (1989). Schizophrenia: Clinical features. In H. I. Kaplan, and B. J. Sadock (Eds.), *Comprehensive textbook of psychiatry* (Vol. I.). Baltimore: Williams & Wilkins.

Growe, G. A., Crayton, J. W., Klass, D. B., and Strizich, E. H. (1979). Lithium in chronic schizophrenia. *American Journal of Psychiatry*, 136:454–455.

Guze, B., Richeimer, S., and Szuba, M. (1995). *The psychiatric drug handbook.* St. Louis: Mosby–Year Book.

Hales, R., Yudofsky, S. C., and Talbott, J. (1994). *Textbook of psychiatry* (2nd ed.). Washington, DC: American Psychiatric Press.

Hatfield, A. B. (1990) *Family Education in Mental Illness.* Guilford Press.

Hatfield, A. B. (1997). Families of adults with severe mental illness: New directions in research. American Journal of Orthopsychiatry, 67(2): 254–260.

Hirayasu, Y. (2000). Management of schizophrenia with comorbid conditions. *American Psychiatric Association 153rd Annual Meeting*, May 17, 2000. Chicago, IL.

Ikeji, O. C. Ohaeri, J. U., Osahon, R. O., Agidee, R. O. (1999). Naturalistic comparative study of outcome and cognitive effects of unmodified electro-convulsive therapy in schizophrenia, mania and severe depression in Nigeria. *East African Medical Journal*, 76(11):644–650.

Johns, C. A. (1996). Managing the refractory patient. *Current Approaches to Psychosis*, 5(10):6.

Jones, P., and Cannon, M. (1998) The new epidemiology of schizophrenia. *Psychiatric Clinics of North America*, 12(1): 1–25.

Jones, R. M. (1994). Negative and depressive symptoms in schizophrenia. *Acta Psychiatrica Scandinavica*, 89(2):81.

Junginger, J. (1995). Common hallucinations and predictions of dangerousness. *Psychiatric Services*, 46(9):911.

Kahn, M. E. (1984). Psychotherapy with chronic schizophrenics: Alliance, transference and countertransference. *Journal of Psychosocial Nursing*, 22(7):20.

Kane, J. M. (1995). Clinical psychopharmacology of schizophrenia. In G. O. Goddard (Ed.), *Treatment of psychiatric disorders* (2nd ed., Vol. 1, pp. 970–986). Washington, DC: American Psychiatric Press.

Kaplan, H. I., and Sadock, B. J. (1995). *Synopsis of psychiatry* (6th ed.). Baltimore: Williams & Wilkins.

Keith, S. (1999). Reviewing outcomes: Schizophrenia comparative trials. *12th Annual U.S. Psychiatric and Mental Health Congress*, Atlanta, GA, 11th–14th, 1999.

Kennedy, R. S. (2000). Novartis issues important change in Mellaril (thioridazine HCL) labeling. *Medscape News*, July 19, 2000 (http://www.medscape.com/psychiatry).

Kissling, W. (1991). *Guidelines for neuroleptic relapse prevention in schizophrenia.* Berlin: Springer-Verlag.

Klausner, M., and Brecher, M. (1995). Risperidone guidelines. *Psychiatric Services*, 46(9):950.

Kolb, L. C., and Brodie, H. K. H. (1982) *Modern clinical psychiatry* (10th ed.). Philadelphia: W. B. Saunders.

Korn, M. L., and Saito, T. (2000). Glutamatergic and GABAergic based issues in schizophrenia. *XXIInd Congress of the Collegium International Neuro-Psychopharmacologicum.* July 9–13, 2000, Brussels, Belgium.

Lamb, R. H., et al. (1986). Families of schizophrenics: A movement in jeopardy. *Hospital and Community Psychiatry*, 37(4): 353.

Lerner, Y., Mintzer, Y., Scheslatzky, M. (1988). Lithium combined with haloperidol in schizophrenia patients. *British Journal of Psychiatry*, 153:359–362.

Levinson, D. F. (1991). Pharmacologic treatment of schizophrenia. *Clinical Therapy*, 13(3):326.

Lieberman, J. A., and Mendelowitz, A. J. (2000). Antipsychotic drugs. In J. A. Lieberman and A. Tassman (Eds.). *Psychiatric drugs.* Philadelphia: W. B. Saunders Company.

Lipton, A. A., and Cancro, R. (1995). Schizophrenia: Clinical features. In H. I. Kaplan and B. J. Sadock (Eds.), *Comprehensive textbook of psychiatry* (6th ed., Vol. 1, pp. 968–986). Baltimore: Williams & Wilkins.

Littrell, K. (1996). Olanzapine: An exciting new antipsychotic. *American Psychiatric Nurses' Association*, 8(4):4.

Marangell, L. B., Yudofsky, S. C., and Sluers, J. M. (1999). Psychopharmacology and electroconvulsive therapy. In R. E. Hales, S. C. Yudofsky, J. A. Talbott (Eds.). *Textbook of Psychiatry.* Washington, DC: American Psychiatric Press.

Marder, S. R., Wirshing, W. C., and Ames, D. (1997). New antipsychotics. In D. L. Dunner and J. F. Rosenbaum (eds.). *Psychiatric Clinics of North America annual of drug therapy.* Philadelphia: W. B. Saunders.

Maxmen, J. S., and Ward, N. G. (1995). *Psychotrophic drugs: Fast facts.* (2nd ed.). New York: W. W. Norton.

McFarlane, E. R. (1995). Families in the treatment of psychotic disorders. *The Harvard Mental Health Letter*, 12(4):4.

McGlashan, T. H., and Hoffman, R. E. (1995). Schizophrenia: Psychodynamic to neurodynamic theories. In H. I. Kaplan and B. J. Sadock (Eds.), *Comprehensive textbook of psychiatry* (6th ed., Vol. 1, pp 957–967). Baltimore: Williams & Wilkins.

Menninger, W. W. (1984). Dealing with staff reactions to perceived lack of progress by chronic mental patients. *Hospital and Community Psychiatry*, 35(8):805.

Metzler, H. Y., Rabinowitz, J., Lee, M. A., et al. (1997). Age onset and gender of schizophrenic patients in relation to neuroleptic resistance. *American Journal of Psychiatry*, (154)4:475.

Mills, J. (2000). Dealing with voices and strange thoughts. In C. Gamble and G. Brennan (Eds.). *Working with serious mental illness: A manual for clinical practice.* London: Bailliere Tindall.

Moller, M. D. (1989). *Understanding and communicating with an individual who is hallucinating* (video). Omaha, NE: NurScience.

Nehart, M. A. (1996). Neurobiology of schizophrenia. *Journal of the American Psychiatric Nurses Association*, 2(5):174.

Peralta-Martin, V., and Cuesta-Zorita, M. J. (1994). Validation of positive and negative symptom scale (PANSS) in a sample of Spanish schizophrenic patients. 22(4):171.

Preston, T., and Johnson, J. (1995). *Clinical psychopharmacology made ridiculously simple*. Miami: Med Master.

Roy, M. A., and DeVrient, X. (1994). Positive and negative symptoms in schizophrenia: A current review. *Canadian Journal of Psychiatry*, 39(7):407.

Saito, T. (2000). New strategies in the neuropathology of schizophrenia. *XXIInd Congress of the Collegium International Neuro-Psychopharmacologicum*. July 9–13, 2000, Brussels, Belgium.

Schatzberg, A. F., and Cole, J. O. (1991). *Manual of clinical psychopharmacology* (2nd ed.). Washington, DC: American Psychiatric Press.

Schiller, L., and Bennett, A. (1994). *The quiet room*. New York: Warner Books.

Schizophrenia (1999). WebMDHealth. Copyright 1999 Nidus Information Services, www.well-connected.com. Well-Connected.

Slately, A. E. (1994). *Handbook of psychiatric emergencies*. Norwalk, CT: Appleton & Lange.

Soyka, Z. (2000). Substance misuse, psychiatric disorder and violent and disturbed behavior. *British Journal of Psychiatry*, 176: 345–350.

Swonger, A., and Matejski, M. P. (1991). *Nursing pharmacology: An integrated approach to drug therapy and nursing practice* (2nd ed.). Philadelphia: J. B. Lippincott.

Taylor, D. M. and McAskill, R. (2000). Atypical antipsychotics and weight gain—A systematic review (in process Citation). *Acta Psychiatric Scandinavia*, 101(6):416–432.

Tollefson, G. (1995). *The neurobiology of schizophrenia*. U. S. Psychiatric and Mental Health Congress Conference and Exhibition, November 17, 1995.

Velligan, D. I., and Miller, A. L. (1999). Cognitive dysfunction in schizophrenia and its importance to outcome: The place of atypical antipsychotics in treatment. *Journal of Clinical Psychiatry*, 60 (23):25–8.

Vidal, G. (1982). *The second American revolution and other essays (1976–1982)*. New York: Random House.

Willick, M. S. (1993). The deficit syndrome in schizophrenia: Psychoanalytic and neurobiological perspectives. *Journal of the American Psychoanalytic Association*, 41(4):1135–1157.

Wright, P., et al. (1993). Genetics and the maternal immune response to viral infection. *American Journal of Medical Genetics*, 48(1):40.

Wuerker, A. K. (2000). The family and schizophrenia. Issues in Mental Health Nursing, 21(1):127–141.

Wyatt, R. J., Kirch, B. G., and Egan, M. F. (1995). Schizophrenia: Neurochemical, viral, and immunological studies. In H. I. Kaplan and B. J. Sadock (Eds.), *Comprehensive textbook of psychiatry* (6th ed., Vol. 1, pp. 927–941). Baltimore: Williams & Wilkins.

Yamada, S. (2000). The role of serotonin in schizophrenia. *XXIInd Congress of the Collegium International Neuro-Psychopharmacologicum*. July 9–13, 2000, Brussels, Belgium.

Yamamoto, B. K., and Meltzer, H. Y. (1995). Basic neuropharmacology of antipsychotic drugs. In G. O. Goddard (Ed.), *Treatment of psychiatric disorders* (2nd ed., Vol. 1, pp. 947–967). Washington, DC: American Psychiatric Press.

Zanriser, J. H., Courey, R. D., and Herghbarger, K. (1991). Individual psychotherapy with schizophrenic outpatients in the public mental health systems. *Hospital and Community Psychiatry*, 42(9):906.

Zerbe, K. J. (1999). *Women's mental health in primary care*. Philadelphia: W.B. Saunders Company.

Outline

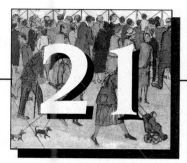

chapter

21

Cognitive Disorders

Elizabeth M. Varcarolis

Key Terms and Concepts

The key terms and concepts listed here also appear in color where they are first defined or discussed in this chapter.

agnosia

agraphia

Alzheimer's disease

amnestic disorder

aphasia

apraxia

cognitive disorder

confabulation

delirium

dementia

hallucinations

hypermetamorphosis

hyperorality

hypervigilance

illusions

perseveration

primary dementia

pseudodementia

secondary dementia

Objectives

After studying this chapter, the reader will be able to

1. Compare and contrast the clinical picture of delirium with the clinical picture of dementia.

2. Discuss three critical needs of a person with delirium and state them in terms of a nursing diagnosis.

3. Formulate three outcomes for clients with delirium.

4. Summarize the essential somatic and psychotherapeutic interventions for a client with delirium.

5. Compare and contrast the signs and symptoms occurring in the four stages of Alzheimer's disease.

6. Demonstrate an example of the following phenomena assessed during the progression of Alzheimer's disease: (a) apraxia, (b) agnosia, (c) aphasia, (d) confabulation, and (e) hyperorality.

7. Formulate at least three nursing diagnoses suitable for a client with Alzheimer's disease and formulate two goals for each.

8. Formulate a teaching plan for an Alzheimer's caregiver, including interventions for (a) communication, (b) health maintenance, and (c) safe environment.

9. Compose a list of appropriate referrals in your community for Alzheimer's persons and their families. Include telephone numbers for at least one support group, hotline, source of further information, and caregiver respite.

*T*he cognitive disorders include delirium, dementia, and amnestic disorder and other cognitive disorders. Cognitive disorders are mental disorders due to general medical conditions and substance-related disorders. See Figure 21–1 for their location on the Mental Health Continuum.

Figure 21–2 identifies the three cognitive disorders and DSM-IV-TR 2000 criteria for each. This chapter addresses the broad categories of delirium and dementia because these are by far the most common conditions that nurses encounter.

PREVALENCE

Delirium "is characterized by a disturbance of consciousness and a change in cognition such as impaired attention span and disturbances of consciousness, that develop over a short period" (DSM-IV-TR 2000, p. 135). Delirium is always secondary to another condition, such as a general medical condition or substance use (drugs of abuse, a medication or toxin exposure), or it may have multiple causes. When the cause cannot be determined, delirium is

coded as **delirium not otherwise specified** (NOS). By definition, delirium is a transient disorder, and if the underlying medical cause is corrected, complete recovery should occur (Goldberg 1998). Delirium secondary to substance abuse is discussed in Chapter 27. This chapter highlights delirium secondary to medical conditions because delirium is one of the most commonly encountered mental disorders in medical practice.

Delirium can affect up to half of all hospitalized and elderly medically ill people at some point (Goldberg 1998). Up to 60% of nursing home residents 75 years of age or older may be delirious at any one time (DSM-IV-TR 2000). Up to 80% of those with terminal illness develop delirium near death (DSM-IV-TR 2000).

Dementia usually develops more slowly and is characterized by multiple cognitive deficits that include impairment in memory. In 80% to 95% of cases, dementias are irreversible (Goldberg 1998). The 5% to 20% of dementias that have a reversible component are **secondary** to other pathological processes (e.g., neoplasms, trauma, infections, and toxic disturbances). When the secondary, or underlying, causes are treated, the dementia often improves. However, most dementias, such as dementias of the

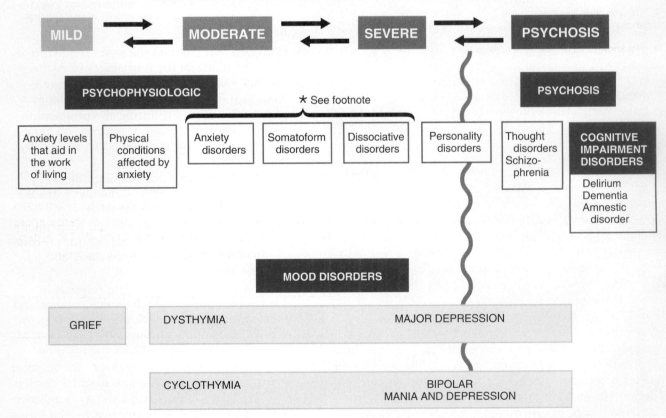

MENTAL HEALTH CONTINUUM FOR COGNITIVE DISORDER

* These disorders are currently classified by presenting clinical symptoms. Previously they were called "neurotic" disorders.

Figure 21–1 Mental health continuum for cognitive disorders.

DSM-IV-TR CRITERIA FOR COGNITIVE DISORDERS

COGNITIVE DISORDERS

DELIRIUM

A. Disturbance of consciousness (i.e., reduced clarity of awareness of the environment with reduced ability to focus, sustain, or shift attention).

B. A change in cognition (memory deficit, disorientation, language disturbance) or the development of a perceptual disturbance that is not better accounted for by a preexisting, established, or evolving dementia.

C. The disturbance develops over a short period of time (usually hours to days) and tends to fluctuate during the course of the day.

Due to:

1. A general medical condition
   or
2. Substance-induced (intoxication or withdrawal)
   or
3. Multiple etiologies (both 1 and 2 above)
   or
4. Not known (not otherwise specified)

AMNESTIC DISORDER

A. The development of memory impairment as manifested by impairment in the ability to learn new information or the ability to recall previously learned information.

B. The memory disturbance causes significant impairment in social or occupational functioning and represents a significant decline from a previous level of functioning.

C. The memory disturbance does not occur exclusively during the course of a delirium or a dementia.

DEMENTIA

A. The development of multiple cognitive deficits manifested by both:

1. **Memory impairment** (impaired ability to learn new information or to recall previously learned information).

2. One (or more) of the following cognitive disturbances:
   (a) **Aphasia** (language disturbance)
   (b) **Apraxia** (impaired ability to carry out motor activities despite intact motor function)
   (c) **Agnosia** (failure to recognize or identify objects despite intact sensory function)
   (d) Disturbance in executive functioning (i.e., planning, organizing, sequencing, abstracting)

B. The cognitive deficits in criteria A1 and A2 each cause significant impairment in social or occupational functioning and represent a significant decline from a previous level of functioning.

Figure 21–2 Diagnostic criteria for delirium, dementia, and amnestic disorder. (Adapted from American Psychiatric Association (2000). *Diagnostic and statistical manual of mental disorders,* 4th ed., Text Revision.) Washington, DC: American Psychiatric Association. Copyright 2000 American Psychiatric Association.)

Alzheimer type, involve a **primary** encephalopathy. Alzheimer's disease accounts for 60% to 80% of all dementias in the US. Vascular dementia (VaD), dementia with Lewy bodies (DLB), and frontotemporal dementia (FTD) together account for 15% to 20% of dementias, with other disorders (hydrocephalus; vitamin B_{12} deficiency) accounting for 5% (Morris 2000). The average lifetime prevalence of Alzheimer's disease is about 5% by age 65, 10% to 15% by 75, and 20% to 40% by age 85 (ADRDA 2000[7/17]). Primary dementias have no known cause or cure; thus, they are progressive and irreversible.

Amnestic disorder is characterized by loss in both short-term memory (including the inability to learn information) and long-term memory, sufficient to cause some impairment in the person's functioning (Goldberg 1998). This memory impairment exists in the absence of other significant cognitive impair-

ments. These amnestic disorders are always **secondary** to underlying causes, such as general medical condition, substance induced; persistent amnestic disorder; and amnestic disorder not otherwise specified. Figure 21–2 identifies the DSM-IV-TR criteria for delirium, dementia, and amnestic disorders.

Delirium

Nurses frequently encounter delirium on medical and surgical units in the general hospital setting. During certain phases of a hospital stay, confusion may be noted (e.g., after surgery or after the introduction of a new drug). The second or third hospital day may herald the onset of confusion for older people and difficulty adjusting to an unfamiliar environment.

Delirium occurs more frequently in elderly than in younger clients. Surgery, drugs, cerebrovascular disease, and congestive heart failure are some of the most common causes. Delirium is also commonly seen in children with fever. Delirium is a common problem in terminally ill clients and, when recognized, is easily treated and may be reversible (deStoutz et al. 1995).

Symptoms of delirium can also be mistaken for depression. A delayed or missed diagnosis can have serious prognostic implications if delirium is not diagnosed in a timely manner (Nicholas and Lindsey 1995). Table 21–1 offers some guidelines to distinguish between delirium, depression, and dementia, since they all are similar.

The essential feature of delirium is a disturbance in consciousness and is generally marked by cognitive difficulties. Thinking, memory, attention, and perception are typically disturbed. The clinical manifestations of delirium develop over a short period (hours to days) and tend to fluctuate during the course of the day.

Since delirious states fluctuate in intensity, nurses may note varying levels of consciousness and orientation during a short period. Delirium is characterized by progressive disorientation to time and place and can be classified as mild to severe. Mild delirium, which becomes more pronounced in the evening, is sometimes referred to as **sundowning.**

Because delirium increases psychological stress, supportive interventions that lower anxiety and reduce manifestations of the delirium can restore a sense of control (Foreman 1990). Clients with delirium may appear withdrawn, agitated, or psychotic. Also, underlying personality traits often become exaggerated; for example, a client may become more paranoid (Goldberg 1998), or a client may become disinhibited.

TABLE 21–1 *Comparison of Characteristics Associated with Delirium, Dementia, and Depression*

	DELIRIUM	DEMENTIA	DEPRESSION
Onset	Sudden	Insidious, relentless, or sporadic	Sudden; related to specific events
Duration	Hours to days	Persistent	Episodic or persistent
Time of day	Worse at night and when drug levels peak; sleep-wake cycle reversed	Stable or no change	Insomnia; sleeps during the day; early morning awakening
Cognitive impairment	Memory, attentiveness, consciousness, calculations	Abstract thinking, judgment, memory, thought patterns, calculations, agnosia, permanent and progressive	Complaints of memory loss, forgetfulness, and inability to concentrate
Activity	Increased or decreased; may fluctuate; may include tremors and spastic movements	Unchanged from usual behavior	Lack of motivation or lethargic; restless or agitated
Speech-language	Slurred or rapid; manic rambling; incoherent	Disordered, rambling, or incoherent; struggles to find words	Slow, sluggish speech; slow processing and response to verbal stimuli
Mood/affect	Rapid mood swings; fearful and suspicious	Depressed, apathetic, uninterested	Extreme sadness, anxiety, and irritability
Delusions/hallucinations	Visual, auditory, tactile; hallucinations and delusions	Delusions but no hallucinations	Delusions about worthlessness; paranoid ideation
Associated factors/triggers	Physical condition, drug toxicity, head injury, change in environment, sensory deficits	Chronic alcoholism, vitamin B_{12} deficiency, Huntington's chorea, vascular disease, human immunodeficiency virus (HIV) infection, Alzheimer's disease	
Reversibility	Potential	No; progressive	Potential

From Seidel, H. M., et al. (1998). *Mosby's guide to physical examination,* 4th ed. St. Louis: C. V. Mosby.

Delirium is always secondary to some physical disorder or drug toxicity. The priorities in medical care are to identify the cause and to make an appropriate medical or surgical intervention. If the underlying disorder is corrected and reversed, complete recovery is possible. If, however, the underlying disorder is not corrected and persists, sustained neuronal damage can lead to irreversible changes, such as dementia and even death.

Therefore, nursing concerns center on

■ assisting with proper health management to eradicate the underlying cause;
■ preventing physical harm due to confusion, aggression, or electrolyte and fluid imbalance; and
■ using supportive measures to relieve distress.

THEORY

Delirium can be caused by any number of pathophysiological conditions. Some of the most common causes of delirium include infections, postoperative states, metabolic abnormalities, hypoxic conditions, drug withdrawal states, and drug intoxications. Multiple drug use, or polypharmacy, is frequently implicated in delirium. Some drugs commonly responsible for delirium states are digitalis preparations and antihistamines, as well as medications used for treatment of hypertension, depression, and Parkinson's disease. Other likely offenders include anticholinergics, benzodiazepines, and analgesics, which induce central nervous system depression (Andresen 1992). Box 21–1 lists common causes of delirium.

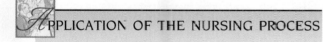

APPLICATION OF THE NURSING PROCESS

ASSESSMENT

Overall Assessment

Problems in accurate assessment of delirium often arise. First, the degree of reversibility can be determined only retrospectively. Second, the relative acuity of the onset depends on how noxious the stimuli are. Third, delirium can occur simultaneously with, or be superimposed on, an irreversible mental syndrome (dementia), thereby further complicating accurate identification.

Generally, the nurse suspects the presence of delirium when a client abruptly develops a disturbance in consciousness that is manifested in reduced clarity of awareness of the environment. The person

may have difficulty with orientation first to time, then to place, and last to person. For example, a man with delirium may think that the year is 1972 instead of the correct year, that the hospital is home, and that the nurse is his wife. Orientation to person is usually intact to the extent that the person is aware of the self's identity. The ability to focus, sus-

BOX 21–1 *Common Causes of Delirium*

POSTOPERATIVE STATES
DRUG INTOXICATIONS AND WITHDRAWALS

■ Alcohol, anxiolytics, opioids, and central nervous system stimulants (e.g., cocaine and crack cocaine)

INFECTIONS

■ Systemic: pneumonia, typhoid fever, malaria, urinary tract infection, and septicemia
■ Intracranial: meningitis and encephalitis

METABOLIC DISORDERS

■ Hypoxia (pulmonary disease, heart disease, and anemia)
■ Hypoglycemia
■ Sodium potassium, calcium, magnesium, and acid-base imbalances
■ Hepatic encephalopathy or uremic encephalopathy
■ Thiamine (vitamin B_1) deficiency (Wernicke's encephalopathy)
■ Endocrine disorders (e.g., thyroidism or parathyroidism)
■ Hypothermia or hyperthermia
■ Diabetic acidosis

DRUGS

■ Digitalis, steroids, lithium, levodopa, anticholinergics, benzodiazepines, central nervous system depressants or tricyclic antidepressants
■ Central anticholinergic syndrome due to use of multiple drugs with anticholinergic side effects

NEUROLOGICAL DISEASES

■ Seizures
■ Head trauma
■ Hypertensive encephalopathy

TUMOR

■ Primary cerebral

PSYCHOSOCIAL STRESSORS

■ Relocation or other sudden changes
■ Sensory deprivation or overload
■ Sleep deprivation
■ Immobilization

tain, or shift attention is impaired. Questions need to be repeated because the individual's attention wanders, or the person might easily get off track and need to be refocused. Conversation is made more difficult because the person may be easily distracted by irrelevant stimuli (APA 1994).

Fluctuating levels of consciousness tend to be unpredictable. Disorientation and confusion are usually markedly worse at night and during the early morning. In fact, some clients may be confused or delirious only at night and may remain lucid during the day. Some clinicians use standardized mental status examinations to screen or follow the progress of an individual with delirium or dementia. A commonly used test that is a quick way to evaluate cognitive function is shown in (Box 21–2).

Nursing assessment should include assessment of

(1) cognitive and perceptual disturbances, (2) physical needs, and (3) mood and behavior.

COGNITIVE AND PERCEPTUAL DISTURBANCES

It may be difficult to engage delirious persons in conversation because they are easily distracted and display marked attention deficits. Memory is often impaired. In mild delirium, memory deficits are noted on careful questioning. In more severe delirium, memory difficulties usually take the form of obvious difficulty in processing and remembering recent events. For example, the person might ask when a son is coming to visit, even though the son has left only an hour before.

Perceptual disturbances are also common. Perception is the processing of information about one's internal and external environment. Various misinter-

---

Box 21–2 *Folstein Mini Mental State Examination*

THE ANNOTATED MINI MENTAL STATE EXAMINATION (AMMSE)

MiniMental LLC

NAME OF SUBJECT _____ Age _____

NAME OF EXAMINER _____ Years of School Completed _____

Approach the patient with respect and encouragement.
Ask: Do you have any trouble with your memory? ☐ Yes ☐ No
May I ask you some questions about your memory? ☐ Yes ☐ No

Date of Examination _____

SCORE   ITEM

5 ( )   **TIME ORIENTATION**
Ask:
What is the year_____(1), season_____(1),
month of the year_____(1), date_____(1),
day of the week_____(1)?

5 ( )   **PLACE ORIENTATION**
Ask:
Where are we now? What is the state_____(1), city_____(1),
part of the city_____(1), building_____(1),
floor of the building_____(1)?

3 ( )   **REGISTRATION OF THREE WORDS**
Say: Listen carefully. I am going to say three words. You say them back after I stop.
Ready? Here they are... PONY (wait 1 second), QUARTER (wait 1 second), ORANGE (wait one second). What were those words?
_____(1)
_____(1)
_____(1)
Give 1 point for each correct answer, then repeat them until the patient learns all three.

5 ( )   **SERIAL 7s AS A TEST OF ATTENTION AND CALCULATION**
Ask: Subtract 7 from 100 and continue to subtract 7 from each subsequent remainder until I tell you to stop. What is 100 take away 7?_____(1)
Say:
Keep Going_____(1)_____(1),
_____(1)_____(1),

3 ( )   **RECALL OF THREE WORDS**
Ask:
What were those three words I asked you to remember?
Give one point for each correct answer_____(1),
_____(1),

2 ( )   **NAMING**
Ask:
What is this? (show pencil)_____(1). What is this? (show watch)_____(1).

For more information or additional copies of this exam, call (617)587-4215
© 1975, 1998 MiniMental LLC

MiniMental LLC

1 ( )   **REPETITION**
Say:
Now I am going to ask you to repeat what I say. Ready? No ifs, ands, or buts.
Now you say that. _____ (1)

3 ( )   **COMPREHENSION**
Say:
Listen carefully because I am going to ask you to do something:
Take this paper in your left hand (1), fold it in half (1), and put it on the floor. (1)

1 ( )   **READING**
Say:
Please read the following and do what it says, but do not say it aloud. (1)

Close your eyes

1 ( )   **WRITING**
Say:
Please write a sentence. If patient does not respond, say: Write about the weather. (1)

_____

_____

1 ( )   **DRAWING**
Say: Please copy this design.

TOTAL SCORE _____   Assess level of consciousness along a continuum

Alert   Drowsy   Stupor   Coma

	YES	NO
Cooperative:	☐	☐
Depressed:	☐	☐
Anxious:	☐	☐
Poor Vision:	☐	☐
Poor Hearing:	☐	☐
Native Language:		

	YES	NO
Deterioration from previous level of functioning:	☐	☐
Family History of Dementia:	☐	☐
Head Trauma:	☐	☐
Stroke:	☐	☐
Alcohol Abuse:	☐	☐
Thyroid Disease:	☐	☐

FUNCTION BY PROXY
Please record date when patient was last able to perform the following tasks.
Ask caregiver if patient independently handles:

	YES	NO	DATE
Money/Bills:	☐	☐	____
Medication:	☐	☐	____
Transportation:	☐	☐	____
Telephone:	☐	☐	____

From "Mini-Mental State." A Practical Method for Grading the Cognitive State of Patients for the Clinician. *Journal of Psychiatric Research* 12(3):189–198, 1975. © 1975, 1988 MiniMental LLC. (For information about how to obtain permission to use or reproduce the MiniMental State Examination, please contact John Gonsalver, Jr., Administrator of the MiniMental LLC, at 31 St James Avenue, Suite 1, Boston, Massachusetts 02116.)

pretations of reality may take the form of illusions or hallucinations.

Illusions are errors in perception of sensory stimuli. For example, a person may mistake folds in the bedclothes for white rats, or the cord of a window blind for a snake. The stimulus is a real object in the environment; however, it is misinterpreted and often becomes the object of the client's projected fear. Illusions, unlike delusions or hallucinations, can be explained and clarified for the individual.

Hallucinations are false sensory stimuli (see Chapter 20). Visual hallucinations are diagnostic of a more cognitive disorder. Tactile hallucinations may also be present. For example, delirious individuals may become terrified when they "see" giant spiders crawling over the bedclothes or "feel" bugs crawling on or under their bodies. Auditory hallucinations occur more often in other psychiatric disorders, such as schizophrenia and depression.

The delirious individual generally possesses an awareness that something is very wrong. For example, the delirious person may state "My thoughts are all jumbled." When perceptual disturbances are present, the emotional response is one of fear and anxiety. Verbal and psychomotor signs of agitation should be noted.

PHYSICAL NEEDS

PHYSICAL SAFETY. A person with delirium becomes disoriented and may try to "go home." Alternatively, a person may think that he or she *is* home and may jump out of a window trying to get away from "invaders." Wandering, pulling out intravenous lines and Foley catheters, and falling out of bed are common dangers that require nursing intervention.

An individual experiencing delirium has difficulty processing stimuli in the environment. Confusion magnifies the inability to recognize reality. The physical environment should be made as simple and as clear as possible. Elevating the head of the bed slightly can maximize orientation to place. Objects such as clocks and calendars can maximize orientation to time. Eyeglasses, hearing aids, and adequate lighting without glare can maximize the person's ability to interpret more accurately what is going on in the environment. Nagley (1986) recommended nurse-client interaction for periods of at least 5 to 10 minutes, when no other nursing actions are being carried out, to help decrease anxiety and increase awareness of reality.

BACTERIOLOGICAL SAFETY. Self-care deficits, injury, or hyperactivity or hypoactivity may lead to skin breakdown and may leave a person prone to infection. Often, this condition is compounded by poor nutrition, forced bed rest, and possible incontinence. These areas require nursing assessment and intervention.

BIOPHYSICAL SAFETY. Autonomic signs, such as tachycardia, sweating, flushed face, dilated pupils, and elevated blood pressure, are often present. These changes must be monitored and documented carefully and may require immediate medical attention.

Changes in the sleep-wake cycle usually occur, and in some cases, a complete reversal of the night-day sleep-wake cycle can occur, as in the sundowner syndrome previously mentioned. The level of consciousness may range from lethargy to stupor or from semicoma to hypervigilance. With hypervigilance clients are extraordinarily alert and their eyes constantly scan the room, they may have difficulty getting to sleep, or may be actively disoriented and agitated throughout the night.

It is also important that the nurse assess all medications because the nurse is in a position to recognize drug reactions or potential interactions before delirium actually occurs.

MOODS AND PHYSICAL BEHAVIORS

The delirious individual's behavior and mood may change dramatically within a short period. Moods may swing back and forth from fear, anger, and anxiety to euphoria, depression, and apathy. These labile moods are often accompanied by physical behaviors associated with feeling states. A person may strike out from fear or anger or may cry, call for help, curse, moan, and tear off clothing one minute and become apathetic or laugh uncontrollably the next. In short, behavior and emotions are erratic and fluctuating. Lack of concentration and disorientation complicate interventions. The following vignette illustrates the fear and confusion a client may experience when admitted to an intensive care unit (ICU).

Vignette

■ A 55-year-old married man, Mr. Arnold, is admitted to the ICU after having a three-vessel coronary artery bypass. Mr. Arnold's surgery has taken longer than usual and has necessitated his remaining on a cardiac pump for 3 hours. He arrives in the ICU without further complications. On awakening from the anesthesia, he hears the nurse exclaim "I need to get a gas." Another nurse answers in a loud voice "Can you take a large needle for the injection?" During this period, Mr. Arnold experiences the need to urinate and asks the nurse very calmly if he can go to the bathroom. Her reply is, "You don't need to go; you have a tube in." He again complains about his discomfort and assures the nurse that if she will let him go to the bathroom, he will be fine. The nurse informs Mr. Arnold that he cannot urinate and that he has to keep the "mask" on so that she can get the "gas" and check his "blood levels." On hearing this, Mr. Arnold begins to implore more loudly and states that he sees the bathroom sign. He assures the *nurse that he will only take a minute. In reality, the sign is an exit sign.*

To prove to him that a bathroom does not exist in the ICU and that the sign does not indicate a bathroom, the nurse takes off the restraints so that his head can be raised to see the sign. He abruptly breaks away from the nurse's grasp and runs toward the entrance to the ICU. He discovers a door, which is the entrance to the nurses' lounge, barricades himself in the room, and pulls out his chest tube, Foley catheter, and intravenous lines. Needless to say, he finds the bathroom that is connected to the lounge. Ten minutes later, the nurses and security personnel break through the barricade and escort Mr. Arnold back to bed.

When he becomes fully alert and oriented a day later, Mr. Arnold tells the nurses his perception of the previous events. Initially, he had thought he had been kidnapped and was being held against his will (the restraints had been tight). When the nurse yelled out about blood gas, he had thought she was going to kill him with noxious gas through his face mask (the reason he did not want to wear the face mask). All he could think about was escaping his tormentor and executioner. In this case, the nurse had not assessed the alteration in Mr. Arnold's mental status and allowed him to get out of bed. The medical jargon and loud voices had perpetuated his confusion and distortion of reality.

What are some more useful interventions the nurse could have used?

What could the nurses have done differently? What would you have done? What initial nursing actions would you have taken in order to assess his bladder?

For example, the nurses could have told Mr. Arnold where he was and that the nursing staff were caring for him; they could have better explained the function of his Foley catheter. Furthermore, the staff could have brought in family members to help calm and orient Mr. Arnold.

Self-Assessment

In many cases, delirium is more easily associated with a medical disease. First, delirium is usually treated on a medical or surgical unit, and second, delirium usually responds to specific medical or surgical interventions, depending on the underlying cause. Frequently, this syndrome reverses within a few days or less when the underlying cause is identified and treated. Because the behaviors exhibited by the client can be directly attributed to temporary medical conditions, intense personal reactions are less likely to occur. In fact, intense conflicting emotions are less likely to occur in nurses working with a client with delirium than in nurses working with a client with dementia, which is discussed later in this chapter.

However, the nurse may find some behaviors associated with delirium especially challenging. Because delirium is predictably more severe and incapacitating during the night and early morning hours, night staff often find that a loud, frightened, agitated, and perhaps aggressive client can take up much of their time. Experienced nurses are aware that even though people with delirium may appear "out of it," they often respond to a calm and caring approach. Maximizing the person's contact with reality during the night can help reduce the anxiety and terror these clients often experience.

However, certain instances may cause staff to have strong negative feelings toward a client with delirium. Such incidents might include withdrawal. For example, nurses working with a client with alcohol withdrawal delirium might think that the client "did it to herself" or is "getting what he deserves." Often, nurses exhibit judgmental attitudes toward people experiencing withdrawal. Unfortunately, negative attitudes by staff serve only to increase the client's anxiety, intensifying feelings of terror, anger, and confusion and defensive behavior.

Assessment Guidelines

ASSESSMENT GUIDELINES: DELIRIUM

1. Assess for fluctuating levels of consciousness, which is key in delirium.
2. Interview family or other caregivers. Identify cognitive behavioral baseline.
3. Assess for past confusional states (e.g., prior dementia diagnosis).
4. Identify other disturbances in medical status (e.g., dyspnea, edema, presence of jaundice).
5. Identify any EEG, neuroimaging, or laboratory abnormalities in client's record.
6. Assess vital signs, level of consciousness, neurological signs.
7. Assess potential for injury (is the client safe from falls, wandering).
8. Assess need for comfort measures (pain, cold, positioning).
9. Are immediate medical interventions available to help prevent irreversible brain damage?
10. Remain nonjudgmental. Confer with other staff readily when questions arise.

NURSING DIAGNOSIS

Safety needs play a substantial role in nursing care. Clients often perceive the environment as distorted. Objects in the environment are often misperceived (illusions) or imagined (hallucinations), and people and objects may be misinterpreted as threatening or harmful. Clients often act on these misinterpretations. For example, if feeling threatened or thinking that common medical equipment is harmful, the client may pull off an oxygen mask, pull out an intravenous or nasogastric tube, or try to flee. In such a case, a person demonstrates a **Risk for injury** related to confusion, as evidenced by sensory deficits or perceptual deficits.

Fever and dehydration may be present; thus, fluid and electrolyte balance may need to be managed. If the underlying cause of the client's delirium results in fever, decreased skin turgor, decreased urinary output or fluid intake, and dry skin or mucous membranes, then the nursing diagnosis of **Fluid volume deficit** is appropriate. Fluid volume deficit may be related to fever, electrolyte imbalance, reduced intake, or infection.

Perceptions are disturbed during delirium. Hallucinations, distractibility, illusions, disorientation, agitation, restlessness, and misperception are often part of the clinical picture. When some of these symptoms are present, **Acute confusion** would be an appropriate nursing diagnosis.

Because disruption in the sleep-wake cycle may be present, the client may be less responsive during the day and may become disruptively wakeful during the night. At no time, either during the day or the night, does the client experience a restful sleep; instead, he or she has a fragmented and fluctuating state of consciousness (McHugh and Folstein 1987). Therefore, **Disturbed sleep pattern** related to impaired cerebral oxygenation or disruption in consciousness is a likely diagnosis.

Sustaining communication with a delirious client is difficult. **Impaired verbal communication** related to cerebral hypoxia or decreased cerebral blood flow, as evidenced by confusion or clouding of consciousness, may be diagnosed.

Other nursing concerns include **Fear, Self-care deficit, Disturbed thought processes,** and **Impaired social interaction.** Fear is one of the most common of all nursing diagnoses, and may be related to illusions, delusions, or hallucinations, as evidenced by verbal and nonverbal expressions of fearfulness.

Table 21-2 identifies nursing diagnoses for any confused client (delirium or dementia).

TABLE 21–2   *Potential Nursing Diagnoses—Confused Client*

SYMPTOMS	NURSING DIAGNOSIS
Wandering, unsteady gait, acts out fear from hallucinations or illusions, forgetting things (leaves stove on, doors open)	Risk for Injury
Awake disoriented during the night (**sundowning**), frightened at night	Disturbed Sleep Pattern Fear
	Acute Confusion
Too confused to take care of basic needs	Self-Care Deficit (specify) Ineffective Coping Functional Urinary Incontinence Imbalanced Nutrition: Less than body requirements Deficient Fluid Volume Disturbed Sensory Perception Impaired Environmental Interpretation Syndrome Disturbed Thought Processes
Sees frightening things that are not there (**hallucinations**), mistakes everyday objects for something sinister and frightening (**illusions**), may become paranoid thinking that others are doing things to confuse them (**delusions**)	
Does not recognize familiar people or places, has difficulty with short- and/or long-term memory, forgetful and confused	Impaired Memory Impaired Environmental Interpretation Syndrome Acute/Chronic Confusion
Difficulty with communication, can't find words, difficulty in recognizing objects and/or people, incoherence	Impaired Verbal Communication
Devastated over losing their place in life as they know it (during lucid moments), fearful and overwhelmed by what is happening to them	Spiritual Distress Hopelessness Situational Low Self-Esteem Grieving
Family and loved ones overburdened and overwhelmed, inability to care for client's needs	Disabled Family Coping Interrupted Family Processes Impaired Home Maintenance Caregiver Role Strain

OUTCOME CRITERIA

The overall outcome criteria is that the client will return to the pre-morbid level of functioning. The client may present various needs; however, **Risk for injury** is usually present. Appropriate outcome criteria might include the following:

■ Client will remain safe and free from injury while in the hospital.
■ During lucid periods, client will be oriented to time, place, and person with the aid of nursing interventions, such as clocks, calendars, and other orienting information.
■ Client's tubes will remain in place (e.g., intravenous, nasogastric, catheter, or oxygen) while confused, with the aid of frequent orientation by nurse, family caregivers, and medications, if necessary.
■ Client will remain free from falls and injury while confused, with the aid of nursing safety measures.
■ Client will respond to external controls if he or she becomes physically aggressive toward self, other clients, or staff.

Because of **fluctuating levels of consciousness,** client needs to be checked for orientation frequently (Johnson et al. 2000).
Client can:

■ Identify self
■ Identify significant other
■ State the current month and year
■ State where he or she is
■ State the season
■ Explain what is going on, during lucid intervals

INTERVENTION

Medical management of delirium involves treating the underlying organic causes. If the underlying cause of delirium is not treated, permanent brain damage may ensue. Judicious use of antipsychotic or antianxiety agents may also be useful in controlling agitation and psychotic symptomatology.

Nursing care involves encouraging one or two significant others to stay with the delirious client to avoid the use of physical restraints (Sullivan et al. 1991). A client in acute delirium should never be left alone. The nurse should promote adequate and accurate sensory input through the use of eyeglasses or hearing aids, if appropriate. Communication should occur face to face and should consist of simple, direct statements. Orientation may be aided by maintenance of familiar objects in the environment and by use of orienting devices, such as calendars

and clocks. Although the use of reality orientation is extremely questionable in clients with chronic confusion, it may prove helpful during lucid periods in clients with acute confusional states, such as delirium.

The nurse should allow clients to care for themselves in areas of competency and should do only what is necessary for the client, while providing continual explanations when physical care is given. Safety may be aided by the use of night lighting and soothing music and by the involvement of significant others in supervising the client. Delirious clients may also try to get out of bed and suffer physical injury due to falls. Confused clients often try to remove necessary treatment equipment (e.g., intravenous lines, oxygen cannulas, drainage tubes) which can result in harm to the client. Whenever possible, it is helpful to have a one-to-one caregiver present when the client is restless or agitated. The client should be orientated in a calm, caring manner using simple, brief statements at periodic intervals. As with any client exhibiting psychotic symptoms, a tolerant, calm, matter-of-fact approach by the nurse has proved to be the most helpful.

The client's environment needs to be as quiet as possible. Placing a "Quiet" sign on the client's door and locating the client's room in the least noisy part of the unit can help prevent startling and confusion for the client. Table 21–3 presents nursing guidelines for caring for a delirious client.

EVALUATION

Long-term outcome criteria for a delirious person include the following:

■ The client will remain safe.
■ The client will be oriented to time, place, and person by discharge.
■ The underlying cause will be treated and ameliorated.

However, the short-term outcomes or goals need constant assessment. For example, are the client's vital signs within normal limits? Are all intravenous and nasogastric tubes, Foley catheters, and hyperalimentation lines intact? Are the client's skin turgor and urine specific gravity within normal limits? Is the client oriented to time and place? Has the client's anxiety level decreased from panic levels to severe or moderate levels? Frequent checking of the parameters of the short-term goals helps monitor successful treatment of the client's underlying medical condition, as well as the client's responses to nursing interventions, and helps prevent possible progression to more profound levels of illness or to irreversible neuronal changes.

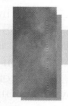

TABLE 21–3 *Guidelines for Caring for a Delirious Client*

INTERVENTION	RATIONALE
Acute Confusion	
1. Work with treatment team to reduce or eliminate factors causing delirium.	1. Underlying factors can lead to dementia if not reversed.
2. Monitor neurological signs on an ongoing basis.	2. Track progression or reversal of neurological disequilibrium.
3. Introduce self and call client by name at the beginning of each contact.	3. With short-term memory impairment, person is often confused and needs frequent orienting to time, place, and person.
4. Maintain face-to-face contact.	4. If client is easily distracted, he or she needs help to focus on one stimulus at a time.
5. Use short, simple, concrete phrases.	5. Client may not be able to process complex information.
6. Briefly explain everything you are going to do before doing it.	6. Explanation prevents misinterpretation of action.
7. Encourage family and friends (one at a time) to take a quiet, supportive role.	7. Familiar presence lowers anxiety and increases orientation.
8. Keep room well lit.	8. Lighting provides accurate environmental stimuli to maintain and increase orientation.
9. Keep head of bed elevated.	9. Helps provide important environmental cues.
10. Provide clocks and calendars.	10. These cues help orient client to time.
11. Encourage family members to bring in meaningful articles from home (e.g., picture or figurines).	11. Familiar objects provide comfort and support and can aid orientation.
12. Encourage client to wear prescribed eyeglasses or hearing aid.	12. Helps increase accurate perceptions of visual auditory stimuli.
13. Make an effort to assign the same personnel on each shift to care for client.	13. Familiar faces minimize confusion and enhance nurse-client relationships.
14. When hallucinations are present, clarify reality, e.g., "I know you are frightened; I do not see spiders on your sheets. I'll sit with you a while."	14. Person feels understood and reassured while reality is validated.
15. When illusions are present, clarify reality, e.g., "This is a coat rack, not a man with a knife. . . . see? you seem frightened. I'll stay with you for a while."	15. Misinterpreted objects or sounds can be clarified, once pointed out.
16. Inform client of progress during lucid intervals.	16. Consciousness fluctuates: client feels less anxious knowing where he or she is and who you are during lucid periods.
17. Ignore consults and name calling, and acknowledge how upset the person may be feeling. For example: **Client:** You incompetent jerk, get me a real nurse, someone who knows what they are doing. **Nurse:** You are very upset. What you are going through is very difficult. I'll stay with you.	17. Terror and fear are often projected onto environment. Arguing or becoming defensive only increases client's aggressive behaviors and defenses.
18. If client behavior becomes physically abusive, first, set limits on behavior, e.g., "Mr. Jones, you are not to hit me or anyone else. Tell me how you feel." or "Mr. Jones, if you have difficulty controlling your actions, we will help you gain control." Second, check orders for use of chemical or physical restraints (e.g., Posey belt).	18. Clear limits need to be set to protect client, staff, and others. Often, client can respond to verbal commands. Chemical and physical restraints are used as a last resort, if at all.

Dementia: Alzheimer's Disease

Severe memory loss is *not* a normal part of growing older. Slight forgetfulness is a common phenomenon of the aging process (age-associated memory loss), but not to the extent that it interferes with one's activities of daily living. Most people who live to a very old age never experience a significant memory loss or any other symptoms of dementia. Most of us know of people in their eighties and nineties who lead active lives, with their intellect intact. Margaret Mead, Pablo Picasso, Duke Ellington, Count Basie,

Ansel Adams, Sonny Coles, and George Burns are all examples of people who were still active in their careers when they died; all were older than 75 years of age (Picasso was 91; George Burns was 100). The slow, mild cognitive changes associated with aging should not impede social or occupational functioning.

Dementia, on the other hand, is marked by progressive deterioration in intellectual functioning, memory, and ability to solve problems and learn new skills. Judgment and moral and ethical behaviors decline as personality is altered. Table 21–4 shows memory changes for normal aging and memory changes seen in dementia, which may reassure some of you.

In dementia, progressive decline in activities of everyday life, the failure of memory and intellect, and the disorganization of the personality occur. A person's declining intellect often leads to emotional changes, lack of self-care, and finally, to hallucinations and delusions (i.e., psychotic symptoms brought on by neurological changes).

A person may have progressive dementia from various causes; dementia of the Alzheimer type (DAT), Pick's disease, Huntington's chorea, multi-infarct dementias, advanced alcoholism (such as in Korsakoff's syndrome), Lewy body dementia, and Creutzfeldt-Jakob disease are a few examples.

Dementias can be classified as primary or secondary. Primary dementia is not reversible, is progressive, and is not secondary to any other disorder. As mentioned, Alzheimer's disease accounts for about 70% of all dementias, and multi-infarct dementia accounts for about 20% of all dementias (Goldberg 1998). Both Alzheimer's and multi-infarct dementias are primary, progressive, and irreversible.

Secondary dementia occurs as a result of some other pathological process (e.g., metabolic, nutritional, or neurological). Acquired immunodeficiency syndrome (AIDS)-related dementia is an example of a secondary dementia that is increasingly seen in health care settings. The exact prevalence of AIDS-related dementia is not known, but it occurs in 20% to 40% of individuals with human immunodeficiency virus (HIV) infection and in up to 90% of clients dying of AIDS (Buzan and Dubovsky 1995). This phenomenon is now commonly referred to as HIV encephalopathy. Other secondary dementias can result from viral encephalitis, pernicious anemia, folic acid deficiency, and hypothyroidism.

Korsakoff's syndrome is an example of secondary dementia caused by thiamine (vitamin B_1) deficiency that may be associated with prolonged, heavy alcohol ingestion. Along with progressive mental deterioration, Korsakoff's syndrome is marked by peripheral neuropathy, cerebellar ataxia, confabulation, and myopathy (DSM-IV-TR 2000).

Some secondary dementias are treatable. In about 5% to 20% of dementia cases, the symptoms of dementia can be reversed when the underlying cause is eliminated (Goldberg 1998). Table 21–5 lists the common causes of dementia.

Alzheimer's disease attacks indiscriminately. Its victims are male and female, black and white, rich and poor, all with varying degrees of intelligence. Although the disease can strike at a younger age (early onset), most victims are 65 years of age or older (late onset). Alzheimer's is "a thief of minds, a destroyer of personalities, wrecker of family finances and filler of nursing homes" (American Association of Retired Persons 1986).

THEORY

Although the cause of Alzheimer's disease is not known, numerous hypotheses regarding its cause exist.

TABLE 21–4 *Memory Deficit: Normal Aging vs. Dementia*

PARAMETER	NORMAL AGING	DEMENTIA
Degree of change	Slowing	More severe and increasing
	Cautiousness	Variable
	Reduced ability to solve new problems	More severe and increasing
	Disengagement	Variable
	Mildly impaired memory	More severe and increasing
	Mildly impaired intelligence	More severe and increasing
Extent of damage	Difficulty in word finding, but no dysphasia, dyspraxia, agnosia	Dysphasia, dyspraxia, agnosia often found
Rate of change	Very slow change over many years	More rapid through gradual changes

TABLE 21–5 *Some Causes of Dementia*

ILLNESS	TYPE OF DAMAGE	TREATMENT AVAILABLE	POTENTIAL TREATMENT
Dementia of Alzheimer type (DAT)	Plaques, tangles, transmitter defects, abnormal amyloid deposition	+ (?)	Anticholinesterases, nerve growth factor
Vascular dementia	Multiple infarcts, stroke, small vessel disease	+ (?)	Aspirin, lower blood pressure, lower cholesterol
Lewy body dementia	Lewy bodies, transmitter defects	+ (?)	Anticholinesterases
Parkinson's disease	Lewy bodies especially in basal ganglia	—	Antiparkinsonian drugs do not help dementia
Frontal lobe dementia	Various, including Pick's	—	
Normal pressure hydrocephalus	Obstructed cerebrospinal fluid flow due to previous damage, e.g., subarachnoid hemorrhage, meningitis	—	Surgery (shunt)
Punch-drunk syndrome	Repeated head injury	+ (?)	Stop the damage
Slow-growing brain tumor	Pressure causes destruction of brain	+	Surgery
Aluminum and other metals	Direct toxic effect	+	Remove the poison
Wilson's disease	Toxicity of copper	+	Penicillamine
Alcohol abuse	Toxic effect and thiamine deficiency	+	Abstinence, thiamine treatment
Huntington's chorea	Genetic abnormality	—	Screening available
Syphilis (GPI)	Infective	+	Antibiotics
AIDS	Infective, secondary infection	+	Anti-AIDS drugs
CJD	Infective (?)	—	
Vitamin (e.g., B_{12}) deficiencies	Toxic (?)	+	Replacement
Hypothyroidism	Toxic (?)	+	Replacement
Parathyroid disorders	Calcium metabolism	+	Medical or surgical

Data from Jacques and Jackson (2000).

Pathological Findings

Alzheimer's Tangles

Alzheimer's disease results in cerebral atrophy and in neuritic plaques and neurofibrillary tangles that are microscopic abnormalities in brain tissue. Beta-amyloid protein is the main component of neuritic plaques, one of the abnormal structures found in the brain of Alzheimer's clients. Beta-amyloid protein continues to be the subject of intense interest in Alzheimer's research. A more detailed description follows:

1. **Neurofibrillary tangles** form mostly in the hippocampus, the part of the brain responsible for recent (short-term) memory as well as emotions. Therefore, memory and emotions are negatively affected.
2. **Senile plaques** are cores of degenerated neuron material that lie free of the cell bodies on the ground substances of the brain. The quantity of

plaques has been correlated with the degree of mental deterioration.
3. **Granulovascular degeneration** is the filling of brain cells with fluid and granular material. Increased degeneration accounts for increased loss of mental function.

Brain atrophy is observable with wider cortical sulci and enlarged cerebral ventricles, as demonstrated by computed tomography and magnetic resonance imaging (APA 2000).

Genetic Findings

Family members of people with DAT have a risk of acquiring the disease that is higher than that of the general population. Numerous twin studies have shown that, on average, a 40% concordance rate exists in monozygotic twins (Masterman et al. 1995).

Recent developments have helped in the understanding of Alzheimer's disease. There are thought to be at least four genes involved with the transmission of Alzheimer's disease (Korn 2000):

■ The amyloid-beta precursor gene (APP)
■ The apolipoprotein (APO) E gene (E-4)
■ The presenility 1 and 2 genes.

A study of sibling pairs (N = 292) who showed evidence of late-onset Alzheimer's disease were studied. Chromosomes which seemed to have the highest hereditary link were on chromosomes 1, 9, 10, and 19 (Korn 2000).

Nongenetic Findings

Until recently, the only risk factors that seemed to play a role in noninherited cases of Alzheimer's disease were increasing age, Down's syndrome, and most likely, head injury. Dobson and Itzhaki (1999) found that herpes simplex type 1 virus (HSV-1) is in the brain of many elderly people and discovered it as a risk factor when in the nervous system of APOE-epsilon 4 allele carriers.

Neurochemical Changes

Some studies have indicated that people with Alzheimer's dementia have drastically reduced levels of the enzyme acetyltransferase, which is needed to synthesize the neurotransmitter acetylcholine. Some theorists propose that the cognitive defects that occur in Alzheimer's disease, especially memory loss, are a direct result of the reduction in acetylcholine available to the brain.

Diagnostic Tests for Dementia

A wide range of problems may masquerade as dementia and may be mistaken for Alzheimer's disease. For example, depression in the elderly and delirium all have similar symptoms. It is important that nurses and other health care professionals be able to assess some of the important differences among depression, dementia, and delirium. See Table 21–1 for important differences between the three phenomena.

Other disorders that often mimic dementia include drug toxicity, metabolic disorders, infections, and nutritional deficiencies. A disorder that mimics dementia is sometimes referred to as a **pseudodementia**. That is, although the symptoms may suggest dementia, a careful examination may reveal another diagnosis altogether. Newbern (1991) emphasized the critical nature of careful evaluation of

tractable conditions and that histories of alcohol abuse and affective disorders must be considered. When a cognitive syndrome is suspected, clinical evaluation includes the following (Perry and Markowitz 1988):

1. Confirm the diagnosis
2. Search for underlying causes
3. Identify psychosocial stressors that may exacerbate related emotional and behavioral problems

The diagnosis of Alzheimer's disease includes ruling out all other pathophysiological conditions through the history and physical and laboratory tests, many of which are identified in Box 21–3.

Computed tomography, positron-emission tomography, and other developing scanning technologies possess diagnostic capabilities because they reveal brain atrophy and rule out other conditions, such as neoplasms. Mental status questionnaires, such as that in Box 21–2, and various other tests to determine mental status deterioration and brain damage are important parts of the assessment.

In addition to a complete physical and neurological examination, the importance of a complete medical history and description of recent symptoms (including questioning significant others) cannot be overestimated (Souder 1992). Gray-Vickrey (1988) recommended a psychiatric history, a dietary evaluation, and a medication evaluation.

As already mentioned, depression in the elderly is the disorder most often confused with dementia. Medical and nursing personnel should be cautioned, however, that dementia and depression or dementia

BOX 21–3 *Basic Work-Up for Dementia*

■ Chest and skull radiographic studies
■ Electroencephalography
■ Electrocardiography
■ Urinalysis
■ Sequential multiple analyzer: 12-test serum profile
■ Thyroid function tests
■ Folate levels
■ Venereal Disease Research Laboratories (VDRL), HIV tests
■ Serum creatinine assay
■ Electrolyte assessment
■ Vitamin B_{12} levels
■ Liver function tests
■ Vision and hearing evaluation
■ Neuroimaging (when diagnostic issues are not clear)

and delirium *can* coexist in the same person. In fact, studies indicate that many people diagnosed with Alzheimer's dementia also meet DSM-IV-TR criteria for a depressive disorder.

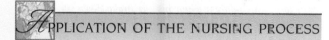

APPLICATION OF THE NURSING PROCESS

ASSESSMENT

Overall Assessment

Alzheimer's disease is commonly characterized by progressive deterioration of cognitive functioning. Initially, deterioration may be so subtle and insidious that others may not notice. In the early stages of the disease, the affected person may be able to compensate for loss of memory. Some people may have superior social graces and charm that give them the ability to hide severe deficits in memory, even from experienced health care professionals. This "hiding" is actually a form of **denial,** which is an unconscious protective defense against the terrifying reality of losing one's place in the world. Family members may also unconsciously deny that anything is wrong as a defense against the painful awareness of deterioration of a loved one. As time goes on, symptoms become more obvious, and other defensive maneuvers become evident. Confabulation (making up stories or answers to maintain self-esteem when the person does not remember) is noticed. For example, the nurse addresses a client who has remained in a hospital bed all weekend:

> **Nurse:** Good morning, Ms. Jones. How was your weekend?
> **Client:** Wonderful. I discussed politics with the President, and he took me out to dinner. *or* I spent the weekend with my daughter and her family.

Confabulation is not the same as lying. When people are lying, they are aware of making up an answer; confabulation is an **unconscious** attempt to maintain self-esteem.

Perseveration (the repetition of phrases or behavior) is eventually seen and is often intensified under stress. The avoidance of answering questions is another mechanism by which the client is able to maintain self-esteem unconsciously in the face of severe memory deficits.

Therefore, (1) denial, (2) confabulation, (3) perseveration, and (4) avoidance of questions are four defensive behaviors the nurse might notice during assessment.

Cardinal symptoms observed in Alzheimer's disease are (DSM-IV-TR 2000):

1. Aphasia (loss of language ability), which progresses with the disease. Initially, the person has difficulty finding the correct word, then is reduced to a few words, and then is finally reduced to babbling or mutism.
2. Apraxia (loss of purposeful movement in the absence of motor or sensory impairment). The person is unable to perform once-familiar and purposeful tasks. For example, in apraxia of gait, the person loses the ability to walk. In apraxia of dressing, the person is unable to put clothes on properly (may put arms in trousers or put a jacket on upside down).
3. Agnosia (loss of sensory ability to recognize objects). For example, the person may lose the ability to recognize familiar sounds (auditory agnosia), such as the ring of the telephone, a car horn, or the doorbell. Loss of this ability extends to the inability to recognize familiar objects (visual or tactile agnosia), such as a glass, magazine, pencil, or toothbrush. Eventually, people are unable to recognize loved ones or even parts of their own bodies.
4. **Memory impairment.** Initially, the person has difficulty remembering recent events. Gradually, deterioration progresses to include both recent and remote memory.
5. **Disturbances in executive functioning** (planning, organizing, abstract thinking).

The degeneration of neurons in the brain is the wasting away of working components in the brain. These cells contain memories, receive sights and sounds, and cause hormones to secrete, produce emotions, and command muscles into motion.

A person with Alzheimer's disease loses a personal history, a place in the world, and the ability to recognize the environment and, eventually, loved ones. Alzheimer's disease robs family and friends, husbands and wives, and sons and daughters of valuable human relatedness and companionship, resulting in a profound sense of grief. Alzheimer's disease robs society of productive and active participants. Because of these devastating effects, it challenges mental health professionals and social agencies, the medical and nursing professions, and researchers looking for possible solutions.

ASSESSING STAGES OF THE DISEASE

Alzheimer's disease has been classified according to the stages of the degenerative process. The number of stages ranges from three to seven, depending on the source. However, four stages, discussed subsequently, are commonly used to categorize the progressive deterioration seen in victims of Alzheimer's disease. Table 21–6 can be used as a guide to the next sections on the four stages of Alzheimer's.

STAGE 1: *MILD ALZHEIMER'S DISEASE.* The loss of intellectual ability is insidious. The person with mild Alzheimer's disease loses energy, drive, and initiative and has difficulty learning new things. Personality and social behavior remain intact, which often influences others to minimize and underestimate the loss of the individual's abilities. The individual may still continue to work, but the extent of the dementia becomes evident in a new or demanding situation. Depression may occur early in the disease but usually lessens as the disease progresses. Activities such as doing the marketing or managing finances are noticeably impaired during this phase.

Vignette

■ *Mr. Collins, 56 years of age, is a lineman for a telephone company. He feels that he is getting old. He keeps forgetting things and writes notes to himself on scraps of paper.*

One day on the job, he forgets momentarily which wires to connect and connects all the wrong ones, causing mass confusion for a few hours. At home, Mr. Collins flies off the handle when his wife suggests they invite the new neighbors for dinner. It is hard for him to admit that anything new confuses him, and he often forgets names (aphasia) and sometimes loses the thread of conversations. Once, he even forgot his address when his car broke down on the highway. He is moody and depressed and becomes indignant when his wife finds 3 months' unpaid bills stashed in his sock drawer. Mrs. Collins is bewildered, upset, and fearful that something is terribly wrong.

The rate of progression varies from person to person. Some individuals with stage 1 Alzheimer's disease decline quickly and may be dead within 3 years. Others, although their condition worsens, may still function in the community with support. And still others may remain at this level for 3 years or more. The average duration of the disease from

TABLE 21–6 *Stages of Alzheimer's Disease*

STAGE	HALLMARKS
Stage 1 (Mild) *Forgetfulness*	Losses in short-term memory; loses things, forgets. Memory aids compensate; lists, routine, organization. Aware of the problem; concerns about lost abilities. Depression common, worsens symptoms. Not diagnosable at this time.
Stage 2 (Moderate) *Confusion*	Memory loss progressive; short-term memory impaired; interferes with all abilities. Withdrawn from social activities. Declines in instrumental activities of daily living (ADLs), e.g., money management, legal affairs, transportation, cooking, housekeeping. Denial common; fear of "losing their mind." Depression increasingly common; frightened because aware of deficits. Cover-up for memory loss through confabulation. Problems intensified when stressed, fatigued, out of own environment, ill. Commonly need day care or in-home assistance.
Stage 3 (Moderate–Severe) *Ambulatory Dementia*	ADL losses (in order): willingness and ability to bathe, grooming, choosing clothing, dressing, gait and mobility, toileting, communication, reading, and writing skills. Loss of reasoning ability, safety planning, and verbal communication. Frustration common; becomes more withdrawn and self-absorbed. Depression resolves as awareness of losses diminishes. Difficult communication; increasing loss of language skills. Evidence of reduced stress threshold; institutional care usually needed.
Stage 4 (Late) *End Stage*	Family recognition disappears; does not recognize self in mirror. Nonambulatory; little purposeful activity; often mute; may scream spontaneously. Forgets how to eat, swallow, chew; commonly loses weight; emaciation common. Problems associated with immobility, e.g., pneumonia, pressure ulcers, contractures. Incontinence common; seizures may develop. Most certainly institutionalized at this point. Return of primitive (infantile) reflexes.

From Hall, G. R. (1994). Caring for people with Alzheimer's disease using the conceptual model of progressively lowered stress threshold in the clinical setting. *Nursing Clinics of North America*, 29(1):129–141.

onset of symptoms to death averages 8 to 10 years but can range from 3 to 20 years (DSM-IV-TR 2000).

STAGE 2: *MODERATE ALZHEIMER'S DISEASE.*

Deterioration becomes evident during the moderate phase. Often, the person with moderate Alzheimer's disease cannot remember his or her address or the date. There are memory gaps in the person's history that may fluctuate from one moment to the next. Hygiene suffers, and the ability to dress appropriately is markedly affected. The person may put on clothes backward, button the buttons incorrectly, or not fasten zippers (apraxia). Often, the person has to be coaxed to bathe.

Mood becomes labile, and the individual may have bursts of paranoia, anger, jealousy, and apathy. Activities such as driving become hazardous; the person may suddenly speed up or slow down for no apparent reason or may go through stop signs. Care and supervision become a full-time job for family members. Denial mercifully takes over and protects people from the realization that they are losing control, not only of their mind but also of their life. Along with denial, people begin to withdraw from activities and others, since they often feel overwhelmed and frustrated when they try to do things that once were easy. The person may also have moments of becoming tearful and sad.

Vignette

■ For a short period, Mr. Collins is transferred to a less complicated work position after his inability to function is recognized. His wife drives him to work and picks him up. Mr. Collins often forgets what he is doing and stares blankly. He accuses the supervisor of spying on him. Sometimes, he disappears at lunch and is unable to find his way back to work. The transfer lasts only a few months, and Mr. Collins is forced to take an early retirement. At home, Mr. Collins sleeps in his clothes. He loses interest in reading and watching sports on television and often breaks into angry outbursts, seemingly over nothing. Often, he becomes extremely restless and irritable and wanders around the house aimlessly.

STAGE 3: *MODERATE TO SEVERE ALZHEIMER'S DISEASE.*

At this stage, the person is often unable to identify familiar objects or people, even a spouse (severe agnosia). The person needs repeated instructions and directions for the simplest tasks (advanced apraxia): "Here is the face cloth, pick up the soap. Now, put water on the face cloth and rub the face cloth with soap. . . . " Often, the individual cannot remember where the toilet is and becomes incontinent. Total care is necessary at this point, and the burden on the family can be emotionally, financially, and physically devastating. The world be-

comes very frightening to the person with Alzheimer's disease because nothing makes sense any longer. Agitation, violence, paranoia, and delusions are commonly seen once the mechanisms of denial and withdrawal are no longer effective. Another problem that is frightening to family members and caregivers is wandering behavior. An estimated 60% of people with Alzheimer's disease may wander and are at risk for becoming lost (ADRDA 2000-B).

Institutionalization may be the most appropriate recourse at this time because the level of care is so demanding, and violent outbursts and incontinence may be crises that the family can no longer handle. Some criteria for placement in a nursing home follow:

- The person wanders.
- The person is a danger to self and others.
- The person is incontinent.
- The person's behavior affects the sleep of others.

Vignette

■ Mr. Collins is terrified. Memories come and then slip away. People come and go, but they are strangers. Someone is masquerading as his wife, and it is hard to tell what is reality and what is memory. Things never stay in the same place. Sometimes, people hide the bathroom where he cannot find it. He in turn has to hide things to keep them safe, but he forgets where he hides them. Buttons and belts are confusing, and he does not know what they are doing there, anyway. Sometimes, he tries to walk away from the terrifying feelings and the strangers. He tries to find something he has lost long ago . . . if he could only remember what it is.

STAGE 4: *LATE-STAGE ALZHEIMER'S DISEASE.*

Late in Alzheimer's disease the following symptoms may occur. Agraphia (inability to read or write), hyperorality (the need to taste, chew, and put everything in one's mouth), blunting of emotions, visual agnosia (loss of ability to recognize familiar objects), and hypermetamorphosis (touching everything in sight) are all associated with this syndrome.

At this stage, the ability to talk, and eventually the ability to walk, are lost. If death due to secondary causes (e.g., infection or choking) has not come, the end stage of Alzheimer's disease is characterized by stupor and coma.

Vignette

■ Mrs. Collins and the children keep Mr. Collins at home until his outbursts become frightening. Once, he is lost for 2 days after he somehow unlocks the front door. Mrs. Collins has her husband placed in a Veterans Administration (VA) hospital. When his wife comes to visit, Mr. Collins sometimes cries. He never talks and is always tied *into his chair when she comes to visit. The staff explain to her that although Mr. Collins can still walk, he keeps getting into other people's beds and scaring them. They explain that perhaps he wants comfort and misses human touch. They encourage her visits, even though Mr. Collins does not seem to recognize her. He does respond to music. His wife brings a radio, and when she plays the country and western music he has always loved, Mr. Collins nods and claps his hands.*

Mrs. Collins is torn between guilt and love, anger and despair. She is confused and depressed. She is going through the painful process of mourning the loss of the man she has loved and shared a life with for 34 years.

Three months after his admission to the VA hospital, and 8 years after the incident of the crossed wires at the telephone company, Mr. Collins chokes on some food, develops pneumonia, and dies.

Self-Assessment

Nurses working in any setting with cognitively impaired clients are aware of the tremendous responsibility placed on the caregivers. Severe confusion, psychotic states, and violent and aggressive behaviors can take their toll on staff and family (Burnside 1988). Taking care of clients who are unable to communicate and who have lost the ability to relate and respond to others is extremely difficult, especially for student nurses or nurses who do not understand dementia or Alzheimer's disease.

Nurses working in facilities for clients who are cognitively impaired (e.g., nursing homes and extended care facilities) need special education and skills. Education needs to include information about the process of the disease and effective interventions, as well as knowledge regarding antipsychotic drugs. Support and educational opportunities should be readily available, not just to nurses but also to nurse's aides, who are often directly responsible for administering basic care.

Burnout of staff can occur. Burnside (1988) identified three possible antidotes to burnout:

1. Revise goals so that they are realistic. Nurses sometimes set goals that are too high and unrealistic. Frustration and discouragement ensue when the goals cannot be met.
2. Refrain from being swept into a hopeless stance. Concentrate on finding satisfaction in small accomplishments (e.g., the client is comfortable, is participating in an activity, or is less delusional than previously). Indeed, for this person, such a situation may mark quite an accomplishment.
3. Research is a prime factor for eliminating staff burnout. Involving nurses in research can increase nurses' knowledge about caring for the de-

mented client and can add a feeling of purpose to a demanding job that requires great patience and maturity.

Assessment Guidelines

ASSESSMENT GUIDELINES: DEMENTIA

1. Identify the underlying cause.
2. How well is the family prepared and informed about the progress of the client's dementia (e.g., the phases and course of Alzheimer's disease, vascular dementia, AIDS-related dementia, multiple sclerosis, lupus, brain injury)?
3. What medications (herbs, complementary agents) is the client currently taking?
4. Evaluate client's current level of cognitive functioning.
5. How is the family coping with the client? What are the main issues at this time?
6. What resources are available to the family? Does the family get help from other family members, friends, and community resources? Is (are) the caregiver(s) aware of community support groups and resources?
7. Obtain the data necessary to provide appropriate safety measures for the client.
8. How safe is the client's home environment (e.g., wandering, eating inedible objects, falls, provocative behaviors toward others)?
9. For what client behaviors could the family use teaching and guidance (e.g., catastrophic reaction, lability of mood, aggressive behaviors, nocturnal delirium; increased confusion and agitation at night; sundowning)?

NURSING DIAGNOSIS

Care for a client with dementia requires a great deal of patience, creativity, and maturity. The needs of such a client can be enormous for nursing staff and for families who care for their loved ones in the home. As the disease progresses, so do the needs of the client and the demands on the caregivers, staff, and family.

One of the most important areas of concern identified by both staff and families is the client's safety. Many people with Alzheimer's disease wander and may be lost for hours or days. Wandering, along with behaviors such as rummaging, may be perceived as purposeful to the person with Alzheimer's disease. Wandering may result from changes in the physical environment, fear caused by hallucinations or delusions, or lack of exercise.

Seizures are common in the later stages of this disease. Injuries from falls and accidents can occur during any stage as confusion and disorientation progress. The potential for burns exists if the client is a smoker or is unattended at the stove. Prescription drugs can be taken incorrectly, or bottles of noxious fluids can be mistakenly ingested, resulting in a medical crisis. Therefore, **Risk for injury** is always present.

As the person's ability to recognize or name objects is decreased, **Impaired verbal communication** becomes a problem. As memory diminishes and disorientation increases **Impaired environmental interpretation syndrome, Impaired memory,** and **Confusion** occur.

During the course of the disease, people show personality changes, increased vulnerability and often inappropriate behaviors. Common behaviors include hoarding, regression, and being overly demanding. Therefore, nurses and family members often intervene in behaviors that signal **Ineffective coping.** Family caregivers may experience compromised or even disabling family coping.

Additional family issues may emerge. Perhaps some of the most crucial aspects of the client's care are support, education, and referrals for the family. The family loses an integral part of its unit. Family members lose the love, the function, the support, the companionship, and the warmth that this person had provided. **Caregiver role strain** is always present, and planning with the family and offering community support is an integral part of appropriate care. **Anticipatory grieving** is also an important phenomenon to assess for and may be an important target for intervention. Helping the family grieve can make the task ahead somewhat clearer and, at times, less painful. Refer back to Table 21–2 for potential nursing diagnoses for confused and demented clients.

OUTCOME CRITERIA

Families who have a member with dementia are faced with an exhaustive list of issues that need addressing. Table 21–7 provides a checklist which

TABLE 21–7 *Problems That May Affect Dementia Sufferers and Their Families*

PROBLEM	EXAMPLES	PROBLEM	EXAMPLES
Memory impairment	Forgets appointments, visits, etc. Forgets to change clothes, wash, go to the toilet Forgets to eat, take tablets Loses things	Repetitiveness	Questions or stories Actions
		Uncontrolled emotion	Distress Anger or aggression Demands for attention
Disorientation	Time: mixes night and day, mixes days of appointments, wears summer clothes in winter, forgets age Place: loses the way around house Person: difficulty recognizing visitors, family, spouse	Uncontrolled behavior	Restlessness day or night Vulgar table or toilet habits Undressing Sexual disinhibition Shoplifting
		Incontinence	Urine Feces Urination or defecation in the wrong place
Needs physical help	Dressing Washing, bathing Toileting Eating Housework Mobility	Emotional reactions	Depression Anxiety Frustration and anger Embarrassment and withdrawal
Risks in the home	Falls Fire from cigarettes, cooker, heating Flooding Letting strangers in Wandering out	Other reactions	Suspiciousness Hoarding and hiding
		Mistaken beliefs	Still at work Parents or spouse still alive Hallucinations
Risks outside	Competence, judgment and risks at work Driving, road sense Gets lost	Decision making	Indecisiveness Easily influenced Refuses help Makes unwise decisions
Apathy	Little conversation Lack of interest Poor self-care	Burden on family	Disruption of social life Distress, guilt, rejection Family discord
Poor communication	Dysphasia		

BOX 21–4 *Suggested Outcome Criteria for Dementia*

INJURY

■ Client will remain safe in the hospital or at home.
■ With the aid of an identification bracelet and neighborhood or hospital alert, client will be returned within 3 hours of wandering.
■ Client will remain free of danger during seizures.
■ With the aid of interventions, client will remain burn free.
■ With the aid of guidance and environmental manipulation, client will not hurt himself or herself if a fall occurs.
■ Client will ingest only correct doses of prescribed medications and appropriate food and fluids.

COMMUNICATION

■ Client will communicate needs.
■ Client will answer yes or no appropriately to questions.
■ Client will state needs in alternative modes when he or she is aphasic (e.g., will signal correct word on hearing it or will refer to picture or label).
■ Client will wear prescribed glasses or hearing aid each day.

CAREGIVER ROLE STRAIN

■ Family members will have the opportunity to express "unacceptable" feelings in a supportive environment.
■ Family members will have access to professional counseling.

■ Family members will name two organizations within their geographical area that can offer support.
■ Family members will participate in ill member's plan of care, with encouragement from staff.
■ Family members will state that they have outside help that allows family members to take personal time for themselves (1 to 7 days) each week or month.
■ Family members will have the names of three resources that can help with financial burdens and legal considerations.

IMPAIRED ENVIRONMENTAL INTERPRETATION: CHRONIC CONFUSION

■ Client will acknowledge the reality, after it is pointed out, of an object or a sound that was misinterpreted (illusion).
■ Client will state that he or she feels safe after experiencing delusions or illusions.
■ Client will remain nonaggressive when experiencing paranoid ideation.

SELF-CARE NEEDS

■ Client will participate in self-care at optimal level.
■ Client is able to follow step-by-step instructions for dressing, bathing, and grooming.
■ Client will put on own clothes appropriately, with aid of fastening tape (Velcro) and nursing supervision.
■ Client's skin will remain intact, despite incontinence or prolonged pressure.

---

*NOT an exhaustive list

---

may help the nurse and families identify areas for intervention. **Risk for injury** is almost always present. Self-care needs, impaired environmental interpretation, chronic confusion, ineffective individual coping, and caregiver role strain are just a few of the areas nurses and other health care members will need to target. See Box 21–4 for some suggestions.

PLANNING

Planning care for a client suffering from dementia is geared toward the client's immediate needs. Refer back to Table 21–7 for help in identifying areas of care needed. Box 21–5 is a Functional Dementia Scale and can be used by families to help plan strategies for immediate needs, and track progression of the dementia.

Identifying level of functioning and assessing caregiver's needs help the nurse identify appropriate community resources. Does the client or family need

■ transport services?
■ supervision and care when primary caregiver is out of the home?
■ referrals to day care centers?
■ information on support groups within the community?
■ meals on wheels?
■ information on respite and residential services
■ telephone numbers for help lines?
■ home health aides?
■ home health services?
■ referral for AA: "Home Safe Program"?
■ additional psychopharmacology for distressing or harmful behaviors?

INTERVENTION

The nurse's attitude of unconditional positive regard is the single most effective tool in caring for demented clients. It induces clients to cooperate with care, reduces catastrophic outbreaks, and increases family members' satisfaction with care.

More than 30% of individuals with dementia have a group of secondary behavioral disturbances, including depression, hallucinations and delusions, agitation, insomnia, and wandering (Corey-Bloom and Galasko 1995). Because these symptoms impair the person's ability to function, increase the need for supervision, and influence the need to institutionalize them, the control of these symptoms is a priority in managing Alzheimer's disease (Corey-Bloom and Galasko 1995). They state

The basic principle underlying all care for the cognitively impaired is to facilitate the highest level of functioning a person is capable of in all areas (e.g., self-care and social and family relationships).

Intervention with family members is critical. The effects of losing a family member to dementia—that is, watching a person who has an important role within the family unit and who is loved and is a vital part of his or her family's history deteriorate—can be devastating. The interventions discussed subsequently are useful.

Communication Guidelines

How nurses choose to communicate with these clients has a major impact on their maintenance of self-esteem and their ability to participate in care.

People with dementia often find it difficult to express themselves. They

■ Have difficulty finding the right words
■ Use familiar words repeatedly

Box 21–5 *Functional Dementia Scale*

Circle one rating for each item:
1. None or little of the time
2. Some of the time
3. Good part of the time
4. Most or all of the time

Client _____
Observer _____
Position or relation to patient _____
Facility _____
Date _____

1	2	3	4	(1)	Has difficulty in completing simple tasks on own (e.g., dressing, bathing, doing arithmetic).
1	2	3	4	(2)	Spends time either sitting or in apparently purposeless activity.
1	2	3	4	(3)	Wanders at night or needs to be restrained to prevent wandering.
1	2	3	4	(4)	Hears things that are not there.
1	2	3	4	(5)	Requires supervision or assistance in eating.
1	2	3	4	(6)	Loses things.
1	2	3	4	(7)	Appearance is disorderly if left to own devices.
1	2	3	4	(8)	Moans.
1	2	3	4	(9)	Cannot control bowel function.
1	2	3	4	(10)	Threatens to harm others.
1	2	3	4	(11)	Cannot control bladder function.
1	2	3	4	(12)	Needs to be watched so doesn't injure self (e.g., by careless smoking, leaving the stove on, falling).
1	2	3	4	(13)	Destructive of materials around him/her (e.g., breaks furniture, throws food trays, tears up magazines).
1	2	3	4	(14)	Shouts or yells.
1	2	3	4	(15)	Accuses others of doing him bodily harm or stealing his/her possessions—when you are sure the accusations are not true.
1	2	3	4	(16)	Is unaware of limitations imposed by illness.
1	2	3	4	(17)	Becomes confused and does not know where he/she is.
1	2	3	4	(18)	Has trouble remembering.
1	2	3	4	(19)	Has sudden changes of mood (e.g., gets upset, angered, or cries easily).
1	2	3	4	(20)	If left alone, wanders aimlessly during the day or needs to be restrained to prevent wandering.

Reprinted with permission from Moore, J. T., et al. (1983). A functional dementia scale. *Journal of Family Practice*, 16:498. Copyright by Appleton and Lange.

TABLE 21–8 *Communication Guidelines for Clients With Dementia*

INTERVENTION	RATIONALE
Chronic Confusion	
1. Always identify yourself and call the person by name at each meeting.	1. Client's short term memory is impaired—requires frequent orientation to time and environment.
2. Speak slowly.	2. Gives client time to process information.
3. Use short, simple words and phrases.	3. Client may not be able to understand complex statements or abstract ideas.
4. Maintain face-to-face contact.	4. Maximizes verbal and nonverbal clues.
5. Be near client when talking, one or two arm-lengths away.	5. This distance can help client focus on speaker as well as maintain personal space.
6. Focus on one piece of information at a time.	6. Attention span of client is poor and easily distracted—helps client focus. Too much data can be overwhelming and can increase anxiety.
7. Talk with client about familiar and meaningful things.	7. Allows self-expression and reinforces reality.
8. Encourage reminiscing about happy times in life.	8. Remembering accomplishments and shared joys helps distract client from deficit and gives meaning to existence.
9. When client is delusional, acknowledge client's feelings and reinforce reality. Do not argue or refute delusions.	9. Acknowledging feelings helps client feel understood. Pointing out realities may help client focus on realities. Arguing can enhance adherence to false beliefs.
10. If a client gets into an argument with another client, stop the argument and get them out of each other's way. After a short while (5 minute), explain to each client matter-of-factly why you had to intervene.	10. Prevents escalation to physical acting out. Shows respect for client's right to know. Explaining in an adult manner helps maintain self-esteem.
11. When client becomes verbally aggressive, acknowledge client's feelings and shift topic to more familiar ground, e.g., "I know this is upsetting for you, since you always cared for others. Tell me about your children."	11. Confusion and disorientation easily increase anxiety. Acknowledging feelings makes client feel more understood and less alone. Topics client has mastery in can remind him or her of areas of competent functioning and can increase self-esteem.
12. Have client wear prescription eyeglasses or hearing aid.	12. Increases environmental awareness, orientation, and comprehension, which in turn increases awareness of personal needs and the presence of others.
13. Keep client's room well lit.	13. Maximizes environmental clues.
14. Have clocks, calendars, and personal items (e.g., family pictures or Bible) in clear view of client while he or she is in bed.	14. Assists in maintaining personal identity.
15. Reinforce client's pictures, nonverbal gestures, Xs on calendars, and other methods used to anchor client in reality.	15. When aphasia starts to hinder communication, alternate methods of communication need to be instituted.

- Invent new words to describe things
- Frequently lose their train of thought
- Rely on nonverbal gestures

Burnside (1988) suggested the following guidelines for implementing interventions or teaching a severely cognitively impaired person:

1. Provide only one visual clue (object) at a time.
2. Know that the client may lack understanding of the task assigned.
3. Remember that relevant information is remembered longer than irrelevant information.
4. Break tasks into very small steps.
5. Give only one instruction at a time.
6. Report, record, and document all data.

Table 21–8 gives special guidelines for nurses and family members to use to communicate with a cognitively impaired person.

Health Teaching

Health teaching and support for families are vital components of care for individuals with dementia. Educating families who have a cognitively impaired member is one of the most important areas for nurses. Families who are caring for a member in the home need to know about strategies for communicating and for structuring self-care activities (Table 21–9).

Most important, families need to know where to get help. Help includes professional counseling and education regarding the process and the progression of the disease. Families especially need to know about, and be referred to, community-based groups that can help shoulder this tremendous burden (e.g., day care centers, senior citizen groups, organizations providing home visits and respite care, and family support groups). A list with definitions of some of the types of services available in the client's community should be provided to the family, as well as the names and telephone numbers of these services.

Scott and colleagues (1986) confirmed in their research that family support was positively associated

TABLE 21–9   Family and Health Care Guidelines for Self-Care

INTERVENTION	RATIONALE
Dressing and Bathing	
1. Always have client perform all tasks within the capacity of the client's present condition.	1. Maintains client's self-esteem and uses muscle groups; impedes staff burnout; minimizes further regression.
2. Always have client wear own clothes, even if in the hospital.	2. Helps maintain client's identity and dignity.
3. Use clothing with elastic, and substitute fastening tape (Velcro) for buttons and zippers.	3. Minimizes client's confusion and eases independence of functioning
4. Label clothing items with client's name and name of item.	4. Helps identify client if he or she wanders and gives client additional clues when aphasia or agnosia occurs.
5. Give step-by-step instructions whenever necessary, e.g., "Take this blouse . . . put in one arm . . . now the next arm . . . pull it together in the front . . . now . . . ."	5. Client can focus on small pieces of information more easily; allows client to perform at optimal level.
6. Make sure that water in faucets is not too hot.	6. Judgment is lacking in client; is unaware of many safety hazards.
7. If client is resistant to doing self-care, come back later and ask again.	7. Moods may be labile, and client may forget but often complies after short interval.
Nutrition	
1. Monitor food and fluid intake.	1. Client may have anorexia or be too confused to eat.
2. Offer finger food that client can take away from the dinner table.	2. Increases input throughout the day; client may eat only small amounts at meals.
3. Weigh client regularly (once a week).	3. Monitors fluid and nutritional status.
4. During period of hyperorality, watch that client does not eat nonfood items (e.g., ceramic fruit or food-shaped soaps).	4. Client puts everything into mouth; may be unable to differentiate inedible objects made in the shape and color of food.
Bowel and Bladder Function	
1. Begin bowel and bladder program early; start with bladder control.	1. Same time of day for bowel movements and toileting—in early morning, after meals and snacks, and before bedtime—can help prevent incontinence.
2. Evaluate use of disposable diapers.	2. Prevents embarrassment.
3. Label bathroom door as well as doors to other rooms.	3. Additional environmental clues can maximize independent toileting.
Sleep	
1. Since client may become awake, be frightened, or cry out at night, keep area well lighted.	1. Reinforces orientation, minimizes possible illusions.
2. Maintain a calm atmosphere during the day.	2. Encourages a calming night's sleep.
3. Nonbarbiturates may be ordered (e.g., chloral hydrate).	3. Barbiturates can have a paradoxical reaction, causing agitation
4. If medications are indicated, neuroleptics with sedative properties may be the most helpful (e.g., haloperidol [Haldol]).	4. Helps clear thinking and sedates.
5. Avoid the use of restraints.	5. Can cause client to become more terrified and fight against restraints until exhausted to a dangerous degree.

with the caregiver's coping effectiveness. Each stage of Alzheimer's disease involves new and different stresses, which can be diminished by professional assistance.

Milieu Therapy

According to Ninos and Makohon (1985), assisting clients to cope with their environment is the basis

TABLE 21–10 *Types of Services That Might Be Available to People With Dementia*	
TYPE OF SERVICE	**SERVICES PROVIDED**
FAMILY/CAREGIVER (Some clients may live by themselves in the community: active case management is **vital** when this is the case.)	Caregivers have a right to: ■ **Easy access to services** ■ **Respite care** ■ **Full involvement in decision making** ■ **Assessment of the needs of the carer as well as those of the sufferer** ■ **Information and referral** ■ **Case Management:** Coordinate community resources and follow-up
Community Services	■ **Adult Day Care:** Provide activities/socialization/ supervision ■ **Physician Services** ■ **Protective Services:** Prevent/eliminate/remedy effects of abuse or neglect ■ **Recreational Services** ■ **Transportation** ■ **Mental Health Services** ■ **Legal Services**
Home Care	■ **Meals on Wheels** ■ **Home Health Aid** ■ **Homemaker Services** ■ **Hospice Services** ■ **Paid Companion/Sitter** ■ **Skilled Nursing** ■ **Personal Care Services:** Assist in basic self-care activities ■ **Telephone Reassurance:** Regular telephone calls to individuals who are isolated and home-bound* ■ **Personal Emergency Response Systems:** Telephone based systems to alert others that a person who is alone is in need of emergency assistance.*

*Vital for those living alone.

for therapy, particularly nursing therapy. Thus, nurses must identify and modify, where possible, specific functional disturbances and must assist clients and families in compensating for such disturbances.

The Alzheimer's Association is a national umbrella agency that provides various forms of assistance to persons with the disease and their families. The Alzheimer's Association has launched Safe Return, the first nationwide program to help locate and return missing people with Alzheimer's disease and other memory impairments. Information regarding housekeeping, home health aides, and companions should also be available. Such outside resources can help prevent the total emotional and physical fatigue of family members. Family members can call (800) 272–3900 to locate the Alzheimer's Association nearest them. Types of resources that might be available in some communities are found in Table 21–10.

Family members need to know where and how to place the ill member when this becomes necessary. Eventually, the ill person's labile and aggressive behavior, incontinence, wandering, unsafe habits, or disruptive nocturnal activity can no longer be appropriately dealt with in the home. Families need information, support, and legal and financial guidance at this time. When the nurse is unable to provide the relevant information, proper referrals by the social worker are needed. Information regarding advance directives, durable power of attorney, guardianship, and conservatorship should be included in the communication with the family (Weiler and Buckwalter 1988). Useful guidelines for families in structuring a safe environment and planning appropriate activities are found in Table 21–11.

Psychopharmacology

COGNITIVE IMPAIRMENT

There is as yet no cure for Alzheimer's disease. There are, however three FDA-approved Alzheimer's disease drugs: tacrine (Cognex), donepezil (Aricept), and rivastigmine (Exelon). All these drugs work to increase the brain's supply of acelylcholine, a nerve communicator that is deficient in people with Alzheimer's. They have shown positive effects not only on cognition but also on behavior and ADL function.

Tacrine (THA, Cognex) was the first cholinesterase inhibitor to be approved by the US Food and Drug Administration (FDA) for the treatment of mild to moderate symptoms of Alzheimer's disease. It has been shown to improve functioning and slow the progress of the disease, particularly in the area of cognition and memory in about 20% to 50% of clients with Alzheimer's disease. Unfortunately, tac-

TABLE 21–11 *Family Guidelines for Care at Home*

INTERVENTION	RATIONALE
Safe Environment	
1. Gradually restrict use of the car.	1. As judgment becomes impaired, client may be dangerous to self and others.
2. Remove throw rugs and other objects in person's path.	2. Minimizes tripping and falling.
If client is in hospital or living with family:	
3. Minimize sensory stimulation.	3. Decreases sensory overload, which can increase anxiety and confusion.
4. If client becomes verbally upset, listen briefly, give support, then change the topic.	4. Goal is to prevent escalation of anger. When attention span is short, client can be distracted to more productive topics and activities.
5. Label all rooms and drawers. Label often-used objects (e.g., hairbrushes and toothbrushes)	5. May keep client from wandering into other client's rooms. Increases environmental clues to familiar objects.
6. Install safety bars in bathroom.	6. Prevents falls.
7. Supervise client when he or she smokes.	7. Danger of burns is always present.
8. If client has history of seizures, keep padded tongue blades at beside. Educate family and observe.	8. Seizure activity is common in advanced Alzheimer's disease
If Client Wanders:	
1. If client wanders during the night, put mattress on the floor.	1. Prevents falls when client is confused.
2. Have client wear Medic-Alert bracelet that cannot be removed (with name, address, and telephone number).	2. Client can easily be identified by police, neighbors, or hospital personnel. Provide police department with recent pictures.
3. Alert local police and neighbors about wanderer.	3. May reduce time necessary to return client to home or hospital.
4. If client is in hospital, have him or her wear brightly colored vest with name, unit, and phone number printed on back.	4. Makes client easily identifiable.
5. Put complex locks on door.	5. Reduces opportunity to wander.
6. Place locks at top of door.	6. In moderate and late DAT, ability to look up and reach upward is lost.
7. Encourage physical activity during the day.	7. Physical activity may decrease wandering at night.
8. Explore the feasibility of installing sensor devices.	8. Provides warning if client wanders.
Useful Activities	
1. Provide picture magazines and children's books when client's reading ability diminishes.	1. Allows continuation of usual activities that the client can still enjoy; provides focus.
2. Provide simple activities that allow exercise of large muscles.	2. Exercise groups, dance groups, and walking provide socialization as well as increased circulation and maintenance of muscle tone.
3. Encourage group activities that are familiar and simple to perform.	3. Such activities as group singing, dancing, reminiscing, and working with clay and paint all help to increase socialization and minimize feelings of alienation.

DAT, dementia of the Alzheimer's type.

rine is associated with a high frequency of side effects, including elevated liver transaminase levels, gastrointestinal effects, and liver toxicity. The hepatic effects, along with the inconvenience of multiple dosing requirement, have reduced the use of this drug (Keltner and associates, 2001).

Donepezil (Aricept) inhibits acetylcholine breakdown and was approved by the FDA in December 1996. It also appears to slow down deterioration in cognitive functions but without the potentially serious liver toxicity attributed to tacrine. In client studies with donepezil, some individuals with Alzheimer's disease did experience diarrhea and nausea. Both tacrine and donepezil have been shown to slow down cognitive deterioration by about 2 months.

Rivastigmine (Exelon), a brain selective acetylcholinesterase inhibitor, was approved in 2000. In clinical trials rivastigmine helped slightly more than half of the people who took it. The most common side effects are nausea, vomiting, loss of appetite, and weight loss. In most cases these side effects were temporary (ADRDA 2000-C).

Other cholinesterase inhibitors are being developed in other countries and are being studied in clinical trials.

Galantamine (Reminyl) is a reversible cholinesterase inhibitor and a fourth drug currently under FDA review. A drug that is currently available in Germany, Memantine, has shown promise in improving cognitive and daily life activities, without changing behavioral symptoms. This drug seems to be useful for people in advanced Alzheimer's disease. This drug works by affecting NMDA receptor, another chemical and structural system involved in memory (ADRDA 2000-D).

Perhaps the most exciting is the start of clinical trials of a **vaccine (AN-1792)** that is hoped will clear the brain of beta amyloid plaques. Scientists have hypothesized that these plaques, found in the brains of Alzheimer's victims, impede nerve cell function and cause nerve cell death in the brains of people with Alzheimer's disease (ADRD 2000-E; Alz Assoc. 2000).

BEHAVIORAL SYMPTOMS

Other medications are often useful in managing behavioral symptoms of individuals with dementia, but these need to be used with severe caution. A rule of thumb for elderly clients—**START LOW AND GO SLOW.** Some of the troubling behaviors experienced by Alzheimer's clients and their caregivers are (1) psychotic symptoms (hallucinations, paranoia), (2) severe mood swings (depression very common), (3) anxiety (agitation), and verbal or physical aggression (combativeness). Table 21–12 lists acceptable medications for these behavioral symptoms.

ALTERNATIVE AND COMPLEMENTARY TREATMENTS

There are a number of **herbal** or **all natural** drugs currently under investigation. However, there is not enough scientific evidence yet concerning their effectiveness or harmfulness. Keep in mind that *all natural* or *herbal* does not mean that a substance is safe. Some alternative treatments being investigated are vitamin E, *Ginkgo biloba*, huperzine A, coenzyme Q 10, and phosphatidyl serine (ADRDA 2000-F). See the SIMON/Varcarolis for Alzheimer's Association website for more on these substances (See Research Findings box).

TABLE 21–12 *Acceptable Medications to Target Specific Problems in Dementia*

SYMPTOM/BEHAVIOR	COMMENTS AND CAUTIONS
Psychotic Symptoms (Delusions and Hallucinations)	
Antipsychotics ■ Haloperidol (Haldol) ■ Olanzapine (Zyprexa) ■ Quetiapine (Seroquel) ■ Risperidone (Risperdal)	The traditional drugs can produce akathisia, with increased restlessness and agitation. Clients can become more incapacitated by the parkinsonian and anticholinergic side effects.
Affective Symptoms (Depression)	
Antidepressants ■ Bupropion (Wellbutrin) ■ Fluoxetine (Prozac) ■ Nefazodone (Serzone) ■ Paroxetine (Pavil) ■ Sertraline (Zoloft) ■ Trazodone (Desyrl)	Agents with high anticholinergic activity should be avoided. The selective serotonin reuptake inhibitors appear to be well tolerated and effective in geriatric clients.
Anxiety	
Buspirone (Buspar)	It has no serious side effects for the elderly and should be considered.
Benzodiazepines ■ Alprazolam (Xanax) ■ Diazepam (Valium) ■ Lorazepam (Ativan)	Have side effects. Produce psychomotor impairment, drowsiness, or cognitive impairment. Shorter-acting agents should be used at doses as low as possible.
Agitated/Combative Behavior	
Antipsychotics	**When the behavior is a consequence of underlying psychotic process only.**
Buspirone	Can decrease episodic agitation in dementia clients (5 mg tid).
Trazodone	Appears to decrease aggressive behavior in agitated demented clients over 3–4 weeks.
Benzodiazepines	May nonspecifically sedate agitated clients; however, oversedation impairs function and can increase cognitive ability and psychomotor impairment.

Data from Goldberg (1998); and Alzheimer's Disease and Related Disorders B Association (2000) B and C.

RESEARCH FINDINGS

The Effectiveness of Ginkgo Biloba on Cognitive Function in Clients with Alzheimer's Disease

Objective

To determine the effectiveness of treatment with ginkgo biloba extract on objective measures of cognitive function in clients with Alzheimer's disease, based on a review of the literature.

Method

The authors attempted to identify all English and non-English articles in which ginkgo biloba extract was given to people experiencing dementia or cognitive impairment. The criteria for inclusion were the following: (1) the clients were either diagnosed with Alzheimer's disease per the DSM-III-R, National Institute of Neurological Disorders and Stroke-Alzheimer's Disease and Related Disorders Association; (2) there were clearly stated study exclusion criteria, that is, those studies that did not have stated exclusions for depression, other neurologic disease, and central nervous system medications were excluded; (3) standardized ginkgo biloba extract was used; (4) the study was randomized, placebo-controlled, and double-blind; (5) at least one outcome measure was an objective assessment of cognitive function; and (6) there was enough statistical information for analysis.

Results

Of the more than 50 identified articles, the overwhelming majority did not meet inclusion criteria, primarily because of lack of clear diagnoses of dementia and Alzheimer's disease. Only four studies met all inclusion criteria. There was a total of 212 subjects in each of the placebo and ginkgo treatment groups. Overall, there was a significant effect size of 0.40 ($P < .0001$), which translated into a 3% difference in the Alzheimer's Disease Assessment Scale cognitive subtest.

Conclusion

Based on a quantitative analysis of the literature, there is a small but significant effect of 3 to 6 months of treatment with 120–240 mg of ginkgo biloba extract on objective measures of cognitive function in Alzheimer's disease. Ginkgo biloba has not had significant adverse effects in clinical trials, but there are two reports of bleeding complications. In Alzheimer's disease, there are limited and inconsistent results that prevent knowing if there are effects on noncognitive behavioral and functional measures. Also, further research will be needed to determine the best dosage and to define which ingredients in the ginkgo biloba extract are producing the demonstrated effects on people with Alzheimer's disease.

From Oken, B.S., Storzbach, D.M., and Kaye, J.A. (1998). The efficacy of ginkgo biloba on cognitive function in Alzheimer's disease. *Archives of Neurology*, 55(11):1409–1415.

EVALUATION

Outcome criteria set for clients with cognitive impairment need to be measurable, be within their capabilities, and be evaluated frequently. As the person's condition continues to deteriorate, outcomes (goals) need to be altered to reflect the person's diminished functioning. Frequent evaluation and reformulation of outcome criteria and short-term goals also help diminish staff and family frustration, as well as minimize the client's anxiety by ensuring that tasks are not more complicated than the person can accomplish. The overall goals in treatment are to promote the client's optimal level of functioning and to retard further regression, whenever possible. Working closely with the family and providing them with the names of available resources and support may help increase the quality of life for both the family and the client. See Case Study 21–1 and Nursing Care Plan 21–1.

Visit the **Evolve** website at
http://evolve.elsevier.com/Varcarolis
for more Case Studies.

CASE STUDY 21–1   *Working With a Person Who Is Cognitively Impaired*

During the past 4 years, Mr. Ludwik has demonstrated rapidly progressive memory impairment, disorientation, and deterioration in his ability to function, related to Alzheimer's disease. He is a 67-year-old man who retired at age 62 to spend some of his remaining "youth" with his wife and to travel, garden, visit family, and finally experience the plans they made over the past 40 years. He was diagnosed with Alzheimer's disease at age 63.

Mr. Ludwik has been taken care of at home by his wife and daughter, Daisy. Daisy is divorced and has returned home with her two young daughters.

The family members find themselves progressively closer to physical and mental exhaustion. Mr. Ludwik has become increasingly incontinent when he cannot find the bathroom. He wanders away from home constantly, despite close supervision. The police and neighbors bring him back home an average of four times a week. Once, he was lost for 5 days, after he had somehow boarded a bus for Pittsburgh, 1000 miles from home. He was robbed and beaten before being found by the police and returned home.

He frequently wanders into his granddaughters' rooms at night while they are sleeping and tries to get into bed with them. Too young to understand that their grandfather is lonely and confused, they fear that he is going to hurt them. Four times in the past 2 weeks, he has fallen while getting out of bed at night, thinking he is in a sleeping bag camping out in the mountains. After a conflicted and painful 2 months, the family places him in a special hospital for people with Alzheimer's disease.

Mrs. Ludwik tells the admitting nurse, Mr. Jackson, that her husband wanders almost all the time. He has difficulty finding the right words for things (aphasia) and becomes frustrated and angry when that happens. Sometimes, he does not seem to recognize the family (agnosia). Once, he thought that Daisy was a thief breaking into the house and attacked her with a broom handle. This story causes Daisy to break down into heavy sobs: "What's happened to my father? He was so kind and gentle. Oh God . . . I have lost my father."

Mrs. Ludwik tells Mr. Jackson that her husband can sometimes participate in dressing himself; at other times, when he appears confused over what goes where, he needs total assistance. At this point, Mrs. Ludwik begins to cry uncontrollably, saying "I can't bear to part with him . . . but I can't do it any more. I feel as if I've betrayed him."

Mr. Jackson then focuses his attention on Mrs. Ludwik and her experience. He states, "This a difficult decision for you." He says that he supports their decision to move Mr. Ludwik to the Alzheimer's unit. However, he is also aware that families usually have conflicting and intense emotional reactions of guilt, depression, loss, anger, and other painful feelings. Mr. Jackson suggests that Mrs. Ludwik talk to other families with a cognitively impaired member. "It might help you to know that you are not alone, and having contact with others to share your grief can be healing." One of the groups he suggests is the Alzheimer's Disease and Related Disorders Association (ADRDA), or simply Alzheimer's Association, a well-known self-help group.

ASSESSMENT

Because, indeed, the family is just as much the client as the family member with Alzheimer's disease, Mr. Jackson tries to take the most pressing immediate needs into consideration. He obtains the following data on initial assessment:

Objective Data

- Wanders away from home about four times a week
- Was lost for 5 days and was robbed and beaten
- Often incontinent when he cannot find the bathroom
- Has difficulty finding words
- Has difficulty identifying members of the family at times
- Has difficulty dressing himself at times
- Falls out of bed at night
- Has memory impairment
- Is disoriented much of the time
- Gets into bed with granddaughters at night when wandering
- Family undergoing intense feelings of loss and guilt

Subjective Data

- "I can't bear to part with him."
- "I feel I've betrayed him."
- "I've lost my father."

CASE STUDY 21–1 *Working With a Person Who Is Cognitively Impaired* (Continued)

SELF-ASSESSMENT

Mr. Jackson has worked on his particular unit for 4 years. It is a unit especially designed for cognitively impaired individuals, which makes nursing care easier than on a regular unit. However, Mr. Jackson would be the first to admit that he has come a long way during the time he has worked on the unit.

Four years ago, he found himself getting constantly frustrated and angry. He had entered this special unit enthusiastically and had worked hard setting goals and trying to implement them. However, he thought no one, especially the clients, cared about what he was doing for them. When the nursing coordinator asked him what made him come to that conclusion, he burst out "Nothing I do seems to make any difference . . . no one listens to me."

Mr. Jackson had a lot to learn about Alzheimer's disease, and he found that the more he learned, the more he understood about why change took so long or, in some cases, could not take place. He, like everyone before him, learned to become more realistic in formulating goals, thereby lessening his frustration.

From his co-workers, he also learned many nursing care strategies that increased competent care and decreased frustration. For example, he learned that he could distract certain clients from inappropriate behaviors (e.g., arguing with others or taking things out of other people's rooms) by engaging them in another, enjoyable activity, such as talking about something they were interested in. This reduced Mr. Jackson's initial response of scolding the client, which had usually resulted in escalating the client's anxiety, confusion, and sometimes aggression, and left Mr. Jackson annoyed and upset.

As time progressed, Mr. Jackson found that he was well suited to this kind of nursing. He has an enthusiastic manner, and his patience, wit, and genuine liking of his clients make him an ideal role model for staff new to the unit. He does a lot of teaching on the unit, both formal and informal. He is compiling a workbook for caregivers of the cognitively impaired.

NURSING DIAGNOSIS

Mr. Jackson evaluates the data. Indeed, many potential nursing diagnoses and several client needs are identified that require intervention by the nursing staff. Mr. Jackson chooses four initially: the first one deals with client safety, two address maintaining an optimal level of functioning and preventing further regression, and the fourth deals with the very real and immediate needs of a family in crisis. Therefore, Mr. Jackson makes the following diagnoses:

1. **Risk for injury** related to confusion, as evidenced by wandering

   ■ Wanders away from home about four times a week
   ■ Wanders despite supervision
   ■ Falls out of bed at night
   ■ Gets into other people's beds
   ■ Wanders at night

2. **Functional urinary incontinence** related to disturbed cognition, as evidenced by inability to find the toilet

   ■ Incontinent when he cannot find the bathroom

3. **Self-care deficit** (self-dressing deficits) related to impaired cognitive functioning, as evidenced by impaired ability to put on and take off clothing

   ■ Sometimes is able to dress with help of wife
   ■ At other times is too confused to dress self at all

4. **Anticipatory grieving** related to loss and deterioration of family member

   ■ "I can't bear to part with him."
   ■ "I feel I've betrayed him."
   ■ "I've lost my father."
   ■ Family undergoing intense feelings of loss and guilt

Case Study continued on following page

CASE STUDY 21–1   *Working With a Person Who Is Cognitively Impaired* (Continued)

OUTCOME CRITERIA

Although Mr. Ludwik has many unmet needs that require nursing interventions, Mr. Jackson decides to focus on the four initial nursing diagnoses. As other problems arise, they will be addressed.

NURSING DIAGNOSIS	LONG-TERM OUTCOME	SHORT-TERM GOALS
1. **Risk for injury** related to confusion, as evidenced by wandering.	1. Client will remain safe in nursing home.	1a. Client will remain in bed injury free. 1b. Client will wander only in protected area. 1c. Client will be returned within 2 hours if he succeeds in escaping from the unit.
2. **Functional urinary incontinence** related to disturbed cognition, as evidenced by inability to find the toilet.	2. Client will experience less incontinence (fewer episodes) by fourth week of hospitalization.	2a. Client will participate in toilet training. 2b. Client will find the toilet most of the time.
3. **Self-care deficit** (self-dressing) related to impaired cognitive functioning, as evidenced by impaired ability to put on and take off clothes.	3. Client will participate in dressing himself 80% of the time.	3a. Client will follow step-by-step instructions for dressing most of the time. 3b. Client will dress in own clothes with aid of fastening tape.
4. **Anticipatory grieving** related to loss and deterioration of family member.	4. All family members will state, in 3 months' time, that they feel they have more support and are able to talk about their grieving.	4a. Family members will state that they have opportunity to express "unacceptable" feelings in supportive environment. 4b. Family members will state that they have found support from others who have a family member with Alzheimer's disease.

PLANNING

Mr. Jackson made a Nursing Care Plan (See Nursing care Plan 21–1) to target the client's and family's immediate needs. The Nursing Care Plans for nursing diagnoses 2, 3, and 4 are on the Simon website.

INTERVENTION

Mr. Jackson gives Mrs. Ludwik the names of two organizations in her community that work with families of a cognitively impaired member. He emphasizes that the Alzheimer's Association support group consists of other family members who are going through similar circumstances. He gives Mrs. Ludwik the name of the social worker and the nurse clinician assigned to the unit, who could give the family information on the disease, answer questions, and provide support and further referrals. Mr. Jackson asks Mrs. Ludwik to let him know after 1 week how things are going, and he says that further plans could be made at that time.

Wandering is a common phenomenon, especially in men with Alzheimer's disease. However, because night wandering may be indicative of cardiac decompensation, Mr. Jackson alerts the medical staff. Mr. Ludwik's mattress is placed on the floor to prevent falls, and there is a large area on the unit where he can wander safely. A bright orange vest is made for Mr. Ludwik with his name, unit, and phone number taped on the back, in case he does wander off the unit. A Medic-Alert bracelet is also made up for him, containing the same information. He is encouraged to participate in activities that encourage the exercise of large muscle groups (e.g., exercise and dance groups). He seems to wander less at night if he has been involved in physical exercise during the day. On the nights that he does wander out of his room, the staff allow him to wander in the safe area. He is offered snacks, and the room is kept well lit. Sometimes, Mr. Ludwik curls up on the couch and falls asleep.

On the unit, Mr. Jackson and the staff begin toilet training Mr. Ludwik (i.e., they take him to the toilet early in the morning, after each meal and snack, and in the evening). On this unit, all the rooms, including the bathrooms, are clearly labeled in large, colorful letters; clocks are placed in every room in clear view, and each

room has a large calendar with Xs marking off the days. In lieu of signs, pictures may be substituted to identify function of room (a bed for bedroom) or picture of the person occupying that room.

Mr. Jackson finds that on most mornings, Mr. Ludwik is able to follow simple step-by-step instructions for dressing, but that he is much better at this after breakfast than in the early-morning hours. Therefore, a schedule is set up that includes toilet, breakfast, toileting, and then dressing. When Mr. Ludwik becomes irritable and refuses to dress, Mr. Jackson involves Mr. Ludwik in another activity and, after 15 or 20 minutes, suggests dressing. This seems to work most of the time. Mr. Ludwik always wears his own clothes, unaltered except for the fastening tape that replaces the original buttons and zippers. This seems to lessen Mr. Ludwik's frustration during dressing.

Mr. Ludwik's love for gardening is sublimated into activities such as finger painting and clay modeling. The activity therapist finds that Mr. Ludwik is most content during these times. Nursing Care Plan 21–1 provides more details on Mr. Ludwik's treatment.

EVALUATION

At the end of 4 weeks, Mr. Ludwik is still free from injuries. Placing his mattress on the floor has solved one potential problem. Mr. Ludwik continues to wander at night, but more often, he naps on the couch after having a snack. He did wander off the unit once, when visitors were coming in, but was returned to the unit by the security guard as Mr. Ludwik prepared to leave the hospital. The familiar orange vest was spotted immediately.

When Mr. Ludwik first came to the unit he had been very disoriented. However, getting used to certain staff members and set routines helped to overcome his disorientation. With the aid of the tape fasteners and constant, short reminders, Mr. Ludwik dresses himself with minimal assistance.

Urinary incontinence shows great improvement over the 4-week period. Although Mr. Ludwik is still incontinent, the episodes now occur only four times a week. He is amenable to the toileting schedule and usually complies without problems.

The family begins short-term counseling together. Counseling sessions not only give Mrs. Ludwik and Daisy an opportunity to express pent-up feelings and receive guidance but also allows Mr. Ludwik's granddaughters time to express their own fears and confusion. Mrs. Ludwik has been to two meetings of an Alzheimer's support group, at which she finds great relief. She says that she has felt isolated for so long. Her daughter Daisy is planning to go with her to the next meeting.

Visit the **Evolve** website at
http://evolve.elsevier.com/Varcarolis
for the other Nursing Care Plan diagnoses and for
more Nursing Care Plans.

NURSING CARE PLAN 21–1   A *Person With* Cognitive Impairment

---

NURSING DIAGNOSIS

Risk for Injury: related to altered cerebral functioning, as evidenced by wandering

Supporting Data

■ Wanders despite supervision
■ Falls out of bed
■ Gets into other people's beds

Outcome Criteria: Client will remain safe

SHORT-TERM GOAL	INTERVENTION	RATIONALE	EVALUATION
1. Client will not fall out of bed at any time.	1a. Spend time with client on admission	1a. Lowers anxiety, provides orientation to time and place. Client's confusion is increased by change.	*GOAL MET*
	1b. Label client's room in big, colorful letters.	1b. Offers clues in new surroundings.	
	1c. Remove mattress from bed and place on floor.	1c. Prevents falling out of bed.	Mattress on floor prevents falls out of bed.
	1d. Keep room well lit at all times.	1d. Provides important environmental clues; helps lower possibility of illusions.	
	1e. Show client clock and calendar in room.	1e. Fosters orientation to time.	
	1f. Keep window shade up.	1f. Allows day-night variations.	
2. Client will wander only in protected area.	2a. At night, take client to large, protected, well-lit room.	2a. Client is able to wander safely in protected environment.	*GOAL MET* Client continues to wander at night; with supervision, keeps out of other clients' rooms most of the time.
	2b. Alert physician to check client for cardiac decompensation.	2b. Possible underlying cause of nocturnal wakefulness and wandering.	

NURSING CARE PLAN 21–1   **A *Person* With Cognitive Impairment** *(Continued)*

SHORT-TERM GOAL	INTERVENTION	RATIONALE	EVALUATION
	2c. Offer snacks when client is up—milk, decaffeinated tea, sandwich.	2c. Helps replace fluid and caloric expenditure.	By fourth week, client starts to nap on couch in large room after snacks during the night.
	2d. Allow soft music on radio.	2d. Helps induce relaxation.	
	2e. Spend short, frequent intervals with client.	2e. Decreases client's feelings of isolation and increases orientation.	
	2f. Take client to bathroom after snacks.	2f. Helps prevent incontinence.	
	2g. During day, offer activities that include use of large muscle groups.	2g. For some clients, helps decrease wandering.	
3. Client will be returned within 2 hours if he leaves the unit.	3a. Order Medic-Alert bracelet for client (with name, unit or hospital, phone number).	3a. If client gets out of hospital, he can be identified.	*GOAL MET* By fourth week, client wanders off unit only once; is found in lobby and returned by security guard within 45 minutes.
	3b. Place brightly colored vest on client with name, unit, and phone number taped on back.	3b. If client wanders in hospital, he can be identified and returned.	
	3c. Check client's whereabouts periodically during the day and especially at night.	3c. Helps monitor client's activities.	

SUMMARY

Cognitive disorder is the term that refers to disorders marked by disturbances in orientation, memory, intellect, judgment, and affect resulting from changes in the brain. Delirium and dementia were discussed in this chapter because they are the cognitive disorders most widely seen by health care workers.

Delirium is marked by acute onset, disturbance in consciousness, and symptoms of disorientation and confusion that fluctuate by the minute, hour, or time of day. Delirium is always secondary to an underlying condition; therefore, it is temporary, transient, and may last from hours to days once the underlying cause is treated. If the cause is not treated, permanent damage to the neurons could result in dementia or death.

A number of nursing diagnoses are suggested for confused and demented clients and are presented in Table 21–1.

The clinical picture of delirium in an intensive care unit was described, and medical and nursing interventions were delineated.

Dementia usually has a more insidious onset than delirium. Global deterioration of cognitive functioning (e.g., memory, judgment, ability to think abstractly, and orientation) is often progressive and irreversible, depending on the underlying cause. If dementia is primary (e.g., Alzheimer's disease, multi-infarct dementia, or Pick's disease, Lewy body dementia), the course is irreversible. However, if the underlying cause is treatable, then the progression of the dementia may be halted or reversed.

Alzheimer's disease accounts for up to 70% of all cases of dementia, and multi-infarct disease accounts for about 20%; however, these percentages may change with the rising incidence of AIDS-related dementia (HIV encephalopathy).

Various theories exist about the cause of Alzheimer's disease; none of these is conclusive, although the genetic theory identifies familial tendencies. In this chapter signs and symptoms were noted during the progression of the disease through four stages: stage 1 (mild), stage 2 (moderate), stage 3 (moderate to severe), and stage 4 (late). The phenomena of confabulation, perseveration, aphasia, apraxia, agnosia, and hyperorality were explained.

No known cause or cure exists for Alzheimer's disease, although a number of drugs that increase the brain's supply of acelylcholine (a nerve communication chemical) have helped some people in the early stages slow down the progress of the disease. A number of drugs are in the pipeline and a drug used in Germany, Mematine, for people in more advanced stages. More encouraging is that clinical trials of vaccine (AN-1792), that clears plaques out of the brain are now underway (Al Assoc, 7/11/2000). Much research is still needed for unraveling the mysteries of this devastating illness. Duffy and colleagues (1989) described a nursing research agenda that included better care and management of clients with Alzheimer's disease and an emphasis on research-based practice.

People with Alzheimer's disease have many unmet needs and present many management challenges to their families, as well as to health care workers, once clients with the disease are institutionalized.

Specific nursing interventions for cognitively impaired individuals for increasing communication, safety, and self-care are given. The need for family teaching and support is stressed.

Visit the **Evolve** website at
http://evolve.elsevier.com/Varcarolis
for a post-test on the content in this chapter.

Visit the **Evolve** website at
http://evolve.elsevier.com/Varcarolis
for additional self-study exercises.

Critical Thinking and Chapter Review

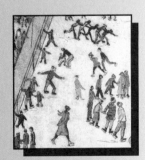

Critical Thinking

1. Mrs. Kendel is a 52-year-old woman who has progressive Alzheimer's disease. She lives with her husband, who has been trying to care for her in their home. Mrs. Kendel often wears evening gowns in the morning, puts her blouse on backward, and sometimes puts her bra on backward outside her blouse.

   She often forgets where things are. She makes an effort to cook but often confuses frying pans and pots and sometimes has trouble turning on the stove.

   Once in a while, she cannot find the bathroom in time, often mistaking it for a broom closet. She becomes frightened of noises and is terrified when the telephone or doorbell rings.

   At other times, she cries because she is aware that she is losing her sense of her place in the world. She and her husband have always been close, loving companions, and he wants to keep her at home as long as possible.

   A. Help Mr. Kendel by writing out a list of suggestions that he can try at home that might help facilitate (a) communication, (b) activities of daily living, and (c) a safe home environment.

B. Identify at least seven interventions that are appropriate to this situation for each of the areas cited above.

C. Identify possible types of resources available for maintaining Mrs. Kendel in her home for as long as possible. Identify the name of one self-help group that you would urge Mr. Kendel to join.

D. Share with your clinical group the name and function of at least three community agencies in your area that could be an appropriate referral for a family in your neighborhood with a member with dementia. (For one, you can call the Alzheimer's Association [800-272-3900] to find a local chapter that might help you with this information; another resource is the Alzheimer's Disease Education and Referral [ADEAR] Center [800-438-4380], website: http://www.alzheimers.org/adear.)

Chapter Review

Choose the most appropriate answer.

1. The nurse assessing a client with suspected delirium will expect to find the client's symptoms developed

   1. over a period of hours to days
   2. over a period of weeks to months
   3. with no relationship to another condition
   4. during the years of life after middle age

2. An outcome that would be appropriate for a client with cognitive impairment related to delirium would be: Client will

   1. participate fully in self-care from admission on
   2. have stable vital signs 6 hours after admission
   3. participate in simple activities that bring enjoyment
   4. correctly interpret reality within 24 hours of admission

3. The nursing diagnosis of highest priority for clients with late Alzheimer's disease is

   1. risk for injury
   2. self-care deficit
   3. self-esteem disturbance
   4. impaired verbal communication

4. Strategies to help staff caring for cognitively impaired clients avoid developing burnout include

   1. setting realistic client goals
   2. insulating self from emotional involvement with clients
   3. sedating clients to promote rest and minimize catastrophic episodes
   4. encouraging family to permit use of restraint to promote client safety

5. Psychobiological interventions showing promise for the treatment of cognitive impairment associated with Alzheimer's disease include

   1. cholinesterase inhibitors
   2. herbals including ginkgo
   3. SSRIs and trazodone
   4. benzodiazepines and buspirone

NURSE, CLIENT, AND FAMILY RESOURCES

Books

Mace, N. L., and Rabins, P. V. (1999). *The 36-hour day: The family guide to caring for persons with Alzheimer's disease, related dementing illnesses, and memory loss in later life.* Baltimore: The Johns Hopkins University Press.

Mathiasen P. (1997). *An ocean of time: Alzheimer's: tales of hope and forgetting.* New York: Scribner.

Medina, J. (1999). *What you need to know about Alzheimer's.* New Harbinger Publications.

Associations

Alzheimer's Disease and Related Disorders Association
919 North Michigan Avenue, Suite 1000
Chicago, IL 60611-1676
1-312-335-8700; 1-800-272-3900
(For caregivers of Alzheimer's clients)

Alzheimer's Disease Education and Referral Center
Hotline: 1-800-438-4380
(Information, referrals, publications regarding clinical trials)

Internet Sites

Alzheimer's Association
http://www.alz.org

Alzheimer Society of Canada
http://www.alzheimer.ca

Family Caregiver Alliance
http://www.caregiver.org

Yahoo's Alzheimer's Disease Links
http://www.yahoo.com

Infoseek's Alzheimer's Disease Links
http://www.infoseek.com

REFERENCES

Alzheimer's Association Newsletter 13(2):4, 1993.

Alzheimer's Disease (Part I). (1992). *The Harvard Mental Health Letter,* 9(3):1.

Alzheimer's Disease and Related Disorders Association, Inc. (2000). Alzheimer's.

Alzheimer's Disease and Related Disorders Association, Inc. (A) (2000). Family caregivers, 7/17/00. http://www.alz.org.

Alzheimer's Disease and Related Disorders Association, Inc. (B) (2000). Treating behavioral symptoms, 6/08/00. http://www.alz.org.

Alzheimer's Disease and Related Disorders Association, Inc. (C) (2000). Treating cognitive symptoms, 5/02/00. http://www.alz.org.

Alzheimer's Disease and Related Disorders Association, Inc. (D) (2000). Experimental therapeutic shows promise for people with moderately severe to severe Alzheimer's disease, 7/12/00. http://www.alz.org.

Alzheimer's Disease and Related Disorders Association, Inc. (E) (2000). Alzheimer's scientists announce initial results of Alzheimer vaccine, 7/11/00. http://www.alz.org.

Alzheimer's Disease and Related Disorders Association, Inc. (F) (2000). Alternative treatments, 3/22/00. http://www.alz.org.

Alzheimer's in the skin (1993). *Discover,* 12:26.

American Association of Retired Persons (AARP) (1986). *Coping and caring: Living with Alzheimer's disease.* Washington, DC: American Association of Retired Persons.

American Psychiatric Association (2000). *Diagnostic and statistical manual of mental disorders* (4th ed., revised). Washington, DC: American Psychiatric Association.

Andresen, G. (1992). How to assess the older mind. *RN,* 55(7):34.

Brennan, P. F., et al. (1995). The effects of a special computer network on caregivers of persons with Alzheimer's disease. *Nursing Research,* 44(3):155.

Burnside, I. (1988). *Nursing and the aged* (3rd ed.). New York: McGraw-Hill.

Buzan, R. D., and Dubovsky, S. L. (1995). Dementia due to other general medical conditions and dementia due to multiple etiologies. In G. O. Gabbard (Ed.), *Treatments of psychiatric disorders* (Vol. 1, pp. 535–554). Washington, DC: American Psychiatric Press.

Caine, E. D., et al. (1995). Delirium, dementia, and amnestic and other cognitive disorders and mental disorders due to a general medical condition. In H. I. Kaplan and B. J. Sadock (Eds.), *Comprehensive textbook of psychiatry* (6th ed., Vol. 1, pp. 705–754). Baltimore: Williams & Wilkins.

Corey-Bloom, J., and Galasko, D. (1995). Adjunctive therapy in patients with Alzheimer's disease: A practical approach. *Drugs and Aging,* 7(2):79.

de-Stoutz, N. D., et al. (1995). Reversible delirium in terminally ill patients. *Journal of Pain and Symptom Management,* 10(3):249.

Dewan, M. J., and Gupta, S. (1992). Toward a definite diagnosis of Alzheimer's disease. *Comprehensive Psychiatry,* 33(4):282.

Dobson, D. B., and Itzhaki, R. F. (1999). Herpes simplex virus type 1 and Alzheimer's disease. *Neurobiology of Aging,* 20(4): 467–468.

Duffy, L. M., Hepburn, K., Christensen, R., and Brugge-Wiger, P. (1989). A research agenda in care for patients with Alzheimer's disease. *Journal of Nursing Scholarship,* 21(4):254.

Eagger, S. A., and Harvey, R. J. (1995). Clinical heterogeneity: Responders to cholinergic therapy. *Alzheimer's Disease and Associated Disorders,* 9(2):37.

Foreman, M. D. (1990). Complexities of acute confusion. *Geriatric Nursing,* 11:136.

Goldberg, R. J. (1998). *Practical guide to the care of the psychiatric patient* (2nd ed). St. Louis: Mosby–Year Book.

Gray-Vickrey, P. (1988). Evaluating Alzheimer's patients. *Nursing 88,* 18:34.

Hall, G. R. (1991). This hospital patient has Alzheimer's. *American Journal of Nursing,* 91(10):44–50.

Hall, G. R. (1994). Caring for people with Alzheimer's disease using the conceptual model of progressively lowered stress threshold in the clinical setting. *Nursing Clinics of North America,* 29(1):129.

Johnson, M., Maas, M., and Moorehead, S. (2000). *Iowa outcomes project:* Nursing outcomes classifications (NOC). St. Louis: Mosby.

Kaufman, D. M. (1995). *Clinical neurology for psychiatrists* (4th ed.). Philadelphia: W. B. Saunders.

Keltner, N. L., Zielinski, A. L., and Hardin, M. S. (2001). Drugs used for the cognitive symptoms of Alzheimer's disease. *Perspectives in Psychiatric Care,* 37(1):31–34.

Korn, M. (2000). Dementia from many perspectives. XXII Congress of the Collegium Internationale Neuro-Psychopharmacologicum, April 29–May 6, 2000, San Diego, CA.

Mace, N. L., and Rabins, P. B. (1981). *The 36-hour day.* Baltimore: Johns Hopkins University Press.

Maier-Lorentz, M. M. (2000). Effective nursing interventions for the management of Alzheimer's disease. *Journal of Neuroscience Nursing,* 32(3):153–157.

Masterman, D. L., et al. (1995). Alzheimer's disease. In G. O.

Gabbard (Ed.), *Treatments of psychiatric disorders* (Vol. 1, pp. 535–554). Washington, DC: American Psychiatric Press.

McHugh, P. R., and Folstein, M. F. (1987). Organic mental disorders. In R. Michels and J. O. Cavenar (Eds.), *Psychiatry* (Vol. I). Philadelphia: J. B. Lippincott.

Minthon, L., et al. (1995). Long-term effects of tacrine on regional cerebral flow changes in Alzheimer's disease. *Dementia*, 6(5):245.

Morris, J. C. (2000). Alzheimer's disease: Unique, differentiable, and treatable. XXII Congress of the Collegium Internationale Neuro-Psychopharmacologicum, April 29–May 6, 2000, San Diego, CA.

Nagley, S. J. (1986). Predicting and preventing confusion in your patients. *Journal of Gerontological Nursing*, 12(3):27.

National Institutes of Health (1997). New drug therapies delay effects of Alzheimer's disease. Washington, DC: NIH Press Release, April 23, 1997.

Newbern, V. B. (1991). Is it really Alzheimer's? *American Journal of Nursing*, 2:51.

Nicholas, L. M., and Lindsey, B. A. (1995). Delirium presenting with symptoms of depression. *Psychosomatics*, 36(5):471.

Ninos, M., and Makohon, R. (1985). Functional assessment of the patient. *Geriatric Nursing*, 6:139.

Parnetti, L. (1995). Clinical pharmacokinetics of drugs for Alzheimer's disease. *Clinical Pharmacokinetics*, 29(2):110.

Perry, S. W., and Markowitz, J. (1988). Organic mental disorders. In J. A. Talbott, R. E. Hales, and S. C. Yudofsky (Eds.), *Textbook of psychiatry*. Washington, DC: American Psychiatric Press.

Powell, L. S., and Courtice, K. (1983). *Alzheimer's disease: A guide for families*. Reading, MA: Addison-Wesley.

Reisberg, B. (1984). Stages of cognitive decline. *American Journal of Nursing*, 84:225.

Scott, J. F., Roberto, K. A., and Hutton, J. T. (1986). Families of Alzheimer's victims: Family support to the caregivers. *Journal of American Geriatrics Society*, 34:348.

Shifu, X., Hequn, Y., and Peifen, Y., and the Cerebrolysin Study Group (2000). Efficacy of FPF 1070 (Cerebrolysin) in patients with Alzheimer's disease. *Clinical Drug Investigation*, 19(1):42–53.

Souder, E. (1992). Diagnosing dementia: Current clinical concepts. *Journal of Gerontological Nursing*, 18(2):5.

Sullivan, E. M., Wanich, C. K., and Kurlowicz, L. H. (1991). Elder care. *AORN Journal*, 53(3):820.

Tacrine update (1993). *Alzheimer's Research Review*, Summer.

Weiler, K., and Buckwalter, K. C. (1988). Care of the demented client. *Journal of Gerontological Nursing*, 14(7):26.

Williams, L. (1986). Alzheimer's: The need for caring. *Journal of Gerontological Nursing*, 12(2):21.

Wilson, H. S. (1990). Easing life for the Alzheimer's patient. *RN*, 53(12):24.

Wolanin, M. O., and Fraelich-Philips, L. R. (1981). *Confusion, prevention and cure*. St. Louis: C. V. Mosby.

Yi, E. S., et al. (1994). Alzheimer's disease and nursing: New scientific and clinical insights. *Nursing Clinics of North America*, 29(1):85.

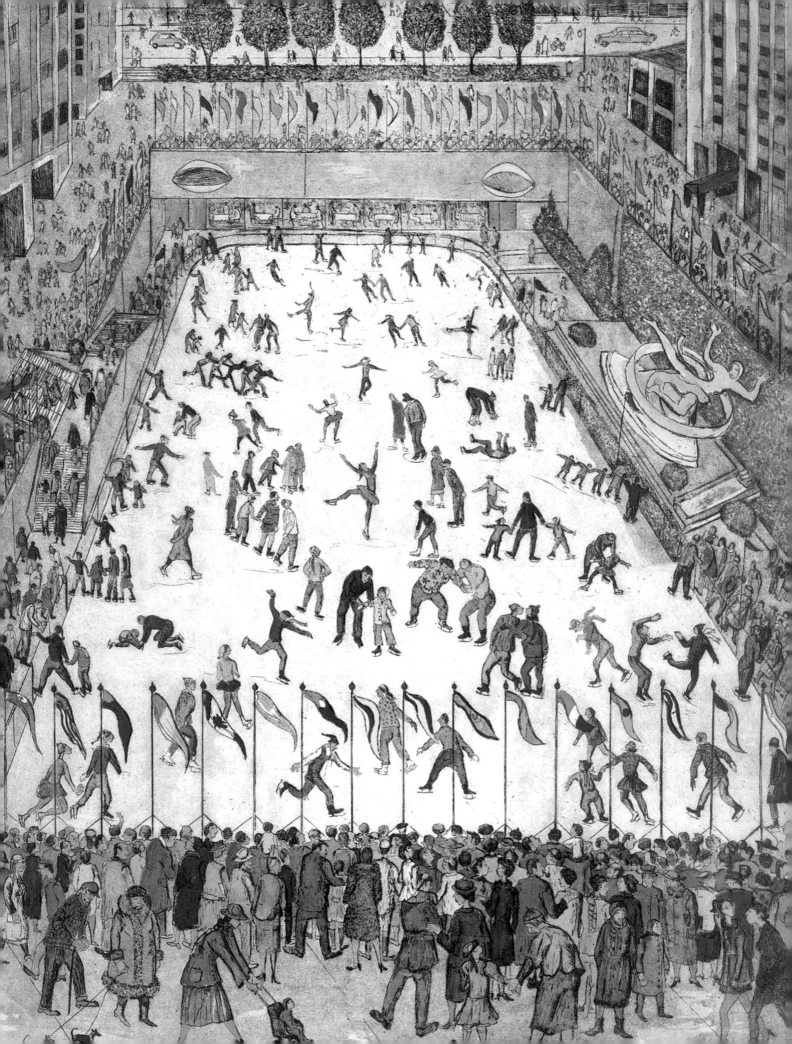

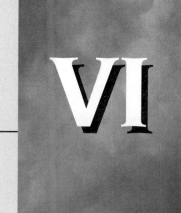
Psychiatric Emergencies

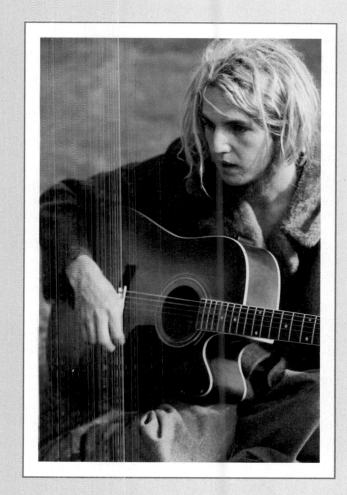

If you treat an individual as he is,
he will stay as he is, but if you
treat him as he ought to be and
could be, he will become as he
ought to be and could be.

JOHANN WOLFGANG GOETHE
(1749–1832)

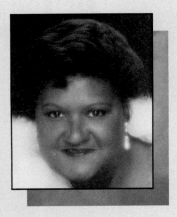

A Nurse Speaks

PATRICIA A. CLAYBROOK

I have been a nurse for the past 27 years. I entered a three-year diploma program after finishing high school. By the age of 20 I had completed my nursing courses and entered the working world. I started out as a surgical nurse. I thought this would be exciting and keep me interested in the field. I felt that I could contribute my skills and knowledge more effectively in the surgical suite. But after one year I was bored with the routine and felt I was not making any impact on people's lives. I then switched to psychiatric nursing. I went from being uninvolved to being totally involved with clients. After working for several years, I felt that I needed more theoretical knowledge to go with my practical knowledge. I returned to school and completed my masters in psychology. But something was missing. I didn't feel that psychology helped me to look at the client as a whole, so I have returned to school and am completing my masters in psychiatric nursing.

When I first entered into mental health nursing, there was only one job and that was being in the psychiatric unit for the severely mentally ill. These jobs were generally in state mental institutions. But like mental health treatment, mental health nursing has changed. The focus today, as in health care today, is the community. The community can have many definitions. But the community in which I find myself practicing mental health nursing is the criminal justice system of the county in which I live. Forensic nursing is a relatively recent and fast-developing specialization within the field of psychiatry. The forensic psychiatric nurse must be a member of the interdisciplinary team working for the overall improvement of the quality of life of inmates. The forensic psychiatric nurse must first explore her/his feelings about the mentally ill offenders.

My role in this setting is one of primary clinician. I am responsible for assessing the mental status of the inmates in my area, and I am responsible for defining their treatment plan in conjunction with the psychiatrist. But sometimes my role becomes one of teacher. This means not only educating the inmate to what his capabilities may be in jail but also to what his limitations for treatment may be in jail, and I may be called upon to educate the custodial staff regarding mental illness and how best to treat the inmate.

I'll never forget a 19-year-old inmate who was in custody for drug possession charges. This inmate had a long history of mental illness. At the age of 11, he poured gasoline on himself and set himself on fire. He had been in the social system from age two, starting in foster care and then going to juvenile institutions. This young man was considered to be a disruptive, manipulating, self-abusing, and combative individual by the custodial staff and some of the other clinicians. They could not see past his behavior to see a young man feeling so bereft of love and caring that any attention received in the jail system meant that someone cared about him. Unfortunately, most of the time the attention was very negative. After working with this young man for a while, he started to share some of his fears of always being alone and not having any one to care about him, or anyone he could care about. He craved attention from me, and I become a mother figure to him. After working with custodial staff, I was able to help them understand and appreciate that this individual was functioning emotionally between the ages of 3 and 5. He was like a child throwing tantrums for attention. We worked together to institute a small reward system for this inmate, i.e., extra cookies with/between meals and extra time out of his cell when he maintained appropriate behavior. With all our efforts we were able to decrease the self-mutilating behavior to once a month. This was significant progress since his pattern in the past had been throwing tantrums every other day. Eventually, this inmate was released with a follow-up plan to get connected with long-term psychiatric care in the community. He eventually was referred to a facility that dealt not only with people with psychiatric problems but also with those who had been in the criminal justice system. It

612

was necessary for me to take on the role of client advocate and case manager for this client, and I had to make numerous calls not only to attorneys but also to the outside agencies.

The inmate just described is not an isolated case. He is but one of the many who, without specialized treatment and intervention, would have become one of the many repeat chronic offenders. It is important that nurses be aware that the power of their knowledge and skills can really make a significant difference in people's lives. Nurses need to increase consistently their knowledge through their practice, research, and further education.

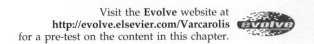
Outline

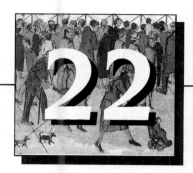

22

Crisis

Elizabeth M. Varcarolis

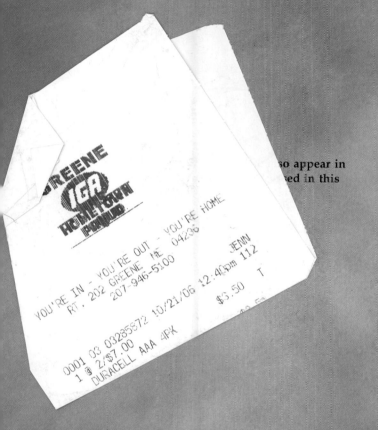

...so appear in
...ed in this

Objectives

After studying this chapter, the reader will be able to

1. Differentiate among the three types of crises discussed in this chapter and give an example of each from your own experience.
2. Delineate at least six aspects of crisis that have relevance for nurses involved in crisis intervention.
3. Develop a handout including areas to assess during crisis, with at least two sample questions for each area.
4. Discuss four common problems health care professionals may have when starting crisis intervention and discuss at least two interventions for each problem.
5. Compare and contrast the differences among primary, secondary, and tertiary intervention, including appropriate intervention strategies.
6. Explain to a classmate four potential crisis situations, common in the hospital setting, that a client may face. Give concrete examples of how they can be minimized.
7. Make a list of at least five resources in your community that could be used as a referral for a person in crisis.

615

EPIDEMIOLOGY

A crisis is an acute, time-limited phenomenon experienced as an overwhelming emotional reaction to a

- Stressful situational event
- Developmental event
- Societal event, or
- Cultural event, or to the perception of that event

We experience crises during our lifetimes. A crisis itself is not a pathological state, and being in crisis is not pathological. It is a struggle for equilibrium and adjustment when problems are perceived as unsolvable. A crisis presents both a danger to personality organization and a potential opportunity for personality growth. The outcome depends on how the individual perceives and deals with the crisis and what outside supports are available at the time the crisis occurs.

Violence in Our Lives

Acts of violence in our society are abysmally high and increase the incidence for individuals, families, and communities with lives shattered by grieving. For example, young men and women currently experience high amounts of violence in dating relationships. Studies have found that 32% to 51% of women and 20% to 30% of men admit to hitting their partners (Stringham 1999).

PEOPLE IN CRISIS. The level of violence aimed at children has reached public health crisis proportions, a chilling trend similar in scope to violence directed at teenagers from street gunfire (Aguilera 1998).

FAMILIES IN CRISIS. Acts of violence at schools across the country committed by gun wielding students happen all too frequently, for example, Jonesboro, AK, on March 24, 1998, and Columbine High School, Littleton, CO, April 20, 1999, which were two well-publicized examples. These and other shooting rampages by youth randomly killing youth resulted in multiple casualties and widespread grieving (Hospital Security and Safety Management, 1999).

COMMUNITIES IN CRISIS. Increase in reported acts of road rage leaving lives in upheaval, deaths, and grief is becoming part of our everyday lives. One nursing study (Coler, et al 2000) was initiated to illustrate that the nursing phenomenon, violence, exists as part of community and that violence should now be classified under community.

COMORBIDITY

"A psychological crisis refers to an individual's inability to solve a problem" (Aguilera, 1998). However, we know there are many factors that limit a person's ability to problem-solve or cope with stressful life events or situations, such as

- The number of other stressful life events with which the person is currently coping
- The presence of other unresolved losses the person may be dealing with
- The presence of concurrent psychiatric disorders
- The presence of concurrent medical problems
- Experiencing excessive fatigue or pain
- The quality and quantity of a person's usual coping skills. Coping skills are often acquired through a variety of sources, for example, cultural responses, modeling others' behaviors, and life opportunities to broaden our experience and acquire new responses.

Chapter 28 discusses the vulnerability of people with severe mental illness and their susceptibility to crisis and crisis interventions. Nurses, perhaps more than any other group, deal with people who are experiencing disruption in their lives. People often undergo increased amounts of stress and anxiety in medical and surgical, formal psychiatric, and community settings.

THEORY

Crisis theory was developed in the early 1940s by **Erich Lindemann**, who conducted a classic study of the grief reactions of close relatives of victims in the Coconut Grove nightclub fire. This study formed the foundation of crisis theory and clinical intervention. Lindemann observed that "acute grief was the normal reaction to a distressing situation." Lindemann showed that preventive intervention in crisis situations could eliminate or decrease serious personality disorganization and devastating psychological consequences from the sustained effects of severe anxiety.

In the early 1960s, Gerald Caplan (1964) defined crisis theory and outlined crisis intervention. Since that time, our understanding of crisis and effective intervention has been refined and enhanced by numerous clinicians and theorists.

In 1961, a report from the Joint Commission on Mental Illness and Mental Health spoke about the need for community mental health centers throughout the country. This report stimulated the establishment of crisis services, which are now an important part of mental health programs in hospitals and communities.

Donna Aguilera and **Janice Mesnick** (1970) provided a framework for nurses in assessment and intervention, which has grown in scope and practice. Aguilera (1998) continues to set a standard in the practice of crisis assessment and intervention.

The following ways of assessing crisis are derived from established crisis theory and constitute a sound knowledge base for the application of the nursing process to a crisis. An understanding of these three areas of crisis theory enables application of the nursing process: (1) types of crisis, (2) phases of crisis, and (3) aspects of crisis that have relevance for nurses.

Types of Crisis

Three basic types of crisis situations have been identified: (1) maturational, (2) situational, and (3) adventitious. People who have pre-existing mental health problems are very vulnerable and prone to crisis. Chapter 28 addresses crisis and rehabilitation of the mentally ill. Psychiatric emergencies (suicide, family violence, sexual assault, uncontrollable anger) are covered in Unit VI: Psychiatric Emergencies. Drug overdoses and alcohol intoxication and withdrawal are covered in Chapter 27.

Maturational Crisis

A process of maturation occurs throughout the life cycle. Erikson identified eight stages of growth and development in which specific maturational tasks must be mastered. The path (stages) to adulthood is stressful and at times can be overwhelming. Erikson says that each of these stages constitutes a crisis in personal growth and development.

Each developmental stage can be referred to as a maturational crisis. When a person arrives at a new stage, formerly used coping styles are no longer appropriate, and new coping mechanisms have yet to be developed. For a time, the person is without effective defenses. This often leads to increased anxiety, which may manifest as variations in the person's normal behavior. Temporary disequilibrium may affect interpersonal relationships, body image, and social and work roles (Hoff 1995). The aging process is an excellent example of a maturational crisis. Successful resolution of these tasks leads to development of basic human qualities. Erikson believed that the way these crises are resolved at one stage affects the ability to pass through subsequent stages, because each crisis provides the starting point for moving to the next stage. If a person lacks support systems and adequate role models, successful resolution may be difficult or may not occur. Unresolved problems in the past and inadequate coping mechanisms can adversely affect what is learned in each developmental stage. When a person is experiencing severe difficulty during a maturational crisis, professional intervention may be indicated.

Alcohol and drug addiction are examples of how progression through the maturational stages can be interrupted. This phenomenon is too often seen among teenagers today. When the addictive behavior is controlled (by the late teens), the young person's growth and development will resume at the point at which it was interrupted. A young person whose addiction is arrested at 19 years of age could have the social and problem-solving skills of a 14-year-old. Often these teenagers do not receive treatment, and their adult coping skills are diminished or absent.

Situational Crisis

A situational crisis arises from an external rather than an internal source. Examples of external situations that could precipitate a crisis include loss of a job, the death of a loved one, abortion, a change of job, a change in financial status, coming out as to homosexual orientation, divorce, the addition of new family members, pregnancy, and severe physical or mental illness.

These situations were first referred to as life events by Holmes and Rahe (1967). Each event is assigned stress points that, when totaled, may predict the risk for illness. A high point count can act as a predictor of physical or psychological illness. Refer to Chapter 12 for the updated Miller and Rahe (1997) Life Events and Social Readjustment Scale.

Some authors refer to these events as critical life problems because these problems are encountered by most people during the course of their lives. Whether these events precipitate a crisis depends on such factors as the degree of support available from caring friends and family members, a person's general emotional and physical status, and a person's ability to understand and cope with the meaning of the stressful event.

As in all crises or potential crisis situations, the stressful event involves a loss or change that threatens a person's self-concept and self-esteem. To varying degrees, successful resolution of a crisis depends on resolution of the grief associated with the loss.

Adventitious Crisis

An adventitious crisis, or crisis of disaster, is not a part of everyday life; it is unplanned and accidental. Adventitious crises may result from (1) a natural disaster (e.g., flood, fire, earthquake), (2) a national disaster (e.g., war, riot, airplane crashes), or (3) a crime of violence (e.g., rape, assault or murder in the workplace or school, bombing in crowded areas, spousal or child abuse).

Recent literature identifies numerous studies related to the psychological sequelae suffered by people after bombings, hurricanes, earthquakes, and the witnessing of traumatic deaths of others. Common phenomena experienced were acute stress disorder (ASD), posttraumatic stress disorder (PTSD), and depression. **The need for psychological first aid (crisis intervention) and debriefing after any crisis situation cannot be overstressed for all age groups (children, adolescents, adults, and the elderly).**

Many people may be experiencing two types of crisis situation simultaneously. For example, a 51-year-old woman may be going through a midlife crisis (maturational) when her husband dies suddenly of cancer (situational). In the example of a 14-year-old girl being forced to move away from her friends because of a parent's job transfer to another state, identify the types of crises involved. If the same 14-year-old girl had to move because of an earthquake, what crises would then be involved?

Phases of Crisis

Caplan (1964) identified four distinct phases of crisis:

Phase 1

A person confronted by a conflict or problem that threatens the self-concept responds with increased feelings of anxiety. The increase in anxiety stimulates the use of problem-solving techniques and defense mechanisms in an effort to solve the problem and lower anxiety. Review the signs and symptoms of anxiety (mild, moderate, severe, panic) and anxiety defenses in Chapter 13.

Phase 2 *Problem Solving + Defense Mech. Fail*

If the usual defensive response fails, and if the threat persists, anxiety continues to rise and produce feelings of extreme discomfort. Individual functioning becomes disorganized. Trial-and-error attempts at solving the problem and restoring a normal balance begin.

Phase 3

If the trial-and-error attempts fail, anxiety can escalate to severe and panic levels, and the person mobilizes automatic relief behaviors, such as withdrawal and flight. Some form of resolution (e.g., compromising needs or redefining the situation to make an acceptable solution) may be made in this stage.

Phase 4

If the problem is not solved, anxiety can overwhelm the person and lead to serious personality disorganization. This maladaptive response can take the form of confusion, immobilization with fear, violence against others, or suicidal behavior, as well as yelling or running about aimlessly (Robinson 1973; Hoff 1989).

Refer to Figure 22–1 for a diagram of the phases of crisis.

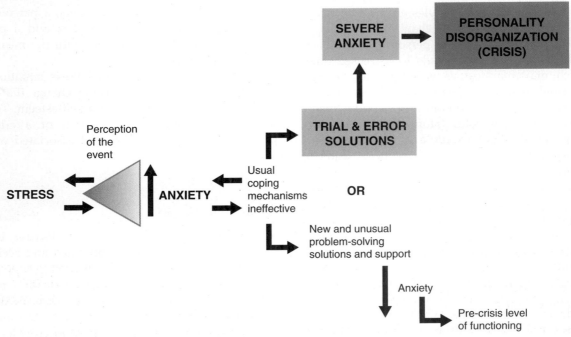

Figure 22–1 Phases in the process of crisis versus stabilization of a potential crisis event.

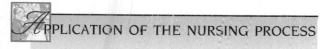

Aspects of Crisis Th_____ _lave Relevance
for Nurses

There are spe_____ects of crisis theory that are
basic to cri___ability of positive crisis outcomes
stated tha__nt____ention (Box 22–1). Hoff (1995)
is enh__t, which closely follow the nursing
crisi__y First.

p___
___social assessment of the individual's or
___y's crisis, including evaluation of victimiza-
___, trauma, and the risk of suicide or assault
___others
___Development of a plan with the person or fam-
ily in crisis
3. Implementation of the plan, drawing on personal, social, and material resources
4. Follow-up and evaluation of the crisis management process and outcomes

BOX 22–1   *Foundation for Crisis Intervention*

1. A crisis is self-limiting and is usually resolved within 4 to 6 weeks.
2. The resolution of a crisis results in one of three different functional levels. The person will emerge at a:

   ■ higher level of functioning,
   ■ the same level of functioning,
   ■ lower level of functioning.

3. The goal of crisis intervention is to maintain the pre-crisis level of functioning.
4. The form of resolution of the crisis depends on the actions of the subject and the intervention of others.
5. During a crisis, people are often more open to outside intervention than they are at times of stable functioning. With intervention, the person can learn different adaptive means of problem solving to correct inadequate solutions.
6. The person in a crisis situation is assumed to be mentally healthy and to have functioned well in the past but is presently in a state of disequilibrium.
7. Crisis intervention deals with the person's present problem and resolution of the immediate crisis only. Dealing with material not directly related to the crisis can take place at a later time. Crisis intervention deals with the "here and now."
8. The nurse must be willing to take an active, even directive, role in intervention, in direct contrast to what occurs in conventional therapeutic intervention techniques, which stress a more passive and nondirective role.
9. Early intervention probably increases the chances for a better prognosis.
10. The client is encouraged to set realistic goals and plan an intervention with the nurse that is focused on the current situation.

𝒜PPLICATION OF THE NURSING PROCESS

ASSESSMENT

Overall Assessment

A person's equilibrium may be adversely affected by one or more of the following: (1) an unrealistic perception of the precipitating event, (2) inadequate situational supports, or (3) inadequate coping mechanisms (Aguilera 1998). It is crucial to assess these factors when a crisis situation is evaluated, because data gained from the assessment are used as guides for both the nurse and the client to set realistic and meaningful goals, as well as to plan possible solutions to the problem situation. Again the reader is referred to Chapter 13 for assessing levels of mild, moderate, and severe to panic anxiety. Refer to Figure 22–2 to understand how these factors affect a crisis situation.

After determining whether there is a need for external controls because of suicidal or homicidal ideation or gestures, the nurse assesses three main areas: the client's (1) perception of the precipitating event, the client's (2) situational supports, and the client's (3) personal coping skills.

ASSESSING THE CLIENT'S PERCEPTION OF THE PRECIPITATING EVENT

The nurse's initial task is to assess the individual or family and the problem. The more clearly the prob-

lem can be defined, the better the chance that an effective solution will be found. A number of authors (Croushore et al. 1981; King 1971) suggest sample questions:

■ Has anything particularly upsetting happened to you within the past few days or weeks?
■ What was happening in your life before you started to feel this way?
■ What leads you to seek help now?
■ Describe how you are feeling right now.

■ How does this situation affect your life?
■ How do you see this event as affecting your future?
■ What would need to be done to resolve this situation?

Vignette

■ Laura, a 15-year-old girl, is brought to the emergency room after slashing her wrists. She was found by her mother, who returned home early from a date. Her mother called the police, and they rushed Laura to the hospital. After Laura is seen by the medical personnel, she is interviewed by the psychiatric nurse working in the emergency

department. The nurse speak... self and tells Laura she would ... her. The nurse states "It looks as ... overwhelming. Is that how you're fee... makes the observation that things mus... Laura wants to kill herself. Laura sits slu... with her hands in her lap and her head ha... There are tears in her eyes. *She introduces herself and spends some time with the nurse*

EXAMPLE: ASSESSING LAURA'S PERCEPTION OF THE PRECIPITATING EVENT

Nurse: Laura, tell me what has happened.
Laura: I can't . . . I can't go home . . . no one

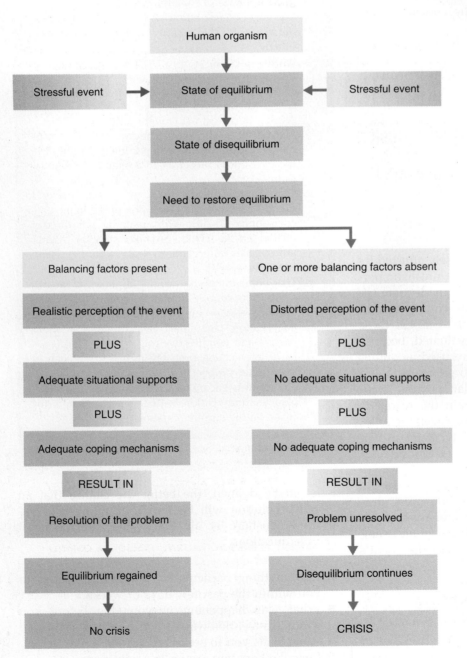

Figure 22–2 The effects of balancing factors in a stressful event. (Redrawn from Aguilera, D. C. (1998). *Crisis intervention: Theory and methodology (8th ed.).* St. Louis: Mosby.)

cares . . . no one believes me . . . I can't go through it again.

Nurse: Tell me what you can't go through again, Laura.

(Laura starts to cry, shaking with sobs. The nurse sits quietly for a while, offers Laura some tissues, then speaks.)

Nurse: Laura, tell me what is so terrible Let's look at it together.

■ *After a while, Laura starts telling the nurse that when she was 9 years old her mother had a boyfriend. When her mother was out of the house, the boyfriend would touch her. Eventually, he forced her to have sex with him. He threatened Laura that if she told anyone he would kill her. When she was 11 years old, the boyfriend moved to another state. Two weeks ago, Laura's mother said the old boyfriend was coming back to live with them. Laura, terrified, told her mother what had happened years ago, but her mother called her a liar. Her mother said that if it came to a choice between Laura and the boyfriend, the mother would take the boyfriend.*

ASSESSING SITUATIONAL SUPPORTS

The client's support systems are assessed to determine the resources available to the person. Does the stressful event involve important people in the support system? Is the client isolated from others, or are there family and friends who can provide the vital support? Family and friends may be called upon to aid the individual by offering material or emotional supports, for example, lending money, offering services, or being available to give affection and understanding. If these resources are not available, the nurse/counselor acts as a temporary support system while relationships with individuals or groups in the community are established. The following are some sample questions to ask:

■ With whom do you live?
■ To whom do you talk when you feel overwhelmed?
■ Whom can you trust?
■ Who is available to help you?
■ Where do you go to worship (or talk to God), to school, or to other community-based activities?
■ During difficult times in the past, who did you want most to help you?
■ Who is the most helpful?

EXAMPLE: ASSESSING LAURA'S SITUATIONAL SUPPORTS

Nurse: Laura, who can you go to? Do you have any other family?

Laura: No My dad left when I was 6. We stay pretty much alone. My mom doesn't allow my brother and me to play with other kids.

Nurse: Do you have anyone you can talk to?

Laura: No I really don't have any friends. All the other kids think I'm stuck-up. I don't fit in too well, I guess. My mom would never let me go out, anyway. There are always things to do at home.

Nurse: What about your place of worship, or your teachers at school?

Laura: The teachers are nice, but I can't tell them things like this. Besides, they wouldn't believe me either.

ASSESSING PERSONAL COPING SKILLS

In crisis situations, it is important to evaluate the person's level of anxiety. Common coping mechanisms may be overeating, drinking, smoking, withdrawing, seeking out someone to talk to, yelling, fighting, or engaging in other physical activity (Croushore et al. 1981). The potential for suicide or homicide must be assessed. If the client is suicidal, homicidal, or unable to take care of personal needs, hospitalization should be considered (Aguilera 1998). Some sample questions to ask are

■ Have you thought of killing yourself or someone else? If yes, have you thought of how you would do this?
■ What do you usually do to feel better?
■ Did you try it this time? If so, what was different?
■ What helped you through difficult times in the past?
■ What do you think might happen now?

■ *The nurse learns that Laura does very well in school, especially in math. Laura explains that when she studies, she can forget her problems and get lost in other worlds. Getting good grades also has another reward: it is the only time her mother says anything nice about her. Her mother boasts to her boyfriends about how bright her daughter is.*

EXAMPLE: ASSESSING LAURA'S PERSONAL COPING STYLE

Nurse: What do you think would help your situation?

Laura: I don't want to die. I just don't know where to turn.

■ *The nurse tells Laura that she wants to work with her to find a solution, and that she is concerned for Laura's safety and well-being.*

SELF-ASSESSMENT

Nurses need to monitor personal feelings and thoughts constantly when dealing with a person in crisis. It is important to recognize one's own level of anxiety to prevent closing off the expression of painful feelings by the client. Because a client's situation or anxiety level may trigger uncomfortable levels of anxiety in the nurse at times, the nurse tends to repress such feelings to maintain personal comfort. When the nurse is not aware of personal feelings and reactions, she or he may unconsciously prevent the expression of the painful feelings in the client that are precipitating the nurse's own discomfort. Thus, closing off feelings in the client can render the nurse ineffective. There may be times when the nurse, for perhaps personal reasons, feels he or she cannot effectively deal with a client's situation at this point in time. Therefore, the nurse might ask another colleague to work with a particular client. This will give the nurse a chance to work out some uncomfortable or painful issues for himself or herself.

Beginning nurses in crisis intervention often face common problems that must be worked through before they become comfortable and competent in the role of a crisis counselor. Four of the more common problems are

1. The nurse's needing to be needed
2. The nurse setting unrealistic goals for clients
3. The nurse having difficulty dealing with the issue of suicide
4. The nurse having difficulty terminating

Refer to Table 22–1 for examples and results of these problems, appropriate interventions, and desired outcomes. It is crucial in beginning crisis intervention that supervision be made available as an integral part of the training process. The supervisor should be an experienced professional, such as a nurse counselor, nursing supervisor, or other.

Nurses working in disaster situations can become overwhelmed by witnessing catastrophic loss of human life (e.g., plane crashes, school shootings) and/or mass destruction of people's homes and belongings (floods, fires, tornadoes) leaving many families bereft of a sense of stability, well-being, and shelter. Disaster nurses need both supportive ties and access to debriefing. Debriefing is an important step for staff in coming to terms with overwhelming violent, or otherwise disastrous situations once they are

over. It helps staff place the crisis in perspective and begin healing themselves. Chapter 23 discusses this further.

Assessment Guidelines

> **ASSESSMENT GUIDELINES: CRISIS**
>
> 1. Identify whether the client's response to the crisis warrants psychiatric treatment or hospitalization to minimize decompensation (suicidal behavior, psychotic thinking, violent behavior).
> 2. Do the nurse and client have a clear understanding of the *precipitating* event?
> 3. Assess the client's understanding of his or her present *situational supports*.
> 4. What *coping styles* does the client usually use? What coping mechanisms may help the situation in the present?
> 5. Are there certain religious or cultural beliefs that need to be considered in assessing and intervening in this person's crisis?
> 6. Is this situation one in which the client needs primary (education, environmental manipulation, or new coping skills), secondary (crisis intervention), or tertiary (rehabilitation) intervention?

NURSING DIAGNOSIS

A person in crisis may exhibit various behaviors that indicate a number of human problems. For example, when a person is in crisis, the nursing diagnosis of ineffective coping is often evident. Because anxiety levels may escalate to moderate or severe levels, the ability to solve problems is usually impaired, if it is present at all. **Ineffective coping** may be evidenced by inability to meet basic needs, inability to meet role expectations, alteration in social participation, use of inappropriate defense mechanisms, or impairment of usual patterns of communication. See Table 22–2 for some signs and symptoms of people in crisis that may be used as a guide for identifying potential nursing diagnoses.

The assessment of Laura's (1) perception of the precipitating event, (2) situational supports, and (3) personal coping skills gives the nurse enough data to formulate two diagnoses and to work with Laura in setting goals and planning interventions.

EXAMPLE: NURSING DIAGNOSIS FOR LAURA

The nurse formulates the following nursing diagnoses:

■ *Anxiety (moderate/severe):* related to rape-trauma syndrome, as evidenced by ineffectual problem solving and feelings of impending doom.

TABLE 22–1 *Common Problems Faced by Beginning Practitioners*

EXAMPLES	RESULTS	INTERVENTIONS	OUTCOME
Problem 1: *Nurse needs to feel needed.* **Feels total responsibility to "care for" or "cure" client's problems**			
Nurse Allows excessive phone calls between sessions Gives direct advice without sufficient knowledge of client's situation Attempts to influence life style of client on a judgmental basis	Client becomes more dependent on nurse and relies less on own abilities Nurse reacts to client's not getting "cured" or taking advice by projecting feelings of frustration and anger onto client	Nurse Evaluates with an experienced professional nurse's needs versus client's needs Discourages dependency by client Encourages goal setting and problem solving by client Takes control only if suicide or homicide is a possibility	Client is free to grow and problem-solve own life crises Nurse's skills and effectiveness grow as comfort with role and own goals are clarified
Problem 2: *Nurse sets unrealistic goals for clients.* **Goals become nurse's goals and not mutually determined goals for the client**			
Nurse Expects physically abused woman to leave battering partner Expects man who abuses alcohol to stop drinking when loss of family or job is imminent	Nurse feels anxious and responsible when expectations are not met; anxiety resulting from feelings of inadequacy are projected onto client in the form of frustration and anger	Nurse Examines with an experienced professional realistic expectations of self and client Re-evaluates client's level of functioning and works with client on his level Encourages setting of goals by client	Nurse's ability to assess and problem-solve increases as anger and frustration decrease Client feels less alienated, and a working relationship can ensue
Problem 3: *Nurse has difficulty dealing with suicidal client*			
Nurse selectively inattends by Denying possible clues Neglecting to follow up on verbal suicide clues Changing topic to less threatening one subject when self-destructive themes come up	Client is robbed of opportunity to share feelings and find alternatives to intolerable situation Client remains suicidal Nurse's crisis intervention ceases to be effective	Nurse Assesses her own feelings and anxieties with help of an experienced professional Evaluates all clues or slight suspicions and acts on them, e.g., "Are you thinking of killing yourself?" If yes nurse assesses Suicide potential Need for hospitalization	Client experiences relief in sharing feelings and evaluating alternatives Suicide potential can be minimized Nurse becomes more adept at picking up clues and minimizing suicide potential
Problem 4: *Nurse has difficulty terminating after crisis has resolved*			
Nurse is tempted to work on other problems in client's life in order to prolong contact with client	Nurse steps into territory of traditional therapy without proper training or experience	Nurse Works with an experienced professional to Explore own feelings regarding separations and termination Reinforce crisis model; crisis intervention is a preventive tool, not psychotherapy Nurse becomes better able to help client with his feelings when nurse's own feelings are recognized	Client is free to go back to his life situation or request appropriate referral to work on other issues of importance to him

Data from Finkleman, A. W. (1977). The nurse therapist: Outpatient crisis intervention with the chronic psychiatric patient. *Journal of Psychosocial Nursing and Mental Health Services*, 8:27; and Wallace, M. A., and Morley, W. E. (1970). Teaching crisis intervention. *American Journal of Nursing*, 7:1484.

■ *Compromised family coping:* related to Laura's perception of inadequate understanding by her mother and fear of renewed sexual assault.

OUTCOME CRITERIA

Planning realistic client outcome is done together with the client or family. Realistic outcomes are made to fit within the person's cultural and personal values. Without the client's involvement, the outcome criteria (goals at the end of 4 to 8 weeks) may be irrelevant or unacceptable solutions to that person's crisis.

For example, a nurse new to crisis intervention who suggests that a woman leave her husband because he beats her may be surprised to find that the woman has different thoughts on what she wants as a final solution. Thus, goals are always made with the client, and they have to be congruent with clients' needs, values, and (in some instances) cultural expectations. The nurse evaluates the overall outcomes and goals for safety and works on contingency plans when necessary.

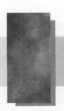

TABLE 22–2 *Potential Nursing Diagnoses for Crisis Intervention*

SYMPTOM	NURSING DIAGNOSIS
Overwhelmed, depressed, states has nothing in life worthwhile, assess self-hate and feelings of being ineffectual	**Risk for Self-Directed Violence** **Chronic Low Self-Esteem** **Spiritual Distress** **Hopelessness** **Powerlessness**
Confused, high anxiety, incoherent, crying, sobbing, extreme emotional pain	**Anxiety (moderate, severe, panic)** **Acute Confusion** **Disturbed Thought Processes** **Sleep Deprivation**
Difficulty with interpersonal relationships, isolated, few or no social supports	**Social Isolation** **Risk for Loneliness** **Impaired Social Interaction**
Unable to function at work/school/home at previous level, difficulty concentrating or completing simple tasks	**Ineffective Coping** **Interrupted Family Processes** **Caregiver Role Strain**
Presents with traumatic, emotionally overwhelming event or loss. Unable to work through overwhelming loss or event	**Risk for Post-Trauma Syndrome** **Rape-Trauma Syndrome** **Dysfunctional Grieving** **Chronic Sorrow**

Johnson et al (2000) in Table 22–3 have identified some outcomes for people having difficulty coping during a crisis.

Vignette

■ *A social worker is called. Laura, the nurse, and the social worker meet together. All agree that Laura should not be in the home if the boyfriend returns. The nurse then meets with Laura and her mother; however, Laura's mother continues to berate Laura for lying. She states that she does not care what Laura says, she has her own life to live. She says if Laura doesn't like it, she can move out.*

EXAMPLE: PLANNING THE INTERVENTION WITH LAURA

The nurse and Laura set four goals together:

1. Laura will return to her pre-crisis state within 2 weeks.
2. Laura and staff will find a safe environment for Laura, before the boyfriend comes to live with Laura's mother.
3. Laura will have at least two outside supports available within 24 hours with aid of staff.
4. Laura will have continued evaluation and support until the immediate crisis is over (6 to 8 weeks).

PLANNING

Nurses are called upon to plan and intervene through a variety of crisis intervention modalities, such as disaster nursing, mobile crisis units, group work, health education and crisis prevention, victim outreach programs, and telephone hotlines.

The nurse may be involved in planning and intervention for an individual (as in physical abuse), group (as in students in a classmate's suicide event or shooting), or community (as in disaster nursing for tornadoes, shootings, and airplane crashes).

A determination is made concerning the following questions (Aguilera 1998):

1. How much has this crisis affected the person's life? Can he or she still go to work? School? Care for family members?
2. How is the state of disequilibrium affecting significant people in his life (wife, husband, children, boss, boyfriend, girlfriend, family members)?

Data from these two questions will guide the nurse as to what kinds of immediate action to take.

TABLE 22-3   Potential Outcome Criteria for Crisis

Definition: Actions to manage stressors that tax an individual's resources

COPING	NEVER DEMONSTRATED 1	RARELY DEMONSTRATED 2	SOMETIMES DEMONSTRATED 3	OFTEN DEMONSTRATED 4	CONSISTENTLY DEMONSTRATED 5
Indicators	1	2	3	4	5
130201 Identifies effective coping patterns					
130202 Identifies ineffective coping patterns	1	2	3	4	5
130203 Verbalizes sense of control	1	2	3	4	5
130204 Reports decrease in stress	1	2	3	4	5
130205 Verbalizes acceptance of situation	1	2	3	4	5
130206 Seeks information concerning illness and treatment	1	2	3	4	5
130207 Modifies life style as needed	1	2	3	4	5
130208 Adapts to developmental changes	1	2	3	4	5
130209 Uses available social support	1	2	3	4	5
130210 Employs behaviors to reduce stress	1	2	3	4	5
130211 Identifies multiple coping strategies	1	2	3	4	5
130212 Uses effective coping strategies	1	2	3	4	5
130213 Avoids unduly stressful situations	1	2	3	4	5
130214 Verbalizes need for assistance	1	2	3	4	5
130215 Seeks professional help as appropriate	1	2	3	4	5
130216 Reports decrease in physical symptoms of stress	1	2	3	4	5
130217 Reports decrease in negative feelings	1	2	3	4	5
130218 Reports increase in psychological comfort	1	2	3	4	5
130219 Other _____ (Specify)	1	2	3	4	5

From Johnson, H., Maas, M., Meriden, M., and Moorehead, S. (2000). *Nursing outcomes classification (NOC)*, (2nd ed., p. 12). St. Louis: Mosby.

During the initial interview, the person in crisis first needs to gain a feeling of safety. Solutions to the crisis may be offered so that the client is aware of other options. Planning crisis intervention requires a creative and flexible approach through the use of traditional and nontraditional therapeutic roles. The nurse may act as educator, advisor, and model. The nurse keeps in mind that it is the client who solves the problem, not the nurse. Important assumptions when working with a person in crisis (Hoff 1995) are that

■ The person is in charge of his or her own life.
■ The person is able to make decisions.
■ The crisis counseling relationship is one between partners.

The nurse helps the client refocus to gain new perspectives on the situation. The nurse supports the client during the process of finding constructive ways to solve or cope with the problem. The client is involved in setting outcomes as well as in planning interventions.

Vignette

■ *After talking with the nurse and the social worker, Laura seems open to the possibility of going to a foster home. She also agrees to talk to a counselor at her school. The nurse sets up an appointment when she, Laura, and the counselor can meet. The nurse will continue to see Laura twice a week.*

INTERVENTION

Overall Interventions

Action is taken with the expectation that if the planned action is taken, the outcome criteria will be met (Aguilera 1998). Crisis intervention has two basic initial goals:

1. **Client safety.** External controls may be applied for protection of the person in crisis if the person is suicidal or homicidal.
2. **Anxiety reduction.** Anxiety reduction techniques are used, so that inner resources can be put into effect.

During the initial interview, the person in crisis first needs to gain a feeling of safety. Solutions to the crisis may be offered, so that the client is aware of other options. Feelings of support and hope will temporarily diminish anxiety. The nurse needs to play an active role by indicating that help is available. Help is conveyed by the competent use of crisis skills and genuine interest and support. It is not conveyed by the use of false reassurances and platitudes, such as "everything will be all right."

Crisis intervention requires a creative and flexible approach through the use of traditional therapeutic and nontraditional therapeutic roles. The nurse may act as educator, adviser, and model. See Table 22-4 for guidelines for nursing interventions.

Counseling Strategies

There are three levels of nursing care in crisis intervention: (1) primary, (2) secondary, and (3) tertiary. Psychotherapeutic nursing interventions in crisis are directed toward these three levels of care.

PRIMARY CARE. Primary care promotes mental health and reduces mental illness in order to decrease the incidence of crisis. On this level the nurse can

1. Work with an individual to recognize potential problems by evaluating the stressful life events the person is experiencing.

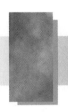

TABLE 22–4   *Overall Guidelines for Nursing Intervention*

INTERVENTION	RATIONALE
1. Assess for any suicidal or homicidal thoughts or plans.	1. Safety is always the first consideration.
2. Initial steps are taken to make the person feel safe and to lower anxiety.	2. When people feel safe and anxiety decreases, the individuals are able to problem-solve solutions with the nurse.
3. Listen carefully (e.g., make eye contact, give frequent feedback to make sure you understand, summarize what the client says at the end).	3. When people believe that someone is really listening, that can translate into someone cares about their situation and help may be available. This offers hope.
4. Crisis intervention calls for directive and creative approach. Initially, the nurse may make phone calls (arrange babysitters, visiting nurse, find shelter, social worker).	4. Initially, a client may be so confused and frightened that usual tasks are not possible at this moment.
5. Identify needed social supports (with client's input) and mobilize the most needed first.	5. Does the person need shelter; help with care for children or elders, medical work-up, emergency medical attention, hospitalization, food, safe housing, self-help group?
6. Identify needed coping skills (problem-solving skills, relaxation, assertiveness, job training, newborn care, self-esteem raising).	6. Increasing coping skills and learning new ones can help with current crisis and help minimize future crises.
7. Plan with the client interventions acceptable to both counselor and client.	7. Increases client's sense of control, self-esteem, and compliance with plan.
8. Plan regular follow-up on client's progress (e.g., phone calls, clinic visits, home visits as appropriate).	8. Evaluation of plan: what works, what doesn't work.

2. Teach an individual specific coping skills, such as decision-making, problem-solving, assertiveness skills, meditation, and relaxation skills, to handle stressful events.
3. Assist an individual to evaluate the timing or reduction of life changes in order to decrease the negative effects of stress as much as possible. This may involve working with a client to plan environmental changes, make important interpersonal decisions, and rethink changes in occupational roles.

SECONDARY CARE. Secondary care establishes intervention during an acute crisis to **prevent** prolonged anxiety from diminishing personal effectiveness and personality organization. The nurse works with the client to assess the client's problem, support systems, and coping styles. Desired goals are explored and interventions planned. Secondary care lessens the time a person is mentally disabled during a crisis. Secondary level care occurs in hospital units, emergency rooms, clinics, or mental health centers, usually during daytime hours.

TERTIARY CARE. Tertiary care provides support for those who have experienced and are now recovering from a disabling mental state. Social and community facilities that offer tertiary intervention include rehabilitation centers, sheltered workshops, day hospitals, and outpatient clinics. Primary goals are aimed at facilitating optimal levels of functioning and preventing further emotional disruptions. People with severe and persistent mental problems are often extremely susceptible to crisis, and community facilities provide the structured environment that can help prevent problem situations. Refer to Chapter 28 for crisis strategies and rehabilitation of people with severe and long-term mental illness.

McCloskey and Bulechek (2000) identify activities that are effective with people in crisis. See Box 22–2.

Vignette

■ *The nurse performs secondary crisis intervention and meets with Laura twice weekly during the next 4 weeks. Laura is motivated to work with the social worker and the nurse to find another place to live. The nurse suggests several times that Laura start to see a counselor in the outpatient clinic after the crisis is over, where she could talk about some of her pain. Laura is not interested, however, and says she will talk to the school counselor if she needs to talk.*

Three weeks after the attempted suicide, foster placement is found for Laura. The couple seems very interested in Laura, and Laura appears happy about the attention she is receiving.

Box 22–2 *Crisis Intervention*

Definition: Use of short-term counseling to help the patient cope with a crisis and resume a state of functioning comparable to or better than the precrisis state.
Activities:

■ Provide an atmosphere of support
■ Determine whether patient presents safety risk to self or others
■ Initiate necessary precautions to safeguard the patient or others at risk for physical harm
■ Encourage expression of feelings in nondestructive manner
■ Assist in identification of the precipitants and dynamics of the crisis
■ Assist in identification of past/present coping skills and their effectiveness
■ Assist in identification of personal strengths and abilities that can be used in resolving the crisis
■ Assist in development of new coping and problem solving skills, as needed
■ Assist in identification of available support system(s)
■ Introduce patient to persons (or groups) who have successfully undergone the same experience
■ Assist in identification of alternative courses of action to resolve the crisis
■ Assist in the evaluation of the possible consequences of the various courses of action
■ Assist patient to decide on a particular course of action
■ Assist in formulating a time frame for implementation of chosen course of action
■ Evaluate with patient whether crisis has been resolved by chosen course of action
■ Plan with patient how adaptive coping skills can be used to deal with crises in the future

From McCloskey, J. C., and Bulechek, G. M (2000). *Nursing intervention classification* (3rd ed. p. 239). St. Louis: Mosby.

EVALUATION

Goals can be short term or long term and are compared with the outcomes for the effectiveness of the crisis intervention. This is usually done 4 to 8 weeks after the initial interview, although it can be done in a shorter time frame (e.g., by the end of the visit the anxiety level will go from severe to moderate). If the intervention has been successful, the person's level of anxiety and ability to function should be at pre-crisis levels. Often, a person chooses to follow up additional areas of concern, and referral to other agencies for more long-term work is arranged. Crisis intervention often serves to prepare a person for further treatment.

Vignette

■ After 6 weeks, Laura and the nurse decide that the crisis is over. Laura remains aloof and distant. The nurse evaluates Laura as being in a moderate amount of emotional pain. Laura feels she is doing well, however, and feels more secure and accepted. The nurse's assessment indicated that Laura had other serious issues (e.g., the issue of her earlier sexual assaults), and the nurse strongly suggests to Laura that she could benefit from further counseling. The decision, however, is up to Laura. Laura says she is satisfied with the way things are, and again states that if she has any problems she will see her school counselor.

Postscript: Two years later, Laura is continuing to do well in school and is planning to go to a local community college for computer programming. Laura gets along well with her foster parents, and plans are being made for adoption. Laura remains aloof. She has no close friends and continues to throw her energy into her studies. For the present, she is getting pleasure from her academic accomplishments, and she has security and warm attention in her new home environment. If at a later date she decides there are other things for her to work out, she knows the resources that are available in her community.

Visit the **Evolve** website at
http://evolve.elsevier.com/Varcarolis
for more Case Studies.

CASE STUDY 22-1   *Working With a Person in Crisis*

Ms. Greg, the psychiatric nurse consultant, was called to the neurological unit. She was told that Mr. Raymond, a 43-year-old man with Guillain-Barré syndrome, was presenting a serious nursing problem, and the staff requested a consult. The disease has caused severe muscle weakness to the point he was essentially paralyzed; however, he was able to breathe on his own.

The head nurse said that Mr. Raymond was hostile and sexually abusive to the nursing staff. His abusive language, demeaning attitude, and angry outbursts were having an adverse effect on the unit as a whole. The other nurses stated that they felt ineffective and angry and that they had tried to be patient and understanding; however, nothing seemed to get through to him. The situation had affected the morale of the staff and, the nurses believed, the quality of their care.

Mr. Raymond, an American Indian, was employed as a taxicab driver. Six months before his admission to the hospital, he had given up drinking after years of episodic alcohol abuse. He was engaged to a woman who visited him every day.

He needed a great deal of assistance with every aspect of his activities of daily living. Because his muscle weakness was so severe, he had to be turned and positioned every 2 hours. He was fed through a gastrostomy tube.

ASSESSMENT

Ms. Greg gathered data from Mr. Raymond and the nursing staff and spoke with Mr. Raymond's fiancée.

Mr. Raymond's Perception of the Precipitating Event

During the initial interview, Mr. Raymond spoke to Ms. Greg angrily, using profanity and making lewd sexual suggestions. He also expressed anger about needing a nurse to "scratch my head and help me blow my nose." He still could not figure out how his illness suddenly developed. He said the doctors told him that it was too early to know for sure if he would recover completely, but that the prognosis was good.

Mr. Raymond's Support System

Ms. Greg spoke with Mr. Raymond's fiancée. Mr. Raymond's relationships with his fiancée and with his American Indian culture group were strong. With minimal ties outside their reservation, neither Mr. Raymond nor his fiancée had much knowledge of outside supportive agencies.

Mr. Raymond's Personal Coping Skills

Mr. Raymond came from a strongly male-dominated subculture in which the man was expected to be a strong leader. His ability to be an independent person with the power to affect the direction of his life was central to his perception of being acceptable as a man.

Mr. Raymond felt powerless, out of control, and enraged. He was handling his anxiety by displacing these feelings onto the environment, namely, the staff and his fiancée. This redirection of anger temporarily lowered his anxiety and distracted him from painful feelings. When he intimidated others through sexual profanity and hostility, he felt temporarily in control and experienced an illusion of power. He used displacement to relieve his painful levels of anxiety when he felt threatened.

Mr. Raymond's use of displacement was not adaptive, because the issues causing his distress were not being resolved. His anxiety continued to escalate. The effect his behavior was having on others caused them to move away from him. This withdrawal further increased his sense of isolation and helplessness.

SELF-ASSESSMENT

Ms. Greg met with the staff twice. The staff discussed their feelings of helplessness and lack of control stemming from their feelings of rejection by Mr. Raymond. They talked of their anger about Mr. Raymond's demeaning behavior and their frustration about the situation. Ms. Greg pointed out to the staff that Mr. Raymond's feelings of helplessness, lack of control, and anger at his situation were the same feelings the staff was experiencing. Displacement of the helplessness and frustration by intimidating the staff gave Mr. Raymond a brief feeling of control. It also distracted him from his own feelings of helplessness.

The nurses became more understanding of the motivation for the behavior Mr. Raymond employed to cope with moderate to severe levels of anxiety. The staff began to focus more on the client and less on personal reactions, and decided together on two approaches they could try as a group. First, they would not take Mr. Raymond's behavior personally. Second, Mr. Raymond's feelings that were displaced would be refocused back to him.

NURSING DIAGNOSIS

On the basis of her assessment, Ms. Greg identified three main problem areas in order of importance and formulated the following nursing diagnoses:

1. **Ineffective coping** related to inadequate coping methods, as evidenced by inappropriate use of defense mechanism (displacement)

   ■ Anger directed toward staff and fiancée
   ■ Profanity and crude sexual remarks aimed at staff

   ■ Frustration and withdrawal on the part of the staff
   ■ Continued escalation of anxiety

2. **Powerlessness** related to cultural differences and lack of control over his health care environment, as evidenced by frustration over inability to perform previously uncomplicated tasks

   ■ Angry over nurses' having to "scratch my head and blow my nose"
   ■ Minimal awareness of available supports in larger community

Case Study continued on following page

3. **Ineffective coping** related to exhaustion of staff supportive capacity toward client, as evidenced by staff withdrawal and limited personal communication with client

■ Staff felt ineffective.
■ Morale of staff was poor.
■ Nurses believed that the quality of their care was adversely affected.

OUTCOME CRITERIA

Ms. Greg spoke to Mr. Raymond and told him she would like to spend time with him for 15 minutes every morning and talk about his concerns. She suggested that there might be alternative ways he could handle his feelings, and community resources could be explored. Mr. Raymond gruffly agreed, saying "You can visit me, if it will make you feel better." They made arrangements to meet at 7:30 AM for 15 minutes each morning.

For each nursing diagnosis the following outcomes were set:

NURSING DIAGNOSIS	SHORT-TERM GOAL
1. **Ineffective coping** related to inadequate coping methods, as evidenced by inappropriate use of defense mechanisms (displacement)	1. Mr. Raymond will be able to name and discuss at least two feelings about his illness and lack of mobility (by the end of the week).
2. **Powerlessness related** to lack of control over health care environment, as evidenced by frustration over inability to perform previous tasks	2. Mr. Raymond will be able to name two community organizations that could offer him information and support (by the end of 2 weeks).
3. **Ineffective coping** related to exhaustion of staff supportive capacity toward client, as evidenced by staff withdrawal and limited personal communication	3. Staff and nurse consultant will discuss reactions and alternative nursing responses to Mr. Raymond's behavior (twice within the next 7 days).

PLANNING

Ms. Greg created a nursing care plan (Nursing Care Plan 22–1) and shared it with the staff.

INTERVENTION

The following morning, Ms. Greg went into Mr. Raymond's room at 7:30 AM and sat by his bedside. At first, Mr. Raymond's comments were hostile.

DIALOGUE	THERAPEUTIC TOOL/COMMENT
Nurse: Mr. Raymond, I'm here as we discussed. I'll be spending 15 minutes with you every morning. We could use this time to talk about some of your concerns.	Nurse offers herself as a resource, gives information, and clarifies her role and client expectations. Night was the most difficult time for Mr. Raymond. In the early morning he would be the most vulnerable and open for therapeutic intervention and support.
Mr. R: Listen, sweetheart, my only concern is how to get a little sexual relief, get it?	

Nurse:	Being hospitalized and partially paralyzed can be overwhelming for anyone. Perhaps you wish you could find some relief from your situation.	Nurse focuses on the process "need for relief" and not the sexual content. Encourages discussion of feelings. Sexual issues are often challenging to new nurses, and discussing your feelings and appropriate interventions with an experienced professional is important for your own growth and to the quality of the care you give.
Mr. R:	What do you know, Ms. Know-it-all? I can't even scratch my nose without getting one of those fools to do it for me . . . and half the time those bitches aren't even around.	
Nurse:	It must be difficult to have to ask people to do everything for you.	Nurse restates what the client says in terms of his feelings. Continues to refocus away from the environment back to the client.
Mr. R:	Yeah . . . the other night a fly got into the room and kept landing on my face. I had to shout for 5 minutes before one of those bitches came in, just to take the fly out of the room.	
Nurse:	Having to rely on others for everything can be a terrifying experience for anyone. It sounds extremely frustrating for you.	Nurse acknowledges that frustration and anger would be a normal and healthy response for anyone in this situation. Encourages the client to talk about these feelings instead of acting them out.
Mr. R:	Yeah . . . it's a bitch . . . like a living hell.	

Ms. Greg continued to spend time with Mr. Raymond in the mornings. He was gradually able to talk more about his feelings of anger and frustration and was less apt to act with hostility toward the staff. As he began to feel more in control, he became less defensive about others caring for him.

After 2 weeks, Ms. Greg cut her visits down to twice a week. Mr. Raymond was beginning to get gross motor movements back but was not walking yet. He still displaced much of his frustration and lack of control on the environment, but he was better able to acknowledge the reality of his situation. He could identify what he was feeling and talk about those feelings briefly.

Case Study continued on following page

CASE STUDY 22-1	*Working With a Person in Crisis* *(Continued)*

	DIALOGUE	**THERAPEUTIC TOOL/COMMENT**
	Nurse: What's happening? Your face looks tense this morning, Mr. Raymond.	Nurse observes the client's clenched fists, rigid posture, and tense facial expression.
	Mr. R: I had to wait 10 minutes for a bedpan last night.	
	Nurse: And you're angry about that.	Nurse verbalizes the implied.
	Mr. R: Well, there were only two nurses on duty for 30 people, and the aide was on her break . . . You can't expect them to be everywhere . . . but still . . .	
	Nurse: It may be hard to accept that people can't be there all the time for you.	Nurse validates the difficulty of accepting situations one does not like when one is powerless to make changes.
	Mr. R: Well . . . that's the way it is in this place.	

EVALUATION	After 6 weeks, Mr. Raymond was able to get around with assistance, and his ability to perform his activities of daily living was increasing. Although Mr. Raymond was still angry and still felt overwhelmed at times, he was able to identify more of his feelings. He did not need to act them out so often. He was able to talk to his fiancée about his feelings, and he lashed out at her less. He was looking forward to going home, and his boss was holding his old job. Mr. Raymond contacted the Guillain-Barré Society, who made arrangements	for a meeting with him. He was still thinking about Alcoholics Anonymous but believed he could handle this problem himself. The staff felt more comfortable and competent in their relationships with Mr. Raymond. The goals had been met. Mr. Raymond and Ms. Greg both believed that the crisis was over, and the visits were terminated. Mr. Raymond was given the number of the crisis unit and encouraged to call if he had questions or felt the need to talk.

Visit the **Evolve** website at
http://evolve.elsevier.com/Varcarolis
for the other Nursing Care Plan diagnoses and for
more Nursing Care Plans.

NURSING CARE PLAN 22–1   A Person in Crisis: Mr. Raymond

NURSING DIAGNOSIS

Ineffective coping: related to inadequate coping methods, as evidenced by inappropriate use of defense mechanisms (displacement).

Supporting Data

- Anger directed at staff and fiancée
- Profanity and crude sexual remarks aimed at staff
- Isolation related to staff withdrawal
- Continued escalation of anxiety

Outcome Criteria: By discharge, Mr. Raymond will state he feels more comfortable discussing difficult feelings.

SHORT-TERM GOAL	INTERVENTION	RATIONALE	EVALUATION
1. Mr. Raymond will be able to name and discuss at least two feelings about his illness and lack of mobility (by the end of the week).	1a. Nurse will meet with client for 15 minutes at 7:30 AM each day for a week.	1a. Night was usually the most frightening for client; in early morning, feelings were closer to surface.	*GOAL MET* Within 7 days, Mr. Raymond was able to speak to nurse more openly about feelings of anger and frustration.
	1b. When client lashes out with verbal abuse, nurse will remain calm.	1b. Client perceives that nurse is in control of her feelings. This can be reassuring to client and can increase client's sense of security.	
	1c. Nurse will consistently redirect and refocus anger from environment back to client, e.g., "It must be difficult to be in this situation."	1c. Refocusing feelings offers client opportunity to cope effectively with his anxiety and decreases need to act out toward staff and fiancée.	
	1d. Nurse will come on time each day and stay for allotted time.	1d. Consistency sets stage for trust and reinforces that client's anger will not drive nurse away.	

Nursing Care Plan continued on following page

NURSING CARE PLAN 22–1   A *Person in Crisis*: Mr. Raymond *(Continued)*

NURSING DIAGNOSIS

Powerlessness: related to health care environment, as evidenced by frustration over inability to perform previous tasks.

Supporting Data

■ Angry over nurses having to "scratch my head and help me blow my nose"
■ Minimal awareness of available supports in larger community

Outcome Criteria: By discharge, Mr. Raymond will have contacted at least one outside community support.

SHORT-TERM GOAL	INTERVENTION	RATIONALE	EVALUATION
1. By end of 2 weeks, Mr. Raymond will be able to name at least two community organizations that can offer information and support.	1a. Nurse will spend time with client and his fiancée. Role of specific agencies and how they may be of use will be discussed.	1a. Both client and fiancée will have opportunity to ask questions with nurse present.	*GOAL MET* By end of 10 days, Mr. Raymond and his fiancée could name two community resources they were interested in. At end of 6 weeks, Mr. Raymond had contacted the Guillain-Barré Society.
	1b. Nurse will introduce one agency at a time.	1b. Gradual introduction allows time for information to sink in and minimizes feeling of being pressured or overwhelmed.	
	1c. Nurse will follow up but not push or persuade client to contact any of the agencies.	1c. Client is able to make own decisions once he has appropriate information.	

SUMMARY

A crisis is not a pathological state but a struggle for emotional balance. It can offer the opportunity for emotional growth, or it can lead to possible personality disorganization. Early intervention during a time of crisis greatly increases the possibility of a successful outcome. There are three types of crisis: maturational, situational, and adventitious, as well as specific phases in its development. Crisis and crisis intervention are based on certain assumptions:

1. A crisis is usually resolved within 4 to 6 weeks.
2. Crisis intervention therapy is short term, from 1 to 6 weeks, and focuses on the present problem only.

3. Resolution of a crisis takes three forms: a person emerges at a higher level, at pre-crisis level, or at a lower level of functioning.
4. Social support and intervention can maximize successful resolution.
5. Crisis therapists take an active and directive approach with the client in crisis.
6. The client takes an active role in setting goals and planning possible solutions.

Traditionally, crisis intervention is aimed at the mentally healthy person who is functioning well but is temporarily overwhelmed and unable to function. However, people who have long-term and persistent mental problems are also susceptible to crisis, and the crisis model can be adapted for their needs also.

The steps in crisis intervention are consistent with the nursing process (assessment, nursing diagnosis, identifying expected outcomes, planning, intervention, and evaluation). Each has specific goals and tasks.

Specific qualities in the nurse that can facilitate effective intervention are a caring attitude, flexibility in planning care, an ability to listen, and an active approach.

Nurses' ability to be aware of their own feelings and thoughts is crucial in working with a person in crisis. The availability of peer supports and supervision to discuss the questions that normally arise is essential for the beginning crisis counselor. Learning crisis intervention is a process, and there are certain problems all health care professionals must deal with to improve their skills.

The basic goals of crisis intervention are to reduce the individual's anxiety level and to support the effort to return to the person's pre-crisis level of functioning.

Visit the **Evolve** website at
http://evolve.elsevier.com/Varcarolis
for a post-test on the content in this chapter.

Visit the **Evolve** website at
http://evolve.elsevier.com/Varcarolis
for additional self-study exercises.

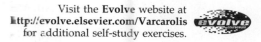

Critical Thinking and Chapter Review

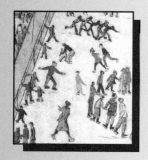

Critical Thinking

Write a short paragraph in response to the following:

1. After you determine whether a person is homicidal or suicidal or both, identify the three important areas in the assessment. Give examples of two questions in each area that need to be answered before planning can take place.

2. Clara, 22, a senior in nursing school, tells her nursing instructor that her mother (aged 45) has just lost her job. Clara's mother has been drinking heavily for years and tells Clara she can't cope anymore; she wants to leave and "find herself." Clara has a 12-year-old sister, Joy, and her mother tells Clara that it is time for Clara to start taking some responsibility and earning a living. Clara's father was killed 8 years ago in a hit-and-run accident by a drunken driver.

   A. How many different types of crises are going on with this family? Discuss the crises in light of each individual in this family.

   B. If this family came for crisis counseling, what areas would you assess and what kinds of questions would you ask in order to assess each member's individual needs and the needs of the family as a unit (perception of event, coping styles, social supports)?

   C. Formulate some tentative goals you might set in conjunction with the family.

D. Identify and name appropriate referral agencies in your area that would be useful if this family were willing to expand their resources and stabilize.

E. How would you set up follow-up visits for this family? Would you see them together, alone, or in a combination during the crisis period (4 to 6 weeks)? How would you decide whether follow-up counseling was indicated?

Chapter Review

1. Which statement about crisis theory will provide a basis for nursing intervention?

   1. A crisis is an acute, time-limited phenomenon experienced as an overwhelming emotional reaction to a problem perceived as unsolvable.
   2. A person in crisis has always had adjustment problems and has coped inadequately in his/her usual life situations.
   3. Crisis is precipitated by an event that enhances the person's self-concept and self-esteem.
   4. Nursing intervention in crisis situations rarely has the effect of ameliorating the crisis.

2. Mrs. T, a single mother of four, comes to the crisis center 24 hours after an apartment fire in which all the family's household goods and clothing were lost. Mrs. T. has no family in the area. Her efforts to mobilize assistance have been disorganized and she is still without shelter. She is distraught and confused. The nurse assesses the situation as

   1. a maturational crisis
   2. a situational crisis
   3. an adventitious crisis
   4. evidence of an inadequate personality

3. Mrs. T, an advertising copywriter and single mother of four, comes to the crisis center 16 hours after an apartment fire in which all the family's household goods and clothing were lost. Mrs. T. has no family in the area. Her efforts to mobilize assistance have been disorganized and ineffectual. She is still without shelter. She is distraught and confused. The intervention that takes priority would be

   1. anxiety reduction
   2. arrange shelter
   3. contact out-of-area family
   4. hospitalize and place on suicide precautions

4. Which belief would be LEAST helpful for the nurse working in crisis intervention to hold?

   1. A person in crisis is incapable of making decisions.
   2. The crisis counseling relationship is one between partners.
   3. Crisis counseling helps the client refocus to gain new perspectives on the situation.
   4. Anxiety reduction techniques are used so client inner resources can be accessed.

5. The priority goal of crisis intervention is

   1. client safety
   2. anxiety reduction
   3. identification of situational supports
   4. teaching specific coping skills that are lacking

NURSE, CLIENT, AND FAMILY RESOURCES

Associations

Emotions Anonymous
P.O. Box 4245
St. Paul, MN 55104-0245
1-612-647-9712
(12-step program of recovery from emotional difficulties)

Workaholics Anonymous
P.O. Box 289
Menlo Park, CA 94026-0289
1-510-273-9253
(12-step program of recovery from compulsive overworking)

Red Cross Disaster Mental Health Services (DMHS)
Contact local Red Cross for information

Internet Sites

Alliance for Psychosocial Nursing
http://www.psychnurse.org

NAMI (National Alliance for the Mentally Ill)
http://www.nami.org

Mental Health Net
http://mentalhelp.net

REFERENCES

Aguilera, D. C. (1998). *Crisis intervention: Theory and methodology* (8th ed.). St. Louis: Mosby.

Aguilera, D., and Mesnick, J. (1970). *Crisis intervention: Theory and methodology* St. Louis: Mosby.

Caplan, G. (1964). *Symptoms of preventive psychiatry*. New York: Basic Books.

Cole, M. S., Fravjo, L. do C., Coehlo, A. A., et al. (2000). Social violence: A case for classification as a sub-phenomenon of community in the ICNP. *International Nursing Review*, 47(1): 8–13.

Croushore, T., et al. (1981). *Using crisis intervention wisely*. Philadelphia: Nursing 3_ Books, Intermed Communications.

Doenges, M., and Moorehouse, M. (1988). *Nurses' pocket guide: Nursing diagnoses with interventions* (2nd ed.). Philadelphia: F. A. Davis.

Donlon, F. T., and Rockwell, D. A. (1982). *Psychiatric disorders, diagnosis and treatment*. Bowie, MD: Robert J. Brady.

Ewing, C. P. (1978). *Crisis intervention as psychotherapy*. New York: Oxford University Press.

Finkelman, A. W. (1977). The nurse therapist: Outpatient crisis intervention with the chronic patient. *Journal of Psychosocial Nursing and Mental Health Services*, 8:27.

Garrison, C. Z., et al. (1995). Posttraumatic stress disorder in adolescents after Hurricane Andrew. *Journal of American Academy of Child and Adolescent Psychiatry*, 34(9):1193.

Goenjian, A. K., et a . (1995). Psychiatric comorbidity in children after the 1988 earthquake in Armenia. *Journal of American Academy of Child and Adolescent Psychiatry*, 34(9):1174.

Hoff, L. A. (1989). *People in crisis: Understanding and helping* (3rd ed.). Menlo Park, CA: Addison-Wesley.

Hoff, L. A. (1995). *People in crisis: Understanding and helping* (4th ed.). San Francisco: Jossey-Bass.

Holmes, T. H., and Masuda, M. (1972). Psychosomatic syndrome. *Psychology Today*, April:72.

Holmes, T. H., and Rahe, R. H. (1967). The social readjustment rating scale. *Journal of Psychosomatic Research*, 11(2):213–218.

Hospital Security and Safety Management. (1999). *Dealing with school shootings, violence: How Jonesboro and Denver hospitals met this new challenge to emergency preparedness*. 20(4):5–10.

Karanci, A. N., and Rustemli, A. (1995). Psychological consequences of the 1992 Erzincan (Turkey) earthquake. *Disasters*, 19(1):8.

King, J. M. (1971). The initial interview: Basis for assessment in crisis intervention. *Perspectives in Psychiatric Care*, 6:247.

Leach, J. (1995). Psychological first aid: A practical aide-memoire. *Aviation, Space and Environmental Medicine*, 66(7):668.

Miller, M. A., and Rahe, R. H. (1997). Life changes scaling for the 1990s. *Journal of Psychosomatic Research*, 43(3):279–292.

Robinson, L. (1973). Psychiatric emergencies. *Nursing* 73(7):43.

Stringham, P. (1999). Domestic violence. *Primary Care*, June, 26(2): 373–384.

Urano, R. J., et al. (1995). Longitudinal assessment of posttraumatic stress disorder and depression after exposure to traumatic death. *Journal of Nervous and Mental Disorders*, 183(1):36.

Wallace, M. A., and Morley, W. E. (1970). Teaching crisis intervention. *American Journal of Nursing*, 7:1484.

Outline

PREVALENCE

COMORBIDITY

THEORY

Psychobiological Factors

Biochemical-Genetic Theories

Application of the Nursing Process

ASSESSMENT

Overall Assessment

Verbal and Nonverbal Clues

Lethality of Suicide Plan

High-Risk Factors

Assessment Tools

Self-Assessment

Assessment Guidelines

NURSING DIAGNOSIS

OUTCOME CRITERIA

PLANNING

INTERVENTION

Overall Guidelines for Nursing Interventions

Hospitalized: Put on Suicide Precautions

Outside the Hospital

Counseling

Community

Hospital

Telephone Hotlines

Health Teaching

Milieu Therapy

Psychobiological Interventions

Psychotherapy

Suicidal Person

Family

Survivors of Completed Suicide: Postvention

Counselors and Nursing Staff: Postvention

EVALUATION

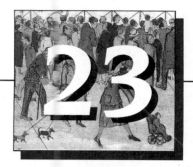

23

Suicide

Elizabeth M. Varcarolis

Objectives

After studying this chapter, the reader will be able to

1. Describe the profile of suicide in the United States, professions at risk, most common psychopathology, and populations at risk.

2. Identify common precipitating events.

3. Role-play two verbal and two nonverbal clues that might signal suicidal ideation.

4. Using the SAD PERSONS scale, explain ten risk factors to consider when assessing for suicide.

5. Describe three expected reactions a nurse may have when beginning work with suicidal clients.

6. Give examples of primary, secondary, and tertiary (postvention) interventions.

7. Distinguish among the interventions that a nurse may carry out (a) in the community, (b) in the hospital, and (c) on a telephone hotline.

8. Formulate a "no-suicide contract."

9. Develop a care plan for a teenage client (a) in the hospital, and (b) in the community.

PREVALENCE

Suicide ranks as the eighth leading cause of death in the United States, and there are about 75 suicides a day, or one every 20 minutes, and more than 30,000 each year (Roy, 1999). The suicide rate remained fairly stable from 1983 to 1998; however, the rate for 15- to 24-year-olds has increased two to threefold. The elderly (age 65 and over) have the highest risk of committing suicide—50% higher than for teenagers or the national average (Roy, 1999). Box 23–1 provides information on prevalence within discrete populations. Figure 23–1 shows the U.S. suicide rate by age, gender, and racial groups.

COMORBIDITY

Suicide is not a disorder per se, but it does appear to have a higher rate of occurrence among a number of psychiatric disorders that can be viewed as a risk factor for suicide:

- Depressive disorders — *MDD Bipolar*
- Schizophrenia
- Alcohol use disorder/substance abuse (e.g., cocaine)
- Borderline and antisocial personality disorder
- Panic disorder (20% of persons with panic disorder have made a suicide attempt at one time [NIMH])
- Organic mental disorder

Some victims of **completed suicide** may have two or more diagnoses according to the *Diagnostic and Statistical Manual of Mental Disorders*, for example, e.g., major depression (MD) and substance abuse. It is, however, important to keep in mind that suicide is not necessarily synonymous with a mental disorder. The act of purposeful self-destruction represented by taking one's own life is usually accompanied by intense feelings of pain and loneliness, coupled with the belief that there are no solutions to the pain and isolation and total hopelessness, as exemplified in the following suicide note:

> I'm sorry for the grief I've caused you. I am just in too much pain to go on—I can't take it anymore. I have no love in my life and I have nothing to live for. I am so sorry. . . .

Box 23–1 *Suicide Facts*

- Suicide is the eighth leading cause of death in the United States.
- Suicide is the third leading cause of death among young people 15 to 24 years of age, following unintentional injuries and homicide.
- Suicide outnumbers homicide by 3 to 2.
- Suicide by firearms is the most common method for both men and women. *including youth*
- More men than women die by suicide.
  - The gender ratio is 4:1.
  - 72% of all suicides are committed by white men.
  - 79% of all firearm suicides are committed by white men.
- The highest suicide rates are for white men over age 85, who had a rate of 65/100,000.
- Suicide is the fourth leading cause of death for children between the ages of 10 and 14 years.
- Professional persons (lawyers, dentists, military men, and physicians) have a higher than average suicide rate.
- Native Americans and Alaskan Natives have long had elevated suicide rates.
- Suicide among African American males aged 15 to 19 years has increased 105% between 1980 and 1996; 100% increase in the group is attributable to firearms.
- Most elderly suicides have visited their primary care physician a month before their suicide.

ATTEMPTED SUICIDES

- No national data on attempted suicides are available; reliable scientific research, however, has found that:
  - More women than men report a history of attempted suicide, with a gender ratio of 2:1.
  - The **strongest risk factors** for attempted suicide in **adults** are depression, alcohol abuse, cocaine use, separation or divorce, and physical illness.
  - The **strongest risk factors** for attempted suicide in **youth** are depression, alcohol or other drug use disorder, and aggressive or disruptive behaviors (antisocial personality disorder).

Adapted from: NIMH Suicide Facts (1997) and Surgeon General's Call to Action to Prevent Suicide 1999 (Dept. of Health and Human Services).

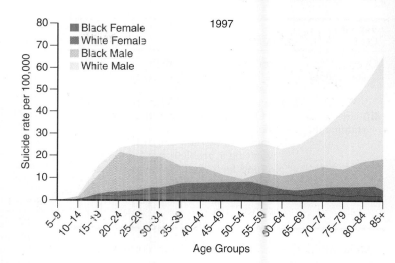

Figure 23–1 U.S. suicide rates by age, gender, and racial group. (From National Institute of Mental Health Data: Centers for Disease Control and Prevention, National Center for Health Statistics.)

THEORY

Psychobiological Factors

A central underlying psychobiological factor to suicide intent is hopelessness (Ghosh and Victor, 1999; Beck, et al. 1990). Contemporary suicidologists believe that the suicidal persons most likely to act out their fantasies are those who (Roy, 1999):

■ Have suffered a loss of love
■ Have suffered a narcissistic injury (humiliation, loss of job, threat of incarceration)
■ Experience overwhelming moods such as rage or guilt
■ Identify with a suicide victim (suicide contagion/copycat suicide)

Group dynamics underlie mass suicides such as those of the Heaven's Gate massacre (March 1997) and the Jonestown tragedy (November 1978).

Biochemical-Genetic Theories

Suicide behavior seems to run in some families. For example, Margaux Hemingway's 1997 suicide death was the fifth suicide among four generations of Ernest Hemingway's family. However, it is difficult to distinguish biochemical or genetic predisposition to suicide from predisposition to depression or alcoholism. Both of these disorders run in families and most likely have a genetic component.

Twin studies and adoption studies suggest the presence of genetic factors in suicide. For example, Roy and associates (1999) demonstrated that the suicide concurrence rate was higher for monozygotic twins than for dizygotic twins. Studies examining biological relatives of adoptees who committed suicide found a significantly higher incidence of suicide than in the biological relatives of control subjects (Schulsinger et al., 1979).

Low levels of the neurotransmitter serotonin (5-HT) are thought to play a part in the decision to commit suicide. Low serotonin levels are related to depressed moods. In a study of people hospitalized for suicide attempts, those with low serotonin levels were more likely to commit suicide than those with normal levels (Roy, 1995). A study by Pandey and colleagues (1995) observed a higher number of serotonin-2 receptors (5-HT-2) in both the brain and platelets of suicidal patients. Therefore, it is possible that 5-HT-2 receptors may represent biological markers for identifying suicide-prone patients. A study of violent suicide attempts demonstrated lower cerebrospinal fluid (CSF) levels of 5-H1AA as well as higher levels of 3-methyl-4-hydroxyphenyl-glycol (MHPG) (Schulsinger et al., 1979).

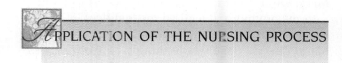

APPLICATION OF THE NURSING PROCESS

ASSESSMENT

Overall Assessment

VERBAL AND NONVERBAL CLUES

Almost all people considering suicide send out clues, especially to people they think of as supportive. Nurses often fit this category. Clues may be verbal, behavioral, somatic, or emotional.

VERBAL CLUES	EXAMPLES
Overt statements	"I can't take it anymore." "Life isn't worth living anymore." "I wish I were dead." "Everyone would be better off if I died."
Covert statements	"It's OK now, soon everything will be fine." "Things will never work out." "I won't be a problem much longer." "Nothing feels good to me anymore, and probably never will." "How can I give my body to medical science?"

Most often it is a relief for people contemplating suicide to finally talk to someone about their despair and loneliness. **Asking someone if he or she is thinking of suicide does *not* "give a person ideas."** Self-destructive ideas are a personal decision. Making covert indications of suicide overt *does* make possible a decrease in isolation and can increase problem-solving alternatives for living. People who attempt suicide, even those who regret the failure of their attempt, are often extremely receptive to talking about their suicide crisis. Often people express gratitude for the opportunity to talk to someone (Rives, 1999). Specific questions to ask include the following (Stevenson, 1988):

■ Are you experiencing thoughts of suicide?
■ Have you ever had thoughts of suicide in the past?
■ Have you ever attempted suicide?
■ Do you have a plan for committing suicide?
■ If so, what is your plan for suicide?

The following dialogue illustrates how the nurse can make covert messages overt:

Nurse: You haven't eaten or slept well for the past few days, Mary.
Mary: No, I feel pretty low lately.
Nurse: How low are you feeling?
Mary: Oh, I don't know. Nothing seems to matter to me anymore. It's all so meaningless. . . .
Nurse: What is meaningless, Mary?
Mary: Life . . . the whole thing . . . nothingness. Life is a bad joke.
Nurse: Are you saying that you don't think life is worth living?
Mary: Well . . . yes. It's all so hopeless anyway.
Nurse: Are you thinking of killing yourself, Mary?
Mary: Oh, I don't know. Well, sometimes I think about it. I probably would never go through with it.
Nurse: Let's talk more about what you are thinking and feeling. Since this is important, Mary, I will need to share your thoughts with other members of the staff.

Be alert for behavioral clues, somatic clues, and emotional clues.

BEHAVIORAL CLUES	EXAMPLES
Sudden behavioral changes may be noted, especially when depression is lifting and when the person has more energy available to carry out a plan.	Signs include giving away prized personal possessions, writing farewell notes, making out a will, and putting personal affairs in order.

SOMATIC CLUES	EXAMPLES
Physiological complaints can mask psychological pain and internalized stress.	Symptoms associated with chronic stress include headaches, muscle aches, difficulty sleeping, irregular bowel habits, unusual appetite, and weight loss.

EMOTIONAL CLUES	EXAMPLES
Various emotions can signal possible suicidal ideation.	Symptoms include social withdrawal, feelings of hopelessness and helplessness, confusion, irritability, and complaints of exhaustion.

LETHALITY OF SUICIDE PLAN

The evaluation of a suicide plan is extremely important in determining the degree of suicidal risk. Three main elements must be considered when evaluating the lethality of a suicide plan: (1) specificity of details; (2) lethality of the proposed method; and (3) availability of means (Farberow, 1967). People who have definite plans for the time, place, and means are at high risk. Someone who is considering suicide but has not thought about when, where, or how is at a lower risk.

The lethality of method, indicating how quickly a person would die by that method, thereby lessening the probability of intervention, also indicates the level of risk. Higher-risk methods, also referred to as "hard" methods, include

■ Using a gun.
■ Jumping off a high place.
■ Hanging.
■ Carbon monoxide poisoning.
■ Staging a car crash.

Example of lower-risk methods, also referred to as "soft" methods, include

■ Slashing one's wrists.
■ Inhaling natural gas.
■ Ingesting pills.

When the means are available, the situation is more serious. For example, a man who has access to a high building and states that he will jump from it, or a woman who has a gun and says that she will shoot herself, is a serious risk. When people are psychotic, they are at high risk regardless of the specificity of details, lethality of method, and availability of means, because impulse control, judgment, and thinking are all grossly impaired. A psychotic person is particularly vulnerable if experiencing command hallucinations.

HIGH-RISK FACTORS

Data gathered from numerous studies have identified risk factors. The act of suicide may be precipitated by many internal, external, and coexisting conditions and events. Studies in the literature find that social isolation and severe life events often precede a suicide attempt.

Teenagers often feel invincible and may act out with risky behavior and may believe they will not die if a chance that could cause death is taken. Some teens may romanticize risk taking without understanding the consequences of their behavior and could die.

Suicide by imitation appears to be particularly marked in sensationalized, insensitive, and inappropriate coverage (CDC, 1994). A workshop sponsored by the CDC (1994) proposed guidelines for responsible and factual presentation and reporting of suicide events. Repetitive, ongoing, and/or prominent coverage of a suicide "tends to promote and maintain preoccupation with suicide among at-risk persons, especially among persons 15–24 years of age" (CDC, 1994). The baseline rate of suicidal behavior may increase for several weeks after the dramatization.

A phenomenon among adolescents and young adults is suicide contagion or copycat suicide. Suicidal behavior increases in adolescents following an extensively publicized story of a suicide (often a public figure or a teen idol), or geographically in a community after a publicized suicide of a younger person (Pataki, 1999).

SOCIAL ISOLATION. Suicidal individuals frequently have difficulty forming and maintaining relationships. Usually there is a high rate of divorce, separation, or single marital status. Norman Cousins maintains that all human history is an endeavor to shatter loneliness. He tells the story of a woman who had committed suicide. She had written in her diary every day during the week before her death, "Nobody called today, nobody called today, nobody called today" (Mowshowitz, 1984).

SEVERE LIFE EVENTS. Severe life events often precede a suicide attempt. Paykel and colleagues (1975) found that people who attempted suicide were four times as likely to suffer severe life events (e.g., divorce, death, sickness, blows to self-esteem,

legal problems, interpersonal discord) in the 6 months before their attempts as people in the general population. Having serious arguments with a spouse, having a new person in the home (baby, elderly parent), and having to appear in court were more frequent occurrences for persons who attempted suicide than for nonsuicidal persons (Hoff, 1995). A study by Parker (1988) found that adolescents attempting suicide experienced more life changes than other adolescents and had a history of emotional illness in the family.

Disadvantageous childhood and family circumstances can lend increased risk and vulnerability to adolescent suicidal behaviors (Fergusson and Lynsky, 1995). Low self-esteem is closely related to feelings of depression and hopelessness and suicidal tendencies. Assessment of adolescents should include an evaluation of self-esteem, and therapies should include the targeting of self-esteem deficits.

An important, previously unrecognized risk factor in jail suicide is the charge of manslaughter or murder, as revealed by a study by Durand and associates (1995).

The Surgeon General's Call to Action to Prevent Suicide 1999 identifies specific risk factors, many of which have been mentioned. The reader is urged to review the protective factors against suicide as well. See Table 23–1 for a summary of risk factors compared with protective factors.

ASSESSMENT TOOLS

Many tools can be used to aid a health care worker in assessing suicidal potential. Patterson and co-workers (1983) devised an assessment aid using a brief acronym (SAD PERSONS scale) to evaluate ten major risk factors for suicide potential (Box 23–2). The SAD PERSONS assessment is a simple, clear-cut, and practical guide for gauging suicide potential. Ten categories are described in the assessment tool, and the person being evaluated is assigned one point for each applicable category. The person's total points are compared with a scale, which assists health care workers in determining whether hospital admission is necessary. The decision to admit someone to a hospital unit depends on many variables, such as whether the person (1) lives alone, (2) has access to a high-risk weapon, or (3) has attempted suicide previously.

The following scale serves as a general guideline:

POINTS	GUIDELINES FOR INTERVENTION
0–2	Treat at home with follow-up care
3–4	Closely follow up and consider possible hospitalization
5–6	Strongly consider hospitalization
7–10	Hospitalize

TABLE 23–1 *Suicide Risk vs. Protective Factors*

RISK FACTORS	PROTECTIVE FACTORS
■ Previous suicide attempt ■ Mental disorders—particularly mood disorders such as depression and bipolar ■ Co-occurring mental and alcohol and substance abuse disorders ■ Family history of suicide ■ Hopelessness ■ Impulsiveness and/or aggressive tendencies ■ Barriers to accessing mental health treatment ■ Relational, social, work, or financial loss ■ Physical illness ■ Easy access to lethal methods, especially guns ■ Unwillingness to seek help because of stigma and/or suicidal thoughts ■ Influence of significant people—family members, celebrities, peers who have died by suicide—both through direct personal contact or inappropriate media representations ■ Cultural and religious beliefs—for instance, the belief that suicide is a noble resolution of a personal dilemma ■ Local epidemics of suicide that have a contagious influence ■ Isolation, a feeling of being cut off from other people	■ Effective and appropriate clinical care for mental, physical, and substance abuse disorders ■ Easy access to a variety of clinical interventions and support for seeking help ■ Restricted access to highly lethal methods of suicide ■ Family and community support ■ Support from ongoing medical and mental health care relationships ■ Learned skills in problem solving, conflict resolution, and nonviolent handling of disputes ■ Cultural and religious beliefs that discourage suicide ■ Employed

U.S. Public Health Service (1999). The Surgeon General's call to action to prevent suicide. Washington, D.C.

BOX 23–2 *Nursing Assessment: SAD PERSONS Scale*

S	Sex	Men kill themselves three times more often than women, although women make attempts three times more often than men.
A	Age	High-risk groups: 19 years old or younger; 45 years or older, especially the elderly of 65 years or older.
D	Depression	Studies report that 35% to 79% of those who attempt suicide manifested a depressive syndrome.
P	Previous attempts	Of those who commit suicide, 65% to 70% have made previous attempts.
E	ETOH	ETOH (alcohol) is associated with up to 65% of successful suicides. Estimates are that 15% of alcoholics commit suicide. Heavy drug use is considered to be in this group and is given the same weight as alcohol.
R	Rational thinking loss	People with functional or organic psychoses are more apt to commit suicide than those in the general population.
S	Social supports lacking	A suicidal person often lacks significant others (friends, relatives), meaningful employment, and religious supports. All three of these areas need to be assessed.
O	Organized plan	The presence of a specific plan for suicide (date, place, means) signifies a person at high risk.
N	No spouse	Repeated studies indicate that persons who are widowed, separated, divorced, or single are at greater risk than those who are married.
S	Sickness	Chronic, debilitating, and severe illness is a risk factor.

Data from Patterson W., et al. (1983). Evaluation of suicidal patients: The SAD PERSONS scale. *Psychosomatics*, 24(4):343; Adam 1989; *Merck manual* 1992; Mueller and Leon, 1996.

Self-Assessment

People who are suicidal present affect and behavior that are difficult for nurses to manage effectively. *All* health care professionals who work with suicidal people need supervision and guidance by a more experienced health care professional. Most people who are suicidal experience extreme hopelessness and helplessness, are withdrawn and keenly sensitive to rejection, are ambivalent, and may be hostile and angry. Affects such as these can stir up strong negative reactions in others. Birtchnell (1983) identified in the literature numerous reactions that often arise in health care workers when working with a client who is suicidal. If these and other intense emotional responses are not made known and discussed with a more experienced practitioner, effective intervention will be limited, especially if these feelings are perceived by the suicidal client.

The universal reactions of anxiety, irritation, avoidance, and denial in any health care worker caring for a suicidal person are discussed hereafter.

ANXIETY. Anxiety may have numerous sources. However, it is important to recognize that two common sources of anxiety are activated when a nurse is working with a suicidal client. First, Birtchnell (1983) states that there are suicidal inclinations in all of us. A suicidal patient has the capacity to arouse these latent emotions and perhaps bring them out more strongly. Second, suicidal behavior or ideations on the part of the client may be interpreted by concerned health care personnel as personal rejection. Both sources of anxiety are usually working at an unconscious level. Nurses must become aware of their own anxiety and attempt to identify the source, or the unmet need or expectation. Personal anxiety can then be reduced and not transferred to the client.

IRRITATION. People who make repeated suicide attempts are often accused by family as well as health care workers of just "trying to get attention" or "looking for sympathy." It is common to hear of friends or family members out of frustration telling a suicidal person to "go ahead and get it over with." Such remarks by family and health providers strip the suicidal person of all hope and act as an encouragement to kill himself or herself. No matter how trivial the suicidal attempt may appear, it is a genuine communication that the person is despairing and is unable to find a way out of a desperate situation or state of mind.

AVOIDANCE. People who are suicidal and people who are psychotic are frequently kept at a distance and "handled with kid gloves" by both medical and nursing personnel (Birtchnell, 1983). Nurses and physicians may get caught up into taking responsibility for the actions of the suicidal person

(rescue fantasy). Then, when things do not go the way the nurse or physician would like them to go, helplessness sets in. Staff then avoid situations or people that stimulate feelings of helplessness and incompetence. When the need to feel in control and responsible for other people's decisions is lessened through experience and supervision, the nurse is better able to refocus energies back to the client.

DENIAL. Denying or minimizing suicidal ideation or gestures is a defense against experiencing the feelings aroused by a suicidal person. Denial can be seen in such statements as "I can't understand why anyone would want to take his own life." Often, family members and health care professionals are unable to acknowledge suicidal tendencies in someone close to them. Denial also occurs when identification with a suicidal person is strong, such as when a colleague commits suicide or a respected figurehead sends forth covert suicidal messages.

Assessment Guidelines

ASSESSMENT GUIDELINES: SUICIDE

1. Assess risk factors, including history of suicide (family, client, friends), degree of hopelessness, helplessness, and anhedonia; and lethality of plan.

2. If there is a history of suicide (client or family), assess

   ■ Intent: Example: Was there a high probability of being discovered or not?
   ■ Lethality: Was the method used highly lethal or less lethal?
   ■ Did the client suffer physical harm (e.g., admission to intensive care unit) or not?
   ■ How high was the lethality of the previous attempt?

3. Does client age, medical condition, or diagnosis of mental disorder (depression/substance abuse/psychosis) put him/her at higher risk?

4. Determine the appropriate level of suicide precautions for the client (physician or nurse clinician), even in the emergency room. If a client is at high risk, hospitalization may be necessary.

5. A red flag goes up if the client suddenly goes from sad/depressed to happy and seemingly peaceful. Often a decision to commit suicide "gives a way out of severe emotional pain."

6. If the client is to be managed on an outpatient basis, then:

   ■ Assess social supports.
   ■ Assess friends' and family's knowledge of signs and symptoms of potential suicide behavior (e.g., increasing withdrawal, preoccupation, silence, and remorse).
   ■ Identify community supports and groups the client and family could use for support.

NURSING DIAGNOSIS

The nursing diagnoses for a person who is suicidal may address many areas. However, the nursing diagnosis with the highest priority is **Risk for Suicide,** which may be evidenced by various emotional states. Feelings of hopelessness, anger, poor impulse control, frustration, abandonment, and rejection are common among people who are suicidal. Suicide is often related to a loss. The loss of a significant person can leave a person feeling isolated, panicky, and confused. Loss of job, status, and money, when combined with sickness, can be overwhelming. Risk for self-harm can also be related to crises in adolescents, adulthood, and the elderly. Table 23–2 identifies a number of nursing diagnoses that may apply to your suicidal client.

OUTCOME CRITERIA

The Nursing Outcome Classification (NOC) group (Johnson and associates 2000) have identified specific outcome criteria to use when working with a suicidal individual. They particularly target the nursing diagnosis **Risk for Suicide** (Table 23–3).

PLANNING

One of the most difficult decisions clinicians must make in planning care is choice of treatment setting. Does the client require hospitalization, or will an aggressive and vigilant outpatient plan provide for safety? Suicidal individuals who plan to take their own life by a specific plan and have no hope for feeling better require immediate hospitalization. The presence of a prior suicide attempt is one of the best indicators of future suicide or suicide attempt, but only a few individuals who complete suicide have made prior attempts (Rives, 1999). Initiation of hospitalization for high-risk suicidal clients and determination of appropriate times for discharge have been drastically affected by managed care systems. Approval for hospitalization may be questioned or denied, and in so doing, the managed case system places the clinician in a legal and ethical dilemma. Wysoker (1999) states that "if in the clinician's professional judgment hospitalization is deemed necessary, then treatment must be pursued with the Managed Care Company" (p. 166). More and more professionals and hospitals are being held liable for their actions in the treatment of suicidal clients. Being knowledgeable about the clinical interventions for suicidal clients and the legal issues surrounding the care of these clients is imperative for psychiatric nurses (Wysoker, 1999).

The plan of care includes a good assessment of the suicidal client's risk factors. Some risk factors can be reduced by interventions for depression and substance abuse. Psychological autopsy studies have consistently shown an association between major mental illness, especially depression and alcoholism, and completed suicide (Rives, 1999). Therefore, aggressive treatment of suicidal clients with depression and/or substance abuse needs to be part of the plan.

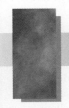

TABLE 23–2   *Potential Nursing Diagnoses—Suicidal Client*

SIGNS AND SYMPTOMS	POTENTIAL NURSING DIAGNOSES
There are overt or covert clues (e.g., I can't stand the pain), has a plan (gun), is in high-risk category on assessment (elderly/teenager, isolated, depressed, has had a recent loss), has a DSM diagnosis (substance abuse, depression, borderline personality disorder, psychosis).	Risk for Suicide
Overwhelmed with situational crises, relies heavily on drugs/alcohol, few supportive systems, poor problem-solving skills, has "tunnel vision," family not available, or crisis in the family, poor family communication.	Ineffective Coping Disabled Family Coping
Lack of hope for the future, belief that nothing can change intolerable situation, intense feelings of isolation, deprivation, lack of love, having nowhere to turn, believes that she has no control over her life or future.	Hopelessness Powerlessness Social Isolation Spiritual Distress Loneliness
Believes that he or she is no good, worthless, ineffective, a burden to others, can't do anything right.	Situational Low Self-Esteem Chronic Low Self-Esteem
Does not know where to turn, doesn't understand age-related crises, feelings of loss, depression, available resources.	Knowledge Deficit

TABLE 23-3 Suicide Self-Restraint

Definition: Self-restraint of own behaviors to avoid abuse and neglect of dependents or significant others

SUICIDE SELF-RESTRAINT	NEVER DEMONSTRATED 1	RARELY DEMONSTRATED 2	SOMETIMES DEMONSTRATED 3	OFTEN DEMONSTRATED 4	CONSISTENTLY DEMONSTRATED 5
Indicators	1	2	3	4	5
1 Expresses feelings					
2 Maintains connectedness in relationships	1	2	3	4	5
3 Seeks help when feeling self-destructive	1	2	3	4	5
4 Verbalizes suicidal ideas if present	1	2	3	4	5
5 Verbalizes control of impulses	1	2	3	4	5
6 Refrains from gathering means for suicide	1	2	3	4	5
7 Does not give away possessions	1	2	3	4	5
8 Does not require treatment for suicidal gestures or attempts	1	2	3	4	5
9 Refrains from using mood-altering substance(s)	1	2	3	4	5
10 Discloses plan for suicide if present	1	2	3	4	5
11 Upholds suicide contract	1	2	3	4	5
12 Maintains self-control without supervision	1	2	3	4	5
13 Does not attempt suicide	1	2	3	4	5
14 Other _____ (Specify)	1	2	3	4	5

Modified from: Johnson, H., Maas, M., Meriden, M., and Moorehead, S. (2000). *Nursing Outcomes Classification (NOC)*, (2nd ed.) (p. 410). St. Louis: Mosby.

Other risk factors that are appropriate for interventions are isolation or a deep sense of loss and grief. However, other factors cannot be changed, for example, previous attempt or easy access to lethal methods, but knowledge of these risk factors can alert others to heightened risk for suicide during periods of crisis (significant stressful life events). What is important is to consider the actual efficacy of various approaches and techniques. There is increased awareness for the necessity to further test and evaluate the effectiveness of interventions specific to discrete populations (e.g., youth, elderly, the medically ill, and persons with mental and substance abuse disorders [U.S. Public Health Service, 1999; Ghosh and Victor, 1999 Roy, 1999]). A plan agreed to by both client and clinician ensures the greatest level of compliance (Eves 1999).

INTERVENTION

The Surgeon General's Call to Action (U.S. Public Health Service, 1999) emphasizes the following factors regarding suicide prevention:

■ Interventions are more likely to be successful if they involve a variety of services and providers.
■ The need to develop and test interventions to provide a "fit." Factors such as age, gender, and ethnic and cultural groups are considerations for effective interventions.
■ Suicide prevention must recognize and affirm the value, dignity, and importance of each person.

Suicide intervention can be divided into three distinct areas: primary, secondary, and tertiary.

Primary intervention includes activities that provide support, information, and education in situations that could otherwise become more serious and even lethal. Primary intervention can be practiced in schools, homes, hospitals, and industrial settings. See Box 23–3 for methods of developing effective suicide prevention strategies.

Secondary intervention is treatment of the actual suicidal crisis. It is practiced in clinics, in hospitals, and on telephone hotlines. Most people who are suicidal do not necessarily want to die; they just do not know how to go on living in an intolerable situation or state of mind. The client's ambivalence is one of the most important tools a nurse has when working with a suicidal person.

Tertiary intervention/postvention can refer to (1) interventions with family and friends of a person who has committed suicide, or (2) interventions with a person who has recently attempted suicide. Tertiary intervention for the latter is geared toward minimizing the traumatic after-effects of the suicide attempt.

Overall Guidelines for Nursing Interventions

HOSPITALIZED: PUT ON SUICIDE PRECAUTIONS

For the hospitalized client put on suicide precautions (Table 23–4):

Box 23–3 *Methodology: Advance the Science of Suicide Prevention*

■ Enhance research to understand risk and protective factors related to suicide, their interaction, and their effects on suicide and suicidal behaviors. Additionally, increase research on effective suicide prevention programs, clinical treatments for suicidal individuals, and culture-specific interventions.
■ Develop additional scientific strategies for evaluating suicide prevention interventions and ensure that evaluation components are included in all suicide prevention programs.
■ Establish mechanisms for federal, regional, and state interagency public health collaboration toward improving monitoring systems for suicide and suicidal behaviors and develop and promote standard terminology in these systems.
■ Encourage the development and evaluation of new prevention technologies, including firearm safety measures, to reduce easy access to lethal means of suicide.

U.S. Public Health Service (1999). *The Surgeon General's call to action to prevent suicide.* Washington, D.C.

■ Suicide precautions range from arm's-length constraint (one-to-one with staff member at arm's length at all times), to one-to-one contact with staff at all times but may attend activities off the unit maintaining one-to-one contact, to knowing the client's whereabouts at all times on the unit and accompanied by staff while off the unit.
■ If there is fear of imminent harm, restraints may be required.
■ Record client's mood, behavior and pertinent verbatim statement, every 15 minutes.
■ *Follow unit protocols and keep detailed records in client's chart.*

OUTSIDE THE HOSPITAL

For the client outside the hospital:

■ If a client is to be managed outside the hospital, the family, significant other, or friends should be alerted to the risk and treatment plan and informed of signs of deepening depression, such as a return or worsening of hopelessness.
■ When the client is to be managed on an outpatient basis (Slaby, 1994), then:

  ■ Social support should be rallied by having clients list three people to call on their suicide contract for support if they become overwhelmed with hopelessness.
  ■ Appropriate psychopharmacotherapy, psychotherapy, or sociotherapy should be initiated.
  ■ Clients and their family and friends should be given the psychiatric clinician's telephone number as well as that of a backup clinician or emergency room where they can go if the clinician is unavailable.
  ■ A return visit (even the next day if it is felt that the decision not to hospitalize may need to be reconsidered) should be scheduled.
  ■ Friends and family should be alerted to signs such as increasing withdrawal, preoccupation, silence, remorse, and sudden change from sad to happy and "worry-free."
  ■ Careful records should be kept in all instances documenting specific reasons why a client was or was not hospitalized.

■ If the client is to be managed on an outpatient basis, then medication should be given in limited amount (e.g., 3–5 day supply with no refill).
■ List support people and agencies to use as outpatient and crisis hotline numbers for clients/family/friends.
■ **If it's an accepted procedure at your facility/clinic,** form a written no-suicide contract with the client, such as "I will not kill myself for any reason, and if I should feel suicidal, I will (a) talk to a staff member, or (b) talk to my therapist."

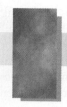

TABLE 23–4   *Suicidal Precautions and Constant One-to-One Observations*

STAFF ASSESSMENT	POSSIBLE CLIENT SYMPTOMS	NURSING RESPONSIBILITIES
Suicidal Precautions		
Client with suicidal ideations and who, after assessment by unit staff, presents clinical symptoms that indicate a suicide potential	1. The client with a concrete suicide plan 2. The client who is ambivalent about making a no-suicide contract 3. The client with minimal insight into existing problems 4. The client with limited impulse control	1. Conduct close observation (i.e., within visual range of staff) while client is awake. Accompany to bathroom. Place client in multiple-client room. Check every 15–30 minutes while client is awake. 2. Chart client's whereabouts, mood, verebatim statements, behavior every 15–30 minutes. 3. Ensure that meal trays contain no glass, metal silverware, or other sharps. 4. The nurse and physician explain to the client what they will be doing and why—Both document this in the chart.
Constant One-to-One Observations		
Client with suicidal ideations or delusions of self-mutilation who, according to assessment by unit staff, presents clinical symptoms that suggest a clear intent to follow through with the plan or delusion.	1. The client who is currently verbalizing a clear intent to harm self 2. The client who is unwilling to make a no-suicide contract 3. The client who presents with no insight into existing problems 4. The client with poor impulse control 5. The client who has already attempted suicide in the recent past by a particularly lethal method (e.g., hanging, gun, carbon monoxide poisoning)	1. Conduct one-to-one nursing observation and interaction 24 hours a day (never out of staff's sight). 2. Maintain arm's length at all times. 3. Chart client's whereabouts, mood, verbatim statements, and behavior every 15–30 minutes. 4. Ensure that meal trays contain no glass or metal silverware. 5. During observations when client is sleeping, **hands should always be in view,** not under the bed covers. 6. The nurse and physician explain to the client what they will be doing and why—Both document this in the chart.

Counseling

Counseling skills used by the nurse working with a client who is suicidal are practiced (1) in the community, (2) in hospitals, and (3) on telephone hotlines. The key element is the establishment of a workable relationship. There is general agreement by workers in this field on the importance of warmth, sensitivity, interest, concern, and consistency on the part of the helping person. Studies indicate that any treatment modality can be effective as long as it (1) includes the establishment of a personal relationship with the suicidal person, (2) encourages more realistic problem-solving behavior, and (3) reaffirms hope (Evans, 1983).

Material from the McKinley Health Center (1996) states that most suicides can be prevented by sensitive response to the person in crisis. You should

■ *Remain calm.* In most instances, there is no rush. Sit and listen—really listen—to what the person is saying. Give understanding and active emotional support for his or her feelings.

■ *Deal directly with the topic of suicide.* Most individuals have mixed feelings about death and dying and are open to help. Don't be afraid to ask or talk directly about suicide.

■ *Encourage problem solving and positive actions.* Remember that the person involved in emotional crisis is not thinking clearly; encourage him or her to refrain from making any serious, irreversible decisions while in a crisis. Talk about the positive alternatives that may establish hope for the future.

■ *Get assistance.* Although you want to help, do not take full responsibility by trying to be the sole counsel. Seek out resources that can lend qualified help, even if it means breaking a confidence. Let the troubled person know you are concerned—so concerned that you are willing to arrange help beyond that which you can offer.

The University of California at Los Angeles (UCLA) suicide prevention experts have summarized the information to be conveyed to the person in crisis as follows:

1. **The crisis is temporary.**
2. **Unbearable pain can be survived.**
3. **Help is available.**
4. **You are not alone.**

COMMUNITY

Usually, people in suicidal crisis are seen in emergency rooms and referred to an outpatient clinic. Indeed, if after initial assessment the person is thought to be at low risk and not in need of hospitalization, referral to a clinic for crisis counseling is always indicated. Hoff (1995) names six techniques that are useful in an outpatient community setting:

TECHNIQUE	ACTION
Relieve isolation.	Arrange for the person to stay with family or friends. If no one is available and the person is highly suicidal, hospitalization must be considered.
Remove all weapons.	Weapons and pills are removed by friends, relatives, or the nurse.
Encourage alternative expression of anger.	Have the person talk freely about feelings, unmet expectations, and disappointments. Plan with the person alternative ways of handling frustration and anger.
Avoid final decision for suicide during crisis.	Assure the person that the suicidal crisis is a temporary state. Encourage the person to avoid a decision until alternatives can be considered during a noncrisis state (see subsequent discussion of no-suicide contract).
Re-establish social ties.	Contact family members. Arrange for family crisis counseling. Activate links to self-help groups: e.g., Widow-To-Widow, Parents Without Partners, and Al-a-Teen.
Relieve extreme anxiety and sleep loss.	After thorough assessment, a tranquilizer may be prescribed to induce sleep and lower anxiety. **Note: Only a 1- to 3-day supply should be given, and only with a return appointment for crisis counseling.**

NO-SUICIDE CONTRACT. All persons receiving crisis counseling for suicidal ideations or actual suicide attempts should be given the opportunity for follow-up counseling or psychotherapy after the immediate crisis is over. A no-suicide contract between a counselor and a suicidal client has been used successfully in numerous settings, such as individual therapy, family therapy, group work, and behavioral therapy. The contract is outlined in clear and simple language. The purpose of the no-suicide contract is to give the counselor time to explore alternatives with the client. Check with your agency if they use a no-suicide contract. When the time of the contract is up, the contract is renegotiated. Examples of entries in a no-suicide contract include the following:

- "I will talk to my counselor if I have thoughts of harming myself."
- "I will wait until next week when I see my counselor before I take any action to harm myself."
- "I will go to the hospital emergency room if I start to have suicidal impulses."
- "I won't kill myself, either on purpose or accidentally, for any reason."

CRISIS COUNSELING. Crisis counseling is imperative for a person who is suicidal. Such a person may be in an acute crisis situation or may be chronically suicidal. A person who is chronically suicidal usually has the following clinical history:

1. Has eliminated all resources—is isolated and withdrawn from significant others.
2. Abuses alcohol, drugs, or both.
3. Has recurrent depression.
4. Has made several previous suicide threats or attempts over a period of several years.
5. Has made numerous bids for help, with little or no relief.
6. Presents with instability in job performance, interpersonal relationships, or both.

Crisis counseling can be effective for the chronically suicidal person; however, it cannot alter personality patterns, such as borderline personality. More research and clinical study are needed in the areas of formulating a treatment plan and intervening successfully with such persons.

HOSPITAL

How and when to use hospitalization is somewhat controversial. **Danger to self or others** is a general guideline. Legalities are often an important consideration. Either too much or too little restraint may be grounds for liability. Too much restraint may be grounds for abridgment of civil rights; too little restraint may be grounds for malpractice. Generally, if the primary counselor (e.g., nurse, social worker, psychologist) determines that the person is highly suicidal, has no immediate supports, and is exhausted and unable to carry out an alternative to suicide, hospitalization is indicated. However, some people are more responsive to treatment when they are not under constant observation.

Even when the decision for hospitalization is made, there are no hospitals that are 100% "suicide proof." Every hospital should have a suicide protocol that attempts to ensure the suicidal client's safety. **Students are advised to become familiar with the suicide protocol in the hospital or community setting with which they are affiliated.** Box 23–4 lists guidelines for minimizing suicidal behavior on a psychiatric unit.

Suicide precautions are meant to provide the client with a sense of security. If the client loses control and makes a suicide attempt, the staff will step in and assume control. Built into the suicide protocol are frequent interactions between staff and the suicidal client, for example, once every 30 minutes or three times a day for 15 minutes. Refer to Chapter 8 for:

■ Uses and contraindicators for seclusion and/or restraints.
■ Legal and ethical procedure to follow.
■ Correct documentation of care.

TELEPHONE HOTLINES

A counselor on a telephone hotline is often a lay person or volunteer who has had special training. At other times, friends, neighbors, relatives, police officers, nurses, and the clergy find themselves at the other end of a telephone cry for help. All volunteers should have professional training, have supervision available, and work in an environment with sufficient staff.

ESTABLISH RAPPORT. Keeping the person on the line as long as possible is the most important thing. As long as the person keeps talking, he or she is not acting out suicidal threats. It is often helpful to acknowledge the person's distress. Although you do not know how people feel, you can tell them that you understand they are in distress and are extremely unhappy. This lets them know that

■ You take their concerns seriously.
■ There is no need to complete the suicidal act to make it clear that they are in distress.
■ Other alternatives are available.

For example, "The fact that you are considering suicide makes it clear that you are feeling overwhelmed and need some assistance, but there is no need for you to hurt yourself without first talking about what can be done to help you."

Establishing rapport may also be contingent on allowing ventilation of the caller's feelings. The helping person often has to accept angry or manipu-

Box 23–4 Guidelines for Minimizing Suicidal Behavior on Psychiatric Unit*

THE CLIENT

1. Suicide precaution, include one-on-one monitoring, having client in view at all times (one arm's-length distance between staff member and client), **when client assessed as actively suicidal.**
   a. Includes during toileting
   b. Includes during the night
2. Suicide observation includes a 15-minute visual check of suicidal client, when client is not assessed to be a particular risk.
3. For each of the above, behavior, mood, and verbatim statements are recorded in the chart every 15 minutes.

THE ENVIRONMENT

1. Use plastic utensils.
2. Do not allow clients to spend too much time alone in their rooms. Do not assign to a private room.
3. Jump-proof and hang-proof the bathrooms by installing break-away shower rods and recessed shower nozzles.
4. Keep electrical cords to a minimal length.
5. Install unbreakable glass in windows. Install tamper-proof screens or partitions too small to pass through. Keep all windows locked.
6. Lock all utility rooms, kitchens, adjacent stairwells, and offices. All nonclinical staff (e.g., housekeepers, maintenance workers) should receive instructions to keep doors locked.
7. Take all potentially harmful gifts (e.g., flowers in glass vases) from visitors before allowing them to see clients.
8. Go through client's belongings with client and remove all potentially harmful objects (e.g., belts, shoelaces, metal nail files, tweezers, matches, razors, perfume and shampoo).
9. Ensure that visitors do not leave potentially harmful objects in client's room (e.g., matches, nail files).
10. Search clients for harmful objects (e.g., drugs, sharp objects, cords) on return from pass.

*ALWAYS FOLLOW YOUR UNIT PROTOCOLS AND CHARTING.

lative communication. The goal is to keep the caller talking and provide a psychological lifeline.

Reinforcing the caller's positive responses is also useful. Any positive responses, thoughts, and actions that the person communicates need to be met with a validation that these were positive and in the person's best interests. For example, if the caller says that he or she was thinking about suicide but decided to call first, this should be reinforced as a positive move: "Your calling me at this time was a very positive move; I am glad you decided to call now."

IDENTIFY THE PROBLEM. The problem needs to be clearly identified. The use of problem-solving approaches is helpful. Problem-solving statements help define the problem and explore avenues of action. For example:

■ To whom have you talked about this problem?
■ How do you think this problem will affect your life?
■ Have you told anyone how you feel?
■ What would keep you from taking your life at this point?
■ What do you think it makes sense to do now?

ASSESS THE LETHALITY OF THE SITUATION

1. If the caller is threatening suicide, evaluate the lethality of the plan.
2. If the caller has already taken pills, determine what kind and how many, whether he or she has been drinking alcohol, and other relevant medical information.
3. Determine whether there is someone nearby—neighbor, bystander, housekeeper, or manager. If the answer is yes, tell the caller that you want to speak to that person right now.
4. If not, try to get the caller's address and explain that you want to get help for him or her.
5. If the caller does not want to give you the address, instruct him or her on first aid:

   ■ Taking pills—induce vomiting.
   ■ Bleeding—apply pressure with bandage.
   ■ Inhalation poisoning—get fresh air, loosen tight clothing.

6. Pass a note to a staff member to attempt to have the call traced. Notify the telephone operator and then the police.

EVALUATE POSITIVE COPING AND ENCOURAGE ALTERNATIVES. Has the caller felt this way in the past? What did he or she do then? What works best? What could the caller do differently in this situation? What does the caller think would help change his or her situation? Give refer-

rals to appropriate places in the community that may help alter the situation.

Health Teaching

Primary intervention in the form of health teaching is an important way to lessen suicidal attempts. The goal is to reach people before they become so overwhelmed that suicide appears to be a rational alternative. Primary intervention relates to the principles of good mental health. The following programs provide support, information, and education:

■ Programs on emotional health in junior and senior high schools, for example, assess for depression and substance abuse, increase availability of mental health professionals.
■ Competently staffed drug and alcohol programs in the community providing aid to adolescents, adults and the elderly and their families.
■ Special programs in industry for drug and alcohol abusers.
■ Seminars for all health care providers on assessment and intervention in suicide, especially for those working in schools, industry, and well-baby clinics.
■ Seminars and group activities for the elderly that focus on (1) physical concerns such as reactions to medications and physical changes, and (2) emotional concerns such as how to cope with loneliness, separation from family, and loss of friends through death.

Milieu Therapy

Hospitalization is sometimes the most therapeutic environment during the acute suicidal phase. Placing a highly suicidal person in a controlled hospital environment can provide structure and control and can give the person time to evaluate his or her situation with professional staff. During hospitalization, the client's suicidal risk and the level of suicidal precaution needed are continually assessed. Refer to Chapter 8 for legally accepted hospital procedures to your affiliating agency's procedure manual. Repeated monitoring of a person's suicidal intent and extent of hopelessness is ongoing. The decision to discontinue suicide precautions is ideally based on clinical observations of nursing staff, physicians, and social workers, as well as on input from the client. Therefore, the decision to continue or discontinue suicide precautions should be based on subjective data and objective clinical observations.

After the acute phase, more long-term goals can be put into place. Because social isolation and withdrawal are often present, active encouragement and advice about contacting significant persons and loved ones needs to be given. Renewal of friendships and important relationships can help foster self-esteem. When the crisis pertains to a significant other (e.g., spouse, parent, child), therapies such as family, couple, or group counseling may be indicated.

Community agencies may be useful in helping a person renew or initiate activities related to work, special interests, hobbies, sports, and other activities that can help enhance self-esteem.

Psychobiological Interventions

Caution is always used when treating suicidal clients in outpatient settings, but the selective serotonin reuptake inhibitors (SSRIs) provide an alternative to hospitalization (Rives, 1999).

In cases in which extreme anxiety and lack of sleep last for several days, the risk of suicide can increase. An anxiolytic will usually take care of both the anxiety and the sleeping problem. If medication is given, the supply should be **for 1 to 3 days only,** with a return appointment scheduled for re-evaluation. Anxiolytics, however, should never be given to a highly suicidal individual. Generally, a lethal dose for anxiolytics is 10 times the normal dose. When a drug is combined with alcohol, however, only half that amount can cause death (Hoff, 1995).

When a coexisting psychiatric condition is present in a person who is suicidal, somatic intervention is dictated according to the psychopathology. For example, a person who is suicidal and also has the diagnosis of schizophrenia may need increased antipsychotic medication. Similar considerations are made for people who are clinically depressed as well as suicidal.

Electroconvulsive therapy can save the life of a seriously depressed and highly suicidal person. It can take 1 to 3 weeks of antidepressant therapy before the person experiences an elevation of mood; therefore, electroconvulsive therapy can have more immediate effects.

Psychotherapy

There is no "suicide specific" psychotherapy, and clinicians are increasingly aware of the value of integrating principles from psychodynamic and cognitive-behavioral therapy (Ghosh and Victor, 1999). Linehan's "dialectical behavior therapy" (DBT) developed specifically to treat chronically suicidal borderline individuals has shown particular promise for individuals with suicidal and parasuicidal behaviors (Linehan, 1997; Linehan et al., 1994).

SUICIDAL PERSON

Initial intervention for a suicidal person consists of crisis intervention. However, all persons should be offered the opportunity for further therapy after the crisis is over.

FAMILY

A variety of family interventions have been applied to the treatment of families with a suicidal member. Carlson and Asarnow (1995) report a cognitive-behavioral model that is a six-session family treatment for adolescent suicide attempters and their families. This approach employs six intervention strategies:

1. Exercises designed to establish a positive family atmosphere
2. Exercises designed to help family members recognize and label their feelings
3. Exercises designed to teach a basic approach to problem solving
4. Use of role playing, scripts, and interactions with feedback to try out new ways of relating
5. Negotiating skills with practice
6. Practicing enjoying pleasant activities and sharing positive feelings

SURVIVORS OF COMPLETED SUICIDE: POSTVENTION

Intervention for family and friends ("survivors") of a person who has committed suicide should be initiated within 24 to 72 hours after the death. Natural feelings of denial and avoidance predominate during the first 24 hours (Thompson, 1996). Mourning the death of a loved one who has committed suicide is painful at all times. The family of a person who has committed suicide is often faced with the process of mourning without the normal informal social supports usually provided. Unfortunately, neighbors, acquaintances, and even family friends are often confused and may blame the family for the death. Families of people who have committed suicide are often stigmatized and cut off and isolated from the usual supports during the time of mourning. Survivors often feel that they are "going crazy." They need to be told that these feelings are normal. Survivors need to find outlets for the undercurrent of anger against the deceased, who is responsible for the trauma, confusion, and pain inflicted on them. Unfortunately, few friends or family members of a person who has committed suicide seek out counseling. Pronounced feelings of anger and guilt are common reactions.

Thompson (1996) states that persons exposed to traumatic events such as suicide or sudden loss often manifest the following posttraumatic stress reactions: irritability, sleep disturbance, anxiety, startle reaction, nausea, headache, difficulty concentrating, confusion, fear, guilt, withdrawal, anger, and reactive depression. The particular pattern of the emotional reaction and type of response will differ with each survivor depending on the relationship of the deceased, circumstances surrounding the death, and coping mechanisms of the survivors. The ultimate contribution of suicide or sudden loss intervention in survivor groups is to create an appropriate and meaningful opportunity to respond to suicide or sudden death.

To reduce the trauma associated with the sudden loss, posttraumatic loss debriefing can help initiate an adaptive grief process and prevent self-defeating behaviors. Stages of posttraumatic loss debriefing are as follows (Thompson 1996):

1. *Introductory stage.* Introduce survivors to the debriefing process.
2. *Fact stage.* Information is gathered to "re-create the event" from what is known about it.
3. *Life review stage.* The opportunity to share "remember when . . . " stories lessens tension and anxiety within the survivor group.
4. *Feeling stage.* Feelings are identified and integrated into the process.
5. *Reaction stage.* Explore the physical and cognitive stress reactions to the traumatic event.
6. *Learning stage.* Assist survivors in learning new coping skills to deal with their grief reactions.
7. *Closure stage.* Wrap up loose ends, answer outstanding questions, provide final assurances, and create a plan of action that is life centered.

Self-help groups have been found to be extremely beneficial for survivors of a suicidal family member or friend. Many people join self-help groups even if the suicide took place 25 to 30 years before.

Self-help groups for the survivors of a family member or friend who committed suicide are similar to all other self-help groups. Essentially, these groups for family survivors are run by people who have lost someone through suicide. When a professional is involved, it is in the role of facilitator, consultant, or educator—not that of leader. Ideally, lay leaders should have some professional training in group processes and awareness of the limitations of the group experience. Professional therapists (e.g., nurses, social workers, psychiatrists, psychologists) should be used as a source of referral and should be available for consulting. Referral for individual and family therapy is advised once individual and family problems have been identified.

COUNSELORS AND NURSING STAFF: POSTVENTION

Staff and therapists who have been working with a client who successfully commits suicide also need support. Staff should have the opportunity to make adequate emotional expression of feelings of self-blame, guilt, and anger. If one of the staff has been closely involved over a long period with the client who has committed suicide, the staff member will also pass through a period of grief. Suicide can be a real possibility for a therapist involved in direct client care. Feelings of anger and guilt, loss of self-esteem, and intrusive thoughts about the suicide are common. Symptoms similar to those of posttraumatic stress disorder were experienced by a significant percentage of psychiatrists who had a client who committed suicide. Peer support and supervision help work through the loss.

A thorough psychological postmortem assessment should be carried out among staff. This can be a traumatic time for staff. Group support and processing the event can be healing. The suicidal event is reviewed to identify overlooked clues, faulty judgments, or changes in protocols that could be useful when evaluating future clients. Discussion during the postmortem should center on piecing together the pressures that led up to the client's taking his or her life.

EVALUATION

Evaluation of a suicidal client is an ongoing part of the assessment. The nurse must be constantly alert to changes in the suicidal person's mood, thinking, and behavior. As mentioned, sudden behavioral changes can signal suicidal intent, especially when the client's depression is lifting and more energy is available to carry out a preconceived plan. A person with a diagnosis of schizophrenia is also at risk when recovering from a psychotic episode. Anniversaries of losses and holiday seasons are particularly difficult times for some people.

Evaluation includes identifying the presence or absence of any clues or thoughts of suicide. The nurse also looks for indications that people are communicating thoughts and feelings more readily and that their social network is widening. For example, if people are able to talk about their feelings and engage in problem solving with the nurse, this is a positive sign. Are the clients increasing their social activities and expanding their interests? Do they state that they have more or fewer suicidal thoughts? Essentially, the nurse evaluates the goals and establishes new ones as different situations arise. Outcome criteria for a client who is in a crisis situation may differ from those for one who is chronically suicidal.

Visit the Evolve website at
http://evolve.elsevier.com/Varcarolis
for more Case Studies.

CASE STUDY 23–1 *Working with a Person Who Is Suicidal*

Thomas Martin, a 46-year-old social worker was brought to the hospital for evaluation after an attempted suicide. When he did not show up for work, his co-worker called to check on him. His landlady stated that his car was still in the driveway and that she would check his room. She found Mr. Martin lying on the bed, beside him an empty bottle of sleeping pills. A strong smell of liquor filled the room and a nearly empty bottle of scotch was on a table by the bed. An ambulance took Mr. Martin to the emergency department, where his stomach was lavaged. He stayed in the emergency room (ER) for 16 hours until he was no longer groggy. He was then seen by a psychiatric nurse, Mrs. Ruiz, for evaluation.

He told Mrs. Ruiz that he had been separated from his wife for 2 years but had seen his 8-year-old son every week during that time. Three days before his suicide attempt, his wife sent him a letter stating that she wanted to remarry and move to Oklahoma with her son and new husband.

ASSESSMENT

Mr. Martin's manner was hostile and sarcastic. He told the nurse that it did not matter what anyone did, he would "do it again," and that next time he would succeed. He sat sneering at the nurse, saying, "I never liked nurses anyway."

DIALOGUE

Nurse: What is it about nurses that you don't like?

Mr. M.: *(mimicking the nurse's tone)* What is it about nurses that you don't like—what drivel. Don't try that therapeutic garbage on me. I don't need help from you or anyone else.

(Silence) You're all castrating bitches . . . all women are. I hate all women.

Nurse: Tell me about one woman who has hurt you.

Mr. M.: *(angrily)* . . . Stop prying into my business with your little therapeutic diddies.

(Silence) Well . . . my wife . . . she . . . she . . . oh God . . . *At this point Mr. Martin starts sighing deeply, then bursts into tears.*

Nurse: *Waits a few minutes.* This situation with your wife and son moving away has upset you deeply.

Mr. M.: I don't want to live if I can't see my son. He is all I have left. He is the only thing that ever mattered to me.

Nurse: You have no friends or family?

Mr. M.: All my family died when I was a kid. As for friends . . . I don't need other people. Anyway, people don't seem to like me much. Look, don't spend time worrying about me. I've got a few more tricks up my sleeve.

Nurse: Do you mean that you will try to kill yourself again?

Mr. M.: What could it possibly mean to you?

Nurse: I *am* concerned about you, Mr. Martin.

Mr. M.: Well . . . isn't that the nurse thing to say. . . . Such great understanding.

Nurse: I do understand that you are very troubled right now and have no one to go to.

Case Study continued on following page

CASE STUDY 23–1   *Working with a Person Who Is Suicidal* (Continued)

Mrs. Ruiz organized her data into objective and subjective components.

Objective Data	Subjective Data
1. Male, age 46, no support systems	1. "I don't want to live if I can't see my son."
2. Impending loss of significant relationship with son	2. "I've got a few more tricks up my sleeve."
3. Possible drinking problem, need more data	3. "He (son) is the only thing that ever mattered to me."
4. Suicide attempt	4. "All my family died when I was a kid."
5. Holds responsible job	5. "I don't need other people."
6. Estranged wife and son moving away from area	6. "People don't seem to like me much."
7. Appears articulate and bright	

SELF-ASSESSMENT

Mrs. Ruiz knew that working with Mr. Martin was going to evoke high anxiety. In talking to her clinical supervisor, it became apparent that the idea of sending Mr. Martin to a male nurse therapist, while logical on the surface, was motivated by Mrs. Ruiz's own anxiety. She was trying to avoid Mr. Martin. "I guess I did try to shove him off. His sarcasm and belittling made me feel put down and angry."

Reviewing that first session with the supervisor clarified a number of important dynamics. First, it became evident that Mr. Martin was experiencing low self-esteem as a result of the impending loss of his son's companionship. Mr. Martin's rage at the loss and his inability to change the situation resulted in intense feelings of helplessness. Second, it appeared from the data that Mr. Martin was extremely isolated. It also seemed that most of this isolation was self-imposed. His sarcasm and belittling remarks appeared to be devices to (1) push people away, (2) temporarily lift sagging self-esteem through "one-upmanship," and (3) divert attention from his own fears. The supervisor and Mrs. Ruiz saw the need to relieve Mr. Martin's isolation without increasing his anxiety to severe levels.

It was important for Mr. Martin to talk about some of his feelings. Identifying and expressing pent-up feelings could have a number of benefits. First, it could minimize feelings of isolation. Second, it could reduce the need to act them out through self-destructive channels. Third, once identified, these feelings could be more positively discharged and worked through.

NURSING DIAGNOSIS

Mrs. Ruiz analyzed her data and set up her nursing diagnoses in order of priority.

Risk for Suicide related to self-harm behavior and belief that he has no reason to live

■ Suicide attempt
■ "I don't want to live if I can't see my son."
■ "He is the only thing that ever mattered to me."
■ "I've got a few more tricks up my sleeve."
■ Is holding a responsible job

Impaired social interaction related to inability to engage in satisfying relationships

■ "He (son) is all I have left."
■ "All my family died when I was a kid."
■ "I don't need other people."
■ "People don't seem to like me much."

Mrs. Ruiz discussed the case with the admitting resident. Because Mr. Martin stated that he wanted to kill himself, had no family or friends that could stay with him, and had access to drugs, the deci-

CASE STUDY 23–1   *Working with a Person Who Is Suicidal (Continued)*

sion was made to hospitalize him for further evaluation. Ordinarily, Mrs. Ruiz would follow him in clinic after discharge. In this case, Mrs. Ruiz told the physician that she thought it best for a male psychiatric nurse to work with Mr. Martin after discharge. Mrs. Ruiz explained that she thought Mr. Martin

would have a strong negative transference with a female nurse, and at this time working with him on alternatives in his life was the main goal. After the immediate crisis was over, working on his interpersonal relationships would take priority.

OUTCOME CRITERIA	Mrs. Ruiz identified the following outcome criteria:

Nursing Diagnosis	Outcome Criteria
Risk for Suicide	**Mr. Martin will not attempt suicide.**
Impaired social interaction	**Mr. Martin will state that he feels less isolated and frightened by people** (on a scale of 1–10, 1 feeling the least isolated).

PLANNING

Mr. Martin was kept in the hospital for 3 days. During that time he was placed on suicide precautions, as outlined in Table 23–4. He was discharged to the community outpatient division of the hospital after the staff thought that he was no longer a suicidal risk. When asked if he wanted a male nurse instead of a female nurse, he stated, "No . . . I'll talk to the little nursie. . . . She's got a thing for me."

PLANNING OUTCOME CRITERIA

The nurse met with Mr. Martin, and both worked out the following goals.

NURSING DIAGNOSIS	LONG-TERM OUTCOME	SHORT-TERM GOALS
1. **Risk for Suicide** related to loss of a son	1. Mr. Martin will state that he wants to live.	1a. Mr. Martin will make a no-suicide contract with the nurse by the end of the first session. 1b. Mr. Martin will talk about painful feelings by (date). 1c. Mr. Martin will look at alternative ways he can keep in touch with his son by (date).
2. **Impaired social interaction** related to social isolation	2. Mr. Martin will state that he feels less isolated and is participating in at least one activity involving other people.	2a. Mr. Martin will discuss feelings of isolation and loneliness by (date). 2b. Mr. Martin will identify three positive aspects of self and job by (date). 2c. Mr. Martin will state that he enjoys one new weekly activity by (date).

Case Study continued on following page

CASE STUDY 23–1   *Working with a Person Who Is Suicidal* (Continued)

INTERVENTION

At first, Mr. Martin was sarcastic, belittling, flirtatious, and hostile. Mrs. Ruiz kept her responses neutral and continued to focus her concern on Mr. Martin's situations and on working with alternatives. She gave him frequent opportunities to talk about his feelings. Initially, Mr. Martin would ridicule the nurse and belittle the idea: "Oh . . . you want to know about my precious painful feelings." Gradually, the testing-out behavior began to diminish. Slowly, and with some reluctance, Mr. Martin began talking about his feelings of loneliness and despair and sense of being a failure as a husband and father. He talked about the pain of his separation from his wife and his feelings of being a failure to his son.

The nurse continued to be neutral, not getting involved with power struggles or becoming defensive. Mrs. Ruiz began to see more clearly how these sarcastic and belittling behaviors helped Mr. Martin to defend against painful feelings of failure and low self-esteem. Refer to Nursing Care Plan 23–1, which follows, for specific interventions used with Mr. Martin.

EVALUATION

After 2 months, Mr. Martin stated that although he missed his son desperately, he no longer thought of suicide. He did not want to leave his son that legacy. He was planning his next vacation in Oklahoma, camping with his son for 2 weeks. His interpersonal relationships were still strained. He was beginning to look at situations that gave rise to his sarcasm and belittling and to relate his actions to feelings that had been unconscious. His sarcasm toward and belittling of Mrs. Ruiz had diminished a great deal, although he still resorted to them when he felt threatened. He spent more time examining his life, his feelings, and where he wanted to go, and less on defensive behaviors. Although by this time the crisis was over, Mr. Martin continued counseling with Mrs. Ruiz. He was able to say that at times he felt more comfortable with his co-workers, although he still did not feel at home with others. He had resumed weekly bowling. He said he was surprised to find that he enjoyed it. He had even started talking to a "fellow there who is also divorced and got a rough deal. He's not a bad guy."

Visit the **Evolve** website at
http://evolve.elsevier.com/Varcarolis
for the other Nursing Care Plan diagnoses and for
more Nursing Care Plans.

NURSING CARE PLAN 23–1   *A Suicidal Client After Discharge:* Mr. Martin

NURSING DIAGNOSIS
Risk for Suicide: Related to loss of son

Supporting Data
- Suicide attempt
- "I don't want to live if I can't see my son."

- "I've got a few more tricks up my sleeve."
- Impending loss of son

Outcome Criteria: Mr. Martin will refrain from further suicide attempts.

NURSING CARE PLAN 23–1 **A Suicidal Client After Discharge: Mr. Martin** (Continued)

SHORT-TERM GOAL	INTERVENTION	RATIONALE	EVALUATION
1. Mr. Martin will make a no-suicide contract with nurse by end of first session.	1a. Assess suicide status.	1a. Ongoing periodic check of suicidal status. Higher rate of suicide for those who have attempted suicide.	*GOAL MET* Mr. Martin signed contract: "I will talk to the nurse if I think about killing myself. If she isn't available, I will call the crisis hotline" (first session).
	1b. Even if Mr. Martin denies suicide, make a no-suicide contract.	1b. Demonstrates concern and offers alternatives if suicidal thoughts return.	
2. Mr. Martin will talk about painful feelings by (date).	2a. Remain neutral in face of hostility and put-downs.	2a. Diminishes power struggles and discourages continuing acting out behaviors.	*GOAL MET* During first to third week, hostile and sarcastic communication was constant. By fourth week, Mr. Martin stated, "You really want to know." Mr. Martin talked of feeling like a failure as a husband and father.
	2b. Refocus attention back to Mr. Martin.	2b. Arguments and power struggles keep attention focused away from important issues.	
	2c. Give frequent opportunities for discussion of feelings through verbal invitation and stated concern.	2c. Aggressive, hostile communications are cover for painful feelings. When client can express feelings in words, there is less need to act them out.	
3. Mr. Martin will look at alternative ways he can keep in touch with his son by (date).	3. Alternative solutions can be problem-solved once feelings and problems are identified.	3. Acceptable alternatives increase a future orientation and decrease hopelessness. Client can experience feelings of control over situation.	*GOAL MET* By fifth week, Mr. Martin talked about taking son on a camping trip during summer recess.

NURSING DIAGNOSIS

Impaired social interaction: Related to social isolation

Supporting Data

■ "He (son) is all I have left."
■ "All my family died when I was a kid."

■ "I don't need other people."
■ "People don't seem to like me much."

Outcome Criteria: Mr. Martin will state that he feels less isolated and less frightened of people by (date) (on a scale of 1–10, 1 feeling the least isolated).

Nursing Care Plan continued on following page

NURSING CARE PLAN 23–1   A *Suicidal Client After Discharge*: **Mr. Martin** (*Continued*)

SHORT-TERM GOAL	INTERVENTION	RATIONALE	EVALUATION
1a. Assess suicide 1. Mr. Martin will discuss feelings of isolation and loneliness by (date).	1. Provide opportunities for Mr. Martin to express feelings and thoughts regarding his self-imposed isolation.	1. Before change can take place, clarification of personal feelings and thoughts is necessary.	*GOAL MET* By fourth week, Mr. Martin spoke of feeling alone—son is only contact to life.
2. Mr. Martin will identify three positive aspects of self and job by (date).	2a. Validate Mr. Martin's strengths. 2b. Encourage self-evaluation of positive as well as negative aspects of Mr. Martin's life.	2a. Positive as well as negative feedback aid in more realistic perception of self. 2b. Client can begin to see himself more clearly, with increase in self-esteem.	By fifth week, Mr. Martin stated that he thinks he is a good worker and is respected (if not liked) by his peers.
3. Mr. Martin will state that he enjoys one new weekly activity with at least one other person by (date).	3a. Review previous activities that Mr. Martin enjoyed before his marriage ended. 3b. Have Mr. Martin choose an activity that he is willing to participate in.	3a. Change focus from negative present to positive aspects of his past. Can help increase hope and self-esteem. 3b. Participating in own problem solving and decision making offers a sense of control and an increase in self-esteem.	*GOAL MET* By seventh week, Mr. Martin stated that he started bowling again and was surprised that he had a good time.

SUMMARY

Suicide is the willful act of ending one's life. People can also hasten their death by covert self-destructive behaviors, such as alcoholism, medical noncompliance, hyperobesity, and anorexia nervosa. Death from such causes is a result of chronic self-destructive behavior. Suicidal behavior can be classified into three categories: (1) completed, (2) attempted, and (3) ideation. Statistics surrounding suicide provide a profile that can be useful when

assessing a person's suicidal intention. Many complex factors contribute to a person's decision to commit suicide, including psychodynamic, sociological, and biochemical elements.

It is imperative for the nurse to assess the client's suicidal intent. The nurse assesses verbal and nonverbal clues, the lethality of the suicide plan, and high-risk factors. Nursing diagnoses may include a number of problem areas; however, **Risk for Suicide** is the most crucial initially. When planning care, the nurse plans specific goals. The nurse's personal reactions to suicide and the suicidal client need to be addressed. Common and expected reactions have been discussed, and supervision with a more experienced health care professional emphasized.

Intervention in suicide can be on a primary, secondary, or tertiary level. Secondary interventions take place in the ER, in a hospital unit, and in community settings and on suicide hotlines. Evaluation is ongoing, especially with a person who has a potential for suicide, because the incidence is often higher when depression is lifting or when a person is recovering from a psychotic episode. Goals are evaluated and reset, according to changes in the assessment and progress by the client toward mutually agreed-upon goals. The case study highlighted nurses' work with a suicidal client.

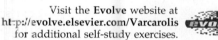

Visit the **Evolve** website at
http://evolve.elsevier.com/Varcarolis
for a post-test on the content in this chapter.

Visit the **Evolve** website at
http://evolve.elsevier.com/Varcarolis
for additional self-study exercises.

Critical Thinking and Chapter Review

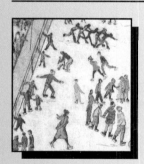

Critical Thinking

1. Read the suicide protocol at your hospital unit/community center. Are there any steps you anticipate having difficulty carrying out? What suggestions do your peers/clinical group have regarding these difficulties that you could implement?
2. How would you respond to a staff person who expresses guilt over the completed suicide of a client on your unit?
3. Identify three common and expected emotional reactions that a nurse might have when initially working with people who are suicidal. How do you think you might react? What actions could you take to process the event and obtain support?

Chapter Review

Choose the most appropriate answer.

1. Charles Brown, 52, lost his wife in an automobile accident 4 months ago. Since that time he has been severely depressed, withdrawn from contacts with family and friends, and has taken to drinking to "numb the pain." Using the SAD PERSONS assessment scale, how many points does Mr. Brown have?

   1. Three
   2. Four
   3. Five
   4. Six

2. Which of the following cannot be relied upon to provide a basis for nursing intervention with a suicidal client?

   1. Most people who are planning suicide give clues.
   2. The nurse should not bring up the subject of suicide with a client.

> 3. When depression is lifting there is more energy to carry out a suicide plan.
> 4. Most people who contemplate suicide are highly ambivalent about dying.

3. Select the example of primary intervention in suicide.

> 1. Working with the family of a recent suicide victim.
> 2. Placing the hospitalized client on suicide precautions.
> 3. Keeping the caller to a crisis hotline on the phone and working out alternatives to suicide.
> 4. Providing a seminar for the elderly focusing on coping with loneliness and physical changes.

4. Miss B. has a concrete plan to commit suicide by hanging. She refuses to make a no-suicide contract because she believes there is no hope for a better life now that her fiancé has left her and God has abandoned her. She believes the breakup with her fiancé was because he found out "how worthless I am." Which of Miss B.'s nursing diagnoses is of highest priority?

> 1. Hopelessness
> 2. Spiritual distress
> 3. Low self-esteem
> 4. Risk for violence—self-inflicted

5. The guideline used to justify hospitalization for a client with suicidal ideation is

> 1. The client is a danger to self or others.
> 2. The client made a prior suicide attempt.
> 3. The client has felt this way in the past.
> 4. The client is unwilling to take anxiolytic medication.

NURSE, CLIENT, AND FAMILY RESOURCES

Associations

American Foundation for Suicide Prevention
120 Wall Street, 22nd Floor
New York, NY 10005
1–888–333–2377; 1–212–363–3500
http://www.afsp.org

American Suicide Foundation
1045 Park Avenue, Suite 3C
New York, NY 10028
1–800–ASF–4042; 1–212–410–1111
(Provides referrals to national support groups for suicide survivors)

American Association of Suicidology
4201 Connecticut Avenue NW, Suite #310
Washington, DC 20008
1–202–237–2280

Friends for Survival
P.O. Box 214463
Sacramento, CA 95821

1–916–392–0664; 1–800–646–7322
(For family, friends, and professionals after a suicide death)

Ray of Hope
P.O. Box 2323
Iowa City, IA 52244
1–319–337–9890

SOSAD (*Save Our Sons and Daughters*)
1–313–361–5200
(For family and friends of survivors of homicide and suicide)

Internet Sites

Suicide Awareness Voices of Education
http://www.save.org

The Samaritans
http://www.samaritans.org.uk/

(If You Are Thinking About) Suicide . . . Read This First
http://www.metanoia.org/suicide/

Suicide @ *rochford.org*
http://www.rochford.org/suicide

REFERENCES

Beck, A.T., et al. (1990). Relationship between hopelessness and ultimate suicide: A replication with psychiatric outpatients. *American Journal of Psychiatry,* 147:190–195.

Birtchnell, J. (1983). Psychotherapeutic considerations in the management of the suicidal patient. *American Journal of Psychotherapy,* 37(1):24.

Carlson, G. A., and Asarnow, J. R. (1995). Mood disorders and suicidal behavior. In G. O. Gabbard (Ed.), *Treatments of psychiatric disorders* (Vol. I, pp 253–285). Washington, DC: American Psychiatric Press.

Centers for Disease Control and Prevention (CDC) (1994). Programs for the prevention of suicide among adolescents and young adults, and suicide contagion and reporting of suicide: Recommendations from a national workshop. *Morbidity and Mortality Weekly Report* 43 (No. RR-6).

Densmore, W. E. (1997). Take caution with "no-suicide contract" (letter). *Journal of Psychosocial Nursing,* 35(5):11.

Durand, C. J., et al. (1995). A quarter century of suicide in a major urban jail: Implications for community psychiatry. *American Journal of Psychiatry,* 152(7):1077–1080.

Evans, D. L. (1983). Explaining suicide among the young: An analytic review of the literature. *Journal of Psychosocial Nursing and Mental Health Services,* 21(5):9.

Farberow, N. L. (1967). Crisis, disaster, and suicide: Theory and therapy. In E. S. Schneidman (Ed.), *Essays in self-destruction.* New York: Jason Aronson.

Fergusson, D. M., and Lynsky, M. T. (1995). Childhood circumstances, adolescent adjustment, and suicide attempts in a New Zealand birth cohort. *Journal of American Academy of Child and Adolescent Psychiatry,* 34(5):612.

Ghosh, T. B., and Victor, B. S. (1999). Suicide. In R. E. Hale, S. C. Yudofsky, and J. A. Talbott (Eds.), *Textbook of psychiatry.* Washington, DC: American Psychiatric Press, Inc.

Hammel-Bissell, B. P. (1985). Suicidal casework: Assessing nurses' reactions. *Journal of Psychosocial Nursing and Mental Health Services,* 23(10):20.

Hoff, L.A. (1995). *People in crisis: Understanding and helping* (4th ed.). San Francisco: Jossey-Bass.

Linehan, M. M. (1997). *Behavioral treatments of suicidal behaviors. Definitional obfuscation and treatment outcomes.* Annals of New York Academy of Science, December 29; 836:302–328.

Linehan, M. M., Tutek, D. A., Heard, H. L., Armstrong, H. E. (1994). Interpersonal outcomes of cognitive behavioral treatment of chronically suicidal borderline patients. *American Journal of Psychiatry,* 151(12):1771–1776.

McKinley Health Center (1996). University of Illinois, Champaign Urbana. Online Psychological Services, 1996.

Mowshowitz, I. (1984). The special role of the pastoral counselor. In N. Linzer (Ed.), *Suicide: The will to live vs. the will to die.* New York: Human Sciences Press.

National Institute of Mental Health (NIMH) (1997). Data: Center for Disease Control and Prevention, National Center for Health Statistics.

Overholser, J. C., et al. (1995). Self-esteem deficits and suicidal tendencies among adolescents. *Journal of American Academic Child Adolescent Psychiatry,* 34(7):919.

Pandey, G. N., et al. (1995). Platelet serotonin-2A receptors: A potential biological marker for suicidal behavior. *American Journal of Psychiatry,* 52(6):850.

Parker, S.D., (1988). Accident or suicide: Do life change events lead to adolescent suicide? *Journal of Psychosocial Nursing,* 152(5):850.

Pataki, C.S. (1999). Mood disorders and suicide in children and adolescents. In H. I. Kaplan and B. J. Sadock (Eds.), *Comprehensive textbook of psychiatry* (7th ed.). Philadelphia: Lippincott, Williams & Wilkins.

Patterson, W., et al. (1983). Evaluation of suicidal patients: The SAD PERSONS scale. *Psychosomatics,* 24(4):343.

Paykel, E. S., et al. (1975). Suicide attempts and recent life events. *Archives of General Psychiatry,* 33:327.

Rives, W. (1999). Emergency department assessment of suicidal patients. *Psychiatric Clinics of North America,* 22(4):779–787.

Roy, A. (1999). Psychiatric emergencies: Suicide. In H. I. Kaplan and B. J. Sadock (Eds.), *Comprehensive textbook of psychiatry* (7th ed.). Philadelphia: Lippincott, Williams & Wilkins.

Roy, A. (1995b). Suicide. In H. I. Kaplan and B. J. Sadock (Eds.), *Comprehensive textbook of psychiatry VI.* Baltimore: Williams & Wilkins

Roy, A., et al. (1995). Attempted suicide among living co-twins of twin suicide victims. *American Journal of Psychiatry,* 152(7): 1075.

Schulsinger, F., Kety, S. S., and Rosenthal, et al. (1979). *A family study of suicide in origin, prevention and treatment of affective disorders.* In M. Schou and E. Stromgren (Eds.), (pp 277–287). New York: Academic Press.

Slaby, A. E. (1994). Handbook of Psychiatric Emergencies. Norwalk, CT: Appleton & Lange.

Stevenson, J. M. (1988). Suicide. In A. Talbott, R. Hales, and S. C. Yudoksky (Eds.), *Textbook of psychiatry.* Washington, DC: American Psychiatric Press.

Thompson, R. (1996). Post-traumatic loss debriefing: Providing immediate support for survivors of suicide or sudden loss. Ann Arbor MI: ERIC Clearinghouse on Counseling and Personnel Services.

U.S. Public Health Service (1999). The Surgeon General's call to action to prevent suicide. Washington, D.C.

Wysoker, A. (1999). Legal and ethical considerations; Suicide: Risk management strategies. *Journal of American Psychiatric Association,* 5(5):164–166

*A*nger and aggression are difficult targets for nursing intervention, particularly if their focus is the nurse, because they imply threat and thereby readily elicit emotional and personal responses. **Anger** is an emotional response to the perception of frustration of desires, threat to one's needs (emotional or physical), or challenge. **Aggression** is harsh physical or verbal action that reflects rage, hostility, and potential for physical or verbal destructiveness. Anger and aggression are the last two stages of a response that begins with feelings of vulnerability and then uneasiness. Clients often communicate their anxiety before escalating to anger. Nursing interventions for anger and aggression begin at these early stages, with accurate assessment of clients' behaviors, appropriate intervention, and care to reassess that the intervention was effective. See Chapters 13 and 14 for interventions that can be used when anxiety is escalating. Impulsive clients and those who are temperamentally predisposed to feelings of irritability and hostility may move quickly through these early stages, so that a display of anger is their first sign of distress. Quick and accurate intervention nevertheless prevents aggression, which in most instances is the physical attempt to take control.

PREVALENCE

Nurses will inevitably be asked to deal with anger and aggression because these are universal emotions. Anger is included in all descriptions of primary emotions and is one of six that can generally be identified across cultures via facial expression (Ekman 1972). In addition, while anger and aggression are more obvious in some people than others, both are responses to perceptions of threat or loss of control; the need for health care and the environments in which health care is typically provided readily precipitate feelings of personal peril and lack of control.

Aggression and violence are usually a result of the unchecked escalation of anger. Checks on this escalation may include use of appropriate anger management skills by the angry individual, internalized societal strictures, external presence of social controls such as teachers or respected others, or active intervention by others such as nurses or therapists. There is some evidence that these checks on aggression are less available now than they have been, leading to an increased incidence of violence that has declined somewhat since 1991. The Centers for Disease Control (CDC) reported more than 50,000 deaths from suicide and homicide between 1985 and 1996. In 1996 the homicide rate was 8.3 per 100,000 individuals in the population, down by 23.1% from a high of 10.8 per 100,000 in 1991. Despite this decline in violent deaths, more than 2,800,000 people are currently victims of violence each year, and the CDC has suggested that its widespread incidence indicates that it is a common part of social interactions in many environments (CDC 1998, 1999a).

Women and children are disproportionately affected by violence. In 1994 more than 500,000 women were seen in emergency rooms for injuries caused by interpersonal violence. Between 1981 and 1991 the annual death rate by homicide for young men between 15 and 19 increased 124%, from 12 to 33 per 100,000. These rates declined somewhat so that by 1996 the homicide rate for this group was 26 per 100,000, still near the highest ever recorded for this age group in this country during peacetime (CDC 1999b). In addition, 9,000,000 children are estimated to witness violence each year at home or at school (CDC 1998). In one study, nearly one third of urban children and 9% of suburban children reported seeing someone shot or stabbed in 1996 (Lurie 1999). The witnessing of violence by children is correlated with later emotional disorders and is one of the risk factors for anger and violence in adolescence and adulthood (Schwab-Stone, 1999).

Research on the effects of culture and ethnicity on prevalence of anger and aggression is limited, and often contradictory; it frequently focuses specifically on criminal populations, with findings that are likely not generalizable to noncriminal members of the same ethnic groups (Lyon et al. 1992; Valdez et al. 1995). Research on domestic violence that has included ethnicity as one of the variables indicated that ethnicity is not a predictor of either more or less violence among couples and families (Gin et al. 1991; Kua and Ko 1991; White and Koss 1991).

COMORBIDITY

Although anger is a universal emotion, at times leading to aggression and violence, evidence exists that it is more prevalent when a variety of co-morbid conditions are present. Many researchers have found a correlation between later quickness to anger and aggression, and hyperactivity, attention deficits, and impulsivity in children, especially male children (Loeber and Southamer-Loeber, 1998; Lipsey and Derzon, 1998). In adults, the incidence of anger has been found to be higher than in the general population when the following sample of illnesses are present: unipolar depression (Mammen, Shear, Pilkonis et al, 1999; Riley, Treiber, Woods, 1989); posttraumatic stress disorder, especially patients who are hospitalized with this disorder (McFall, Fontana, Raskind et al, 1999); mania (McElroy, 1999); personality disorders, including avoidant, dependent, borderline, narcissistic, and antisocial personality disorders, especially when depression is also present (Fava, 1998); and Tourette's disorder (Bruun and Budman, 1998).

In a review of studies of mental illnesses in violent offenders, one author found higher incidences of the major mental illnesses than in the general population. Schizophrenia was nearly three times more prevalent, major depression three to four times more prevalent, and bipolar disorder seven to fourteen times more prevalent in these particular incarcerated groups (Monahan, 1992). Most people with psychiatric illnesses are not violent. However, anger and aggression can be products of the disordered thinking and the disturbances of perception and cognition that are symptoms of these illnesses.

Anger and hostility are also risk factors for cardiovascular disease, including ischemic heart disease and cerebral vascular attacks (CVA). Levels of hostility have been shown to increase adrenocorticotropin and cardiovascular responses to stress and, in longitudinal studies, to increased illness (Davis et al. 2000; al'Absi et al. 2000; Everson et al. 1999).

THEORY

Another Look at an Old Theory

Early theories of aggression, developed from preexisting theories of drive (Freud 1933) and instinct (Lorenz 1966), led to therapies in which clients were encouraged to express their anger. Expression (i.e., "getting it all out") became the therapeutic focus, rather than a search for solutions and resolution (Rappaport 1967).

Research has since shown that simple expression of anger is not beneficial to clients. Rather, expression of anger can lead to increased anger and to negative physiological changes. Similar affective and physiological correlates were seen when subjects articulated angry thoughts while discussing provocative events (Davison et al. 1991).

The physiological changes associated with anger expression are significant because they reflect cardiac reactivity in men that has been shown to be associated with coronary heart disease. In other research, the opposite approach to anger—repression—has been associated with essential hypertension and cardiac reactivity in women (Gentry 1985; Julius et al. 1985; Manuck et al. 1985; Anderson and Lawler 1995; Siegman et al. 2000). These changes

were strongest in African Americans, who had longer lasting cardiac reactivity to anger than white research subjects (Fredrickson et al. 2000). In addition, men with high levels of expressed anger have been shown to have twice the risk of cerebral vascular attacks (CVA) as men with the lowest levels; this was true even when other risk factors such as smoking were controlled for (Everson et al. 1990). Negative cardiovascular effects do not occur when provocative events are handled assertively or when participants respond reflectively, constraining anger while trying to solve the underlying problem (Harburg et al. 1991; Anderson and Lawler 1995). Total repression of anger without the use of constructive outlets, however, has been linked with immunological problems and some forms of cancer (Esterling et al. 1990; Jensen 1987; Temoshok 1987).

Finally, family therapists have suggested that the venting of anger in ongoing relationships solves nothing and may serve to maintain dysfunctional interaction patterns. The possibility of developing more constructive interactional strategies is then diminished (Burman et al. 1993).

Clearly, the simple expression of anger is not useful. However, other anger management techniques that can be taught have been shown to be beneficial. These techniques are derived from two theoretical bases.

Behavioral Theory

Early behaviorists held that emotions, including anger, were learned responses to environmental stimuli (Skinner 1953). Social learning theorists adapted this theory through research that showed that children learn aggression by imitating others and that people repeat behavior that is rewarded (Bandura 1973). Thus, children who watch television violence learn violent ways of resolving problems. Not only is television violence portrayed as an option for resolving conflict, but 73% of violent acts are also shown without negative consequences (National Television Violence Study Council 1996). When parents are not present or are too preoccupied to teach their children alternative ways of dealing with problems, the range of skills learned by the children for managing frustration remains limited. Similarly, children who grow up in angry families learn to respond to frustration with anger and violence. Anger and aggression in the family and on television have two intrinsic rewards: (1) frequently, they accomplish the purpose of keeping the angry person in control while those around the person are intimidated; (2) they also provide for the relief of pent-up distress. Children and young adults with mental problems may be unable to process anger management skills taught by parents and schools.

Bandura's research suggested that emotional arousal would have an increased probability of expression as aggression when the context predisposed to aggression; this has implications for the psychiatric milieu in particular. Staff attitudes have been shown to set the context within which emotional arousal occurs. For example, a rigid intolerance of affect and an authoritarian style by nurses have been associated with assault (Soloff 1983; Cooper and Mendonca 1989; Durivage 1989). Alternatively, a client may receive increased status and approval from other clients because of intimidation and threats that remain unaddressed by staff. The milieu is in this way predisposed to reward arousal when it is discharged via anger or aggression.

Cognitive Theory

Novaco's research (1976, 1985) described how cognitions drive anger. Individuals appraise events as threatening, and this cognition leads to the emotional and physiological arousal necessary to take action. Although threat is usually understood as an alert to physical danger, Beck (1976) noted that perceived assault on areas of personal domain, such as values, moral code, and protective rules, can also lead to anger. For example, anger and aggression are generated around moral issues, such as whether women have a right to abortion. People with frequent anger are often those who are vigilant for signs of threat, such as gang members who scan their environment for signs of disrespect. Such signs are cognitively interpreted as threats to status. In addition, people who are temperamentally predisposed to irritability and hostility are more likely to interpret stressful or ambiguous events as threats.

For example, clinic clients who have been kept waiting for long periods of time without explanation may interpret this as neglect and a lack of respect. Anger may escalate when the initial appraisal is followed by cognitions such as "They have no right to treat me this way. I am a person too." These additional cognitions become the drivers of the escalation, until successful interventions are used or until those who are angry take action. As Novaco (1985) noted, cognition and mood interact and can become mutually reinforcing; the later cognitions increase the anger, which validates the cognitions. The resulting action may take the form of assault. In some individuals, the period of escalation can be rapid.

In contrast, clients less predisposed to anger might interpret the wait as a sign that the clinic is busy. These clients might be frustrated by the situation, but in the absence of anger they might access and utilize skills such as asking how much longer the wait is likely to be, finding distractions in the environment, or rescheduling the appointment.

Novaco stated that "there is no direct relationship between external events and anger. The arousal of anger is a cognitively mediated process" (1985, p. 210). An event may generate fear, hurt, humiliation, or powerlessness in some individuals (however, subsequent cognitions may then generate anger as a response to "being made to feel this way"), while generating anger in others. An event is more likely to lead to anger and then to aggression if the event is perceived as threatening (Beck 1976). This function is thus adaptive and ideally leads to self-preservation in circumstances of genuine danger (e.g., war). This adaptive function is likely the reason that anger is a primary and universal emotion. However, problems result when the same escalation process of cognition-emotion-action, or cognition-emotion-cognition-more emotion-action, occurs in social settings where physical danger is not present.

Nurses, of course, are not immune to anger. A client who is shouting angrily may reasonably be appraised as a potential threat. This appraisal may lead to anger on the nurse's part, as well as an impulse for self-protection. One study found that the nurse's response to anger from a client varied according to the interpretation given to the client's anger and to the nurse's self-appraised ability to manage the situation. Only when self-efficacy was perceived as adequate did the nurse move to help the client. When self-efficacy was not seen as adequate, nurses showed a decreased ability to process the client's message and a decreased ability to problem-solve (Smith and Hart 1994).

Neurobiology of Anger and Aggression

Brain Abnormalities

Many neurological conditions are associated with anger and aggression. For example, certain brain tumors, Alzheimer's disease, temporal lobe epilepsy, and traumatic injury to certain parts of the brain result in changes to personality that include increased violence. Twenty-five percent of people with brain injury have severe behavior disorders, including aggression, that disrupt their lives (Jacobs 1987).

Serotonin

Studies have shown a relationship between impulsive aggression and low levels of the neurotransmitter serotonin (Brown et al. 1989; Kavoussi et al. 1997). There is also preliminary evidence for a genetic disturbance in serotonergic function that may predispose individuals to impulsive aggressive behaviors (Kavoussi et al. 1997).

Specific Areas of the Brain and Anger

One site known to be associated with aggression is the limbic system, which mediates primitive emotion and behaviors that are necessary for survival. The limbic system contains several structures that appear to have a role in the production of aggression. The area of the brain called the *amygdala* mediates anger experiences, judging events as either aversive or rewarding (Foster 1996). For example, in animal studies, stimulation of the amygdala produces rage responses, while lesions in the same structure produce docility. The temporal lobe of the brain shares some structures with the limbic system. Here, in the temporal lobe, memory is thought to be integrated; memory of previous insult is important in the cognitive appraisal of threat in the face of new stimuli. This lobe is also the source of complex partial seizures, which include aggressive behavior. Interestingly, high violence scores correlate with CT scan and EEG abnormalities in the temporal lobes of maximum security patients (Kavoussi et al. 1997).

While the amygdala has been implicated in rage, other portions of the brain are activated with anger. These areas include the left orbitofrontal cortex, the right anterior cingulate cortex, and as noted previously, the temporal lobes. The left orbitofrontal cortex has been suggested as having a role in inhibiting responses and mediating behavior according to the social context. Thus, studies showing activation of this area during anger may be showing the brain's prevention of an angry response while the anger is being experienced (Dougherty et al. 1999).

Genetics

Finally, research findings indicate that violence is a function of both genetics and childhood environment. For example, researchers have noted that family dynamics affect the disposition of infant members; disorganized, unpredictable families, or those high in conflict, tend to have more irritable infants than families that are stable (Brackbill et al. 1990; Eisenberg et al. 1997). Similarly, anger in toddlers has been seen to be related to child-rearing variables in their mothers, with nonconflictual parent-child relationships most highly correlated with low toddler anger (Brook et al. 1999). Of course, family dynamics may themselves reflect genetic variables.

Genetic Studies: Criminal Proband. One review of adoption studies concluded that genetic factors explain more of the difference in antisocial behaviors than environmental factors. In general, when an adopted child had either an alcoholic or an antisocial biological parent, the presence of a poor adoptive environment resulted in a greater increase in antisocial behavior, including violence, than would be expected from the simple sum of the two effects (Cadoret 1982; Cadoret et al. 1985). In another study, adoptees with criminality in both their biological and their adoptive parents were 14 times more likely to be criminal than those without this parental history (Cloninger et al. 1982). Such studies have looked at three factors that are typically associated with aggression and violence: alcoholism, criminality, and antisocial personality disorder. Results in this research area have been similar and consistent (Dahl 1994; DiLalla and Gottesman 1991).

Genetic Studies: General Population. Other research has attempted to look at genetic factors implicated in anger that is not criminal. Generally this research looks at anger as a function of temperament. Researchers have measured temperamental factors such as fear, anger, frustration, and positive affect in infants, and have found their results to be predictive of temperament in preschool and middle childhood. Anger seen as a part of temperament at six and ten months of age predicted anger and frustration at seven years of age (Rothbart et al. 2000). A study of anger in adolescents found that trait anger, or anger that is a relatively enduring part of personality, explained more episodes of anger than did simple stress or state anger, generated by specific context (Yarcheski et al. 1999).

Clearly, some individuals are biologically more predisposed than others to respond to life events with irritability, easy frustration, and anger. This predisposition may be a function of genetics or of neurological development that occurs in the context of certain infant and childhood environments. The combination of these two risk factors appears to be exponential. Nevertheless, if all the dimensions of anger are centrally mediated, then successful interventions can be designed to target any of its manifestations. This is likely the reason biologic, pharmacologic, behavioral, and cognitive strategies have all proven effective in the management of anger and aggression.

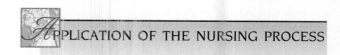

APPLICATION OF THE NURSING PROCESS

ASSESSMENT

Overall Assessment

Accurate and early assessment can identify client anxiety before it escalates to anger and aggression. Such assessment also leads directly to the appropriate nursing diagnosis and intervention. Client expressions of anxiety and of anger generally look similar. Both may involve increased rate and volume of speech, increased demands, irritability, frowning, redness of face, pacing, and twisting of hands or clenching and unclenching of fists. Box 24–1 identifies presenting signs and symptoms for the risk of escalating anger leading to aggressive behavior. Simple observation of these signs, however, does not provide the information necessary to drive the appropriate intervention. Taking an accurate history of the client's background and usual coping skills, as well as gathering the client's perception of the issue (if possible), are required.

Clients' perceptions, such as the belief that they are being made to wait unnecessarily in a clinic waiting room, often provide a useful point of intervention. In this example, the nurse may apologize for the wait (thereby validating the client's distress), explain the reason, and offer to provide updates at regular and predictable intervals. In other situations, the client's perception may be vague, constantly changing, or otherwise of less use. For example, a client recently admitted to an inpatient medical unit may have multiple complaints, all of which are communicated in a loud and angry voice. Additional client history can let the nurse know if this client has generally useful coping skills that either are not readily available or have failed in the crisis of the acute illness, or it can let the nurse know if the client has a limited range of coping at baseline. For example, if a history reveals that the client generally responds to stress by jogging or working out, the nurse might empathize with this additional loss brought about by the hospitalization and work with the client to devise another strategy for the length of the admission, or might work with the physical therapy department to create a program of modified physical activity that would not harm the client. If the client's usual coping skills are poor, different types of interventions must be designed.

A brief anger-aggression questionnaire that takes little time to complete can also be used as an evaluation tool before, during, and after anger management skills training to evaluate client change.

Self-Assessment

The nurse's ability to intervene safely in situations of anger and potential violence depends on his or her awareness of self. Without this awareness, nursing interventions are marked by impulsive or emotion-based responses, which are generally nontherapeutic and may be harmful. Self-awareness includes knowledge of personal responses to anger and aggression, of norms brought from the nurse's own family, and of norms brought from the larger society. In addition, staff must be aware of personal dynamics that may trigger emotions and reactions that are not therapeutic with specific clients. Finally, nurses must assess situational factors (e.g., fatigue) that may decrease normal competence in the management of complex client problems. Self-assessment introduces objectivity and awareness into nurse-client interactions, which are prerequisites for planned, theory-based interventions.

Nurses' responses to angry or threatening clients can escalate along a continuum similar to that of clients. Depending on their level of comfort, nurses may respond with professional concern, sympathy, anxiety, fear, or anger of their own. However, the more a nursing intervention is prompted by emotion, the less likely it is to be therapeutic. For example, a nurse who interprets client anger as a threat and becomes frightened may respond with flight or with inappropriate aggression before assessing the situation and the self's competence to deal with it.

Box 24–1 *Presenting Signs and Symptoms of Violence*

1. Violence is usually (BUT NOT ALWAYS) preceded by:*
   a. Hyperactivity: most important predictor of imminent violence (e.g., pacing, restlessness.
   b. Increasing anxiety and tension: clenched jaw or fist, rigid posture, fixed or tense facial expression, mumbling to self (client may have shortness of breath, sweating, and rapid pulse).
   c. Verbal abuse: profanity, argumentativeness
   d. Loud voice, change of pitch, or very soft voice forcing others to strain to hear.
   e. Intense eye contact or avoidance of eye contact.
2. Recent acts of violence, including property violence
3. Stone silence
4. Alcohol or drug intoxication
5. Carrying a weapon or object that may be used as a weapon (e.g., fork, knife, rock).
6. Milieu conducive to violence:
   a. Overcrowding
   b. Staff inexperience
   c. Staff provocative/controlling
   d. Poor limit setting
   e. Arbitrarily taking away privileges

---

*Sometimes violence may be perceived to come from "out-of-the-blue."

From Varcarolis, E.M. (2000). *Psychiatric nursing clinical guide: assessment tools and diagnoses.* Philadelphia: W.B. Saunders.

In addition, facial expression is the quickest marker of emotional activation and can communicate the emotion to others before the person is aware he or she is experiencing it. This expression of emotion can activate the same feeling in others, a process called emotional contagion (Hatfield et al. 1994). When the nurse and the client are responding to each other from emotion and impulse, the potential exists for a mutually reinforcing cycle of anger and aggression.

Nurses' responses may also reflect norms from their families of origin. In some families, anger is responded to with attempts at peacemaking; in others, anger is responded to aggressively, with attempts to maintain domination. Some families ignore anger, leaving its antecedents and consequences unaddressed, while others respond to it with strict rules of allowed and forbidden behaviors. These responses are usually learned early (Bandura 1973) and are often unexamined; many people remain unaware that alternative responses exist that are both possible and permissible. Even those who, in adulthood, have altered their approach to the presence of anger may find old patterns resurfacing when their stress is increased. These unexamined responses by nurses can strongly influence their limit-setting styles as well as their impulsive reactions when they feel threatened.

Similarly, nurses have personal issues that they bring to potential conflict. Certain types of clients may lead to feelings of dislike, irritability, or fear. Certain types of interactions or settings may trigger intense personal feelings. If these precipitants to discomfort are known in advance, the nurse is less surprised when they occur and can also develop a self-management strategy for their occurrence.

Finally, situational events can affect nursing interventions. Staff may be dealing with such issues as sleep deprivation, fatigue, conflict with co-workers, and burnout. Acknowledging these issues allows the nurse to re-examine the response to a client or to negotiate a reassignment of clients for a time.

Self-assessment ideally promotes calm, theory-based responses to client anger and potential aggression. These responses are further supported by the following techniques:

■ Deep breathing
■ Relaxation of muscles that are not in use
■ Empathetic interpretation of the client's distress
■ Review of intervention strategies

In settings in which staff can reasonably expect episodes of client anger and aggression, staff must have regular teaching and practice of verbal and nonverbal interventions. This fosters increased confidence in the nurse's own abilities and those of co-workers.

Assessment Guidelines

ASSESSMENT GUIDELINES: ANGER AND AGGRESSION

1. A history of violence is the simple best predictor of future violence.
2. Clients who are hyperactive, impulsive, or predisposed to irritability are at higher risk for violence.
3. Assess client risk for violence:

   ■ Has a wish or intent to harm?
   ■ Has a plan?
   ■ Has availability to carry out plan?
   ■ Consider demographics: sex (male), age (14–24), socioeconomic status (low), and support system (low)

4. Aggression by clients occurs most often in the context of limit-setting by the nurse.
5. Clients with a history of limited coping skills, including lack of assertiveness or use of intimidation, are at higher risk to use violence.
6. Assess self for personal triggers and responses likely to escalate client violence, including client characteristics or situations that trigger impatience, irritation, or defensiveness.
7. Assess personal sense of competence when in any situation of potential conflict; consider asking for the assistance of another staff member.

NURSING DIAGNOSIS

Two nursing diagnoses are important when potential aggression is identified. These are Ineffective coping and Risk for self-directed violence or Risk for other-directed violence. First we'll look at Ineffective coping, overwhelmed, and Ineffective coping, maladaptive. These two types of ineffective coping represent two major ways clients become anxious and angry. Clients may have coping skills that are adequate for day-to-day events in their lives but are overwhelmed by the stresses of illness or hospitalization. Other clients may have a pattern of maladaptive coping, which is marginally effective and consists of a set of coping strategies that have been developed to meet unusual or extraordinary situations (e.g., abusive families).

Ideally, intervention occurs at the point of ineffective individual coping. Nurses work with clients to support or teach ways of coping that will decrease anxiety and distress. However, client behavior may escalate quickly, or the client may mask early signs of distress; nurses may be distracted and may miss those early signs, even when they are visible. Other clients may be acutely intoxicated and not amenable to early nursing interventions. In these situations, the problem with anger may not be resolved before the **Risk for violence** exists. When this diagnosis is used, de-escalation of anger is the primary nursing intervention. Seclusion, restraint, or psychopharmacology may be necessary to ensure the safety of clients and staff.

OUTCOME CRITERIA

Having clearly defined outcome criteria (goals) when interventions are planned for angry and aggressive clients is important for identifying the behaviors that staff would encourage and identify if

their interventions have been successful. Specific outcome criteria have been outlined by Johnson and colleagues (2000) for use with angry and aggressive clients.

See Table 24–1 for potential outcomes for aggressive behaviors (NOC 2000).

PLANNING

Planning interventions necessitates having a sound assessment, e.g., past history (previous acts of violence, comorbid disorders), evaluation of present

TABLE 24–1 *Nursing Outcomes: Aggression and Control*

Definition: Self-restraint of assaultive, combative, or abusive behaviors toward others

AGGRESSIVE CONTROL	NEVER DEMON- STRATED 1	RARELY DEMON- STRATED 2	SOMETIMES DEMON- STRATED 3	OFTEN DEMON- STRATED 4	CONSISTENTLY DEMONSTRATED 5
Indicators					
1. Refrains from verbal outbursts	1	2	3	4	5
2. Refrains from violating others' personal space	1	2	3	4	5
3. Refrains from striking others	1	2	3	4	5
4. Refrains from harming others	1	2	3	4	5
5. Refrains from harming animals	1	2	3	4	5
6. Refrains from destroying property	1	2	3	4	5
7. Communicates needs appropriately	1	2	3	4	5
8. Communicates feelings appropriately	1	2	3	4	5
9. Verbalizes control of impulses	1	2	3	4	5
10. Identifies when angry	1	2	3	4	5
11. Identifies when frustrated	1	2	3	4	5
12. Identifies situations that precipitate hostility	1	2	3	4	5
13. Identifies responsibility to maintain control	1	2	3	4	5
14. Identifies when feeling aggressive	1	2	3	4	5
15. Identifies alternatives to aggression	1	2	3	4	5
16. Identifies alternatives to verbal outbursts	1	2	3	4	5
17. Vents negative feelings appropriately	1	2	3	4	5
18. Upholds contract to restrain aggressive behaviors	1	2	3	4	5
19. Maintains self-control without supervision	1	2	3	4	5
20. Other _____ (Specify)	1	2	3	4	5

From: Johnson, H., Maas, M., Meriden, M., and Moorehead, S. (2000). *Nursing outcomes classification (NOC)* (2nd ed.). St. Louis: Mosby, p. 112.

coping skills, and willingness on the part of the client to learn alternative and nonviolent ways of handling angry feelings.

Does the client:

1. Have good coping skills but is presently overwhelmed?
2. Have marginal coping skills and uses anger/violence as a way to cover other feelings and gain a sense of mastery or control?
3. Have a neuropsychotic or chronic psychotic disorder and is prone to violence?
4. Have cognitive deficits that predispose to anger in the form of misinterpretation of environmental stimuli?

Does the situation call for:

1. Psychotherapeutic approaches to teach the client new skills for handling anger?
2. Immediate intervention to prevent overt violence (de-escalation techniques, restraints/seclusion, and/or psychopharmacy)?

Approaches that have been proved particularly effective in the management of anger are (a) behavioral and (b) cognitive-behavioral techniques used in individual, family, couple, or group formats.

INTERVENTIONS

Interventions are best developed from research-based theory. However, the form the intervention takes will vary by client presentation and history, pre-existing client coping skills, co-occurring mental disorders, and setting.

General Hospital Settings

ANGRY CLIENTS WITH HEALTHY COPING WHO ARE OVERWHELMED

A careful assessment, with history and information from family, determines whether client anger is a usual or an unusual way of managing stress. Interventions for clients whose usual coping strategies are healthy involve finding ways to re-establish or substitute similar means of dealing with the hospitalization. This problem solving occurs in collaboration with the client, in which the nurse acknowledges the client's distress, validates it as understandable under the circumstances, and indicates a willingness to search for solutions. Validation includes making an apology to the client when appropriate, such as when a promised intervention (e.g., changing a dressing by a certain time) has not been delivered.

This collaboration cannot occur unless nurses recognize their own self-protective responses to angry clients, including the wish to avoid contact with them, impatience, and frustration. Unrecognized, these understandable but unhelpful responses on the part of nurses can result in negative cycles of staff-client conflict in which the client feels increasingly misunderstood and ignored, and therefore increasingly hostile, while staff wish to further avoid or to punish. These negative interactive cycles interfere with the provision of empathic care; they ultimately lead to burnout in nurses.

Finally, clients who have become angry may be unable to moderate this emotion enough to problem-solve with their nurses; others may be unable to communicate the source of their anger. Often, the nurse, knowing the client and the context of the anger, can make an accurate guess at what feeling is behind the anger. Naming this feeling can lead to a dissipation of the anger, can help the client to feel understood, and can lead to a calmer discussion of the distress. Some of the feelings that can precipitate anger are listed in Box 24–2. An example of nursing interventions that are helpful in dissipating anger in a hospital situation follows:

Vignette

■ A 41-year-old woman with a long history of peripheral vascular disease and of surgeries for vascular grafts and repair of graft occlusions is admitted to the hospital with severe pain in her left foot. Tests reveal that vessels to the foot are occluded. Additional surgery is ruled out, and

BOX 24–2   Feelings That May Underlie Anger

Discounted
Embarrassed
Frightened
Found out
Guilty
Humiliated
Hurt
Ignored
Inadequate
Insecure
Not heard
Out of control of the situation
Rejected
Threatened
Tired
Vulnerable

medication is prescribed. Unfortunately, the medication is ineffective, and the foot begins to become necrotic. Physicians then discuss amputation with the client. The client refuses the surgery, demands a series of unproven alternative therapies, and is extremely angry with all members of the hospital staff. The treatment team becomes increasingly impatient to schedule further surgery before the necrosis worsens, and the client begins to experience systemic signs of infection. This impatience aggravates the client's feelings of being out of control and erodes her belief that she is a competent partner in her treatment.

Intervention. The nurse is aware that before her disability from progressive vascular disease, the client was employed for many years as a buyer at a local department store. The nurse knows, too, that the client's family lives some distance from the hospital and is unable to visit regularly. Finally, the nurse understands that when the client was admitted, she had expected medical intervention once more to save her leg. Nursing intervention is twofold. First, the client's anger and unwillingness to discuss her condition end when the nurse names her feelings of fear and being out of control. Once the client's anger is reduced, the nurse is able to help her negotiate more time for the final decision; this allows the client to complete her anticipatory grieving (including stages of denial, anger, and bargaining). In this interval, the client's wish to explore alternative therapies is addressed via second and third medical opinions; she is also able to consult further with her family.

ANGRY CLIENTS WITH MARGINAL COPING SKILLS

Clients whose coping skills were marginal before hospitalization need a different set of interventions than those with basically healthy ways of coping. Clients with maladaptive coping are poorly equipped to use alternatives when their initial attempts to cope are unsuccessful or are found to be inappropriate. Such clients frequently manifest anger and aggression. For some, anger and intimidation are primary strategies used to obtain their short-term goals of feelings of control/mastery. For others, the anger occurs when limited or primitive attempts at coping are unsuccessful and alternatives are unknown. For these clients, anger is a particular risk in inpatient settings.

This is especially true for hospitalized clients with chemical dependence who may be anxious about being cut off from their substance of choice; they may have well-founded concerns that any physical pain will be inadequately addressed. Many clients with marginal coping also have personality styles that externalize blame. That is, they see the source of their discomfort and anxiety as being outside themselves; relief must therefore also come from an outside source (e.g., the nurse/medication).

Again, an adequate nursing history allows for early identification of clients who need special care plans. This recognition also decreases the potential for staff frustration by altering expectations of clients' coping abilities.

Initial client anxiety can be addressed with a respectful approach that establishes a sense of mutual collaboration. Respect can be maintained if nurses operate from the following assumptions (Linehan 1993a):

■ Clients are doing the best they can.
■ Clients want to improve.
■ Client behaviors make sense within their world view.

In addition, baseline anxiety can be moderated by the provision of comfort items before they are requested (e.g., decaffeinated coffee, deck of cards); this can build rapport and acts symbolically to reassure. Anxiety can also be minimized by reducing ambiguity. This strategy includes clear and concrete communication. Providing clarity about what the nurse can and cannot do is most usefully ended with an offer of something within the nurse's power to provide (i.e., leaving the client with a "yes").

Interventions for anxiety might also include the use of distractions, such as magazines, action comics, and video games. Generally, distractions that are colorful and do not require sustained attention work best, although this varies according to the client's interests and abilities. Finally, clients with a high level of baseline anxiety and limited coping skills are helped when their interactions with the treatment team are predictable; this might include speaking with the physician at a specific time each day or having the client see a single spokesperson from the treatment team each day.

Because these clients have limited coping skills, nursing interventions include teaching alternative behaviors and strategies. For clients who externalize blame, such teaching may best be preceded by a gentle challenge. The challenge serves to engage the client's interest in teaching that might otherwise be seen as irrelevant (Doren 1996).

Vignette

■ *A 21-year-old man who was in an automobile accident is bedridden with a pelvic fracture. During his first day of admission, he yells at each nurse who walks by his room, using expletives in his demands that the nurse enter the room.*

Intervention. The nurse who is assigned to the client for the evening stops in his doorway after he yells at her and asks in mild disbelief: "Is this working for you? Do nurses really come in here when you yell at them that way?" The client responds sullenly, justifying his behavior by complaining about his care. However, the nurse's challenge has caught his attention, and she goes on to suggest (i.e., teach) alternative strategies for contacting her and other nurses. The strategies are immediately put into use by the client.

This intervention is also important in that the nurse has taught a couple of strategies, providing the client with choices and thus with more control.

Often, anger may be communicated via long-term verbal abuse. If attempts to teach alternatives have not been successful, three interventions can be used.

1. The first is to leave the room as soon as the abuse begins; the client can be informed that the nurse will return in a specific amount of time (e.g., 20 minutes) when the situation is calmer. A matter-of-fact, neutral manner is important because fear, indignation, and arguing are gratifying to many verbally abusive clients. Alternatively, if the nurse is in the midst of a procedure and cannot leave immediately, the nurse can break off conversation and eye contact, completing the procedure quickly and matter-of-factly before leaving the room.

2. Withdrawal of attention to the abuse is successful only if a second intervention is also used. This step requires attending positively to nonabusive communication by the client. Interventions can include discussing non–illness-related topics, responding to requests, and providing emotional support.

3. Clients who are regularly verbally abusive may respond best to the predictability of routine, such as scheduled contacts with the nurse (e.g., every 30 minutes or every 60 minutes). Use of such contacts provides nursing attention that is not contingent on the client's behavior and therefore does not reinforce the abuse. This intervention works only to the extent that the nurse maintains the scheduled contacts as agreed on. In addition, other staff members must be informed of the care plan so that they do not inadvertently sabotage it by responding to incidental requests by the client. Of course, the client's illness or injury may sometimes require nursing visits for assessment or intervention outside the scheduled contact times. These visits can be carried out in a calm, brief, matter-of-fact manner. This care plan is best negotiated with the client and can be presented as supportive in that it attempts to address client anxiety about getting needs met (anxiety that is

reflected in the verbal abuse and also manifested by frequent angry demands) through the predictability of the nurse's contacts.

Appropriate interventions can be difficult when the nurse is feeling threatened. Remaining matter of fact with clients who habitually use anger and intimidation can be difficult because these people are often skillful at making personal and pointed statements. It is important for the nurse to remember that clients do not know their nurses personally and thus have no basis on which they can make accurate judgments. Nurses can also vent their own responses elsewhere, with other staff or family members or via critical incident debriefing.

Inpatient Psychiatric Settings

It is important to know that not all psychiatric clients are potentially violent, and aggression appears to be correlated less with certain illnesses than with certain client characteristics. For example, the best single predictor of violence is a history of violence in a particular client (Davis 1991; Davis and Boster 1983). A second significant risk factor is impulsivity (Rossi et al. 1986; Berkowitz 1982, 1983).

The context of anger and aggression has also been reported as a factor. In one study, clients identified conflict with staff as the most common reason for violence (Sheridan et al. 1990). In another study, impulsive behavior by psychotic clients was not a function of symptoms such as hallucinations and delusions but was a result of interactions with staff that involved setting of limits or imposition of rules (Gallop et al. 1992).

Given these factors, research on the relationship of client anger to nursing styles of limit setting is pertinent. In one study, six interpersonal styles were studied: (1) authoritarian, (2) platitudes, (3) solutions provided without options, (4) solutions provided with options, (5) empathy without options, and (6) empathy with options. An authoritarian style of limit setting might be simply telling an angry client that she or he is (i.e., the behavior is) *inappropriate*. Providing solutions without options might be telling a client to take a time-out away from others. Empathy with options might consist of acknowledging the client's anger followed by asking whether the client would be helped by a time-out or whether talking the issue out with a staff member would be more useful.

This study found that nursing styles of setting limits were powerful moderators of situational anger, regardless of the client's diagnosis or impulsivity. For all clients, an authoritarian style was more likely to precipitate anger than were other styles. Empathy with options was the strategy that was least likely to generate anger. For nonimpulsive clients, three styles were effective without causing anger:

1. solutions with options,
2. empathy without options, and
3. empathy with options.

For clients with high levels of impulsivity, however, only the third style kept anger at a low level. Interestingly, with these clients, empathy alone (i.e. without options) was not sufficient (Lancee et al. 1995).

If staff can identify clients who have a potential for violence, early intervention becomes possible. Nurses can work with the clients to recognize their early signs of anger and can teach them strategies to manage the anger and to prevent aggression. Because anger has a strong cognitive component, cognitive interventions are helpful. Cognitive techniques can be taught in groups (Gerlock 1994) or individually (Reeder 1991). Both state and trait anger have been decreased via the use of cognitive therapy groups. While anger is often an attempt to regain or maintain control, it generally works only for the short term. Cognitive therapy can provide an alternative means of control that works for the long term as well.

Vignette

■ *A 19-year-old man has a 2-year history of quadriplegia. This client also has a history of drug abuse that began in grade school, an inability to set or work toward long-term goals, and a primary coping style of anger and intimidation. The client is admitted to an inpatient psychiatric unit because of increasing suicidal ideation. He clearly communicates to staff that his preferred means of coping with anger is to "cuss people out" and run into them with his wheelchair. However, in the hospital, the consequence of wheelchair assaults is that the client is secluded in his room, which he finds intolerable. The client requests that someone work with him on anger management, so that he can have the increased control afforded by the ability to develop alternatives.*

Intervention. Via cognitive therapy, this client is taught to identify the thoughts and beliefs he uses to drive his anger. These typically relate to feeling unheard by the staff; secondarily, he often believes that staff purposely act to increase their control at his expense. The client is taught to look at each situation to find proof for and against his beliefs (e.g., in neutral observations of a particular staff member, did this person act like a "control freak"?). He then learns to substitute more reality-based interpretations of events and interactions. Finally, the client is taught to generate options for action in the situation; he then lists the pros and cons of those

options. These are interventions developed by Beck (Beck 1976; Beck et al. 1979) and Beck and Freeman (1990). Because cognitive therapy is a specialized therapy learned in part through supervised clinical practice, cognitive interventions would be enhanced by the consultation of an advanced practice nurse with expertise in this modality.

Response. Because this client is intelligent and motivated to gain increased personal control, he learns these techniques quickly. In addition, once it becomes clear that issues of feeling unheard and out of control underlay most episodes of anger, the client is able to target those issues for problem solving. He rapidly develops effective and appropriate ways to make himself heard and understood. He also becomes adept at communicating when he feels out of control and at finding ingenious ways of negotiating control on issues that are particularly important to him. The client's suicidal impulses, which occur when he is frustrated, also diminish.

In the absence of clear markers for clients who are at risk for violence, nurses are left with their clinical judgment and intuition. While expert intuition is valuable, bias may occur. For example, one study looked at how well client ethnicity correlated with the accuracy of staff prediction of violence. Clients of color and male clients were found to be the groups in which violence was overpredicted most often (McNiel and Binder 1995).

Clients With Cognitive Deficits

A client group that is particularly at risk for acting aggressively is that with cognitive deficits. Such deficits may result from delirium, brain injury, or illnesses associated with aging (e.g., Alzheimer's disease, multi-infarct dementia). Delirium is a side effect of certain metabolic dysfunctions, such as electrolyte imbalance; it is time limited, ending when the underlying disorder is treated. Delirium is marked by clouded consciousness; decreased ability to shift, focus, and sustain attention to environmental stimuli; and disorientation. Hallmark symptoms include a short onset and waxing and waning of symptoms (American Psychiatric Association 2000).

Alzheimer's disease and multi-infarct dementia are progressive diseases of brain deterioration. The onset is slow, and these diseases are ultimately fatal. Brain injury may be traumatic or the result of illnesses such as carcinoma. Although symptoms and prognoses of such injuries are highly variable, depending on the cause and the affected area, they often have the following elements in common with delirium and illnesses such Alzheimer's disease: decreased impulse control, emotional lability, and decreased ability to interpret information from the environment. Clients who are unable to understand their environment can become anxious, frightened, angry, and assaultive. Their situation is analogous to that of an individual who remembers falling asleep at home but awakens in the morning in a train station in another country, surrounded by strangers and noise, with no recollection of coming there.

Traditional approaches to disorientation and to the agitation that it can cause have relied heavily on reality orientation and medication. Reality orientation consists of providing the correct information to the client about place, date, and current life circumstances. For many clients, this is comforting because it reminds them of pertinent information and helps them feel grounded. For others, reality orientation does not work and may cause further escalation. A client who does not understand the environment may also not be able to recognize or trust the caregiver. If the client is feeling frightened and threatened, information from a seeming stranger is suspect and becomes part of the confusion. Some disoriented clients believe that they are young and feel the need to return to important tasks that are specific to those earlier years. For example, an elderly woman may insist that she has babies at home that she needs to care for. This client is likely to become more agitated if the nurse tries to tell her that her babies have grown up and that there is no home to return to. A woman who believes that she is 23 years old and has babies at home would not be calmed by being told that she is 78 and has no babies. It is often more helpful in such a case to try to reflect back to clients their feelings and to show understanding and concern for their plight. For example:

Nurse: "Mrs. Green, you miss your children, and this can be a lonely place."

Sedating medication may calm agitation, but it also acts to further cloud a client's sensorium, making disorientation worse. A negative spiral of disorientation, agitation, medication, clouded consciousness, and further disorientation that leads to additional agitation and more medication may result. The outcome of such a spiral is generally oversedation—and possibly a hastened death from diseases related to inactivity.

Alternative interventions exist. Orientation aids, such as a calendar and a clock, can provide easy reference and increased autonomy; they must be prominent and must be easily read by clients with diminished eyesight. Because such clients have difficulty interpreting environmental stimuli, another set of interventions involves making the environment as simple, predictable, and comfortable as possible. Simplicity includes decreasing sensory stimuli. In the hospital, this might include placing the client's bed away from doorways that enter onto the hall

and choosing not to turn on the television. Predictability can be provided by making each day's activity schedule as much like that of the previous day as possible; the day's schedule can be prominently posted in the client's room. Comfort might include familiar photographs, familiar objects from home, and a rocking chair; the latter can provide a rhythmic source of self-soothing.

If a client becomes agitated, a calm and unhurried approach is important to avoid further increasing the client's fear. A client who is uncertain of the surroundings feels further threatened by the rush toward him or her of one or more strangers who also appear agitated (i.e., staff). The steps for making contact with an agitated, disoriented client (catastrophic reaction) are listed in Box 24–3.

Episodes of agitation have been decreased in number and in intensity for clients with age-related dementias and in clients with head injuries as the result of identification of the antecedents and consequences of such episodes (Teri and Logsdon 1990; Uomoto and Brockway 1992). Once antecedents are understood, interventions are often obvious.

Vignette

■ An 81-year-old woman with Alzheimer's disease always becomes agitated during her morning care; this comes to be a time dreaded among her caregivers. Careful observation of the antecedents to episodes of agitation reveals a natural course to the morning problems. The client is initially calm when care begins. However, one staff person gives morning care to the client and her roommate at the same time, moving between the two. Observation of the process reveals that the client becomes distracted by cues being given to her roommate and often startles when the caregiver returns to her. As this process continues over several minutes, the client becomes increasingly distressed and then agitated. When her care is provided by one person who remains with her throughout the process, the client's morning agitation ends.

Consequences of agitation may also be a factor if they serve to reinforce the behaviors. For example, an elderly man who loves ice cream and who becomes calm when it is given to him becomes agitated more often when ice cream is routinely used to stop his angry behaviors.

Finally, clients who misperceive their setting or life situation may be calmed by **validation therapy** (Feil 1992). This intervention begins where clients are and grounds them where they feel most secure. Rather than attempting to re-orient the client, the nurse asks him or her to further describe the setting or situation that the client has reported as a problem (e.g., the need to return home). During the conversa-

BOX 24–3 *Cognitive Deficits*

THE CATASTROPHIC REACTION: MAKING CONTACT

Cognitive deficits result in:

A decreased ability to interpret sensory stimuli.
A decreased ability to tolerate sensory stimuli.

Striking out represents fear or the feeling that the environment is out of control.

A second agitated person (e.g., staff) leads to increased agitation.

Therefore:

1. Face the client from within 2 feet, remaining as calm and unhurried as possible.
2. Say the client's name.
3. Gain eye contact.
4. Smile.

5. Repeat (2) through (4) several times if necessary, to gain and maintain contact.
6. Use gentle touch, keep voice soft (the person often matches this tone and lowers his or her voice also).
7. Ask the client if he or she needs the bathroom.
8. Help the client regain a sense of control—ask what he or she needs.
9. Validate the client's feelings: "You look upset. This can be a confusing place."
10. Use short, simple sentences; complex explanations just represent more noise.
11. Decrease sensory stimulation.
12. Use rhythmic sources of self-stimulation, e.g., humming, a rocking chair.

Adapted from Rader, J., Doan, J., Schwab, M. (1985). How to decrease wandering, a form of agenda behavior. *Geriatric Nursing,* 6(4):196–199.

tion, the nurse can comment on what appears to be underlying the client's distress, thus validating it. For example, the elderly woman who believes that she needs to return home to care for her children is asked to tell the nurse more about her children. The nurse may note that the client misses her children and that the current setting gets lonely at times. As nurses show interest in aspects of the client's life,

they establish themselves as safe, understanding persons. In turn, the client often becomes calmer and more open to redirection. As clients reminisce in this fashion, they often bring themselves into the present: "Of course, they're all grown and doing well on their own now." Refer to Chapter 21 for more on interventions for people with cognitive impairments. Box 24–4 provides a framework for

BOX 24–4 *Cognitive Deficits: Validation Therapy*

This therapy lets you begin emotionally where the client is.

This therapy "grounds" the client where he or she feels most secure.

Reality orientation is the first intervention. Resistance to this may represent an increased feeling by the client that the environment makes no sense.

Therefore:

1. Make a connection with the person as outlined in Box 24–3.
2. Repeat some part of what the client has said: "You need to go home to fix dinner for your children?"
3. Reflect what seems to be the underlying feeling

(usually related to a lack of connectedness or security): "You miss your children. And this can be a lonely place."
4. Continue to talk with the client about the topic (e.g., the children); this establishes you as a safe, understanding person.
5. As the client becomes calmer and more secure, redirect him or her (e.g., back to the client room).
6. Provide a parting reinforcer (e.g., food, rocking chair), an esteem-enhancing comment, or a reassuring comment.
7. Provide orienting information again only if the person requests it.

Adapted from Rader, J., Doan, J., Schwab, M. (1985). How to decrease wandering, a form of agenda behavior. *Geriatric Nursing,* 6(4):196–199.

validation therapy. Refer to Chapter 33 for more on the use of validation reminiscent therapeutic modalities for the elderly.

Interventions for Aggressive or Violent Clients

At times, the best early assessment and intervention, whether behavioral or medicinal, is unsuccessful in calming an aggressive client. If that client presents risk to self or others, seclusion or restraint is necessary. Use of seclusion or restraint in these circumstances demonstrates the value of human life by preventing clients from harming themselves or others. Interventions here reflect a nursing diagnosis of **Risk for violence directed at others (or self).** The rule of thumb is always to use the least restrictive approach that the situation warrants.

DE-ESCALATION TECHNIQUES

Refer to Box 24–5 for some guidelines for de-escalation techniques.

PSYCHOBIOLOGICAL INTERVENTIONS

Medication for anger and aggression best targets the underlying cause of the anger. For example, antipsychotic medication is used for clients whose halluci-

> **Box 24–5** *De-escalation Techniques: Practice Principles*
>
> 1. Maintain the client's self-esteem and dignity
> 2. Maintain calmness (your own and the client's)
> 3. Assess the client and the situation
> 4. Identify stressors and stress indicators
> 5. Respond as early as possible
> 6. Use a calm, clear tone of voice
> 7. Invest time
> 8. Remain honest
> 9. Establish what the client considers to be his or her need
> 10. Be goal oriented
> 11. Maintain a large personal space
> 12. Avoid verbal struggles
> 13. Give several options
> 14. Make clear the options
> 15. Utilize a non-aggressive posture
> 16. Use genuineness and empathy
> 17. Attempt to be confidently aware
> 18. Use verbal, non-verbal, and communication skills
> 19. Be assertive (not aggressive)
> 20. Assess for personal safety
>
> _____
>
> From Mason, T., and Chandley, M. (1999). *Management of violence and aggression* (p. 73). Philadelphia: Churchill Livingstone.

nations, delusions, or thought disorders drive their anger. Similarly, manic clients who are irritable and show poor impulse control are helped by treatment with mood-stabilizing medications, such as lithium. In both these examples, benzodiazepines may be used until the primary medication has reached a therapeutic blood level or has had sufficient time to take effect.

In the absence of psychotic symptoms, antipsychotic medications are not the best choice for the treatment of aggression. This use relies solely on the sedative effects of the drug and it places clients at risk for side effects, including the permanent and disfiguring tardive dyskinesia.

Benzodiazepine use for aggression is always short term. With long-term use, clients develop tolerance to its sedative effects, are at increased risk for side effects, and may develop psychological dependence on the drug. In a small number of clients, benzodiazepines have led to paradoxical rage responses, indicating that careful observation is necessary when these drugs are used for calming agitated, aggressive clients.

Unfortunately, the psychological mechanisms contributing to anger are not always clear. In many cases, nurses rely on empirical research about the effects of medication on anger in various client populations. For example, fluoxetine has been seen to decrease anger in clients with borderline personality disorder, depression, and post-traumatic stress disorder. The decreases occurred independent of changes in clients' depressed mood (Fave et al. 1993; Salzman et al. 1995; Rubey et al. 1996). This effect is likely a function of the role serotonin has been found to play in impulsive aggression. Similarly, risperadone has been reported to decrease irritable aggression in patients with Axis I disorders, likely because of its effects on serotonin receptors (Monnelly and Ciraullo, 1999).

Impulsive anger related to brain injury, either from trauma or illnesses such as stroke, has been found to respond to beta blockers (e.g., propranolol). In many of the clinical trials reported with these clients, beta blockers were successful after multiple failed attempts with antipsychotics, benzodiazepines, anticonvulsants, and lithium. Improvement was marked or moderate in as many as 75% of clients in some reports (Williams et al. 1982; Greendyke et al. 1984). An 8-week trial may be necessary with beta blockers. In addition, these drugs can increase blood levels of certain antipsychotic medications, leading to increased side effects or toxicity. Other common side effects are bradycardia, hypotension, and occasional depression.

All psychoactive drugs must be used with caution, and with elderly clients, drugs are usually given in doses lower than what would normally be considered therapeutic. Elderly clients are often sensitive to psychiatric medications; they experience side effects and toxic effects more quickly than younger clients. Treatment effects can regularly be seen at lower-than-usual doses. For these clients, pharmacotherapy is best begun slowly and dosages raised gradually.

Similarly, clients of differing ethnic groups and of differing national origin respond differently from each other in both the treatment effects and the side effects of medications, including psychiatric medications. These differences are in part a function of differing drug effects at the cellular level and are thought to result from both genetic and environmental factors (e.g., diet). Pharmacotherapy is again best begun slowly, with dosages raised gradually; several drug trials may be required before the most useful regimen is found. As with all clients, concern must be taken for client reports of effects and side effects; translators and experts in the client's culture may be necessary for these reports to be obtained most accurately (Lin et al. 1995).

Maxmen and Ward (1995) stated that it is important to identify whether the presenting behavior is acute aggression or chronic aggression. Acute aggression can be medically managed best by short-term use of medications with rapid onset of action (Maxmen and Ward 1995; Marangell 1999).

Chronic aggression is a more common problem, and aggression may diminish only after a therapeutic dose of the appropriate medication is used for 4 to 8 weeks. Clients should be informed about this time lag. Drugs used to treat clients with chronic aggression include propranolol, anticonvulsants (carbamazepine, valproic acid), lithium, and buspirone. Caution is taken when chronic aggression is treated with antipsychotics (risk of tardive dyskinesia, hypotension, oversedation), and benzodiazepines, which rarely halt chronic violence and may trigger paradoxical rage reaction (Maxmen and Ward 1995).

A summary of medications used in the treatment of persistent/chronic aggression is given in Table 24–2.

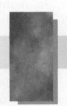

TABLE 24–2   *Psychotropic Treatment of Chronic Aggression*

GENERIC GROUP	INDICATIONS	COMMENTS
Beta blockers, e.g., propranolol	Recurrent or chronic aggression in organically based violence, e.g., Alzheimer's disease Stroke Huntington's disease Psychosis in which aggression is unrelated to psychotic thought	Often used in high doses (120–240 mg/day). Consistent and effective results may take 4–8 weeks.
Anticonvulsants	Bipolar disorder Borderline personality disorder Conduct disorder Episodic dyscontrol Posttraumatic stress disorder (PTSD) Central nervous system disorder	Carbamazepine—monitor bone marrow suppression and blood abnormalities. Valproic acid—monitor liver function and platelets.
Lithium	Mania-associated violence Uncontrolled rage triggered by nothing or minor stimuli, e.g., borderline personality disorder, PTSD	Effective for violence in prisoners and mentally retarded. Does not affect aggressive behavior until therapeutic blood levels are reached.
Buspirone (BuSpar)	Cognitively impaired populations and possibly prison populations	Nonsedating and nonaddicting. Effectiveness takes 4–10 weeks to decrease aggression.
Nadolol	Diminishes assaultiveness in chronic paranoid schizophrenia	Few reports.
Trazodone	Aggression and agitation in demented and mentally retarded (does not impair cognition).	Do not use in males who cannot report priapism. Monitor for orthostatic hypotension.

Adapted from Maxmen, J. S., and Ward, N. G. (1995). *Psychotropic drugs fast facts* (2nd ed., pp. 233–236). New York: W. W. Norton. Copyright © 1995 by Nicholas J. Ward and the Estate of Jerrold S. Maxmen. Copyright © 1991 by Jerrold S. Maxmen. Reprinted by permission of W. W. Norton & Company, Inc.

SECLUSION OR PHYSICAL RESTRAINTS

Seclusion is the involuntary confinement of a client alone in a room, which the client is prevented from leaving, for a specific period of time. The goal of seclusion is never punitive. Rather, as noted earlier, *the goal is safety of the client and others.* Certain clients are able to control their aggression without restraint as long as they are alone or are in an environment of very low stimulation. Other clients may be coming out of a period of time in restraints and may need a period of time in seclusion in order to make a successful transition back onto the unit or into the normal living environment. As a part of this transition, clients may be placed on a schedule that alternates periods of seclusion with increasing time in the ward community (e.g., 45 minutes in seclusion, alternating with 15 minutes out, followed by 30 minutes in seclusion and 30 minutes out).

Seclusion or physical restraint is not used unless alternative interventions have been considered, including verbal intervention, behavioral care plan, medication, decrease in sensory stimulation, removal of a particular problematic stimulus, presence of a significant other, frequent observation, and use of a sitter. Seclusion or restraint is used in circumstances in which the client

- Presents a clear and present danger to self.
- Presents a clear and present danger to others.
- Has been legally detained for involuntary treatment and is thought to be an escape risk.
- Requests to be secluded or restrained. (APNA, 2000)

The mechanism for placing an aggressive client in restraints requires having an adequate number of staff available, all of whom have been trained in restraint procedures. Staff who work in areas where potentially aggressive clients are regularly treated, such as emergency departments (EDs) and psychiatric units, are required to have regular training and practice in restraint procedures. Such training and practice increase staff proficiency in the use of restraints and decrease the possibilities of injury to clients or staff.

Clients may not be held in seclusion or restraint without a physician's order. Once in restraint, clients must be directly observed and formally assessed at frequent, regular intervals for level of awareness, level of activity, safety within the restraints, hydration, toileting, nutrition, and comfort. The frequency of observation is mandated by licensing and accreditation agencies. Refer to Chapter 8 for more on the legalities of seclusion and restraints and Chapter 19 for more on the procedure.

Guidelines for mechanical restraints are given in Table 24–3.

TABLE 24–3 *Some Guidelines for Mechanical Restraint*

Indications for use	To protect the patient from self-harm
	To prevent the patient from assaulting others
Legal requirements	Multidisciplinary involvement
	Physician's signature
	Patient advocate/relative notification
	Patient agreement
Clinical assessments	Patient's mental state
	Risks to the patient
	Need for restraints
Observations	Nurse in constant attendance
	Written record every 15 minutes
	Release limb from restraint every 2 hours
	Stretch limb through range of movement
	Monitor vital signs
	Observe blood flow
	Observe the restraint is not rubbing
	Provide for nutrition, hydration, and elimination.
Release procedure	Limit on time in restraint
	Behaviors required before release
	Release procedure
	Terminating restraints
Documentation	Restraint documentation
	Patient's record
	Day report

Adapted from Mason, T., and Chandley, M. (2000). *Management of violence and aggression.* Philadelphia: Churchill Livingstone, p. 179.

EVALUATION

Evaluation of the care plan is essential for clients who are potentially angry and aggressive. A well-considered plan has specific outcome criteria goals (e.g., see Table 24–1). Evaluation provides information about whether the interventions have met these goals; if they have not, the plan must be revised. The plan is also individualized. For example, an initial care plan may include assessment of the environmental stimuli that precede a client's agitation. Once these have been identified, the plan provides interventions that are specific to those stimuli. However, the plan can work only if staff evaluate the effectiveness of this approach by noting whether the agitation has decreased or disappeared. Evaluation may reveal that the client's agitation has decreased except for specific situations. The plan can then be revised to include these situations.

SUMMARY

Angry emotions and aggressive actions are difficult targets for nursing intervention. Since these two phenomena are universal, nurses benefit from an understanding of how the angry and aggressive client should be handled. An understanding of client cues to escalating aggression, appropriate goals for intervention for individuals in a variety of situations, and helpful nursing interventions are important for nurses in any setting.

Numerous theories exist that help explain why anger for some gets out of control; the theories can help us understand what triggers and escalates aggression in various individuals. As opposed to older beliefs, it has been found that "getting it all out" is not, after all, a useful way to diminish anger. On the contrary, it has been found that the expression of anger can lead to increased anger and to negative physiological changes. There are, however, two theories of anger and aggression that have led to useful management techniques that are beneficial for clients who escalate out of control. These two theories are the (1) behavioral theory and (2) cognitive theory of anger and aggression. A third theory of anger and aggression is biological theory, which helps explain why some people are more prone to anger and aggressive behavior than others in terms of genetic inheritance and some medical conditions (temporal lobe epilepsy, traumatic head injury, Alzheimer's disease).

It is helpful for providers of care to know what cues should be looked for and what should be assessed when a client's anger is escalating (verbal cues, nonverbal cues that include facial expression, breathing, body language, and posture). A client's past aggressive behavior is also an important indicator to future aggressive episodes.

Working with angry and aggressive clients is a challenge for all nurses, and a careful understanding and recognition of one's personal responses to angry or threatening clients can be crucial. We all possess personal dynamics that may trigger emotions and reactions that are not therapeutic with specific clients. Unexamined responses to angry clients, even though they reflect those of society or the nurse's personal culture, may strongly influence unhelpful or even provocative responses to threatening clients. Certain types of clients may evoke feelings of dislike, irritability, or fear in the nurse. If these feelings remain unexamined, they can influence interactions that may precipitate or even escalate aggressive or angry behavior.

Many approaches are effective in helping clients de-escalate and maintain control. Different interventions exist for clients who are overwhelmed than for those who have marginal patterns of coping. For clients with cognitive deficits, a whole different set of interventions can be extremely useful in allaying a client's anxiety and minimizing aggressive behavior. When a client's anger is escalated to potential for violence, other modalities may prove helpful, employing the least restrictive whenever possible. Guidelines for de-escalation are given. Next, specific medications may be useful, and at other times, usually as a last resort when other interventions have been tried and failed, restraints may be needed to protect the safety of the client as well as other clients and the staff. Each unit has a clear protocol for the safe administration of restraints and for the humane management of care during the time the client is restrained, as well as clear guidelines for understanding and protecting the client's legal rights. Refer to Chapter 8 for a full discussion of clients' legal rights.

Visit the **Evolve** website at
http://evolve.elsevier.com/Varcarolis
for a post-test on the content in this chapter.

Visit the **Evolve** website at
http://evolve.elsevier.com/Varcarolis
for additional self-study exercises.

Critical Thinking and Chapter Review

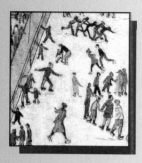

Critical Thinking

1. A 24-year-old man with mania is admitted to an inpatient unit. Staff notes that the client is irritable and has a history of assault. What interventions should be built into the care plan?
   a. Identify appropriate responses the nurse can take with the client.
   b. Identify at least three long-term outcomes to consider when planning care.
2. Identify some assessment data that can be used as predictors of potential violence.
3. What are the four indicators for the use of seclusion and restraint rather than verbal interventions?

Chapter Review

Choose the most appropriate answer.

1. Which is a clinical example of the use of predictability when caring for an anxious, angry client who possesses limited coping skills? The nurse

   1. refocuses conversation to minimize client tangentiality.
   2. empathizes with the client's underlying fear and anxiety.
   3. agrees to meet with the client for 10 minutes every 2 hours
   4. teaches the client techniques to manage auditory hallucinations

2. In planning intervention for an angry client, the nurse must understand that withdrawal of attention to verbally abusive behaviors works only if the strategy is accompanied by

   1. attending positively to nonabusive communication
   2. requiring the client to wait before granting requests
   3. large doses of antipsychotic medication
   4. empathic communication

3. To act to prevent displays of anger and aggression the nurse must understand that anger and aggression are preceded by feelings of

   1. vulnerability
   2. depression
   3. elation
   4. isolation

4. Which data are most useful to the nurse planning intervention for an angry client?

   1. client facial expression
   2. client body language
   3. client medical diagnosis
   4. client perception of the situation

5. The intervention of choice for a client with the nursing diagnosis ineffective individual coping, psychotic who is demonstrating early signs of escalation of anger is

   1. physical restraint or seclusion
   2. short acting antipsychotic medication
   3. making contact with client during calm times
   4. pointing out that the client's behavior is inappropriate

NURSE, CLIENT, AND FAMILY RESOURCES

Books

Mason, T. and Chandley, M. (1999). Managing Violence and Aggression: A Manual for Nurses and Health Care Workers. Edinburgh, UK: Churchill Livingstone.

Fava, M. (Ed.) (1997). Anger, aggression, and violence. The Psychiatric Clinics of North America, 20(2). Philadelphia: W. B. Saunders.

Internet Sites

Anger Management
www.angermgmt.com

CDC—Anger Website
www.cdc.gov/hcipc/dvp/dvp/htm

Stopping School Violence
www.ncpc.org/2schvio.htm

REFERENCES

al'Absi, M., Bongard, S., and Lovallo, W. (2000). Adrenocortico-tropin responses to interpersonal stress: Effects of overt anger expression style and defensiveness. *International Journal of Psychophysiology*, 37(3):257.

American Psychiatric Association (1994). *Diagnostic and statistical manual of mental disorders* (4th ed.). Washington, DC: American Psychiatric Association.

American Psychiatric Nurses Association (2000). Position statement on the use of seclusion and restraint. *www.apna.org* 1–15.

Anderson, S., and Lawler, K. (1995). The anger recall interview and cardiovascular reactivity in women: An examination of context and experience. *Journal of Psychosomatic Research*, 39(3): 335–343.

Bandura, A. (1973). *Aggression: A social learning analysis.* New York: Prentice Hall.

Beck, A. (1976). *Cognitive therapy and the emotional disorders.* New York: International Universities Press.

Beck, A., et al. (1979). *Cognitive therapy of depression.* New York: Guilford Press.

Beck, A., and Freeman, A. (1990). *Cognitive therapy of personality disorders.* New York: Guilford Press.

Berkowitz, L. (1982). Aversive conditions as stimuli to aggression. In L. Berkowitz (Ed.), *Advances in experimental psychology.* San Diego: Academic Press.

Berkowitz, L. (1983). In R. G. Green and E. I. Donnerstein (Eds.), *Aggression: Theoretical and empirical views* (Vol. 1). New York: Academic Press.

Blue, H., and Griffith, E. (1995). Sociocultural and therapeutic perspectives on violence. *Psychiatric Clinics of North America*, 18(3):571–587.

Brackbill, W., White, M., Wilson, M., Kitch, D. (1990). Family dynamics as predictors of infant disposition. *Infant Mental Health Journal*, 11:113–126.

Brook, J., Whiteman, M., and Brook, D. (1997). Transmission of risk factors across three generations. *Psychological Reports*, 85(1): 227–241.

Brown, C., et al. (1989). Blood platelet uptake of serotonin in episodic aggression. *Psychiatry Research*, 27(1):5–12.

Bruun, R., Budman, C. (1998). Paroxetine treatment of episodic rages associated with Tourette's disorder. *Journal of Clinical Psychiatry*, 59(11):581–584.

Burman, B., Margolin, G., and John, R. (1993). America's angriest home videos: Behavioral contingencies observed in home reenactments of marital conflict. *Journal of Consulting and Clinical Psychology*, 61(1):28–39.

Cadoret, R. (1982). Genotype-environmental interaction in antisocial behavior. *Psychological Medicine*, 12:235–239.

Cadoret, R., et al. (1985). Alcoholism and antisocial personality disorder: Interrelationships, genetic and environmental factors. *Archive of General Psychiatry*, 42:161–167.

Centers for Disease Control. (1998). *MMWR Morbidity and Mortality Weekly Report*, 47:1–89.

Centers for Disease Control. (1999a). Facts about violence among youth and violence in schools. *Media Relations*, 404.

Centers for Disease Control. (1999b). *Healthy People 2000 Review, 1998–1999*. Available at www.cdc.gov/nchs/data/hp2k99.pdf.

Cloninger, C., et al. (1982). Predisposition to petty criminality in Swedish adoptees: II. Cross-fostering analysis of gene-environment interaction. *Archives of General Psychiatry*, 39:1242–1249.

Cooper, A., and Mendonca, J. (1989). A prospective study of patients' assaults on nursing staff in a psychogeriatric unit. *Canadian Journal of Psychiatry*, 34(5):399–404.

Dahl, A. (1994) Heredity in personality disorders: An overview. *Clinical Genetics*, 46:138–143.

Davis, D., and Boster, L. (1988). Multifaceted therapeutic interventions with the violent psychiatric inpatient. *Hospital and Community Psychiatry*, 39(8):867–869.

Davis, M., Matthews, K. and McGrath, C. (2000). Hostile attitudes predict elevated vascular resistance during interpersonal stress in men and women. *Psychosomatic Medicine*, 62(1):17–25.

Davis, S. (1991). Violence by psychiatric inpatients: A review. *Hospital and Community Psychiatry*, 42:585–590.

Davison, G., et al. (1991). Relaxation, reduction in angry articulated thoughts, and improvements in borderline hypertension and heart rate. *Journal of Behavioral Medicine*, 14(5):453–468.

DiLalla, L., and Gottesman, I. (1991). Biologic and genetic contributors to violence: Widom's untold tale. *Psychological Bulletin*, 109(1):125–129.

Doren, D. (1996). *Understanding and treating the psychopath.* Northvale, NJ: J. Aronson.

Dougherty, D., Shin, L., Alpert, N., Pitman, R., Orr, S., Lasko, M., Macklin, M., Fischman, A., Rauch, S. (1999). Anger in healthy men: A PET study using script-driven imagery. *Biological Psychiatry*, 46:466–472.

Durivage, D. (1989). Assaultive behavior: Before it happens. *Canadian Journal of Psychiatry*, 34(5):393–397.

Eisenberg, N., Fabes, R., Shepard, S., Murphy, B., Guthrie, I., Jones, S., Friedman (1997). Contemporaneous and longitudinal prediction of children's social functioning from regulation and emotionality. *Child Development*, 68:642–664.

Ekman, P. (1972). *Darwin and facial expression: A century of research in review.* New York: Academic Press.

Ekman, P., Levenson, R., and Friesen, W. (1983). Autonomic nervous system activity distinguishes among emotions. *Science*, 221(4616):1208–1210.

Esterling, B., et al. (1990). Emotional repression, stress disclosure responses, and Epstein-Barr viral capsid antigen titers. *Psychosomatic Medicine*, 52(4): 397–410.

Eversor, S., Kaplan, G., Goldberg, D., Lakka, T., Sivenius, J., Salonen, J. (1999). Anger expression and incident stroke: Prospective evidence from the Kuopio ischemic heart disease study. *Stroke*, 30(3):523–528.

Fava, M., et al. (1993). Anger attacks in unipolar depression: I. Clinical correlates and response to fluoxetine treatment. *American Journal of Psychiatry*, 150(8):1158–1163.

Fava, M. (1998). Depression with anger attacks. *Journal of Clinical Psychiatry*, 15(Suppl. 59):18–22.

Feil, N. (1992). *Validation: The Feil method.* Cleveland: Edward Feil Productions.

Feinberg, T., et al. (1986). Facial discrimination and emotional recognition in schizophrenia and affective disorders. *Archives of General Psychiatry*, 43(3):276–279.

Fredrickson, B., Maynard, K., Helms, M., Haney, T., Siegler, I., Barefoot, J. (2000). Hostility predicts magnitude and duration of blood pressure responses to anger. *Journal of Behavioral Medicine*, 23(3):229–243.

Freud, S. (1933). *New introductory lectures on psychoanalysis*. New York: Morton.

Gallop, R., McCay, E., and Esplen, M. (1992). The conceptualization of impulsivity for psychiatric nursing practice. *Archives of Psychiatric Nursing*, 6(6):366–373.

Gentry, W. (1985). Relationship of anger-coping styles and blood pressure among black Americans. In M. A. Chesney and R. H. Roseman (Eds.), *Anger and hostility in cardiovascular and behavioral disorders* (pp. 139–147). Washington, DC: Hemisphere Publishing.

Gerlock, A. (1994). Veterans' responses to anger management intervention. *Issues in Mental Health Nursing*, 15(4):393–408.

Gin, N., et al. (1991). Prevalence of domestic violence among patients in three ambulatory care internal medicine clinics. *Journal of General Internal Medicine*, 6(4):317–322.

Greendyke, R., Schuster, D., and Wooten, J. (1984). Propranolol in the treatment of assaultive patients with organic brain disease. *Journal of Clinical Psychopharmacology*, 4:282–285.

Harburg, E., et al. (1991). Anger-coping styles and blood pressure in black and white males: Buffalo, New York. *Psychosomatic Medicine*, 53(2):153–164.

Hatfield, E., Cacioppo, J., and Rapson, R. (1994). *Emotional contagion*. New York: Cambridge University Press.

Jacobs, H. (1987). The Los Angeles head injury survey: Project rationale and design implications. *Journal of Head Trauma Rehabilitation*, 2(3):37–50.

Jensen, M. (1987). Psychobiological factors predicting the course of breast cancer. *Journal of Personality*, 55(3):317–342.

Johnson, M., Mass, M., Moorehead, S. (2000). *Nursing outcomes classification (NOC)*. St. Louis: Mosby.

Julius, S., Schneider, R., and Egan, B. (1985). Suppressed anger in hypertension: Facts and problems. In M. A. Chesney and R. H. Rosenman (Eds.), *Anger and hostility in cardiovascular and behavioral disorders* (pp. 127–135). Washington, DC: Hemisphere Publishing.

Katz, P., and Kirkland, F. (1990). Violence and social structure on mental hospital wards. *Psychiatry*, 53:262–277.

Kavoussi, R., Armstead, P., and Coccaro, E. (1997). The neurobiology of impulsive aggression. *Psychiatric Clinics of North America*, 20(2):395–401.

Kua, E., and Ko, S. (1991). Family violence and Asian drinkers. *Forensic Science International*, 50(1):43–46.

Lancee, W., et al. (1995). The relationship between nurses' limit-setting styles and anger in psychiatric inpatients. *Psychiatric Services*, 46(6):609–613.

Levenson, R., Ekman, P., and Friesen, W. (1990). Voluntary facial action generates emotion-specific autonomic nervous system activity. *Psychophysiology*, 27(4): 363–384.

Lin, K., Anderson, D., and Poland, R. (1995). Ethnicity and psychopharmacology: Bridging the gap. *Psychiatric Clinics of North America*, 18(3):635–648.

Linehan, M. (1993a). *Cognitive-behavioral treatment of borderline personality disorder*. New York: Guilford Press.

Linehan, M. (1993b). *Skills training manual for treating borderline personality disorder*. New York: Guilford Press.

Lipsey, M. and Derzon, J. (1998). Predictors of violence or serious delinquency in adolescence and early adulthood: A synthesis of longitudinal research. In, Loeber, R. and Farrington, D. (Eds.), *Serious and Violent Juvenile Offenders* (pp. 86–106). Thousand Oaks, CA: Sage Publications.

Loeber, R. and Southamer-Loeber, M. (1998). Development of juvenile aggression and violence: Some common misconceptions and controversies. *American Psychologist*, 53:242–259.

Lorenz, K. (1966). *On aggression*. New York: Bantam Books.

Lyon, J., Henggeler, S., and Hall, J. (1992). The family relations, peer relations, and criminal activities of Caucasian and Hispanic-American gang members. *Journal of Abnormal Child Psychology*, 20(5):439–449.

Lurie, S. (1999). Child psychiatrists address problem of youth violence. *JAMA*, 282(20):1906–1907.

Mammen, O., Shear, M., Pilkonis, P., Kolko, D., Thase, M., Greeno, C. (1999). Anger attacks: Correlates and significance of an under-recognized symptom. *Journal of Clinical Psychiatry*, 60(9):633–642.

Manuck, S., et al. (1985). Behavioral factors in hypertension: Cardiovascular responsivity, anger, and social competence. In M. A. Chesney and R. H. Rosenman (Eds.), *Anger and hostility in cardiovascular and behavioral disorders* (pp. 149–172). Washington, DC: Hemisphere Publishing.

Marangell, L.B., Silver, J.M., Yudofsky, S.C. (1999). Pharmacology and electroconvulsive therapy. In R.E. Hales, S.C. Yudofsky, and J.A. Talbott (Eds.) *Textbook of psychiatry*. Washington, D.C.: American Psychiatric Press.

Maxmen, J. S., and Ward, N. G. (1995). *Psychotropic drugs fast facts* (2nd ed.). New York: W. W. Norton.

McElroy, S. (1999). Recognition and treatment of DSM-IV intermittent explosive disorder. *Journal of Clinical Psychiatry*, 60 Suppl. 15:12–16.

McFall, M., Fontana, A., Raskind, M., Rosenheck, R. (1999). Analysis of violent behavior in Vietnam combat veteran psychiatric inpatients with post-traumatic stress disorder. *Journal of Traumatic Stress*, 12(3):501–517.

McNeil, D., and Binder, R. (1995). Correlates of accuracy in the assessment of psychiatric inpatients' risk of violence. *American Journal of Psychiatry*, 152(6):901–906.

Monahan, J. (1992). Mental disorder and violent behavior: Perceptions and evidence. *American Psychologist*, 47:511–521.

Monnelly, E., and Ciraulo, D. (1999). Risperadone effects on irritable aggression in posttraumatic stress disorder. *Journal of Clinical Psychopharmacology*, 19(4):377–378.

National Television Violence Study Council (1996). National violence study: Council statement. Studio City, CA: MediaScope.

Novaco R. (1976). The functions and regulations of the arousal of anger. *American Journal of Psychiatry*, 133(10):1124–1127.

Novaco, R. (1985). Anger and its therapeutic regulation. In M. A. Chesney and R. H. Rosenman (Eds.), *Anger and hostility in cardiovascular and behavioral disorders* (pp. 203–222). New York: McGraw-Hill.

Oster, C. (1976). Sensory deprivation in geriatric patients. *Journal of the American Geriatrics Society*, 24(10):461–463.

Outlaw, F. (1993). Stress and coping: The influence of race on the cognitive appraisal processing of African-Americans. *Issues in Mental Health Nursing*, 14:399–409.

Rappaport, D. (1967). *The collected papers of David Rappaport*. New York: Basic Books.

Reeder, D. (1991). Cognitive therapy of anger management: theoretical and practical considerations. *Archives of Psychiatric Nursing*, 5(3):147–150.

Riley, W., Treiber, F., Woods, M. (1989). Anger and hostility in depression. *Journal of Nervous and Mental Disease*, 177:668–674.

Rossi, A., et al. (1986). Characteristics of psychiatric patients who engage in assaultive or other fear-inducing behaviors. *Journal of Nervous and Mental Disease*, 174(3):154–160.

Rothbart, M., Evans, D., and Ahadi, S. (2000). Temperament and personality: Origins and outcomes. *Journal of Personality and Social Psychology*, 78(1):122–135.

Rubey, R., Johnson, M., Emmanuel, N., Lydiard, R. (1996). Fluoxetine in the treatment of anger: An open clinical trial. *Journal of Clinical Psychiatry*, 57(9):398–401.

Ryan, J., and Poster, E. (1989). The assaulted nurse: Short-term and long-term responses. *Archives of Psychiatric Nursing*, 3(6): 323–331.

Salzman, C., et al. (1995). Effect of fluoxetine on anger in symptomatic volunteers with borderline personality disorder. *Journal of Clinical Psychopharmacology*, 15(1):23–29.

Schwab-Stone, M., Chen, C., Greenberger, E., Silver, D., Lichtman, J., Voyce, C. (1999). No safe haven. II: The effects of violence exposure on urban youth. *Journal of the American Academy of Child and Adolescent Psychiatry*, 38(4):359–367.

Sheridan, M., et al. (1990). Precipitants of violence in a psychiatric inpatient setting. *Hospital and Community Psychiatry*, 41(7):776–780.

Siegman, A. (1993). Cardiovascular consequences of expressing, experiencing, and repressing anger. *Journal of Behavioral Medicine*, 16(6):539–569.

Siegman, A., Anderson, R., and Berger, T. (1990). The angry voice: Its effects on the experience of anger and cardiovascular reactivity. *Psychosomatic Medicine*, 52(6):631–643.

Siegman, A., Townsend, S., Civelek, A., Blumenthal, R. (2000). Antagonistic behavior, dominance, hostility, and coronary heart disease. *Psychosomatic Medicine*, 62(2):248–257.

Skinner, B. (1953). *Science and human behavior*. New York: Macmillan.

Smith, M., and Hart, G. (1994). Nurses' responses to patient anger: From disconnecting to connecting. *Journal of Advanced Nursing*, 20(4):643–651.

Soloff, P. (1983). Seclusion and restraint. In J. Lion and W. Reid (Eds.), *Assaults within psychiatric facilities* (pp. 241–264). New York: Grune & Stratton.

Suedfeld, P. (1969). Introduction and historical background. In J. P. Zubeck (Ed.), *Sensory deprivation: 15 years of research* (p. 4). New York: Appleton-Century-Crofts.

Temoshok, L. (1987). Psychoimmunology and AIDS. *Clinical Immunology Newsletter*, 9:113–116.

Teri, L., and Logsdon, R. (1990). Assessment and management of behavioral disturbances in Alzheimer's disease. *Comprehensive Therapy*, 16(5):36–42.

Uomoto, J., and Brockway, J. (1992). Anger management training for brain injured patients and their family members. *Archives of Physical Medicine and Rehabilitation*, 73(7):674–679.

Valdez, A., et al. (1995). Illegal drug use, alcohol and aggressive crime among Mexican-American and white male arrestees in San Antonio. *Journal of Psychoactive Drugs*, 27(2):135–143.

Varcarolis. E.M. (2000). *Psychiatric nursing clinics guide*. Philadelphia: W.B. Saunders.

Virkkuner, M., et al. (1994). CSF biochemistries, glucose metabolism, and diurnal activity rhythms in alcoholic, violent offenders, fire setters, and healthy volunteers. *Archives of General Psychiatry*, 51(20):20–27.

White, J., and Koss, M. (1991). Courtship violence: Incidence in a national sample of higher education students. *Violence and Victims*, 6(4):247–256.

Williams, D., et al. (1982). The effect of propranolol on uncontrolled rage outbursts in children and adolescents with organic brain dysfunction. *Journal of the American Academy of Child Psychiatry*, 21:129–135.

Wolkowitz, O., and Pickar, D. (1991). Benzodiazepines in the treatment of schizophrenia: A review and reappraisal. *American Journal of Psychiatry*, 148(6):714–726.

Yarcheski, A., Mahon, N., and Yarcheski, T. (1999). An empirical test of alternate theories of anger in early adolescence. *Nursing Research*, 48(6):317–323.

Outline

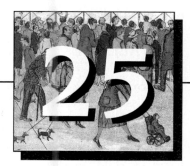

25

Family Violence

KATHLEEN SMITH-DIJULIO

Key Terms and Concepts

The key terms and concepts listed here also appear in color where they are first defined or discussed in this chapter.

crisis situation
economic maltreatment
emotional violence
family violence
health care record
neglect
perpetrator
physical violence

primary prevention
safety plan
secondary prevention
sexual violence
shelters/safe houses
tertiary prevention
vulnerable person

Objectives

After studying this chapter, the reader will be able to

1. Discuss the epidemiological theory of violence in terms of stresses on the perpetrator, vulnerable person, and environment that could escalate anxiety to the point at which violence becomes the relief behavior.

2. Contrast and compare three characteristics of perpetrators with three characteristics of a vulnerable person.

3. Name three indicators of (a) physical violence, (b) sexual violence, (c) neglect, and (d) emotional violence.

4. Describe four areas to assess when interviewing a person who has experienced family violence.

5. Formulate four nursing diagnoses for the survivor of violence and list supporting data from the assessment.

6. Write out a safety plan, including the essential elements, for an abused spouse.

7. Compare and contrast primary, secondary, and tertiary levels of intervention, giving two examples of intervention for each level.

8. Identify two common emotional responses you might experience when faced with a person subjected to family violence.

9. Describe at least three possible referrals for a violent family (child, adult, elder) and write down the telephone numbers of the corresponding agencies in your community.

10. Name and discuss three psychotherapeutic modalities that are useful for violent families.

PREVALENCE

Violence is among America's most important public health issues. A violent family is one in which at least one family member is using physical or sexual force against another, resulting in physically or emotionally destructive injury, or both. The true prevalence of child, spouse/couple, elder abuse is not known because of underreporting and variability of reporting methods, instruments, sites, and reporters.

It has been estimated that half of all Americans have experienced violence in their families. A substantial percentage of childhood injuries are due to abuse (Reece and Sege 2000; DiScala 2000). It is estimated that one million Americans age 60 or older are abused in domestic settings each year (Tatara 1997). One type of violence is a fairly strong predictor of another. This connection calls for more coordinated efforts of prevention and intervention.

Violence can also occur in gay and lesbian relationships. Domestic violence is the third largest health problem for gay men, following substance abuse and AIDS. Violence between siblings is one of the most common and unrecognized forms of domestic violence. Another alarming and often unreported form of domestic violence is that of children toward parents. Although often not reported or even discussed, violence toward men by women also occurs and also goes unrecognized as a problem. In fact, according to the 1998 Department of Justice reports on the National Violence Against Women survey, 37.5% of victims each year are men (Tjaden and Thoennes 1998).

COMORBIDITY

The secondary effects of violence, such as anxiety, depression, and suicide, are health care issues that can last a lifetime. Family violence is common in childhood histories of juvenile delinquents, runaways, violent criminals, prostitutes, and those who in turn are violent toward others. Exposure to violence can adversely affect children's development because the energy needed to successfully accomplish developmental tasks goes to coping with violence (Lawson 1998; Beauchesne et al. 1997). Abused adolescents report more psychopathological changes, poorer coping and social skills, a higher incidence of dissociated identity disorder, and poorer impulse control than do other adolescents. Women who are victims of prolonged childhood sexual abuse are more likely to develop major psychiatric distress. When health care providers do not routinely assess for history of sexual abuse, symptoms arising in

times of crisis may be labeled with adult psychopathology and not understood as possible post-trauma response (Creedy et al. 1998). Box 25–1 identifies some of the sequelae of family violence.

Social factors that reinforce violence include the wide acceptance of the hitting of children (corporal

BOX 25–1 *Long-Term Effects of Family Violence*

People involved in family violence are found to have higher levels of

- Depression
- Suicidal feelings
- Self-contempt
- Inability to trust
- Inability to develop intimate relationships in later life

Victims of severe violence are also at higher risk for experiencing recurring symptoms of posttraumatic stress disorder:

- Flashbacks
- Dissociation—out-of-body experiences
- Poor self-esteem
- Compulsive or impulsive behaviors (e.g., substance abuse, spending money, gambling, and promiscuity)
- Multiple somatic complaints

Children who witness violence in their homes

- After the age of 5 or 6 years show an indication of identifying with the aggressor and losing respect for the victim
- Are at greater risk for developing behavioral and emotional problems throughout their lives

Some mental and behavioral disorders are associated with violence in childhood:

- Depressive disorders
- Posttraumatic stress disorder
- Somatic complaints
- Low self-esteem
- Phobias (agoraphobia, social and specific phobias)
- Antisocial behaviors
- Child or spouse abuse

Adolescents are more likely to have behavioral symptoms such as

- Failing grades
- Difficulty forming relationships
- Increased incidence of theft, police arrest, and violent behaviors
- Seductive or promiscuous behaviors
- Running away from home

punishment); the celebration of increasingly violent movies, video games, the internet, and comic books; the violent themes in rap music; and the increase in the total volume of pornography (which is strongly associated with physical abuse of women).

THEORY

Family violence refers to physical injury or mental anguish (e.g., putdowns, demeaning actions toward partners, controlling) inflicted by one family member upon another and the omission or deprivation of essential services by a caregiver. To be more effective in working with victims, the nurse needs an understanding of conditions for violence and types of maltreatment. Fundamental to this entire discussion is self-understanding, which is addressed under the Self-Assessment section.

Conditions for Violence

Abuse occurs across all segments of American society and is reinforced by the society and the culture. The actual occurrence of violence requires (1) a perpetrator; (2) someone who by age or situation is vulnerable, i.e., children, women, men, the elderly, and the mentally ill or physically challenged person; and (3) a crisis situation.

The Perpetrator

The propensity for violence is rooted in childhood and manifested by a general lack of self-regard, dissatisfaction with life, and inability to assume adult roles. Often the abuser lacked good role models and was deprived of learning and problem-solving skills. Witnessing family violence, experiencing family violence, and neglectful or abusive parenting are contributing factors.

Perpetrators, those who initiate violence, often consider their own needs to be more important than anyone else's and look toward others to meet their needs. Specific characteristics of violent parents and those who maltreat elders are listed in Boxes 25–2 and 25–3, respectively.

Since recent surveys suggest that 37.5% of victims are men, and the results of a Journal of the American Medical Association study showed equal numbers of men and women victims, the principles discussed in this chapter apply to any member of a household who is violent toward another member (e.g., siblings, same sex partners, extended family members). Violence toward children and older adults will be considered separately.

BOX 25–2 *Characteristics of Violent Parents*

- A history of violence, neglect, or emotional deprivation as a child
- Family authoritarianism: raise children as they were raised by their own parents
- Low self-esteem, feelings of worthlessness, depression
- Poor coping skills
- Social isolation (may be suspicious of others): few or no friends, little or no involvement in social or community activities
- Involved in a crisis situation: unemployment, divorce, financial difficulties
- Rigid, unrealistic expectations of child's behavior
- Frequent use of harsh punishment
- History of severe mental illness, such as schizophrenia
- Violent temper outbursts
- Looking to child for satisfaction of needs for love, support, and reassurance (often unmet because of parenting deficits in family of origin)
- Projection of blame onto the child for their "troubles" (e.g., stepparent may project hostility toward new mate onto a child)
- Lack of effective parenting skills
- Inability to seek help from others
- Perception of the child as bad or evil
- History of drug or alcohol abuse
- Feeling of little or no control over life
- Low tolerance for frustration
- Poor impulse control

Data from Warner, C. G. (Ed.). (1981). *Conflict intervention in social and domestic violence.* Bowie, MD: Robert J. Brady.

Vignette

- A 53-year-old man came to the ambulatory care clinic looking very fatigued and complaining of pain in his left shoulder "since last night." Holding his left arm close to his side, he averted his eyes from those of the receptionist, nurse, and doctor. When asked if anything had occurred that might have caused the pain, he answered, "I fell." Asked why he had not sought care last night, he stated, "I . . . I . . . thought it would go away overnight."

  Upon further examination and x-ray, it was determined that the patient had sustained a fractured clavicle. Additional direct, supportive questioning elicited the information that the patient had been injured when pushed down the stairs by his 17-year-old stepson.

> ### Box 25–3 *Characteristics of Elder Abusers*
>
> **PHYSICAL AND PSYCHOLOGICAL VIOLENCE**
>
> The perpetrator may have
>
> - A history of mental illness
> - A recent decline in mental status
> - Recent medical problems
> - A financial dependence on the victim
> - Shared living arrangements with the victim
> - A history of alcohol or drug abuse
> - Pathological family dynamics
>
> **NEGLECT**
>
> The perpetrator may
>
> - Abuse alcohol or drugs
> - Not live with the victim
> - Not have a decline in mental status
> - Not have recent medical problems
> - Not experience the victim as a source of stress
>
> **FINANCIAL MALTREATMENT**
>
> The perpetrator may
>
> - Abuse alcohol or drugs
> - Be a distant relative
> - Be financially dependent on the victim
> - Be greedy
>
> ---
>
> Data from Wolf, R. S., and Pillemer, K. A. (1989). *Helping elderly victims: The reality of elder abuse.* New York: Columbia University Press; and Wolf, R. S. (1990). Elder abuse: Scope, characteristics, and treatment. *Nurse Practitioner Forum*, 1(2):102.

Men and women who are violent are found in all segments of society. Men who abuse believe in male supremacy, being in charge, and being dominant. Some reasons they give for being abusive are believing their partner was not sensitive to their needs (46%) or not listening to them (43%), or that their partner was being verbally abusive (38%) (Hoff 1999). "Acting out" physically makes them feel more in control, more masculine, and more powerful. Parent-child interactions, peer-group experiences, observations of the partner dyad, and the influence of the media (television, comics, video games, movies) all support the same message: males can expect to be in a position of power in relationships and may use physical aggression to maintain that position.

Extreme pathological jealousy is characteristic of an abuser. Many refuse to allow their partners to work outside the home; others demand that their partners work in the same place as they do so that they can monitor activities and friendships. Many accompany their partners to and from all activities and forbid them to have personal friends or to participate in recreational activities outside the home. When this is not possible, a man or woman may restrict mobility by monitoring the odometer and keeping clock watches. Even with such restrictions, abusers accuse their partners of infidelity. Many perpetrators maintain their possessiveness by controlling the family finances to the extent that there is barely enough money for daily living. These abusive men and women may appear to outsiders as ordinary doctors, nurses, machinists, lawyers, salesmen, executives, and plumbers—or even police officers, judges, and politicians. It is important to recognize there are a wide variety of cultural norms dictating male-female relationships, some of which might appear to be abusive. Learning about the cultural backgrounds of patients can prevent mistaking common cultural norms for abuse (Campbell and Campbell 1996). Misunderstandings frequently exist regarding traditional culture-bound health practices and the knowledge level of health care providers caring for specific populations (Davis 2000).

Individuals are more likely to engage in family violence with use of substances. Alcohol and other drugs (illicit or prescribed) may play a disinhibitory role in disregarding social rules that prohibit violence against children, women, and the elderly, whom perpetrators view as weak and inferior. The consumption of alcohol and drugs is often used as a rationalization by the victim to excuse the behavior ("He was drunk, and he didn't know what he was doing"). In fact, when drug and alcohol use is reduced or eliminated, family violence still occurs.

Both male and female perpetrators perceive themselves as having poor social skills. They describe their relationships with their spouses as being the closest they have ever known, which is typical in enmeshed and co-dependent relationships. They lack supportive relationships outside the marriage.

The Vulnerable Person

The **vulnerable person** is the one in the family unit on whom violence is perpetrated. In some situations, violence does not occur until after the legal marriage of couples who have lived together or dated for a long time.

Pregnancy often serves to increase violence even further (Parker et al. 1999). An estimated 15% to 25% of women experience violence during pregnancy. One reason may be that the husband resents the added responsibility that a baby requires, or he may resent the relationship that the baby will have with his mate. Violence also escalates when the wife makes a move toward independence, such as visiting friends without permission, getting a job, or going back to school. Victims are at greatest risk for violence when they attempt to leave the relationship.

Children are most likely to be abused if they are under 3 years of age; are perceived as being different because of temperamental traits, congenital abnormalities, or chronic disease; remind the parents of someone they do not like (perhaps an ex-spouse); are different from the parents' fantasy of what the child should be like; or are a product of an unwanted pregnancy. Interference with emotional bonding between parents and child (e.g., with a premature birth or prolonged illness requiring hospitalization) has also been found to increase the risk of possible future abuse. Adolescents are abused at least as frequently as children, yet are often overlooked.

Elder adults may become vulnerable because of being in poor mental or physical health or being disruptive (e.g., a person with Alzheimer's disease). The dependency needs of elderly persons are usually what puts them at risk for abuse. The typical victim is female, over 75 years of age, white, living with a relative, and having a physical and/or mental impairment. Dealing with the problems of the elderly can be stressful for adult caregivers at the best of times, but in families in which violence was a coping strategy, the potential for abuse is great. Other scenarios are the elder male cared for by a daughter whom he abused as a child, and who now is abusive toward him, or the elderly woman abused by her husband as part of a long-standing abusive relationship (Brandl and Raymond 1997). Many caregivers become angry because of failing health of a loved one.

The Crisis Situation

Anyone may be at risk for abuse in a crisis situation, one that puts stress on a family with a violent member. Stressful life events tax coping skills, leaving the perpetrator incapable of dealing with what is going on. A person with good impulse control who can solve problems and has a healthy support system is less likely to resort to violence. Social isolation caused by frequent moves or an inability to make friends contributes to ineffective coping during crisis situations. Refer to Chapter 22 for more on crisis and crisis intervention.

The Cycle of Violence

The intensity of violence alternates with periods of safety, hope, and trust. This pattern has been described as a process of escalation/de-escalation.

The **tension-building stage** is characterized by minor incidents such as pushing, shoving, and verbal abuse. During this time the victim does not say that the abuse is unacceptable, for fear more severe abuse will follow. Abusers then rationalize that their abusive behavior is acceptable.

As the tension escalates, both spouses may try to reduce it. The batterer may try to reduce the tension with the use of alcohol or drugs. The vulnerable person may try to reduce the tension by minimizing the importance of the incidents ("I should have had the house neater . . . dinner ready"). The abused may also try to reduce the tension by somatizing, thus perpetuating the "poor-me" image.

During the **acute battering stage,** the perpetrator releases the built-up tension by brutal and uncontrollable beatings. He is unable to control the degree of destructiveness inflicted on the victim. Severe injuries can and do result. The perpetrator may have amnesia and may not remember what happened during the battering. The victim usually depersonalizes the incident and is able to remember the beatings in detail. After the beatings, both are in shock.

The **honeymoon stage** may be characterized by kindness and loving behaviors. The perpetrator, at least initially, feels remorseful and apologetic and may bring presents, make promises, and tell the victim how much she is loved and needed. The victim usually believes the promises, feels needed and loved, and drops any legal proceedings or plans to leave that may have been initiated during the acute battering stage. Unfortunately, without intervention the cycle will repeat itself. The honeymoon stage will fade away as tension starts to build.

When **escalation/de-escalation** occurs, conditions of anger and fear escalate until an incident of violence occurs, after which there is a diffusion of tension and a brief feeling of safety. Over time, the periods of calmness and safety are briefer and the periods of anger and fear are more intense. There are periods of stability, but the violence increases over time. With each repeat of the pattern, the self-esteem of those experiencing the violence becomes more and more eroded. The victim either believes the violence was deserved or accepts the blame for it. This can lead to feelings of depression, hopelessness, immobilization, and self-deprecation.

Types of Maltreatment

Five specific types of maltreatment have been identified: (1) physical violence, (2) sexual violence, (3) emotional violence, (4) neglect, and (5) economic maltreatment.

1. *Physical Violence.* **Physical violence** is infliction of physical pain or bodily harm (e.g., slapping, punching, hitting, pushing, restraining, biting, throwing, burning).

2. *Sexual Violence.* **Sexual violence** is any form of sexual contact or exposure without consent, or when the victim is incapable of giving consent. Childhood sexual abuse destroys an individual's positive self-concept and can interfere with the learning of self-care skills. Sexual abuse of adults is usually referred to as sexual assault, or rape, and is discussed in Chapter 26.

3. *Emotional Violence.* **Emotional violence** is the infliction of mental anguish (e.g., threatening, humiliating, intimidating, and isolating). It can take the form of

   - Terrorizing an individual through verbal threats.
   - Demeaning an individual's worth/putdowns.
   - Blatant or subtle hostility and hatred directed toward an individual—or omissions.
   - Persistently ignoring an individual and her or his needs.
   - Consistently belittling and criticizing an individual.
   - Withholding warmth and affection from an individual.
   - Threatening an individual with abandonment or institutionalization (nursing home, psychiatric hospital).

4. *Neglect.* **Neglect** can be physical, developmental, or educational. **Physical neglect** is failure to provide the medical, dental, or psychiatric care needed to prevent or treat physical or emotional illnesses. **Developmental neglect** is failure to provide emotional nurturing and the physical and cognitive stimulation needed to ensure freedom from developmental deficits. **Educational neglect** occurs when a child's caretakers deprive the child of the education available in accordance with the state's education laws.

5. *Economic Maltreatment.* **Economic maltreatment** is illegal or improper exploitation of funds or other resources for one's personal gain or withholding support.

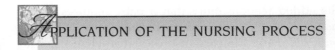

APPLICATION OF THE NURSING PROCESS

ASSESSMENT

Self-Assessment

In all areas of psychiatric nursing and counseling, the nurse should be aware of personal emotions and thoughts. Strong negative feelings can cloud one's judgment and interfere with assessment and intervention, no matter how well the nurse tries to cover or deny feelings. Intense and overwhelming feelings may be aroused by working with those experiencing violence. The nurse may also have come from a violent environment and thus identify too closely with the victim; old personal issues around the abuse may surface, further clouding judgment (Moore et al. 1998). Many nurses do not feel educated well enough or have not had enough supervisory experience to intervene in cases of family violence (Ellis 1999). Supervision needs to be made available to nurses when working with victims of violence. These situations are often complex and entail multifaceted interventions and follow-up when possible.

Nurses with a personal history of abuse and those working with family violence need a source of psychological support. Interdisciplinary team conferences can be especially helpful in clarifying reactions and neutralizing intense emotions. Information from physicians, psychologists, nurses, and social workers can assist in refocusing efforts to work constructively with a family in crisis. Sharing perceptions and feelings with other professionals can help reduce feelings of isolation and discomfort for nurses.

Awareness of personal feelings in response to those experiencing violence stimulates examination of personal views toward violence and the status of children, women, and elders. This is most effectively done through professional or peer supervision. Common responses of health care professionals to violence are listed in Box 25–4.

Overall Assessment

Persons experiencing violence present in every health care setting, including outpatient clinics, community health centers, emergency departments, general hospitals, physicians' offices, nursing homes, and during home health visits. Complaints may be vague and can include insomnia, abdominal pain, hyperventilation, headache, or menstrual problems. Attention to the process and setting of the interview are important to facilitate accurate assessment of physical and behavioral indicators of family violence (Fishwick 1998). All assessments should include a

BOX 25–4   Common Responses of Health Care Professionals to Violence

FEELING	SOURCE
Anger	Anger may be felt toward the person responsible for the violence, toward those who allowed it to happen, and toward society for condoning its occurrence through attitudes, traditions, and laws.
Embarrassment	The victim is a symbol of something close to home: the stress and strain of family life unleashed as uncontrollable anger.
Confusion	Our cherished view of the family as a haven of safety and privacy is challenged.
Fear	A small percentage of perpetrators are dangerous to others.
Anguish	The nurse may have experienced family violence.
Helplessness	The nurse may want to do more, to eliminate the problem, to cure the victim.
Discouragement	Discouragement may result if no long-term solution is achieved.
"Blame the victim" mentality	Lay people as well as health care workers can get caught up in "blaming the victim" for not having the house neat, food on time, clothes neat. There is never an excuse for violence, and no one has the right to hurt another person. "Blaming the victim" can occur when health care professionals feel overwhelmed. Supervision is a must for therapeutic intervention.

history of sexual abuse, family violence, and drug use or abuse. The assessment should be completed with the victim alone.

THE PROCESS AND SETTING OF THE INTERVIEW

Important and relevant information about the family situation can be gathered by routine assessment conducted with tact, understanding, and a calm, relaxed attitude. Important interviewing guidelines are listed in Box 25–5. A person who feels judged or accused of wrongdoing is most likely to become defensive, and any attempts at changing coping strategies in the family are thwarted. It is better to ask about ways of solving disagreements or methods of disciplining children rather than use the words *abuse* or *violence.*

When interviewing, sit near the abused client and spend some time establishing trust and rapport before focusing on the details of the violent experience. Reassure the client that he or she did nothing wrong. The interview should be nonthreatening and supportive. The person who experienced the violence should be allowed to tell the story and not be interrupted. Establishing trust is crucial if the client is to feel comfortable enough to self-disclose. Verbal approaches may include the following:

■ Tell me about what happened to you.
■ Who takes care of you? (for children and dependent elders)
■ What happens when you do something wrong? (for children) *or* How do you and your partner/

BOX 25–5   Interview Guidelines

DO

■ Conduct the interview in private
■ Be direct, honest, and professional
■ Use language the client understands
■ Ask the client to clarify words not understood
■ Be understanding
■ Be attentive
■ Inform the client if you must make a referral to Children's/Adult Protective Services, and explain the process
■ Assess safety and help reduce danger (at discharge)

DON'T

■ Do *not* try to "prove" abuse by accusations or demands
■ Do *not* display horror, anger, shock, or disapproval of the perpetrator or situation
■ Do *not* place blame or make judgments
■ Do *not* allow the client to feel "at fault" or "in trouble"
■ Do *not* probe or press for answers the client is not willing to give
■ Do *not* conduct the interview with a group of interviewers
■ Do *not* force a child or anyone to remove clothing

caregiver resolve disagreements? (for women and the elderly)

■ What do you do for fun?
■ Who helps you with your child(ren), parent?
■ What time do you have for yourself?

Questions that are open-ended and require a descriptive response can be less threatening and elicit more relevant information than questions that are direct or can be answered "yes" or "no." Here are some examples of how to approach parents:

■ What arrangements do you make when you have to leave your child alone?
■ How do you discipline your child?
■ When your infant cries for a long time, how do you get him or her to stop?
■ What about your child's behavior bothers you the most?

When trust has been established, openness and directness about the situation can strengthen the relationship with those experiencing violence. The Nursing Research Consortium on Violence and Abuse has developed a five-question assessment tool (Box 25–6) that has been used extensively to assist in the routine identification of domestic violence. It can be used in clinical settings without requesting permission. The following Vignette illustrates the key points for assessing a woman in crisis at the initial interview, as well as suggested follow-up.

Vignette

■ *Darnell Peters is a 42-year-old married woman in a relationship she describes as "bad for a long time. We don't communicate." She is brought to the emergency department by ambulance with lacerations to her face and swollen eyes, lips, and nose. She tells the nurse that her husband had been in bed asleep for hours before she joined him. On getting into bed, she attempted to redistribute the blankets. Suddenly, he leaped from the bed, started punching her in the face, and began to throw her against the wall. She called out to her 11-year-old son to call the police. The police arrived, called an ambulance, and took Mr. Peters to jail.*

The nurse takes Mrs. Peters to an individual examination room (to emphasize confidentiality) to assess the whole problem. Mrs. Peters states that their relationship is always stormy. "He is always putting me down and yelling at me." He started hitting her 5 years ago when she became pregnant with her second and last child. The beatings have increased in intensity over the past year, and this emergency department visit is the fifth this year. Tonight is the first time she has ever called the police.

BOX 25–6   *Abuse Assessment Screen*

1. Have you ever been emotionally or physically abused by your partner or someone important to you?
   Yes _____ No _____
   If yes, by whom? _____
   Number of times _____
2. Within the past year, have you been hit, slapped, kicked, or otherwise physically hurt by someone?
   Yes _____ No _____
   If yes, by whom? _____
   Number of times _____
3. Since you have been pregnant, have you been hit, slapped, kicked, or otherwise physically hurt by someone?
   Yes _____ No _____
   If yes, by whom? _____
   Number of times _____
4. Within the past year, has anyone forced you to engage in sexual activities?
   Yes _____ No _____
   If yes, by whom? _____
   Number of times _____
5. Are you afraid of your partner or anyone listed above?
   Yes _____ No _____

The Abuse Assessment Screen was developed by the Nursing Research Consortium on Violence and Abuse, 1989. Its reproduction and use is encouraged.

Mrs. Peters has visibly lost control. Periods of crying alternate with periods of silence. She appears apathetic and depressed. The nurse remains calm and objective. After Mrs. Peters has finished talking, the nurse explores alternatives designed to help her reduce the danger when she is discharged. "I'm concerned that you will be hurt again if you go home. What options do you have?" Acknowledging the escalating intensity of the violence, Mrs. Peters is able to make arrangements with a shelter to take her and her two children in until after she has secured a restraining order.

The nurse charts the abuse referrals. Careful and complete records help ensure that Mrs. Peters will receive proper follow-up care, and will assist Mrs. Peters when and if she pursues legal action (see the later section, "Maintaining Accurate Records").

When determining the need for further help, it is also useful to assess (a) violence indicators, (b) levels of anxiety and coping responses, (c) family coping patterns, (d) support systems, (e) suicide potential, (f) homicide potential, and (g) drug and alcohol use.

ASSESSING TYPES OF MALTREATMENT

PHYSICAL VIOLENCE. A series of minor complaints, such as headaches, "back trouble," dizziness, and "accidents," especially falls, may be covert indications of violence. Overt signs of battering include bruises, scars, burns, and other wounds in various stages of healing, particularly around the head, face, chest, arms, abdomen, back, buttocks, and genitalia. Injuries seen in emergency departments, clinics, and offices that should arouse the nurse's suspicion are listed in Box 25–7. If the explanation does not match the injury seen, or if the client minimizes the seriousness of the injury, violence may be suspected. The key to identification is a high index of suspicion.

Nonspecific bruising in older children is common. Any bruises on an infant under 6 months of age should be considered suspicious. A specific type of abuse to which young children are susceptible is **shaking.** The baby who has been shaken may often present with respiratory problems. If the pulmonary examination is not normal, the possibility of rigorous shaking must be considered. Full bulging fontanelles and a head circumference greater than the 90th percentile are also suggestive. Shaking can cause intracranial hemorrhage leading to cerebral edema and death (Spicknell 1998).

Ask clients directly, but in a nonthreatening manner, whether the injury has been caused by someone close to them. Observe the nonverbal response, such as hesitation or lack of eye contact, as well as the verbal response. Then ask specific questions, such as "When was the last time it happened?" "How often does it happen?" "In what ways are you hurt?"

Along with recognition of the indicators of physical violence, nurses note the alleged method of injury. Inconsistent explanations serve as a warning that further investigation is necessary. Vague explanations, such as "She fell from a chair (a lap, down the stairs)," "He was running away," or "The hot water was turned on by mistake," should alert the nurse to possible violence.

SEXUAL VIOLENCE. Patients with a history of sexual abuse often display various psychopathologies (Garber et al. 1997). Childhood sexual violence is likely to be a significant factor in the development of depression for many women (Horsfall 1997). It is estimated that one in four females and one in six males will be sexually abused as children and is common across cultures (Heritage 1998). Sexual abuse of boys appears to be common, underreported, underrecognized, and untreated (Holmes and Slap 1998).

BOX 25–7 *Presenting Problems of Victims of Family Violence in the Emergency Department*

EMERGENCY DEPARTMENT

■ Bleeding injuries, especially to head and face
■ Internal injuries, concussions, perforated eardrums, abdominal injuries, severe bruising, eye injuries, strangulation marks on neck
■ Back injuries
■ Broken or fractured jaws, arms, pelvis, ribs, clavicle, legs
■ Burns from cigarettes, appliances, scalding liquids, acids
■ Psychological trauma, anxiety, attacks of hyperventilation, heart palpitations, severe crying spells, suicidal tendencies
■ Miscarriages

AMBULATORY CARE SETTINGS

■ Perforated eardrums, twisted or stiff neck and shoulder muscles, headache
■ Depression, stress-related conditions (e.g., insomnia, violent nightmares, anxiety, extreme fatigue, eczema, loss of hair)
■ Talk of having "problems" with husband or son, describing him as very jealous, impulsive, or an alcohol or drug abuser
■ Repeated visits with new complaint
■ Bruises of various ages and specific shapes (fingers, belt)

IN BOTH SETTINGS

■ Observe for signs of stress due to family violence: emotional, behavioral, school, or sleep problems and increased aggressive behavior
■ Injuries to a pregnant woman
■ Recurrent visits for injuries attributed to being "accident prone"

Vignette

■ Ms. Randall, 83, is admitted from an adult foster home for evaluation of deterioration in her mental status. She is confused and disoriented to time and place and is unable to give a coherent history. Blood and urine are collected for diagnostic evaluation. The laboratory report notes semen in the urine. Adult Protective Services is called to begin an investigation into the adult family home.

EMOTIONAL VIOLENCE. Whenever physical or sexual violence is occurring, emotional violence also occurs It may also exist alone. When there is emotional violence, low self-esteem, anguish and isolation are instilled in place of love and acceptance. Emotional violence is less obvious and more difficult to assess than physical violence.

NEGLECT. Neglected children and elders often appear undernourished, dirty, and poorly clothed. Neglect is also manifested by inadequate medical care, such as lack of immunizations or untreated medical conditions.

ECONOMIC MALTREATMENT. Failure to provide for the needs of the victim even when adequate funds are available is a sign of economic maltreatment. Another sign is unpaid bills when another person is supposed to do so, resulting in the heat or electricity being turned off (Hogstel and Curry 1999).

ASSESSING THE LEVEL OF ANXIETY AND COPING RESPONSES

Nonverbal responses to history taking can be indicative of the victim's anxiety level. The identification of anxiety levels is described in Chapter 14. Hesitation, lack of eye contact, and vague statements, such as "It's been rough lately," indicate that the situation is difficult to talk about.

Agitation and anxiety bordering on panic are often present in victims experiencing violence. Because they live in terror, battered individuals remain vigilant, unable to relax or sleep. Signs of the effect of living with chronic stress and severe levels of anxiety may be present (e.g., hypertension, irritability, gastrointestinal disturbances).

Vignette

■ A *woman coming to the walk-in clinic with bilateral corneal abrasions raised the index of suspicion of an astute nurse who noted the vague responses to history questions and the client's unrelenting checking of the clock followed by urgently stating, "I've got to get home." Upon further questioning, the woman revealed that she was often quite fatigued because of caring for her five children under 7 years of age. Yet her husband, who worked until 2 AM, expected her to be awake when he came home from work and have a warm meal ready in the oven. "He hits me if I'm asleep." She had taped her eyes open so that even if she were lying down when he came home she would look awake. "I didn't even think about taking my contacts out."*

The coping mechanisms many battered individuals employ to live in violent and terrifying situations often prevent the dissolution of the marriage. These coping mechanisms present in the form of beliefs or myths (Table 25–1). Because of feelings of confusion, shame, despair, and powerlessness, victims may withdraw from interaction with others.

ASSESSING FAMILY COPING PATTERNS

When assessing family violence, the nurse should show a willingness to listen and avoid any judgmental tone. Questioning about memories of early family relationships can provide additional information about attitudes in the home and the way they might influence coping. Living with children and older adults in the same household can cause frustration, stress, and anger. Unless there are appropriate outlets for stress, violence can occur. Box 25–9 is a useful guide for assessing the risk of elder abuse in the home.

ASSESSING SUPPORT SYSTEMS

The person experiencing violence is usually in a dependent position, relying on the perpetrator (spouse, parent, other family member, or caregiver) for basic needs. Such situations foster isolation from others. Children's options are especially limited, as are those of the physically and mentally challenged. Assessing for support should focus on intrapersonal, interpersonal, and community resources (e.g., the school system for school-age victims).

ASSESSING SUICIDE POTENTIAL

A person experiencing violence may feel so trapped in a detrimental relationship, yet so desperate to get out, that suicide may seem the only answer. The threat of suicide may also be used by an emotionally violent person in an attempt to manipulate the partner or spouse into caving in to demands ("Don't leave me or I'll kill myself" or "I took all my pills . . . I said I would the next time you were late").

A suicide attempt may be the presenting symptom in the emergency department. It has been estimated that at least 10% of abused women attempt suicide. With sensitive questioning conducted in a caring manner, the nurse can elicit the history of violence. Often the overdose is with a combination of alcohol and other central nervous system depressants, tranquilizers, or sleeping medications that have been prescribed in previous visits to physicians' offices, clinics, or emergency departments.

When the crisis of the immediate suicide attempt has been resolved, careful questioning to determine lethality is in order. (See Chapter 23 for suicide assessment.) For example, if the client still feels that life is not worth living, has a suicide plan, and has the means to carry it out, admission to an inpatient psychiatric unit must be considered. On the other hand, if the client is talking about future plans and hanging in there "for the sake of the children," outpatient referrals are appropriate.

TABLE 25–1   *Myth Versus Fact: Family Violence*

MYTH	FACT
1. 95% of abuse victims are women.	1. Recent surveys report that from 30% to 40%, perhaps 50%, of abuse victims are men.
2. The victim's behavior often causes violence.	2. The victim's behavior is *not* the cause of violence. Violence is the abuser's pattern of behavior, and the victim cannot learn how to control it.
3. Men have the right to keep their wives/children in line.	3. No person has the right to beat or hurt another person.
4. Spouse abuse is a minor problem.	4. There is a *real* danger that a woman may be killed by a violent partner.
5. Battered women are masochistic and like to be beaten. (The abuse cannot be that bad or they would leave.)	5. Women do not like, ask, or deserve to be abused. Economic considerations are usually the only reason they stay.
6. Family violence is most prevalent in those from poor working-class backgrounds who are usually poorly educated.	6. Violence occurs in families from all socioeconomic, religious, cultural, and educational backgrounds.
7. The family is sacred and should be allowed to take care of its own problems.	7. Intervention in family violence is justified because it always escalates in frequency and intensity, can end in death, and is passed on to future generations.
8. Victims of abuse tacitly accept the abuse by trying to conceal it, by not reporting it, or by failing to seek help.	8. When attempting to disclose their situation, many women are met with disbelief. This discourages them from persevering.
9. Myths abused women believe: "I can't live without him." "If I hadn't done . . . . it wouldn't have happened." "He will change." "I stay for the sake of the children." "His jealousy and possessiveness prove he really loves me."	9. These myths are coping mechanisms women use to allay panic in a situation of random and brutal violence. They give the illusion of control and rationality.
10. Alcohol and stress are the major causes of physical and verbal abuse	10. This myth offers an explanation of and tolerance for verbal abuse/battering. There are no excuses and it is not acceptable behavior. Abuse is a learned behavior, not an uncontrollable reaction. People are abusive because they have acquired the belief that violence and aggression are acceptable and effective responses to real or imagined threats.
11. Violence occurs only between heterosexual partners.	11. Gay and lesbian partners experience violence for reasons similar to those in heterosexual partners.
12. Pregnancy protects a woman from battering.	12. Battering frequently begins or escalates during pregnancy.

ASSESSING HOMICIDE POTENTIAL

Inquire whether the client feels safe to go home, and if so, whether a safety plan is in place for when the violence recurs. Certain factors place a vulnerable person at greater risk for homicide from continuing and escalating violence:

■ The presence of a gun in the home
■ Alcohol and drug abuse
■ The perpetrator also being violent in other situations (harmed pets, beat a spouse when she was pregnant, forced sex upon her)
■ The perpetrator being extremely jealous and obsessive about his relationship with the victim and trying to control all her daily activities (Campbell 1995)

Persons victimized by violence should be asked if they have ever felt like killing the perpetrator, and if so whether they have the current desire and means to carry it out. If the answer is "yes," intervention is required.

ASSESSING DRUG AND ALCOHOL USE

A person experiencing violence may self-medicate with alcohol or other drugs as a way of escaping a dreadful situation. The drugs are usually central nervous system depressants (e.g., benzodiazepines) prescribed by physicians in response to the battered person's presentation with vague complaints, which are often stress related (e.g., insomnia, gastrointestinal upsets, feeling jittery, difficulty concentrating).

The level of intoxication can be determined by history, physical examination, and blood alcohol level. If the battered woman is intoxicated on presentation, allow her to sober up before instituting referral. Referral information will not be understood or assimilated if she is intoxicated. She should not be discharged with her husband.

Assess for a chronic alcohol or drug problem (refer to Chapter 27) and provide appropriate treatment referrals. Choices of treatment can include both inpatient and outpatient options.

MAINTAINING ACCURATE RECORDS

Because of the possibility of legal action, it is essential that the health care record contain an accurate and detailed description of the victim's medical history, the psychosocial history of the family, and observations of the family interactions during the interviews. Especially important in documenting findings from initial assessment are (1) verbatim statements of who caused the injury and when it occurred; (2) a body map to indicate size, color, shape, areas, and types of injuries, with explanations; and (3) physical evidence, when possible, of sexual abuse. Procedures for evidence collection must be carefully followed or legal action can be thwarted. If the beating has just occurred, ask the client to return in a day or two for more photos; bruises may be more evident at that time. The client must be assured of the confidentiality of the record and of its power should legal action be initiated. Even if intervention does not occur at this time, the record is begun; the next provider will not have to stumble across the problem and will be in a better position to offer support.

Assessment Guidelines

ASSESSMENT GUIDELINES: FAMILY VIOLENCE

During your assessment and counseling, maintain an interested and empathetic manner. Refrain from displaying horror, anger, shock, or disapproval of the perpetrator or the situation. Assess for:

1. Presenting signs and symptoms of victims of family violence
2. Potential problem in vulnerable families. For example, some indicators of vulnerable parents who might benefit from education and effective coping techniques
3. Physical, sexual, and/or emotional abuse and neglect and economic maltreatment in the case of elders

4. Family coping patterns
5. Client's support system
6. Drug or alcohol use
7. Suicidal or homicidal ideas
8. Posttrauma syndrome
9. If the client is a child or an elder, identify the protection agency in your state that will have to be notified.

NURSING DIAGNOSIS

Nursing diagnoses are focused on the underlying causes and symptoms of family violence (Carlson-Catalano 1998). **Risk for injury, Risk for violence, Anxiety,** and **Fear** are nursing diagnoses that apply. **Disabled family coping, Powerlessness,** and **Caregiver role strain** are others. Feelings of helplessness, hopelessness, and powerlessness contribute to the diagnosis of **Body image disturbances** and **Chronic low self-esteem.** The crisis of family violence precipitates **Interrupted family process** or **Impaired parenting** as the family system becomes less able to meet the emotional, physical, or security needs of its members.

Pain related to physical injury or trauma would most certainly take high priority and need immediate attention. See Table 25–2 for a list of potential nursing diagnoses for family violence.

TABLE 25–2 *Potential Nursing Diagnoses for Family Violence*

SIGNS AND SYMPTOMS	POTENTIAL NURSING DIAGNOSES
Bruises, cuts, broken bones, lacerations, scars, burns, wounds in various phases of healing, particularly when explanations don't match injury, or explanations vague	Risk for Injury Pain Risk for Infection Impaired Skin Integrity Risk for Post Trauma
Isolated, fearful, feelings of shame and low self-esteem, feelings of worthlessness, depression, being helpless	Powerlessness Ineffective Coping Fear Risk for Self-Directed Violence Self-Esteem Disturbance Helplessness Spiritual Distress
Vaginal-anal bruises, sores, discharge, peritoneal pain, positive VDRL	Rape Trauma Syndrome Risk for Infection

The identification of desired outcomes and designing of nursing interventions that facilitate achieving those outcomes should be developed as much as possible in collaboration with the survivor and primary support person. These outcomes should be continually reassessed and revised as new information about the survivor's needs emerges. A comprehensive plan can also be the coordinating framework for the work of an interdisciplinary team.

OUTCOME CRITERIA

Johnson and Colleagues (2000) in their Nursing Outcome Classification (NOC) identify the following outcome criteria for abuse cessation (Table 25–3; scale of 1–5, 1 = no evidence, 5 = extensive evidence):

■ Cessation of abuse reported by victim
■ Physical abuse has ceased
■ Emotional abuse has ceased
■ Sexual abuse has ceased
■ Neglect has ceased
■ Financial exploitation has ceased

Table 25–4 may be used as a guideline for specific outcome criteria for child, spouse, elder abuse and for the abuser, along with short and intermediate goals.

PLANNING

Family violence is all too common, and nurses and other health care workers encounter it frequently in community health clinics, emergency rooms, on home visits, doctors' offices, obstetrical units, in schools, nursing homes, and home health, or in any other arena where nurses meet the public. You may even find that your neighbor, a colleague, your best friend, your sister-in-law, or other member of your family is involved in abusive situations (either as the abused or the abuser).

Violence within families is seldom recognized by outsiders, including nurses. Yet the nurse is often the first point of contact for people experiencing family violence and thus is in an ideal position to contribute to prevention, detection, and effective intervention. The Joint Commission on Accreditation of Healthcare Organizations (JCAHO) requires staff education in family violence as well as standards of care to guide clinical practice (Capezuti 1997). The Nursing Network on Violence Against Women encourages the development of a nursing practice that focuses on health issues relating to the effects of violence on women's lives. Altering the pattern of violence against women can also affect child abuse, because the main predictor of violence toward children is violence toward their mothers. Ultimately, the general tolerance of violence in the United States must be addressed if long-lasting changes are to be made.

Most hospitals and community centers have protocols for child, spouse, or elder abuse that may or may not meet all the needs of your client(s). Unless it is a case of child abuse in which the child has been removed from the home, most interventions, after needed emergency care, will take place within the community. Plans should center around the client's safety first and, whenever possible, or in the best interest of the client, should be discussed with the client (partner/spouse, parents or elder). Planning needs to also take into consideration the needs of the abuser, e.g., parents, caretakers, spouse abuser, if they seem willing to learn violent-free alternatives to frustration and aggression.

INTERVENTION

Nurses have a legal responsibility and are mandated to report suspected or actual cases of child and elder abuse. The appropriate agency may be the state or county child welfare agency, law enforcement agency, juvenile court, or county health department. Each state has specific guidelines for reporting, including whether the report can be oral or written, or both, and specifying the time that can elapse after suspicion of abuse or neglect (immediately, 24 hours, or 48 hours). Every battered person is a crime victim, and assault with a weapon is reportable in most states. Also, approximately 40 states have marital rape statutes. An example follows of a case to report.

Vignette

■ *Two nurses who work in a family practice clinic are suspicious of child abuse. A 12-year-old girl has recurrent urinary tract infections. She is always accompanied to clinic visits by her father, who even goes into the bathroom with her when she is producing urine samples. He answers all questions for her even when they are directed toward her. He has recently refused the next diagnostic test for attempting to ascertain the reason for the recurrent infections.*

After pressure by the nurses, the physician agrees to ask the girl some questions in private. The nurses think the physician has discounted the problem, asked superficial questions, and dismissed their concerns. They attempt to get the girl alone for a discussion, but to no avail. After consultation with clinical resources, they decide to report their concerns to Children's Protective Services. They in-

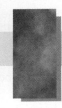

TABLE 25–3   *Abusive Behavior Self-Control*

Domain—Psychosocial Health (III)
Class—Self-Control (O)
Scale—Never demonstrated to Consistently demonstrated (m)
Definition: Self-restraint of own behaviors to avoid abuse and neglect of dependents or significant others

ABUSIVE BEHAVIOR SELF-CONTROL	NEVER DEMONSTRATED 1	RARELY DEMONSTRATED 2	SOMETIMES DEMONSTRATED 3	OFTEN DEMONSTRATED 4	CONSISTENTLY DEMONSTRATED 5
Indicators	1	2	3	4	5
1 Avoids physically abusive behavior					
2 Avoids emotionally abusive behavior	1	2	3	4	5
3 Avoids sexually abusive behavior	1	2	3	4	5
4 Avoids neglect of dependent's basic needs	1	2	3	4	5
5 Uses alternative coping mechanisms for stress	1	2	3	4	5
6 Discusses the abusive behavior	1	2	3	4	5
7 Identifies factors contributing to abusive behavior	1	2	3	4	5
8 Expresses feelings about victim	1	2	3	4	5
9 Identifies available community resources for help	1	2	3	4	5
10 Expresses frustrations	1	2	3	4	5
11 Uses nurturing behavior toward victim	1	2	3	4	5
12 Demonstrates self-esteem	1	2	3	4	5
13 States expectations congruent with developmental level	1	2	3	4	5
14 Applies appropriate caregiving techniques	1	2	3	4	5
15 Uses support network	1	2	3	4	5
16 Expresses empathy for victim	1	2	3	4	5
17 Demonstrates impulse control	1	2	3	4	5
18 Demonstrates knowledge of correct role behaviors	1	2	3	4	5
19 Seeks treatment as needed	1	2	3	4	5

From: Johnson, H., Maas, M., Meriden, M., and Moorehead, S. (2000). *Nursing Outcomes Classification (NOC)*, 2nd ed., St. Louis: Mosby.

TABLE 25-4 *Specific Outcome Criteria*

OUTCOME CRITERIA	SHORT AND INTERMEDIATE GOALS
Child	
CHILD WILL: 1. Know what plans are made for his or her protection and state them to the nurse. 2. Demonstrate renewed confidence and feelings of safety during follow-up visits.	1. Be safe until adequate home and family assessment is made by (date). 2. Be treated by nurse practitioner or physician and receive medical care for injuries within 1 hour. 3. Participate with therapists (nurse, social worker, counselor) for purpose of ongoing therapy and emotional support (art, play, group, other) within 24 hours.
Spouse Abuse Client	
CLIENTS WILL: 1. Within 3 weeks, state that they believe that they do not deserve to be beaten. 2. Within 3 weeks, state they have joined a support group or are receiving counseling (family, couples, individual). 3. State that their living conditions are now safe from spouse abuse or potential abuse; or 4. Within 2 months, state that they have found safe housing for self and children.	1. Have timely access to medical care for fractures, wounds, burns, and other injuries 2. After initial interview, name four community resources they can contract (hotlines, shelters, support groups, neighbor(s), crisis center, legal guidance, or spiritual advisors), who do not support violence. 3. After initial interview, describe a safety plan to be used in future violent situations 4. State their right to live in a safe environment by (date).
Elder Abuse	
CLIENTS WILL: 1. State that caregiver has provided adequate food, clothing, housing, and medical care by (date). 2. Be free of physical signs of abuse by (date). 3. Demonstrate control of personal finances by (date). 4. Demonstrate control of legal matters. 5. Demonstrate control of personal possessions.	1. State that they feel safer and more comfortable by (date) using a scale of 1–5 (1 being the safest) or: 2. Ask to be removed from violent situation by (date). 3. Name and recite the phone numbers of two people who can be called for if in need of help. 4. Have access to the names and phone numbers of at least two lawyers who can help them with legal matters and securing their finances/possessions.
Abuser	
ABUSER WILL: 1. Avoid physical, sexual, emotional, neglectful or sexually abusive behaviors. 2. Use alternative coping mechanisms for stress. 3. Identify factors contributing to abusive behavior. 4. Identify community resources for help. 5. Use support network. 6. Demonstrate impulse control.	1. State he or she is willing to work on living in a violence-free environment by (date). 2. Attend anger management training (AMT) course within 2 weeks. 3. Demonstrate at least three new alternative methods for relieving frustration, anger, and aggression. 4. Attend and participate in support group/parenting group/men's group/caregiver support group. 5. Identify two community supports that can help family minimize stress and isolation (parenting classes, respite, housekeepers, men's groups, women's groups).

form the father, who becomes outraged at their accusations and threatens to change doctors The nurses try to reassure him about the nature of the referral, to no avail Subsequent investigation confirms the likelihood of sexual abuse, and the child is placed in temporary foster care with follow-up counseling. The father refuses treatment and 4 months later leaves the family.

This case illustrates that a reasonable basis for suspecting maltreatment, not proof, is all that is required to report. Nurses must attempt to maintain both an appropriate level of suspicion and a neutral, objective attitude. One can be too concerned and jump to conclusions (which is what the physician in this case thought the nurses were doing) or not concerned enough and rationalize an incomplete examination to avoid confrontation (which is what the nurses thought the physician was doing). Given these opposing stances, the case was reported, as required by law and ethical standards, and Children's Protective Services was given the opportunity to sort it out.

Competency may be a consideration in a situation of elder mistreatment. Unless incompetency has been established legally, elders have the right to self-determination. Some institutions and health care agencies have developed guidelines for dealing with actual or suspected situations of mistreatment. These protocols list possible behaviors or conditions of the elderly and the most appropriate intervention. The establishment of such protocols is highly recommended because it gives support to the nurse's actions.

Quality nursing care for those experiencing violence must be culturally sensitive (Campbell and Campbell 1996). The nurse must be aware of the cultural issues that may affect response to violence and to intervention. For example, Cambodian women control their responses to stress and violence through nonconfrontation and withdrawal, which are designed to restore equilibrium. Culture is important because it is central to how people organize their experience. Even the most acculturated people have a tendency to revert to their cultural past in organizing coping strategies after a stressful event (Campbell et al. 1993). If there is a language barrier, the nurse should speak slowly and clearly in English, without using jargon, and allow time for the response. If no English is spoken, a trained medical interpreter should be provided. A family member should *not* be used, to ensure confidentiality and to protect the person from future retaliation.

Primary prevention consists of measures taken to prevent the occurrence of family violence (Beauchesne et al. 1997). Identifying people at high risk, providing health teaching, and coordinating supportive services to prevent crises are examples of primary prevention. Specific strategies include (1) reducing stress, (2) reducing the influence of risk factors, (3) increasing social support, (4) increasing coping skills, and (5) increasing self-esteem. Community health nurses are also in a position to assess family functioning in the home during visits for such matters as assisting children with chronic health problems. In addition, the community health nurse and clinic nurse maintain contact with the family over time, which allows for assessment of changes. They are also in an excellent position to connect parents to appropriate resources in the community that can meet their needs.

Secondary prevention involves early intervention in abusive situations to minimize their disabling or long-term effects. Nurses can establish screening programs for individuals at risk, participate in the medical treatment of injuries resulting from violent episodes, and coordinate community services to provide continuity of care (Davidhizer et al. 1997). Stress and depression can be reduced with supportive psychotherapy, support groups, pharmacotherapy, and telephone numbers to safe houses. Social dysfunction or lack of information can be addressed by counseling and education. Caregiver burden can be reduced by assistance in caregiving, nursing, or housekeeping or (in cases in which caregiving needs exceed even optimized caregiver capacity) placement of the patient in a more appropriate setting. The following Vignette illustrates a successful secondary prevention effort.

Vignette

■ *Billy, age 4, is brought into the physician's office by 15-year-old Mary, the children's babysitter, with second-degree burns on his right hand. Mary frequently babysits for Billy and his younger brother Jimmy, age 2, and older brother Tom, age 6. Mary appears apprehensive and says she is very concerned. Mary tells the nurse that the children have told her in the past that Billy's mother has threatened them with burning if they do not behave. Billy told her that his mother once held his hands on a cold stove and told him that if he was bad, she would burn him. Mary is shocked that Billy's mother would do such a thing, but at the same time she mentions she feels guilty for "telling on Ms. J."*

Mary also states that the older brother told Mary what had happened but was afraid that if his mother found out, she would burn him also. Mary says she is aware that the mother hits the children, but she did not believe that anyone would burn her own child.

The nurse reports what happened to the physician, and the mother is called and asked to come to the office.

Billy appears frightened and in pain. The nurse asks Mary to come with Billy while she examines him.

Nurse: Tell me about your hand, Billy. *Billy looks down and starts to cry.*
Nurse: It's OK if you don't want to talk about it, Billy.
Billy: *Not looking at the nurse, he says softly,* My mommy burned my hand on the stove.
Nurse: Tell me what happened before that happened.
Billy: Mommy was mad because I didn't put my toys away.
Nurse: What does your mommy usually do when she gets mad?
Billy: She yells mostly; sometimes she hits us.
Mommy is going to be so mad at Tommy for telling.
Nurse: Tell me about the hitting.

Billy: Mommy hits us a lot since Daddy left us. *Billy starts to cry to himself.*

On examination, the nurse notices a ringed pattern of burns across Billy's right palm like the burner of an electric stove. There are blisters on the fingers. Billy appears well-nourished and properly dressed. He is at his approximate developmental age except for some language delay.

Because of the physical evidence and history, there is strong suspicion of child abuse. Children's Protective Services is notified, and the family situation is evaluated for possible placement of Billy in protective custody. The initial evaluation concludes that there is no indication of serious potential harm to the child and that Billy should return home.

The mother, who was initially defensive, starts to cry and states, "I can't cope with being alone and I don't know where to turn." The intervention that the nurse facilitates centers around caring for Billy's immediate health needs; finding supports for the mother to help her cope with crises; providing a counseling referral for the mother to learn alternative ways of expressing anger and frustration; informing the mother of parents' groups; providing referrals to play groups or day care for the children to help increase their feelings of self-esteem and security; and providing a break, and perhaps some instruction in parenting, for the mother.

Tertiary prevention involves nurses facilitating the healing and rehabilitative process by counseling individuals and families; providing support for groups of survivors; and assisting survivors of violence to achieve their optimal level of safety, health, and well-being (Chiocca 1998). Tertiary interventions often occur in mental health settings.

Communication Guidelines

Counseling interventions include crisis intervention and the promotion of growth. It is useful to emphasize that people have a right to live without fear of violence or physical harm, and without fear of assault. The role of the nurse is to support the victim, counsel about safety, and facilitate access to other resources as appropriate. By listening, giving support, discussing options, and describing other ways of living, the nurse initiates an awareness of other possibilities.

All women experiencing violence should be counseled about developing a safety plan, a plan for a fast escape when violence recurs. They should be asked to identify the signs of escalation of violence and to pick a particular sign that will tell them in the future that "now is the time to leave." If chil-

dren are present, they can all agree on a code word that, when spoken by their mother, means "it is time to go." If she plans ahead, she may be able to leave before the violence occurs. She should plan where she is going and how she will get there. The nurse should suggest that she have a bag already packed for herself and her children with the items designated in Box 25–8. The packed bag should be kept in a place where the perpetrator will not find it.

If the battered person chooses to leave, shelters or safe houses (for both sexes) are available in many communities (although, sadly, only at half the rate of animal shelters—a reflection of our social values). They are open 24 hours a day and can be reached through hotline information, hospital emergency rooms, YWCAs, or the local office of the National Organization for Women (NOW). The address of the house is usually kept secret to protect the women from attack by their mates. Besides protection, many of these safe shelters provide important education and consciousness-raising functions. The woman should be given the number of the nearest available shelter, even if she decides for the present to stay with her partner. Referral phone numbers may be kept for years before the decision to call is made. Having the number and a contact person all that time contributes to thinking about options.

Case Management

Community mental health centers are becoming increasingly involved in the delivery of services to victims and perpetrators of domestic violence. Nurses working in these settings have the opportunity to be case managers to coordinate community, medical, criminal justice, and social systems in order to provide comprehensive services for violent families. Strategies must encompass needs for housing, child care, economic stability, physical and emotional safety, counseling, legal protection, career development or job training, education, ongoing support groups, and health care. The myriad of agencies and people that those seeking help have to reach can be daunting and confusing. A nurse functioning in a case manager role can assist the client in choosing the best options for her and coordinating the interventions of several agencies. Suggestions for interventions for common assessment domains and community resources are listed in Table 25–5.

Milieu Therapy

Interventions are geared toward stabilizing the home situation and maintaining a violence-free environment. The interventions offered should leave options for growth, increase in self-esteem, and a

BOX 25–8 *Personalized Safety Guide*

**SUGGESTIONS FOR INCREASING SAFETY—
IN THE RELATIONSHIP**

■ I will have important phone numbers available to my children and myself.

■ I can tell _____ and _____ about the violence and ask them to call the police if they hear suspicious noises coming from my home.

■ If I leave my home, I can go (list four places) _____ , _____ , _____ , or _____ .

■ I can leave extra money, car keys, clothes, and copies of documents with _____ .

■ If I leave, I will bring _____ (see checklist next page).

■ To ensure safety and independence, I can: keep change for phone calls with me at all times; open my own savings account; rehearse my escape route with a support person; and review safety plan on __ (date).

**SUGGESTIONS FOR INCREASING SAFETY—
WHEN THE RELATIONSHIP IS OVER**

■ I can: change the locks; install steel/metal doors, a security system, smoke detectors, and an outside lighting system.

■ I will inform _____ and _____ that my partner no longer lives with me and ask them to call the police if he or she is observed near my home or my children.

■ I will tell people who take care of my children the names of those who have permission to pick them up. The people who have permission are: _____ , _____ and _____ .

■ I can: tell _____ at work about my situation and ask _____ to screen my calls.

■ I can avoid stores, banks, and _____ that I used when living with my battering partner.

■ I can obtain a protective order from _____ . I can keep it on or near me at all times as well as have a copy with _____ .

■ If I feel down and ready to return to a potentially abusive situation, I can call _____ for support or attend workshops and support groups to gain support and strengthen my relationships with other people.

IMPORTANT PHONE NUMBERS

Police _____
Hotline _____
Friends _____
Shelter _____

ITEMS TO TAKE CHECKLIST

Identification
Birth certificates for me and my children
Social security cards
School and medical records
Money, bankbooks, credit cards
Keys to house/car/office
Driver's license and registration
Medications
Change of clothes
Welfare identification
Passport(s), green cards, work permits
Divorce papers
Lease/rental agreement, house deed
Mortgage payment book, current unpaid bills
Insurance papers
Address book
Pictures, jewelry, items of sentimental value
Children's favorite toys and/or blankets

---

higher quality of life for all family members (Lawson 1998). Some mental health agencies have family-based units where a caseworker or clinician comes to the home instead of the family going to the agency. Providing and maintaining a therapeutic environment in the home ideally involves three levels of help for violent families:

1. Provide the family with economic support, job opportunities, and social services, such as family service agencies.

2. Arrange social support in the form of a public health nurse, lay home visitor, day care teacher, school teacher, social worker, respite worker, or any other potential contact person who has a good relationship with the family.

3. Encourage and provide family therapy.

Self-Care Activities

The primary goal of intervention is empowerment (Hattendorf and Tollenrud 1997). Supporting the cli-

TABLE 25–5 *Victims of Violence—Nursing Needs Assessment and Intervention*

	ASSESSMENT	INTERVENTION	
Domain	**Nursing Assessment**	**Nursing Education/ Intervention**	**Community Agencies**
Physiological	Brief head-to-toe assessment	Appropriate medical follow-up	Community clinics Medical staff referrals
	Nutritional habits	Healthy dietary practices Basic food groups Food availability	WIC (Women, Infants, Children) services Community food shelves
	Sleep patterns	Impact of sleep deprivation	Counseling, crisis nursery
	Chemical dependency/use	Encourage access to counseling/support groups	Referrals to AA, counselors, community agencies supporting rehabilitation
	Sexual assault	Assess for immediate physical needs	Sexual assault advocates
Psychological/ sociocultural	Self-esteem	Affirm: You don't deserve it/ You didn't cause it	Battered women's resources
	Coping needs/skills	Need to take care of self	Community women's courses, groups, public library
	Support system (family, friends)	Emphasize need to access Provide opportunity to call Help identify support services	Support groups Stress management classes Crisis nursery Battered women's groups and shelters
	Depression	Offer support Validate: It is part of the abuse cycle Evaluate severity: candidate for posttraumatic stress disorder?	Counseling, psychotherapy Resources at place of employment
Educational	Understanding/perception of abuse	Definitions/characteristics: What constitutes abuse, escalating characteristics	Battered women's resources
	Literacy		Community education
	Language/hearing barriers		Interpreter services, hearing society
Financial	Is there need for money? (transportation, food, medical care, basic needs)		Social services Battered women's resources Counseling, employment, clothing community resources Medical assistance/AFDC
Legal	Desire for legal action	Facilitate contact of law enforcement Advise of resources available	Battered women's advocates Law enforcement
	Legal questions		Judicare or local attorney resources Legal clinics Battered women's resources
Safety	Fear level	Safety plan: ■ Self-defense ■ Emergency numbers ■ Self-protection during abuse; curl into ball, hold head, scream loudly ■ Have children or neighbors call 911	Community self-defense classes Women's shelter and advocates

Table continued on following page

TABLE 25–5 *Victims of Violence—Nursing Needs Assessment and Intervention* (Continued)

	ASSESSMENT	INTERVENTION	
Domain	**Nursing Assessment**	**Nursing Education/Intervention**	**Community Agencies**

	Safety level:
	■ Does she feel safe?
	■ Has there been a recent increase in violence?
	■ Has she been "choked"
	■ Is there a weapon in the house?
	■ Has he used/threatened to use a weapon?
	■ Has he threatened to harm the children?
	■ Has he threatened to kill her?
		Counsel regarding long-range plans:
		■ Discuss potential for escalation and increased risk
		■ Discuss awareness of options, considering risk
		Escape plan:
		■ Where will she go?
		■ How will she get there?
		■ What does she need to leave?
		■ Hide an "escape kit" that is easily accessible:
		  papers, money, documents
		  phone numbers, including number of women's shelter
		  clothing, glasses, medications
		  keys
			Child protection
			Women's shelter and advocates

	Safety of children	Presence of child abuse	Child protection

AFDC, Aid to Families with Dependent Children.
Developed by Marlene Jezierski, R. N. From Jezierski, M. (1994). Abuse of women by male partners: Basic knowledge for emergency nurses. *Journal of Emergency Nursing,* 20(5):361.

ent to act on her own behalf can decrease feelings of helplessness and hopelessness. The initial phase of recovery begins when a woman first makes steps to leave the relationship (Landenburger 1998). Giving referral numbers and providing an opportunity for her to call from your office, or inquiring at the next visit whether she was successful in reaching the appropriate agency, demonstrates confidence in her ability to take care of herself.

Specific referrals regarding emergency money and legal counseling should be made available to each woman. Vocational counseling is another referral that may be appropriate. Battered women should be given referrals to parenting resources that enable them to explore alternative approaches to discipline (i.e., no hitting, slapping, or other expressions of violence).

Health Teaching

In families at risk for violence, health teaching includes meeting with both the client and the family and discussing associated risk factors. The client, caregiver, and family need to learn to recognize behaviors and situations that might trigger violence.

Normal developmental and physiological changes should be explained to enable family members to gain a more positive view of the victim and the crisis situation. Gaining a more complete understanding can help family members broaden their insight and thus increase their compassion. They may then begin to anticipate new stress situations and be able to prepare for them before a crisis occurs. Refer to Chapter 35 for family interventions.

Nurses who work on a maternity unit are often in a position to spot potential violence in new families and initiate appropriate interventions, including education about effective parenting as well as coping techniques. Information about these interventions should be shared with the client's ambulatory care nurse for appropriate monitoring and follow-up. Parents who are candidates for special attention include

■ New parents whose behavior toward the infant is rejecting, hostile, or indifferent.
■ Teenage parents, most of whom are children

themselves and who require special help and guidance in handling the baby and discussing their expectations of the baby and their support systems.

■ Retarded parents, for whom careful, explicit, and repeated instructions on caring for the child and recognizing the infant's needs are indicated.

■ Parents who grew up watching their mother being beaten. This is the biggest risk factor for perpetuation of family violence.

Nurses can also recognize the vulnerable child. When it is known that specific children are at risk, referrals to community resources are in order. These may include emergency child care facilities, emergency telephone numbers, numbers of 24-hour crisis centers or hotlines, and respite programs in which volunteers take the child for an occasional weekend so that parents can get some relief. Public health nurses can make home visits; such visits allow assessment of potential violence in the crucial first few months of life. This early period is when the style of parent-child interactions is set for later life. Important factors for the public health nurse to assess are noted in Box 25-9. Such observations made by nurses in clinic and public health settings are fundamental in case finding and evaluation.

Psychotherapy

Psychotherapy is carried out by a nurse who is educated at the master's level in psychiatric nursing and certified or eligible for certification. Therapy is most effective after crisis intervention, when the situation is less chaotic and tumultuous. A variety of therapeutic modalities are available for violent families.

INDIVIDUAL THERAPY

The goals of individual therapy for a survivor are empowerment and practice in recognizing and selecting productive life options and developing a solid sense of self (Hattendorf and Tollerud 1997). People who experienced violence as a child or who have left a violent relationship may choose individual therapy to work out symptoms of depression, anxiety, somatization, or posttraumatic stress disorder. Many of the psychological symptoms shown by battered women can be understood as complex survival strategies and responses to violence. This constellation of symptoms has been referred to as the "battered woman syndrome" (the posttraumatic stress disorder category in DSM-IV-TR).

Individual therapy is often indicated for the perpetrator also, particularly when an individual psychopathological process is identified. Many perpetrators meet the DSM-IV criteria for intermittent

BOX 25-9   *Factors to Assess During a Home Visit*

FOR CHILD

Responsiveness to infant's crying
Responsiveness to infant's signals related to feeding
Caregiver's facial expressions in response to infant
Holding of child
Playfulness of caregiver with infant
Type of physical contact during feeding
Temperament of infant: average, quiet, or active
Parent's attitudes signaling possible warnings:

■ Complaints of inadequacy as a parent
■ Complaints of inadequacy of child
■ Fear of "doing something wrong"
■ Attribution of badness to newborn
■ History of a destructive childhood
■ Misdirected anger
■ Continued evidence of isolation, apathy, anger, frustration, projection
■ Adult conflict

Environmental conditions:

■ Sleeping arrangements
■ Child management
■ Home management
■ Use of supports (formal and informal)

Need for immediate services for situational (economics, child care), emotional, or educational information:

■ Sharing information about hotlines, babysitters, homemakers, parent groups
■ Sharing information about child development
■ Child care and home management

FOR ELDER

Environmental conditions:

■ House in poor repair
■ Inadequate heat, lighting, furniture, cooking utensils
■ Presence of garbage or vermin
■ Old food in kitchen
■ Lack of assistive devices
■ Locks on refrigerator
■ Blocked stairways
■ Victim lying in urine, feces, or food
■ Unpleasant odors

Medication:

■ Medication not being taken as prescribed (e.g., not available, confused about procedure, physically unable)

Data from Galbraith 1986; Elder abuse 1991.

explosive disorder, which involves repeated episodes of assault or destruction of property out of proportion to precipitating stressors that cannot be accounted for by another mental disorder, the physiological effects of a substance, or a general medical condition. Therapy for the perpetrator is most effective when it is court mandated, because then the perpetrator is more likely to stay the course of treatment.

FAMILY THERAPY

Because family violence is a symptom of a family in crisis, each part of the family system needs attention. Also, because change in one member of the family system affects change in the whole system, support and understanding are needed by all members. Family interventions may maximize positive interactions among family members. Family therapy should take place *only* if the violence is recent and if *both* partners to be involved. The perpetrator should have taken steps to control violent behavior that are verified by the survivor.

Expected outcomes are that the perpetrator will recognize inner states of anger and learn alternative ways of dealing with anger. Intermediate goals are that members of the family will openly communicate and learn to listen to each other.

GROUP THERAPY

Therapy groups provide assurances that one is not alone and that positive change is possible. Because many survivors have been isolated over time, they have been deprived of validation and positive feedback from others. Working in a group can help diminish feelings of isolation, strengthen feelings of self-esteem and self-worth, and increase the potential for realistic problem solving in a supportive atmosphere.

Self-help groups serve a vital function for many people. Hotlines provide emergency resources and information on how to contact self-help groups within the community, such as Parents Anonymous.

The real problem in a violent relationship is the perpetrator. Nurses engaged in therapy with perpetrators have a duty to warn potential victims if they conclude that the perpetrator is a danger. Refer to Chapter 8 for legal guidelines. In groups for perpetrators, the men are taught to recognize signs of escalating anger and learn ways of channeling their anger nonviolently. Men who have never discussed problems with anyone before are encouraged to discuss their thoughts and feelings. Group therapy can help create a community of healing and restoration.

EVALUATION

Failures in interventions with abusive families are often due not to our lack or theirs but to deficits in the social, economic, and political systems in which we live. A very real problem is that of social exclusion by which multidimensionally disadvantaged individuals are prohibited from obtaining formal helping services (Hilbert and Krishnan 2000). Nurses can direct their interventions to the social environment and can question, among other things, the acceptance of corporal punishment as a technique for guiding behavior in children, the unequal burden of caregiving responsibilities placed on women, the low priority given to education and preparation for parenthood, and the belief that one has little social value if one is elderly.

Evaluation of brief interventions can be based on whether the survivor acknowledges the violence, is willing to accept intervention, and/or is removed from the violent situation. With more long-term intervention, evaluation should be made by all members of the health care team on an ongoing basis. Because violence is a symptom of a family in distress, diagnosis, interventions, and evaluation should ideally be carried out by a multidisciplinary team that includes a physician, a nurse, a social worker, an attorney, and perhaps a psychiatrist. Follow-up is crucial in helping defray the frequency of family violence.

The following is a case study of family violence.

Visit the **Evolve** website at
http://evolve.elsevier.com/Varcarolis
for more Case Studies.

CASE STUDY 25–1   *Working With a Family Experiencing Violence*

Mrs. Rob, a recently widowed 84-year-old woman, moved to her son's apartment 3 months ago. She had been living alone in her third-floor walk-up in the city.

Because of her declining health, crime in the neighborhood, and three flights of stairs to climb, and with her son John's encouragement, she went to live with him.

He and his wife, Judy, who have been married for almost 20 years, have five children 6 to 18 years of age, all living in a rather cramped three-bedroom apartment.

Mrs. Rob was being cared for by the visiting nurse, who monitored her blood pressure and adjusted her medication. Over a series of visits, the nurse, Ms. Green, noticed that Mrs. Rob was looking unkempt, pale, and withdrawn. While taking her blood pressure, the nurse observed bruises on Mrs. Rob's arms and neck. When questioned about the bruises, Mrs. Rob appeared anxious and nervous. She said that she had slipped in the bathroom. Mrs. Rob became increasingly apprehensive and stiffened up in her chair when her daughter-in-law, Judy, came into the room asking when the next visit was. The nurse noticed that Judy avoided eye contact with Mrs. Rob.

When the injuries were brought to Judy's attention, she responded by becoming angry and agitated, blaming Mrs. Rob for causing so many problems. She would not explain the reason for the change in Mrs. Rob's behavior or the origin of the bruises to the nurse. She merely commented, "I have had to give up my job since my mother-in-law came here. It's been difficult and crowded ever since she moved in. The kids are complaining. We are having trouble making ends meet since I gave up my job. And my husband is no help at all."

ASSESSMENT

Ms. Green suspected that Mrs. Rob was experiencing mistreatment and spoke of the case with her team at the visiting nurse center. The nurse identified objective and subjective data that supported suspected elder mistreatment.

NURSE'S FEELINGS AND SELF-ASSESSMENT

Ms. Green has been in a number of situations with violent families, but this was the first time she encountered elder maltreatment. She discussed her reactions with the other team members. She was especially angry at Judy, although she was able to understand the daughter-in-law's frustration. The team concurred with Ms. Green that there seemed to be potential for positive change with this family. If abuse did not abate, more drastic measures would need to be taken and legal services contacted.

Objective Data

1. Physical symptoms of violence (i.e., bruises, unkempt appearance, withdrawn attitude)
2. Stressful, crowded living conditions
3. No eye contact between Mrs. Rob and her daughter-in-law
4. Economic hardships leading to stress
5. No support for the daughter-in-law from rest of family for care of Mrs. Rob
6. Mrs. Rob unable to make decisions

Subjective Data

1. Mrs. Rob states she "slipped in the bathroom," but physical findings do not support explanation.
2. Daughter-in-law states, "It's been difficult and crowded ever since she moved in."
3. Mrs. Rob exhibits withdrawn and apprehensive behavior.

NURSING DIAGNOSIS

On the basis of the data, the nurse formulated the following nursing diagnoses:

1. **Risk for injury** related to increase in family stress, as evidenced by signs of violence.

   ■ Mrs. Rob states she slipped in the bathroom, but physical findings do not support that explanation
   ■ Physical symptoms of violence present (bruises, unkempt appearance, withdrawn attitude)
   ■ Stressful, crowded living conditions

2. **Ineffective individual coping** related to helplessness, as evidenced by inability to meet role expectations.

   ■ Mrs. Rob appears unkempt, anxious, depressed
   ■ Mrs. Rob exhibits withdrawn and apprehensive behavior
   ■ Mrs. Rob is unable to make decisions

Case Study continued on following page

CASE STUDY 25–1   *Working With a Family Experiencing Violence* (Continued)

3. **Risk for violence** related to increased stressors within a short period, as evidenced by probable elder abuse and feelings of helplessness verbalized by primary caregiver.

   ■ Judy states, "It's been difficult and crowded ever since she moved in"
   ■ No eye contact between Judy and Mrs. Rob
   ■ Signs and symptoms of physical abuse on elder
   ■ "My husband is no help at all"

4. **Caregiver role strain** related to extreme feelings of being overwhelmed and of helplessness.

   ■ Family not helping with care of mother-in-law; burden of care on Judy
   ■ Economic hardships leading to stress when Judy gave up job to care for Mrs. Rob

OUTCOME CRITERIA

1. Client will be well nourished and free from signs of physical abuse by (date).
2. Client will have definite plans for alternatives to present living situation within 1 month.
3. Abuser will demonstrate control over her feelings by (date) and is not abusing Mrs. Rob.
4. Client and family members will meet together and discuss mutual expectations and actions they wish to share.
5. Family members will share the responsibility of caring for Mrs. Rob.

PLANNING

The nurse discusses several possible goals with members of her team, giving attention to the priority of goals and to whether they are realistic in this situation.

INTERVENTION

Violence toward elders is a signal of a family in crisis. Ms. Green knew she had to address the needs of the whole family to effect change within the family system. She focused on Mrs. Rob's physical safety first, then on Mrs. Rob's strengths to work within the family system. It was evident that Judy was overwhelmed with multiple stressors, and interventions for her and the rest of the family were vital for effective change.

Ms. Green continued to meet with the family on a weekly basis. Interventions were mapped out, with input from the family. Although it was difficult at first to get the husband involved, he became more active when his feelings of helpless-

ness and guilt began to fade. Ms. Green encouraged the children to participate, and many useful suggestions came from their observations and ideas.

This family seemed motivated to change their circumstances because all members were feeling overwhelmed and helpless. Although suggestions regarding outside services were initially met with some resistance, other services were contacted. Judy stated that she found weekly counseling a great help. The Friendly Visitors Service allowed Judy some time to herself each week. Refer to Nursing Care Plan 25–1 for specific interventions for this family.

EVALUATION

Eight weeks after the nurse's initial visit, Mrs. Rob appeared well groomed, friendly, and more spontaneous in her conversation. She commented, "Things are better

with my daughter-in-law." No bruises or other signs of physical violence were noticeable. She was considerably more outgoing and even took the initiative to con-

CASE STUDY 25–1 Working With a Family Experiencing Violence (Continued)

tact an old friend. She had talked openly with her son and daughter-in-law about stress in the family. Mrs. Rob said that she went out for a walk when her daughter-in-law, Judy, appeared tense, and returned to find the tension had lessened. Neither Mrs. Rob nor her family had initiated plans for alternative housing.

As a further result of the nurse's intervention, Judy was more in control of her emotions. Although she did on occasion yell at her mother-in-law, she felt this was no longer the same uncontrolled, explosive anger. Verbalizing her feelings to her husband helped alleviate her frustrations. Judy was seeing a counselor at the community center and was planning to look for a part-time job to "get out of the house."

The family members gradually began to communicate with one another. Mrs. Rob's other son and his family were contacted for assistance. Although this son had not yet offered to share some of the responsibility for taking care of his mother, he did agree to give some financial support. The family continued to meet with the nurse.

Visit the **Evolve** website at
http://evolve.elsevier.com/Varcarolis
for the other Nursing Care Plan diagnoses and for
more Nursing Care Plans.

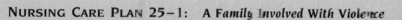

NURSING CARE PLAN 25–1: A Family Involved With Violence

NURSING DIAGNOSIS

Risk for injury: related to increase in family stress, as evidenced by signs of abuse

Supporting Data

- States that she slipped in the bathroom
- Physical symptoms of abuse (bruises, unkempt appearance, withdrawn attitude)
- Stressful, crowded living conditions

Outcome Criteria: Client will be well nourished and free from signs of physical abuse by (date).

SHORT-TERM GOAL	INTERVENTIONS	RATIONALE	EVALUATION
1. Client will state that abuse has decreased using a scale from 1–5 (1 being the least abuse) by (date)	1a. Follow state laws and guidelines for reporting elder abuse. 1b. Assess severity of signs and symptoms of abuse.	1a. Provide maximum protection under the law. Provide data for future use. 1b. Accurate charting (body map, pictures with permission, verbatim statements) helps follow progress and provides legal data.	1. Goal met, client states that after family talked to the nurse and planned strategies, physical abuse no longer occurs.

Nursing Care Plan continued on following page

NURSING CARE PLAN 25–1:   A *Family Involved With Violence* (Continued)

SHORT-TERM GOAL	INTERVENTIONS	RATIONALE	EVALUATION
	1c. Do a careful Home Assessment to identify other areas of abuse and neglect.	1c. Check food is adequate, presence of vermin, blocked stairways, medication safety, etc. All indicate abuse and neglect. Determine the kinds of problems in the home in order to plan intervention. Identify community resources that could help the elder and caregivers.	
	1d. Discuss with client factors leading to abuse and concern for safety.	1d. Identify family stressors and potential areas for intervention. Validates situation is serious and increases client's knowledge base.	
2. In 1 week client will name and have the telephone numbers or two people she can call in case of further abuse.	2. Discuss with client support services such as hotlines, and crisis units to call in case of emergency situations.	2. Maximizes client's safety through use of support systems.	2. Client has been talking to two old friends who she had stopped talking to because of shame and depression. She has called the hotline once to get information on transportation to the senior center in town.
3. Within 1 week, family and nurse will identify four interventions that could help decrease family stress and feelings of helplessness.	3a. Discuss with family members their feelings and identify at least four areas that are the most difficult for the various family members.	3a. Listening to each family member and identifying unmet needs, helps family as well as nurse identify areas that require changing and interventions.	3. Over time, the nurse and family have identified several areas where community intervention will help.

NURSING CARE PLAN 25–1: A Family Involved With Violence *(Continued)*

SHORT-TERM GOAL	INTERVENTIONS	RATIONALE	EVALUATION
	3b. Identify potential community supports, skills training, respite places, homemakers, financial aids etc. that might help meet family's unmet needs.	3b. When stressed, individuals solve problems poorly, and do not know about or cannot manage to organize outside help. Finances are often a problem.	The daughter-in-law was glad to get out of the house for anger-management classes, and the son stated he would try to take on more responsibility, but he often felt guilty and angry, too. Reluctantly he and his wife agreed to try a support group with other caregivers in similar situations.

SUMMARY

Family violence occurs across all age groups and can be predicted with some accuracy by examining the characteristics of perpetrators, vulnerable people, and situations in which violence is likely. Maltreatment can be physical, sexual, emotional, economic, or caused by neglect. Assessment includes identifying indicators of mistreatment, levels of anxiety, coping mechanisms, support systems, and suicide and homicide potential as well as alcohol and drug abuse.

Visit the **Evolve** website at
http://evolve.elsevier.com/Varcarolis
for a post-test on the content in this chapter.

Visit the **Evolve** website at
http://evolve.elsevier.com/Varcarolis
for additional self-study exercises.

Critical Thinking and Chapter Review

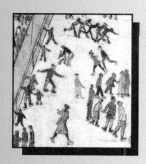

Critical Thinking

1. How would you respond to a colleague who has witnessed a child being abused and stated, "I don't think it's any of our business what people do in the privacy of their own homes"? What would you do? Legally? Ethically?
2. Congratulations! You successfully convinced your colleagues to routinely assess for family violence. Now they want to know how to do it. How would you go about teaching them to assess for child abuse? Spouse abuse? Elder abuse?
3. Your HMO's routine health screening form for adolescents, adults, and elders has just been changed to include questions about family violence. How would

716 **UNIT VI ■** *Psychiatric Emergencies*

you respond to patients who indicate on this form that family violence occurs in their home?

4. Write out a safety plan that could be adopted with other clients.
5. Identify at least four referrals in your community for a battered person.
6. Identify two referrals in your community for a violent person, partner, or parent.

Chapter Review

1. Identifying people at high risk and providing health teaching about recognizing behaviors and situations that might trigger violence are examples of

   1. primary intervention
   2. secondary intervention
   3. tertiary intervention
   4. nonintervention

2. Which example of thinking is not a myth that would keep a woman locked into an abusive relationship?

   1. "If I'm patient, he'll change."
   2. "I deserved to be beaten."
   3. "I'll stay for the sake of the children."
   4. "No adult has the right to control or harm another."

3. When making assessments the nurse should bear in mind that a common characteristic of an abusing parent is

   1. being a female
   2. having poor coping skills
   3. having realistic expectations of child behavior
   4. abstaining from use of chemical substances of abuse

4. A "red flag" for suspected physical violence during assessment of a client is

   1. client explanation does not match the injury
   2. client has no history of stress-related physical problems
   3. client mentions having a concerned, supportive spouse
   4. client is anxious but open and direct explaining complaint/injury

5. Which nursing diagnosis should be considered for the Jones family? The husband is disabled, unable to work, drinks episodically, and abuses the two preschool children at these times. The wife works outside the home.

   1. powerlessness
   2. caretaker role strain
   3. self-esteem disturbances
   4. ineffective family coping: disabling

NURSE, CLIENT, AND FAMILY RESOURCES

Associations

Family Violence Sexual Assault Institute (FUSAI)
1300 Clinic Drive
Tyler, TX 75701
1-903-595-6600 (voice); 1-904-595-6799 (fax)

National Domestic Violence Hotline (NDV Hotline)
3616 Far West Boulevard, Suite 101-297
Austin, TX 78731-3074
1-800-799-SAFE (Hotline)

Batterers Anonymous
8485 Tamarind #D
Fontane, CA 92335
1-909-355-1100
(For men who wish to control their anger and eliminate their abusive behavior)

Child Abuse Prevention—Kids Peace
1-800-257-3223

Child Help USA Hotline
1-800-422-4453 (24 hours)

Youth Crisis Hotline
1-800-HIT-HOME

Runaway Hotline
1-800-231-6946

Internet Sites

National Coalition Against Domestic Violence
http://www.ncadv.org

National Clearinghouse Child Abuse and Neglect Information
1-800-394-3366
http://www.calib.com/nccanch

Prevent Child Abuse America Home Page
http://www.childabuse.org

Child Abuse Prevention Network
http://child.cornell.edu

Victim Services Domestic Violence Shelter Tour
http://www.dvsheltertour.org

David Baldwin's Trauma Information Page
http://www.trauma-pages.com/
Site focuses on emotional trauma and traumatic stress

National Committee to Prevent Child Abuse
200 Michigan Avenue
17th Floor
Chicago, IL 60604
312/663-3520
http://www.childabuse.org

American Academy of Pediatrics
http://www.aap.org

SAVE: Stop America's Violence Everywhere
AMA Alliance
http://www.ama-assn.org/ad-com/alliance/shelter/shelter.htm

Especially for Men

Men Who Have Experienced Sexual Abuse (NOMSV)
http://www.malesurvivor.org/

Men's Rape Prevention Project
http://www.mrpp.org
(Helping men who rape)

REFERENCES

Beauchesne, M. A., et al. (1997) Violence prevention: a community approach. *Journal of Pediatric Health Care*, 11(4):155.

Brandl B., and Raymond, J. (1997). Unrecognized elder abuse victims. *Journal of Case Management*, 6(2):62.

Campbell, J. C., and Campbell, D. W. (1996). Cultural competence in the care of abused women. *Journal of Midwifery*, 41(6):457.

Campbell, J. C. (1995). Prediction of homicide of and by battered women. In J. C. Campbell (Ed.), *Assessing dangerousness*. Thousand Oaks, CA: Sage.

Campbell, D., and Campbell, J. (1993). Nursing care of families using violence. In J. C. Campbell and J. Humphreys (Eds.), *Nursing care of survivors of family violence* (2nd ed.) (p. 290). St. Louis: C. V. Mosby.

Capezuti, E. et al. (1997). Reporting elder mistreatment. *Journal of Gerontological Nursing*, 23(7):24.

Carlson-Catalano, J. (1998). Nursing diagnoses and interventions for post–acute-phase battered women. *Nursing Diagnosis*, 9(3):101.

Chiocca, E. M. (1998). The nurse's role in the prevention of child abuse and neglect: Part II. *Journal of Pediatric Nursing*, 13(3):194.

Creedy, D., Nizette, D., Henderson, K. (1998). A framework for practice with women survivors of childhood sexual abuse. *Australian/New Zealand Journal of Mental Health Nursing*, 7(2):67–73.

Davis, R. E. (2000). Cultural health care of child abuse: The Southeast Asian practice of cao gio. *Journal of American Academy of Nurse Practitioners*, 12(3):89–95.

Davidhizer, R., et al. (1997). Elder abuse: The American experience. Part 2. *Elderly Care*, 9(5):9.

DiScala, C. (2000). Child abuse and unintentional injuries: A 10-year retrospective. *Archives of Pediatric and Adolescent Medicine*, 154(1):16.

Ellis, J. M. (1999). Barriers to effective screening for domestic violence by registered nurses in the emergency department. *Critical Care Nursing Quarterly*, 22(1):27.

Fishwick, N. J. (1998). Assessment of women for partner abuse. *Neonatal Nursing*, 27(6):661.

Garber, A., et al. (1997). Assessing for sexual abuse. *Journal of Psychosocial Nursing and Mental Health Services*, 35(3):26.

Hattendorf, J., and Tollerud, T. R. (1997). Domestic violence-counseling strategies that minimize the impact of secondary victimization. *Perspectives in Psychiatric Care*, 33(1):14.

Heritage, C. (1998). Working with childhood sexual abuse survivors during pregnancy, labor, and birth. *Journal of Obstetrics, Gynecological and Neonatal Nursing*, 27(6):671.

Hilbert, J. C. and Krishnan, S. P. (2000). Addressing barriers to community care of battered women in rural environments: Creating a policy of social inclusion. *Journal of Health and Social Policy*, 12(1):41–52.

Hoff, B. H. (1999). Why women assault: Review of Fiebert and Gonzalez, College women who initiate assaults on their male partners and the reasons offered for such behavior. *MenWeb on-line Journal* (ISSN: 1095-5240 http:www.vix.com/menmag/fiebert3.htm) January 1, 1999.

Hogstel, M. O., and Curry, L. C. (1999). Elder abuse revisited. *Journal of Gerontological Nursing*, 25(7):10.

Holmes, W. C., Slap, G. B. (1998) Sexual abuse of boys: definitions, prevalence, correlates, sequelae, and management. *Journal of the American Medical Association* 280(21):1855–1862.

Horsfall, J. (1997) Women's depression: nursing theory and practice. *Contemporary Nurse*, 6(3/4)–129.

Johnson, M., Mass, M., Moorehead, S. (2000). *Iowa outcomes project: Nursing outcomes classification (NOC)*. St. Louis: Mosby.

Landenburger, K. M. (1998). The dynamics of leaving and recovering from an abusive relationship. *Journal of Obstetrics, Gynecological and Neonatal Nursing*, 27(6):700.

Lawson, L. (1998). Milieu management of traumatic youngsters. *Journal of Child and Adolescent Psychiatric Nursing*, 11(3):99.

Mayer, B. (1998). Dilemmas in mandatory reporting of domestic violence: carative ethics in emergency rooms. *Nursing Connections*, 11(4):5–21.

Monk, M. (1998). Interviewing suspected victims of child maltreatment in the emergency department. *Journal of Emergency Nursing,* 24(1):31.

Moore, M. L. (1998). Attitudes and practices of registered nurses toward women who have experienced abuse/domestic violence. *Journal of Obstetrics, Gynecological and Neonatal Nursing,* 27(2):175.

Parker, B., et al. (1999). Testing an intervention to prevent further abuse to pregnant women. *Research in Nursing and Health,* 22(1): 59.

Reece, R. M., and Sege, R. (2000). Childhood head injuries: accidental or inflicted? *Archives of Pediatric and Adolescent Medicine,* 154(1):11.

Smart, J. D. (1999). Public health nursing in children's protective services. *Public Health Nursing,* 16(6):390.

Spicknell, K. (1998). Shaking babies. *Nursing Times,* 94(12):34.

Tatara, T. (1997). *Summaries of the statistical data on elder abuse in domestic settings for FY 95 and FY 96.* Washington, DC: National Center on Elder Abuse.

Thobaben, M. (1996). Elder abuse and neglect. *Home care provider,* 1(5):267.

Tjaden, P. G., and Thoennes, N. (1998). *Prevalence, Incidence and Consequences of Violence Against Women: Findings from the National Violence Against Women Survey,* U.S. Department of Justice, National Institute of Justice and Centers for Diseases Control and Prevention Research in Brief series, November, 1998, NCJ 172837.

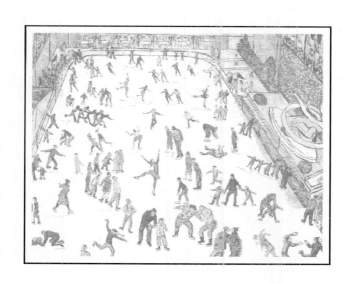

Outline

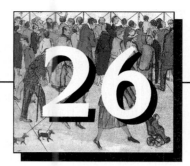

26

Sexual Assault

KATHLEEN SMITH-DIJULIO

Key Terms and Concepts

The key terms and concepts listed here also appear in color where they are first defined or discussed in this chapter.

acquaintance/date rape

acute phase

blame

compound reaction

controlled style of coping

expressed style of coping

long-term reorganization phase

rape-trauma syndrome

silent reaction

spousal/marital rape

Objectives

After studying this chapter, the reader will be able to

1. Define sexual assault (rape).

2. Discuss the reasons that rapes go unreported.

3. Distinguish between the acute and long-term phases of the rape-trauma syndrome and identify some common reactions during each phase.

4. Identify and give examples of five areas to assess when working with a person who has been sexually assaulted.

5. Formulate two long-term and two short-term outcomes for the nursing diagnosis **Rape-trauma syndrome.**

6. Analyze your thoughts and feelings regarding the myths about rape and its impact on survivors.

7. Identify six overall guidelines for nursing interventions.

8. Describe the role of the sexual assault nurse examiner to a colleague.

9. Discuss the responsibilities of the nurse when a rape survivor is discharged from the emergency department, citing specific referrals from your community.

10. Develop a handout delineating the nurse's role when staffing a rape-crisis hotline.

11. Discuss the long-term psychological effects of sexual assault that might lead to a survivor's seeking psychotherapy.

12. Identify three outcome criteria that would signify successful interventions for a person who has suffered a sexual assault.

*S*exual assault (rape) is an act of violence, and sex is the weapon used by the perpetrator. Rape engulfs its victims in fear, causing severe panic reactions. After being traumatized, the person raped often carries an additional burden of shame, guilt, fear, anger, distrust, and embarrassment.

Rape, often referred to as **sexual assault,** is nonconsensual vaginal, anal, or oral penetration, obtained by force, by threat of bodily harm, or when a person is incapable of giving consent. It is usually men who rape, and most of those raped are women. However, the percentage of sexual assaults occurring in men who present to an emergency room (ER) is now more than 10% (Pesola, Westfal, and Kuffner 1999). When men are raped, the rape is generally perpetrated by a heterosexual male.

A male who is raped is more likely to have physical trauma and to have been victimized by several assailants than is a female. Reported homosexual rape occurs primarily in closed institutions, such as prisons and maximum-security hospitals. The psychodynamics are the same as those of heterosexual rape, and males experience the same devastation and sequelae as do females.

According to recent national studies, 1 in 6 women and 1 in 33 men will experience an attempted or completed rape during their lifetime (Linden 1999). Since women are more frequently assaulted sexually, this chapter uses the female pronoun throughout; however, the principles discussed apply to anyone who is raped.

THEORY

Stranger rape is what most people envisage when they think of sexual assault, yet this is the least common type. Notable subtypes that occur much more frequently are spousal/marital rape and acquaintance/date rape. In recent years the courts have recognized spousal/marital rape, in which the perpetrator (nearly always the male) is married to the person raped. With acquaintance/date rape, the perpetrator is known to, and presumably trusted by, the person raped. The incidence of rape peaks among females 16 to 19 years of age. Nonetheless, many thousands of women over 50 years of age are raped every year. The psychological and emotional sequelae of rape seem to vary depending on the level of intimacy of the perpetrator. Sexual distress is more common among women who have been sexually assaulted by intimates; fear and anxiety are more common in those assaulted by strangers; depression occurs in both groups.

There is a growing awareness of spousal rape in the United States. Feminists have done a great deal to raise the consciousness of individuals and of American society as a whole to the fact that women are people, not property, and should be accorded the same rights and privileges as men. This change is evidenced in laws such as those that allow a wife to bring rape charges against her husband. Formerly it was believed that a man was entitled to sex in a relationship, no matter how he obtained it.

Date/acquaintance rape has increased in the United States in recent years with drugs, often combined with alcohol, used to commit sexual assault. Gamma-hydroxybutyrate, flunitrazepam, and ketamine are purported to facilitate acquaintance rape (Smith 1999). Often these drugs are slipped unknowingly to the victim (e.g., "the new Mickey Finn"). Once ingested, victims lose their ability to ward off attackers, develop amnesia, and are unreliable witnesses. Since the symptoms mimic alcohol, victims are not always screened for these drugs (Smith 1999). Legislative efforts at the state and federal levels have been initiated to limit the use of and access to these drugs.

Most people who are raped suffer severe and long-lasting emotional trauma. Long-term psychological effects of sexual assault may include the development of depression, suicide, anxiety, and fear; difficulties with daily functioning; low self-esteem; sexual dysfunction; and somatic complaints. Incest victims may experience a negative self-image, depression, eating disorders, personality disorders, self-destructive behavior, and substance abuse. Timely intervention can greatly help to minimize the devastating sequelae of rape. A history of sexual abuse in psychiatric clients is associated with a characteristic pattern of symptoms that may include depression, anxiety disorders, chemical dependency, suicide attempts, self-mutilation, compulsive sexual behavior, and psychotic-like symptoms.

The **rape-trauma syndrome** is a variant of posttraumatic stress disorder and consists of (1) an acute phase and (2) the long-term reorganization process that occurs after an actual or attempted sexual assault. Each phase has separate symptoms. Refer to Chapter 14 for more on posttraumatic stress disorder (PTSD).

Acute Phase of Rape-Trauma Syndrome

The **acute phase** of the rape-trauma syndrome occurs immediately after the assault and may last for a couple of weeks. This is the stage seen by emergency department personnel. Nurses are the clinicians most involved in dealing with these initial reactions. During this phase, there is a great deal of

TABLE 26-1   *Acute Phase of Rape-Trauma Syndrome*

IMPACT REACTION	SOMATIC REACTION	EMOTIONAL REACTION
Expressed Style Overt behaviors ■ Crying, sobbing ■ Smiling, laughing, joking ■ Restlessness, agitation, hysteria ■ Volatility, anger ■ Confusion, incoherence, disorientation ■ Tenseness **Controlled Style** Covert reactions ■ Confusion, incoherence, disorientation ■ Masked facies ■ Calm, subdued appearance ■ Shocked, numb, confused, disbelieving appearance ■ Distractibility, difficulty making decisions	Evidenced within first several weeks after a rape **Physical Trauma** ■ Bruises (breasts, throat, or back) ■ Soreness **Skeletal Muscle Tension** ■ Headaches ■ Sleep disturbances ■ Grimaces, twitches **Gastrointestinal** ■ Stomach pains ■ Nausea ■ Poor appetite ■ Diarrhea **Genitourinary** ■ Vaginal itching ■ Vaginal discharge ■ Pain or discomfort	■ Fear of physical violence and death ■ Denial ■ Anxiety ■ Shock ■ Humiliation ■ Fatigue ■ Embarrassment ■ Desire for revenge ■ Self-blame ■ Lowered self-esteem ■ Shame ■ Guilt ■ Anger

Data from Burgess A. W. (1995). Rape trauma syndrome: A nursing diagnosis. *Occupational Health Nursing*, 33(8):405; and Burgess, A. W., and Holstrom, L. L. (1974). The rape victim in the ER. *American Journal of Nursing*, 73(10):1740.

disorganization in the person's life style, and somatic symptoms are common. This disorganization can be described in terms of impact reactions, somatic reactions, and emotional reactions (Table 26–1).

The most common initial reaction is shock, numbness, and disbelief. Outwardly, the person may appear self-contained and calm and may make remarks such as "It doesn't seem real" or "I don't believe this really happened to me." Sometimes, cognitive functions may be impaired, and the traumatized person may appear extremely confused and have difficulty with concentrating and decision making. Alternatively, the person may become hysterical or restless, or may cry or even smile. These reactions to crisis are typical and reflect cognitive, affective, and behavioral disruptions.

People who have experienced an emotionally overwhelming event may need to deny its impact. Examples of such denial may be found in statements such as "I don't want to talk about it" or "I just want to forget what happened." Behaviors that minimize the magnitude of the event include reluctance to seek medical attention and failure to follow up with legal counsel.

Long-Term Reorganization Phase of Rape-Trauma Syndrome

The long-term reorganization phase of rape-trauma syndrome occurs two or more weeks after the rape.

Nurses who initially care for the survivors can help them anticipate and prepare for the reactions they are likely to experience. These include the following:

■ **Intrusive thoughts** of the rape break into the survivor's conscious mind during the day and during sleep. These thoughts commonly include anger and violence toward the assailant, flashbacks (re-experiencing the traumatic event), dreams with violent content, and insomnia.

■ **Increased motor activity** follows, such as moving, taking trips, changing telephone numbers, and making frequent visits to old friends. This activity stems from the fear that the assailant will return. Anxiety, mood swings, crying spells, and depression are likely to be observed.

■ **Fears and phobias** develop as a defensive reaction to the rape. Typical phobias include
Fear of the indoors (if the rape occurred indoors).
Fear of the outdoors (if the rape occurred outdoors).
Fear of being alone (common for most women after an assault).
Fear of crowds—"Any person in the crowd might be a rapist."
Fear of sexual encounters and activities. Many women experience acute disruption of their sex life with partners. Rape is especially disruptive for those with no previous sexual experience.

As mentioned, the consequences of sexual assault may be severe, debilitating, and long term. Intervention and support for the survivor can help prevent some of the sequelae mentioned: anxiety, depression, suicide, difficulties with daily functioning and interpersonal relationships, sexual dysfunction, and somatic complaints.

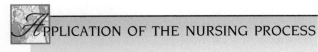

APPLICATION OF THE NURSING PROCESS

ASSESSMENT

Once the rape survivor is at the emergency department, the attention received depends on the protocol of the particular hospital. Ledray and Arndt (1994) suggest the following interventions:

■ Treatment and documentation of injuries
■ Treatment and evaluation of sexually transmitted diseases (STDs)
■ Pregnancy risk evaluation and prevention
■ Crisis intervention and arrangements for follow-up counseling
■ Collection of medicolegal evidence while maintaining the proper chain of evidence

The nurse talks with the survivor, the family or friends who accompany the survivor, and the police to gather as much data as possible for assessing the crisis. The nurse then assesses the survivor's (1) level of anxiety, (2) coping mechanisms used, (3) available support systems, (4) signs and symptoms of emotional trauma, and (5) signs and symptoms of physical trauma. Information obtained from the assessment is then analyzed, and nursing diagnoses are formulated. The independent nursing role of sexual assault nurse examiner or forensic nurse specialist successfully accomplishes all of these activities (Ledray 1998).

Overall Assessment

ASSESSING THE LEVEL OF ANXIETY

A client who is experiencing severe to panic levels of anxiety will not be able to problem-solve or process information. The nurse uses approaches that can lower the client's anxiety so that mutual goals can be set and information can be assimilated. Support, reassurance, and appropriate therapeutic techniques can help diminish anxiety. Refer to Chapters 12 and 13 for more discussion on levels of anxiety and therapeutic interventions.

ASSESSING COPING MECHANISMS USED

The same coping skills that have helped the survivor through other difficult problems will be used in adjusting to the rape. In addition, new ways of getting through the difficult times may be developed, for both the short- and long-term adjustment.

Behavioral responses include crying; withdrawing; smoking; wanting to talk about the event; acting hysterical, confused, disoriented, or incoherent; or even laughing or joking. These behaviors are examples of an expressed style of coping (see Table 26–1).

Cognitive coping mechanisms are the thoughts people have that help them deal with high anxiety levels. If thoughts are verbalized, the nurse will know what the survivor is thinking. If not, the nurse can ask questions, such as "What do you think might help?" or "What can I do to help you in this difficult situation?"

ASSESSING SUPPORT SYSTEMS AVAILABLE

The availability, size, and usefulness of a survivor's social support system need to be assessed. Often partners or family members do not understand the survivor's feelings about the sexual assault, and they may not be the best supports available. Pay careful attention to verbal and nonverbal cues of the survivor that may communicate the strength of her social network.

Vignette

■ Ms. Ruiz, age 18, is brought to the emergency department by a concerned neighbor. She was found wandering aimlessly outside her house, sobbing, and muttering "He had no right to do that to me." Because of Ms. Ruiz's distraught appearance and her statement, the triage nurse suspects sexual assault and brings the victim to the office of the psychiatric nurse, Ms. Wong. Ms. Wong introduces herself, explains her role, and states that she is there to help. Ms. Wong then asks Ms. Ruiz what happened. After careful, sensitive, nonthreatening questioning, Ms. Ruiz divulges that she had been out with her boyfriend, who took her to a "rave" party and then raped her. She got a ride back home but no one else was at home. She was so upset and afraid, she did not go inside, and the neighbor, Ms. Green, had seen her outside.

After the entire history and examination are completed, plans for discharge are discussed. Ms. Ruiz states that no one will be home until Sunday night, two days away, and that she does not feel comfortable calling any friends because she does not want them to know what has happened. The neighbor, Ms. Green, had told the nurse earlier that Ms. Ruiz could stay with her family.

Nurse: Earlier, your neighbor, Ms. Green, told me that you are welcome to spend the weekend with her family.

Ms. Ruiz: *(Loudly, sharply, with eyes wide)* Oh, no, I couldn't do that.

Nurse: You don't seem to like that idea.

Ms. Ruiz: Oh, I just wouldn't want to bother them.

Nurse: Ms. Green seems quite concerned about your welfare.

Ms. Ruiz: Oh, yes, she's very nice. *(Pause)*

Nurse: But not someone you would want to spend the weekend with?

Ms. Ruiz: Her children are too noisy. I've got homework to do.

Nurse: You might not get the quiet you need to study. *(Pause)* Yet you also do not want to be alone?

Ms. Ruiz: *(Wringing a tissue in her hands, head hanging, soft voice)* I can't go in that house anymore.

Nurse: Something about being in that house disturbs you?

Ms. Ruiz: Mr. Green *(deep sigh, pause)* used to . . . uh . . . take advantage of me when I used to babysit his children.

Nurse: Take advantage?

Ms. Ruiz: Yes . . . *(sobbing)* he used to force me to have sex with him. He said he'd blame it on me if I told anyone.

Nurse: What a frightening experience that must have been for you.

Ms. Ruiz: Yes.

Nurse: I can see why you would not want to spend the night there. Let's continue to explore other options

A suitable place to stay is finally arranged. Ms. Ruiz is given counseling referrals that will help her deal with the process of reorganization after the current rape experience as well as begin to explore her feelings about past sexual abuse she has suffered at the hands of her neighbor.

ASSESSING SIGNS AND SYMPTOMS OF EMOTIONAL TRAUMA

Nurses work most frequently with sexual assault survivors in the emergency department soon after the rape has occurred. Rape is a psychological emergency and should receive immediate attention. Some emergency departments provide the services of sexual assault nurse examiners or clinician who are specially trained to meet the myriad needs of the sexual assault survivor (Cornell 1998).

The extent of the psychological and emotional trauma sustained may not be readily apparent from behavior, especially if the person uses the controlled style of coping during the acute phase of the rape trauma (see Table 26–1).

A nursing history should be conducted and properly recorded. When obtaining a history, the nurse needs to determine only the details of the assault that will be helpful in addressing the immediate physical and psychological needs of the victim. Allow the survivor to talk at a comfortable pace. Pose questions in nonjudgmental, descriptive terms. Refrain from asking "why" questions. Relating the events of the rape will most likely be traumatic and embarrassing.

If suicidal thoughts are expressed, the nurse should assess what precautions are needed by asking direct questions, such as "Are you thinking of harming yourself?" and "Have you ever tried to kill yourself before this attack occurred?" If the answer is yes, the nurse must make a thorough suicide assessment (plan, means to carry it out) as described in Chapter 23.

ASSESSING SIGNS AND SYMPTOMS OF PHYSICAL TRAUMA

Practitioners must provide psychological support while collecting and preserving potentially crucial legal evidence such as hair, skin, and semen samples. The most characteristic physical signs of sexual assault are injuries to the face, head, neck, and extremities. Any noted injuries should be carefully documented, preferably on a body map (Girardin 1997).

The nurse takes a brief gynecological history, including date of last menstrual period, the likelihood of current pregnancy, and any history of venereal disease. If the survivor has never undergone a pelvic examination, the steps will need to be explained. The nurse plays a crucial role in giving support and minimizing the trauma of the examination. The survivor may feel that it is another violation to her body Recognizing this, the nurse can explain the examination procedure in a way that will be reassuring and supportive. Allowing the survivor to participate in all decisions affecting care helps her regain a sense of control over her life.

The survivor has the right to refuse either a legal or a medical examination. **Consent forms must be signed for photographs, pelvic examination, and whatever other procedures might be needed to collect evidence and provide treatment.** The correct preservation of body fluids and swabs is essential because DNA (genetic) fingerprinting may identify the rapist. A shower and fresh clothing should be available to the survivor immediately after the examination, if possible.

It is a common practice to treat prophylactically for syphilis, chlamydiosis, and gonorrhea, according to guidelines from the Centers for Disease Control and Prevention.

Human immunodeficiency virus (HIV) exposure is an ever-growing concern of sexual assault survivors. The concern should always be addressed and the rape survivor given the information needed to evaluate the likely risk. With this information the person and her sexual partner(s) can make educated choices about HIV testing and safer-sex practices until testing can be done.

About 3% to 5% of women who are raped become pregnant as a result. Pregnancy prophylaxis can be offered in the emergency department or at follow-up, after the results of the pregnancy test are obtained.

All data must be carefully documented, including verbatim statements by the survivor, detailed observations of emotional and physical status, and all results from the physical examination. All laboratory tests performed should be noted and findings recorded as soon as they are available. The Emergency Nurses Association (1998) has a position statement on forensic evidence collection.

Self-Assessment

Nurses' attitudes influence the physical and psychological care administered to rape survivors. Knowing the myths and facts surrounding sexual assault can increase nurses' awareness of their personal beliefs and feelings regarding rape. Nurses who examine their personal feelings and reactions before encountering a rape survivor are better prepared to give empathetic and effective care. Nurses must also examine their feelings about abortion because a client might choose to abort a fetus produced as a result of rape. It is the patient's choice and if an individual nurse is too conflicted to work with the patient, she should switch duties with another nurse. It is better to ask for help with a client than to make the client uncomfortable. The process is the same as that described for caring for survivors of other types of violence (see Chapter 25). Table 26–2 compares rape myths and facts.

TABLE 26–2   *Myth vs. Fact: Rape*

MYTH	FACT
1. Many women really want to be raped.	1. Women do not ask to be raped—no matter how they are dressed, what their behavior is, or where they are at any given time. Studies show that violence toward women in the media leads to attitudes that foster tolerance of rape.
2. Most rapists are oversexed.	2. Sex is used as an instrument of violence in rape. Rape is an act of aggression, anger, or power.
3. Most women are raped by strangers.	3. The majority (57%) of rape victims are raped by someone they know and who is a part of their extended family.
4. No healthy adult female who resists vigorously can be raped by an unarmed man.	4. Most men can overpower most women because of differences in body build. Also, the victim may panic, making her actions less effective than usual.
5. Most charges of rape are unfounded.	5. There is no evidence to show that there are more false reports for rape than for other crimes. Most rape victims do not even report the rape.
6. Rapes usually occur in dark alleys.	6. Over 50% of all rapes occur in the home.
7. Rape is usually an impulsive act.	7. Most rapes are planned; over 50% involve a weapon.
8. Nice girls don't get raped.	8. Any woman is a potential rape victim. Victims range in age from 6 months to 90 years.
9. There was not enough time for a rape to occur.	9. There is no minimal time limit that characterizes rape. It can happen very quickly.
10. Do not fight or try to get away because you will just get hurt.	10. There are no verifiable data to substantiate the theory that a victim will be injured if she tries to get away.
11. Only females are raped.	11. There is a growing number of male rape victims—not necessarily just men in prisons or in the homosexual community.
12. Rape is a sexual act.	12. Rape is a violent expression of aggression, anger, and need for power.

ASSESSMENT GUIDELINES: SEXUAL ASSAULT

1. Assess physical trauma. Use a body map and ask permission to take photos.
2. Assess psychological trauma. Write down verbatim statements of client.
3. Assess available support system. Often partners or family members do not understand the trauma of rape, and they may not be the best supports to rally at this time.
4. Assess level of anxiety. If clients are in severe to panic levels of anxiety, they will not be able to problem-solve or process information.
5. Identify community supports (e.g., attorneys, support groups, therapists that work in the area of sexual assault.
6. Encourage clients to tell their story. *Do not* press them to.

NURSING DIAGNOSIS

Rape-trauma syndrome is the nursing diagnosis that applies to the physical and psychological effects resulting from an episode of sexual assault. It includes an acute phase of disorganization of the survivor's life style and a long-term phase of reorganization.

RAPE-TRAUMA SYNDROME: COMPOUND REACTION. Compound reaction includes

- All symptoms listed under rape-trauma syndrome (see Table 26–1)
- Reliance on alcohol or other drugs
- Reactivated symptoms of previous conditions, such as physical or psychiatric illness

RAPE-TRAUMA SYNDROME: SILENT REACTION. Silent reaction is a complex stress reaction to rape, in which an individual is unable to describe or discuss the rape. Symptoms include

- Abrupt changes in relationships with men
- Nightmares
- Increasing anxiety during the interview, such as blocking of associations, long periods of silence, minor stuttering, or physical distress
- Marked changes in sexual behavior
- Sudden onset of phobic reactions
- No verbalization of the occurrence of rape

OUTCOME CRITERIA

Long-term outcome includes the absence of any residual symptoms after the trauma.

Examples of short-term goals are as follows:
Rape-trauma syndrome: acute phase. The survivor will

- Begin to express reactions and feelings about the assault before leaving the emergency room.
- Have a short-term plan for handling immediate situational needs.
- List common physical, social, and emotional reactions that often follow a sexual assault before she leaves the emergency department.
- Speak to a community-based rape-victim advocate in the emergency department.
- State the results of the physical examination completed in the emergency department.
- State that she will keep a follow-up appointment with the nurse, rape-victim advocate, or social worker on (date).

Examples of long-term goals are as follows:
Rape-trauma syndrome: long-term reorganization phase. The survivor will

- Discuss the need for follow-up crisis counseling and other support by (date).
- State that the acuteness of the memory of the rape subsides over time and is less vivid and less frightening within 3 to 5 months.
- State that the physical symptoms (e.g., sleep disturbances, poor appetite, and physical trauma) have subsided within 3 to 5 months.

PLANNING/INTERVENTION

The circumstance of rape can be the most devastating experience in a person's life and constitutes an acute adventitious crisis. Typical crisis reactions reflect cognitive, affective, and behavioral disruptions. For survivors to return to their previous level of functioning, it is necessary for them to fully mourn their losses, experience anger, and work through their terrifying fears. Table 26–3 provides overall guidelines for planning interventions.

Communication Guidelines

The rape survivor may be too traumatized, ashamed, or afraid to come to the hospital. Cultural definitions of what constitutes rape may also affect the decision to seek treatment. For these reasons, most communities provide telephone hotlines on a 24-hour basis. The most effective approach for counseling in the emergency department or crisis center is to provide nonjudgmental care as well as optimal emotional support. Displays of shock, horror, disgust, surprise, or disbelief are not appropriate. Confidentiality is crucial. The most helpful things the nurse can do are to listen and let the survivor talk. A woman who feels understood is no longer alone; she then feels more in control of her situation.

TABLE 26–3 *Overall Guidelines for Nursing Interventions*

INTERVENTION	RATIONALE
1. Follow your institution's protocol for sexual assault.	1. Protocols set standard procedures for safe and effective treatment guidelines
2. Do not leave the person alone.	2. Prevents increase in isolation and escalation of anxiety.
3. Maintain a nonjudgmental attitude.	3. Decreases emotional burden.
4. Provide nonjudgmental care.	4. Lessens feelings of shame and embarrassment.
5. Ensure confidentiality.	5. Encourages sharing the event and protects a person's self-concept and sense of control.
6. Encourage the person to talk through empathetic listening.	6. Helps the person sort out thoughts and feelings. Anxiety is lowered by reducing feelings of isolation.
7. Keep accurate records of ■ Physical trauma ■ Verbatim statements ■ Photos (need the person's permission)	7. Can be used in a court of law for her defense.
8. Obtain medico-legal specimens with client's written permission	8. Specimens and DNA testing increases likelihood of identifying perpetrator.
9. Engage the support system (e.g., family and friends) when appropriate.	9. Provides warmth and feelings of safety when shock wears off and the acute disorganization phase begins. The focus should remain on returning the victim to psychological well-being.
10. Emphasize that the person did the right thing to save her life.	10. Helps reduce guilt and maintain self-esteem.
11. Arrange for support follow-up.	11. Acknowledges that healing takes time.

It is especially important to help the survivor and her significant others separate issues of vulnerability from **blame.** Although the person may have made choices that made her more vulnerable, she is not to blame for the rape, no matter what she did. She may, however, decide to avoid some of those choices in the future (e.g., walking alone late at night or excessive use of alcohol). Focusing on one's behavior (which is controllable) allows the survivor to believe that similar experiences can be avoided in the future.

Vignette

■ *Mary has come to see that it was not her fault that she was raped. However, she is now adamant about not walking from the bus stop alone late at night, and from now on will take a cab, get a lift from a friend, or take a safer alternative route when going home.*

If the survivor consents, involve her support system (e.g., family or friends) and discuss with them the nature and trauma of sexual assault and possible delayed reactions that may occur. One survivor expressed it this way:

It takes a few days to hit you. It was bad. It was really rough for my husband. I needed to be reassured. I needed to be told that there was nothing I could do to prevent it. Understanding helps.

Social support effectively moderates somatic symptoms and subjective health ratings. The survivor who is able to confide comfortably in one or two friends or family members, especially immediately after the assault, is likely to experience fewer somatic manifestations of stress. Family and friends may need support and reassurance as much as the survivor does. This is especially true for those from traditional cultures. The long-standing cultural myth that women are the property of men still prevents some people from empathizing with the woman's severe psychic injury and from being supportive. She is, instead, often thought of as devalued.

Self-Care Activities

When preparing the survivor to go home, give all referral information and follow-up instructions in writing, detailing likely physical concerns and emotional reactions, legal matters, victim compensation, and ways that family and friends can help. This is important, since the amount of verbal information the patient can retain will likely be limited owing to anxiety. Written material can be referred to repeatedly over time. Legal referrals (i.e., names of attorneys who specialize in rape cases and options for low-cost legal assistance) can also be given.

Case Management

Caring for the survivor is not completed in a single visit. Her emotional state and other psychological needs should be reassessed by phone or personal contact within 24 to 48 hours after discharge from the hospital. Repeat referrals should be made for needed resources or support services at this time. Effective crisis intervention and continuity of care require outreach activities and services beyond the emergency medical setting.

Survivors may seek help from medical professionals rather than from mental health professionals because medical treatment is more socially sanctioned and they are likely to be experiencing the physical sequelae of stress. Aware of this, the office nurse can make a more focused assessment of stress-related symptoms and/or depression and ascertain the need for mental health referral. Reporting symptoms and seeking medical treatment are adaptive coping behaviors and can be reinforced as such.

Follow-up visits should occur at least 2, 4, and 6 weeks after the initial evaluation. At each visit, the survivor should be assessed for psychological progress, venereal disease, and pregnancy.

Counseling on the Crisis Hotline

The trained phone counselor talks briefly with the person to determine where she is, what has happened, and what kind of help she needs. The counselor provides empathic listening and the survivor is further encouraged to go to the hospital. The main focus of the telephone contact is on the immediate steps the survivor may take. The counselor provides the necessary information for the woman to make decisions.

Psychotherapy

SURVIVOR

Most rape survivors are eventually able to resume their previous lives after supportive services and crisis counseling. However, many carry with them a constant emotional trauma: flashbacks, nightmares, fear, phobias, and other symptoms associated with posttraumatic stress reaction (PTSD) (see Chapter 14). Some people who survive rape may be susceptible to a psychotic episode or an emotional disturbance so severe that hospitalization is required. Others, whose emotional life may be so overburdened with multiple internal and external pressures, may require individual psychotherapy.

Depression and suicidal ideation are frequent sequelae of rape. Depression is more common in those who do not disclose the assault to significant others because of concerns about being stigmatized, having children living at home, or having a pending civil lawsuit. Any exposure to stimuli related to the traumatic event may activate a reliving of the traumatic state.

Rape survivors are likely to benefit from group therapy or support groups. These modalities may be particularly beneficial for survivors from cultures that are group oriented rather than individualistic, and for women who derive much of their self-definition from cultural norms. Group therapy can make the difference between a person coming out of the crisis at a lower level of functioning or gradually adapting to the experience with an increase in coping skills.

RAPIST

Psychotherapy is essential for rapists' behavior if change is to occur. Unfortunately, most rapists do not acknowledge the need for behavior change and there is no single method or program of treatment that has been found to be totally effective. If a nurse is in the situation of having to counsel the rapist, awareness of her own feelings and reactions will be crucial so as not to interfere with the therapeutic process.

EVALUATION

Rape survivors are recovered if they are relatively essentially free of any signs or symptoms of PTSD, that is, if they are

- Sleeping well, with very few instances of episodic nightmares or broken sleep.
- Eating as was their pattern before the rape. (Clients may respond to the crisis of rape by undereating or overeating.)
- Calm and relaxed or only mildly suspicious, fearful, or restless.
- Getting support from family and friends. Some strain might still be present in relationships, but it should be minimal.
- Generally positive about themselves. On occasion, doubts about self-worth may occur.
- Free from somatic reactions. If mild symptoms persist and minor discomfort is reported, the survivor should be able to talk about it and feel in control of the symptoms.

In general, the closer the survivor's life style is to the pattern that was present before the rape, the more complete the recovery has been.

Visit the **Evolve** website at
http://evolve.elsevier.com/Varcarolis
for more Case Studies.

CASE STUDY 26–1 *Working with a Person Who Has Been Raped*

Latisha Smith, a 36-year-old single mother of two, went out one evening with some friends. Her children were at a slumber party and she "needed to get away and have a little rest and relaxation." She and her friends had gone bowling. Later in the evening, Latisha was tired and ready to go home. A man who had joined the group offered to take her home. She had seen the man at the bowling alley before but did not know much about him. Not in the habit of going home alone with men she did not know, she hesitated. A friend whom she trusted encouraged her to go with James because he was a nice man.

James drove Latisha home. He then asked if he could come into her house to use the bathroom before driving the long distance to his house. She reluctantly agreed and sat on the living room couch. After using the bathroom, James sat next to Latisha and began to kiss her and fondle her breasts. As she protested, James became more forceful in his advances. Latisha was confused and frightened. She managed to get away from him briefly, but he began grabbing, squeezing, and biting her. He told her gruffly, "If you don't do what I say, I'll break your neck." She screamed, but he proceeded to rape her. James became nervous that the noise would alert the neighbors and raced out of the house. A neighbor did in fact arrive just after James fled. The neighbor called the police and then brought Latisha to the local hospital emergency department for a physical examination, crisis intervention, and support.

In the emergency department, Latisha was visibly shaken. She kept saying, over and over, "I shouldn't have let him take me home. I should have fought harder, I shouldn't have let him do this."

The nurse took Latisha to a quiet cubicle. She didn't want Latisha to stay alone and asked the neighbor to stay with her. The nurse then notified the doctor and the rape-victim advocate. When the nurse came back, she told Latisha that she would like to talk to her before the doctor came. Latisha looked at her neighbor and then down. The nurse asked the neighbor to wait outside for a while and said she would call her later.

Latisha: It was horrible. I feel so dirty.
Nurse: You have had a traumatic experience. Do you want to talk about it?
Latisha: I feel so ashamed, I should have never let that man take me home.
Nurse: You think that if you hadn't gone home with a stranger this wouldn't have happened?
Latisha: Yes . . . I shouldn't have let him do it to me anyway, I shouldn't have let him rape me.
Nurse: You mentioned that he said he would break your neck if you didn't do as he said.
Latisha: Yes, he said that . . . he was going to kill me, it was awful.
Nurse: It seems you did the right thing in order to stay alive.

As the nurse continued to talk with Latisha, her anxiety level seemed to lessen. The nurse talked to Latisha about the kinds of experiences rape victims often have after the rape, and explained that the reactions she might have 2 or 3 weeks from now are normal in these circumstances. The nurse continued to collect the necessary information. She said that the doctor would want to examine Latisha, and explained the procedure to her. She then asked Latisha to sign a consent. While preparing Latisha for examination, the nurse noticed bite marks and bruises on both breasts. She also noted Latisha's lower lip, which was cut and bleeding. The nurse kept detailed notes on her observations and drew a body map. After the examination, Latisha was given clean clothes and a place to shower.

ASSESSMENT

The nurse organized her data into subjective and objective components.

Objective Data
1. Crying and sobbing
2. Bruises and bite marks on each breast
3. Lip cut and bleeding
4. Rape reported to the police

Subjective Data
1. "He was going to kill me."
2. "It was horrible. I feel so dirty."
3. "I shouldn't have let him rape me."

SELF-ASSESSMENT

The nurse had worked with rape survivors before and had helped develop the hospital protocol. It took a while for her to be able to remain neutral as well as responsive, because her own anger at rapists had initially interfered. She also

CASE STUDY 26–1 Working with a Person Who Has Been Raped (Continued)

remembers a time when a woman came in stating that she was raped but was so calm, smiling, and polite that the nurse initially did not believe her story. She had not, at that point, examined her own feelings or dealt with the popular societal myths regarding rape. It was only later, when she had talked to more experienced health care personnel, that she learned that crisis reactions can seem bizarre, confusing, and contradictory.

The nurse learned that staying with the survivor, encouraging her to express her reactions and feelings, and listening were effective methods of reducing feelings of anxiety. Once the nurse learned through supervision and peer discussion to let go of her personal anger at the attacker and her ambivalence toward the survivor, her care and effectiveness improved greatly. All of this growth took time and support from more experienced nurses and other members of the health care team.

NURSING DIAGNOSIS

The nurse formulated the following diagnosis:

1. Rape-trauma syndrome

   ■ "I shouldn't have let him rape me."
   ■ "He was going to kill me."

   ■ Crying and sobbing.
   ■ Bruises and bite marks on both breasts.
   ■ Rape reported to the police.
   ■ "It was horrible. I feel so dirty."

OUTCOME CRITERIA

Latisha will be free of signs of PTSD. Note: This is often a long-term process. The nurse devised a plan of care for Latisha, based on the nursing diagnosis and the nurse's training as a crisis counselor.

NURSING DIAGNOSIS	LONG-TERM OUTCOME	SHORT-TERM GOALS
Rape-trauma syndrome	1. Within 5 months Latisha will state that she thinks less about the rape, is sleeping better, feels safer, and is functioning at her previous level.	1a. Latisha will begin to express emotional reactions and feelings before she leaves the emergency department. 1b. Latisha will be able to list possible socioemotional reactions following sexual assault. 1c. Latisha will have written referrals for legal, medical, and crisis counseling before she leaves the emergency department.

Case Study continued on following page

CASE STUDY 26-1   *Working with a Person Who Has Been Raped* (Continued)

NURSING DIAGNOSIS	LONG-TERM OUTCOME	SHORT-TERM GOALS
		1d. Latisha will have a follow-up appointment with the gynecology clinic and the rape advocate-counselor for weekly meetings before she leaves the emergency department.
		1e. Latisha's anxiety level will go from severe to moderate before she leaves the emergency department.

INTERVENTION

Latisha stated that she felt more comfortable after taking a shower and talking to the nurse. She seemed less confused and better able to concentrate, and she began to discuss what she would tell her children. Specific interventions are found in Nursing Care Plan 26–1.

It was decided that Latisha's neighbor would stay with her overnight. Latisha had an appointment the following week with the nurse counselor and with a women's health nurse practitioner in the outpatient clinic. She was also given written information about legal counseling, crisis groups, and other community follow-up services for rape survivors.

The nurse documented Latisha's physical and emotional status, including verbatim responses, as well as the results of the physical examination and tests. The nurse called Latisha the next morning and encouraged her to call back if she had any further questions.

EVALUATION

Latisha kept her counseling appointment with the nurse counselor at the community mental health center as well as her appointment with the women's health nurse practitioner. She continued with the counseling for several months. For a time, she experienced acute anxiety attacks when she went out at night, and she had new locks put on all her windows and doors. After 3 months, she expressed interest in a group that was forming in the next town for women who had been raped; however, she said that she didn't know if she could go because it started at 6 PM. The counselor told her that arrangements could be made for a volunteer to take her there and back until she felt safer going out at night.

After 4 months, Latisha stated that she did feel safer and had been out at night twice in the past week. She was not comfortable yet, but said she was making progress. She told the counselor that she was not ready to date. The group had been a great help to her. She continued to call the nurse counselor about once every 2 weeks to report on her progress.

Latisha said she was functioning well as a mother and in her job. After 5 months, the flashbacks ceased and she started sleeping throughout the night without nightmares.

Visit the **Evolve** website at
http://evolve.elsevier.com/Varcarolis
for the other Nursing Care Plan diagnoses and for
more Nursing Care Plans.

NURSING CARE PLAN 26–1   Rape Survivor

SHORT-TERM GOAL	INTERVENTION	RATIONALE
1. Survivor will begin to express emotional reactions and feelings before she leaves the emergency room.	1a. Nurse remains neutral and nonjudgmental and assures survivor of confidentiality.	1a. Lessens feelings of shame and guilt and encourages sharing of painful feelings.
	1b. Nurse does not leave survivor alone.	1b. Deters feelings of isolation and escalation of anxiety.
	1c. Nurse allows negative expressions and behavioral self-blame while using reflective techniques.	1c. Fosters feelings of control.
	1d. Nurse assures survivor she did the right thing to save her life.	1d. Decreases burden of guilt and shame.
	1e. When anxiety level is down to moderate, nurse encourages problem solving.	1e. Increases survivor's feeling of control in her own life (when in severe anxiety, a person cannot problem-solve.)
2. Survivor will be able to list possible socioeconomic reactions following sexual assault.	2. Nurse tells survivor of common reactions experienced by people in long-term reorganization phase, e.g., phobias, flashbacks, insomnia, increased motor activity.	2. Helps survivor anticipate reactions and understand them as part of recovery process.
3. Survivor will state that she will keep a follow-up appointment with the gynecology clinic and rape advocate or counselor before she leaves the emergency room.	3a. Nurse explains emergency room procedure to survivor.	3a. Lowers anticipatory anxiety.
	3b. Nurse explains physical examination.	3b. Allows for questions and concerns; victim may be too traumatized and may refuse.
	3c. Nurse has survivor sign consent form.	3c. Follows legal protocol.
	3d. Nurse (or female rape-victim advocate) stays with survivor during examination.	3d. Often decreases isolation and anxiety.
	3e. Nurse explains role of rape-victim advocate.	3e. Awareness of supports and why they are needed.
	3f. Nurse gives results of gynecological and physical examination to survivor.	3f. Enables survivor to participate in decision and to understand need for follow-up care.

Nursing Care Plan continued on following page

3. Many rapes go unreported. A reason the client may choose to report a rape is

   1. The victim knows the rapist.
   2. The victim hopes to obtain justice.
   3. Taboos exist against talking about sex.
   4. The victim as well as the rapist goes on trial.

4. An intervention that would be useful when working with a person in the ER who has been sexually assaulted is

   1. Interact in a cool and reserved fashion.
   2. Help client separate issues of vulnerability from blame.
   3. Structure communication to minimize expression of strong feelings.
   4. Expect family and friends to provide majority of emotional support for client.

5. Identify the data which, if found in the medical record of a sexual assault victim, would indicate that reorganization after a rape crisis is not yet complete.

   1. Free from somatic reactions.
   2. Generally positive about self.
   3. Calm and relaxed during interactions.
   4. Episodic nightmares frequently experienced.

NURSE, CLIENT, AND FAMILY RESOURCES

Rape, Abuse, Incest National Network (RAINN)
1-800-656-HOPE
http://www.feminist.com/rainn.htm

Sexual Abuse Survivors Anonymous (SASA)
PO Box 241046
Detroit, MI 48224
(12-step program for survivors of rape, incest, or sexual abuse)

Survivors of Incest Anonymous (SIA)
PO Box 26870
Baltimore, MD 21212
1-410-282-3400
(12-step program for survivors of incest)

REFERENCES

Boutcher, F., and Gallop, R. (1996). Psychiatric nurses' attitudes toward sexuality, sexual assault and rape, and incest. *Archives of General Psychiatric Nursing*, 10(3):184.

Burgess, A. W. (1995). Rape trauma syndrome: A nursing diagnosis. *Occupational Health Nursing*, 33(8):405.

Burgess, A. W., and Holstrom, L. L. (1974). The rape victim in the ER. *American Journal of Nursing*, 73(10):1740.

Cornell, D. H. (1998). Helping victims of rape: A program called SANE, Sexual Assault Nurse Examiner. *New Jersey Medicine*, 95(2):43–46.

Girardin, B. W., et al. (1997). *Color atlas of sexual assault*. St. Louis: Mosby.

Emergency Nurses Association (1998). Emergency nurses association position statement. Forensic evidence collection. *Journal of Emergency Nursing*, 24(5):38A.

Ledray, L. E. (1998). SANE development and operation guide. *Journal of Emergency Nursing*, 24(2):197–198.

Ledray, L. E., and Arndt, S. (1994). Examining the sexual assault victim: A new model for nursing care. *Journal of Psychosocial Nursing and Medical Health Services*, 32(2):7–12.

Linden, J. A. (1999). Sexual assault. *Emergency Medical Clinics of North America*, 17(3):685–697.

Pesola, G. R., Westfal, R. E., and Kuffner, C. A. (1999). Emergency department characteristics of male sexual assault. *Academy of Emergency Medicine*, 6(8):792–798.

Smith, K. M. (1999). Drugs used in acquaintance rape. *Journal of American Pharmacological Association*, 39(4):519–525.

TABLE 27–1   Drug Information: Physical Complications Related to Drug Abuse (Continued)

DRUG	PHYSICAL COMPLICATIONS
Route: Ingestion	
Caffeine	Gastroesophageal reflux Peptic ulcer Increased intraocular pressure in unregulated glaucoma Tachycardia Increased plasma glucose and lipid levels
Phencyclidine piperidine (PCP)	Respiratory arrest
Route: Smoking, Ingestion	
Marijuana	Impaired lung structure Chromosomal mutation—increased incidence of birth defects Micronucleic white blood cells—increased risk of disease due to decreased resistance to infection Possible long-term effects on short-term memory
Route: Smoking, Chewing	

Nicotine	*Heavy chronic use associated with*
	    Emphysema
	    Cancer of the larynx and esophagus
	    Lung cancer
	    Peripheral vascular diseases
	    Cancer of the mouth
	    Cardiovascular disease
	    Hypertension

Route: Intravenous,* Smoking	
Heroin	Constipation Dermatitis Malnutrition Hypoglycemia Dental caries Amenorrhea
Route: Sniffing, Snorting, Bagging (Fumes Inhaled From a Plastic Bag), Huffing (Inhalant-Soaked Rag in the Mouth)	
Inhalants	Respiratory arrest Tachycardia Arrhythmias Nervous system damage

*Note: The complications listed can result from any drug taken intravenously.

depressants act on gamma-aminobutyric acid (GABA). This finding helps explain the addictive and cross-tolerance effects that occur when the use of alcohol is combined with barbiturates and benzodiazepines.

New studies demonstrate that inactivating both the dopamine and the serotonin transporters in the brains of mice drastically reduces their experience of cocaine's reward system (NIH 2001).

Psychological Theories

Although no known addictive personality type exists, associated psychodynamic factors exist, including

■ An intolerance for frustration and pain
■ Lack of success in life
■ Lack of affectionate and meaningful relationships

- Low self-esteem; lack of self-regard
- Risk-taking propensity

A person uses substances to feel better. The habit of using a substance in response to psychological needs then becomes reinforced, and over time, the behavior develops into an addiction.

Sociocultural Theories

Sociocultural theories attempt to explain differences in the incidence of substance use in various groups. Social and cultural norms influence when, what, and how a person uses substances. For example, in Asian cultures, the prevalence rate is relatively low. This is due in part to a deficiency in about 50% of the population of aldehyde dehydrogenase, the chemical that breaks down alcohol acetaldehyde. With this first step in alcohol breakdown a severe flush and palpitation may occur (APA 2000b). This reaction effectively keeps many Asians from drinking.

Another theory correlates substance use with the degree of socioeconomic stress people experience. Being a drug addict can give a person a place of acceptance in his or her subculture. This is most true in economically deprived and unstable environments, where drugs may be taken to provide a person with a sense of belonging and identity. The dominance of the drug subculture in highly stressed communities can make it almost impossible not to develop a problem.

Women in general are diagnosed with lower rates of substance use than men. Addicted women are viewed much more negatively than addicted men in many cultural groups. This negative attribution may lead to avoidance of the diagnosis, and thus a lack of treatment services.

In summary, there is no single cause of substance abuse. Multiple factors contribute to substance use, abuse, and addiction in any individual. For example, a child of an alcoholic parent may have a biochemical deficiency predisposing him or her to alcoholism and may grow up with low self-esteem in a society that has no rituals governing alcohol use. Because of complex biological, psychological, and sociocultural factors, this person is at risk for developing alcoholism.

DEFINITIONS

The diagnostic scheme in the *Diagnostic and Statistical Manual of Mental Disorders, fourth edition* (DSM-IV-TR) (APA 2000b) focuses on the behavioral aspects and the pathological patterns of use, emphasizing the physical symptoms of tolerance and withdrawal. An overview of DSM-IV-TR diagnostic criteria for substance abuse and dependence is shown in Figure 27–1.

Tolerance and Withdrawal

The concept of substance dependence includes the concepts of tolerance and withdrawal. Tolerance is a need for higher and higher doses to achieve the desired effect. Withdrawal occurs after a long period of continued use, so that stopping or reducing use results in specific physical and psychological signs and symptoms. Since alcohol is still the most common drug of abuse in the United States and poses the greatest withdrawal danger, DSM-IV-TR diagnostic criteria for alcohol intoxication, withdrawal, and delirium are highlighted in Figure 27–2. Information on signs and symptoms of intoxication and withdrawal from substances of abuse are identified later in this chapter.

Other terms are frequently used in reference to substance abuse. Flashbacks, synergistic effects, and antagonistic effects are briefly discussed here, although they are seen in many situations, not just substance abuse.

Flashbacks

Flashbacks are a common effect of hallucinogenic drugs. Flashbacks are transitory recurrences in perceptual disturbance caused by a person's earlier hallucinogenic drug experiences when he or she is in a drug-free state (APA 2000b). Such experiences as visual distortions, time expansion, loss of ego boundaries, and intense emotions are reported. Flashbacks are often mild and perhaps pleasant, but at other times, individuals experience repeated recurrences of frightening images or thoughts.

Synergistic Effects

Some drugs when taken together intensify or prolong the effect of either or both of the drugs. For example, combinations of alcohol plus a benzodiazepine, alcohol plus an opiate, and alcohol plus a barbiturate all produce a synergistic effect. All these drugs are CNS depressants. Two of these drugs taken together result in far greater CNS depression than the sum of the effects of each drug added to-

SUBSTANCE ABUSE vs. DEPENDENCE

SUBSTANCE ABUSE

Maladaptive pattern of substance use leading to clinically significant impairment or distress, manifested by one or more of the following within a 12-month period:

1. Inability to fulfill major role obligations at work, school, and home.

2. Participation in physically hazardous situations while impaired (driving a car, operating a machine, exacerbation of symptoms, e.g., ulcers).

3. Recurrent legal or interpersonal problems.

4. Continued use despite recurrent social and interpersonal problems.

SUBSTANCE DEPENDENCE

Maladaptive pattern of substance use leading to clinically significant impairment or distress, manifested by three or more of the following within a 12-month period:

1. Presence of tolerance to the drug.

2. Presence of withdrawal syndrome.

3. Substance is taken in larger amounts/for longer period than intended.

4. Unsuccessful or persistent desire to cut down or control use.

5. Increased time spent in getting, taking, and recovering from the substance. May withdraw from family or friends.

6. Reduction or absence of important social, occupational, or recreational activities.

7. Substance used despite knowledge of recurrent physical or psychological problems or that problems were caused or exacerbated by one substance.

Figure 27–1 DSM-IV-TR criteria for substance abuse and dependence. (Adapted from American Psychiatric Association (2000). *Diagnostic and statistical manual of mental disorders* (4th ed., text revision) *(DSM-IV-TR)*. Washington, D.C.: American Psychiatric Association Press. Copyright 2000 American Psychiatric Association.)

ALCOHOL-RELATED DISORDERS

ALCOHOL INTOXICATION

1. Recent ingestion.

2. Clinically significant, maladaptive behavior or psychological changes (sexual, aggressive, mood, and judgment).

3. At least one of the following:
   - Slurred speech
   - Incoordination
   - Unsteady gait
   - Nystagmus
   - Impairment in attention or memory
   - Stupor or coma

4. Symptoms not due to another medical/mental condition.

ALCOHOL WITHDRAWAL

1. Cessation (reduction) of ETOH use that has been heavy or prolonged.

2. Two (or more) of the following:
   - Nausea or vomiting
   - Anxiety
   - Transient visual, tactile, or auditory hallucinations or illusions
   - Autonomic activity (sweating, increased pulse over 100)
   - Psychomotor agitation
   - Insomnia
   - Grand mal seizures
   - Increased hand tremor

SUBSTANCE INDUCED DELIRIUM

1. Impaired consciousness (reduced awareness of environment).

2. Changes in cognition (memory, disorientation, language, visual or tactile hallucinations, illusions).

3. Develops over short period of time — hours to days — and fluctuates over a day.

4. Evidence of substance use (history, physical, laboratory findings) and symptoms developed during withdrawal.

Figure 27–2 DSM-IV-TR criteria for alcohol-related disorders. ETOH, ethyl alcohol. (Adapted from American Psychiatric Association (2000). *Diagnostic and statistical manual of mental disorders* (4th ed., text revision) *(DSM-IV-TR)*. Washington, D.C.: American Psychiatric Association Press. Copyright 2000 American Psychiatric Association.)

gether. Many unintentional deaths have resulted from lethal combinations of drugs.

Antagonistic Effects

Many people may take a combination of drugs to weaken or inhibit the effect of another drug. For example, cocaine is often mixed with heroin (speed-ball). The heroin (CNS depressant) is meant to soften the intense letdown of cocaine (CNS stimulant) withdrawal. Naloxone (Narcan), an opiate antagonist, is often given to people who have over-dosed on an opiate (usually heroin) to reverse respiratory and CNS depression. Since the duration of naloxone action may be less than that of the narcotic that was taken, further monitoring and possible additional doses of naloxone may be needed.

Co-dependence

Co-dependence is a cluster of behaviors once thought to exist only in alcohol addiction. People who are codependent usually have a constellation of maladaptive thoughts, feelings, behaviors, and attitudes that effectively prevent them from living full and satisfying lives. Symptomatic of co-dependence is valuing oneself by what one does, what one looks like, and what one has, rather than by who one is (Box 27-1).

Living with a substance abusing or alcoholic individual is a source of stress and requires family system adjustments. People who are co-dependent often exhibit overresponsible behavior—doing for others what they could just as well do for themselves. Talking in terms of extremes of overresponsibility or underresponsibility points to a need for behavioral change rather than the need for recovery from a disease. Table 27-2 offers some guidelines for a person in a co-dependent relationship.

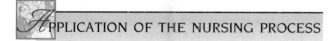

APPLICATION OF THE NURSING PROCESS

ASSESSMENT

Assessment is becoming more complex because of the increase in the simultaneous use of many substances (**polydrug abuse**), the co-existence of psychiatric disease with substance abuse (**dual diagnosis**), and associated comorbid physical illnesses, includ-

ing HIV infection, the acquired immunodeficiency syndrome (AIDS), dementia, and encephalopathy.

Sensitivity to multicultural and racial issues is important in interpreting symptoms, making diagnoses, providing clinical care, and designing prevention strategies.

Overall Assessment

INTERVIEW GUIDELINES

An overall assessment is outlined in Table 27-3. Please review the overall areas.

When assessing past substance use behavior, the nurse assesses all drugs taken, the amount, the length of use, the route, and the drug preference. It is important to determine how the drugs were used—that is, whether they were taken intravenously, intramuscularly, intradermally (skin-popped), or intranasally

Box 27-1   Overresponsible (Co-dependent) Behaviors

Co-dependent individuals find themselves

1. Attempting to control someone else's drug use.
2. Spending inordinate time thinking about the addicted person.
3. Finding excuses for the person's substance abuse.
4. Covering up the person's drinking/drugging or lying.
5. Feeling responsible for the person's drug use.
6. Feeling guilty for the addicted person's behavior.
7. Avoiding family and social events because of concerns or shame about the addicted member's behavior.
8. Making threats regarding the consequences of the alcoholic's/drug abuser's behavior and failing to follow through.
9. Eliciting promises for change.
10. Feeling like they are "walking on eggshells" on a routine basis to avoid causing problems, especially in relation to alcohol or drug use.
11. Allowing moods to be influenced by those of the addicted person.
12. Searching for, hiding, and destroying the abuser's source of drug or alcohol supply.
13. Assuming the alcoholic's/substance abuser's duties and responsibilities.
14. Feeling forced to increase control over the family's finances.
15. Often bailing the addicted person out of financial or legal problems.

mas, subdural hematomas, and other conditions can go unnoticed if symptoms of acute alcohol intoxication and withdrawal are not distinguished from the symptoms of a brain injury. Therefore, neurological signs (pupil size, equality, and reaction to light) should be assessed, especially with comatose clients suspected of having traumatic injuries. In addition, questions about alcohol abuse should be asked as part of the assessment of any non–sports-related trauma (Israel 1996).

A urine **toxicology screen** and/or **blood alcohol level (BAL)** can be useful for assessment purposes.

Assessment strategies include data collection pertaining to both substance dependence and psychiatric impairment. Problem areas in assessment that are of particular relevance in a population with comorbidity include the masking of withdrawal by the subtle symptoms of psychiatric impairment (e.g., irritability, depression, restlessness). A further complication is the difficulty in differentiating normal aspects of the substance abuse recovery process from psychiatric impairment, such as major depression (Brady 1999).

Tolerance and progression of substance use and abuse also may be difficult to assess. Individuals with comorbid illnesses often follow a pattern of sporadic abuse with bingeing. These individuals are often poor historians and may have impaired capacities for honesty, recall, and insight.

Individuals with previously established psychiatric impairment may be experiencing substance abuse or dependence if they exhibit increasing frequency of symptoms, exacerbation without obvious reason, chronic noncompliance with treatment regimens, and self-medication or use of a substance in response to symptomatology secondary to psychiatric impairment or social stressors (Boyd and Hauenstein 1997). Substance abuse can go undetected in those who are depressed, suicidal, or anxious unless a thorough history is taken. Similarly, the understanding and treatment of substance-dependent people are enhanced by inquiries about symptoms of depression and anxiety.

ASSESSMENT TOOLS

There are a number of helpful tools that nurses can use to assess if the individual has an alcohol or drug problem. Two that may be very useful are

1. *Alcohol*: The Brief Version of the Michigan Alcohol Screening Test (MAST) (Box 27–2).
2. *Other substances of abuse*: The Drug Abuse Screening Test (DAST) (Box 27–3).

Once specific data are obtained, it is helpful to know if the person is abusing a substance, or ac-

tively dependent on the substance(s). Figure 27–2 (DSM-IV-TR) gives guidelines for this distinction.

PSYCHOLOGICAL CHANGES

Certain psychological characteristics are associated with substance abuse, including denial, depression, anxiety, dependency, hopelessness, low self-esteem, and various psychiatric disorders. It is often difficult to determine which came first, psychological changes or substance abuse. Some people self-medicate to cope with psychiatric symptoms. For these people, symptoms of psychological difficulty remain, even after months of sobriety. Psychological changes that occurred as a result of drinking resolve quickly with sobriety.

Substance-abusing people are threatened on many levels in their interactions with nurses. *First*, they are concerned about being rejected. They are acutely aware that not all nurses are equally willing to care for addicted people, and in fact, many clients may have experienced instances of rejection in past en-

BOX 27–2 *Michigan Alcohol Screening Test (MAST) Brief Version*

Scoring Yes to 3 or more indicates alcoholism

1. Do you feel you are a normal drinker?
2. Do friends or relatives think you are a normal drinker?
3. Have you ever attended a meeting of Alcoholics Anonymous?
4. Have you ever gotten in trouble at work because of drinking?
5. Have you ever lost friends or girlfriends/boyfriends because of drinking?
6. Have you ever neglected your obligations, your family, or your work for 2 or more days in a row because of your drinking?
7. Have you ever had delirium tremens (DTs), severe shaking, or heard voices or seen things that were not there after heavy drinking?
8. Have you ever gone to anyone for help about your drinking?
9. Have you ever been in a hospital because of your drinking?
10. Have you ever been arrested for drunken driving or other drunken behavior?

From Pokorny A. D., Miller B. A., and Kaplan, H. B. (1972). The brief MAST: A shortened version of the Michigan Alcohol Screening Test. *American Journal of Psychiatry*, 129:342–345. Reprinted by permission. Copyright 1972 American Psychiatric Association.

BOX 27–3   Drug Abuse Screening Test (DAST)

The following questions concern information about your involvement with drugs *not including alcoholic beverages* during the past 12 months.

In the statements, "drug abuse" refers (1) to the use of prescribed or OTC drugs in excess of the directions and (2) any nonmedical use of drugs. The various classes of drugs may include cannabis, solvents, antianxiety drugs, sedative-hypnotics, cocaine, stimulants, hallucinogens, and narcotics. Remember that the questions *do not include alcoholic beverages.*

Have you used drugs other than those required for medical purposes?   Yes ____ No ____

Do you abuse more than one drug at a time?   Yes ____ No ____

Are you always able to stop using drugs when you want to?   Yes ____ No ____

Have you had "blackouts" or "flashbacks" as a result of drug use?   Yes ____ No ____

Do you ever feel bad about your drug abuse?   Yes ____ No ____

Does your spouse (or parents) ever complain about your involvement with drugs?   Yes ____ No ____

Have you neglected your family because of your use of drugs?   Yes ____ No ____

Have you engaged in illegal activities in order to obtain drugs?   Yes ____ No ____

Have you ever experienced withdrawal symptoms (felt sick) when you stopped taking drugs?   Yes ____ No ____

Have you had medical problems as a result of your drug use (e.g., memory loss, hepatitis, convulsions, bleeding, etc.)?   Yes ____ No ____

Scoring: one positive response warrants further evaluation   Yes ____ No ____

From Skinner, H. A. (1982). Drug Abuse Screening Test (DAST) (p. 363). Langford Lance, England: Elsevier Science Ltd. Reprinted with kind permission from Elsevier Science Ltd., The Boulevard, Langford Lance, Kidlington OX5, United Kingdom. Copyright 1982.

---

counters with nursing personnel. *Second,* substance abusers may be anxious about recovering because to do so they must give up the substance they think they need to survive. *Third,* addicts are concerned about failing at recovering. Addiction is a chronic relapsing condition. In fact, relapse is one of the criteria for diagnosing addiction. Most addicts have tried recovery at least once before and have re-

lapsed. As a result, many become discouraged about their chances of ever succeeding.

These concerns can threaten the addict's sense of security and sense of self, increasing anxiety levels. To protect against these feelings, the addict establishes a **predictable defensive style.** The elements include defense mechanisms (denial, projection, rationalization), as well as characteristic thought processes (all-or-none thinking, selective attention) and behaviors (conflict minimization and avoidance, passivity, and manipulation) (Table 27–4). The substance abuser is not able to give up these maladaptive coping styles until more positive and functional skills are learned (Wing 1996).

Assessing Signs of Intoxication and Withdrawal

CNS DEPRESSANTS

This class of drugs includes alcohol, benzodiazepines, and barbiturates. Symptoms of intoxication, overdose, and withdrawal, along with possible treatments, are presented in Table 27–5.

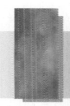

TABLE 27–4   Three Defensive Styles of Coping That Contribute to Substance Abuse Maintenance

Rationalization	Falsifying an experience by giving a contrived, socially acceptable, and logical explanation to justify an unpleasant experience or questionable behavior. *Examples:* "Sure I got a little angry with my boss. Everyone comes in late to work, so why does he have to pick on me all the time? "My wife made such a big deal about me not showing up for our son's graduation. I had some business entertaining to do that night and we ran late. That happens to everyone."
Projection	Attributing an unconscious impulse, attitude, or behavior to someone else (blaming or scapegoating). *Example:* "Look, if it wasn't for the fact I can't find a job and my boyfriend is uncaring, I wouldn't need coke to get through the day."
Denial	Escaping unpleasant realities by ignoring their existence. *Example:* "I'm sick of everyone thinking I drink too much. I can control my drinking whenever I want . . . and stop whenever I want."

Alcohol and other CNS depressant withdrawal re-actions are associated with severe morbidity and mortality, unlike withdrawal from other drugs. The syndrome for alcohol withdrawal is the same for the entire class of CNS depressant drugs. Alcohol is used here as the prototype. The time intervals are delayed when other CNS depressants are the main drugs of choice or are used in combination with alcohol. In addition, as clients age, their symptoms of withdrawal continue for longer periods and ap-pear to be more severe than in younger clients.

Multiple drug and alcohol dependencies can re-sult in simultaneous withdrawal syndromes that present a bizarre clinical picture and may pose problems for safe withdrawal. Family and friends may help provide important information that can assist in care planning. The DSM-IV-TR (APA 2000b) identifies two alcohol withdrawal syndromes: (1) al-cohol withdrawal and (2) the more severe alcohol withdrawal delirium (see Fig. 27–2).

ALCOHOL WITHDRAWAL. The early signs of withdrawal develop within a few hours after cessa-tion or reduction of alcohol (ethanol) intake; they peak after 24 to 48 hours and then rapidly and dra-matically disappear, unless the withdrawal pro-gresses to alcohol withdrawal delirium.

TABLE 27–5   CNS *Depressants*

		OVERDOSE		WITHDRAWAL	
DRUG	**INTOXICATION**	**Effects**	**Possible Treatments**	**Effects**	**Possible Treatments**
Barbiturates Benzodiaze-pines Chloral hy-drate Glutethimide Meprobamate Alcohol (ETOH)	*Physical* Slurred speech Incoordination Unsteady gait Drowsiness Decreased blood pressure *Psychological-perceptual* Disinhibition of sexual or aggres-sive drives Impaired judgment Impaired social or occupational function Impaired attention or memory Irritability	Cardiovascular or respiratory de-pression or ar-rest (mostly with barbitu-rates) Coma Shock Convulsions Death	*If awake* Keep awake Induce vomiting Give activated charcoal to aid absorp-tion of drug Every 15 min-utes check vi-tal signs (VS) *Coma:* Clear airway; endotracheal tube Intravenous (IV) fluids Gastric lavage with activated charcoal Frequent VS checks for shock and cardiac arrest after client is stable Seizure precau-tions Possible hemo-dialysis or peritoneal di-alysis Flumazenil (Romazicon) IV	*Cessation of pro-longed-heavy use* Nausea-vomiting Tachycardia Diaphoresis Anxiety or irrita-bility Tremors in hands, fingers, eyelids Marked insom-nia Grand mal seizures *After 5–15 years of heavy use:* Delir-ium	Carefully titrated detoxification with similar drug **NOTE: Abrupt withdrawal can lead to death**

Data from American Psychiatric Association (2000b). *Diagnostic and statistical manual of mental disorders* (4th ed., revised) (DSM-IV-TR). Washington, DC: American Psychiatric Association, and Bohn, M. J. (2000). Alcoholism. *Psychiatric Clinics of North America,* 16(4):679.

Early signs of withdrawal include anxiety, anorexia, insomnia, and tremor. The person may appear hyper-alert, manifest jerky movements and irritability, startle easily, and experience subjective distress often described as "shaking inside." The person may also report transient, poorly formed hallucinations, illusions, or vivid nightmares. Nausea and vomiting may also occur.

A kind, warm, and supportive manner on the part of the nurse can allay anxiety and provide a sense of security. Consistent and frequent orientation to time and place may be necessary. Encouraging the family (one at a time) or close friends to stay with the client in quiet surroundings can also help increase orientation and minimize confusion and anxiety. **Illusions** are usually terrifying for the client. Illusions are misinterpretations of objects in the environment, usually of a threatening nature. For example, a person may think that spots on the wallpaper are blood-leaching ants. However, illusions can be clarified; this reduces the client's terror: "See, they are not ants, they are just part of the wallpaper pattern." If a person experiencing withdrawal is argumentative, hostile, or demanding, it is often because of this deep-seated anxiety as well as feelings of guilt and shame. The nurse can help the client overcome these feelings, making relief and hope possible by demonstrating an accepting attitude and showing strong support for efforts at recovery.

Pulse and blood pressure are usually elevated. Grand mal seizures may also develop; these usually appear 7 to 48 hours after cessation of ethanol intake, particularly in people with a history of seizures.

Careful assessment followed by appropriate medical and nursing interventions can prevent the more serious withdrawal reaction of delirium.

ALCOHOL WITHDRAWAL DELIRIUM. Alcohol withdrawal delirium is considered a medical emergency and has a mortality rate of up to 5% to 10% even if treated (Weinrieb and O'Brien 1997). Death is usually due to myocardial infarction, fat emboli, peripheral vascular collapse, electrolyte imbalance, aspiration pneumonia, or suicide. The state of delirium usually peaks 2 to 3 days (48 to 72 hours) after cessation or reduction of intake (can occur later) and lasts 2 to 3 days.

Along with anxiety, insomnia, anorexia, and delirium, additional features include

- Autonomic hyperactivity (e.g., tachycardia, diaphoresis, elevated blood pressure)
- Severe disturbance in sensorium (e.g., disorientation, clouding of consciousness)

- Perceptual disturbances (e.g. visual or tactile hallucinations)
- Fluctuating levels of consciousness (e.g., ranging from hyperexcitability to lethargy)
- Delusions (paranoid), agitated behaviors, and fever (100°F to 103°F).

Vignette

■ After her divorce, Mary started having a few drinks after coming home from work. She initially found that these drinks helped her relax and "put me in a good mood." Over time, Mary found that two drinks no longer did the trick and that she required three and then four drinks to achieve the relaxed feeling and mild euphoria she sought. Mary's body was building up a tolerance for the drug, and it took larger and larger doses to get the desired effect. The body is able to adjust to gradually increased doses of certain drugs over time and begins to require a certain level of the drug to function "normally." After 10 years, Mary was having a couple of drinks at lunch, before dinner, and during the evening. However, on first glance, the effects of alcohol did not show. Mary was able to appear normal with a high blood alcohol level. Mary eventually developed the habit of taking a drink every morning to settle the "shakes" and prevent tremulousness. She drank in the morning not to feel good but to prevent feeling bad.

In the spring of 2000, after suffering an acute attack of pancreatitis, Mary was hospitalized; she was given intravenous fluids and had a nasogastric tube in place. After 3 days, Mary became extremely agitated. She screamed that she was being held hostage by Iranian terrorists. She mistook her water carafe for a time bomb (**illusion**). She became terrified at night, believing that she saw giant ants on the walls.

Mary's blood pressure increased from 120/70 mm Hg on admission to 150/100 mm Hg. Her pulse increased from 88 to 140. She thought it was the winter of 1985, about the time of her divorce.

After alcohol withdrawal delirium was diagnosed, Mary was given 100 mg of chlordiazepoxide hydrochloride (Librium) intravenously and then orally every 4 hours. Her pulse and blood pressure were monitored every hour. She was given 100 mg of thiamine intramuscularly, prophylactically against encephalopathy, as well as magnesium sulfate. Mary had normal skin turgor, and her urine specific gravity was within normal limits; therefore, fluids were not forced.

Her terror at seeing large ants was reduced by the nurse's presence and assurances that the nurse did not see the ants. Once the nurse showed her the carafe and poured some of the water into a glass, Mary understood that it was not a bomb.

Mary's agitation and aggressiveness became worse at night, and a friend stayed with her, talking in a calm manner and orienting her to the surroundings. When the nurses came to give medication and check vital signs and urinary output, they carefully explained everything they were going to do beforehand to allay misinterpretation of their actions by Mary.

Mary was placed in a private, well-lit room. A minimal amount of environmental stimuli was allowed (e.g., no radios or television, one visitor at a time). A clock was placed in clear view. The head of her bed was kept elevated to increase environmental orientation, and her bed faced the window to provide further orientation to time of day.

Three days later, Mary was fully oriented although still taking chlordiazepoxide. The episode had frightened her. She agreed to go to an Alcoholics Anonymous meeting and learn about other available avenues to sobriety.

Immediate medical attention is warranted (see the section on Pharmacology for Treatment in Substance Abuse for a full discussion of medical treatments).

Alcohol, however is the only drug for which objective measures of intoxication exist. The relationship between blood alcohol level (BAL) and behavior in a nontolerant individual is shown in Table 27–6. Knowledge of the BAL assists the nurse in determining the level of intoxication, the level of tolerance, and whether the person accurately reported recent drinking during the nursing history. These factors are also assessed by means of behavioral cues. As tolerance develops, a discrepancy exists between BAL and expected behavior. A person with tolerance to alcohol may have a high BAL but minimal signs of impairment, as indicated in the following vignette.

Vignette

■ Clarence presents in the emergency department with a BAL of 0.51 mg%. He is stuporous and ataxic and has slurred speech. The fact that he is still alive indicates a high tolerance for alcohol. A nursing history conducted as the client sobers up revealed an extensive drinking history. When the blood alcohol level is this high, assessing for withdrawal symptoms is important.

The nursing history, physical examination, and laboratory tests are methods used to gather data about drug-related physical problems (Conway and Fairbrother 1999; Meehan et al. 1998). The extent of impairment depends on individual susceptibility as well as on amount of drug used and route of administration. Each class of drugs has its own physiological signs and symptoms of intoxication, which are summarized in the tables for each substance class of abuse.

CNS STIMULANTS

Table 27–7 outlines the physical and psychological effects of intoxication from abuse of amphetamines and other psychostimulants, possible life-threatening results of overdose, and emergency measures for both overdose and withdrawal. All stimulants accelerate the normal functioning of the body and affect the CNS. Common signs of stimulant abuse include dilation of the pupils, dryness of the oronasal cavity, and excessive motor activity.

When a person who has ingested a stimulant experiences chest pain, has an irregular pulse, or has a history of heart trouble, the person should be taken to an emergency department immediately.

COCAINE AND CRACK. Cocaine is a naturally occurring stimulant extracted from the leaf of the

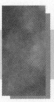

TABLE 27–6 *Relationship Between Blood Alcohol Levels and Behavior in a Nontolerant Drinker*

BLOOD ALCOHOL LEVELS	BLOOD ALCOHOL ACCUMULATION	BEHAVIOR
0.05 mg%	1–2 drinks	Changes in mood and behavior; judgment is impaired
0.10 mg%	5–6 drinks	Voluntary motor action becomes clumsy; **legal level of intoxication in most states**
0.20 mg%	10–12 drinks	Function of entire motor area of the brain is depressed, causing staggering and ataxia; emotional lability is present
0.30 mg%	15–18 drinks	Confusion; stupor
0.40 mg%	20–24 drinks	Coma
0.50 mg%	25–30 drinks	Death due to respiratory depression

TABLE 27-7 *Stimulants*

DRUG	INTOXICATION	OVERDOSE		WITHDRAWAL	
		Effects	Possible Treatments	Effects	Possible Treatments
Cocaine-crack (short-acting) *Note:* High obtained: snorted for 3 min; injected for 30 sec; smoked for 4–6 sec (crack) Average high lasts cocaine 15–30 min; crack 5–7 min	*Physical* Tachycardia Dilated pupils Elevated blood pressure Nausea and vomiting Insomnia *Psychological-perceptual* Assaultive Grandiose Impaired judgment Impaired social and occupational functioning Euphoria	Respiratory distress Ataxia Hyperpyrexia Convulsions Coma Stroke Myocardial infarction Death	Antipsychotics Medical and nursing management for Hyperpyrexia (ambient cooling) Convulsions (diazepam) Respiratory distress Cardiovascular shock Acidify urine (ammonium chloride for amphetamine)	Fatigue Depression Agitation Apathy Anxiety Sleepiness Disorientation Lethargy Craving	Antidepressants (desipramine) Dopamine agonist Bromocriptine
Amphetamines (long-acting) Dextroamphetamine Methamphetamine Ice (synthesized for street use)	Increased energy *Severe effects* Resembles paranoid schizophrenia Paranoia with delusions Psychosis Visual, auditory, and tactile hallucinations Severe to panic levels of anxiety Potential for violence NOTE: Paranoia and ideas of reference may persist for months afterward	Same as above	Same as above	Same as above	Same as above

Data from American Psychiatric Association (2000b). *Diagnostic and statistical manual of mental disorders* (4th ed. text revision) (DSM-IV-TR). Washington, DC: American Psychiatric Association Press; O'Connor P. G., Samet J. H., Stein M. D. (1994). Management of hospitalized drug users: Role of the internist. *American Journal of Medicine*, 96:551; Bell K (1992). Identifying the substance abuser in clinical practice. *Orthopedic Nursing*, 11(2):29.

coca bush. Crack is a cheap, widely available alkalinized form of cocaine. When crack is smoked, it takes effect in 4 to 6 seconds. Dependence on crack develops rapidly. The fleeting high obtained from crack (lasting 5 to 7 minutes) is followed by a period of deep depression that reinforces addictive behavior patterns and guarantees continued use of the drug.

Cocaine is classified as a schedule II substance—"high abuse potential with some recognized medical use." People who sniff cocaine have problems that relate to deterioration of the nasal passages: sores, hoarseness, and throat infections. Those who smoke the drug can have lung damage, upper gastrointestinal tract problems, and throat damage from the harsh smoke. Intravenous users may experience endocarditis, heart attacks, angina, and needle-related diseases, such as hepatitis and HIV.

Cocaine exerts two main effects on the body, both anesthetic and stimulant. As an anesthetic, it blocks the conduction of electrical impulses within the nerve cells that are involved in sensory transmissions, primarily pain. It also acts as a stimulant for both sexual arousal and violent behavior. Cocaine produces an imbalance of neurotransmitters (dopamine and norepinephrine) that may be responsible for many of the physical withdrawal symptoms reported by heavy chronic cocaine users: depression, paranoia, lethargy, anxiety, insomnia, nausea and vomiting, and sweating and chills—all signs of the body struggling to regain its normal chemical balance.

NICOTINE AND CAFFEINE. Most people ingest caffeine by way of coffee, tea, or cola drinks. People ingest coffee as a drug: "I've got to have two cups in the morning to function"; for social reasons: "Let's get together for coffee"; or as a reward: "After I finish this job, I'm going to take a coffee break."

Nicotine can act as a stimulant, depressant, or tranquilizer. Nicotine can also be chewed (smokeless tobacco), which adds cancer of the mouth to the list of dangers; cancer of the lungs is highly correlated with smoking tobacco. Nicotine is addicting, and treatments to comfortably withdraw without severe cravings are often unsuccessful. Wellbutrin (Zyban)

has been a successful treatment for many individuals during nicotine withdrawal.

OPIATES

This drug class includes opium, morphine, heroin, codeine, fentanyl and its analogs, methadone, and meperidine. Use of heroin by American teenagers is increasing according to national and statewide surveys (Schwartz 1998). Heroin is becoming cheaper and more potent, and novices are starting with nasal administration (Schwartz 1998). Table 27–8 lists signs and symptoms of intoxication, overdose, withdrawal, and possible treatments.

MARIJUANA (CANNABIS SATIVA)

Cannabis sativa is an Indian hemp plant. **Tetrahydrocannabinol (THC)** is the active ingredient found in the resin secreted from the flowering tops and leaves of the cannabis plant. THC has mixed depressant and hallucinogenic properties. Marijuana, the leaves of the cannabis plant, is generally smoked ("joint," "reefer," "roach"), but it can be ingested. It is the most widely used illicit drug in the United States. Desired effects include euphoria, detachment, and relaxation. Other effects include talkativeness, slowed perception of time, inappropriate hilarity, heightened sensitivity to external stimuli, and anxiety or paranoia. Long-term dependence on cannabis

---

TABLE 27–8 *Opiates*

DRUG	INTOXICATION	OVERDOSE Effects	OVERDOSE Possible Treatments	WITHDRAWAL Effects	WITHDRAWAL Possible Treatments
Opium (paregoric)	*Physical* Constricted pupils	Pupils may be dilated due to anoxia	Narcotic antagonist, e.g., naloxone	Yawning Insomnia	■ Methadone tapering ■ Clonidine-naltrexone
Heroin	Decreased respiration	Respiratory depression-arrest	(Narcan), quickly	Irritability	detoxification
Meperidine (Demerol)	Drowsiness		reverses central	Runny nose (rhinorrhea)	■ Buprenorphine substitution
Morphine	Decreased blood pressure	Coma	nervous system	Panic	stitution
Codeine	Slurred speech	Shock	depression	Diaphoresis	
Methadone (Dolophine)	Psychomotor retardation	Convulsions		Cramps	
Hydromorphone (Dilaudid)	*Psychological-perceptual* Initial euphoria followed	Death		Nausea-vomiting	
Fentanyl (Sublimaze)	by dysphoria and impairment of attention-judgment-memory			Muscle aches ("bone pain")	
Fentanyl analogs	Impaired judgment			Chills Fever Lacrimation Diarrhea	

Definition: An opiate is a derivative or synthetic that affects the central nervous system and the autonomic nervous system. Medically used primarily as an analgesic (pain killer). Consistent use causes tolerance and distressing withdrawal symptoms.

Data from American Psychiatric Association (2000b). *Diagnostic and statistical manual of mental disorders* (4th ed., text revised) (DSM-IV-TR). Washington, DC: American Psychiatric Association Press; O'Connor, P. G., Samet, J. H., and Stein, M. D. (1994). Management of hospitalized intravenous drug users: Role of the internist. *American Journal of Medicine*, 96:551; Bell K. (1992). Identifying the substance abuser in clinical practice. *Orthopedic Nursing* 11(2):29.

can result in lethargy, anhedonia, difficulty concentrating, and loss of memory for some people.

Overdose and withdrawal (other than craving) rarely occur. Medical indications exist for the use of THC (e.g., control of chemotherapy-induced nausea, reduced intraocular pressure in glaucoma, and appetite stimulation in AIDS wasting syndrome).

HALLUCINOGENS

Hallucinogens are drugs that alter one's mental state in a short period.

LSD AND LSD-LIKE DRUGS. LSD (lysergic acid diethylamide, also known as "acid"), **mescaline** (peyote), and **psilocybin** (magic mushroom) are hallucinogens. Mescaline and the mushroom *Psilocybe mexicana* (from which psilocybin is isolated) have been used for centuries in religious rites by Native Americans living in the southwestern United States and northern Mexico. The hallucinogenic experience produced by LSD is called a "trip."

PHENCYCLIDINE PIPERIDINE (PCP). PCP (phencyclidine piperidine) is also known as angel dust, horse tranquilizer, or peace pill. The route of administration plays a significant role in the severity of PCP intoxication. The onset of symptoms from oral ingestion occurs about 1 hour later. When taken intravenously, sniffed, or smoked, the onset of symptoms may occur within 5 minutes. The signs and symptoms of PCP intoxication range from acute anxiety to acute psychosis. The cardinal signs include a blank stare, ataxia, muscle rigidity, vertical and horizontal nystagmus, tendency toward violence, and generalized anesthesia that lessens the sensations of touch and pain, making staff interventions difficult. High doses may lead to hyperthermia, agitated and repetitive movements, chronic jerking of the extremities, hypertension, and kidney failure. Persons with PCP intoxication may become stuporous with their eyes open, may be comatose, or may experience status epilepticus or respiratory arrest (Table 27–9).

Suicidal ideation is always assessed, especially in cases of toxicity or coma. If the client appears to be suicidal, the nurse should determine whether previous suicide attempts have occurred. Information regarding suicide history of family members is also elicited.

Long-term use of PCP can result in long-term effects such as dulled thinking, lethargy, loss of impulse control, poor memory, and depression.

Inhalants

About 19% of adolescents in the United States say that they have sniffed inhalants—usually volatile solvents, such as spray paint, glue, cigarette lighter fluid, and propellant gases used in aerosols—at least once in their lives (Espeland 2000). Types of inhalants, signs of intoxication, and side effects are given in Table 27–10. Inhalant use may be an early marker of substance abuse and should be the focus of increased prevention and early diagnosis and treatment (Espeland 2000).

RAVE AND TECHNO DRUGS/DATE RAPE DRUGS

Raves or techno dances are all-night dance parties attended by large numbers of youth, sometimes in excess of 20,000 (Weir 2000). This phenomenon is international in scope. These techno dances are distinguished by hypnotic electric music and liberal use of techno drugs such as **ecstasy** (MDMA), **GHB** (gamma-hydroxybutyrate), and **ketamine.**

Ecstasy (3,4-methylenedioxymethamphetamine, MDMA, also called "Adam"), is a prototype of a class of substituted amphetamines that also includes MDA (methylenedioxyamphetamine, "Love") and MDE ("Eve"). These recreational drugs produce subjective effects resembling those of amphetamine and lysergic acid diethylamide, and in that sense, MDMA and similar drugs may represent a distinct category of drugs (entactogens) Jaffe 1999).

After taking a usual dose (100 to 150 mg) of MDMA, subjective side effects include euphoria, increased energy, increased self-confidence, increased sociability, and feeling close to people (Jaffe 1999; Liberg et al. 1998). Due to its psychostimulant and psychedelic effects, ecstasy and the others are increasingly abused especially within the rave subculture.

These are not innocent drugs, and adverse effects such as hyperthermia, rhabdomyolysis, acute renal failure, hepatotoxicity, depression, panic attacks, and psychosis may occur (Jaffe 1999, Liberg et al. 1998). Other reported toxicities include cardiovascular collapse, and a number of deaths have occurred. Morgan (2000) states there is growing evidence that chronic, heavy, recreational use of ecstasy is associated with sleep disorders, depressed mood, persistent elevation of anxiety, impulsiveness, and hostility as well as selective impairment of episodic memory, weakening memory, and attention.

The drugs most frequently used to facilitate a sexual assault (rape) are flunitrazepam (Rohypnol), a fast-acting benzodiazepine, and gamma-hydroxybutyrate and its congeners (Schwartz et al. 2000). Perpetrators use these drugs because they rapidly produce disinhibition and relaxation of voluntary muscles; they also cause the victim to have lasting anterograde amnesia for events that occur. Alcohol potentiates the effects of these drugs.

Self-Assessment

Although you may identify with, and have empathy for, clients addicted to caffeine or tobacco, your re-

TABLE 27–9   *Hallucinogens*

| DRUG | INTOXICATION | | OVERDOSE | |
	Physical	Psychological-Perceptual	Effects	Possible Treatments
Hallucinogens **Lysergic acid diethylamide (LSD)** **Mescaline (peyote)** **Psilocybin**	Pupils dilated Tachycardia Diaphoresis Palpitations Tremors Incoordination Elevated temperature, pulse, respiration	Fear of going crazy Paranoid ideas Marked anxiety-depression Synesthesia, e.g., colors are heard; sounds are seen Depersonalization Hallucinations occur although sensorium is clear Grandiosity, e.g., thinking one can fly	Psychosis Brain damage Death	Keep client in room with low stimuli—minimal light, sound, activity Have one person stay with client; reassure client, "talk down client" Speak slowly and clearly in low voice. Give diazepam or chloral hydrate for extreme anxiety/tension
Phencyclidine piperidine (PCP)	Vertical or horizontal nystagmus Increased blood pressure, pulse, and temperature Ataxia Muscle rigidity Seizures Blank stare Chronic jerking Agitated, repetitive movements Belligerence, assaultiveness, impulsiveness, Impaired judgment, impaired social and occupational functioning	*Severe effects* Hallucinations, paranoia Bizarre behaviors, e.g., barking like a dog, grimacing, repetitive chanting speech Regressive behavior **Violent bizarre behaviors** Very labile behaviors	Psychosis Possible hypertensive crisis/cardiovascular accident Respiratory arrest Hyperthermia Seizures	*If alert* *Caution:* Gastric lavage can lead to laryngeal spasms or aspiration Acidify urine (cranberry juice, ascorbic acid); in acute stage, ammonium chloride acidifies urine to help excrete drug from body—may continue for 10–14 days Room with minimal stimuli **Do *not* attempt to talk down!** Speak slowly, clearly, and in low voice ■ Diazepam ■ Haloperidol may be used for severe behavioral disturbance (*not* a phenothiazine) *Medical intervention for* Hyperthermia High blood pressure Respiratory distress Hypertension

Definition: A hallucinogen produces *abnormal mental phenomena* in the cognitive and perceptual spheres; for example, distortion in space and time, hallucinations, delusions (paranoid or grandiose), and synesthesia may occur.

Data from American Psychiatric Association (2000b). *Diagnostic and statistical manual of mental disorders* (4th ed., text revised) (DSM-IV-TR). Washington, DC: American Psychiatric Association Press; Bell K. (1992). Identifying the substance abuser in clinical practice. *Orthopedic Nursing*, 11(2):29.

sponses to clients who abuse substances may not be so empathetic. A client who has overdosed on heroin or cocaine, or who comes in with complications from ecstasy or other techno drugs, may be met with disapproval, intolerance, and condemnation or may be considered morally weak. Also, manipulative behaviors often seen in these clients may lead

you to feel angry and exploited. You might want to help but may perceive the client who abuses drugs to be willful, uncooperative, and unworkable.

In some areas of the United States, the recreational use of cocaine, marijuana, and amphetamine is so common that a nurse may view this occurrence of intoxication or overdose as normal and may not have much emotional reaction. This attitude is a detrimental as strong emotional disapproval because the nurse may underestimate the importance of supportive measures and client education and the need for follow-up psychotherapeutic intervention.

Perhaps the most detrimental attitude in nurses and other health care workers is that of enabling. Enabling is supporting, or denying the seriousness of, the client's physical or psychological substance dependence. Behaviors that signal enabling by the nurse include

■ Encouraging denial by agreeing that the client only drinks or takes drugs socially or when he or she is a little nervous
■ Ignoring cues to possible dependency by steering away from drugs to topics that are more comfortable for the nurse (e.g., anxiety or depression)
■ Demonstrating sympathy for the client's reasons (e.g., work, family, or financial problems) for abusing drugs rather than pointing out that these difficulties are often the result of—not the cause of—substance abuse
■ Preaching that the problem can be overcome by

will power, thus minimizing the fact that the person is physically or psychologically chemically dependent and has lost control over the use of the drug

To come to a true personal understanding means that you must examine your own attitudes, feelings, and beliefs about addicts and addiction. It often means that you must examine your own substance use and that of others, and this is not always pleasant work.

A history of substance abuse in a nurse's own family can overshadow the nurse's interactions with addicts. The negative or positive experiences a nurse has had with addicted family members can influence interpersonal interactions with present or future clients.

Therefore, it is important that you attend to personal feelings that arise when you work with addicts. All health care professionals require supervision if they are not experienced in this area. Nurses who do not attend to, and work through, expected negative feelings that arise during treatment have power struggles with the clients and the therapeutic

TABLE 27–10   Drug Information: Inhalants

DRUG	INTOXICATION	SIDE EFFECT-OVERDOSE	TREATMENT
Volatile Solvents (Gases or liquids that vaporize at room temperature) ■ Butane ■ Paint thinner ■ Paint and wax removers ■ Propellant gases used in aerosols, e.g., whipped cream dispensers, hair spray ■ Airplane glue ■ Nail polish remover ■ Dry cleaning fluid	Excitation followed by drowsiness, disinhibition, staggering, lightheadedness, and agitation	Damage to the nervous system Death	Support affected systems
Nitrates ■ Room deodorizers (less common because products containing butyl and propyl were banned in 1991)	Enhance sexual pleasure		Neurological symptoms may respond to vitamin B_{12} and folate.
Anesthetics ■ Gas—especially nitrous oxide ■ Liquid ■ Local	Giggling, laughter Euphoria	Chronic users may experience polyneuropathy and myelopathy	

From National Institute on Drug Abuse Research Report Series (1993). *Inhalant abuse* (NIH Publication No. 94-3818). Washington, D.C.: U.S. Department of Health and Human Services.

process is generally ineffective. Cultural sensitivity and competence are also important when working with addicted clients (Allen 1998). But what about the nurse who has a substance abuse problem?

CHEMICALLY IMPAIRED NURSE

Substance dependency in nurses is a serious problem for both the nurse and those under the nurse's care. Nurses have a 32% to 50% higher rate of chemical dependency than the general population. Among practicing nurses, estimates of nurses who are chemically dependent range from 10% to 20%. Helping the chemically impaired nurse is difficult but not impossible. The choices for actions are varied, and the only choice that is clearly wrong is to do nothing.

Without intervention or treatment, the problems associated with the chemical dependency escalate, and the potential for patient harm increases. Without intervention, co-workers are left feeling helpless, hopeless, and staff morale continues to plummet. Without intervention, the impaired nurse is not forced to seek treatment and perhaps save his or her own life or professional career (Smith et al. 1998).

Some early indicators of a substance abuse problem that can alert peers (nurses) and nurse-managers who are sensitive to job performance problems include

- Changing a life style to focus on activities that encourage substance use
- Showing inconsistency between statements and actions
- Displaying increasing irritability
- Projecting blame on others
- Isolating oneself from social contacts
- Showing deteriorating physical appearance
- Having frequent episodes of vaguely described illness
- Having frequent tardiness and absenteeism
- Manipulating possession of the narcotic keys for a particular shift (e.g., night shift)
- Having deepening depression

Often, the impaired nurse volunteers to work additional shifts to be nearer to the source of the drug. The nurse may leave the unit frequently or spend a lot of time in the bathroom. When the impaired nurse is on duty, more clients may complain that their pain is unrelieved by their narcotic analgesic or that they are unable to sleep, despite getting sedative medications. Increases in inaccurate drug counts and vial breakage may occur.

Once indicators of impaired practice are observed, clear and concise documentation is vital (specific dates, times, events, consequences). The documentation needs to be all factual. If possible, having an-

other co-worker witness the impaired nurse's actions and behaviors provides validation.

Once there is clear documentation, it needs to be reported to the nurse-manager. Intervention is the responsibility of the nurse-manager; however, clear documentation by co-workers is crucial. The nurse-manager's major concerns are with job performance and client safety. Once the nurse-manager has been informed, the legal and ethical responsibilities for in-house reporting have been met (Smith et al. 1998). If the impaired nurse continues to remain in the situation, and the same problems persist, and no action is taken by the nurse-manager, then the information needs to be taken to the next level in the chain of command (Smith et al. 1998). These measures can prevent harm to clients under the impaired nurse's care and can save a colleague's professional career or even life.

Reporting an impaired colleague is not easy, even though it is our responsibility. In order not to "see" what is going on, nurses may deny or rationalize, thus **enabling** the impaired nurse to potentially endanger lives while becoming sicker and more isolated. Box 27–4 can be used as a guide to evaluate one's own coping styles.

Referral to a treatment program should always be an option. Programs for chemically dependent nurses have been developed in some states in response to a policy statement issued by the American Nurses' Association. Some state boards of nursing allow impaired nurses to avoid disciplinary action if they seek treatment. The aim of these programs is to protect clients and to keep the nurse in active practice (perhaps with limitations) or to return the nurse to practice after suspension and professional help. Nurses who continue to show signs of impaired practice should not be returned to direct patient care.

Vignette

- *Elyse, a 34-year-old recently divorced registered nurse, is brought into the hospital emergency department by two friends who had gone to her apartment after a frantic call from her. When she didn't answer the door, they had the superintendent let them in. They state that they found Elyse lying on the couch with a half-empty bottle of vodka as well as an empty bottle of diazepam pills. When her friends tried to talk to Elyse, she responded with slurred speech. When she attempted to walk, her gait was unsteady. The friends report that when they questioned Elyse about her condition, she became extremely irritable. They say that as they sat with Elyse, they became increasingly alarmed and took her to the emergency room. The following initial interview takes place there after she is treated and determined to be stable.*

BOX 27-4   *Have I Enabled?*

Have I

Excused	or ignored behaviors in a peer that may be suggestive of impairment and justified those behaviors as "just having a bad day" or "stress"?
Never	told the supervisor about possible behaviors indicative of impairment that I observed because I was afraid of being wrong and did not want anyone to get angry at me?
Accepted	responsibility for my colleague's unfinished work and at times attempted to counsel and solve his or her problem?
Believed	that nurses do not use drugs or alcohol to the point of practice impairment and that substance use can be stopped at any time unless the person is morally weak?
Liked	to use drugs or alcohol myself to relax or enjoy with friends? I do not want anyone to look at me. In fact, I have used a few discontinued drugs from work myself. Doesn't everyone?
Exonerated	a peer's irresponsible actions by covering for attendance or tardiness? Have I co-signed wastes I have not truly witnessed or corrected the narcotic count to account for a discrepancy?
Defended	a colleague when it was suggested there may be a problem with impairment?

From Smith, L., Taylor, B. B., and Hughes, T. L. (1998). Effective peer response to impaired nursing practice. *Nursing Clinics of North America*, 33(1):105–118.

DIALOGUE	THERAPEUTIC TOOL/ COMMENT
Nurse: Elyse, I get the impression that life must have been getting very difficult for you lately.	Validating and empathizing
Elyse: (Silence) . . . I don't think you would understand.	
Nurse: I guess sometimes it feels as if no one understands, but I would like to try.	Reflecting/empathizing
Elyse: At times . . . I feel I can't go on any more . . . so many losses.	
Nurse: Loss is difficult. Elyse, tell me about your losses.	Encouraging the client to share her painful feelings
Elyse: My brother's sudden death . . . We were so close . . . I depended on him so much.	
Nurse: It must have been difficult for you to lose him so suddenly.	Empathizing
Elyse: (Silence) . . . No one knows . . . then Harry, he left . . . (*Elyse starts to cry*)	
Nurse: Tell me what you are feeling right now.	Encouraging the expression of feelings while feelings are close to the surface
Elyse: I don't know . . . angry maybe . . . why does everyone leave me? . . . Oh, I hate them . . . Oh, I wish I had a Valium now . . .	
Nurse: And what does the Valium do to help you?	Beginning to explore the drug dependence in a gently nonthreatening manner

Elyse becomes less defensive as time goes on and seems to relate best to the nurse. The nurse tells Elyse about a Narcotics Anonymous (NA) group that is made up of chemically impaired people from the health care professions. She states that substance abuse disorders among nurses and doctors are a widespread, recognized problem. Elyse has a tendency to minimize her drug dependence. Elyse's nurse-manager and a representative from the Employee Assistance Program (EAP) discuss Elyse's dependence on substances.

Elyse agrees to go for evaluation and treatment. She also agrees to take her vacation time and some leave of absence and be evaluated at a later date. Elyse understands that if she is successful with treatment, she will be monitored for a period of time by nursing management and others when she returns to caring for patients.

Assessment Guidelines

ASSESSMENT GUIDELINES: CHEMICALLY IMPAIRED CLIENTS

1. Is immediate medical attention warranted for a severe or major withdrawal syndrome? For example, alcohol and sedatives can be life threatening during a major withdrawal.
2. Is the client experiencing an overdose to a drug/ alcohol that warrants immediate medical attention? For example, opioids or depressants can cause respiratory depression, coma, and death. Consult Tables 27–6 and Tables 27–8 to 27–10 for symptoms of drug overdose and treatments.
3. Does the client have any physical complications related to drug abuse (e.g., AIDS, abscess, tachycardia, hepatitis)?
4. Does the client have suicidal thoughts, or indicate through verbal or nonverbal cues a potential for self-destructive behaviors?
5. Does the client seem interested in doing something about his or her drug/alcohol problem?
6. Do the client and family have information about community resources for alcohol/drug withdrawal (detoxify safely) and treatment, for example:
   ■ Support groups
   ■ Treatment for psychiatric comorbidities
   ■ Family treatment to address enabling behaviors, and provide support for families and friends

NURSING DIAGNOSIS

Appropriate nursing diagnoses depend on accurate assessment. Whereas DSM-IV-TR criteria emphasize patterns of use and physical symptoms, nursing diagnoses identify how dependence on substances of abuse interferes with a person's ability to meet the activities and demands of daily living.

Nursing diagnoses for clients with psychoactive substance use disorders are many and varied as a result of the large range of physical and psychological effects of drug abuse or dependence on the user and his or her family. Potential nursing diagnoses for people with substance use disorders are listed in Table 27–11.

OUTCOME CRITERIA

WITHDRAWAL

■ Remains free from injury while withdrawing from substance

■ Remains free from injury during multiple withdrawals from drugs
■ Evidence of stable condition within 72 hours

INITIAL AND ACTIVE DRUG TREATMENT

■ Maintains abstinence from chemical substances
■ Demonstrates acceptance for own behavior at the end of 3 months
■ Continues attendance for treatment and maintenance of sobriety (e.g., AA, CA, NA, or group therapy, cognitive-behavioral therapy, or other)
■ Attends a relapse prevention program during active course of treatment
■ Verbalizes cues or situations that pose increased risk of drug use
■ States he or she has a stable group of drug-free friends and socializes with them at least three times a week
■ Demonstrates new skills in dealing with troubling feelings (anger, loneliness, cravings, anxiety)

HEALTH MAINTENANCE

■ Demonstrates responsibility in taking care of health care needs as evidenced by keeping appointments and adherence to medications and treatment
■ Client's medical tests will demonstrate a reduced incidence of medical complications related to substance abuse after 6 months.

PLANNING

Planning care requires attention to the client's social status, income, ethnic background, sex, age, substance use history, and current condition. It is safest to propose abstinence as a treatment goal for all addicts. Abstinence is strongly related to good work adjustments, positive health status, comfortable interpersonal relationships, and general social stability. Planning must also address the client's major psychological, social, and medical problems as well as the substance-using behavior. Involvement of appropriate family members is essential.

Unfortunately, deterioration in a person's social status and social relations often occurs as a result of addiction. Job demotion or loss of job, with resultant reduced or nonexistent income, may occur. Meeting basic needs for food, shelter, and clothing is thereby hampered. Marriages and other close relationships deteriorate and fail, and the person is often left alone and isolated. The lack of interpersonal and social supports is a complicating factor in treatment planning for the addict.

TABLE 27-11 *Potential Nursing Diagnoses: Substance Abuse*

SIGNS AND SYMPTOMS	NURSING DIAGNOSES
Vomiting, diarrhea, poor nutritional and fluid intake	**Imbalanced Nutrition: Less than body requirements** **Deficient Fluid Volume**
Audiovisual hallucinations, impaired judgment, memory deficits, cognitive impairments related to substance intoxication/withdrawal (problem solving, ability to attend to tasks, grasp ideas)	**Disturbed Thought Processes** **Disturbed Sensory Perception**
Changes in sleep-wake cycle, interference with stage IV sleep, not sleeping or long periods of sleeping related to effects of or withdrawal from substance	**Disturbed Sleep Pattern**
Lack of self-care (hygiene, grooming). Not caring for basic health needs	**Ineffective Health Maintenance** **Self-Care Deficit** **Nonadherence to Health Care Regimen**
Feelings of hopelessness, inability to change, feelings of worthlessness, life has no meaning or future	**Hopelessness** **Spiritual Distress** **Situational Low Self-Esteem** **Chronic Low Self-Esteem** **Risk for Violence: Self-Directed** **Risk for Suicide**
Family crises and family pain, ineffective parenting, emotional neglect of others, increased incidence of physical and sexual abuse toward others, increased self-hate projected to others	**Interrupted Family Processes** **Impaired Parenting** **Risk for Violence: Other-Directed**
Excessive substance abuse affects all areas of a person's life: loses friends, poor job performance, illness rates increase, prone to accidents and overdoses	**Ineffective Coping** **Impaired Verbal Communication** **Social Isolation** **Risk for Loneliness** **Anxiety** **Risk for Suicide**
Increased health problems related to substance used and route of use, as well as overdose	**Activity Intolerance** **Ineffective Airway Clearance** **Ineffective Breathing Pattern** **Impaired Oral Mucous Membrane** **Risk for Infection** **Decreased Cardiac Output** **Sexual Dysfunction**
Total preoccupation and time consumed with taking and withdrawing from drug	**Delayed Growth and Development** **Ineffective Coping** **Impaired Social Interaction** **Dysfunctional Family Processes: Substance Dependence**

INTERVENTION

The aim of treatment is self-responsibility, not compliance. A major challenge is improving treatment effectiveness by matching subtypes of clients to specific types of treatment. Although addicts share some characteristics and dynamics, significant differences exist within the addict population in regard to physiological, psychological, and sociocultural processes. These differences influence the recovery process, either positively or negatively.

Often, the choice of inpatient or outpatient care depends on cost and whether insurance coverage is available. Outpatient programs work best for employed substance abusers who have an involved social support system. People who have no support and structure in their day often do better in inpatient programs when these programs are available.

In addition, neuropsychological deficits have been associated with long-term alcohol abuse. Impairment has been found in abstract reasoning ability, ability to use feedback in learning new concepts, attention and concentration spans, cognitive flexibility, and subtle memory functions. These deficits undoubtedly have an impact on the process of alcoholism treatment.

At all levels of practice, the nurse can play an important role in the intervention process by recognizing the signs of substance abuse in both the client and the family and by knowing available resources to help with the problem.

Communication Guidelines

Communication strategies involve working with behaviors that almost all substance abusers have in common, including dysfunctional anger, manipulation, impulsiveness, and grandiosity. The nurse's ability to develop a warm, accepting relationship with an addicted client can assist the client in feeling safe enough to start looking at problems with some degree of openness and honesty. If the nurse has not worked through strong negative feelings related to the use of substances, the nurse should refer the client to another staff person who has dealt with these issues and can begin promoting recovery. The client-counselor relationship is often considered to be more important than the type of treatment pursued (Franklin and Frances 1999).

Franklin and Frances (1999) identify some characteristics of a counselor that can facilitate work with substance users:

- Knowledge of addiction
- Ability to form caring relationships
- Capacity to tolerate anxiety and depression
- Persistence and patience
- Capacity to listen
- Honesty

Principles behind interventions include the following:

1. *Expect abstinence/sobriety.* The distortions, memory loss, and confusion that occur as a result of drug intoxication make communication and intervention ineffective when the person is intoxicated.
2. *Individualize goals and interventions.*
3. *Set limits on behavior* and on conditions under which treatment will continue.
4. *Support and redirect defenses* rather than attempting to remove them.
5. *Recognize that the process of recovery is carried out in stages.*

6. *Look for therapeutic leverage.* Make abstinence and sobriety worthwhile for the substance abuser (e.g., keeping one's job, family, friends).

The following dialogue demonstrates the use of therapeutic leverage in addressing the role of drug use in the client's life. It is presented as a dialogue between a nurse and a 17-year-old young man. His parents are divorced, and his father abuses him when drinking. He was picked up three times during the preceding 7 months for possession of cocaine.

DIALOGUE	THERAPEUTIC TOOL/ COMMENT
Nurse: I understand you entered the treatment program yesterday afternoon following your court appearance.	Placing the event in time and sequence, validating the precipitating event
Frank: Yeah—it was my Dad's idea.	
Nurse: Well, what do you think of the idea?	Encouraging evaluation (actions first, thoughts, then feelings).
Frank: I don't like it. I don't need this place. I'm not a junkie—I just use cocaine, that's all. I can handle it.	
Nurse: From what I've heard, your involvement with cocaine has gotten you into trouble.	Pointing out realities
Frank: Yeah, well, I guess I can't deny that . . . but I still don't think I need this place.	
Nurse: Are you saying that you don't think you need a treatment program?	Validating the client's perception
Frank: Well, I don't know, I guess maybe I am messed up a bit.	
Nurse: "Messed up."	Restating
Frank: Yeah.	
Nurse: What is one thing about you that's messed up?	Encouraging client to be specific rather than global
Frank: *(Silence)* I guess I feel like I don't belong anywhere.	
Nurse: Talk more about that.	Clarification

A useful tool for helping the resistant addict develop a willingness to engage in treatment is known as the intervention. The concept behind the intervention is that addiction is a progressive illness and rarely goes into remission without outside help. The steps in an intervention are outlined in Box 27–5.

Intervention Strategies

PRIMARY PREVENTION

Primary prevention through health teaching can have an important impact on how youngsters and adolescents choose to solve problems and relate interpersonally. Elderly individuals who are experiencing stressful life events are often at risk. Targeting this population is an approach to preventing

alcohol abuse in the elderly (Cowart and Sutherland 1998).

Young people who participate in groups such as scouting, 4-H clubs, school clubs, and organized church activities are at a lower risk for substance abuse. Activities such as these help develop self-confidence and self-esteem in young people. Part-time job placement can be an important alternative to substance abuse. Earning money on one's own can increase feelings of self-worth and confidence.

Primary prevention of HIV infection in the drug population is facilitated by needle exchange programs, in which addicts return their used needles for sterile ones. One of three people with AIDS in the United States is an intravenous drug user or the sexual partner of an intravenous drug user. Reducing needle sharing can reduce the spread of HIV. This is a controversial issue in many cities. Nurses may support this intervention in a public health issue to address the AIDS problem health crisis.

BRIEF INTERVENTIONS

Use of brief interventions to effect behavior change allows the nurse to take advantage of any interaction with a substance-abusing client and use it as an opportunity for managing associated behaviors. Key interventions can be remembered by using the acronym, FRAMES. The elements are (Dyehouse and Sommers 1998; Fingfeld 1999).

■ Feedback
■ Responsibility
■ Advice
■ Menu (options)
■ Empathy
■ Self-efficacy

A case manager focuses on these elements when conducting a comprehensive needs assessment to (1) identify presenting problems, (2) develop an individualized plan including client goals and a plan to reach those goals, (3) link clients with various treatment providers, (4) monitor the treatment process and its progress, and (5) serve as the client's advocate when needed (Allen 1998).

Motivational interviewing is a communication technique designed to help patients identify and acknowledge substance abuse behaviors and to move toward cessation. Motivational interviewing relies on nonconfrontational approaches to integrate behavior change (Compton et al. 1999). Inherent in this approach is (1) acceptance facilitates change and (2) ambivalence is normal. Five general principles to motivate change include

1. Express empathy
2. Develop discrepancy

Box 27–5   Steps in the Intervention

1. All the people concerned about, and affected by, the person's drinking are gathered together to present their case. The intervention must be rehearsed before it is actually carried out, usually with the support and guidance of a counselor.
2. Specific evidence related to the drinking is presented by each person, and it is written down so that each person does not have to rely on memory in a tense situation.
3. Timing must be right:

   ■ There must be current evidence available.
   ■ It must take place after a crisis is precipitated by alcohol use and *not* when the person is intoxicated or in severe withdrawal.

4. The intervention requires privacy. It is held in a place where no interruptions can occur.
5. Anticipate the use of defenses. Do not react to them.
6. Demonstrate genuine, but firm, concern.
7. Understand alcoholism as a disease.
8. Present treatment alternatives.
9. Prepare responses to possible outcomes. The goal is to get the affected person treatment. If the alcoholic person agrees to get treatment, then he or she is taken immediately to a detoxification unit, where arrangements have been previously made. If the person refuses, then family members state that his or her decision must force them to make decisions of their own because they are no longer willing to live with the alcoholic person's behavior.

Adapted from Johnson, V. E. (1986). *Intervention: How to help someone who doesn't want help.* Minneapolis: Johnson Institute.

3. Avoid argumentation
4. "Roll" with resistance
5. Support self-efficacy

Psychotherapy

Nurses with advanced training may be involved in psychotherapy with substance-using clients. Psychotherapy assists clients in identifying and using alternative coping mechanisms to reduce reliance on substances. Eventually, psychotherapy can assist recovering addicts to become increasingly comfortable with sobriety.

Evidence-based practice and data indicate that cognitive-behavioral therapies, psychodynamic/interpersonal therapies, group and family therapies, and participation in self-help groups are all effective with selected substance use disorders (APA 2000a).

Confidentiality must be maintained throughout therapy except when this conflicts with events that require mandatory reporting (e.g., child abuse).

Many critical issues arise during the first 6 months of sobriety. These include the following:

■ Physical changes take place as the body adapts to functioning without substances.
■ Numerous signals occur in the client's internal and external world that previously were cues to drinking and drug use. Different responses to these cues need to be learned.
■ Emotional responses (feelings that were formerly diluted with substances) are now experienced full strength. Because they are so unfamiliar, they can produce anxiety.
■ Responses of family and co-workers to the client's new behavior must be addressed. Sobriety disrupts a system, and everyone in that system needs to adjust to the change.
■ New coping skills must be developed to prevent relapse and ensure prolonged sobriety.

Psychotherapy needs to be directive, open and honest, and caring. The therapeutic process involves teaching the client to identify the physical and emotional changes that are occurring in the here and now. The nurse-therapist can then assist in the problem-solving process.

INDIVIDUAL THERAPY

Individual psychotherapy may be a significant and sometimes essential contribution to the recovery process. Often, the best time for a recovering alcoholic to engage in insight psychotherapy is after 2 to 5 years of sobriety—once defenses have been loosened. Therapy can play an important role in relapse prevention.

RELAPSE PREVENTION

Relapses are common during a person's recovery. The goal of relapse prevention is to help the person learn from those situations so that periods of sobriety can be lengthened over time and so that lapses and relapses are not viewed as total failure. Relapse can result in a renewed and refined change effort.

Vignette

■ Bill, *a 20-year-old single man, is brought to the emergency department in a coma. He is accompanied by his mother, with whom Bill lives in a small apartment. Bill had been in his room at home. When his mother was not able to arouse him, she dialed 911 for an ambulance. A syringe and some white powder were found next to Bill.*

Bill's breathing is labored, and his pupils are constricted. Vital signs are taken; his blood pressure is 60/40 mm Hg, and his pulse is 132. Bill's situation is determined to be life threatening.

Bill's mother is extremely distressed, but she is able to report to the staff that Bill has a substance abuse problem and had been taking heroin for 6 months before entering a methadone maintenance program.

It is determined at this point to administer a narcotic antagonist, and naloxone is given intramuscularly. After this, Bill's breathing improves, and he responds to verbal stimuli.

Bill's mother later tells staff that Bill has been in the methadone maintenance program for the past year but has not attended the program or received his methadone for the past week. At their urging, she calls the program, which arranges to send an outreach worker, Mr. Rodriguez, to talk to her and Bill. Bill makes an appointment with Mr. Rodriguez for the following Monday.

Mr. Rodriguez knows that Bill's future ultimately rests with Bill. On Monday, Mr. Rodriguez talks to Bill regarding Bill's perceptions of his situation, where Bill wants to go, and what Bill thinks he needs to get there.

DIALOGUE	THERAPEUTIC TOOL/ COMMENT
Mr. Rodriguez: I was in the emergency room Friday afternoon when you were brought in by ambulance.	Placing the event in time and sequence, validating the precipitating event
Bill: Were you? I guess a lot of people thought it was over for me.	
Mr. Rodriguez: It certainly looked quite serious.	Emphasizing the reality—prevents minimizing situation

Bill: Yeah. I should never have left the program. I was doing better, and I just didn't think I needed it anymore.

Mr. Rodriguez: You said you were doing well.   Reflecting

Bill: Yeah. I had a job, and I was beginning to save some money. Wow! I can't believe I blew this whole thing.

Mr. Rodriguez: I don't know that you really did. Your counselor for the program phoned your doctor this morning to find out how you were doing.   Pointing out reality

Bill: Do you think they will take me back?

Mr. Rodriguez: Why don't we talk some more, and after we finish, I'll speak with the other staff about your situation. If you would like to get back into the program, you can call your counselor and we'll support your decision.   Gathering information

---

After reviewing Bill's history, the health care team decides that the self-help, abstinence-oriented recovery treatment might be the most helpful program. Bill has not been taking drugs a long time, he has a job, and he appears motivated. Naltrexone (Trexan) will be given in conjunction with relapse prevention training and regular attendance at Narcotics Anonymous meetings

---

General strategies for relapse prevention are cognitive and behavioral: recognizing and learning how to avoid or cope with threats to recovery; changing life style; learning how to participate fully in society without drugs; and securing help from other people, or social support. Box 27–6 identifies strategies that are instrumental in relapse prevention.

GROUP THERAPY

Group therapy has been helpful for many people recovering from addiction. The advantages of group therapy are

■ Social isolation is decreased.
■ Newly recovering addicts have role models in people with longer histories of sobriety.

■ Addicts are encouraged to seek support and encouragement from a variety of people.
■ The therapist can observe the interpersonal behavior of the clients without always being directly involved.

Groups can be closed or open, homogeneous or mixed, education oriented or therapy oriented. Cli-

BOX 27–6 *Relapse Prevention Strategies*

BASICS

1. Keep the program simple at first; 40% to 50% of clients who abuse substances have mild to moderate cognitive problems while actively using.
2. Review instructions with health team members.
3. Use a notebook and write down important information and telephone numbers.

SKILLS

Take advantage of cognitive-behavioral therapy to increase your coping skills. Identify which important life skills are needed

1. Which situations do you have difficulty handling?
2. Which situations are you managing more effectively?
3. In which situations would you like to develop more skills to act more effectively?

RELAPSE PREVENTION GROUPS

Become a member of a relapse prevention group. These groups work on

1. Rehearsing stressful situations using a variety of techniques.
2. Finding ways to deal with current problems or ones that are likely to arise as you become drug free.
3. Providing role models to help you make necessary life changes.

INCREASE PERSONAL INSIGHT

Therapy—group, individual, or family therapy—can help you gain insight and control over a variety of psychological concerns, for example:

1. What drives your addictions?
2. What constitutes a healthy supportive relationship?
3. Increasing your sense of self and self-worth.
4. What does your addictive substance give you that you think you need and cannot find otherwise?

Adapted from Zerce, K. J. (1999). *Women's mental health in primary care* (pp. 94–95). Philadelphia: WB Saunders. Reprinted with permission.

ents should be screened for admission to the group, and the therapist should maintain good record keeping throughout. Ground rules must be developed that include commitments to the following points:

- Minimal stay in the group
- Expectations of regular attendance or advance notice of absences
- Advance notice to the group if the client is considering leaving
- Abstinence and willingness to talk about fears of drinking or actual lapses should they occur
- Communication about other difficult issues in the client's life
- Communication about group dynamics
- Confidentiality

Goals for therapy include

- Maintaining sobriety
- Developing motivation to continue to grow and change
- Recognizing and identifying behavior patterns that led to drinking
- Learning new ways to handle old problems
- Developing an emergency plan for high-risk situations that might lead to relapse
- Recognizing and identifying feelings (especially guilt, anger, depression, fear)
- Learning to enjoy life without psychoactive substances
- Physical exercise (Ermalinski et al. 1997)

FAMILY THERAPY

Family therapy for substance abusers is based on the premise that the addiction is a family illness because all members are affected. Family members of substance abusers lack trust in each other, lack nurturing closeness, and inadequately solve problems. Children become used to extra and inappropriate responsibilities. Parental role models are distorted. In fact, family equilibrium is established around the substance use. Therefore, removal of the substance-using behavior becomes a threat.

As with any form of therapy, abstinence must be a goal. The family must begin to learn healthy ways to solve problems. Children of substance users are at high risk for developing their own addiction. This risk should be discussed openly at family therapy sessions.

Family members are usually concerned about the client's return to substance use. Members frequently walk on eggshells, not talking about substance use or other problems in an attempt to prevent a relapse. Ongoing therapy helps family members change roles as the need for control is lessened.

(Spouses frequently are reluctant to give up the position of power they had when their spouse was intoxicated.) Responsibility needs to be renegotiated. Children's roles and changes in behaviors also need to be examined.

MARITAL THERAPY

For the married couple, issues about time spent at home and about sex are prominent. The substance-abusing client may not have much libido as she or he begins to recover. Sex is not a paramount urge. Having felt deprived in many areas, the spouse may want gratification of unmet needs soon after recovery begins. Couples need further education in the recovery process to deal with major changes in marital functioning. For example, the wife may not understand the anger of the recovering husband. She may balk at his attendance at 12-step meetings or his kindness to people he meets there. She may feel rejected and not needed. These issues predominate in the early months of recovery.

SELF-HELP GROUPS FOR CLIENT AND FAMILY

Counseling and support should be encouraged for all families with a drug-dependent member. Al-Anon and Al-a-Teen are self-help groups that offer support and guidance for adults and teenagers, respectively, in families with a chemically dependent member. Others include Adult Children of Alcoholics (AcoA), Pills Anonymous (PA), and Narcotics Anonymous (NA), to name but a few.

TWELVE-STEP PROGRAMS

The most effective treatment modalities for all addictions have been the 12-step programs. Alcoholics Anonymous (AA) is the prototype of all 12-step programs that were subsequently developed for any number and types of addictions. Three basic concepts are fundamental to all 12-step programs:

1. Individuals with addictive disorders are powerless over their addiction, and their lives are unmanageable.
2. Although individuals with addictive disorders are not responsible for their disease, they are responsible for their recovery.
3. Individuals can no longer blame people, places, and things for their addiction; they must face their problems and their feelings.

The 12 steps are considered the core of treatment (Box 27–7). Using the 12 steps is often referred to as "working the steps." They are designed to help a person refrain from addictive behaviors as well as to foster individual change and growth. They offer the behavioral, cognitive, and dynamic structure needed in recovery. In addition to AA, other 12-step pro-

Box 27–7 *The Twelve Steps of Alcoholics Anonymous*

1. We admitted we were powerless over alcohol—that our lives had become unmanageable.
2. Came to believe that a power greater than ourselves could restore us to sanity.
3. Made a decision to turn our will and our lives over to the care of God **as we understood Him.**
4. Made a searching and fearless moral inventory of ourselves.
5. Admitted to God, to ourselves, and to another human being the exact nature of our wrongs.
6. Were entirely ready to have God remove all these defects of character.
7. Humbly asked Him to remove our shortcomings.
8. Made a list of all persons we had harmed, and became willing to make amends to them all.
9. Made direct amends to such people whenever possible, except when to do so would injure them or others.
10. Continued to take personal inventory, and when we were wrong, promptly admitted it.
11. Sought through prayer and meditation to improve our conscious contact with God, **as we understood Him,** praying only for knowledge of His will for us and the power to carry that out.
12. Having had a spiritual awakening as the result of these steps, we tried to carry His message to alcoholics, and to practice these principles in all our affairs.

The Twelve Steps are reprinted with permission of Alcoholics Anonymous World Services Inc. Permission to reprint the Twelve Steps does not mean that AA has reviewed or approved the contents of this publication, nor that AA agrees with the views expressed herein. AA is a program of recovery from alcoholism *only*—use of the Twelve Steps in connection with programs and activities that are patterned after AA, but that address other problems, or in any other non–AA context, does not imply otherwise.

grams include Pills Anonymous, Narcotics Anonymous, Cocaine Anonymous (CA), and Valium Anonymous. Self-help groups help family members deal with many common issues. Al-Anon and Narc-Anon are support groups for spouses and friends of alcoholics or addicts. Al-Anon, like AA, Al-a-Teen, and Adult Children of Alcoholics work through a combination of educational and operational principles centered around acceptance of the disease model of addiction, including pragmatic methods for avoiding enabling behaviors.

Milieu Therapy

Most addicted people do not come readily for treatment. The motivation of an addicted client, like that of anyone else who is facing changes in life style, is mixed. Whatever motivation is there can be encouraged. It is part of the nurse's job to help clients become receptive to the possibility of change. This can occur in the context of the therapeutic environment.

Substance abusers often seem indifferent to the destruction they bring on themselves and their families. They also show marked dependency on others (most often loved ones) to solve their problems. This characteristic can give the family and friends an effective means of motivating the substance-abusing person toward treatment. When family and friends refuse to solve the person's problems, the individual is forced to face the consequences of his or her behavior.

RESIDENTIAL PROGRAMS

Residential treatment programs are best suited for individuals who have a long history of antisocial behavior. The goal of treatment is to effect a change in life style, including abstinence, development of social skills, and elimination of antisocial behavior. Follow-up studies suggest that clients who stay 90 days or longer exhibit a significant decrease in illicit drug use and recorded arrests and an increase in legitimate employment. Length of stay increases with family-focused treatment (McComish et al. 2000). Synanon, Phoenix House, and Odyssey House are three of the more familiar names among the 300-plus therapeutic communities in the United States.

INTENSIVE OUTPATIENT PROGRAMS

Most treatment for substance-abusing clients takes place in the community. Clinical Pathway 27–1 is an example of the steps addicted people follow in an intensive outpatient program, including a variety of psychotherapeutic and pharmacologic interventions along with behavioral monitoring.

Intensive outpatient treatment programs are becoming more popular because they are viewed as flexible, diverse, cost-effective, and responsive to the specific individual needs of a person.

OUTPATIENT DRUG-FREE PROGRAMS AND EMPLOYEE ASSISTANCE PROGRAMS

Outpatient drug-free programs are better geared to the polydrug-abusing or alcoholic client rather than to the client who is heavily addicted to heroin. These centers may offer vocational education and placement, counseling, and individual or group psychotherapy. Employee assistance programs (EAP) have been developed to provide the delivery of

CLINICAL PATHWAY 27–1   *Intensive Outpatient Program for Substance Abuse*

	FIRST 4 WEEKS	NEXT 6 WEEKS	NEXT 2 WEEKS
Assessment	Evaluation (CAC) H&P (MDs), NPs, PAs	Initial treatment plan completed Diagnostic summary completed First treatment plan review	Continue ongoing monitoring of abstinence Conduct second treatment plan review
Diagnostic Studies	Routine lab tests* Complete or partial physical examination	Review laboratory results	Repeat follow-up labs and workup as needed
Medications	Written orders	Medication monitoring, prn Routine laboratory and medication levels*	
Treatment Activity	Individual counseling, psychoeducational groups, random drug screens—monitoring of results; random alcohol saliva tests—monitoring of results; attendance at AA/NA meetings.	⟶	⟶
Teaching	Disease concept of alcoholism/addiction explained Family education sessions begin; rules and regulations explained	Education on feelings, 12 steps, relapse prevention, post–acute withdrawal symptoms, anger management, spirituality of recovery	⟶
Discharge Planning	Initial assessment of discharge needs	Discharge status reviewed	Revise discharge needs Transfer patient to aftercare phase
Consults	Psychiatric evaluations Subspecialists or legal authorities*	⟶	⟶
Patient Outcomes	Verbalizes understanding of concept	Verbalizes feeling states Verbalizes relapse triggers	Presents 1st step Receives peer evaluation
	Attends 12-step AA meetings 3 times per week	⟶	Gives life story
	Abstains from all mood-altering substances	⟶	Gives peer goals to complete Presents completed peer goals to peers
		Develops strategies to avoid relapse Prepares 1st step: relapse prevention	Graduates to aftercare phase of program

*As indicated.
CAC, community alcohol center; H&P, history and physical; prn, as needed; AA, Alcoholics Anonymous; NA, Narcotics Anonymous; MDs, physicians; NP, nurse practitioner; PA, physician's assistant.
Modified from Mary T. Pfister, RN, MHA, Mountainside Hospital, Glen Ridge/Montclair, NJ.

mental health services in occupational settings. Many hospitals and corporations offer their employees counseling and support as an alternative to being terminated when the employee's work performance is negatively affected by his or her impairment.

Psychopharmacology and Drug Addictions

The predominant somatic therapies are for detoxification (management of withdrawal) or for attempts to alter drug use (e.g., disulfiram [Antabuse], methadone, and naltrexone).

ALCOHOL WITHDRAWAL

Not all people who stop drinking require management of withdrawal. This decision depends on the length of time and the amount the client has been drinking, the prior history of withdrawal complications, and the overall health status. Medication should not be given until the symptoms of with-

drawal are seen. Early withdrawal symptoms are tremors, diaphoresis, rapid pulse (>100), elevated blood pressure (>150/90 mm Hg), and occasional transient tactile or visual hallucinations. Grand mal seizures can occur and are self-limited. The withdrawal process, not the seizure, needs to be treated. Drugs that are useful in treating alcohol withdrawal delirium are listed in Table 27-12.

Cross-dependent sedatives (chemical equivalents) are temporarily useful for reducing symptoms. Cross-dependent sedatives work by controlling the overactivity of the sympathetic nervous system. Chemical equivalents to alcohol that are used for this purpose include the benzodiazepines, such as oxazepam (Serax) or lorazepam (Ativan). These two drugs are not metabolized in the liver and are perhaps the best choice for alcoholic clients (Haack 1998; Weinrieb and O'Brien 1997). Other drugs include diazepam (Valium) and chlordiazepoxide hydrochloride (Librium), or alprazolam (Xanax).

TABLE 27-12 *Treatment of Alcohol Withdrawal Delirium*

DRUG	DOSE	PURPOSE
Sedatives *Benzodiazepines* Chlordiazepoxide (Librium) drug of choice	25-100 mg PO q4h tapered to zero over 5-7 days	Chlordiazepoxide and diazepam are cross-addicting, provide *safe* withdrawal, and have *anticonvulsant* effects
Diazepam (Valium)	5-10 mg PO q2-4h in tapering doses	Has anticonvulsant qualities
Oxazepam (Serax) or lorazepam (Ativan)	30-90 mg PO qid and 45 mg at bedtime and tapered to zero over 5-7 days.	Not metabolized in the liver
Thiamine (Vitamin B₁) Given intramuscularly or intravenously before glucose loading	100 mg PO qd for 3 days	Prevents Wernicke's encephalopathy
Magnesium Sulfate Especially if history of seizures	1 g IM q6h for 2 days	Increases effectiveness of vitamin B₁. Helps reduce status postwithdrawal seizures
Anticonvulsant Phenobarbital		For seizure control
Folic Acid	1 mg PO qid	Most effective in short time. Takes days to reach therapeutic level
Multivitamins	1 daily	Malabsorption due to heavy long-term alcohol abuse causes deficiencies in many vitamins

PO, orally; qd, every day; qid, four times a day.
From Weinrieb, R. M., and O'Brien, C. P. (1997). Diagnosis and treatment of alcoholism. In D. L. Dunner (Ed.), *Current psychiatric therapy II* (pp. 153–156). Philadelphia: W. B. Saunders; Franklin, J. E., and Frances, R. F. (1999). Alcohol and other psychoactive substances use disorders. In Hales, R. E., Yudofsky, S. C., and Talbott, J. A. (Eds.). *The American Psychiatric Press textbook of psychiatry* (3rd ed.). Washington, DC: American Psychiatric Press.

The pulse and blood pressure should be checked hourly for the first 8 to 12 hours after admission, at least every 4 hours during the first 48 hours, and then four times a day thereafter. The pulse is a good indication of progress through withdrawal. Elevated pulse may indicate impending alcohol withdrawal delirium, signaling the need for more rigorous sedation. Thiamine (vitamin B_1) deficiency is often present and thiamine should be given routinely. Thiamine replacement is given in order to prevent Wernicke's syndrome (encephalopathy). Wernicke's syndrome is characterized by nystagmus, ptosis, ataxia, confusion, coma, and possible death.

Hypomagnesemia is another condition found in people with long-term drinking problems. Magnesium sulfate may be given to increase the body's response to thiamine and to raise the seizure threshold.

Anticonvulsants may or may not be used. Diazepam or phenobarbital may be used on a short-term basis to control seizures and prevent status epilepticus. Phenytoin (Dilantin) is only used if the person has a history of primary seizure disorder, not related to alcohol withdrawal.

Fluid and electrolyte replacements may be necessary, especially if the client is vomiting, has diarrhea, and is experiencing diaphoresis. In these cases, the client may be dehydrated and may need proper fluid and electrolyte replacement (e.g., potassium). However, caution is warranted. Diuresis occurs when BALs rise, but fluid retention may occur as BALs fall; therefore, a person in withdrawal may be overhydrated. Rigorous fluid therapy could cause serious complications, such as congestive heart failure.

ALCOHOL TREATMENT

NALTREXONE (TREXAN, REVIA). Naltrexone (an agent used for narcotic addiction) is also used with success for some people in the treatment of alcoholism, especially for people with high levels of craving and somatic symptoms (Freed 1997). Naltrexone works by blocking opiate receptors, thereby blocking the mechanism of reinforcement and reducing or eliminating alcohol preference.

DISULFIRAM (ANTABUSE). Disulfiram (Antabuse) is used on motivated clients who have shown the ability to stay sober. Disulfiram works on the classical conditioning principle of inhibiting impulsive drinking because the client tries to avoid the unpleasant physical effects from the alcohol-disulfiram reaction. These effects consist of facial flushing, sweating, throbbing headache, neck pain, tachycardia, respiratory distress, a potentially serious decrease in blood pressure, and nausea and vomiting. The adverse reaction usually begins within minutes to a half hour after drinking and may last 30 to 120

minutes. These symptoms are usually followed by drowsiness and are gone after the person naps.

Disulfiram must be taken daily. The action of the drug can last from 5 days to 2 weeks after the last dose. It is most effectively used early in the recovery process while the individual is making the major life changes associated with long-term recovery from alcoholism. Disulfiram should always be prescribed with the full knowledge and consent of the client. The client needs to be told about the side effects and must be well aware that any substances that contain alcohol can trigger an adverse reaction. Three primary sources of hidden alcohol exist—food, medicines, and preparations that are applied to the skin. People also need to be careful to avoid inhaling fumes from substances that might contain alcohol, such as paints, wood stains, and stripping compounds. Unfortunately, voluntary compliance with the disulfiram regimen is often poor and studies have failed to find different treatment outcomes between subjects taking disulfiram and those taking placebo (Weinreib and O'Brien 1997).

OPIOID TREATMENT

METHADONE (DOLOPHINE). Methadone (Dolophine) is a synthetic opiate that at certain doses (usually 40 mg) blocks the craving for, and effects of, heroin. It has to be taken every day, is highly addicting, and when stopped produces withdrawal. To be effective, the client must take a dose that will prevent withdrawal symptoms, block drug craving, and block any effects of illicit use of short-acting narcotics through the development of tolerance and cross-tolerance (National Institute on Drug Abuse [NIDA] 1994a).

A methadone maintenance program is not considered to be an effective treatment in itself. At times, it keeps the client out of the illegal drug subculture, but, to be successful, programs must include counseling and job training (Sees et al. 2000). Methadone maintenance reduces heroin addicts' risk of infection with HIV by reducing the occurrence of drug injection.

Methadone is the only medication currently approved for the treatment of the pregnant opioid addict. The clinical studies available demonstrate that methadone maintenance at the appropriate dose, when combined with prenatal care and a comprehensive program of support, can significantly improve fetal and neonatal outcome.

L-ALPHA ACETYLMETHADOL. As an alternative to methadone, LAAM is effective for up to 3 days (72 to 96 hours), so clients need to come to an outpatient service for their medication only three times a week. This regimen makes it easier for clients to keep jobs and gives them more freedom than is available with methadone maintenance. LAAM is also an addictive narcotic: its therapeutic effects and side effects are the same as those of morphine.

NALTREXONE (TREXAN, REVIA). Naltrexone is a relatively pure antagonist that blocks the euphoric effects of opioids. It has low toxicity with few side effects. A single dose provides an effective opiate blockade for up to 72 hours. Taking naltrexone three times a week is sufficient to maintain a fairly high level of opiate blockade. For many clients, long-term use results in gradual extinction of drug-seeking behaviors. Naltrexone does not produce dependence. As previously mentioned, it has also been approved for the treatment of alcoholism because it decreases the pleasant, reinforcing effects of alcohol.

CLONIDINE. Clonidine was initially marketed for high blood pressure, but it is also an effective somatic treatment for some chemically dependent individuals when combined with naltrexone. Clonidine is a nonopioid suppresser of opioid withdrawal symptoms. It is also nonaddicting.

BUPRENORPHINE. Buprenorphine is a partial opioid agonist. At low doses (2 to 4 mg per day sublingually), the drug blocks signs and symptoms of opioid withdrawal. In experimental studies, buprenorphine has been shown to suppress heroin use in both inpatient and outpatient settings (APA 2000a).

NICOTINE PATCH

Transdermal nicotine doubles long-term abstinence rates. It is preferred over nicotine gum because of its improved compliance, steadier blood levels, little long-term dependence, and less complicated instructions.

EVALUATION

Treatment outcome is judged by increased lengths of time in abstinence, decreased denial, acceptable occupational functioning, improved family relationships, and, ultimately, ability to relate normally and comfortably with other human beings.

The ability to use existing supports and skills learned in treatment is important for ongoing recovery. For example, recovery is actively viable if, in response to cues to use the substance, the client calls his or her sponsor or other recovering persons; increases attendance at 12-step meetings, aftercare, or other group meetings; or writes feelings in a log and considers alternative action. Continuous monitoring and evaluation lead to a better chance for prolonged recovery.

Visit the **Evolve** website at
http://evolve.elsevier.com/Varcarolis
for more Case Studies.

CASE STUDY 27-1   *Working With a Person Dependent on Alcohol*

Mr. Young, aged 49 years, and his wife arrive in the emergency department one evening, fearful that he has had a stroke. His right hand is limp and he is unable to hyperextend his right wrist. Sensation to the fingertips in his right hand is impaired.

Mr. Young looks much older than his stated age; in fact, he looks to be about 65. His complexion is ruddy and flushed. History taking is difficult. Mr. Young answers only what is asked of him, volunteering no additional information. He states that he took a nap that afternoon and that when he awakened, he noticed the problems with his right arm.

Mr. Young reveals that he has been unemployed for 4 years because the company he worked for went bankrupt. He has been unable to find a new job but has a job interview in 10 days' time. His wife is now working full time, so the family finances are okay. They have two grown children who no longer live at home.

He denies any significant medical illness except for high blood pressure, just diagnosed last year. His family history is negative for illness, with the exception of alcoholism. His mother is a recovering alcoholic. Ms. Dee, the admitting nurse, asks Mr. Young questions about his use of alcohol, including quantity, frequency, and withdrawal experiences. In general, he denies any significant alcohol involvement. Ms. Dee shares with him the fact that the disease of alcoholism runs in families. She asks Mr. Young whether (1) he knows this and (2) if it concerns him with regard to his own drinking. Mr. Young says that he knows and that he does not want to think about it.

Ms. Dee then speaks with Mrs. Young about the events of the day. Ms. Dee states that she spoke with Mr. Young and that she is concerned that he might have an alcohol problem. Ms. Dee shares the impressions that led her to that tentative conclusion and asks Mrs. Young to describe her husband's involvement

Case Study continued on following page

with alcohol. Mrs. Young's shoulders slump; she sighs and says, "I have spent the entire day talking to a counselor at the local treatment center to see if I can get him in. He won't admit that he has a problem." Mrs. Young then recounts a 6-year history of steadily increasing alcohol use. She says that for a while she could not admit to herself that her husband was an excessive drinker. "He tried to hide it, but gradually I knew. I could tell from little changes that he was intoxicated. I couldn't believe it was happening because he had been through the same thing with his mother and we'd always had such a good relationship. I thought I knew him. Actually, I guess I did when he was a working man. Being unemployed and unable to find a job has really floored him. And now he's even going to job interviews intoxicated."

Mrs. Young recounts how her husband's drinking worsened dramatically with unemployment and how she tried ridding their home of liquor, only to find bottles hidden in their mobile home one day when she went to clean it. She describes her feelings, which are like an emotional roller coaster—elated and hopeful when he seems to be doing okay; dejected and desperate on other occasions, such as the time that she found the

alcohol in their mobile home. Mrs. Young hates going to work for fear of what he might do while she is gone. She says she is terrified that one day her husband will crack up the car and kill himself, because he often drives when intoxicated. Ms. Dee discusses with Mrs. Young her own involvement as part of the family system. Options for Mrs. Young and her husband are discussed.

Meanwhile, the physician in the emergency department has examined Mr. Young. The diagnosis is radial nerve palsy. Mr. Young most likely passed out while lying on his arm. Because Mr. Young was intoxicated, he had not felt the signals that his nerves sent out to warn him to move (numbness, tingling). Mr. Young continued to lie in this position for so long that the resultant cutting off of circulation was sufficient to cause some temporary nerve damage.

Mr. Young's BAL is 0.31 mg%. This is three times the legal limit for intoxication in many states (0.1 mg%). Even though he has a BAL of 0.31 mg%, Mr. Young is alert and oriented, not slurring his speech or giving any other outward signs of intoxication. The difference between Mr. Young's BAL and his behavior indicates the development of tolerance, a symptom of physical dependence.

ASSESSMENT	Ms. Dee organizes her data into objective and subjective components. **Objective Data** ■ Drives when intoxicated ■ Nerve damage due to having passed out while lying on arm ■ Increased alcohol use during stress of unemployment ■ Capacity to obtain employment impaired by alcohol use	■ Disruption in marital relationship caused by alcohol use ■ Unable to see effects of his drinking ■ Family history of alcoholism ■ BAL three times the legal limit of intoxication; has developed tolerance **Subjective Data** ■ Denies he has an alcohol problem
SELF-ASSESSMENT	The denial the alcoholic client exhibits often results in rejection by nurses, who feel that the alcoholic causes his or her own problems. Nurses generally feel sympathetic toward spouses and other family members but have a sense of helplessness about ability to effect change. Feelings of rejection, sympathy, and helplessness impair the nurse's ability to facilitate change. True, some alcoholic persons do maintain their denial and effectively resist intervention, but many others welcome the opportunity to begin to learn different ways of coping with life	problems. Before dismissing alcoholic clients as "not wanting help" or being "the only ones that can change things," nurses need to ask themselves if they have done all that they can in an attempt to engage the client in the change process. Ms. Dee has seen many clients with the disease of alcoholism make radical changes in their lives, and she has learned to view alcoholism as a treatable disease. She is aware also that it is the client who makes the changes, and she no longer feels responsible when a client is not ready to make that change.

CASE STUDY 27–1   *Working With a Person Dependent on Alcohol (Continued)*

NURSING DIAGNOSIS	From the data, the nurse formulates the following nursing diagnosis: **Ineffective coping** related to alcohol use, as evidenced by ■ Increased alcohol use during stressful period of unemployment	■ Capacity to obtain employment impaired by alcohol use ■ Disruption in marital relationship caused by alcohol use ■ Unable to see effect of his drinking on his life functioning

PLANNING OUTCOME CRITERIA

It is decided to allow Mr. Young to sober up in the emergency department because it is difficult to discuss goals when the client is intoxicated. When the client is sober, the nurse establishes goals with the client that are realistic, appropriate, and measurable.

NURSING DIAGNOSIS	LONG-TERM OUTCOME	SHORT-TERM GOALS
1. **Ineffective coping** related to alcohol use	1. Client will abstain from alcohol.	1a. Client will identify the role of alcohol in his life and his risk for alcoholism, given his family history. 1b. Client will agree to remain sober until his job interview 10 days hence. To assist in this effort, he agrees to ■ Obtain an appointment at a community alcohol center. ■ Attend at least one AA meeting each day. ■ Call his sponsor when he feels the need for a drink. 1c. Client will state two alternative behaviors to engage in when he experiences the urge to drink. 1d. Client will name two ways to begin to rebuild trust in his relationship with his wife.

Case Study continued on following page

CASE STUDY 27–1   *Working With a Person Dependent on Alcohol* (Continued)

INTERVENTION	Ms. Dee suggests that Mrs. Young attend Al-Anon meetings and gives her information on where she can find groups in her area. She also urges Mrs. Young to discuss what is going on with her grown children and tells her about the problems that adult children of alcoholics often experience. She encourages Mrs. Young to let her children know of support groups they can go to if they feel the need.

Ms. Dee also urges Mrs. Young *not* to go in the car with her husband if he is driving while intoxicated. Ms. Dee states that she should not protect him from the results of his drinking (e.g., bail him out of jail if he is arrested for driving while intoxicated or make excuses for him). Ms. Dee adds that Al-Anon could offer crucial support for Mrs. Young and could assist her in minimizing her enabling behaviors, which family members often exhibit.

Ms. Dee outlines an initial care plan for Mr. Young (Nursing Care Plan 27–1). Attending AA is a central part of the treatment program, along with a variety of other interventions, such as skills training, education, medical intervention, family counseling, and evaluation for naltrexone therapy.

EVALUATION

Mr. Young's willingness to become actively involved in planning short-term goals is evidence that the goals are realistic and appropriate. In this case, the main opportunity for evaluating the short-term goals is when and if Mr. Young calls back to report on steps he has taken to meet those goals. At that time, he should be supported and validated for the progress he has made and encouraged to "keep up the good work." Other referrals may be given if indicated.

Mr. Young does continue with AA. His denial persists, but he is highly motivated to keep his marriage. He gradually accepts a variety of referrals; as time progresses, he finds that the positive feedback and support from others increases his self-esteem, decreases his feelings of isolation, and reinforces his long-term goal of sobriety.

Visit the **Evolve** website at
http://evolve.elsevier.com/Varcarolis
for the other Nursing Care Plan diagnoses and for
more Nursing Care Plans.

NURSING CARE PLAN 27–1   *A Person with Alcoholism: Mr. Young*

NURSING DIAGNOSIS

Ineffective Coping: related to alcohol use

Supporting Data

- Alcohol use increases in response to the stress of job loss, lowered role status.
- Alcohol use has impaired client's capacity to obtain employment.

- Alcohol use is causing disruptions in relationship with wife.
- Family history of alcoholism exists.

Outcome Criteria: Client will abstain from alcohol.

NURSING CARE PLAN 27–1   A Person with Alcoholism: Mr. Young (Continued)

SHORT-TERM GOAL	INTERVENTION	RATIONALE	EVALUATION
1. Client will identify the role of alcohol in his life and his risk for alcoholism, given his family history.	1a. Point out relationship between no job and increased alcohol use 1b. Provide information on the disease of alcoholism. 1c. Point out the factors placing person at risk for alcoholism. 1d. Communicate concern, empathy, nonjudgmental acceptance, warmth.	1a. Use assessment data to clarify behavior patterns. 1b. Emphasizing alcoholism as a disease can lower guilt and help increase self-esteem. 1c. Children with alcoholic parents are at a greater risk for developing alcoholism themselves. 1d. Helps establish a therapeutic relationship based on understanding and provides an atmosphere of openness and support. Helps client maintain self-esteem.	*GOAL MET* Client listens to nurse—admits that going to job interviews intoxicated would lower the chance of getting a job. States that he felt so down that he needed alcohol to feel better.
2. Client will state two alternative behaviors that he can exercise when experiencing the urge to drink by (date).	2a. Evaluate client's situation by using a crisis intervention model, i.e., assessing precipitating events, support systems, and coping skills. 2b. Explore alternative coping skills. Skills training may be needed (e.g., assertiveness, socialization, problem solving).	2a. Identifies high-risk situations and opportunities for change. 2b. Behavior change is a learning process. Relapse prevention can be practiced.	*GOAL MET* After 3 weeks, client states that he has attended AA every day. He is learning to identify situations that trigger the urge to drink and is learning new coping behaviors. After 5 weeks, client has a slip and drinks for 2 days; he decides to try naltrexone.

Nursing Care Plan continued on following page

NURSING CARE PLAN 27–1 **A *Person with Alcoholism*: Mr. Young** *(Continued)*

2c. Encourage participation in AA, group therapy, or other appropriate modalities.	2c. Provides support and minimizes feelings of isolation while client is learning new skills.
2d. Referral to a physician for complete physical examination; possible naltrexone (ReVia) use.	2d. Naltrexone can help block cramping in some people.

SUMMARY

Substance use and dependence occur on a continuum, and the development of addiction and dependence is a time-related phenomenon. Various theories attempt to explain why some people develop a substance abuse problem and others do not. Because no clear consensus exists about the nature of alcoholism and other drugs, notions about treatment are also inconsistent. The more closely clients are matched to a range of treatment alternatives, the greater the likelihood that sobriety or drug-free behavior will be achieved and overall life functioning will be improved.

Nurses encounter people with alcohol and drug problems in all areas of practice and thus must be prepared to assess, implement, and evaluate nursing care of their clients. Interview guidelines are given. Assessment tools are provided along with overall assessment guides. Psychological changes can occur with substance abuse and each drug has its own signs of intoxication and withdrawal. Self-assessment is vital. Some nursing diagnoses applicable to alcoholic clients include ineffective denial, risk for injury, hopelessness, risk for infection, altered family process, risk for self-harm, and many more.

Principles and specific examples of psychotherapeutic interventions include behavior therapy; individual, group, family, and marital therapy; and self-help groups, such as AA. Psychopharmacology may be used in treatment; various outpatient modalities were discussed. Whatever techniques are used, the nurse must make clear to the client what expectations are reasonable. Issues common in early treatment are discussed, as are some general approaches to relapse prevention.

Nurses and other health care workers are at an even higher risk for chemical dependency than non–health care workers. Specific interventions and guidelines can help protect clients who are under an impaired nurse's care and can save the nurse's future livelihood—if not the impaired nurse's life.

Visit the **Evolve** website at
http://evolve.elsevier.com/Varcarolis
for a post-test on the content in this chapter.

Visit the **Evolve** website at
http://evolve.elsevier.com/Varcarolis
for additional self-study exercises.

Critical Thinking and Chapter Review

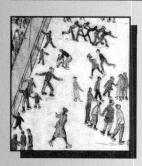

Critical Thinking

1. Write a paragraph regarding your possible reactions to a drug-dependent client to whom you are assigned.

   a. Would your response differ, depending on the substance, for example, alcohol versus heroin; marijuana versus cocaine? Give reasons for your answers.

   b. Would your response be different if the substance-dependent person were a professional colleague? How?

2. Rosetta Seymour is a 15-year-old teenager who has started using heroin nasally.

   a. Briefly discuss the trend in heroin use among teenagers.

   b. When Rosetta asks you why she needs to take more and more to get "high," how would you explain to her the concept of tolerance?

   c. If she had just taken heroin, what would you find on assessment of physical and behavioral/psychological signs and symptoms?

   d. If she came into the emergency room with an overdose of heroin, what would be the emergency care? What might be effective long-term care?

3. Tony Garmond is a 45-year-old mechanic. He has a 20-year history of heavy drinking and he says he wants to quit drinking but needs help.

   a. Role-play with a classmate an initial assessment. Identify the kinds of information you would need to have to plan holistic care.

   b. Mr. Garmond tried stopping by himself but is in the emergency room with delirium tremens. What are the dangers for Mr. Garmond? What are the appropriate medical interventions?

   c. What are some possible treatment alternatives for Mr. Garmond when he is safely detoxified? How would you explain to him the usefulness and function of Alcoholics Anonymous? What are some additional treatment options that might be useful to Mr. Garmond? What is available as referrals for Mr. Garmond in your community?

Chapter Review

1. When intervening with a client who is intoxicated from alcohol, it is useful for the nurse to first

   1. Let the client sober up.
   2. Decide immediately on care goals.
   3. Ask what drugs other than alcohol the client has recently used.
   4. Gain compliance by sharing personal drinking habits with the client.

2. A principle of counseling intervention that should be observed by the nurse caring for a chemically dependent client is

   1. Look for therapeutic leverage.
   2. Communicate that relapses are expected.

3. Recognize that recovery is considered complete and absolute.
4. Remove unhealthy defenses, then assist client to build new ones.

3. As the nurse evaluates the client's progress, which treatment outcome would indicate a poor general prognosis for long-term recovery from substance abuse?

1. Client demonstrates improved self-esteem.
2. Client demonstrates enhanced coping abilities.
3. Client demonstrates improved relationships with others.
4. Client demonstrates positive expectations for ongoing drug use.

4. Which statement provides a basis for planning care for a client who has abused CNS stimulants?

1. Symptoms of intoxication include grandiosity, paranoia, hallucinations.
2. Medical management focuses on removing the drugs from the body.
3. Withdrawal is simple and rarely complicated.
4. Postwithdrawal symptoms include fatigue and depression.

5. The provision of optimal care for clients withdrawing from substances of abuse is facilitated when the nurse understands that severe morbidity and mortality are often associated with withdrawal from

1. Alcohol and CNS depressants.
2. CNS stimulants and hallucinogens.
3. Narcotic antagonists and caffeine.
4. Opiates and inhalants.

NURSE, CLIENT, AND FAMILY RESOURCES

Associations

Alcoholics Anonymous World Services
475 Riverside
New York, NY 10115
1-212-870-3400

Narcotics Anonymous World Services Office
P.O. Box 9999
Van Nuys, California 91409
1-818-773-9999

Al-Anon Family Group Headquarters, Inc.
(for Al-Anon, Al-a-teen, Al-a-tots, ACoA)
1600 Corporate Landing Parkway
Virginia Beach, VA 23454
1-888-4AL-ANON

National Clearinghouse for Alcohol and Drug Information
P.O. Box 2345
Rockville, MD 20856
http://www.health.org

CSAT (Center for Substance Abuse Treatment)
National Drug Hotline (bilingual)
1-800-662-4357
http://www.samhsa.gov/csat/csat.htm

National Institute on Drug Abuse (NIDA)
American Self-Help Clearinghouse
1-201-625-7101
http://mentalhelp.net/selfhelp/

Internet Sites

National Addiction Technology Transfer Centers Home Page
http://www.nattc.org

Addiction Research Foundation/Center for Addiction and Mental Health
http://www.arf.org

REFERENCES

Allen K. (1998). Essential concepts of addiction for general nursing practice. *Nursing Clinics of North America*, 33(1):1.
American Psychiatric Association. (2000a). *Practice guidelines for the treatment of psychiatric disorders compendium 2000*. Washington, DC: American Psychiatric Association.
American Psychiatric Association. (2000b). *Diagnostic and statistical manual of mental disorders—text revision* (4th ed). Washington, DC: American Psychiatric Association Press.
Bell, K. (1992). Identifying the substance abuser in clinical practice. *Orthopedic Nursing*, 11(2):29.
Boyd, M. R., and Hauenstein, E. J.: (1997). Psychiatric assessment and confirmation of dual disorders in rural substance abusing women. *Archives of Psychiatric Nursing*, 11(2):74.

Brady, K. T. (1999). *New frontiers in the assessment and treatment of dual diagnosis.* The American Psychiatric Association 152nd Annual Meeting, Washington, DC.

Compton, P., Monahan G., and Simmons-Cody, H. (1999). Motivational interviewing: An effective brief intervention for alcohol and drug abuse patients. *Nurse Practitioner,* 24(11):27.

Conway, R., and Fairbrother, G. (1999). Substance-use assessment for hospital inpatients. *Professional Nursing,* 14(7):458.

Cowart, M. E., and Sutherland, M. (1998). Late-life drinking among women. *Geriatric Nursing,* 19(4):214.

Dyehouse, J. M., and Sommers, M. S (1998). Brief intervention after alcohol-related injuries. *Nursing Clinics of North America,* 33(1):93.

El-Mallakh, P. (1998). Treatment models for clients with co-occurring addictive and mental disorders. *Archives of Psychiatric Nursing,* 12(2):71.

Ermalinski, E. et al. (1997). Impact of a body-mind treatment component on alcoholic inpatients. *Journal of Psychosocial Nursing,* 35(7):39.

Espeland, K. E. (2000). Inhalant abuse. *Lippincott's Primary Care Practice,* 4:336.

Fingfeld, D. L. (1999). Use of brief interventions to treat individuals with drinking problems. *Journal of Psychosocial Nursing,* 37(4):23.

Fink, A., et al. (1996). Alcohol-related problems in older persons: Determinants, consequences, and screening. *Archives of Internal Medicine,* 156(11)

Flagler, S., Hughes, T. L., and Kovalesky, A. (1997). Toward an understanding of addiction. *Journal of Obstetric and Gynecological Neonatal Nursing,* 26(4):441.

Franklin, J. E., and Frances, R. F. (1999). Alcohol and other psychoactive substances use disorders. In Hales, R. E., Yudofsky, S. C., and Talbott, J. A. (Eds.). *The American Psychiatric Press textbook of psychiatry* (3rd ed.). Washington, DC: American Psychiatric Press.

Freed, P. E., and Yolk, L. N. (1997). Naltrexone: A controversial therapy for alcohol dependence. *Journal of Psychosocial Nursing,* 35(7):24.

Galloway, G. P., et al. (2000). Abuse and therapeutic potential of gammahydroxybutyric acid. *Alcohol,* 20(3):263–269.

Haack, M. R. (1998). Treating acute withdrawal from alcohol and other drugs. *Nursing Clinics of North America,* 33(1):75.

Hegadoren, K. M., Baker, G. B., and Bourin, M. (1999). 3,4-Methylenedioxy analogues of amphetamine: Defining the risk to humans. *Neuroscience Behavioral Review,* 23(4):539–553.

Israel, Y., et al. (1996). Screening for problem drinking and counseling by the primary care physician–nurse team. *Alcohol Clin Exp Res,* 20(8):1443.

Jaffe, J. H. (1999). Amphetamine (or amphetamine-like) -related disorders. In B. J. Sadock and V. A. Sadock (Eds). *Kaplan and Sadock's Comprehensive Textbook of Psychiatry,* 7th ed. (Vol I, pp. 971–982). Philadelphia: Lippincott Williams & Wilkins.

Jessup, M. (1997). Addiction in women: Prevalence, profiles and meaning. *Journal of Obstet Gynecol Neonatal Nurs,* 26(4):449.

Kutlenios, R. M. (1998). Genetics and alcoholism—implications for advanced practice psychiatric/mental health nursing. *Archives Psychiatric Nursing,* 12(3):154.

Liberg, J. P., Howca, K. E., Nordby, G., and Jacobsen, D. (1998). Ecstasy: Cool dope with long-lasting effects? *Tidsskr Norlaegeforen,* 118(28):4384–4387.

McComish, J. F., et al. (2000). Survival analysis of three treatment modalities in a residential substance abuse program for women and children. *Outcomes Management for Nursing Practice,* 4(2):71.

Meehan, A. J., Carey, N., and Haynes, D. E. (1998). A clinical pathway for the secondary diagnosis of alcohol misuse: Implications for the orthopaedic patient. *Orthopaedic Nursing,* 17(6):49.

Morgan, M. J. (2000). Ecstasy (MDMA): A review of possible persistent effects. *Psychopharmacology (Berlin),* 152(3):230–241.

Mynatt, S. (1999). Effectiveness of intervention into substance abuse disorders in women with comorbid depression. *Journal of Psychosocial Nursing,* 37(5):16.

National Institute on Drug Abuse Clinical Report Series: Relapse prevention (NIH Publication No. 94-3845). Washington, DC: US Department of Health and Human Services, 1994a.

National Institute on Drug Abuse Research Report Series: Inhalant abuse (NIH Publication No. 94-3818). Washington, DC: US Department of Health and Human Services, 1994b.

National Institute on Drug Abuse. Study clarifies brain mechanisms of cocaine's high, April 23, 2001. HHSPRESS@LIST.NIH.GOV.

O'Connor, P. G., Samet, J. H., and Stein, M. D. (1994). Management of hospitalized drug users: Role of the internist. *American Journal of Medicine,* 96:551.

Patterson, D. G., MacPherson, J., and Brady, N. M. (1997). Community psychiatric nurse aftercare for alcoholics: A five-year follow-up study. *Addiction,* 92(4):459.

Schwartz, R. H., Milteer, R., and LeBeaur, M. A. (2000). Drug facilitated sexual assault ("date rape"). *South Med J,* 93(6):558–561.

Schwartz, R. H. (1998). Adolescent heroin use: A review. *Pediatrics,* 102(6):1451–1466.

Sees, K. L., et al. (2000). Methadone maintenance vs. 180-day psychosocially enriched detoxification for treatment of opioid dependence: A randomized controlled trial. *Journal of American Medical Association,* 283(10):1303.

Smith, L. L., Taylor, B. B., and Hughes, T. L. (1998). Effective peer response to impaired nursing practice. *Nursing Clinics of North America,* 33(1):105–118.

Thomas, H. (1993). Psychiatric symptoms in cannabis users. *British Journal of Psychiatry,* 163:141.

Trkulja, V., and Lackovic, Z. (1997). Ecstasy. *Lijec Vjesn,* 119(5–6):158–166.

Weinrieb, R. M. and O'Brien, C. P. (1997). Diagnosis and treatment of alcoholism. In D. L. Dunner (Ed.), *Current psychiatric therapy II* (pp. 153–156). Philadelphia: W. B. Saunders.

Weir, E. (2000). Raves: A review of the culture, the drugs and the prevention of harm. *Canadian Medical Association Journal,* 162(13):1829–1830.

Wing, D. M. (1996). A concept analysis of alcoholic denial and cultural accounts. *Advanced Nursing Science,* 19(2):54.

Outline

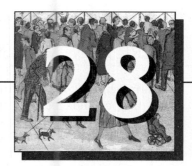

Severe Mental Illness: Crisis Stabilization and Rehabilitation

Elizabeth M. Varcarolis

Key Terms and Concepts

The key terms and concepts listed here also appear in color where they are first defined or first discussed in this chapter.

de-institutionalization

dual diagnosis

psychoeducation

severe mental illness (SMI)

social skills training

supportive group therapy

vocational rehabilitation programs

Objectives

After studying this chapter, the reader will be able to

1. Discuss the behavioral and psychological manifestations of severe mental illness as it relates to the person's daily functioning, non-adherence to treatment, and family and other interpersonal relationships.

2. Describe the reciprocal relationship between the family and the mentally ill member.

3. Explain the role of case manager in the care of the severely mentally ill person.

4. Explain the role of the nurse in the care of the severely mentally ill person.

5. Develop an outline for a psychoeducational teaching plan for a person with severe mental illness. (Choose one of your clients or one in a facility you use in your clinical experience).

6. Defend the use of the newer atypical antipsychotics in the treatment of severe mental illness. How do they affect the person regarding:
   - Side effects
   - Cognitive and negative symptoms
   - Ability to relate to others
   - Relapse rate
   - Quality of life
   - Long-term cost to the community

7. Analyze why it is important for a severely mentally ill person to work (either sheltered workshop or other). How does it benefit the person? How does it benefit the community?

SEVERE MENTAL ILLNESS

The term **chronic mental illness** refers to mental illness that extends beyond the acute stage into a long-term stage that is marked by persistent impairment of functioning. Almost all mental illnesses are chronic, with remissions and exacerbations of varying lengths. This decrease in functioning pervades a person's abilities to perform in all, or nearly all, aspects of daily living. Skill deficits range from an inability to prepare meals to an inability to cope with everyday stressors. Here we will use the term **severe mental illness** (SMI), which is essentially synonymous with **seriously and persistently mentally ill.**

Grob (1994) states that the seriously mentally ill include individuals with quite different disorders, prognoses, and needs, whose outcomes vary considerably over time. Often the severity and course of the illness are influenced by poverty, racism, and substance abuse.

The severely mentally ill population are at risk for multiple physical, emotional, and social problems. Indeed, the person with a mental illness often has impairments in well-being and functioning that exceed those in people with chronic physical problems (Hays et al. 1995).

Precise calculation of the extent of severe and persistent mental illness in the United States is difficult. Before de-institutionalization, the mentally disabled population was easier to quantify. People with severe mental illness were hospitalized, sometimes for the remainder of their lives. With the move to community-based mental health centers, and after changes within the population itself, there is no way to tabulate this group accurately. However, it is estimated that two thirds of those with major mental illness have persistent physical and emotional problems (Worley et al. 1990). NAMI (2000a) contends that we are still experiencing the negative effects of de-institutionalization due to chronic underfunding of public programs and a shift of public mental health resources away from programs serving the most severely ill consumer.

Chronicity can occur in persons of any gender, age, culture, or geographical location. However, this population includes two subgroups with unique characteristics: (1) those old enough to have experienced institutionalization (before approximately 1975) and (2) those young enough to have been hos-pitalized only during acute exacerbations of their disorders.

Older Populations

Before the move in 1975 to de-institutionalize the severely mentally ill, psychiatric hospitals were the long-term residences for many people. Medical paternalism was a pervasive philosophical stance at that time. The health care approach to the severely mentally ill person was that of making all their decisions. The daily institutional routine left little room for a person to exercise what social and problem-solving skills remained. Much of a person's behavior became a combination of the disease process and the decreased sense of self that resulted from the lack of autonomy.

Vignette

■ *Marian was a resident at a facility for the severely and persistently impaired during her adolescence and young adulthood. On discharge, she moved to a community home, where she spent long periods sitting in front of the living room window. Marian did not ask to go out into the garden she watched for so many hours. Indeed, she rarely asked for anything, including snacks or recreational activities. The caregivers worked with Marian for several months to help her to recognize her needs of the moment and then to articulate or act on them. There was a major celebration the day that she walked into the kitchen and made a peanut butter sandwich of her own volition. Some of the dependency caused by the institutionalization was being positively altered.*

Younger Populations

People young enough never to have been institutionalized may not have the problems of passivity and lack of autonomy that long-term hospitalization causes. However, lack of experience with formal treatment may contribute to the person's not truly believing that there is a problem. Denial, often coupled with the use of recreational drugs that further impair already faulty judgment and impulse control, puts severely ill young adults at particular risk for many additional problems, including brushes with the law and frequent loss of employment after short periods.

In addition, an increasingly large proportion of the general population is coming of age in families affected by mental health issues such as depression, violence, addictions, and chronic mental illness. As these children develop, their world view may be

The editor would like to thank Anne Cowley Herzog and Peggy H. Miller for their contributions to this chapter in the third edition of *Foundations of Psychiatric Mental Health Nursing.*

distorted. Frequently, social interaction and coping skills are compromised. In the presence of major stressors, many youths who are vulnerable may develop their own problems with mental illness. This sets the stage for their own persistent long-term mental illness.

Vignette

■ *Joshua, 26 years old, has had several short hospitalizations for treatment of schizophrenia. Between admissions, he lives in unstable short-term settings, varying from rooming houses to his car. He no longer lives with his mother or siblings; his mother has been imprisoned for drug dealing and his siblings are in foster homes. He has been jailed several times for misdemeanors such as shoplifting and creating a public nuisance (e.g., loud arguments in stores). He has difficulty finding and keeping jobs as a laborer.*

DEVELOPING A SEVERE MENTAL ILLNESS

The term severe mental illness refers to people with major mental illness (e.g., schizophrenia, schizo-affective disorder, bipolar disorder, or major depression) and the social, vocational, and functional impairment that often are a result of these chronic and severe illnesses (Lamb 1999).

Severe mental illness has much in common with persistent long-term physical illness. The original problem sets in motion an erosion of basic coping mechanisms and compensatory processes. As the disorder extends beyond the acute stage, more and more of the neighboring systems are involved. For example, with chronic congestive heart failure the lungs and kidneys begin to deteriorate. However, the disability of severe mental illness may go much further in destroying a person's quality of life. In the case of an illness such as schizophrenia, a person's thought processes, ability to maintain contact with others, and ability to stay employed frequently deteriorate. For example, a person may have difficulty thinking clearly about even ordinary things such as self-care and relations with others. This causes the person's interactions to be perceived as bizarre, unsatisfying, and anxiety provoking by both self and others. In turn, the person, friends, and even family members will hesitate to seek out interactions. Problematic communications escalate the tensions in relationships and erode the person's self-image.

People with severe mental illness often miss out on making friends and sharing social activities that are so important to us all. Social skills training and supportive interventions mentioned later in the chapter can make a positive difference in many of these people's lives. In the case of a business relationship between supervisor and employee, the person's ability to remain productive and employed is endangered. These stressors strain an already vulnerable person and can precipitate further deterioration in function.

Another similarity between physical illness and mental illness is the unpredictability of the disease course. Not knowing when the problem will exacerbate contributes additional stress. There is a major deficit in adequate coping mechanisms for stress in those with a severe and persistent mental disorder. The fear of relapse and avoidance of stress can cause a withdrawal from life that eventually heightens the person's social isolation and apathy, just as is the case with a physical dysfunction such as incontinence.

Exacerbations may decrease in frequency and intensity through careful attention to both the history of the disease itself and awareness of daily functioning. Assessment in these areas requires thorough and regular evaluation by an interdisciplinary psychiatric team (nurse, physician, social worker, occupational therapist). In this way, subtle impairments may be noted before the onslaught of more dramatic deterioration. As in the aphorism "A stitch in time saves nine," assessing an early symptom or sign and initiating treatment can decrease the severity of the exacerbation and the accompanying disruption of the person's life.

Rehabilitation is a critically important concept for people with serious mental illness. Through rehabilitation, disabilities and inabilities resulting from long-term mental illness can be attended to, in the hope that they may be lessened or eradicated. Just as in medical-surgical nursing, the best mental health rehabilitation begins on the first day of acute care and continues after discharge from the facility. This can take place in a variety of community centers and programs.

Unfortunately, people with severe mental illness have a high level of economic and social disadvantages. Barriers to effective treatment and rehabilitation are substantial. Lack of insurance leads the list, and public insurance programs are the major points of leverage for improving access (McAlpine and Mechanic 2000). Again, unfortunately, the problems of adequate care for the severely mentally ill are exacerbated by the managed care trend to reduce the intensity of treatment and fund the more traditional drugs, which do not target important symptoms, have more severe and dangerous side effects, but cost less for the managed care systems (NAMI 2000a).

PSYCHOLOGICAL AND BEHAVIORAL EFFECTS OF SEVERE MENTAL ILLNESS

Insufficient Housing

Housing is the first need of the seriously mentally ill once they are discharged from a hospital setting. Families are not always able to provide shelter, and there is no hope of recovering from any illness on the streets. These people also need a place where they can belong—a refuge or haven.

People with severe mental illness often cannot understand what others say, nor can they communicate to others their thoughts or needs. Some may retreat in confusion, others may have grandiose ideas of their abilities, and most cannot make sound judgments. Without careful discharge planning and a strong social support system in place, many of the seriously mentally ill become homeless or missing. They often leave behind distraught families, who are desperate for their return (NAMI 2000b). Studies consistently show that between 25% to 40% of homeless individuals have severe mental illness, not including people who have a primary diagnosis of substance abuse (NAMI 2000b).

Adults with severe mental illness are increasingly using temporary homeless shelters and local jails and prisons as permanent housing resources. What is even more disturbing is that on any given night, 338,000 people with mental disabilities are using the public streets, sidewalks, parks, bus stations, and public libraries as places to live (NAMI 2000b).

There is a strong relationship between life without a home and mental disorder. Life on the street or in a shelter, whether temporary or not, can have a very negative influence on a person's self-esteem. Homelessness on top of a fragile mental status may be all that is necessary to provoke a crisis or exacerbate an existing mental disorder.

Safe, acceptable housing is critical if people with severe mental illness are to maintain themselves within the community. Rehabilitative efforts are doomed unless affordable, adequate housing is available (Lieberman et al. 1999).

Nonadherence to Medication

The newer medications, when taken, do work. Treatment success rate is (NAMI 2000a)

- Bipolar disorder: 80%
- Major depression: 65%
- Schizophrenia: 60%

There are many reasons people are noncompliant with their medication: cost is a factor, distressing side effects are a factor, confusion about how to take medications and unsatisfactory relationships with health care professionals also play a role for many clients. See Table 28–1 for factors that contribute to nonadherence to medications.

However, there are other issues as well. National studies highlight the disparity between treatment standards and actual medical practice for the person with severe mental illness (NAMI 2000a).

- Only one third of individuals with schizophrenia are receiving appropriate doses (Lehman et al. 1998).
- Forty percent of depressed individuals receive subtherapeutic doses of medication (Fallon Healthcare System 1998).
- Long-term medication monitoring is inadequate (Fallon Healthcare System 1998).

Perhaps the most serious factor is that although the newer medications are more effective in treating a wider variety of symptoms with fewer short-term and long-term problems, cost is usually the consideration used by health care and managed care plans. Controlling cost through the use of less expensive traditional medications conflicts with most recent clinical treatment guidelines (NAMI 2000a).

> As someone with schizophrenia, finding the right medication has been a critical component of my recovery. It's a modern form of torture to give a medication with irreversible side effects when alternatives are available (*Moe Armstrong, M.A., M.B.A., Director, Consumer and Family Affairs*).

Adequate monitoring of medication efficacy by a community-based health care provider is often difficult. Often a psychiatric social worker is the primary contact. Because the physical issues of pharmacotherapeutics are often subtle, they are frequently missed until they have mushroomed and caused dramatic problems. For example, constant smacking of the lips by a client may be assessed by a nonmedical person as a manifestation of agitation and anxiety and not as an early sign of tardive dyskinesia. Neuroleptic malignant syndrome, agranulocytosis, and liver dysfunction may also result from the use of medications, especially the traditional, less expensive medications. Without early detection and treatment, a person is at high risk for possible permanent impairment or even death. For this reason, it is imperative for the person with a severe mental illness to see a psychiatric nurse or physician regularly for monitoring of medications and possible side effects. Psychiatric social workers are often not

TABLE 28–1 *Selected Factors That Contribute to Nonadherence to Medical Regime*

FACTOR	SUGGESTED INTERVENTIONS
Use of power struggles to gain a sense of control	Devise ways to give client more control over regimen by giving alternate effective treatment options.
Reluctance to give up a behavior that is a usual coping mechanism (e.g. smoking, diet, drugs/alcohol)	Teach client alternative coping strategies (relaxation, exercise, creative pursuits) and demonstrate role play that ceases the negative coping behavior and replaces it with a more productive one.
Secondary gains from the "sick" role	Teach family and staff to give positive reinforcement for healthy behavior and use of healthy coping skills, and draw away from giving attention to problem behavior.
Self-destructive behavior (suicide, anorexia, bulimia, drugs)	Perform good nursing assessment and work or refer client to competent specially trained clinician.
Negative family influence related to denial, lack of understanding, or need for client to maintain sick role	Family teaching and possibly family therapy can clarify issues, identify long-range consequences of nonadherence, and involve them in treatment plan.
Lack of economic resources (can't afford medications or time off to keep appointments)	Refer to social services; identify community resources that may be helpful
Lack of transportation	Refer to social services.
Unsatisfactory relationships with health care personnel	Work to establish partnership with client showing concern and interest; avoid power struggles.
Cultural and/or religious beliefs	Identify specific concerns. Emphasize what can happen when regimen is not followed. Attempt to engage client, family and friends to problem-solve alternative solutions.
Language problems, inability to read or understand instructions	Obtain an interpreter, and involve other members of the family who may have more facility with English. Have written instructions in client's primary language.
Uncomfortable side effects	Encourage client and family to share untoward reactions to drug so adjustments can be made before client stops taking medication or treatment.
Lack of skills to adhere to treatment regimen	Assess and identify needed skills, such as decision-making skills, relaxation skills, assertiveness training skills, relapse prevention techniques.
Conflict with self-image, especially children and adolescents (e.g., taking medication or imposing limits on activity)	Refer and encourage client to join a group with others grappling with similar issues.
Confusion about (1) taking the medication, (2) when to take, or (3) if he or she has already taken medication	Set up a concrete system for taking medications (cross-off chart, pillbox with separate compartments). Try to enlist help from family or others if available.

Data from Gorman L. M., Sultan, D. F., and Raines M. L. (1996). Davis' manual of psychosocial nursing for general patient care. Philadelphia: F. A. Davis; and Shultz J. M., and Videbeck, S. D. (1998). Lippincott's manual of psychiatric nursing care plans. Philadelphia: J. B. Lippincott.

trained properly to monitor psychiatric medications, whereas advanced practice psychiatric nurse specialists and psychiatric nurses have the appropriate education and training.

Coexisting Substance Abuse

There is a higher prevalence of substance abuse among people with severe mental illness than other populations (RachBeisel et al. 1999). Severely mentally ill persons suffer serious adverse consequences from substance use disorder. Research has demonstrated that integrated treatment programs that combine mental health and substance abuse interventions offer more promise of success than the traditional model in which separate services for severely mentally ill persons were offered (Drake and Mueser 2000). A person with severe mental illness coupled with a substance abuse problem is often referred to as having a **dual diagnosis.**

Clinical implications of substance abuse among the severely mentally ill include (Ryrie 2000)

■ Poor medication adherence
■ Increased rates of suicidal behavior
■ Increased rates of violence
■ Homelessness
■ Worsening of psychotic symptoms
■ Increase in HIV infection
■ Increased use of institutional services

OVERVIEW OF RESOURCES

Although the trend in health care is based on the concept of a national network of strong, community-based health care centers that work to maintain a client's ability to function independently out of the hospital setting, the reality still has yet to be realized (NAMI 2000a). A well-coordinated, comprehensive, and cost-effective community-based system of care that is individualized and available to all in need would be the ideal situation.

The goal of community-based health care programs is to provide broad community mental health services that will prevent psychiatric hospitalization, maintain stability in a community setting, and achieve the highest possible level of functioning. **Adult outpatient services** provide evaluation for possible psychiatric hospitalization, both voluntary and involuntary; initiate mental health treatment when necessary; respond to crisis calls and walk-in requests for services; and coordinate psychiatric emergency responses with hospitals, police, and other community service providers. **Day care services** are designed to provide alternatives to 24-hour care and to supplement other modes of treatment and residential services. **Case managers** serve as coordinators to ensure the integration and cooperation of the various elements of the system and to act as advocates for the clients in the system.

A variety of services are focused on the mentally ill who are also diagnosed with alcohol-related problems. Regional outpatient clinics provide therapeutic and **rehabilitative services for alcoholics and drug abusers** and their families. Services include medical and psychosocial assessment, detoxification, crisis intervention, and monitored disulfiram (Antabuse) administration. Similar services are available for mentally ill persons who abuse drugs, including direct treatment, referral, community education, and crisis intervention.

Community mental health services are also designed to provide outreach and case management for the persistently and seriously mentally disabled who are also homeless. Client participation in the program is voluntary. **Community outreach programs** send professional and nonprofessional workers into streets, parks, temporary shelters, bus stations, beaches, and anywhere else the mentally ill may be found. A team approach is used to gain access to clients and to connect them with the various services available to meet their needs. The role of the outreach worker is to be an advocate in all areas of client need, to foster client independence, and to terminate outreach services when appropriate.

Temporary shelters do not provide the ideal living situation but are usually a safe and supportive environment for individuals who have no other option. The mentally ill do need a place to live, even if it is temporary. A life can go either way in a public shelter. A person may become more chronically entrenched or may take steps toward improving quality of life. Often, the longer people stay in a shelter setting, the less likely they are to emerge from it.

Multiservice centers collaborate with the outreach unit in implementing individualized service plans for the persistently mentally ill. They supply hot meals, laundry and shower facilities, clothing, social activities, transportation to and from shelters, access to a telephone, and a mailing address for the person.

A study by Murray and Baier (1995) found that by using a transitional residential program, 48% of the residents who were formerly homeless and severely mentally ill were able to maintain permanent housing and a disability pension or a job.

Vignette

■ *Carl, a 36-year-old man, is admitted to the Specialized Shelter Program in March. He has recently moved from Salt Lake City, Utah, where he resided with his sister. Carl is diagnosed as a paranoid schizophrenic and is also mildly developmentally disabled. He is a pleasant man who wants to stay in Los Angeles because of the mild climate. He has never been homeless before but finds himself without funds to rent an apartment. Because Carl is an affable person who is eager to please, he is very easy to manipulate, which increases his vulnerability on the streets. His mental health case manager requests close monitoring via shelter placement. With the support of his case manager and the Specialized Shelter Program, Carl realizes his goals to move into a hotel, where he can be taught additional independent living skills, and to obtain his own apartment eventually.*

Refer to Chapter 6 for a discussion of community mental health resources.

Unfortunately, there are not enough quality community-based health care systems in the country and it is often the poorest and most seriously ill clients who fall through the cracks.

That is not to say there are not model systems run by professionally competent health care workers; there are. However, there need to be more that are governed by the current standards of care that are research based, and there needs to be a change in the public policies of managed care companies.

Ian Falloon started his Optimal Treatment Project (OTP) in 1993. The goal of the OTP project is "to make sure that all people receive optimal treatment as soon as a psychotic disorder is suspected, and

Box 28–1 *Evidence-Based Treatment for the Severely Mentally Ill Used in the Optimal Treatment Project*

■ Early detection and intervention, oriented at minimizing the impact of the disease.
■ Continuous goal-oriented assessment so that the continuous changing needs of the patient can be matched with the individualized treatment plan.
■ Assertive case management, making sure outreach is part of treatment as well as helping with daily needs and activities.
■ Education of the patient about the disorder and its treatments, including information about optimal doses of neuroleptic medications, with education about compliance and early recognition of warning signs and side effects.
■ Biomedical strategies, emphasizing a comprehensive approach that includes behavioral, social, and pharmacologic interventions.
■ Stress management using resource groups.
■ Activities of daily living skills training.
■ Ongoing therapy, such as pharmacologic or cognitive-behavioral therapy for maintenance.

From Ulf, M., Ivarson, E., and Falloon, I. (2000). A two-year controlled study on the efficacy of integrated care in schizophrenia. Presented at the *World Association for Psychosocial Rehabilitation;* VIIth World Congress; May 7–10, 2000, Paris. Summary prepared by Sadler, P., *www.medscape.com/medscape/CNO/2000/WAPR/WAPR-01.html.*

this treatment continued until all signs of the disorder and its associated disabilities and handicaps have resolved.' (Ulf et al. 2000). The treatment is evidence based, and Box 28–1 identifies some of the strategies used in the OTP.

CASE MANAGEMENT

Whether as a broker of services or as a therapist, the case manager can provide entrance into the system of care. Severely and persistently mentally ill people often have a variety of needs that span many different categories. One major problem is their frequent inability to 'access or accept services that may help them to attain and maintain a maximum level of independence or a reasonable quality of life" (Melzer et al. 1991). Casually made multiple referrals can be beyond the coping capabilities of the chronically mentally ill. With one person coordinating services, help can be more efficient. In addition, the basic needs of the person (food, shelter, clothing) are more likely to be addressed (Lapierre and Padgett 1992).

Case managers are required to coordinate a wide range of community support and rehabilitative services. People with serious mental illness may need intermittent crisis stabilization throughout the course of their illness to help prevent relapse and keep them out of the hospital and in the community. An important area to identify is those individuals who are living alone with aged caregivers (Research Findings).

RESEARCH FINDINGS

Planning by Older Mothers for the Future Care of Offspring with Serious Mental Illness

Objective

This study examined the permanency planning by older mothers for their adult offspring with long-term mental illness. The study looked at residential and financial planning, the desire for future family care, and perceived need for and use of services to assist with planning.

Method

Mail surveys were completed by 157 mothers (mean age 67 years old) and covered 41 states. The mean age (average age) of the offspring with severe mental illness was 38 years old. The primary diagnosis was schizophrenia or schizoaffective disorder (60%), multiple diagnoses (20%), or bipolar disorder (16%).

Results

Out of the 157 completed questionnaires, only 11% of mothers had reported definite plans for future residence for their offspring. Two thirds of the respondents had completed financial plans. Some had done little or no planning. Seventy-five percent stated they hoped that another family member would care for their offspring in the future, while only one quarter thought such arrangements would actually occur. More than two thirds expressed the need for services to help with planning, although less than one third had used such services.

offspring's future. Assistance should focus on mechanisms such as estate planning to enable case management and other services after parents' death. The involvement of nondisabled siblings in planning should be encouraged.

From Smith, G. C., Hatfield, A. B., and Miller, D. C. (2000). *Psychiatric Services*, 51(9):1162–1166.

Conclusion

Older parents of adults with long-term mental illness need professional help with planning for

OVERVIEW OF REHABILITATION

The overall long-term outcomes of rehabilitation for severely mentally ill clients are for them to

■ Retain positive coping strategies during times of stress and crisis with the aid of the nurse, family, or friends.
■ Maintain optimum level of functioning in
Work
Home
Community
■ Function in the community with minimal need for inpatient services.
■ Maintain stable functioning between episodes of exacerbations.

In the following sections we discuss

■ Crisis stabilization
■ Client and family psychoeducation
■ Social skills training
■ Vocational rehabilitation programs
■ Supportive group therapy
■ Cognitive-behavioral therapy of psychotic symptoms

Crisis Stabilization

People with a severe mental illness frequently experience crises. The incidence of crises may be increased in this population because of the nature of their vulnerability to stress, poor cognitive functioning, and lack of adequate problem-solving skills. Crisis theory and intervention can be adapted successfully with people who have long-term mental illness. Five characteristics of people with a severe mental illness have been identified (Finkelman 1977):

1. Inadequate problem-solving ability
2. Inadequate communication skills
3. Low self-esteem
4. Poor success with endeavors such as work, school, family, and social relationships
5. Inpatient or outpatient treatment for at least 2 years

Although the client's illness is long term, there are healthy as well as unhealthy aspects of the client's personality. It is important to emphasize healthy aspects, rather than solely the pathological aspects, during assessment of this client. Some of the major differences between the person who has long-term and severe difficulties in cognitive functioning and the mentally healthy person are outlined in Table 28–2.

Potential Crisis Situations

People usually have a number of coping responses they use when stressed in their everyday world. Any kind of change in our routines or lives constitutes some degree of stress. For the person with limited abilities, even slight change might increase the potential for a full-blown crisis. Four common potential crisis situations for the severely and persistently mentally ill client have been identified (Finkelman 1977):

1. Change in treatment approaches, such as change in routine of treatment, therapist's absence due to vacation or illness, or change in appointment time.
2. Problems or changes at work, at school, or with the family, and anniversaries of significant or traumatic events in the person's life.
3. Lack of money, inadequate transportation, and problems meeting basic needs.

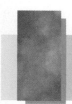

TABLE 28–2 Mentally Healthy Versus a Severely and Persistently Mentally Ill Person in Crisis

SEVERELY MENTALLY ILL PERSON	MENTALLY HEALTHY PERSON
Because of chronically high anxiety state, potential crisis event is usually distorted by minimizing or maximizing the event.	Has realistic perception of potential crisis event.
Inadequate sense of personal boundaries. Cognitive functioning assumes inadequate problem-solving abilities; nurse becomes more active in assisting person with this task.	Has healthy sense of personal boundaries, good problem-solving abilities.
Person often has no family or friends and may be living an isolated existence.	Usually has adequate situational supports.
Because cognitive functioning in people with severe mental illness is poor, coping mechanisms are usually inadequate or poorly used.	Usually has adequate coping mechanisms. Defense mechanisms can be used as support to lower anxiety.

Data from Finkleman, A. W. (1977). The nurse therapist: Outpatient crisis intervention with the chronic psychiatric patient. *Journal of Psychosocial Nursing and Mental Health Services*, 8:27.

4. Sexual relationships for people unsure about their own sexual identity are always a source of anxiety. These feelings can be compounded in severely and persistently ill clients if there are other complications (e.g., pregnancy, impotence).

Adapting the Crisis Model

Traditionally, crisis intervention refers to disequilibrium in the functioning of otherwise mentally healthy persons. The goal is to prevent temporary difficulty in functioning from progressing to severe personality disorganization. Intervention and support can help people find the way back to their previous level of functioning. People with severe and long-term mental health problems, however, are readily susceptible to crisis. The nurse must be able to adapt the crisis model to this group. These adaptations include focusing on the client's strengths, modifying and setting realistic goals with the client, taking a more active role in the problem-solving process, and using direct interventions, such as mak-

ing arrangements the person would ordinarily be able to make. See Chapter 22 for crisis intervention.

Client and Family Psychoeducation

An important need of families caring for the severely and persistently mentally ill is education to help them understand the disease process. Families need to be prepared to meet the many concerns related to safety, communication, medication compliance, and symptom and behavior management. This should include written instruction and supportive follow-up by phone or home visits. Resources for respite and day care should also be made available when appropriate. "Providing families with knowledge and information has been associated with a decrease in fear, anxiety, and confusion—and helps them cope with the illness and all its ramifications" (Feternelj-Taylor and Hartley 1993).

The need to provide multiple types of support for families cannot be overemphasized. Without ties to family, the confusion, alienation, poverty, and lack of coping and communication skills can lead to another person's joining the ranks of the homeless: girls and boys, men and women, the elderly, and even entire families.

Health care personnel are becoming increasingly aware of the overwhelming impact a mentally ill member has on the family unit. Dealing with a family member who has a mental illness is a major crisis for the family that pervades all aspects of family life. Chronic mental illness presents substantial burden, stigma, and isolation to families (Lieberman et al. 1999). It is important that professionals not only recognize the problems facing the family but also identify the strengths from which the family can plan support.

There seems to be no question that a burden does exist for the family caring for a severely mentally ill member at home. Family life can become disorganized, household routines are upset, and family members fear unexpected psychotic episodes (Loukissa 1995). Extreme degrees of stress are often experienced by families attempting to cope with a family member who is disorganized in thinking and unpredictable in behavior. Economic and human burdens mount, along with increased responsibilities. Research on these stresses and the strain on family members did not begin until the 1960s, when the effect of specific client behaviors and the impact of short hospitalizations on the family were studied (Grad and Sainsbury 1993). Today, research is focused on caregiver characteristics such as kinship and gender. There is also greater awareness of the importance of exploring social support and educating the family about all aspects of their ill member's disease and care.

An examination of the issues of family burden makes clear the need to give adequate care and attention to caregivers. Often the family becomes the most accurate source of information for use in diagnosis and client management. Cooperative planning and respect for family members are essential in providing individualized client care as well as support for the caregivers. In this way, clients can develop coping skills to assist them throughout the lengthy and unpredictable course of the disease. Evidence from a study conducted by Cuijpers and Stam (2000) concluded that psychoeducation should concentrate on helping relatives to cope with the strain on the relationship with the severely mentally ill individual and with that individual's disrupting behavior.

The psychoeducational model has five basic aims (Lieberman et al. 1999):

1. *The treatment team must develop a genuine working relationship with the family members and other supportive persons.* Family members and supportive persons need coping skills and social support, and active engagement in the educational process is encouraged.
2. *A structured and stable teaching plan.* The plan (Table 28–3) should meet the family's needs and should incorporate input from the family, the ill member, as well as the health care provider (Pollio, et al. 1998). For example:

- What is known scientifically about the severe mental illness
- Medication teaching
- Signs of relapse
- Available treatment centers
- Available support groups

3. The assumption is made that family members are doing the best that they can do. Setbacks are received as lack of knowledge or treatment services or lack of skills. *The family's tendency to be self-critical and demoralizing is actively minimized.* The goal is to strengthen the alliance so that the family can move forward.
4. *Develop step-by-step communication and problem solving skills.* For example:

- Active listening
- Giving positive feedback
- Making a positive request
- Steps in problem solving

Family psychoeducation can be viewed as a specific form of skills training, using the family system as a vehicle for targeting goals and skills.

5. *Helping the family develop a network* of involved, understanding, and supportive people and resources (e.g., National Alliance for the Mentally Ill, NAMI). Important resources may include

- Residential support services
- Transportation services
- Intensive case management
- Psychosocial rehabilitation
- Peer support

TABLE 28–3   *Topical Outline for Client and Family Psychoeducation*

BOTH CLIENTS AND FAMILY	CLIENTS	FAMILY
■ Understanding nature of illness, etiology, and treatment	Monitoring stress, balancing stimulation with caution about adding stressors	Maintaining simple, structured, consistent environment
■ Discovering relationship of illness and stress	Self-regulating specific symptoms of illness	Managing specific behavioral problems
■ Identifying early symptoms of acute episodes of illness	Learning to understand others, empathy development	Realizing importance of low-key, noncritical attitude and communication
■ Understanding medications, their purpose and importance	Developing social and leisure skills, balancing with constructive activity	Including the patient in activities
■ Learning from aftercare visits, using staff for consultation on problems	Learning to live with stigma, taking part in self-help groups for the mentally ill	Understanding importance of developing own life
■ Honing communication and problem-solving skills		Taking part in support groups for families, advocacy for mentally ill

*Education is tailored to the needs of individual patients and families, but includes information in these areas when appropriate.
Modified from Holmes, H., et al. (1994). Nursing model of psychoeducation for the seriously mentally ill. *Issues in Mental Health Nursing,* 15:93.

■ Consumer-run services
■ Round-the-clock crisis services
■ Outpatient services with mobile capabilities

International studies have validated that family stress—reflected in criticism and emotional overinvolvement with the mentally ill relative—is the most positive indicator of relapse in schizophrenia and mood disorders (Lieberman et al. 1999).

Lam (1991) has identified three factors that underlie better outcomes for clients who receive family intervention:

1. Lower negative family emotional affect (EE—expressed emotion)
2. Improved adherence with medication
3. Better monitoring of the client by the treatment team

Unfortunately, fewer than 10% of families with a schizophrenic member receive education and support, even though the vast majority of families are in regular contact with their schizophrenic relative (NAMI 1998).

Social Skills Training

The advent of the newer (atypical) antipsychotics (e.g., clozapine [Clozaril], risperidone [Risperdal], and olanzapine [Zyprexa] and others) has brought with them the potential for the enhancement in cognitive ability and increased learning capacity for individuals with severe and enduring mental illness. Therefore, more than ever before, these clients are better able to learn social skills and adapt them into their personal, social, and work lives.

Social skills training involves using a variety of learning techniques to teach clients discrete skills. Social skills training can include independent living skills, conversation skills, dating, job seeking and social perception skills, stress management, affect regulation (temper impulsivity/anger) assertiveness and conversational skills, recreational, interpersonal and social problem skills, and symptom and medication management (Midence 2000). Table 28–4 identifies areas that may be used to assess the need for specific skills in the three areas of living, learning, and working.

TABLE 28–4 *Living, Learning, and Working Skills for Psychiatrically Disabled Clients*

PHYSICAL	EMOTIONAL	INTELLECTUAL
Living Skills		
Personal hygiene	Human relations	Money management
Physical fitness	Self-control	Use of community resources
Use of public transportation	Selective reward	Goal setting
Cooking	Stigma reduction	Problem development
Shopping	Problem solving	
Cleaning	Conversational skills	
Sports participation		
Using recreational facilities		
Learning Skills		
Being quiet	Speech making	Reading
Paying attention	Question asking	Writing
Staying in seating	Volunteering answers	Arithmetic
Observation skills	Following directions	Study skills
Punctuality	Asking for directions	Hobby activities
	Listening	Typing
Working Skills		
Punctuality	Job interviewing	Job qualifying
Use of job tools	Job decision making	Job seeking
Job strength	Human relations	Specific job tasks
Job transportation	Self-control	
Specific job tasks	Job keeping	
	Specific job tasks	

From Anthony, W. A. (1980). *Principles of psychiatric rehabilitation.* Baltimore: University Park Press.

Overall, research findings support the effectiveness of social skills training. Strong evidence exists for the acquisition and maintenance of social skills, moderate evidence for the generalization of social skills training into other areas of the client's life, and weak evidence for reduction of symptoms, relapse, or rehospitalization (Smith, et al. 1996).

Vocational Rehabilitation Programs

Even though competitive employment may be a realistic objective for clients who have high motivation and favorable preconditions, vocational programs should be an integral part of the treatment of people with chronic mental illness (Reker et al 2000). A study conducted by Reker and colleagues (2000) of 471 chronically ill individuals with histories of re-peated and long-term hospitalization supported the argument for giving clients opportunities to learn and improve vocational skills. After 3 years, 11% were in competitive employment, 67% remained in sheltered employment, 7% in outpatient work therapy programs, and only 15% were unemployed.

Bozzer and colleagues (1999) demonstrated in a study that those clients with severe mental illness who completed a vocational rehabilitation program demonstrated significant improvement on measures of assertiveness and work behaviors, and they had decreased depression and improved income and employment status.

There are a number of vocational rehabilitation models. Box 28–2 identifies some successful models.

Once again, sufficient vocational rehabilitation is lacking (e.g., only about 22.6% of those with schizo-

---

Box 28–2   *Some Vocational Rehabilitation Models*

SUPPORTED EMPLOYMENT PROGRAMS (SE)

This model has proven to be most successful in assisting persons with the most serious disabilities to attain and maintain an attachment to the workforce. It is individualized and provides on-site, one-on-one supports, job coaching services, and occurs in competitive, "real work" settings; job coach services are gradually faded and removed.

TRANSITIONAL EMPLOYMENT PROGRAMS (TE)

This model offers a temporary work experience to individuals offering the same supports and services as SE. TE positions are contracted to a service program that fills openings and staffs positions to meet contractual obligations. No individual participants receive permanent TE positions: they must move on to competitive employment within an agreed-on length of time. Staff often cover contract positions, working in the job for a day in cases of illness or with changes in participants' schedules.

CLUBHOUSES

Programs are "member directed," with members defined as individuals with serious mental illness. Clubhouse services and supports are provided to members according to the structure of the "work-ordered day." Members have individual daily responsibilities and schedules to fulfill as preparation for entry or re-entry into the world of work. Membership in a clubhouse is lifelong and members provide each other ongoing support.

JOB CLUBS

There are two main types: in-house clubs and postprogram graduate clubs. Members discuss issues, uncertainties, and problems that they may face while seeking employment or maintaining employment gains. In-house clubs can provide practical guidelines in resume writing, guidelines for work exploration, opportunities to practice interviewing skills, and, in some cases, vocational assessment and interest identification. Postprogram graduate clubs provide essential off-site support services, such as working with new co-workers, adjusting to job requirements, handling issues of stigma and disclosure, and feelings of isolation.

PEER AND NATURAL SUPPORTS

These circles of support are central to the continued success of individuals with serious psychiatric conditions who are attaining and maintaining employment. Circles expand connections beyond the usual family and friends to include wider community links to religious organizations, recreational and activity groups, public libraries, volunteer activities, peer support activities (such as job clubs, support groups that meet regularly, one-on-one relationships, "warm lines" for crisis intervention and supports, and Internet chat rooms).

Adapted from Donegan, K. R., and Palmer-Erbs, V. K. (1998). Promoting the importance of work for persons with psychiatric disabilities, *Journal of Psychosocial Nursing*, 36(4):13–23. Reprinted with permission.

TABLE 28–5	*Supportive Group Therapy for the Severely Mentally Ill Client*		

TARGET POPULATION	GOALS	THERAPIST'S ACTIVITY
■ Schizophrenic clients ■ Psychotic clients ■ Severe mentally ill clients ■ Clients with cognitive disorders	*Overall goal:* Better adaptation to environment 1. Decrease isolation. 2. Increase involvement in group activities. 3. Promote discussion relative to immediate life events and feelings in the group. 4. Detect problems early. 5. Focus on reality testing.	1. Strengthens existing defenses. 2. Is actively involved in the group process. 3. May give advice and direction. 4. Models appropriate behavior. 5. Creates a safe environment.

phrenia are involved in an employer assistance program [NAMI 1998]). This is despite the fact that studies have consistently demonstrated that vocational rehabilitation may replace day treatment or partial hospitalization (NAMI 1998).

Supportive Group Therapy

A helpful form of therapy for persons with a severe long-term mental illness is therapy in a supportive group. In supportive group work, the goals are to help the clients better adapt to the environment by focusing on reality and to help them learn new behaviors to decrease isolation. The therapist needs to note early indications of the emergence of psychotic symptoms; such symptoms may indicate a need to change the client's treatment program. For example, nursing interventions aimed at decreasing anxiety may be implemented, or antipsychotic medication regimens may need to be changed.

Supportive group therapy may include teaching, for example, self-esteem, medication education, nutritional education, or work on areas of expression such as art, music recreation, or other activities (Garrison 1997). Table 28–5 identifies some goals and the group leader's approach when running a supportive group for severely mentally ill clients.

Cognitive-Behavioral Therapy with Psychotic Symptoms

A useful remediation strategy is the use of cognitive restructuring and the use of behavioral learning principles to help reduce psychotic symptoms. Strategies have been successfully applied to treat hallucinations, delusions, and negative symptoms. Common useful strategies include distraction (listening to music or humming when auditory hallucinations occur) or reframing or verbally challenging the person's delusional beliefs (Lieberman et al 1999). Refer to Chapter 20 on schizophrenia for use of cognitive-behavioral techniques with psychotic symptoms.

Visit the **Evolve** website at
http://evolve.elsevier.com/Varcarolis
for more Case Studies.

CASE STUDY 28–1	*A Person with Severe and Persistent Mental Illness*

Evelyn is a 42-year-old woman who was originally diagnosed with schizophrenia approximately 20 years ago. During the last 2 decades, she has been hospitalized several times in acute care psychiatric facilities. Her last admitting diagnosis was borderline personality disorder. Evelyn married for the first time at age 20 and was divorced a few years later. She has been divorced and remarried and has had more informal relationships several times since. She has a 10-year-old daughter, Marie. Evelyn states that she doesn't have any friends: "There just aren't any people who want to be friendly."

During her last separation and divorce, which took place 2 years ago, Evelyn's clinical presentation became

Case Study continued on following page

CASE STUDY 28–1   A *Person with Severe* and *Persistent Mental Illness* (Continued)

more exaggerated. She had worked intermittently up to that time as a temporary clerical worker through a local personnel agency. However, her overreactions to office stress and her manipulating behaviors became so pronounced that she was fired.

Evelyn and Marie live in a dirty motel room. Marie is in and out of foster care homes. She attends school occasionally, but says she hates it "because the kids are so mean and I'm so stupid." She can read on a first-grade level.

Evelyn is seeking admission because "there's a man down the street who says he's going to hurt me. There are a lot of nasty, mean people out there. You just can't get away from them. You've got to let me in!" Although the weather is cold and rainy, she wears no coat. Both her clothes and her body are dirty. She has a large leg ulcer and says, "My leg gets real tired sometimes. I don't remember when my leg got sore like that."

In addition to her psychiatric difficulties, Evelyn has medical problems: a large weeping ulcer (5 cm, stage 3) on a swollen left ankle (4+/4+ to midcalf), high blood pressure (right arm, 154/96; left arm, 160/98), and a serum glucose level of 263. The nurse is unable to get Evelyn to undress because of her agitation. The nurse does, however, feel protruding bones under Evelyn's clothes. Evelyn's skin is dry and flaky, with multiple scars, abrasions, and bruises. Her feet are calloused and cracked. Her heart rate is 98 and her respiration rate 22. She refuses to have her temperature taken. She tells the nurse, "I'm so tired and hungry."

ASSESSMENT

The nurse assessed the following.

Objective Data

1. Several psychiatric admissions over 20 years
2. Multiple short-term relationships with men
3. Difficulty maintaining relationships with others
4. Has a 10-year-old daughter
5. Jobless and underhoused for 2 years
6. Poor hygiene
7. Clothes inappropriate for weather
8. Large leg ulcer, hypertension, hyperglycemia
9. Undernourished
10. Multiple signs of past injuries
11. Difficulty keeping focused during intake interview

Subjective Data

1. "A man . . . says he's going to hurt me."
2. "I'm so tired and hungry."
3. "Marie is in school today. I got scared and couldn't wait for her."
4. "My leg gets real tired sometimes."
5. "There are a lot of nasty, mean people out there. You just can't get away from them."
6. "I don't remember when my leg got sore like that."

SELF-ASSESSMENT

Most nurses become skilled in dealing with both the medical and psychosocial needs of the hospital's population. Through close work with case managers and social workers, help can often be made available after discharge. However, dealing with child neglect and abuse is often difficult for nursing staff. Neglected and abused children do not learn or experience healthy bonding, and they do not develop effective social skills, problem-solving techniques, competencies necessary for employment, self-esteem, and many other skills needed to succeed in life. To care adequately for Evelyn, and indirectly for Marie, the staff realized that the social worker would be an important resource person, providing access and referrals to meet some of this family's needs.

NURSING DIAGNOSIS

The following nursing diagnoses were formulated.

1. **Disturbed thought processes** related to psychiatric dysfunction as evidenced by distractibility and cognitive defects.

   - ■ "A man says he's going to hurt me"
   - ■ Difficulty staying focused
   - ■ "I don't remember when my leg got sore like that"
   - ■ Inability to obtain and retain a job
   - ■ Inability to provide a clean home for self and daughter (Marie)
   - ■ No preparation for Marie's care during the hospitalization

2. **Disabled family coping** related to psychiatric dysfunction and poverty, as evidenced by neglect of daughter.

   - ■ Jobless and underhoused for 2 years
   - ■ Motel room dirty
   - ■ Marie's infrequent school attendance and poor academic function
   - ■ Evelyn's not being where Marie expects to find her after school

   - ■ No preparation for Marie's care during the hospitalization

3. **Impaired tissue integrity** related to venous stasis and impaired cellular function, as evidenced by large ulcer on left ankle.

   - ■ 5-cm, stage 3 ulcer
   - ■ 4+/4+ edema to midcalf on left leg
   - ■ "My leg gets real tired sometimes"

Other nursing diagnoses that deserve attention are

1. **Self-care deficit: Bathing hygiene** related to homelessness and decreased cognitive function and poverty, as evidenced by dirty, torn clothing and dirty hair and skin.

2. **Imbalanced nutrition: Less than body requirements** related to impaired glucose metabolism and poverty, as evidenced by emaciation.

3. **Risk for injury** related to decreased cognitive function and hyperglycemia.

OUTCOME CRITERIA

DIAGNOSES	OUTCOME CRITERIA	SHORT-TERM GOALS
1. **Disturbed thought processes** related to psychiatric dysfunction and hyperglycemia, as evidenced by distractibility and cognitive defects.	1. Evelyn will demonstrate improved thought processes during this admission, as evidenced by decreased distractibility and increased ability to problem-solve care for herself and her daughter.	1a. Evelyn will demonstrate ability to concentrate on learning and/or therapy activities for at least 10 minutes.
		1b. Evelyn will identify three appropriate actions that can be taken to decrease anxiety in the event of stress.
		1c. Evelyn will demonstrate ability to plan and execute three aspects of self-care.

Case Study continued on following page

CASE STUDY 28–1 **A *Person with Severe and Persistent Mental Illness*** *(Continued)*

	DIAGNOSES	OUTCOME CRITERIA	SHORT-TERM GOALS
	2. **Disabled family coping:** related to psychiatric dysfunction and poverty, as evidenced by neglect of daughter.	2. Evelyn will demonstrate improved nurturing behavior toward daughter by discharge, as evidenced by awareness of how to access support for basic needs and education, as well as specified nurturing behaviors.	2a. Evelyn will verbalize an appropriate plan for care of Marie during Evelyn's hospitalization. 2b. Evelyn will discuss with social worker how to access benefits and programs for Marie's support and education by discharge. 2c. Evelyn will demonstrate nurturing behaviors toward Marie during visits throughout this hospitalization.
	3. **Impaired tissue integrity** related to venous stasis and impaired cellular function, as evidenced by large ulcer on left ankle.	3. Evelyn's ulcer will decrease from 5 cm to 1 cm by discharge.	3a. Evelyn's ulcer will no longer exude serosanguineous drainage. 3b. Evelyn's ulcer will be free from infection.

INTERVENTION

Initially, during the first few hours, the focus was on lowering Evelyn's anxiety so that she would accept needed care. Meeting some of her physiological needs (e.g., food, euglycemia) gave the staff the opportunity to make contact with Evelyn. The social worker, Mr. Todd, was contacted and informed that Marie would return from school and not be able to find her mother. Mr. Todd located Marie at school and explained the problem. He then brought her to the hospital to see Evelyn before taking her to an emergency foster home. This activity was necessary not only to protect Marie but also to emphasize to Evelyn how important such interventions were to Marie's well-being.

EVALUATION

Evelyn's psychosocial and medical health improved slowly during the short admission. Her ability to think increased modestly. Her leg ulcer began to show signs of granulation. The edema decreased to 1/4+ and remained at ankle level. Her serum glucose level remained between 140 and 180. Evelyn articulated plans for job training and living at a halfway house during the training period. She also talked about keeping Marie in a stable foster care home until she was working and had a proper home for the two of them. Evelyn agreed to continuing parenting classes through the child welfare agency. However, Marie was demonstrating various acting out behaviors both in the foster home and at school. She stated, "My mother loves me and I want to be with her now. The way we lived was just fine." Her therapist felt considerable resistance from her.

SUMMARY

People with severe mental illness have dysfunctions that pervade their ability to perform all aspects of daily life as well as interfere with their relationships with those around them. The seriously mentally ill include individuals with different disorders, prognoses, and needs whose outcomes vary over time. However, often the severity and course of the illness are influenced by poverty, racism, and substance abuse.

People with severe mental illnesses have numerous deficits. Their interpersonal problems with family members, and their relationships at work and even with those in the health care system can lead to alienation, isolation, fear, and in too many cases, homelessness. Follow-up care with community-based psychiatric treatment centers and rehabilitation helps keep people out of the hospital, in the community, in many cases working, and experiencing their optimum quality of life with relatives and friends. Unfortunately appropriate health care is not always available, and managed care systems do not often support current standards of care for severe mental illness.

Insufficient housing, nonadherence to medications, and co-existing substance abuse can negatively impact on rehabilitation and stabilization of the illness. There are a number of resources within the community that ideally are available to help people maintain stability and prevent relapse. Unfortunately, these are not always available, nor are there a plethora of community services staffed by competent staff following current standards of care. Managed care and insurance policies often dictate the use of medications, using drugs that are the most cost-effective. At other times, some managed care companies may disallow needed follow-up care and services for many of the severely mentally ill people in the United States.

Case managers are a pivotal resource for people with severe mental illness. They are in a position to individualize care for clients with severe mental illness and their families, since family support and education are vital for successful outcomes. Rehabilitation services include crisis stabilization, psychoeducation, social skills training, vocational rehabilitation programs, and supportive group therapies. These are briefly discussed here. Cognitive and behavioral approaches to care are addressed in the discussion on schizophrenia (see Chapter 20).

Visit the **Evolve** website at
http://evolve.elsevier.com/Varcarolis
for a post-test on the content in this chapter.

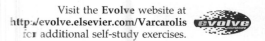

Visit the **Evolve** website at
http://evolve.elsevier.com/Varcarolis
for additional self-study exercises.

Critical Thinking and Chapter Review

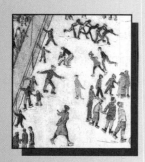

Critical Thinking

Lin Yang, age 42, just moved into town with his mother who is now 70 years old. Lin has a severe mental illness and has a dual diagnosis (schizophrenia and alcohol plus marijuana abuse). Mrs. Yang brings Lin into the community mental health clinic, and you are doing an initial assessment. Mrs. Yang tells you that she has been caring for her son at home since Lin was 15; however, with the move to a new part of the country, she is at a complete loss how best to handle her son and at knowing what is available in the community. Lin is currently taking haloperidol (Haldol), but Mrs. Yang says that Lin often does not take the drug owing to the muscle rigidity and sexual side effects. Mrs. Yang says they have tried many of the traditional antipsychotics. Mrs. Yang tells you that they are currently living in an apartment, and her younger brother is coming to live with them in 6 months.

1. With an understanding of the problems inherent in a person with a severe mental illness, what are some areas of Lin's life you might want to explore in your psychosocial assessment? Consider relationships, employment history, cognitive ability, behaviors, and such. How would knowledge in these areas help your long-term planning?

2. After assessing Lin's medication history, how could you be a client advocate in terms of Lin's nonadherence to traditional antipsychotics? What are some of the problems in adherence for a client with severe mental illness and dual diagnosis? What approach seems to hold out the best chance of success?

3. Of the resources mentioned in this chapter, what are some of the resources that might be potentially appropriate for Lin (assuming a careful psychosocial and medical assessment has been performed, and that all resources are available in your community)?

4. Identify five basic aims of psychoeducation.

5. Make up a structured teaching plan for Mr. Yang (see #2). Use your own community in identifying available treatment centers and available support groups.

6. Using the research update as a guide, what further assessments might you include in long-range planning?

Chapter Review

1. Care planning is facilitated when the nurse understands that a cornerstone of treatment for maintaining the individual with severe mental illness within the community is

   1. Intense psychotherapy.
   2. Medication compliance.
   3. Respite care to ease family burden.
   4. Referrals to numerous community resources.

2. The community mental health nurse believes a particular client would profit from a medication change to a new atypical neuroleptic. The chief barrier to the use of a newer medication to treat this client with severe mental illness who is living in the community is

   1. Cost.
   2. Ineffective case management.
   3. The poor side effect profile of many of the newer drugs.
   4. Inability to provide psychoeducation for clients and families.

3. When planning care for a client with a dual diagnosis the nurse should consider that clients with dual diagnoses require

   1. Less assistance in resolving situational crises.
   2. Minimal training in activities of daily living skills.
   3. Treatment for severe mental illness and substance abuse.
   4. Intermittent therapy given at times when least cognitively impaired.

4. For what reason is short hospitalization for crisis stabilization more often recommended for a client with severe and persistent mental illness than for a client having a crisis who is essentially mentally healthy? The client with severe and persistent mental illness

   1. Often has inadequate situational supports.
   2. Has a good sense of personal boundaries.
   3. Has a realistic perception of the crisis event.
   4. Can mobilize coping defenses to lower anxiety.

5. What topic would be LEAST important to include in psychoeducation for severely mentally ill clients and their families?

1. Understanding medications.
2. Monitoring levels of stress.
3. Improving communication skills.
4. Impact of de-institutionalization.

REFERENCES

Bozzer, M., Samsom, D., and Anson, J. (1999). An evaluation of a community based rehabilitation program for adults with psychiatric disabilities. *Canadian Journal of Community Mental Health*, 18(1):165–179.

Center for Mental Health Services (1995). *Making a difference—interim status report of the McKinney demonstration program for homeless adults with serious mental illness*. Rockville, MD: Center for Mental Health Services.

Cuijpers, P., and Stam, H. (2000). Burnout among relatives of psychiatric patients attending psychoeducational support groups. *Psychiatric Services*. 51(3):375–379.

Drake, R. E., and Wallach, M. A. (1989). Substance abuse among the chronic mentally ill. *Hospital and Community Psychiatry*, 40(10):1041.

Drake, R. E., and Mueser, K. T. (2000). Psychosocial approaches to dual diagnosis. *Schizophrenia Bulletin*, 26(1):105–118.

Fallon Healthcare System, DomCare, and RX Innovations (1998, November). Case studies presented at the Institute for Behavioral Healthcare workshop, *Managing mental health pharmaceutical costs and risk in primary care settings*. St. Louis, Mo.

Finkelman, A. W. (1977). The nurse therapist: Outpatient crisis intervention with the chronic psychiatric patient. *Journal of Psychosocial Nursing and Mental Health Services*, 8:27.

Gorman, L. M., Sultan, D. F., and Raines, M. L. (1996). *Davis' manual of psychosocial nursing for general patient care*. Philadelphia: F. A. Davis.

Grad, J., and Sainsbury, P. (1993). Mental illness and the family. *Lancet*, (1):544.

Grob, G. N. (1994). Mad, homeless and unwanted: A history of the care of the chronic mentally ill in America. *Psychiatric Clinics of North America* 17(3):541.

Hays, R. D., et al. (1995). Functioning and well-being outcomes of patients with depression compared with chronic general medical illnesses. *Archives of General Psychiatry*, 52(1):11.

Lam, D. H. (1991). Psychosocial family intervention in schizophrenia: A review of empirical studies. *Psychological Medicine*, 21(2):423–441.

Lamb, H. R. (1999). Psychic psychiatry and prevention. In R. Hales, S. C. Yudofsky, and J. A. Talbotts (Eds.), *American Psychiatric Press textbook of psychiatry*. Washington, DC: American Psychiatric Press.

Lapierre, E. D., and Padgett, J. (1992). What does a nurse need to know and do to maintain an effective level of case management? *Journal of Psychosocial Nursing and Mental Health Services*, 30(3):35.

Lehman, A., et al. (1998). Patterns of usual care for schizophrenia: Initial results from the Schizophrenia Patient Outcomes Research Team (PORT) client survey. *Schizophrenia Bulletin*, 24:11–20.

Lieberman, R. P., Kopelowicz, A., and Smith, T. E. (1999). Psychiatric rehabilitation. In B. J. Sadock and V. A. Kaplan (Eds.). *Kaplan and Sadock's comprehensive textbook of psychiatry*, (7th ed., Vol. II). Philadelphia: Lippincott Williams & Wilkins.

Lipton, F. R., Seigel, C., Hannigan, A., and Samuels, J., and Baker.

(2000). Tenure supportive housing for homeless persons with severe mental illness. *Psychiatric Services*, 51(4):479–486.

Loukissa, D. A. (1995). Family burden in chronic mental illness: A review of research studies. *Journal of Advanced Nursing*, 21:248.

McAlpine, D. D., and Mechanic, D. (2000). Utilization of specialty mental health care among persons with severe mental illness: The roles of demographics, need, insurance, and risk. *Health Services Research*, 35(1 pt 2):277–292.

Melzer, D., et al (1991). Community care for patients with schizophrenia one year after hospital discharge. *British Medical Journal*, 303:1023

Midence, K. (2000). An introduction to and rationale for psychosocial interventions. In C. Gamble and G. Brennan (Eds.), *Working with serious mental illness: A manual for clinical practice*. London: Baillière Tindall.

Murray, R. L., and Baier, M. (1995). Evaluation of a transitional residential program for homeless chronically mentally ill people. *Journal of Psychiatric and Mental Health Nursing*, 2(1):3.

NAMI (1998). Millions with schizophrenia not getting basic treatment: Landmark study shows care lags far behind science. National Alliance for the Mentally Ill. http://www.nami.org/pressroom/980324102700.html.

NAMI (2000a). Access to effective medications: A critical link to mental illness recovery. National Alliance for the Mentally Ill. http://www.nami.org/update/000709b.html.

NAMI (2000b). NAMI offers testimony on homeless program consolidation legislation. www.nami.org/update/000609.html.

Peternelj-Taylor, C. A., and Hartley, V. L. (1993). Living with mental illness: Professional-family collaboration. *Journal of Psychosocial Nursing*, 31(3):23.

Polko, D. E., North, C. S., and Foster, D. A. (1998). Content and curriculum in psychoeducation groups for families of persons with severe mental illness. *Psychiatric Services*, 49(6):816–822.

RachBeisel, J., Scott, J., and Dixon, L. (1999). Co-occurring severe mental illness and substance use disorders: A review of recent research. *Psychiatric Services*, 50(11):1427–1434.

Recker, T., Hornung, W. P., Schonaur, K., and Eikelmann, B. (2000). Long term psychiatric patients in vocational rehabilitation programme: A naturalistic follow-up study over 3 years. *Acta Psychiatric Scand*, 101(6):457–463.

Ryrie, L. (2000). Coexistent substance use and psychiatric disorders. In C. Gamble and G. Brennan (Eds.), *Working with serious mental illness: A manual for clinical practice*. London: Baillière Tindall.

Schultz, J. M., and Videbeck, S. D. (1998). *Lippincott's manual of psychiatric nursing care plans*. Philadelphia: J. B. Lippincott.

Smith, T. E, Bellack, A. S., and Lieberman, R. P. (1996). Relatives and patients as partners in the management of schizophrenia: The development of a service model. *British Journal of Psychiatry*, 156:654–660.

Ulf, M., Ivarson, B., and Falloon, I. (2000). A two-year controlled study of the efficacy of integrated care in schizophrenia. Presented at the World Association for Psychosocial Rehabilitation, VIIth World Congress. May 7–10, 2000, Paris.

Worley, N. K., Drago, L., and Hadley, T. (1990). Improving the physical health–mental health interface for the chronically mentally ill: Could nurse case managers make a difference? *Archives of Psychiatric Nursing*. 4(2):108.

Outline

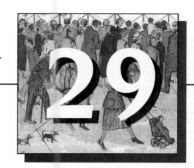

29

Psychological Needs of the Medically Ill

ELIZABETH M. VARCAROLIS

Key Terms and Concepts

The key terms and concepts listed here also appear in color where they are first defined or discussed in this chapter.

coping strategies

holistic assessment

holistic approach

human rights abuses

psychiatric liaison nurse

psychosocial issues of HIV
  infection

quality-of-life assessment

stigmatized medically ill
  persons

Objectives

After studying this chapter, the reader will be able to

1. Describe at least four common responses people experience when faced with a serious medical illness.

2. Analyze how stress can intensify to symptoms of medical disease.

3. Discuss the potential uses of and the rationale for the teaching of relaxation training and coping skills by nurses.

4. Perform psychosocial (psycho-social-spiritual) nursing assessment.

5. Assess your client's coping skills: (a) identify areas for teaching; (b) identify areas of strengths.

6. Apply knowledge of psychological responses to illness in nonpsychiatric settings.

7. Explain how a consultation with a psychiatric liaison nurse could have been useful for one of your medical/surgical patients.

*T*he nurse's view of the individual as a complex blend of many parts is consistent with our holistic approach to nursing care. Nurses who care for people with physical illnesses who are receiving physical treatments need to maintain a holistic view that involves an awareness of psychological, social, cultural, and spiritual issues (Dossey et al. 1995).

A mentally healthy person who experiences psychological, social, cultural, and spiritual problems as a result of situational or maturational problems may be experiencing a crisis. Usually, some time-limited crisis intervention or brief supportive counseling is sufficient to bolster the person's already adequate coping skills until the crisis is past. However, when the situational crisis is a persistent life-threatening or disabling disease, or when a permanent change occurs in the person's situation, long-term interventions may be required. It helps us give more thorough and compassionate care when we are aware of the complex issues people face when faced with a serious medical illness.

PSYCHOLOGICAL RESPONSES TO SERIOUS MEDICAL ILLNESS

People's responses can be many and varied when they find themselves faced with a serious medical problem:

■ Will I be disfigured?
■ Will I have a long-term disability?
■ Will I be able to function as a (wife/husband, parent)
■ Will I be able to continue to work?
■ Will I suffer pain?

People who face the crisis of serious medical diagnoses need the kind of emotional support that allows them to face their burdens without censure or fear of judgment (Zerbe 1999). Strong emotional supports and social ties may not be available. Other questions may arise:

■ How will I cope?
■ How will this affect my life?
■ Will I retain some quality of life?

The editor would like to thank Michelle Conant Dan-El for her contribution to this chapter in the third edition of *Foundations of Psychiatric Mental Health Nursing*.

Emotional Responses

Psychological sequelae of medical illness can be severe and can account for a higher rate of disruption in functional ability than just the medical illness alone would indicate. Among the most common psychological responses to physical illness are depression, anxiety, substance use, denial, and anger.

These and more are all phenomena that can result from experiencing a serious medical condition. For example, the lifetime prevalence rates of substance abuse for those with a medical illness is 9.4% higher than non–medically ill individuals (NIMH 1991).

On the other hand, a psychological condition may supersede or be comorbid with a medical condition. Schuyler (2000) states that depression typically co-occurs with serious medical illness. If depression is present (either occurring before or associated with the medical diagnosis), it can have a profound effect on the client's medical condition. Depression, if not recognized and treated, can affect the severity and functional ability of the client (Schuyler 2000).

Depression

Depression is a risk factor for medical noncompliance. A study by DíMatteo and colleagues (2000) found that the odds are three times greater that depressed clients will be noncompliant with medical treatment recommendations than will nondepressed patients. Stewart and Atlas (2000) state that depression can amplify the pathophysiology of endocrine and cardiac disease and diminish functional ability. A study by Meyer and colleagues (2000) found that individuals who scored higher on the depression component of the Hospital and Anxiety Depression Scale (HADS) were rated higher by physicians in terms of the severity of their illness and their functional impairment.

Anxiety

Anxiety accompanies every illness, especially when pain, disability, hospitalization, economic loss, or fear of death is present. Verbalizing is an effective outlet for anxiety, but the ability to verbalize may be compromised by cultural expectations, disability, or lack of a listener. Helplessness often accompanies anxiety in the person who feels a loss of control over events, such as when awaiting surgery or undergoing invasive treatments. In this case, defense mechanisms may be used with greater frequency, or compulsive behaviors may surface. Self-centeredness characterized by unreasonable requests of caregivers may also be a cover for feelings of inadequacy.

The following vignette shows how acute anxiety can affect a person's ability to take in information, threaten his or her self-esteem ("I should be able to do this without help"), and trigger expected, and at this point adaptive, denial.

Vignette

■ At 27, Ted tests positive for human immunodeficiency virus (HIV). During the posttest counseling session with the public health nurse at the health department, Ted is given referrals and information regarding the virus. The nurse notes that Ted is having difficulty focusing on details and needs to have information repeated several times as he writes copious notes. The nurse gives Ted the opportunity to explore his feelings, but Ted has difficulty in this area because he was raised to believe that dealing with crisis alone is a strength. Ted is also experiencing a great deal of denial in this initial period of loss (see the discussion about the stages of death and dying in Chapter 30). For these reasons, the nurse anticipates the most common and immediate concerns that might be facing a person who has just discovered that he is HIV positive and gently leads Ted into discussing those concerns over a period of several weeks, with the use of reflective statements and silence. This approach gives Ted the opportunity to verbalize his feelings and begin to unburden himself in a safe environment.

Long-term and pervasive anxiety or an anxiety disorder that precedes a medical disorder can actually be a risk factor for a medical disorder. A study of the relationship between an anxiety disorder and the later development of medical morbidity was made by Bowen and associates (2000). Their study, which spanned a 10-year period, found that the anxiety cohort (those with anxiety disorders) had a significantly higher relative risk of developing a medical disease than did the control group (those without anxiety disorders). The highest relative risk was for cerebrovascular disease.

So, from relevant research, it seems important that health care workers such as nurses and physicians need to be diligent in their initial assessments, identifying any coexisting or resulting psychological response or disorder. In most cases of physical illness, the focus is on the complaints of physical symptoms, and minimal attention is given to the psychological responses of the client.

Grief and Loss

Very often, an individual suffers from feelings of grief and loss. Any type of treatment or procedure intended to treat a physical illness that creates a major permanent change is accompanied by feelings of loss. The dynamics involved in coping with these feelings are similar to those operating in a person who is dealing with his or her own death or the death of a loved one. The person must grieve for this loss, just as the dying person must work through the confusion and darkness until a degree of acceptance and relative peace is achieved. Negotiating the loss of physical well-being involves movement through feelings of frustration, vulnerability, and sadness to become a whole person once again. This journey encompasses spiritual as well as emotional changes and, as such, requires spiritual assessment of the client as well as a focus on psychosocial issues. See Chapter 30.

Denial

As an unconscious defense mechanism, denial is a common response to physical illness. A person may believe that the pain is really nothing or will go away (even though it is severe and lasts for long periods) or may minimize dramatic bodily changes. Even after hearing a diagnosis with a poor prognosis, a person in denial may hear only the more positive or hopeful message and may block out the negative. This is a protective measure, and it is necessary in the early stages of loss but can interfere with treatment if it continues for too long. When a person minimizes physical complaints, the nursing staff may unwittingly collude in the denial by not performing a complete assessment and by accepting the person's subjective statements at face value.

Vignette

■ After a car accident, Carol is being assessed by the triage nurse in the emergency department for possible injuries. She complains of a slight headache and dizziness but denies having any other pain or symptoms. Carol is preoccupied with seeing that her 2-year-old son, who was also in the car, is being examined, so she denies her own need for medical attention. Carol's blood pressure is 86/50 mm Hg, and her body posture indicates that she is guarding her abdomen. These observations are reported to the examining physician immediately because they indicate possible internal bleeding and danger of shock. Carol is eventually taken to the operating room so the bleeding may be stopped.

Fear of Dependency

Responses to being dependent might be exhibited as the inability to accept warmth, nurturing, or tenderness from caregivers or as refusal to accept treatment or medical advice. This reaction is strongest in those who have unmet dependency needs and those who have had negative experiences when help was sought in the past. Anger with caregivers may mask acute embarrassment over being in a dependent position by one who needs to project an independent image.

Others find themselves becoming fearful of not having their dependency needs met and do not express any negative feelings to caregivers. These people need to be "good" clients out of fear that they will be abandoned if perceived to be difficult. Any anxiety or anger they suppress may be exhibited through increased somatic complaints.

Vignette

■ *Lillian is a 47-year-old woman who is being treated with hemodialysis and has been complaining of frequent tension headaches and occasional stomach upsets before her treatment appointments. The hemodialysis nurse has always been impressed by Lillian's patience and compliant attitude in spite of her debilitating illness, which has robbed her of a normal family life. For this reason, the nurse suspects that Lillian's physical complaints could be a way of dealing with emotions, so the nurse makes a point of spending more time with Lillian to allow her to talk about her frustrations. Lillian expresses anger and some feelings of hopelessness. She resents others who are healthy, including the people who care for her. Frequent opportunities to verbalize these feelings gradually result in the lessening of her somatic complaints and a decrease in her sense of powerlessness and isolation.*

Even though procedures may extend or promote life, they often take their toll on the client's physical state because of the high degree of anxiety they evoke. Educating a client regarding the specific treatment, identifying an anxious client and referring him or her to community supports, and evaluating coping strategies and teaching more effective skills have all been shown to affect a client's recovery positively. Focusing on a client's strengths and reinforcing and teaching coping skills (e.g., prayer, hobbies, relaxation techniques) are important nursing interventions.

PSYCHOSOCIAL FACTORS IN MEDICAL ILLNESS

The mind-body connection has been extensively researched and is discussed in greater depth in Chap-

ter 12. Hans Selye (1956) was the first to introduce the concept of stress into the field of medicine and physiology. As you know from Chapter 12, stress can lead to changes in physical and mental health in many ways. Cannon's (1914) fight-or-flight response and Selye's general adaptation syndrome (GAS) provided insight into the biological and molecular reactions to stressors in the sympathetic nervous system, the pituitary-adrenocortical axis, and the immune system (Lowery and Houldin 1996). Extensive studies have left little doubt that psychosocial stress can affect the course and severity of illness.

For example, Hemingway and Marmot (1999) reviewed 30 studies that confirmed that an adverse psychosocial environment (stress, depression, and loneliness) can increase a person's risk of heart disease. What is more, an adverse psychosocial environment may even be a predictor of mortality (Hofland 2000). Lesperance and Smith (2000) state that depression alone affects up to 30% of hospitalized individuals with coronary artery disease. If depression is not recognized and treated and if it lasts as long as 1 year after discharge, the person is at higher risk for mortality.

Turks and Bellisimo (1991) state that stressors are "events in which demands of the internal and external environment challenge or exceed the adaptive resources of the individual." Vogel and Romano (1999) state that this definition allows for an understanding of the role of coping so as to moderate the effect of stressors and adapt to environmental demands. There are many healthy ways people can cope with the stress surrounding their illnesses, and these should be encouraged. There are also unhealthy ways people cope with the stresses surrounding their illnesses. These less effective **coping strategies** can be assessed, and new and effective coping skills (cognitive, behavioral, and psychosocial) can be taught.

Numerous medical disorders have been extensively studied in terms of the effects of stress on the course of illness. Although personality traits or life style may very well affect the course of disease, few of the earlier studies support the idea that a specific personality type causes or is an integral part of the cause of a medical disorder. Table 29–1 identifies some physical illnesses that benefit from stress reduction and support. In actual fact, anyone facing a serious medical condition needs a variety of supports and may benefit from learning new coping skills.

Therefore, nurses will be best prepared if they are able to do a thorough holistic assessment of their medically ill client.

TABLE 29–1	*Commonly Known Medical Conditions Negatively Affected by Stress*			
MEDICAL CONDITION	**INCIDENCE**	**GENETIC AND BIOLOGICAL CORRELATES**	**COMMON PRECIPITATING FACTORS**	**HOLISTIC THERAPIES IN ADDITION TO MEDICAL MANAGEMENT**
Cardiovascular Disorder				
Coronary heart disease (CHD)	Higher in males until age 60 Higher in white population than in black population	Family history of cardiac disease a risk factor Other risk factors include hypertension, increased serum lipid levels, obesity, sedentary life style, and cigarette smoking. Psychosocial factors (stress, depression, loneliness) High anxiety risk in client with prior cardiac events	Often, myocardial infarction (MI) occurs after sudden stress preceded by a period of losses, frustration, and disappointments	Relaxation training, stress management, group social support, and psychosocial intervention Support groups for type A personalities and type A modification helpful When indicated, anxiolytics (benzodiazepines) and antidepressants are prescribed
Peptic Ulcer				
Helicobacter pylori	Occurs in 12% of men, 6% of women (more prevalent in industrialized societies)	Infection with *H. pylori* is associated with 95–99% of peptic ulcers Both peptic and duodenal ulcers cluster in families, but separately from each other	Periods of social tension and increased life stress After losses; often after menopause	Antibodies that target *H. pylori* can erode immune system Biofeedback can alter gastric acidity; cognitive-behavioral approaches are used to reduce stress (stress management
Cancer				
	Men: most common in lung, prostate, colon, and rectum Women: most common in breast, uterus, colon, and rectum Death rate higher in men (especially black men) than in women	Genetic evidence suggests dysfunction of cellular profusion Familial patterns: breast cancer, colorectal cancer, stomach cancer, melanoma	Prolonged and intensive stress Stressful life events, e.g., separation from or loss of significant other 2 years before diagnosis Feelings of hopelessness, helplessness, and despair (depression) may precede the diagnosis of cancer	Relaxation, e.g., meditation, autogenic training, self-hypnosis Visualization Psychological counseling Support groups Massage therapy Stress management

Table continued on following page

TABLE 29–1   *Commonly Known Medical Conditions Negatively Affected by Stress* (Continued)

MEDICAL CONDITION	INCIDENCE	GENETIC AND BIOLOGICAL CORRELATES	COMMON PRECIPITATING FACTORS	HOLISTIC THERAPIES IN ADDITION TO MEDICAL MANAGEMENT
Tension Headache				
	Occurs in 80% of population when under stress Begins at end of workday or early evening		Associated with anxiety and depression Begins suboccipitally; usually bilateral	Psychotherapy usually prescribed for chronic tension headaches Learning to cope or avoiding tension-creating situations or people Relaxation techniques, stress management, cognitive restructuring techniques
Essential Hypertension				
	Higher in males until age 60	Family history of cardiac disease and hypertension	Life changes and traumatic life events Stressful jobs, e.g., air traffic controller Hypothesized to be found more in areas of social stress and conflict	Behavioral feedback, stress reduction techniques, meditation, yoga, hypnosis. *However, pharmacological treatment is considered primary for the treatment of hypertension.*

HOLISTIC ASSESSMENT OF A CLIENT'S NEEDS

Psychosocial factors are more commonly being recognized as relevant to the course of disease. It is now accepted by health care professionals that the way a person thinks and feels—whether a person feels cared for and nurtured and has a sense of meaning in life—has a profound effect on the course of disease (Barnett and Chambers 1996).

How can a health care worker know what a client thinks or feels unless the client's psychosocial situation is assessed? Although lip service is always paid to providing a holistic approach to care, the managed care environment often leaves little time for evaluating what could be pivotal information in finding out what a client needs to best cope with illness. It is vital to understand how a client's illness affects his or her life and how the client copes with adversity. Since the best indicator of future behavior is past behavior, ineffective coping strategies used in the past can be changed by learning more adaptive skills. Nurse clinicians are in a primary position to effect change in the quality of life of a client with medical illness and help that client to find the best way to heal or to deal with the illness. An effective nurse-client, or clinician-client, relationship may depend on a shared understanding of the psychosocial stresses the client is experiencing (e.g., troubled family relationships, job pressures, problems with children) and any psychosocial impairment the client may be experiencing (e.g., substance abuse, lack of social supports). Nurses and other health care workers are becoming more and more aware of the role spirituality or religion plays in many clients' lives and how important it is as a source of peace and nourishment. A study by Gioiella and associates (1998) supported the inclusion of spirituality in routine patient assessment and interventions and "associated with a personal perspective on death can help decrease the patient's level of psychosocial distress." In Chapter 9, too, nurses are encouraged to ask about spiritual or religious practices when assessing personal supports. A client may need to be encouraged to verbalize spiritual concerns. Support for the client by a priest, pastor, rabbi, or other religious leader may be indicated, especially in a case of spiritual distress. Many people derive a great deal of comfort and strength from their spiritual beliefs.

An understanding of how a client has dealt with adversity in the past is important in caring effectively for that client. Assessing usual coping skills gives professional health care workers information about which coping skills they will support and encourage and an understanding of what kinds of coping skills may help a client to cope better with a serious medical or surgical situation. The possible effective coping skills offered can be many and varied (e.g., assertiveness training, cognitive reframing, problem-solving skills, social supports). Since it is known that several leading causes of death, including heart disease, stroke, and cancer, are largely preventable by a change in behavior (Barnett and Chambers 1996), a nurse is in a key position to educate and support a client with medical illness in trying out healthier ways of looking at and dealing with illness.

For interventions to be most effective, it is necessary to understand how a person's medical condition affects the quality of life. For example, how is the medical illness affecting the client's ability to function in the home? At work or in school? How is the client's feelings about the illness (depression, anxiety, hopelessness) affecting his or her relationships and ability to function?

A holistic assessment can be a useful tool. A holistic assessment of physical needs includes

- Psychosocial assessment
- Assessment of usual coping strategies
- Overall quality-of-life assessment
- Activities of daily living (ADLs)
- Social activities
- Social supports
- Perception of quality of life
- Feelings
- Pain

Psychosocial Assessment

When working with someone who is medically ill, it is important to know something about the person's life.

- Does the person have someone who can share his or her concerns and who cares for him or her?
- Does the person have friends and supports in the community?
- Does the person have any co-existing conditions that could impede adjustment to the illness, the course of the illness, adaptation to the illness, ability to heal? For example,
    Depression
    Substance abuse
    Compulsive behaviors (gambling, eating, cybersex)
    Personality disorders
- Does the person's cultural view of health and illness help or impede the process of seeking adequate care?

Table 29–2 provides an outline for a psychosocial assessment of a medically ill client. A psychosocial assessment is done in tandem with a thorough physical workup and mental status examination (Chapter 21).

Assessment of Usual Coping Strategies

A person who undergoes a life-threatening disease or chronic illness most often deals with distressing physical side effects and changes in body image. For example, a person who is given a colostomy to avoid death resulting from cancer or ulcerative colitis is left with complex emotional as well as physical dilemmas. This is especially true for women, as Zerbe (1999) points out. A client not only has to learn techniques of dealing with the stoma but also has to learn to deal with the life-long consequences and how they will affect the person's concept of body image, appearance, and relationships. When an individual is faced with chronic physical illness, distressing side effects, and possible disfigurement, many real and legitimate concerns arise (Zerbe 1999).

- Will my partner still be attracted to me?
- Will I continue to be interested in sexual relationships?
- Will I be embarrassed by my friends' reactions to my situation?

TABLE 29–2 *Psychosocial Assessment for Medically Ill Clients*

SOCIAL SUPPORTS	AREAS TO ASSESS
Family	The effects of the client's illness, treatments, and recovery on the family in the past
Friends	With whom can the client share painful feelings?
	Does the client have friends to joke and laugh with?
	Are there people the client believes would stand by him or her?
Religious/Spiritual	Does the client find comfort and support in spiritual practices?
	Is the client a member of a spiritual or religious group in the community (church, temple, place of worship)?
	Does the client find inner peace and strength in religious/spiritual practices?
	■ The following statements may be used in performing a spiritual assessment of a client:
	I believe that life has value, meaning, and direction.
	Often Sometimes Seldom
	I feel a connection with the universe.
	Often Sometimes Seldom
	I believe in a power greater than myself.
	Often Sometimes Seldom
	I believe that my actions make a difference.
	Often Sometimes Seldom
	I believe that my actions express my true self.
	Often Sometimes Seldom
Cultural Beliefs	Does the client use specific culture-oriented treatments or remedies for his or her condition?
	Do the client's cultural beliefs allow for adequate treatment by Western medical standards?
Work	Are there colleagues at work on whom the client can count for support?
Physical Pain	Is the client in pain?
	■ How does the client cope with it?
	■ Is the pain disabling?
	■ Are there pain-reducing techniques that might help?
Major Illness	Does the client have a co-occurring major illness that will negatively affect his or her current condition?
	Is the client undergoing treatments that are affecting daily life more than expected?
	Are there interventions that would help the client to better cope with the sequelae of the illness and treatments?
	Has the client been hospitalized in the past?
	■ How many times?
	■ For what?
	■ How did the client cope?
Addictions/Mental Health	Does the client have a co-occurring mental health problem (depression, anxiety, compulsions)?
	Has the client suffered a mental disease in the past?
	Does the client participate in any compulsive behavior (e.g., smoking, working, spending, gambling, cybersex)?
	Does the client abuse substances (alcohol, drugs [illicit, over-the-counter, prescription])?

■ Will people still think of me and relate to me the way they did before this illness?

Breast cancer survivors have been helped by the camaraderie of other survivors who openly share their techniques of learning to deal with appliances or prostheses; they also can help patients respond to well-intended but probing or embarrassing questions. Women who have previously traveled the same path are the best resources for helping patients establish appropriate boundaries regarding intrusive questions such as "Are you wearing a wig because you lost all your hair as a result of chemotherapy?" (Zerbe 1999).

So it is important to know if a client has the coping skills and social supports to help him or her through the serious and often overwhelming consequences of a medical illness.

Table 29–3 is an assessment tool that highlights some of the characteristics that make people good copers and notes characteristics that may be changed or improved upon through psychosocial interventions or cognitive-behavioral approaches.

Overall Quality-of-Life Assessment

It is helpful for health care workers to understand overall how an illness can affect a person's quality of life. There are a number of quality-of-life assessment questionnaires that can be very helpful. Not only initially but also intermittently, questions such as these can be used to help evaluate the direction of the client's quality of life and how well psychosocial and medical interventions have been in effecting positive changes.

Such questions as the following are included:

QUESTION	YES	SOME	A LITTLE	NO
Has your physical or emotional health limited your social activities?				
Was someone there to help you when you needed or wanted someone?				
Have you been feeling (anxious, irritable, depressed, downhearted)?				

The health survey (SF-12) is useful for identifying the degree to which physical or emotional symptoms are interfering in an individual's life.

TABLE 29–3 *Assessment of Coping Skills*

EFFECTIVE COPING BEHAVIORS	INEFFECTIVE COPING BEHAVIORS
Has optimistic attitude	Sees glass as being half empty instead of half full
Confronts the issues; acts accordingly	Forgets it happened; minimizes critical health status or signals
Seeks information; gets guidance	Shows tendency to find escape or withdraw
Shares concerns; finds consolation	Blames someone, something else
Has capacity for healthy denial	Denies as much as possible; prolonged denial
Redefines the situation, reviews alternatives, examines consequences	Feels things are hopeless, were meant to be; "what's the use?"
Constructive use of distractions: keeping busy, maintaining positive emotional ties with family, friends, community	Withdraws, broods, is overwhelmed with self-pity, anger, envy, guilt about having caused the illness

INTERVENTION STRATEGIES

Ideally, a multidisciplinary team of caretakers, including a psychiatric liaison nurse, should be involved in the treatment of clients with serious medical illness. Using the data from the holistic assessment, nurse clinicians in tandem with a physician are in a position to provide useful and effective interventions from all areas.

People who are medically ill are vulnerable to a variety of psychosocial stresses. How they cope with these stresses may make the difference between living with an acceptable quality of life or giving in to despair, withdrawal, or helplessness and hopelessness. It is a fact that people with serious medical illnesses, especially those that are long-term, are at risk for psychological distress or even worse—depression, substance abuse problems, nonadherence to the medical regime, and worse.

Nurses are in a position to assess and understand clients' psychosocial stressors, identify needed coping skills, and teach stress management techniques. Nurses can play a very important role not only in clients' immediate medical care but also in helping clients to improve their abilities to cope and improve the quality of life during the course of a chronic medical illness.

Does the client have sufficient social supports (family, friends, and religious or spiritual help) to enable him or her to share thoughts and feelings in safety? Would the client benefit from a medical support group? (Most people do.)

Is the pain management program used by the client working? Would complementary approaches (e.g., hypnosis, guided imagery, biofeedback) be helpful in augmenting the client's pain control regime? Does the client have a co-existing mental disorder? Anxiety, depression, substance abuse, and other disorders are treatable. However, if mental disorders are not treated, severe psychological responses or mental health phenomena can increase the severity of the disease and negatively affect functional ability and quality of life.

How does the client cope with stress? Chapter 12 provides tools for measuring levels of stress and suggestions for holistic approaches to stress management. Consider teaching a variety of relaxation techniques, such as meditation, guided imagery, breathing exercises, and others. Behavioral techniques are useful, and nurses with special training can offer their clients progressive muscle relaxation (PMR) or biofeedback. Chapter 12 also identifies a variety of cognitive approaches to help people reduce undue stress, such as journal keeping, restructuring and setting priorities and goals, cognitive reframing, and assertiveness training.

Relaxation techniques, stress management, supportive education, and stress monitoring (e.g., health survey SF-12) should be part of the care of the medically ill client regardless of the medical diagnosis.

There is growing evidence that psychotherapy can help people endure medical illness (Zerbe 1999). Beneficial psychotherapy approaches include

- Cognitive-behavioral psychotherapy
- Guided imagery, biofeedback, acupressure, and hypnosis
- Psychodynamic psychotherapy

Table 29–4 is a guideline for clients and their families for coping with a major medical illness.

HUMAN RIGHTS ABUSES OF THE STIGMATIZED MEDICALLY ILL

Some consumers of health care and some health care providers have voiced the need for examination of human rights abuses of persons stigmatized by the health care system. These stigmatized medically ill persons include those who have mental illness, those who are HIV positive, and those who have been recipients of transgender surgeries or treatments. These are abuses that can result in inadequate care and lead to undue stress, worsening of physical illness, and even death. By assuming that persons with certain illnesses are bad, disgusting, or even just unusual, health care workers fail to acknowledge and understand that the psychosocial issues of these people are similar to those of others and that the same nursing interventions for anger, anxiety, or grief are applicable. Examples of human rights abuse include

TABLE 29–4   *Client and Family Guidelines for Coping With a Major Medical Illness*

Learn all you can about your illness	Knowledge reduces anxiety. Keeping your anxiety at manageable levels helps you understand your options and helps you make decisions you believe are right for you.
Practice healthy behaviors	Good sleep hygiene, diet, and exercise are always good policies. Even if you are physically limited, exercise promotes a positive state of well being. Lack of sleep can increase pain, irritability, and fatigue. Proper nutrition in the face of a medical illness can preserve or promote a healthy immune system.
Take advantage of medical support groups	Support groups that focus on your medical issue can help give you information, help you learn how to handle difficult situations related to your illness, reduce isolation, and offer a safe place to share difficult thoughts and feelings.
Consider entering therapy	There is growing evidence that therapy helps people endure medical illness. Benefits include less pain, better coping skills, and even longer survival, in some situations.
Find a way to express your feelings	Studies have examined the profound healing power of putting upsetting experiences in words, e.g., writing them down, keeping a journal. Acknowledging thoughts and feelings can help your nervous system relax.
Seek additional help if you become depressed, demoralized, anxious, or panicky or have unremitting pain	Your clinician might not be aware of these changes and there are approaches (e.g., acupuncture, acupressure, biofeedback) that can give people control over their physiological responses and reduce the need for high doses of medication.
Find a creative outlet	Poetry or prose, painting or making collages, playing an instrument or singing (anything creative) are powerful tools in working with the fear, anger, and loss that are stirred by illness.
If you are a caregiver, do not neglect your own self-care	Take time for rest and restoration, time to renew yourself in important life interests and activities. If you become depleted, you cannot give to another what is depleted and you no longer possess.

Data from Zerbe, K. J. (1999). *Women's mental health in primary care.* Philadelphia: W.B. Saunders.

- Neglect to fully investigate somatic complaints made by emergency department clients with a history of psychiatric illness.
- Avoidance of contact with, or refusal to care for, persons who are stigmatized, which results in worsening illness or death.
- Hasty labeling with a psychiatric diagnosis and prescription of antipsychotics for persons who have the normal emotional responses (e.g., sadness, anger) to chronic physical illness.
- Inappropriate psychiatric admission of persons who are on medical units or in nursing homes based on the financial needs of the institution or on the staff's inability to manage emotional responses to physical illness or the aging process.

These situations may occur more frequently in the cases of persons who lack family support or the personal resources to advocate for themselves (e.g., those from the lower socioeconomic classes, newly arrived immigrants, those living "unacceptable" alternative life styles).

Vignette

- *Cynthia Bruce was critically injured in a car accident on Monday, August 7, at 50th and C Streets, SE. The accident occurred at approximately 3:30 p.m. Numerous witnesses report that when the fire department personnel working on Cynthia discovered she was biologically a male, they temporarily stopped treatment and made disparaging remarks and jokes about the victim. Cynthia was apparently semiconscious during this time. Cynthia died a short time later at D.C. General Hospital. (Renaissance News & Views, Vol. 9, No. 9, September 1995.)*

The key to increasing awareness of human rights issues in mental health care may be the integration of these concepts into nursing curricula. However, humanitarian values are often sown early in life, and nurses hesitate to confront employers regarding accepted practices that violate human rights. A committee composed of nurses who do not experience a conflict of interest while in the role of client advocates, as well as other hospital employees, could be formed to review such cases and make recommendations to the hospital administration. In this age of managed care and cuts in hospital budgets, human rights is one of nursing's greatest challenges.

Stigmatization of People with HIV Infection

The psychosocial issues of HIV infection are sometimes overwhelming both for nurses and for their clients. The psychological impact of hearing that one has been infected with HIV or the fear that one may test positive for the virus in the future because of past behaviors has led to a new focus by health care professionals who work with populations seeking HIV testing. The nurse now has the role of counselor, which requires an extreme sensitivity to the personality style and coping style of the individual as well as an appreciation of the ramifications of the decision to be tested. The reaction to a positive test result may be so devastating to the person that face-to-face counseling must be given before the test is performed and again after the results are received. Even receiving a negative test result, if it is not accompanied by adequate health education, can produce a false sense of security and negative health behaviors. Tough questions like Who should be tested? and Should HIV-positive women become pregnant? are being addressed by mental health professionals in many settings, and position statements are being formalized by professional associations and other committees. The controversial end-of-life issues, including nurses' responses to persons who request assisted suicide, are confronting nurses in the community who are caring for persons with HIV illnesses. A guideline to interventions for some common issues faced by people with HIV infection is shown in Table 29–5.

HIV encephalopathy (acquired immunodeficiency virus dementia) and the central nervous system infections of cryptococcosis and toxoplasmosis have created a need for psychiatric instruction for emotionally and physically depleted caretakers. The fact that many young people are HIV positive has contributed to the devastation that society experiences as the lives of children and young adults are ended before they can realize their goals. The middle-aged population, who are often caretakers for their children and for their parents, have special needs for support and respite.

ROLE OF THE PSYCHIATRIC LIAISON NURSE

Psychiatric liaison nursing is a relatively new subspecialty of psychiatric nursing that was initiated in the early 1960s. Usually, the psychiatric liaison nurse is a nurse with a master's degree and a background in psychiatric and medical-surgical nursing. A psychiatric liaison nurse functions as a nursing consultant in managing psychosocial concerns and as a clinician in helping the client deal more effectively with physical and emotional problems. Throughout the steps of the nursing process, a psychiatric liaison

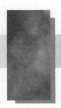

TABLE 29–5   *Common Issues Faced by People With HIV*

INTERVENTION	RATIONALE
Feelings of Isolation, Social Isolation	
Assess social supports: Who are the individuals in the client's network? Are they reliable and a available? Does the client feel they are supportive?	Social support can buffer the effects of physical and psychological stress.
Determine which local agencies and resources would be useful and available to the client. For example, National AIDS Coalition Hotline (1-800-342-AIDS), People with AIDS Coalition Hotline (1-800-828-3280)	The client may be unaware of sources of specific help and emotional support.
Encourage and facilitate the client's verbal expression of concerns, questions, and fears.	When others show genuine concern for the client's experience, his or her anxiety may decrease, along with feelings of alienation.
What to Tell Others	
Assist and support the client in sharing information with significant others regarding his or her HIV-positive status. For example, role play what the client wants to say to family, lover, and close friends.	The client may want family and close friends to know of his or her HIV status. Role playing helps the client become comfortable in disclosing the diagnosis.
Assess whether the client wants others, e.g., employer and casual friends, to know the diagnosis.	The dentist and general practitioner need to know the HIV status. Telling employer and casual friends may be risky; the potential for losing a job is real.
Being Overwhelmed and Anxious	
Encourage the client to participate in determining goals and in decision making regarding his or her care.	This promotes a sense of control and may reduce anxiety.
Provide accurate information about procedures, tests, transmission, and hospital routines. When health care workers are unsure, they should contact the infectious disease department in the hospital or the local health department for up-to-date information.	People often misinterpret the rationale or the reason for procedures and tests. Up-to-date information can reduce anxiety.
Continue to discuss transmission and ways to avoid infecting others.	When anxiety is high, retention of information is diminished.
Clarify misperceptions.	Understanding helps reduce anxiety, thereby facilitating retention of information.
Maintain continuity of nursing care throughout each phase of hospitalization.	Continuity helps the client maintain trust of the nurse and his or her environment.
Feeling Anger and Denial	
Assess the client for maladaptive coping strategies, e.g., prolonged denial.	Prolonged denial interferes with the client's accepting the diagnosis and obtaining treatment.
Avoid false reassurances, e.g., implying that the cure for HIV disease may be at hand.	Stories of clients who have adjusted to their diagnoses successfully encourage realistic hope.

Help the client deal with anger. The nurse can
  Assess the reasons for the client's anger
  Avoid personalizing the client's verbal abuse
  Encourage realizations that will assist the client in resolving angry feelings
  Use nursing peers to discuss personal feelings and frustrations and provide a clear perspective.
	Anger is an expected response; however, excess hostility that alienates all support networks is maladaptive. The client's anger often comes from lack of control over the situation, fear of isolation, or fear of losing employment.

Data from McGrough, K. N. (1990). Assessing social support of people with AIDS. *Oncology Nursing Forum*, 17(1):31; Nyamathi, A., & Van Servellen, G. (1989). Maladaptive coping in critically ill patients with acquired immune deficiency syndrome: Nursing assessment. *Heart and Lung*, 18(2):113.
AIDS, acquired immunodeficiency syndrome; HIV, human immunodeficiency virus.

nurse assists the nursing and medical staff in caring for hospitalized, medically ill clients with mental health concerns. Often these individuals present management problems or have problems that impede their care. Therefore, the psychiatric liaison nurse is a resource for the members of a nursing staff who feel unable to intervene therapeutically with a client.

The psychiatric liaison nurse first meets with the nurse who initiated the consultation. The liaison nurse then reviews the medical records, talks with the physicians, and interviews the client. After interviewing the client, the liaison nurse discusses the assessment and suggestions with the referring nurse. If a psychiatric consultation is warranted, the psychiatric liaison nurse initiates the consultation by contacting the client's medical doctor. A case conference is sometimes needed to enhance communication and consistency in the care of a particular client.

SUMMARY

Just as physical illness is accompanied by emotional responses, so emotions often exacerbate the severity of physical symptoms. The holistic philosophy of nursing dictates that all nurses, regardless of their roles or specialties, maintain a view of clients as having a number of psychosocial needs as well as strengths that can be identified through a holistic assessment. Applying the theories and concepts of psychiatric mental health nursing to the care of all clients is not only a challenge to nurses but is also required by today's health care consumer. Illness disrupts the lives of clients and their families on many levels. By understanding a client's psychosocial needs and knowing when to intervene and where to refer the client, the nurse really practices holistic care and more effectively promotes health.

A growing concern about clients is the state of their spiritual lives. Including this dimension in the holistic nursing assessment allows nurses to see inner strengths in their clients that might be overlooked by a more traditional approach. Interventions coming from this holistic perspective may be more creative, as Eastern and Western approaches are united. Self-assessment allows nurses to explore their own inner strengths and how to use them in their professional lives in the service of clients who challenge nurses most—those who confront nurses with values, life styles, or beliefs that conflict with the nurse's own. It is incumbent on nurses not only to care for clients but also to advocate for them in this ever-changing health care system so that their psycho-social-spiritual needs are not overlooked.

The psychiatric liaison nurse is a nurse clinician who is in the key position of being able to help others to look at their clients in a holistic manner and being able to help those who care for them to understand other issues that are impeding medical progress.

Visit the **Evolve** website at http://evolve.elsevier.com/Varcarolis for a post-test on the content in this chapter.

Visit the **Evolve** website at http://evolve.elsevier.com/Varcarolis for additional self-study exercises.

Critical Thinking and Chapter Review

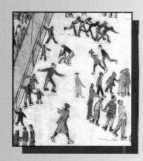

Critical Thinking

Vincent Parello, 58, is being discharged from the hospital after a serious myocardial infarction. His wife died a year ago of cancer and he says he still feels down about it. He talks to his two children on a weekly basis, but he sees them only once a year for a few days around the holidays. He is a hard worker and complains, "I've got so much stress . . . but I am the only one who can do this job." He finds it hard to talk about his thoughts and feelings. "I'll be fine," he says, but the nurse notices that he appears anxious and admits to being lonely "with everyone out of the house." Although overly busy with work, he does go to church every week, and sometime he says he gets sad because it brings back memories of church social events he shared with his family and old friends in the past. When he is told of some limitations on his physical activities, he reacts in a belligerent manner: "I can do anything I used to do." But underneath, the nurse believes he is frightened and is feeling very alone.

1. How would you evaluate this man's social support system?

   a. What other information would you like to know about his situation that might help in your assessment?
   b. What do you need to know about his cultural beliefs and illness?
   c. What recommendations or referrals could you make for him?
   d. How would you approach these recommendations with this particular person?

2. From what you know of Mr. Parello, identify the strengths he has that you would support and encourage.

   a. What cognitive-behavioral coping skills have been proven useful for a client with cardiac problems (CHD)?
   b. What changes in Mr. Parello's approach to his work and life might help lessen his self-driven behaviors?
   c. Which cognitive-behavioral techniques would you choose to teach Mr. Parello?
   d. Would you include any medically related support groups in the information you would give him?

3. Discuss how you would approach the physician regarding Mr. Parello's need to be evaluated for depression. What are some of the compelling reasons depression (and any co-existing mental condition) should be treated in any and all seriously ill medically clients?

Chapter Review

1. Which psychological response to serious mental illness can the nurse expect to find in nearly all clients?

   1. Anger
   2. Anxiety
   3. Depression
   4. Substance abuse

2. While the psychiatric liaison nurse conducts the psychosocial assessment of Mrs. Peters, a client who has been receiving hemodialysis for 3 months, the client reports that she finds herself feeling angry whenever it is time for her dialysis treatment. The nurse can probably attribute this to

   1. Organic changes in Mrs. Peters' brain
   2. A flaw in Mrs. Peters' personality
   3. A normal response to grief and loss
   4. Denial of the reality of a poor prognosis

3. The psychiatric liaison nurse who assesses Mrs. J. realizes that depression is a complicating factor in the client's adjustment to newly diagnosed adult-onset diabetes. To what problem should the nurse advise clinic staff to be particularly alert?

   1. Development of agoraphobia
   2. Treatment noncompliance
   3. Frequent hypoglycemic reactions
   4. Silent urinary tract infections

4. Which client is least likely to be the victim of human rights abuse?

   1. Miss Y., who is HIV positive and being treated for a pulmonary infection
   2. Miss H., who has received transgender surgery and has cholecystitis
   3. Mr. A., who is severely and persistently mentally ill and is being treated for cellulitis
   4. Mr. C., who has Duchenne muscular dystrophy and is experiencing adult respiratory distress syndrome

5. Which client would the nurse assess as having ineffective coping skills?

   1. Mrs. A., who has breast cancer and who confronts her health problem and devises an appropriate plan of action
   2. Miss B., who has MS and keeps herself busy and maintains positive emotional ties with family and friends
   3. Mr. C., who is HIV positive and expresses guilt about his sexual behavior and broods about the hopelessness of his situation
   4. Mr. D., who has AODM and actively seeks information about management of his illness

REFERENCES

American Psychiatric Association. (1980). Diagnostic and statistical manual of mental disorders (3rd ed.). Washington, DC: American Psychiatric Association.

American Psychiatric Association (1994). Diagnostic and statistical manual of mental disorders (4th ed.). Washington, DC: American Psychiatric Association.

Barnett, L., and Chambers, M. (1996). Reiki: Energy medicine. Rochester, VT: Healing Arts Press.

Barry, P. (1984). Psychosocial assessment and intervention. Philadelphia: J. B. Lippincott.

Bowen, R. C., Senthilselvan, A., and Barale, A. (2000). Physical illness as an outcome of chronic anxiety disorders. Canadian Journal of Psychiatry, 45(5) 459–464.

Burke, F. M., Jr. (1991) Triage of disaster-related neuro-psychiatric casualties, Psychiatric Aspects of Emergency Medicine 9(1):87–104.

Cummings, J. L. (1994). Depression in neurological diseases. Psychiatric Annals, 24(10):525–531.

DiMatteo, M. R., Lepper, H. S., Croghan, T. W. (2000). Depression is a risk factor for noncompliance with medical treatment: Meta-analysis of the effects of anxiety and depression on patient adherence. Achives of Internal Medicine, 160(14):2101–2107.

Dossey, B., et al. (1995). Holistic nursing: A handbook for practice. Gaithersburg, MD: Aspen Publishers.

Gioiella, M. E., Berkman, B., and Robinson, M. (1998). Spirituality and quality of life in gynecological oncology patients. Cancer Practice, 6(6):3338.

Hemingway, H., and Marmot, M. (1999). Evidence based cardiology: Psychosocial factors in the aetiology and prognosis of coronary heart disease. Systemic review of prospective cohort studies. British Medical Journal, 19(7214):917–918.

Hofland, P. (2000). Psychosocial factors increasingly recognized as relevant in heart disease. 2000 Reuters Ltd. http://www.mediscape.com/reuters/prof/2000/08/08/20000830epid002.html.

Jenkins, D. (1984). A model depicting the interaction of stress and the organism. In P. D. Barry (Ed.), Psychosocial nursing assessment and intervention. Philadelphia: J. B. Lippincott.

Katon, W. (1984). Depression: Relationship to somatization and chronic medical illness. Journal of Clinical Psychology, 45:4–11.

Lewis, S., et al. (1989). Manual of psychosocial nursing interventions. Philadelphia: W. B. Saunders.

Lesperance, F., and Frasure-Smith, N. (2000). Journal of Psychosocial Research, 48(4–5):379–391.

Lowery, , and Houldin, (1996).

Meyer, T., Klemme, H., and Herrmann, C. (2000). Depression but not anxiety is significant predictor of physicians' assessment of medical status in physically ill patients.

Minuchin, S. (1978) Psychosomatic families: Anorexia nervosa in context. Cambridge, MA: Harvard University Press.

Robinson, E. F., and Asnis, G. M. (1989). Major depression: Masks, misconceptions, and nosologic ambiguities. Psychiatric Annals, 19(7):360–364.

Schuyler, D. (2000). Depression comes in many disguises to the providers of primary care: Recognition and management. Journal of South Carolina Medical Association, 96(6):267–275.

Selye, H. (1956). The stress of life. New York: McGraw-Hill.

Selye, H. (1974). Stress without distress. Philadelphia: J. B. Lippincott.

SF-12 Quality Metric, Inc. All Rights Reserved. SF-12 is the registered trademark of the Medical Outcomes Trust Medical Outcomes Trust and John Ware, Jr—All Rights Reserved. http://www.generic.com/products/Assessments

Stewart, T. D., and Atlas, S. A. (2000). Syndrome X, depression and chaos: Relevance to medical practice. Connecticut Medicine, 64(5):343–345.

Turks, E., and Bellisimo, A. (1991). Behavioral medicine: Concepts and procedures. New York: Pergamon Press.

Vogel, M. E., and Romano, S. E. (1999). Behavioral medicine. In M. Stewart and J. A. Lieberman (Eds.), Primary care clinics in office practice, 26(2):385–400.

Weisman, A. (1984). The coping capacity: On the nature of being mortal. New York: Human Sciences Press.

Zerbe, K. J. (1999). Women's mental health in primary care. Philadelphia: W. B. Saunders.

8. Apply some of the guidelines for helping people to cope with loss of a patient, friend, family member, or classmate.

9. Discuss at least seven behavioral outcomes that indicate a successful bereavement.

10. Identify situations and circumstances that could impact a person coming to terms with loss.

Care for the Dying
Kathy A. Kramer-Howe

Caring for the terminally ill challenges caregivers in deep and personal ways. Intuitively, everyone realizes that death awaits, somewhere far down the road of life, it is hoped. In caring for the dying, nurses are called on both to find acceptance for their clients' deaths and to find a new relationship with their own mortality. The dominant culture offers precious little support for the awareness and acceptance of dying. Life is exalted for its own sake, as though it exists as a process independent of death. Youth, strength, possibilities, growth, change, and newness are prized, and death can appear merely to short-circuit and destroy all of these. It can seem unthinkable that science and technology cannot or will not someday defeat aging, illness, and death itself. Some people foresee that mastery of the human genome or improvements in cryonics ultimately will prevail over the mortal limits of the human body. Yet human wisdom throughout the ages has shown that the very preciousness of living is due to its finite nature. Living well and dying well are two sides of the mortal experience, and the ways in which people face death can shape the ways in which they embrace their lives. Thus, there are many lessons to be gained in caring for the terminally ill, and many gifts to be given and shared with the client and family.

In recent years, the burgeoning hospice and palliative care movement has begun to shed light on the experience of dying in America. The realities can be grim. Studies show that people fear becoming a burden, being abandoned, being in pain, becoming impoverished, and becoming undignified in how they look and smell. These fears are all too well grounded in reality. Physical pain is poorly addressed and often uncontrolled. The chances of dying in pain increase for people who do not speak English or who are poor, black, Hispanic, elderly, or female (Byock 1997). Medicare, insurance policies, and employers do not adequately provide for caregiving in the last year of life, with high social costs resulting from time off work and health problems for caregivers.

On the subjective level, most people confront the realities of life-threatening illness with only the slimmest sense of adequacy. In our pragmatic, how-to culture, it is unsettling to know so little about how to be a person with incurable cancer, how to comfort grieving, worried relatives, how to take leave of one's own health, independence, autonomy, control—and of one's very life. What is helpful in order to have a "good death"? Edwin Shneidman (1980) proposes the metaphor of a rutter (or routier), that is, a ship pilot's personal journal of how to make an uncharted journey safely. These were essential in the early days of exploration. Treacherous shoals and reefs, dangerous islanders, safe harbors, and fruitful landings were vital information for the next captain and craft making the journey. As society engages in a new dialogue about the business of dying, there are more rutters available to help guide the dying. Each life and each death that is witnessed by caring people contributes to a language and taxonomy about dying that can make the journey more bearable. Each life and each death becomes a new rutter for everyone else.

Professional caregivers can become advocates for this vulnerable population. The terminally ill have the right to honest answers to difficult questions; the right to have control over as much of their medical care and living situation as possible; the right to have advance directives completed and followed, including suspending or withholding curative efforts; the right to receive excellent palliative care and to be comfortable; the right to be perceived as fully living; and the right to die as they wish. Caregivers need to understand as much as possible about end-of-life issues so they can help to protect these rights against individual and institutional ignorance, indifference, and neglect. They are called to offer their human and professional support, embodying a vision of possibilities for comfort, dignity, personal control, and even spiritual growth at the end of life. This chapter provides an overview of end-of-life care, with an emphasis on clinical strategies and interventions with clients and families.

HOSPICE AND PALLIATIVE CARE

Before the hospice movement began in England in the 1960s, dying people were routinely shunted into hospital rooms with phrases like, "We're sorry, there's nothing more we can do for you," and with doctor's orders for routine doses of pain medications. Despite the ministrations of caring health professionals and visits from helpless relatives, people who were dying were often neglected, isolated, and in pain. In 1967, Dame Cicely Saunders established St. Christopher's Hospice in London to remedy this state of neglect (Stolberg 1999). In her hospice house, clients' physical comfort was aggressively pursued with round-the-clock pain medication so that they could respond to other pressing issues and enjoy optimal quality of life. Effective management of physical symptoms restored meaningful quality of life to many, and all lived their time as they saw fit. Some took care of legal and financial matters, some went shopping, some said their goodbyes and restored damaged relationships, some aligned themselves with their God, and most were at peace with their lives.

In the United States, Dr. Elisabeth Kübler-Ross began actively listening to the terminally ill, and out of her groundbreaking work came a construct of the human response to death that has entered the popular mainstream. She identified distinctive phases, or cycles, in people's responses to terminal illness: denial, anger, bargaining, depression, and acceptance (Kübler-Ross 1969). She also realized that personal growth did not cease in the last stages of life but on the contrary, often accelerated. Encouraged by her findings, volunteer hospices began to appear in the 1970s. St. Christopher's comprehensive model was adapted, and an interdisciplinary team evolved to include a physician, nurse, social worker, pastor or chaplain, home health aide, and volunteer. Medicare instituted a per diem reimbursement for the hospice team in 1983, and many commercial insurers have followed suit. Hospice organizations have proliferated, mostly nonprofit but also for-profit and governmental organizations. As of 1999, the National Hospice Organization counted over 3100 operating or planned hospices located in the 50 states. Approximately 540,000 patients were served by hospices in the United States in 1998, the great majority dying in their own homes (Hospice Fact Sheet 1999).

Palliative care is a medical specialty that has grown out of the hospice movement and the increasing national awareness of the need for better care for the dying. "Defined by the World Health Organization in 1990, palliative care seeks to address not only physical pain, but also emotional, social, and spiritual pain to achieve the best possible quality of life for patients and their families" (Hospice Fact Sheet 1999). Palliation focuses on aggressive comfort care when the goal is no longer cure. Medications and treatments may be offered and combined in unusual ways, given in different dosages, or used for nonstandard purposes until the patient experiences relief. With rare exceptions, people who have access to expert palliation need not fear pain and discomfort at the end of life or in the chronic phases of their illness. Most of the symptoms associated with cancer, liver and renal failure, dementia, neuropathic diseases, cardiac and pulmonary diseases, and many others can be successfully ameliorated with available medications. For those who do not elect hospice care, more hospitals nationwide offer palliative expertise.

Vignette

■ *Mrs. Dolly is 101 years old, a pleasantly confused old lady whose hair and nails are done every other week in the nursing home where she has lived for the past 6 years. Aside from osteoporosis, weight loss, and chronic constipation, she is quite healthy. The staff is fond of Mrs. Dolly, and when she appears to have a bowel obstruction and is sent to the hospital, people are worried. Unfortunately, she is not a good candidate for anything offered at the hospital. She has a living will and a doctor's order not to resuscitate and is sent back to the nursing home to die. Now having severe abdominal distention and breathing problems, her symptoms are becoming dire and grave. The physician and family oppose any measures to alleviate her abdominal distention and labored breathing. The staff feels helpless and distressed.*

Vignette

■ *Mr. Spence contracted amyotrophic lateral sclerosis at the age of 52. He lived at home until his care overwhelmed his family and has now been in a care center for 9 months. He is almost totally paralyzed but can still use a letter board with a head-mounted laser pointer. He has a warm smile and a very present gaze. He is having shooting pains in his legs and more difficulty swallowing and breathing. The staff worries about losing all communication with him and about his suffering at the end of life. He has rejected a feeding tube or any heroic measures. Will he starve to death? Will he be frightened once he can no longer communicate? Will he linger?*

In each of these vignettes, hospice care offers an antidote to the sense of helplessness and anxiety surrounding these two people. For Mrs. Dolly, the hospice nurse would focus on providing physical relief from her worsening symptoms. After assessing her, the nurse would discuss palliative medicine in appropriate dosages with Mrs. Dolly's doctor, talk with the family, and obtain orders for pain and anxiety-relieving medication. The hospice nurse/social worker would talk with Mrs. Dolly, if possible, and to her family about their perceptions of Mrs. Dolly's current crisis, their expectations based on their history, and their readiness to face her death, both emotionally and practically. Are there funeral plans and are they known to both the hospice and the care center? Are her advance directives in place and visible? Does she want a visit from a rabbi, minister, or chaplain? The home health aide would clean and apply lotion for Mrs. Dolly and make her as comfortable as possible. The staff would be given emotional support and preparation for Mrs. Dolly's death.

For Mr. Spence, a hospice evaluation would also be in order. The hospice nurse and social worker would talk with him about his wishes as his condition declined. They would address his control of eating and his fears of starvation. Breathing and any fears of choking or strangling toward the end of his life would also be discussed. Increased medication and types of care would be talked about so that he could control as much as possible of the process of his illness and dying. Emotional, spiritual, and educational support would be offered to the family and staff about the course of the illness, anticipatory grieving, and ways of using the time remaining to nurture their relationships.

Hospice care is available to everyone, regardless of age or the ability to pay. It is a benefit covered under Medicare Part A and mirrored, to some extent, by most commercial insurance companies. It covers the cost of medications related to the terminal diagnosis, durable medical equipment, basic hygiene supplies, nursing, social worker and home health aid visits, as well as counseling for spiritual issues and bereavement. Volunteers are available for respite visits and general helpfulness. Limited physical, dietary, and occupational therapy are covered. Many hospices will cover the costs of limited palliative treatments such as radiation, chemotherapy, and transfusions. Hospices are under the guidance of a medical director, but the patient's own physician usually remains primary. Physicians often recommend a particular hospice. However, commercial or governmental managed care companies sometimes specify certain contracted hospices. If a person is on Medicaid or a commercial plan, it is best to verify which hospice is to be used.

Hospice care is appropriate when an individual is in the endstages of virtually any disease. The patient does not have to be in the last few days of life. Hospice care can be a supportive presence for many weeks and months of life as long as curative therapies are no longer a goal for the patient and doctor.

In 1998, the average length of stay in hospices nationally was 51.3 days (the median length of stay was 25 days) (Hospice Fact Sheet 1999). Medicare has issued diagnostic criteria for many diseases to help determine the appropriateness of hospice care. The hospice evaluation will help in that determination, and the person's primary doctor will need to sign a certification of terminal illness. This includes the doctor's best guess as to a life expectancy of 6 months or less.

Hospice care is designed to bring comprehensive palliative care to clients where they are residing. It does not pay for 24-hour care, custodial care, or routine room and board. Although freestanding hospice homes are rare, most hospices do offer skilled nursing settings for short-term symptom management and caregiver respite at no cost to the family. More than a physical place, hospice is a philosophy of care. It is founded on the principles of

■ Client dignity and respect
■ Treating the client *and* family and significant others
■ Supporting a peaceful, pain-free death
■ Client control and choice
■ Viewing the client holistically
■ Bereavement support for the family after the death.

NURSING GOALS IN END-OF-LIFE CARE

Nursing the terminally ill requires shifts in expectations by the nurse, both of herself or himself and of the client. For example, the nurse's sense of competency and effectiveness often comes from helping patients get better, stronger, and more independent. The terminally ill are going to grow weaker and sicker and ultimately die. With curable illness it is common to keep a client's spirits up by pointing to improvements and advancement toward long-term goals. A dying person's goals become increasingly short-term and more modest. They may shift from goals centered on physical improvement to adjustments in lifestyle, to relationships, or to spiritual comfort. With the dying, the health care professional is confronted with loss of control, and this can result in feelings of inadequacy or frustration. The nurse is not in control of the processes going on within the client, and neither is the client. In fact, the experience of multiple and inexorable losses can be one of the most grievous for the dying and their loved ones. As a compassionate health care provider, the nurse may also grieve these losses and experience premourning of the client. Premourning is grieving the loss of a person before that person has died, but with the knowledge that death is inevitable (Shneidman 1980). Thus, many emotions are stirred up in the nurse and they deserve acknowledgment and support. The questions in Box 30–1 can provide nurses with insight into their beliefs about death and dying. The following shifts in orientation can help nurses to adjust to this kind of caretaking.

Avoid Seeing a Dichotomy Between the Living and the Dying

Those living with terminal diagnoses are very much alive, and often vibrantly so. They are often working hard to retain and adjust their personal identities to encompass the life-threatening diagnosis. At a time

---

Box 30–1 *Self-Assessment of Your Beliefs About Death and Dying*

THIS SELF-ASSESSMENT DOES NOT GIVE YOU ANY CUTE NICKNAMES OR TELL YOU HOW WELL-ADJUSTED YOU ARE. WHAT IT DOES DO IS GIVE YOU INSIGHT INTO YOUR ATTITUDE ABOUT DEATH.

■ To the best of your memory, at what age were you first aware of death?
  ■ Under the age of three
  ■ Age 3 to 5
  ■ Age 5 to 10
  ■ Age 10 and up
  ■ Other
■ When you were a child, how was death talked about in your family?
  ■ Openly
  ■ As though death were a forbidden subject
  ■ With some discomfort
  ■ Don't remember any talk about death
  ■ Only when necessary, and not in front of the children
■ Which of the following most influences the way you think about death now?
  ■ Death of someone close
  ■ TV, movies, radio
  ■ Things you have read
  ■ Length of time family members have lived
  ■ Religion
  ■ Funerals
  ■ Own health
■ Has religion played an important part in the way you think about death?
  ■ Very important
  ■ Important
  ■ Not very important
  ■ No part at all
■ How often do you think about your own death?
  ■ At least once a day
  ■ Often
  ■ Not more than once a year
  ■ Sometimes

■ Never or almost never
■ Other
■ What does death mean to you?
  ■ The end of life
  ■ The end of physical life; the spirit lives on
  ■ Endless sleep and peace
  ■ Don't know
  ■ A new beginning, life after death
  ■ Other
■ What aspect of your own death bothers you the most?
  ■ I could no longer have any experiences
  ■ I am afraid of what might happen to my body after death
  ■ I am not sure what will happen to me if there is life after death
  ■ I could no longer provide for my family
  ■ My family and friends would grieve
  ■ The process of dying might be painful
  ■ Other
■ What do you believe causes most deaths?
  ■ Most deaths happen because the person wants to die
  ■ Most deaths happen because of the way the person uses or fails to use things such as tobacco, alcohol, medicines, or seat belts
  ■ Most deaths just happen
  ■ Other
■ If your doctor knew that you would die from a disease and had a limited time left to live, would you want the doctor to tell you?
  ■ Yes
  ■ No
  ■ Depends on the circumstances
■ If it were possible, would you want to know the exact date on which you were going to die?
  ■ Yes
  ■ No
  ■ Other

For the meanings of your answers, check the website: http://dying.about.com/health/dying/blasses.htm
From The Mining Company: Death and Dying, 7/8/98. © 1998 General Internet Inc. All rights reserved. General Internet, The Mining Co. and Guidesite are trademarks of General Internet Inc., v3.0. For the rules of use see The Mining Co. User Agreement. Having a Problem? Report It Here http://dying.about.com/health/dying/blasses.htm
Developed at Medical Innovations, 1994, by Michael Seago, adapted by Trudy Weathersby.

when they are reflecting on their lives, their loved ones tend to perceive them as patients in need of special handling. One dying older man poignantly remarked, "For 55 years I had a wife; for the last year I have had a nurse." They experience all the emotional states and often need to talk about them. Some of the reactions they experience are "stoicism, rage, guilt, terror, cringing, fear, surrender, heroism, dependency, ennui, need for control, fight for autonomy and dignity, and denial" (Schneidman 1980). When the nurse takes time to acknowledge all that is well about clients, their uniqueness and strength, without imposing a personal agenda, it can be very welcome to patients.

Understand That There Is No "Right" Way to Die

Most nurses have an idea of what constitutes a "good" death. Certainly, most wish people to arrive at some acceptance and peace about their death. Every individual will die in a uniquely personal way. A fairly good predictor of how a person will die is how that person has reacted to other crises and times of high stress in life (Schneidman 1980). However, not all people die as they have lived. Some people have deaths that are surprising, often in a positive way. It is helpful to be aware of one's own ideas about death and to remain open-minded about each client's experience.

Strive for Increased Physical and Psychological Comfort

With comfort as the primary nursing goal, medications must be given in ways that are effective for that person at that moment. As Ira Byock, MD, writes, "The right amount of pain medication is the amount that works" (Byock 1997). Pain is both physical and psychological, and it is important to assess for emotions and thoughts that may be exacerbating physical discomfort. Active listening and empathy are helpful. Basic breathing and relaxation exercises can help both client and family. Acceptance and even resolution of painful or incomplete aspects of a life can be encouraged, and small changes magnified. Validating who the person is in honest and open exchanges can assist him or her in coming to terms with a lifetime of experience. Pain and pain management of the terminally ill are covered in Chapter 33.

Learn to Follow the Person's Lead

The nurse has a lot to offer and will use many skills and aids. However, nursing the dying is more facili-

tative than directive. Because goals are limited and short term, the nurse needs to be flexible and responsive. A regimen that worked yesterday may need adjustment today, as the client's body systems change. Dying is an active process of change, and both the terminally ill person and the nurse need to be guided by the process. The nurse's ideas of what might work well have to be modified and even abandoned, according to the client's physical and personal responses. In addition, a terminally ill person typically vacillates in ability to face his or her illness and prognosis. It is common for a client to speak about his or her death and then shortly afterwards make comments about getting better or attending some future event. In most cases, there are times when a client wants to talk about how much time he or she has or what death will be like. Following the client's lead instead of confronting a person with unwanted information or avoiding the answers to questions is one way of respecting the client's dignity and autonomy. Sometimes, open-ended questions are helpful, such as

- "Tell me what you are thinking about. What is going on with you now?"
- "What did the doctor tell you about your condition?"
- "What are you hoping for?"
- "What are you looking forward to?"
- "Do you have questions about what is happening with you?"

Relationships Are of Prime Importance

The terminally ill are running out of time, and this may spur them to relate to others with increased emotional honesty. However, they may lack the experience or vocabulary to articulate their needs. The nurse's own degree of honesty and vulnerability to the process can be a model and an encouragement to clients and families. Caregivers often attempt to protect the dying from experiencing afflictive emotions. They may do this by keeping information from them about their illness or by withholding their own feelings of fear, sorrow, or concern. Yet this is a time when emotional honesty and the closeness it can bring are of vital importance to all. The health care professional can play a vital role by inviting clients and their families to be as honest as possible. Families can be reassured that displays of grief or worry by loved ones may actually reassure dying people that their families are facing the inevitable. Family members do not want to think they are causing each other emotional pain, but pain and grief usually accompany separation and loss. Anger, worry, and tears may be tolerated more easily if they are described as expressions of love and grief. Statements such as, "When I think about your not being around, I feel so sad" can often be more easily accepted by clients than such statements as, "Don't be silly, you're not going anywhere" or "Don't leave me!" Finding a metaphor for death and dying can open up dialogue about the dreaded event. One client whose beloved spouse had predeceased her spoke of her death as "going dancing with my honey." The family could embrace that image and use it to speak more openly about death.

Assess for Multiple Diagnoses

People facing terminal illness are often sad, anxious, angry, or withdrawn. Some may have severe or chronic mental illness or addictions. It can be challenging to distinguish among situational responses and clinical conditions deserving of treatment.

Vignette

■ Mrs. Jake is a 79-year-old mother and grandmother with metastasized breast cancer. She received aggressive treatment for more than 2 years but can no longer tolerate such therapies. She lives at home and is being cared for by her elderly husband. Mrs. Jake is vague about pain and other symptoms, although she frequently wrinkles her brow and moans. She can slowly ambulate with a walker, but spends most of the day and night in the back bedroom curled on her side. The curtains are drawn and the TV is on, and the client sleeps a lot. When visitors come, she struggles up and sits briefly on the edge of the bed. She is alert and oriented but does not initiate or sustain conversation. When asked about her feelings she often says she is "disgusted."

Is Mrs. Jake in a lot of discomfort that she cannot articulate? Is she sad, disgusted, or discouraged by her illness and the failure of the treatments? Are there afflictive spousal or familial relationships? Is she clinically depressed?

In the case of Mrs. Jake, the hospice nurse and social worker decided to assess for clinical depression and requested an antidepressant from Mrs. Jake's doctor. She was started on Paxil, and after 2 or 3 weeks began to come alive again. She brightened, smiled, and accepted visitors with more enthusiasm. She was able to provide better information about her pain and discomfort. The curtains were opened and the TV turned off more frequently. She still has a life-threatening illness, but she is now able to talk about her thoughts and feelings.

Vignette

■ Mrs. Johnson is in her late 80s and has been admitted to hospice care because she has stopped eating and is dwindling. It is discovered during a thorough assessment that she had a bad fall within the past few weeks. After that, she became fearful of walking by herself, fearful of being alone, and convinced that she was going to die. Hospice recommends treatment for posttraumatic effects, and the family puts Mrs. Johnson under a psychiatrist's care. Once on an effective antianxiety medication, she slowly loses her crippling fear of living. Hospice provides short-term physical and occupational therapy to teach Mrs. Johnson how to do simple daily tasks, and over a period of weeks she regains some appetite and mobility. She is later discharged from hospice with the plan of moving into an assisted living facility.

Sometimes life-threatening symptoms can be created or exacerbated by psychological states, as in the story of Mrs Johnson. Her terror of falling had generalized into fear of moving at all. This became a conviction that she was about to die, and she began saying her goodbyes and withdrawing from friends and society. Once hospice had verified that she had no life-threatening physical disease process, it could turn its attention to drawing Mrs. Johnson back into living. Hospice coordinated efforts with the family to use a variety of therapies, including teaching the family simple behavioral modification techniques to encourage Mrs. Johnson to do more for herself as they did progressively less and less. The hospice chaplain got involved in providing brief counseling to this Roman Catholic woman to reconnect her to her church community.

MAINTAINING THE CAREGIVER'S EMOTIONAL HEALTH

Nurses working with the dying are bound to be challenged as caregivers at a deep level. This is because each person has a complex unconscious relationship to loss, grief, death, and dying. In these domains, much is unknown. Many confusing feelings and reactions will be triggered. For example, terminally ill patients may be younger than the caregiver; they may resemble the nurse or a loved person in troubling ways; their diseases and symptoms may be reminiscent of significant others who have died, or they may threaten the nurse's sense of safety and acceptability. In addition, their grief and mourning may stimulate the nurse's own grief so that she or he is not sure of the source of the sadness felt. Also, a nurse can have powerful reactions to the client and the family relationships and living conditions. For example, the nurse may disapprove of families who are inattentive caregivers or of spouses or adult children who seem overly controlling or take on exaggerated responsibility for the dying family member. The nurse may be frightened or disgusted by the differing ways people live, for example when they are homeless, drug addicted, or messy and disorganized.

It is critically important that the nurse pay attention to his or her own emotional health in all areas of life, but especially so in these circumstances because the population being treated is so stressed-filled and vulnerable. They cannot be expected to meet the nurse's needs. They are facing one of life's greatest crises—impending death. When the nurse interacts with the client and family, an effort is made to bring emotional health and stability into their chaotic world and to try to "be there" in healthy ways to validate their feelings, their strengths, and their coping. It is hoped that the nurse will offer a sense of positive and unconditional acceptance of what is happening, not false hope or phony cheerfulness. Instead, the nurse takes professional expertise and human nurturing into the client's home. There will be times when a client meets the nurse's needs, and the nurse feels particularly appreciated. However, this should be seen as a special gift, not a steady diet.

Being a caregiver for the sick, grieving, and dying challenges personal boundaries. The nurse can over-identify with the clients and family with the result of feeling drained and helpless or can over-protect himself or herself from them and fail to empathize with their human dilemma. Instant intimacy can grow when caring for the dying because time is short, and the nurse often sees the new relationships as precious and fleeting. Strong enmities can also appear, as people can act very different from the way the nurse wants them to and can thereby disappoint expectations. Box 30–2 provides guidelines to help the health care professional maintain emotional health when working with death and the dying.

COMMUNICATING WITH THE DYING AND THEIR FAMILIES

A dying client and the family are facing a cataclysmic event with very little knowledge and expertise. Whether it's an expected death that ends a long and debilitating illness or a sudden and unwelcome terminal diagnosis, facing death is disruptive and

stressful. Family systems tend to destabilize and break down under the strain. People seek information, context, and understanding of what is normal so as to make sense of what is happening. In stress-

Box 30–2 *Guidelines for Self-Care by Health Care Professionals When Caring for the Dying*

1. Remind yourself that what is happening to your patients and their families is not happening to you. This is their life drama, right now, but not your own.
2. When you notice that you are having a particularly strong emotional reaction, either positive or negative (countertransference), take it as a signal to explore your deeper issues or needs by talking with a trusted friend, counselor, or colleague.
3. Protect your private life by practicing time management, avoiding overwork and working outside of normal hours, not giving out your pager or home telephone number, and taking regular days off and vacations.
4. Clearly state what you can and cannot do for your patients so that your human and professional limitations are known up front.
5. Expect the unexpected. This work can grab your heart at times and spin you around. It is vital and unpredictable work that exists on the very edge of human existential meaning.
6. Practice humility. The border at which life becomes death is beyond control and mastery. There is much you can do, but there is also much that is unknown and unknowable.
7. Do your own mourning when your heart is touched and you need to acknowledge the importance of others in your life. Even after a person has died, he or she continues a relationship with you in your memory. Attend funerals or create grieving rituals when this happens.
8. Create a healthy, balanced private life by releasing stress. This work creates stresses at many levels. As a human being, you are built for stress, but only when you can regularly discharge the stress and regain the homeostasis of the organism. Otherwise, your body can gradually go out of balance and various symptoms and illnesses can result. Methods of discharging stress are well known and are endlessly paraded in the press and media. The challenge is to work them into your busy schedule and stay on course. Foremost among these methods are regular exercise, a balanced diet, adequate rest, vacations, fun and laughter, loving and accepting relationships, and a connection to spirituality.

ful times, two factors seem to make things more bearable: the ability to have control and the ability to predict changes. The nurse or professional caregiver can help in several ways.

Convey Information

Both the client and the family often want to know how to interpret physical symptoms that are occurring. The nurse can share medical expertise about the normal progression of the disease, effects of medication, reasons for changes in drug regimens, and how to provide comfort care and safety if the client is at home. Information dispels many myths and fears and strengthens a sense of control. However, information should be repeated many times, written down, and reviewed frequently. Communication experts say that, under stress, people need at least six reiterations in order to understand and retain new information.

Make Limited But Realistic Predictions

Families facing the death of a loved one are often caught in a dilemma. They are preparing themselves for the time of death as best they can. However, they also need to continue to rearrange their lives and provide care as though the client will live for an indefinite period. They must live in extraordinary ways with the dual realities of impending death and continued life. It is commonplace for family members to admit privately, with guilt or resentment, that they wish this could be over. However, the inability to make sound predictions can create a sense of interminable suffering, both for themselves and for the client. The nurse can interpret physical changes in terms of typical prognostication and give the families realistic updates. When families ask, "How long?" nurses can point to advancing symptoms as signs that there is indeed movement in the disease process. Conversely, when family members fervently deny the severity of an illness, the nurse's predictions can provide some preparation for what is to come.

The nurse must tread carefully in the land of prognostications. Families and clients often probe the medical professional for a time line, with a mixture of dread and desperation. They imagine that medical expertise must have insights they themselves lack. Often, they have been told by a medical person to expect a specific number of months or weeks of life. If this number is exceeded, they can feel they have triumphed over death and the experts. If it is not reached, they can feel betrayed. A two-pronged approach can be helpful:

■ One is to focus the family and client on the here and now, or short-term goals, and on life as it is today.

■ The second is to describe what is being seen and found during physical examination, to paint a picture from which family members can draw their own conclusions.

Comments about such indicators as the client's pulse and heart rate, color, blood pressure, weakness, appetite, and level of consciousness can guide the family toward interpretations they can accept. Unfortunately, until the client has begun to show signs and symptoms of actually dying, it is not possible to predict accurately within short periods of time.

There are times when the expected trajectory of an illness is unrealistic. Some clients, upon hearing that they cannot be cured, expect to die within a few days. One elderly man heard the news and went home to settle all his affairs. He notified his children and friends, bought funeral plans and a plot, arranged all his paperwork, and sat down to await death. In reality, he had several months of life remaining. As time went on, he felt more and more angry, betrayed by the physician, embarrassed to have outlived his friends' and family's expectations, and acutely uncomfortable with his children's attempts to console or take care of him. In another instance, the wife of a man diagnosed with large-cell lung cancer would not accept that he was not imminently dying. She convinced him to reject treatment, did not want to take him home, and managed to convince him that his life was almost over. He became depressed, and she was frightened (Prichard 1979). In these cases, the role of the nurse is crucial to educate and support both client and family as they struggle with the implications of a more accurate prognosis.

Enhance the Competency of the Family

The family is faced with numerous challenges to its sense of competency in seeing this process through. One is learning how to be helpful to the dying person. Establishing a stable environment for the person, keeping things in the same place, and developing routines and daily rhythms can increase comfort. Caregivers can be shown how to assist the person in getting from place to place, bathing, dressing, and other activities of daily life. Another challenge is coping with disruptions in the family members' personal lives. The nurse can educate the caregivers about the necessity for respite and relief, about sharing the burdens and asking for help, and about the urgency for caregivers to take care of their own health.

Families often need continuing reassurance that they are doing a good job, and that what they are experiencing is normal under these conditions. The nurse can help to distinguish between stress and crisis. Stress is normal and unavoidable when caring for a dying loved one. Crisis, however, can be determined by an assessment of the family members' "responses, including perceptual distortion, cognitive disorganization, a spread of inability to take action in other areas of the life space, overwhelming helplessness, extensive denial, and so forth" (Wijnberg and Schwartz 1977). To forestall the possibility of crises, the nurse can help the family member to stay connected with others in his or her support system and can clarify the threats to accustomed roles, habits, life styles, and self-identities posed by death. The painful process of detachment known as anticipatory grief can be explained and supported.

Teach Communication Skills

The journey through terminal illness makes most people feel like strangers in a strange land. Each life, each relationship, is uniquely important. The loss of an important relationship confronts people with a forest of unknowns. Terminal illness separates everyone from familiar roles and daily routines and turns the everyday habits of a lifetime upside down. Everyone is grappling with losses, and it is normal for family members to try to protect each other from their own strange and unwelcome experiences and emotions. Each person has the right to talk about these issues in his or her own time, but often there is an avoidance of sharing that makes things harder than they have to be. The nurse can ask open-ended questions that invite the client and the family to share honestly.

A common family assumption is that the person does not want to talk about death because to do so might undo his or her fighting spirit and hasten the end. In these cases, the family is less sensitive to the person's overtures to talking. A dying mother might say, "I won't be here for my next birthday," and be responded to by her daughter with, "Of course you will, Mother, don't talk like that." In such a situation, the nurse can gently urge the daughter to invite her mother's thoughts and feelings about not being here. A person often speaks in a kind of code, perhaps in order to test the family's readiness to face the dreadful loss ahead (Kelley and Callahan 1992). The person may talk about coming events, about giving away possessions, about hopes for various family members and may say one thing but indicate the opposite in body language. One mother of three was weighing where she wanted to end her days. She repeated her choices (a care center, her

home, or an assisted living facility) several times as if they were all equal, but her head shook with two names and nodded slightly with the third choice. In their eagerness to help her keep her options open as long as possible, the adult children missed the body language.

Certain approaches can be helpful when inviting a terminally ill person to talk. One is to reassure him or her that you are willing to talk about anything at all. Another is to say, "If there were a catastrophe tomorrow, say the roof fell in, and you only had 15 minutes to live, what would be going through your mind as you lay dying? What would be left undone? Is there anything you haven't done or anything you haven't said to someone important?" (Byock 1997) This question can give the client a non-threatening look through the door of death, and focus him or her on resolving any lingering concerns. Another question is "How are you feeling within yourself?" This question usually produces a description of the inner state of soul, heart, or being. It can lead to an exploration of that crucial dimension, so seldom addressed in families. The client and the family can be asked, "How do you understand what the doctors have told you?" to see how each one is interpreting the condition of the client. "What are you expecting, or hoping for, in the next week (or month)?" "Is there anything we haven't talked about that you would like to discuss?"

Counsel About Anticipatory Grieving

As families and clients struggle through the process of ending a life, they may need to understand the effects of anticipatory grieving. The time for good-bye has not arrived, yet emotionally, family members can be detaching from the client. Shock, loss, emptiness, fear, confusion, and mourning are being felt, yet it may not seem appropriate to share these experiences with the person or even with others. Rather than face and share all this, the less involved family members may pull away from the person prematurely in order to forestall their own grief and pain. This can create extra burdens on the immediate caregiver as well as isolate the person. The primary caregiver may find that concentrating on daily tasks is easier than acknowledging the storm of feelings within. In these cases, the nurse can offer to facilitate a family meeting. During these meetings, everyone is encouraged to talk initially without interruption. People are to refrain from trying to "fix" each other or defend themselves. When feelings and circumstances have been shared, problem solving can begin. Families can be counseled about the normalcy of anticipatory grief. Just hearing some of its symptoms and effects can be immensely reassuring.

They can be taught about journaling, talking with a trusted friend, and venting strong feelings in whatever ways suit the individual personality. They can be urged to include the dying person in the sharing of their daily lives by calling, visiting, and doing the ordinary things that show caring like hairbrushing, shaving, applying lotion, and chatting. They can be reminded that the person, also, is undergoing anticipatory grief about the impending separation and might feel reassured to know that others share the experience.

Vignette

■ Jaime is the young wife of a much older man who is dying of cancer. He is carrying on with daily life as if nothing is wrong, even to the point of making up stories about his capabilities. He dresses every day and imagines he is going through his accustomed routines. Thus, Jaime does not feel she can talk with him about his very obvious weight loss and decline. She grows more careful, quiet, and spacy each day. She cannot remember appointments or even what was said 5 minutes before. When the visiting nurse describes anticipatory grief she almost weeps with relief. "You mean it is normal to feel completely crazy? Empty? Lost? Nothing at all?" She is reassured that this strange and unwelcome state will pass, and that it even has a usefulness in protecting her from the full effects of this crisis. After that, Jaime is able to confide regularly in the nurse and accept comfort.

Anticipatory grief is genuine mourning, with symptoms. See Box 30–3 for signs of anticipatory grief.

Anticipatory grief "does not decrease or increase the amount of emotion generated by the loss, yet it can help work through feelings in advance and resolves unfinished business before the separation actually occurs" (Shearer and Davidhizer 1994, p. 62).

To have these experiences named and normalized does not take them away, but it can reduce their frightfulness. This premourning can be described to families as a way to prepare themselves for the loss of their loved one little by little. No one is ever fully prepared. The shock of death cannot be anticipated, but the loss of that important person can be foreseen and imagined. One 29-year-old wife of a dying 32-year-old husband coped by courageously imagining his funeral again and again. Perhaps this helped desensitize her to its inevitable arrival. Others might label such thoughts as morbid, but they are not unusual for people going through an extraordinary trial. People often report that the anticipatory grief process makes the time of bereavement a little eas-

ier, especially if the time leading up to death has been used to say goodbye and comfort each other. The nurse can be of great help in guiding families through this process.

THE FOUR GIFTS OF RESOLVING RELATIONSHIPS

Vignette

■ Mrs. Piati is the aging matriarch of a large clan. She is tiny and frail, in her mid '90s, but still dominates the emotional lives of her seven children and some of her grandchildren. Disagreements about caregiving, money and property, and family history are beginning to create deep resentments among some of the children. The hospice nurse and social worker call a family meeting during which many of the practical matters are resolved satisfactorily. Then the nurse speaks about this opportunity to bring each of their relationships with their mother to a peaceful and loving end. She describes something called "The Four Gifts for Resolving Relationships." The mood quiets and deepens and some of the children have tears in their eyes. One of them blurts out, "This is true. I know because I have never forgiven my father for leaving us when I was young, and I've never been able to feel love for him either, or let him go." She begins to cry, as do two of her siblings. They start talking among themselves about things they love about their mother, and even laugh about her quirks. There is a sense of gentle healing in the group.

Box 30–3 Signs of Anticipatory Grief

- Feelings of emptiness or of being lost
- A sense of being numb and fatigued
- A feeling of unreality and disbelief
- Periods of weeping or raging
- A desire to run away from the situation
- A need to oversee every detail of the patient's care in order to protect her or him from suffering and death
- Fears of the future and the unknown
- Anger at the patient or the medical professionals or both
- Pronounced clinging to or dependency on the patient or other family members
- Fear of going crazy

The deep, vital connections among family members are often unspoken, expressed at a wordless level by our very presence with each other over many years. These bonds are threatened, shaken, and attacked by the impending death of a family member. Very often these deep, underground disruptions show themselves in arguments, family rifts, resentments, disagreements, or distancing. They are masked by anger and irritation or by silence and withdrawal. Families can be shown simple tools for identifying their distress and for expressing it in healthy ways. "The Four Gifts for Resolving Relationships" is one of these tools.

The concept of the Four Gifts was interpreted from the writings of Elisabeth Kübler-Ross and used with her consent by Beverly Ryan, LCSW, of the Hospice of the Twin Cities in Minnesota. Dr. Kübler-Ross observed many couples and families in her workshops for the terminally ill and saw how often relationships shifted from being distant, cold, or angry to becoming warm, loving, and close. The change followed a predictable sequence of emotional communications, and this sequence was eventually formulated into the Four Gifts. Family members can be encouraged to write down their thoughts and feelings and to read them to the dying person, if appropriate, or simply to sit down one-to-one and talk from the heart. Likewise, clients can be invited to share these gifts with the important people in their lives. The gifts work both ways. When done with sincerity and simplicity, they invariably precipitate a healing shift in relationships.

1. **Forgiveness** ("I'm sorry"; "I forgive you"): The first step is to admit to the wrongs and hurts experienced at the hands of the other person. This can be frightening to do because it makes a person vulnerable to fresh injury. The other person may have no idea the speaker has been harboring a resentment or hurt, and may respond with disbelief, defensiveness, or silence. The intention here is to forgive and release the hurt, and that must be the context in which this conversation takes place. Bear in mind two important caveats. One is that sometimes a face-to-face encounter is not possible (as when the client is sedated, comatose, or demented) and sometimes it is not advisable (as when there is conviction that this would cause more distress than it would relieve). In such cases, the effect can still be achieved by writing down the message and reading it to another person or simply by telling another, who acts as a stand-in for the client. The other caveat is that forgiveness does *not* mean that a truly injurious or abusive action has been condoned or accepted. It does not make a wrong right. What it does is signal a desire to let go of blame and anger, to release one's heart from the chains of resentment. As such, it is a gift to the one who offers forgiveness as much or more than it is a gift to the one receiving it.

   The willingness to say, "I forgive you," is accompanied by the question, "Is there anything I have done, or not done, for which I need to say I am sorry?" Being open to hearing about another person's injuries and asking him or her for forgiveness is the other side of the coin of this gift. The art of giving and receiving forgiveness is rarely overt in many families, so most people have had no experience with this remarkably healing practice. They may feel awkward and phony using the words. Doubtless this practice entails taking emotional risks. However, it is the gateway to the other three gifts. Time is running out, and families know it. With some practice and encouragement, many take the chance.

2. **Love** ("I love you"): The second gift is to express love to each other. It is astonishing how many children have never heard their parents say, "I love you." In many long-term marriages, these words have faded away, to be replaced by daily togetherness and the practical caring of a shared life. The end of life is a wonderful time for people to fully express what they mean to each other. Especially meaningful are the many memories of things learned from another, such as values, attitudes, and beliefs. Ultimately, the message is that all people are loved for being just who they are, and they are loved just for being, rather than for what they have done or achieved.

3. **Gratitude** ("Thank you"): This is the moment to take the time to thank each other for what each has been in the other's life. People look back over life together and remember the good times and the tough times. They can take out photo albums, show videos, reminisce, listen again to the client's or family members' favorite stories. Perhaps the rarest commodity in this culture is full attention; to receive a person's undivided attention is precious. It is especially important to acknowledge the things that the patient took for granted. Many fathers and husbands have never been thanked for going to work every day for 30 to 40 years. Many wives and mothers would never expect thanks for all the laundry, mending, and help with school projects. Many exhausted caregivers weep when they are told they really are doing a good job and are appreciated.

4. **Farewell** ("Good-bye, I'll be okay"): Many people say that they hate good-byes. "I don't do good-byes," they may say. It is resisted for several reasons. Saying good-bye brings up feelings of grief

and finality. Also, one hesitates to say goodbye before someone is actually leaving. It may appear to be rushing the person or even causing the departure. Yet when the final separation of death awaits us, the act of saying good-bye is deeply appropriate and meaningful. Survivors feel its absence when there was no chance to say good-bye and usually have to wrestle with it during bereavement. When one acknowledges the coming separation, one both gives and receives permission for the death to occur. The person who is dying knows that the loved one is facing the death and will survive it. The person giving permission loosens his or her grasp and begins to surrender to the inevitability of the death. The phrases one uses can be softened. "I know the time will come when we'll have to part, and these are some of my feelings and thoughts . . ." "I am thinking about having to go on without you, and I know I am going to make it." "Thinking about saying good-bye makes me so terribly sad." However one finds the words, this final gift is a way of acknowledging and honoring the importance of the relationship in one's life and it should be encouraged and even rehearsed if necessary.

The simplest way for a nurse to help the family or client is to simply describe these communications in sequence, and say that they have been found to help many people feel better about what they are going through. People usually grasp the emotional logic of the Four Gifts, and they also feel anxious about the feelings they bring up. The nurse can encourage them by role playing or simply by saying, "I want you to try these, right from the heart, and take the risk that some feelings will arise. That is really okay and very understandable in these circumstances."

Vignette

■ *Tom is a 28-year-old developmentally disabled man with bipolar disorder. He arrived at his dying father's home to see him for the last time, and the nurse told him about the Four Gifts. The young man lived in a group home and had not seen his family for many months. The last time he visited, he had not taken his medication and his misbehavior had estranged his family. The young man sadly entered his father's bedroom and sat on the bed. He said, "Dad, I know you are going to die and I want you to know that I am so sorry for the ways I have acted before now, and the trouble I have caused. Please forgive me, Dad. You have always looked out for me, and I shouldn't have gone off my meds. I love you, Dad. You've never given up on*

me. Thank you for finding me the place where I live and people to love me and look after me. Thanks for being my Dad. I know I have to say good-bye. I promise I will keep on taking my meds so I will behave right. I promise I'll listen to my counselors and have a good life. I love you so much, Dad. Good-bye." He wept with his father who held him for a little while. Then he came out of the room with a tear-streaked face, knowing he would never see his father again alive. He felt complete, however. He had said the important things with courage and taken proper leave of his father.

DEVELOPMENTAL OPPORTUNITIES AT THE END OF LIFE

Our culture is only beginning to offer insight into the period of life that precedes dying. Largely as a result of hospice involvement by thousands of families and clients, paradigms are emerging for more successful approaches to dying well. Many ancient cultures and religions have more highly developed models of how to have a good death. Tibetan Buddhists and ancient Egyptians created long treatises and guidebooks on death and dying. Chief Joseph, a Native American, is often quoted as having said, "Today is a good day to die, because today my whole life is before me." He is said to have spoken these words at the age of 14. Cicely Saunders was asked by a reporter, "Have you thought about how you want to die?" She replied, at the age of 80, "Everybody else says they want to die suddenly, but I say I'd like to die of cancer, because it gives me time to say I'm sorry, and thank you, and good-bye" (Stolberg 1999).

For those who have the gift of time, awareness, and support, this period offers opportunities for continued growth as a person. The possibilities may not be obvious, however, because there is no cultural articulation about or support for this period of life. Instead, families and friends tend to focus more on the disease, treatment options and effects, daily comfort, and encouraging pep talks. Some clients have asked what so many others simply ponder or worry over: "How do I live as a person with cancer (or other disease)? Who am I supposed to be?" A nurse or medical caregiver can be of great help in suggesting some of the possible things to be done during this period, if the client appears to have sufficient energy and presence of mind. Ira Byock (1997) explores and articulates the following developmental possibilities for the dying; completion of worldly affairs; closure of personal and professional relationships; learning the meaning of one's life; love of oneself and of others; acceptance of the finality of life; sense of a new self beyond personal loss; recognition of a transcendent realm.

Completion of Worldly Affairs

There are many legal and financial steps that can be taken to ensure that the patient's wishes are fulfilled. Among these are the completion of a last will and testament, the assignment of durable power of attorney, and the possibility of estate planning.

Closure of Personal and Professional Relationships

Whether the patient has days, weeks, or months to live, the process of bringing completion to important relationships can begin. If the patient is forthright about this, others often feel more comfortable following suit and talking more openly along the lines of "The Four Gifts for Resolving Relationships." In discussions with the patient, the nurse can simply ask who needs to be thanked, forgiven, reconciled with, or told about the patient's love and affection.

Learning the Meaning of One's Life

When confronted with the reality of life's end, most people naturally look back and reminisce. In doing so, they distill and extract the meaning of a lifetime in order to answer the existential question, "Was my life worth living?" This sifting and retelling of stories is called, in the hospice lexicon, life review. It can sound like everyday conversation, but the context of mortality suggests a deep process of evaluation. A nurse can facilitate this process by asking to hear about life's most important moments, such as the first time the patient fell in love or met the future spouse, about achievements and disappointments, about struggles and strengths.

Love of Oneself and Others

There is no requirement that people come to the end of their lives in a state of psychological grace, it has been said. Human beings bring to the end of their days the imperfections and emotional wounds of a lifetime, and many are poorly equipped to heal themselves at a time when they are tired, sick, and disabled. As people review their lives, they may see broken relationships, missed or failed opportunities, and wasted years. They may feel angry, defensive, controlling, or blaming as well as depressed and despairing. Listening to these stories, one might struggle to find values and choices of which to feel proud. However, virtually everyone has loved someone or something, and everyone needs to be loved. A nurse can pay close attention to these relationships and maintain the hope that meaning and resolution might flow from this source.

Acceptance of the Finality of Life

The diagnosis of an incurable, terminal condition confronts people with the unthinkable: that their personal life really will end. People grapple with this existential crisis using a variety of defenses, such as denying the diagnosis or prognosis, bargaining with the self, God, or others, becoming angry, feeling sad and depressed. When nothing removes or ameliorates the crisis, most people arrive at an acceptance of the reality that accompanies all of us from birth—the reality that everyone's life will come to an end, and that now this unique and individual life is going to end. This acceptance does not preclude people from retaining a fighting spirit. People can fight for the most independence possible, for small triumphs, for graceful adaptations to change. However, acceptance that life is coming to an end usually brings an underlying peacefulness and an interest in bringing about the best possible closure.

Sense of a New Self Beyond Personal Loss

Vignette

■ Ed was a dapper 85-year-old widower who had been diagnosed with terminal lung cancer. He lived alone, but in the past few months had enjoyed a new relationship with a woman, which revitalized and delighted him. His diagnosis precipitated the loss of this relationship. He trusted and confided in his hospice nurse and social worker, who stood by him as he cycled through depression, hopelessness and despair, and wave after wave of grief over the loss of his new-found happiness. He was able to weep openly and speak feelingly about the epiphanies and disappointments of his life. Meanwhile, he continued to enjoy what pleasures he could, such as hosting his friends at fine restaurants. Candid about his fears about the unknown, he opened up to people around him in an unprecedented way. After a few *weeks, he seemed to have resolved his struggles and fears and entered a permanent state of joy. He described this as intense happiness upon waking each day. People in his presence felt loved and appreciated. He radiated unconditional affection and delight. Every night, he placed a note by his bed: "If I die during the night, know that I died a happy man." For the remaining 3 weeks of his life, he remained in this state of joy and serenity, making an unforgettable impression on those who cared for him. Ed's new self-defined role was to spread sunshine to all those around him. He had discovered a gift hidden in this end-stage of life—an intense love of life and of others in the present moment. When he died, his womanfriend and sons were holding his hands.*

Recognition of a Transcendent Realm

Vignette

■ *Elka was a single, childless, and highly intelligent woman in her late 70s who followed the teachings of a mystical Christian sect. She believed wholeheartedly that death would liberate her spirit into realms of growth and evolution, and she welcomed the coming event. She completed all her affairs and good-byes, gave everything away, and moved into an adult foster home for the last week of her life. Her body was to be donated for scientific research. Despite her growing weakness and discomfort, she maintained an attitude of celebration about her "transition." Her joyful anticipation and inner peace inspired those who took care of her. After her peaceful death, each of her friends and caregivers received a death card from her, expressing her delight that she had moved on, and also that she had had the last word.*

Some people are able to invest death and dying with transcendent meaning. For them, dying is the next great adventure in a life already guided by eternal principles. Hospice workers speak of the inner light that shines from certain people who are close to death. Instead of fear or sadness, they radiate loving kindness and peaceful anticipation. Acknowledgment and support of the spiritual dimensions of death and dying are integral to hospice care. Chaplains are offered to all hospice families, as are complementary therapies, when available. These include music and art therapy, harp playing, therapeutic touch, aroma therapy, and massage. Offering to pray with a sick person or exploring the person's spiritual views is often an appropriate intervention. As a health care provider, it is important to realize that some people regard dying as a perfectly nor-mal, acceptable, welcome, and even exciting part of life.

Care for Those Who Grieve
Elizabeth Varcarolis

Loss is part of the human experience, and grief and bereavement are the normal responses to loss. The loss may be of a relationship (divorce, separation, death, abortion), of health (a body function or part, mental or physical capacity), of status or prestige, of security (occupational, financial, social, cultural), of self-confidence, of a dream, or of self-concept, or loss can be of a symbolic nature. Other losses include changes in circumstances, such as retirement, promotion, marriage, and aging. All losses affect a person's self-concept. People undergoing therapy may grieve as they give up old and familiar—even if maladaptive—ways of viewing the world. A loss can be real or perceived. Although grief and loss are universal experiences, loss through death is a major life crisis. A person grieves because he or she has become attached to the dying person and is committed to that person. Not to commit is to do without shared joy, security, satisfaction, growth, and comfort (Tschudin 1997).

Bereavement is, on the whole, a physically painful experience (Tschudin 1997). Losses of various kinds can hurt and diminish the part of life that is shared with and related to others, but it can also hurt and diminish one's inner life, which is not so readily shared (Tschudin 1997). Since loss is a part of life, everyone is an expert in loss and bereavement. The catch is that not everyone is expert at coping with losses or at coping well with losses.

REACTIONS TO DEATH AND DYING

Normal grief reactions include depressed mood, insomnia, anxiety, poor appetite, loss of interest, guilt feelings, dreams about the deceased, and poor concentration. Psychological states include shock, denial, and yearning and searching for the deceased. The acute grief reaction lasts from 4 to 8 weeks, the active symptoms of grief usually last from 3 to 6 months, and the complete work of mourning may take from 1 to 2 years or more to complete.

It is important for nurses to understand that cultural influences may dictate how people experience death and dying. The term *bereavement* refers to the social experience of dealing with the loss of a loved one through death. The term *mourning* refers to a culturally patterned behavioral response to loss (Bateman 1999). Sensitivity to the ethnic, cultural, spiritual, and religious beliefs of a diverse cultural population can help nurses more effectively identify a person's needs (Bateman 1999).

Denial and fear of death are strong in the American culture. This denial and fear affect the behavioral responses of the bereaved, the family, and those who support the family in the face of death. Nurses are affected by cultural myths in the same way the rest of society is; when they are faced with a person who is dying, nurses remember their own losses. Difficult memories and unresolved feelings are often awakened. When staff members have not been able to resolve their own conflicts with death, their ability to help others is minimized. Psychological support should be available to help staff better understand the grieving process. When nurses examine their own feelings and their personal experiences of loss, verbal and nonverbal clues to the needs of grieving family members of a dying client become more apparent (Marks 1976). Answers to the questions in Box 30–1, Self-Assessment of Your Beliefs about Death and Dying, should be reviewed.

Sometimes, nurses grieve with family members at the death of a person they have cared for and become fond of. Sometimes, an entire staff may mourn the death of a client. After clients die, nurses manage bereavement tasks, such as making sense of the death, managing mild to intense emotions, and realigning relationships. When multiple deaths are encountered, these tasks become more difficult. Understanding theories, models, tasks, and other factors can help nurses to facilitate their own grief and reduce bereavement overload (Saunders and Valente 1995).

FRAMEWORKS FOR UNDERSTANDING LOSS

Bereavement is a distinct psychological process that involves disengaging strong emotional ties from a significant relationship and reinvesting those ties in a new and productive direction. This reinvestment of emotional energy into new relationships or creative activities is necessary for a person's mental health and ability to function in society. When the mourning process is successfully completed, the griever is released from one interpersonal relationship and is able to form new relationships. The entire process of mourning may take a year or more to complete.

As mentioned earlier, Elisabeth Kübler-Ross (1969) identified distinct phases in a person's response to death and dying (denial, anger, bargaining, depression, and acceptance). These phases do not always occur in a specific order; in fact, they may go through all phases in the space of a few minutes, over and over again (Tschudin 1997, p. 119).

In a study of the grief responses of elderly widows, Hegge and Fischer (2000) found that the grief work followed an erratic cycle, with peaks and valleys, spurts and relapses, through the various phases mentioned in the literature concerning loss and bereavement. Studies of grief and loss by Parkes (1970, 1975), Caplan (1974), Engel (1964), Kübler-Ross (1969), and others identify various phases of bereavement that proceed in orderly sequences within time frames. In reality, these phases overlap, and regression to previous phases is common and is usually marked by the erratic peaks and valleys mentioned.

The various frameworks for grieving and phases of grief are useful models for helping people to understand the deeply felt and disturbing phenomena people experience when confronting profound loss. Denial and shock, anger and guilt, emotional turmoil, disorganization, panic, depression, loneliness and, eventually, acceptance of the loss are all common during bereavement.

The nurse's focus when facilitating bereavement holistically is on helping the bereaved with the many factors of importance to them at particular points in time. Models and frameworks help organize the experience of loss, but models are not the focus of care when facilitating the process of mourning. Often the nurse or other caregiver can best serve the grieving just by being present, listening with interest, and encouraging talk and the telling of meaningful stories.

Many theorists have studied the grief process. Some of the most widely known are George Engel, Colin Parkes, Erich Lindemann, John Bowlby, and Edgar Jackson. Although each theorist uses different terminology, the process all of them outline is fundamentally the same. Each describes commonly experienced psychological and behavioral characteristics. These characteristics follow a pattern of response:

1. Shock and disbelief
2. Sensation of somatic distress
3. Preoccupation with image of the deceased
4. Guilt
5. Anger

6. Change in behavior (e.g., depression, disorganization, or restlessness)
7. Reorganization of behavior directed toward a new object or activity

People react within their own value and personality structures as well as within their social environments and cultural patterns. Most people have been preprogrammed to respond to death in particular ways. Distinct characteristics, however, may be identified throughout the grieving process.

The process of mourning is often divided into stages (phases). The stages discussed here have been identified by Engel (1964) as (1) acute and (2) long term. All frameworks address the same phenomena.

Acute Stage

The acute state (4 to 8 weeks after the death) involves shock and disbelief, developing awareness, and restitution.

Shock and Disbelief

The bereaved's first response is that of **denial.** The person is emotionally unable to accept his or her painful loss. Denial functions as a buffer against intolerable pain and slowly allows the person to acknowledge the reality of death. The mourner may appear to be functioning like a robot. Often, the bereaved person feels numb. A death may be accepted intellectually during this stage—"It's just as well, she was suffering"—although the emotional responses are still repressed. Denial is a needed defense that lasts for a few hours or a few days. Denial that persists longer than a few days may become dysfunctional, making it difficult to move through the process of mourning.

Development of Awareness

As denial fades, painful feelings begin to surface. The finality of the loved one's death becomes more of a reality. Waves of anguish and pain are experienced and may be localized in the chest or the epigastric area. **Anger** often surfaces at this time. Doctors and nurses are often the subjects of blame. Awareness by staff that anger is often displaced onto people in the hospital environment may decrease defensive staff behaviors. **Guilt** is often experienced, and the bereaved blames himself or herself for taking or for failing to take specific actions. Impulsive and self-destructive acts by the mourner,

such as smashing a hand through a window or beating the head against a wall, may be seen. **Crying** is a common phenomenon during this stage. "It is during this time that the greatest degree of anguish or despair, within the limits imposed by cultural patterns, is experienced or expressed" (Engel 1964). Crying can afford a welcome release from pent-up anguish and tension. Assessment of cultural patterns is important to making clinical judgments about the appropriateness of the bereaved's behavior. Failing to cry can be the result of cultural influences or environmental restraints. The person may cry in private. Inability to cry, however, may be the result of a high degree of ambivalence toward the deceased. A person who is unable to cry may have difficulty in successfully completing the work of mourning.

Restitution

Restitution is the formal, ritualistic phase of mourning during the acute stage. It is the institutionalization of mourning: it brings friends and family together in the rites of the funeral service, and serves to emphasize the finality of death. The viewing of the body, the lowering of the casket, and the various religious and cultural rituals all help the bereaved shed any residual denial in an atmosphere of support. Every human society has its own moral and cultural standards according to which the rituals of mourning take place. The gathering in ritualistic farewell to the deceased provides support and sustenance for the family.

Long-Term Stage

After the acute stage has been completed, the main work of mourning goes on intrapsychically during the long-term stage, which lasts for 1 to 2 years or longer. The various phenomena experienced during bereavement are described in Table 30–1.

Most bereaved persons come to terms with their losses with support from family and friends. However, more than 30% may require professional support (Lloyd-Williams 1995). Unresolved grief reactions have been called the hidden disease and may account for many of the physical symptoms seen in doctors' offices and hospital units. The existence of the broken-heart syndrome is supported by statistics that show that surviving spouses die within a year at a much higher rate than do members of control groups (Carr 1985). Suicide is higher among people who have had a significant loss, especially if losses are multiple and grieving mechanisms are limited (Gregory 1994).

TABLE 30–1 *Phenomena Experienced During Bereavement*

SYMPTOMS	EXAMPLES
Sensations of Somatic Distress	
Tightness in throat, shortness of breath, sighing, mental pain, exhaustion; food tastes like sand; things feel unreal. Pain or discomfort may be identical to the symptoms experienced by the dead person. Normally, symptoms are brief.	A woman whose husband died of a stroke complains of weakness and numbness on her left side.
Preoccupation with the Image of the Deceased	
The bereaved brings up and thinks and talks about numerous memories of the deceased. The memories are positive. This process goes on with great sadness. The idealization of the deceased lets the bereaved relive the gratifications associated with the deceased and helps resolve any guilt the bereaved feels concerning the deceased. The bereaved may also take on many of the mannerisms of the deceased through identification. Identification serves the purpose of holding on to the deceased. Preoccupation with the dead person can continue for many months before it lessens.	A man whose wife has just died states, "I just can't stop thinking about my wife. Everything I see reminds me of her. We picked up this seashell on our honeymoon. I remember every wonderful moment we had together. The pain is so great, but the memories just keep coming." His friends notice that when he talks, his hand gestures and expressions are very like those of his recently deceased wife.
Guilt	
The bereaved reproaches himself or herself for real or fancied acts of negligence or omissions in the relationship with the deceased.	"I should have made him go to the doctor sooner." "I should have paid more attention to her, been more thoughtful."
Anger	
The anger the bereaved experiences may not be toward the object that gives rise to it. Often the anger is displaced onto the medical or nursing staff. Often it is directed toward the deceased. The anger is at its height during the first month but is often intermittent throughout the first year. The overflow of hostility disturbs the bereaved, resulting in the feeling that he or she is "going insane."	"The doctor didn't operate in time. If he had, Mary would be alive today." "How could he leave me like this . . . how could he?"
Change in Behavior: Depression, Disorganization, Restlessness	
A person may exhibit marked restlessness and an inability to organize his or her behavior. A depressive mood during routing activities is common, decreasing as the year passes and the intensity of the grief declines. Absence of depression is more abnormal than its presence. Loneliness and aimlessness are most pronounced 6 to 9 months after the death.	Six months after her husband died, Mrs. Faye stated, "I just can't seem to function. I have a hard time doing the simplest tasks. I can't be bothered with socializing." "I feel so down . . . so, so empty."
Reorganization of Behavior Directed Toward a New Object or Activity	
Gradually, the person renews his or her interest in people and activities. The grieving thus releases the bereaved from one interpersonal relationship, and new ones are free to take its place.	Twenty months after her husband's death, Mrs. Faye tells a friend, "I'll be away this weekend. I am going fishing with my brother and his friend. This is the first time I've felt like doing anything since Harry died."

In some cases, bereaved persons become disorganized, neglect themselves, do not eat, use alcohol or drugs, and are susceptible to physical disease. Several studies have shown that the health of widows and close relatives declines within 1 year of bereavement, and medical and psychiatric problems increase (Bowlby and Parkes 1970; Carr 1985).

Health care workers are not immune to grief reactions. A study by Feldstein and Gemma (1995) found that oncology nurses scored higher than the norm in despair, social isolation, and somatization.

Table 30–2 identifies the common phenomena experienced during grief and pathological intensification and indicates appropriate signals for counseling.

HELPING PEOPLE COPE WITH LOSS

Prolonged and serious alterations in social adjustment, as well as medical diseases, may develop if the phases of mourning are interrupted or if needed support is not available. Listening is the most important support for acute grief. The helping person should keep his or her own talking to a minimum.

Telling the story over and over is therapeutic for the bereaved. Listening, **really listening,** not just to the words but to the whole person, can assist in healing. Tschudin (1997, p. 105) states that "listening and not talking, not interrupting, being comfortable

TABLE 30–2   *Common Experiences During Grief and Their Pathological Intensification*

PHENOMENON	TYPICAL RESPONSE	PATHOLOGICAL INTENSIFICATION
Dying	Emotional expression and immediate coping with the dying process	Avoidance; feeling overwhelmed, dazed, confused; feeling self-punitive; feeling inappropriately hostile
Death and outcry	Outcry of emotions with news of the death and turning for help to others or isolating self with self-soothing	Panic; dissociative reactions, reactive psychoses
Warding off (denial)	Avoidance of reminders and social withdrawal, focusing elsewhere, emotional numbing, not thinking of implications to self or of certain themes	Maladaptive avoidances of confronting the implications of death; drug or alcohol abuse, counterphobic frenzy, promiscuity, fugue states, phobic avoidance, feeling dead or unreal
Re-experience (intrusion)	Intrusive experiences, including recollections of negative experiences during relationship with the deceased, bad dreams, reduced concentration, compulsive re-enactments	Being flooded with negative images and emotions; uncontrolled ideation, self-impairing compulsive re-enactments, night terrors, recurrent nightmares, distraught feelings resulting from the intrusion of anger, anxiety, despair, shame, or guilt; physiological exhaustion resulting from hyperarousal
Working through	Recollection of the deceased and a contemplation of self with reduced intrusiveness of memories and fantasies and with increased rational acceptance, reduced numbness and avoidance, more "dosing" of recollections, and a sense of working it through	Feeling an inability to integrate the death with a sense of self and continued life; persistent warded-off themes may manifest as anxious, depressed, enraged, shame-filled, or guilty moods and psychophysiological syndromes
Completion	Reduction in emotional swings and a sense of self-coherence and readiness for new relationships; ability to experience positive states of mind	Failure to complete mourning may be associated with inability to work or create, to feel emotion or positive states of mind

From Horowitz, M. J. (1990). A model of mourning: Change in schemas of self and others. *Journal of the American Psychoanalytic Association*, 38(2), 297–324.

TABLE 30-3 *Guidelines for Helping People in Acute Grief*

INTERVENTION	RATIONALE
1. Employ methods that can facilitate the grieving process (Robinson 1997): a. Give your full presence: use appropriate eye contact, attentive listening, and appropriate touch.	a. Talking is one of the most important ways of dealing with acute grief. Listening patiently helps the bereaved express all feelings, even ones they feel are "negative." Appropriate eye contact helps to convey the awareness that you are there and are sharing their sadness. Suitable human touch can express warmth and nurture healing. Inappropriate touch can leave a person confused and uncomfortable.
b. Be patient with the bereaved in times of silence. Do not fill silence with empty chatter.	b. Sharing painful feelings during periods of silence is healing and conveys your concern.
2. Know about and share with the bereaved information about the normal phenomena that occur during the normal mourning process, because they may concern some people (intense anger at the deceased, guilt, symptoms the deceased had before death, unbidden floods of memories). Give bereaved support during the occurrence of these phenomena and a written handout to refer to.	2. Although the knowledge won't eliminate the emotions, it can greatly relieve a person who is thinking there is something wrong with having these feelings.
3. Encourage the support of family and friends. If no supports are available, refer the client to a community bereavement group. (Bereavement groups are helpful even when a person has many friends or much family support.)	3. There are routine matters that friends can help with. For example a. Getting food into the house b. Making phone calls c. Driving to the mortuary d. Taking care of kids or other family members
4. Offer spiritual support and referrals when needed.	4. Dealing with an illness or catastrophic loss can cause the most profound spiritual anguish (Zerbe 1999).
5. When intense emotions are in evidence, show understanding and support. (Refer to Box 30–4 for guidelines.)	5. Empathetic words that reflect acceptance of a bereaved individual's feelings are healing (Robinson 1997).

with silence when indicated, and using prompts like 'go on,' etc., to encourage the person to continue talking" are the most helpful behaviors.

Talking can release negative emotions. When a person is faced with loss, strong feelings of anger, guilt, and hate are normal reactions that have to be expressed in order to facilitate the process of mourning. It is important that someone listen and encourage the expression of feelings surrounding the person's loss or anticipated loss.

Banal advice and philosophical statements are useless. Unhelpful responses by others, such as "He's no longer suffering" or "You can always have another child" or "It's better this way," can lead the bereaved to believe that others do not understand the acute pain being suffered and that the personal impact of the loss is being minimized. Such statements can compound feelings of isolation.

More helpful responses are "His death will be a terrible loss" or "No one can replace her" or "He will be missed for a long time." Statements such as these validate the bereaved person's experience of loss and communicate the message that the bereaved is understood and supported. Table 30–3 provides guidelines for helping people grieve. Box 30–4 offers guidelines for what to say to a person suffering a profound loss.

Some people find comfort and support in grief counseling or support groups. Six to ten sessions of psychotherapy have been found to be helpful during the crisis period. At a later stage, the use of 15 sessions or more has been found to have a good outcome. More complicated or pathological patterns of grief may require special techniques, such as re-grief work (Middleton and Raphael 1992). One study demonstrated that highly religious clients with grief and bereavement issues tended to improve faster when religious psychotherapy was added to a cognitive-behavioral approach (Azhar and Varma 1995).

Table 30–4 offers guidelines that can help people and their families cope with catastrophic grief.

BOX 30-4   Guidelines for Communicating with a Bereaved Person

When you sense an overwhelming *sorrow*	"This must hurt terribly."
When you hear *anger* in the bereaved's voice	"I hear anger in your voice. Most people go through periods of anger when their loved one dies. Are you feeling angry now?"
If you discern *guilt*	"Are you feeling guilty? This is a common reaction many people have. What are some of your thoughts about this?
If you sense a *fear* of the future	"It must be scary to go through this."
When the bereaved seems *confused*	"This can be a bewildering time."
In almost any *painful situation*	"This must be very difficult for you."

Adapted from Robinson, D. (1997). *Good intentions: The nine unconscious mistakes of nice people.* New York: Warner Books, p. 249. Reprinted with permission. Copyright © 1997 by Duke Robinson.

TABLE 30-4   Guidelines for Dealing with Catastrophic Loss

Take the time you need to grieve.	The hard work of grief uses psychological energy. Resolution of the numb state that occurs after loss requires a few weeks at least. A minimum of 1 year, to cover all the birthdays, anniversaries, and other important dates without your loved one is required before you can learn to live with your loss.
Express your feelings.	Remember that anger, anxiety, loneliness, and even guilt are normal reactions and that everyone needs a safe place to express them. Tell your personal story of loss as many times as you need to—this repetition is a helpful and necessary part of the grieving process.
Establish a structure for each day and stick to it.	Although it is hard to do, keeping to some semblance of structure makes the first few weeks after a loss easier. Getting through each day helps to restore the confidence you need to accept the reality of loss.
Don't feel that you have to answer all the questions asked you.	Although most people try to be kind, they may be unaware of their insensitivity. Down the road, you may want to read books about how others have dealt with similar circumstances. They often have helpful suggestions for a person in your situation.
As hard as it is, try to take good care of yourself.	Eat well, talk with friends, get plenty of rest. Be sure to let your primary care clinician know if you are having trouble eating or sleeping. Make use of exercise. It can help you let out pent-up frustrations. If you are losing weight, sleeping excessively or intermittently, or still experiencing deep depression after 3 months, be sure to seek professional assistance.
Expect the unexpected.	You may begin to feel a bit better, only to have a brief emotional collapse. These are expectable reactions. Moreover, you may find that you dream about, visualize, think about, or search for your loved one. This, too, is a part of the grieving process.
Give yourself time.	Don't feel that you have to resume all of life's duties right away.
Make use of rituals.	Those who take the time to say good-bye at a funeral or a viewing tend to find it helps the bereavement process.
If you do not begin to feel better within a few weeks, at least for a few hours every day, be sure to tell your doctor.	If you have had an emotional problem in the past (e.g., depression, substance abuse), be sure to get the additional support you need. Losing a loved one puts you at higher risk for a relapse of these disorders

From Zerbe, K. J. (1999). *Women's mental health in primary care* (pp 207–208). Philadelphia: W. B. Saunders.

UNRESOLVED AND DYSFUNCTIONAL GRIEF

Acute grief can be a time of exacerbation of any pre-existing medical or psychiatric problems. A history of depression, substance abuse, or post-traumatic stress disorder can complicate grief and certainly deserves specific treatment (Prigerson et al. 1995).

Some indications that a person may have the potential for **dysfunctional grieving** may be gleaned by understanding some things about the bereaved:

■ Does the bereaved person exhibit some of the characteristics that can complicate bereavement?
Was the bereaved heavily dependent on the deceased?
Were there persistent unresolved conflicts between the bereaved and the deceased?
Was the deceased a child (often the most profound loss)?
Does the bereaved have a meaningful relationship or support system?
Has the bereaved experienced a number of previous losses?
Does the bereaved person have sound coping skills?

Box 30–5 *Presenting Symptoms of Dysfunctional Grief*

1. Prolonged and severe symptoms lasting 2 to 3 months or longer
2. Limited response to support
3. Profound and persistent feelings of hopelessness
4. Completely withdrawn or fear of being alone
5. Inability to work, to create, to feel emotion or positive states of mind
6. Maladaptive behaviors in response to the death, for example
   ■ Drug or alcohol abuse
   ■ Promiscuity
   ■ Fugue states
   ■ Feeling dead or unreal
   ■ Suicidal ideation
   ■ Aggressive behaviors
   ■ Compulsive spending
7. Recurrent nightmares, night terrors, compulsive re-enactments
8. Exhaustion resulting from lack of sleep and hyperarousal
9. Prolonged depression, panic attacks
10. Self-neglect

■ Was the deceased's death associated with a cultural stigma (e.g., AIDS, suicide)?
■ Was the death unexpected or associated with violence (murder, suicide)?
■ Has the bereaved had difficulty resolving past significant losses?
■ Does the bereaved have a history of depression, drug or alcohol abuse, or other psychiatric illness?
■ If the bereaved is young, are there indications for special interventions?

Box 30–5 highlights some symptoms of dysfunctional grief. **Dysfunctional grieving** essentially means that the grief work is unresolved. Depression is the most common response to unresolved grief. Disturbances in mood are associated with biological changes in the body during stress-related depressive illness. Some examples include electrolyte disturbance, nervous system alterations dysfunction, and faulty regulation of the autonomic nervous system. Always assess the potential for suicide. Someone who is having difficulty negotiating the work of mourning and is suffering can benefit from counseling, as mentioned earlier.

SUCCESSFUL MOURNING

Worden (1991) identified a task-based model that attempts to describe tasks that are involved in the process of mourning:

■ Accept the reality of the loss
■ Share in the process of working through the pain of grief
■ Adjust to an environment in which the deceased is missing
■ Restructure the family's relationship with the deceased and reinvest in other relationships and life pursuits.

Were these tasks accomplished? The work of mourning is over when the bereaved can remember realistically both the pleasures and the disappointments of the lost loved one. Brief periods of intense emotions may still occur at significant times, such as holidays and anniversaries, but the person or family members have energy to reinvest in new relationships that bring shared joys, security, satisfaction, and comfort. If, after a normal period of time (12 to 24 months), a person has not completed the grieving process, reassessment and re-evaluation are indicated. Johnson et al. (2000) formulated a tool for evaluating the resolution of grief; see Table 30–5.

TABLE 30–5 *Grief Resolution Outcomes*

GRIEF RESOLUTION	NOT AT ALL 1	TO A SLIGHT EXTENT 2	TO A MODERATE EXTENT 3	TO A GREAT EXTENT 4	TO A VERY GREAT EXTENT 5
Expresses feelings about loss	1	2	3	4	5
Expresses spiritual beliefs about death	1	2	3	4	5
Verbalizes reality of loss	1	2	3	4	5
Verbalizes acceptance of loss	1	2	3	4	5
Describes the meaning of loss or death	1	2	3	4	5
Participates in planning funeral	1	2	3	4	5
Maintains current will	1	2	3	4	5
Maintains advance directives	1	2	3	4	5
Discusses unresolved conflicts	1	2	3	4	5
Reports absence of somatic distress	1	2	3	4	5
Reports decreased preoccupation with loss	1	2	3	4	5
Maintains living environment	1	2	3	4	5
Maintains grooming and hygiene	1	2	3	4	5
Reports absence of sleep disturbance	1	2	3	4	5
Reports adequate nutritional intake	1	2	3	4	5
Reports normal sexual desire	1	2	3	4	5
Identifies alternatives to verbal outbursts	1	2	3	4	5
Seeks social support	1	2	3	4	5
Shares loss with significant others	1	2	3	4	5
Reports involvement in social activities	1	2	3	4	5
Progresses through stages of grief	1	2	3	4	5
Expresses positive expectations about the future					
Other	1	2	3	4	5

Note: Grief resolution is defined as adjustment to actual or impending loss.
From Johnson, H., Maas, M., and Moorehead, S. (2000). *Nursing outcomes classification (NOC)* (2nd ed.). St. Louis: Mosby.

SUMMARY

Care for the terminally ill challenges health care providers in deep and personal ways. The hospice movement offers compassionate care for those who are dying. Hospice care focuses on patients' physical and emotional comfort and offers support for dying persons and their families. More and more hospitals are offering palliative expertise for end-of-life care, but in many hospitals, conflict continues to exist between the wishes of dying persons and their families and the medical model of treatment that focuses on the prolongation of life as opposed to the quality of life.

When working with the terminally ill, nursing goals include providing physical and emotional comfort, helping with adjustments in lifestyle and relationships, and offering spiritual support. Health care workers need to shift their thinking so as to avoid seeing a dichotomy between the

3. He is at moderate risk
4. He is at high risk because he was dependent on his mother, demonstrated ambivalence toward her, and has a limited support system

4. Which statement about palliative care could serve as a basis for the information a nurse gives to a client?

1. Palliation focuses on aggressive comfort care when cure is no longer the goal
2. Clients receiving palliative care can realistically expect discomfort at life's end
3. Palliation addresses emotional and spiritual pain more than physical pain
4. Clients receiving palliative care are relieved of the responsibility of making care decisions

5. Which nursing strategy will be disruptive to the provision of nursing care for terminally ill clients?

1. seeing a dichotomy between the living and the dying
2. understanding that there is no "right" way to die
3. learning to follow the client's lead
4. maintaining one's emotional health

NURSE, CLIENT, AND FAMILY RESOURCES

Organizations

Academy of Hospice Nurses
32478 Dunford Road
Farmington Hills, MI 48334
303-432-5482

American Academy of Hospice and Palliative Medicine
P.O. Box 14288
Gainesville, FL 32604-2288
352-377-8900
Web Site: http://www.ahp.org

American Hospice Foundation
1130 Connecticut Avenue, N.W., Suite 700
Washington, DC 20036-4101
202-223-0204

Choice in Dying, Inc.
200 Varick Street
New York, NY 10014-4810
1-800-939-WILL
Web Site: http://www.choices.org

Hospice Nurses Association, National Office
5512 Northumberland Street
Pittsburgh, PA 15217
412-687-3231

Books

For People with a Terminally Ill Family Member
Callahan, M., and Kelley, P. (1997). *Final gifts: Understanding the special awareness, needs, and communication of the dying.* New York: Poseidon.

For Survivors of Suicide
Chance, S. (1992). *Stronger than death.* New York: W. W. Norton.

For Widows
Brothers, J. (1990) *Widowhood.* New York: Ballantine Books.
Caine, L. (1988). *Being a widow.* New York: Penguin Books.

For Bereaved Parents
Rosof, B. D. (1994). *The worst loss: How families heal from the death of a child.* New York: Henry Holt.

For Children
Lionni, L. (1995). *Little blue and little yellow.* New York: Mulberry.

About Death
O'Gorman, S. (1998). Death and dying in contemporary society: An evaluation of current

attitudes and rituals associated with death and dying and their relevance to recent understandings of health and healing. *Journal of Advanced Nursing,* 27: 1127–1135.

Educational Resources About Dying

National Hospice Organization
1700 Diagonal Road
Suite 300
Alexandria, VA 22341
1-800-646-6460

Internet Sites

American Academy of Hospice and Palliative Medicine
http://www.aahpm.org

Approaching Death: Improving Care at the End of Life
http://books.nap.edu/html/approaching/ (online publication)

Webster's Death, Dying and Grief Guide
http://www.katsden.com/death/index.html

Hospice Foundation of America
http://www.hospicefoundation.org

National Institute of Aging
http://www.nih.gov/nia

REFERENCES

Azhar, M. Z., and Varma, S. L. (1995). The religious psychotherapy as management of bereavement. *Acta Psychiatrica Scandinavica,* 91(4):233.
Bateman, A. L. (1999). Understanding the process of grieving and loss: A critical social thinking perspective. *Journal of the American Psychiatric Nurses Association,* 5(5):139–147.
Bowlby, J., and Parkes, C. (1970). Separation and loss within the family. In E. J. Anthony and C. Koupernik (Eds.), *Child in his family.* New York: John Wiley.
Byock, I. (1997). *Dying well: Peace and possibilities at the end of life.* New York: Riverhead Books.
Caplan, G. (1974). *Support systems and community mental health. Lectures on concept development.* New York: Behavioral Publications.
Carr, A. L (1985). Grief, mourning, and bereavement. In H. I. Kaplan and B. J. Sadock (Eds.), *Comprehensive textbook of psychiatry* (4th ed.). Baltimore: Williams & Wilkins.
Engel, G. L. (1964). Grief and grieving. *American Journal of Nursing,* 64(9):93.
Feldstein, M. A., and Gemma, P. B. (1995). Oncology nurses and chronic compounded grief. *Cancer Nursing,* 18(3):228.
Gregory, R. J. (1994) Grief and loss among Eskimos attempting suicide in western Alaska. *American Journal of Psychiatry,* 15(12):1815.
Hegge, M., and Fischer, C. (2000). Grief response of senior and elderly widows: Practice implications. *Journal of Gerontological Nursing,* 26(2):35–43.

Hospice Fact Sheet (1999). National Hospice Organization (http://www.nho.org)

Jackson, E. N. (1967). *Understanding grief: Its routes, dynamics and treatment*. New York: Abingdon Press

Johnson, M., Maas, M., and Moorhead, S. (2000). *Nursing outcome classificaions* (2nd ed.). St. Louis: Mosby.

Kelley, P., and Callahan, M. (1992). *Final gifts*. New York: Poseidon Press.

Kübler-Ross, E. (1969). *On death and dying*. New York: Macmillan.

Lloyd-Williams, M. (1995). Bereavement referrals to a psychiatric service: An audit. *European Journal of Cancer Care*, 4(1):17.

Marks, M. J. (1976). The grieving patient and family. *American Journal of Nursing*, 76:1488.

Middleton, W., and Raphael, B. (1992). Bereavement. In E. S. Paykel (Ed.), *Handbook of affective disorders* (2nd ed.) (pp 619–634). New York: Guilford Press.

Parkes, C. M. (1970). The first year of bereavement: a longitudinal study in the reaction of London widows to the death of their husbands. *Psychiatry* 33(4):444–467.

Parkes, C. M. (1975). *Bereavement: studies of grief in adult life*. Hammonds world, UK: Penguin.

Prichard, E. R., et al. (1979). *Home care: Living with dying*. N.Y.: Columbia University Press.

Prigerson, H. G., et al. (1995). Complicated grief and bereavement-related depressions as distinct disorders: Preliminary empirical validation in elderly bereaved spouses. *American Journal of Psychiatry*, 152:22–30.

Robinson, D. (1997). *Good intentions: The nine unconscious mistakes of nice people*. New York: Warner Books.

Saunders, J. M., and Valente, S. M. (1995). Nurses' grief. *Cancer Nursing*, 17(4):318.

Shneidman, Edwin. (1980). *Voices of death: Letters, diaries and other personal documents from people facing death that provide comforting guidance for each of us*. New York: Harper & Row.

Shearer, R., and Davidhizar, R. (1994). It can never be the way it was. *Home Health Care Nurse*, 12(4):60–65.

Stolberg, S. G. (1999). A conversation with Dame Cicely Saunders: Reflecting on a life of treating the dying. *The New York Times*. May 11, 1999, Tuesday; Health and Fitness Section.

Tschudin, V. (1997). *Counseling for loss and bereavement*. London: Bailliere Tindall.

Wijnberg, M., and Schwartz, M. C. (1977). Competence or crisis: The social work role in maintaining family competency during the dying period. In E. Prichard (Ed.), *Social work with the dying patient and the family* (pp 97–112). New York: Columbia University Press.

Worden, W. (1991). *Grief counseling and grief therapy* (2nd ed.). New York: Springer.

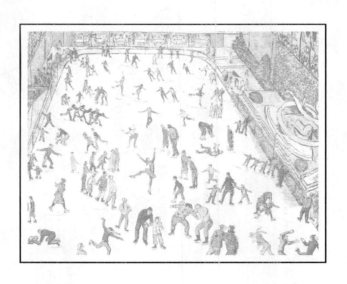

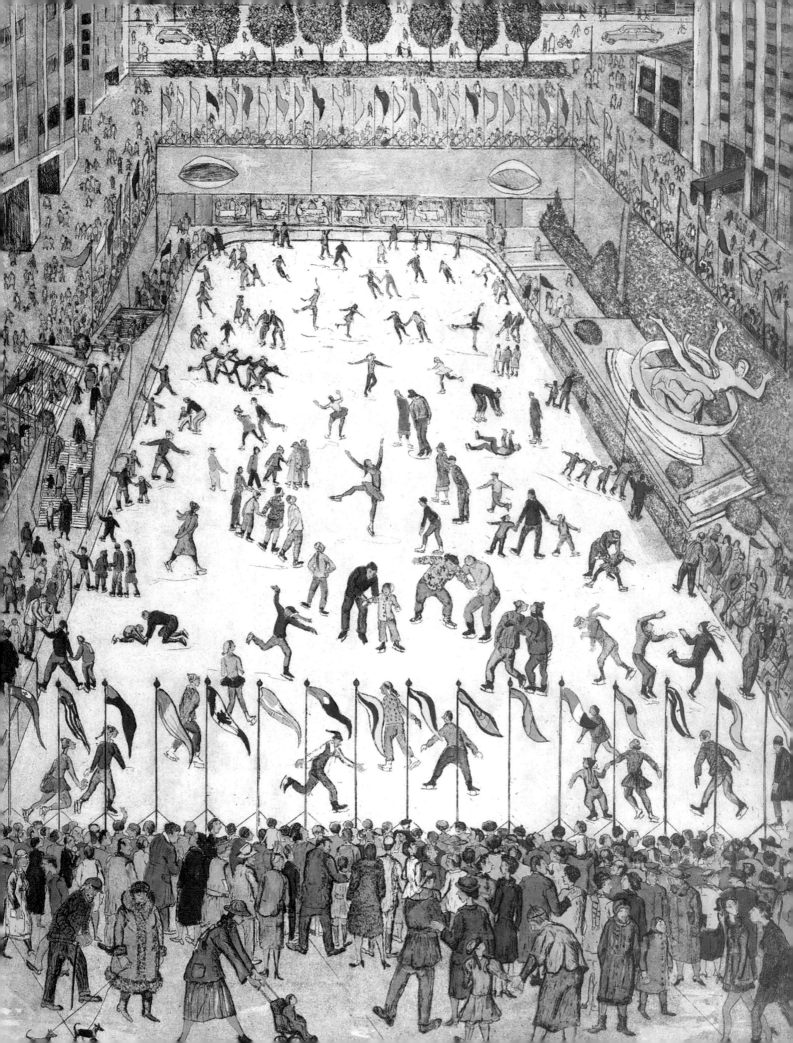

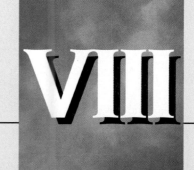

Lifespan Issues and Interventions

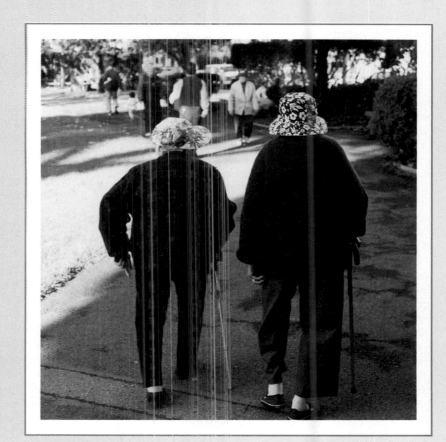

Those who love deeply never grow old; they may die of old age, but they die young.

PINERO

MaryAnn Feldstein

My own career has taken many twists and turns and I have enjoyed adapting to new challenges. After graduating from college I was a medical-surgical nurse working on surgical units and in an intensive care unit where I became interested in how clients and families managed the stress of serious illness. I entered graduate school to study psychiatric mental health nursing so that I could return to an acute care hospital setting and help clients, their families, and the nursing staff deal with the stress of a serious illness. However, graduate school courses and clinical placements piqued my curiosity in doing psychotherapy so I sought and found a position as a psychotherapist for children and adolescents at a community mental health center. Working with children made me realize that you had to work with their families, and I went on for postgraduate training in family therapy first at the Ackerman Institute for Family Therapy in New York and later at the Training Institute of the Philadelphia Child Guidance Clinic. Along the way I started teaching in a graduate program in Psychiatric Mental Health Nursing and eventually did get around to doing some liaison work first, as part of my academic position at Columbia University, at Babies Hospital at Columbia Presbyterian Hospital and later at Memorial Sloan Kettering Cancer Center. At some point I started a small private practice and began doctoral studies in family therapy.

Managed care has changed private practice for everyone. As professionals we have moved from being independent practitioners to becoming subcontractors for insurance surrogate companies. The mental health industry has rapidly changed to one in which our work is increasingly monitored where others have substantial input about the quantity and quality of the treatment we render. These changes mimic similar ones that managed care brought to medical health care practitioners years ago. The goal of most managed care companies is to expedite the treatment process by moving the client through treatment as quickly as possible. (Poynter, 1994)

I went from being a full-time academic with a small fee-for-service private practice to satisfy my clinical interests to a full-time private practitioner with a 40% fee-for-service and 60% managed care private practice. I am professionally happiest when I am in my office working with clients. My introduction to becoming a provider for a managed care company came at the request of a client who asked me if I would be willing to become a provider solely for her if her managed care company elected to cover me. I agreed and submitted my credentials to them for review and was accepted. The managed care company later asked me if I would be willing to accept more referrals; other managed care companies asked me to consider

becoming a provider with them and my referral base grew. I provide the same kind of therapy to clients whether they pay me my full fee or their ten dollar copay. Let me say that I have very mixed feelings regarding managed care. It does provide some therapy for clients who probably could not afford it without this benefit which is positive. It creates an inordinate amount of paperwork for the professional who must complete treatment summaries to request additional sessions every five to eight sessions depending on the managed care company. Lastly, your fee is significantly reduced in my case by more than 50%. Most importantly for the client with managed care:

1. **Privacy is compromised:** managed care companies require therapists to provide detailed information about a client's history and symptoms. Generally, the client and the therapist do not know who has access to this information or how the information may limit his/her future insurability. Anywhere from one to four pages of information are requested by the managed care company anywhere from every three to ten weeks. This information generally has to be faxed to the managed care company. It is not unusual for a managed care company to claim that it never received the faxed information. Typically a therapist is authorized anywhere from three to ten sessions before he needs to resubmit an additional treatment request. In the course of therapy papers with detailed information are submitted to the managed care company repeatedly. Neither the therapist nor the client has any control over who sees these records, how many people see them, how they are handled and how securely they are stored, and what ultimately happens to them.
2. **Choice of therapists is usually limited.** Managed care companies usually only pay for therapy with therapists on their provider panels, and a company can drop any provider whose treatment decisions are at odds with the company policy.
3. **Therapist has a contract first with the managed care company** and then with his client, meaning the therapist may not be able to advocate for a client without jeopardizing his or her listing on the provider panel.
4. **Treatment decisions are influenced by company policy** and treatment is authorized only if it conforms with company policy.
5. **Company policies are apt to encourage very brief treatment** and the use of medication in order to reduce costs and increase profits. (Connecticut Psychotherapists Guild, 1999)

A client calls his or her managed care company and is given the names of a few therapists in his or her zip code based on the presenting problem. Therapists, during the credentialing process, need to list the kinds of problems/issues they consider themselves expert in treating or in some instances are credentialed to treat.

Most of the managed care referrals that I received were in the phase of the family life cycle which family systems therapists refer to as single/unattached. Other referrals, less significant in number, included couples for marital therapy in the married with young children phase of the life cycle. One must determine an appropriate diagnosis for clients in the managed care system. Diagnosis is a reality that exists in the world of mental health care and is a necessity for reimbursement. As a family systems thinker it was hard for me to bridge the large divide that separates family systems thinking from the DSM-IV-TR criteria. To illustrate this dilemma in caring for clients dealing with what I perceived as family life span issues let me offer the reader a few clinical examples.

Aya, age 32, called requesting an appointment because of mood swings. She told me she wanted some insight into why she was having these mood swings. Aya had moved to the United States from Israel in 1992 after feeling pressure to marry. She married and with her husband moved to California. She divorced after a few years and is now living with a man she loves and hopes to marry. She is extremely dependent on him because she has no network of support here. The relationship is her only source of support. She works very long hours for a large accounting firm. She now feels pressure from her family to marry and have children.

Aya did not meet the criteria for a diagnosis of a mood disorder; instead she met the criteria for an adjustment disorder (309.24). She would benefit from some family work in the form of coaching and some help in expanding her social network. As we are nearing the completion of treatment, Aya has done a good deal of family of origin work and less on expanding her social network. Because she only meets the criteria for an adjustment disorder diagnosis, she will only be allowed 20 sessions and the managed care company has told me that they usually allow less for adjustment disorder diagnoses.

Barbara, age 25, comes referred because she is angry because her boyfriend of 8 months has moved to Arkansas to attend graduate school. She feels abandoned as she did when her Dad left when her parents divorced when she was 14 years old. Barbara's mother is an alcoholic. She has two siblings: a sister three years older and a brother four years younger. Barbara had no relationship with her father when I met her and had limited contact with her siblings. I helped her to deal with her feelings surrounding her boyfriend's move and linked them to feelings that she had toward members of her family of origin. Barbara needed to repair her relationship with her father, change her relationship with her mother and reconnect with her siblings. In treatment we addressed these relationships and she began to do this work. Diagnostically she met the criteria for one of the adjustment disorders, 309.28. Her managed care company recommended she see a psychiatrist for a medication evaluation. While I did not agree with this recommendation I needed to tell Barbara that

her managed care company wanted her to do this. She was not considered a candidate for medication and after 16 sessions I was told that they would not authorize any more sessions for an adjustment disorder diagnosis.

Sarah, a 39-year-old single woman in a high-powered media position, came to see me for a medical presenting problem according to the paper work that I received from her managed care provider. Indeed Sarah has Chronic Fatigue Syndrome with debilitating physical and psychological symptoms compromising her functioning for some seven years. She was able to go to work but do little else in her life leaving her feeling normally depressed and anxious. At the age of 39 she was dealing with the probability that she would never marry or have children. Sarah is the oldest of two siblings from an upper middle class Jewish family. Her brother is a physician and is also single. Sarah spends most of her weekends at her parents' home resting. Much of her vacation time is spent at her parents' winter home in Florida; since I have been seeing her, she has taken two vacations with her mother rather than with friends because her mother understands that she can do "very little physically."

In thinking about Sarah's situation and getting to know her a bit better, I felt that Sarah came from an overly close family where young adults had difficulty leaving home. Having a chronic illness kept Sarah close to her parents and made it difficult for her to develop the kinds of relationships necessary in adulthood. The managed care company expected that I would do short-term therapy with Sarah helping her to find ways to manage the stress of a chronic illness. While we were able to do some of this work, the family situation that organizes Sarah's response to her illness and possibly her illness too requires family systems intervention and longer term treatment than most managed care companies are willing to provide.

Sarah met the criteria for a diagnosis of Dysthymia (300.40). It was recommended that she be evaluated for medication. She was evaluated and no medication was recommended however, after 30 sessions her managed care company said she had met the limit for treatment. (Most policies have upper limits of 30 sessions per year.) Sarah asked me if I would appeal this decision which I did telling the managed care company that people with chronic illnesses can benefit from ongoing treatment and support.

Managed care has had a definite impact on psychotherapy. Initially we had hoped that managed care might work well and make therapy available to more people which it probably does. However, the available therapy is dependent on the plan and how many sessions it allows for a particular diagnosis. As a therapist, I find myself frustrated by the limitations of managed care having to terminate therapy with clients before we are ready to say goodbye.

REFERENCE

William L. Poynter. (1994). The Preferred Provider's Handbook. New York: Brunner Mazel. Connecticut Psychotherapists Guild 1998/1999 Directory.

Outline

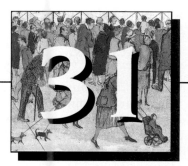

31

Disorders of Children and Adolescents

CHERRILL COLSON

Key Terms and Concepts

The key terms and concepts listed here also appear in color where they are first defined or discussed in this chapter.

adjustment disorder

attention-deficit
  hyperactivity disorder

bibliotherapy

conduct disorder

mental status assessment

oppositional defiant
  disorder

pervasive developmental
  disorder

play therapy

posttraumatic stress
  disorder

resilient child

separation anxiety disorder

social phobic

temperament

therapeutic drawing

therapeutic games

therapeutic holding

time out

Tourette's disorder

Objectives

After studying this chapter, the reader will be able to

1. Explore the various factors and influences involved with child and adolescent disorders and how they contribute to multimodal intervention strategies for these young clients.

2. Explain how the characteristics of resilience can mitigate against etiological influences.

3. Identify characteristics of mental health in children and adolescents.

4. Discuss various components that are involved in constructing a holistic assessment of a child or adolescent.

5. Explore areas concerning the assessment of suicide that may be unique to a child or adolescent.

6. Describe the clinical features and behaviors of at least three child and adolescent psychiatric disorders and identify useful intervention strategies for each.

7. Compare and contrast at least six treatment modalities for children and adolescents.

8. Formulate three nursing diagnoses stating client outcomes with corresponding interventions for at least three child and adolescent psychiatric disorders discussed in this chapter.

PREVALENCE

Of every 5 children in the United States, 1 lives in poverty and 12 million are without health insurance. Foster care rolls have jumped 35% since 1990, with 547,000 in foster care as of March 1999 (Children's Defense Fund 2000). The Methodology for Epidemiology of Mental Disorders in Children and Adolescents (MECA) study estimates that 21% of U.S. children ages 9 to 17 have diagnosable mental or addictive disorders and 11% (4 million) have a major mental illness with significant functional impairment. The most common diagnoses are anxiety disorders, followed by disruptive disorders and mood disorders (Shaffer et al. 1996).* Public recognition of the mental health problems of children and adolescents is long-standing, but the development and funding of child and adolescent services have always been slow. The federal government's recognition of these mental health problems and efforts toward effective treatments were recently identified in *Mental*

---

*Important psychiatric disorders in youth such as mood disorders, anxiety disorders, schizophrenia, and substance abuse are described elsewhere in this text. These are conditions that may be present during childhood or adolescence, but are most often diagnosed when a child reaches maturity. Anxiety and depression are introduced here, as they relate specifically to the child and adolescent.

Health: A Report of the Surgeon General (NIMH 1999). Refer to Table 31–1 for the prevalence of common child and adolescent mental health disorders.

COMORBIDITY

Emotionally disturbed children often meet the criteria for more than one diagnostic category. For example, two thirds of children and adolescents with major depression also have associated disorders such as dysthymia, anxiety disorders, conduct disorders, and substance abuse (Anderson and McGee 1994). Between 40% and 70% of children with attention-deficit hyperactivity disorder (ADHD) have a coexisting diagnosis of conduct disorder (Popper and West 1999). ADHD is also a prominent comorbid feature, occurring in 90% of individuals with juvenile-onset bipolar disorder, along with 90% oppositional defiant disorder and 50% conduct disorder (Inder 2000). Childhood depression is associated with a high incidence of comorbidity, with 20%–80% of children having conduct or oppositional disorders, 30%–75% having anxiety disorders, and 5%–60% displaying symptoms of ADHD (Inder 2000). Multiple services are needed for dual or coexisting diagnoses, such as when depression and suicidal

TABLE 31–1   *Prevalence Rates of Some Child and Adolescent Disorders*

DISORDER	PREVALENCE	MALE:FEMALE RATIO
Autism	3–5 per 10,000	3:1–4:1
Asperger's disorder	0.5–10 per 10,000	3:1–4:1
Rett's disorder	0.5–1.5 per 10,000	All female
Attention-deficit hyperactivity disorder	3%–7% School-age children 2%–20% Grade school children	5:1
Conduct disorder	3%–5% Lifetime prevalence 9% Males, 2% females in children younger than 18 years old	3:1–5:1

Depressive disorders	*Major depression (MM)*
	   Children 0.4%–2.5%
	   Adolescents 0.4%–8.3%
	*Dysthymic depression**
	   Children 0.6%–1.7%
	   Adolescents 1.6%–8.0%
		Children 1:1
		Adolescents 2:1

Anxiety disorders	*Separation anxiety* School age 3%–4% Adolescents 1% *Posttraumatic stress disorder* General population 0.1%–1.3% Children who have suffered sexual abuse 32%–53%	1:1–2:1
Tourette's disorder	5–30 per 10,000	

*Depression persists into adulthood with recurrence rates estimated to be 60%–70%.

ideation coexist with substance abuse, conduct disorders, or ADHD.

Mental illness can become severe and persistent without effective early intervention. Between 20% and 50% of depressed children and adolescents have a family history of depression (Kovacs et al. 1997). A child raised by a depressed parent has an increased risk of developing anxiety disorder, conduct disorder, and alcohol dependence (Weissman et al. 1997). The depressed parent's inability to model effective coping strategies leads to learned helplessness, which leaves the child anxious or apathetic and unable to learn how to master the environment. Another result may be the child's inability to make an emotional attachment when the depressed parent is emotionally unavailable. A child with a conduct disorder may go on to develop an antisocial personality and end up in the criminal justice system.

Abused and neglected children are at great risk for developing emotional, intellectual, and social handicaps as a result of their traumatic experiences (*Mental Health: A Report of the Surgeon General 2000*). Abused children are also at risk for identifying with the aggressor and becoming the neighborhood bully, becoming an abuser in adulthood, or developing dysfunctional behavior patterns in close interpersonal relationships. See Chapter 26 for information about child abuse.

THE CHILD AND ADOLESCENT PSYCHIATRIC NURSE

The first roles the child psychiatric nurse generalist assumed were parental surrogate, socializing agent, teacher, counselor, manager of a therapeutic milieu, and member of a multidisciplinary team (Christ et al. 1965; Middleton and Pothier 1970). More recently, the combined child and adult *Scope and Standards of Psychiatric-Mental Health Nursing Practice* of the American Nurses' Association (ANA 2000) identified the basic-level functions. (See inside front cover.)

Inpatient child and adolescent psychiatric nursing has changed dramatically. There was a substantial increase in the number of children and adolescents treated in inpatient facilities during the 1980s owing to the availability of third-party reimbursement, an increase in the number of psychiatric beds, competition among providers, few treatment alternatives to hospitalization, and the increasing social problems of drugs and violence (Carbray and Rogers Pitula 1991). Now, in response to managed care directives and budget cuts, inpatient psychiatric care has been modified to brief treatment. This change means that the child psychiatric nurse must work with more

acutely ill clients in a shorter time, which makes it more difficult to achieve a therapeutic alliance and to bring about lasting behavioral changes (Delaney 1992).

In addition to there being more acutely ill inpatients, the kinds of childhood disorders seen in the inpatient population have changed. In urban areas, most children are diagnosed with conduct disorder, and fewer than one third come from an intact family (Jemerin and Phillims 1988). These children have been referred to as functional orphans because adequate parenting has never been available. The lack of a family support system limits the nurse's ability to work with caregivers on parenting issues and to ensure that the gains made in treatment are sustained.

Today, much of psychiatric care has moved from inpatient to outpatient facilities and into the community. Mental health nurses have become an integral part of home care and hospice teams, proving their ability to work with children and adolescents in the home. Advanced practice nurses have established school-based primary prevention and treatment programs for children and adolescents (Conley et al. 1996). Therapeutic work is also being carried out in nontraditional settings such as homeless shelters (Gorzka 1999).

Meeting the mental health needs of children and adolescents is a challenge as their needs increase and funding resources and access to specialty care diminish. The scope of the nurse's responsibility for assessment and early intervention in the mental health problems of youths and their families continues to increase. This chapter describes the assessment and interventions for selected mental disorders in children and adolescents and available treatment modalities available through the nursing process.

THEORY

The causes of mental illness in children and adolescents encompass multiple factors. Distinguishing among the genetic, organic, and environmental causes of mental illness makes diagnosis difficult. Increasing numbers of children are born with, or develop, disordered brain function related to malnutrition, lead poisoning, human immunodeficiency virus (HIV), fetal alcohol syndrome (FAS), drug addiction, and traumatic experiences such as child abuse. (See Chapter 27 for issues related to substance abuse.) Younger children are far more difficult to diagnose than older children, as the boundaries between normal and abnormal behaviors are less distinct. Pediatricians and parents often have to wait to see whether some symptoms are the result of developmental lag that will eventually correct itself or something more serious. Therefore, intervention may be delayed until the child reaches school age (St. John Seed 1999). Commonly, a number of factors influence a child's or adolescent's mental health, so interventions need to be multimodal—that is, a variety of interventions may be needed to improve the child's psychological, social, physical, and spiritual well-being and improve the child's or adolescent's quality of life.

There are numerous neurobiological and psychosocial factors that put children and adolescents at risk for emotional and mental disorders. A child's vulnerability to psychopathology is the result of complex, multilayered interactions among the child's characteristics (biological, psychological, and genetic), trauma, disease, interpersonal experiences, environment, and cultural factors, all of which interact to shape the child's development (Jenson 1998). The degree of vulnerability changes over time. The resiliency of the growing child and the presence of positive environmental factors enable a child to continue learning and adapting, which in turn decreases the vulnerability to mental disorders.

Genetic Influences

Heredity factors have been implicated in a number of mental disorders, including autism, bipolar disorders, schizophrenia, and attention-deficit problems (National Institute of Mental Health 1998). For example, genetic studies of ADHD indicate an 80% inheritability factor (Inder 2000). Vulnerability to these disorders exists even when a child is not being raised by the natural parents (Barker 1995). Since not all vulnerable children develop mental disorders, it is assumed that constitutional resilience and a supportive environment play roles in keeping the disorder from developing. According to the *Diagnostic and Statistical Manual of Mental Disorders*, 4th ed., Text Revision (APA 2000), some disorders have a direct genetic link, such as the mental retardation in Tay-Sachs disease, phenylketonuria, and fragile X syndrome. These conditions may become manifest whenever the gene is passed to the child.

Biochemical Factors

Alterations in neurotransmitters play a role in causing child and adolescent disorders. Decreases in norepinephrine and serotonin levels are related to depression and suicide; elevated levels are related to mania. Abnormalities in dopamine receptors and in dopamine transporters have been implicated in ADHD (Inder 2000).

The role of elevated testosterone levels in aggressive behavior has been studied and may have a mediating effect on the ways a child responds to environmental stresses (Lewis 1994).

Temperament

Temperament, according to Thomas and Chess (1977), is the style of behavior a child habitually uses to cope with the demands and expectations of the environment. Temperament is a constitutional factor and is thought to be genetically determined. It may be modified by the parent-infant relationship, with positive or negative results. In the case of the difficult-child temperament, if the caregiver is unable to respond positively to the child, there is a risk of insecure attachment, developmental problems, and future mental disorders.

Social and Environmental Factors

External factors in the environment put stress on children and adolescents and shape their development. Rutter (1987) identified the following familial risk factors as correlating with child psychiatric disorders: (1) severe marital discord, (2) low socioeconomic status, (3) large families and overcrowding, (4) parental criminality, (5) maternal psychiatric disorders, and (6) foster care placement. The greater the number of stressors, the greater the incidence of mental disorders.

The abuse of children and stressful life events are known to relate to the increased incidence of accidental injuries, anxious children, depression, and suicidal behaviors (Kelley 1992). Traumatic life events can lead to insecure attachments, posttraumatic stress disorder (PTSD), conduct disorders, delinquency, and impaired social and cognitive function (Lovrin 1999; Smetana and Kelly 1989). Physical and sexual abuse of young children puts them at risk for developing a dissociative identity disorder as a defense against the overwhelming anxiety associated with the abuse (see Chapters 14 and 25) (Ross 1989; Spiegel and Maldonado 1999).

Cultural and Ethnic Factors

Culture shock and cultural conflicts related to assimilation issues put immigrant children at risk for a variety of problems. Siantz (1993) noted that a disproportionate number of minority children are labeled with mental and learning disorders and suffer from this stigma throughout life. Canino and Spurlock (1994) proposed that the lack of cultural role models can put minority children at risk. Cultural beliefs and values that are at odds with the majority may also put these children at risk. Ogbu (1981) noted differences among minority groups in academic and economic success. Some groups (e.g., Mormons, Amish, Jews) have successful cultural role models and are not considered to be as oppressed as other groups. Other immigrant minorities (e.g., Asian Americans) emigrated to improve their social and economic status, valuing hard work and academic achievement. The American culture has been hostile to some cultural groups (e.g., African Americans, American Indians, and to some extent Native Hawaiians, Mexican Americans, and Puerto Ricans) in their attempts to acculturate into the European-American norm. This can lead to the belief that individual effort, academic success, and acculturation will not advance one's status. The differences in cultural expectations, stresses, and support or lack of support by the dominant culture have profound effects on a child's development and the risk of mental, emotional, and academic problems.

Resiliency

Most children who grow up at risk are able to develop normally, without mental problems. They have a resilience that enables them to handle the stresses of a difficult childhood. The term **resilience** has been associated with the relationship between a child's constitutional endowment and environmental factors. Studies have shown that a resilient child has the following characteristics: (1) a temperament that can adapt to changes in the environment, (2) the ability to form nurturing relationships with other adults when a parent is not available, (3) the ability to distance himself or herself from the emotional chaos of the parent or family, (4) good social intelligence, and (5) the ability to use problem-solving skills (Anthony and Cohler 1987). Other studies have identified the cushioning effects of family stability in the face of poverty and adversity. The nurse's role is to foster these characteristics and environmental supports to keep the at-risk child from developing emotional and mental problems.

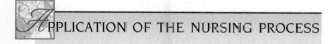

APPLICATION OF THE NURSING PROCESS

OVERALL ASSESSMENT

Mental Health vs. Mental Illness

A mentally disturbed child or adolescent is one whose progressive personality development is interfered with, or arrested by, a variety of biopsychoso-

cial factors, resulting in impairments in the capacities expected of a child of his or her age and physical and cognitive endowment. In comparison, the personality development of a mentally healthy child or adolescent progresses with only minor regressions as the individual masters developmental tasks and learns to love, work, and play with satisfaction (Box 31–1).

Assessment Data

The type of data collected to assess mental health depends on the setting, the severity of the presenting problem, and the availability of resources. The nurse is often the first health care professional to have contact with the child and should be aware of the types of data that can be collected. Box 31–2 identifies assessment data concerning the history of the present illness, the medical history, developmental history, and family history and a developmental assessment, mental status assessment, and neurological assessment. Agency policies determine which data are collected and how they are documented, but a nurse in a primary care setting makes an independent judgment about what to assess and how to do it on the basis of a child's presenting problem and the situation. In all cases, a physical examination is part of a complete work-up for serious mental problems.

Data Collection

Methods of collecting data include interviewing, screening, testing (neurological, psychological, intelligence), observing, and interacting with the child or adolescent. Histories are taken from parents, caregivers, the child (when appropriate) or adolescent, and other family members.

Structured questionnaires and behavior checklists

Box 31–1   *Characteristics of a Mentally Healthy Youth*

■ Trusts others and sees his or her world as being safe and supportive
■ Can correctly interpret reality (reality test) and make accurate perceptions of the environment
■ Has a positive, realistic self-concept and identity
■ Copes with anxiety and stress using age-appropriate behavior
■ Can learn and master developmental tasks
■ Expresses self in spontaneous and creative ways
■ Develops and maintains satisfying relationships

BOX 31–2   *Types of Assessment Data*

HISTORY OF PRESENT ILLNESS

- Chief complaint
- Development and duration of problems
- Help sought and tried
- Effect of problem on child's life at home and school
- Effect of problem on family and siblings' lives

DEVELOPMENTAL HISTORY

- Pregnancy, birth, neonatal data
- Developmental milestones
- Description of eating, sleeping, and elimination habits and routines
- Attachment behaviors
- Types of play
- Social skills and friendships
- Sexual activity

DEVELOPMENTAL ASSESSMENT

- Psychomotor
- Language
- Cognitive
- Interpersonal and social
- Academic achievement
- Behavior (response to stress, to changes in environment)
- Problem-solving and coping skills (impulse control, delay of gratification)
- Energy level and motivation

NEUROLOGICAL ASSESSMENT

- Cerebral functions
- Cerebellar functions
- Sensory functions
- Reflexes
- Cranial nerves

Functions can be observed during developmental assessment and while playing games involving a specific ability, e.g., "Simon says, touch your nose."

MEDICAL HISTORY

- Review of body systems
- Trauma, hospitalization, operations, and child's response
- Illnesses or injuries affecting central nervous system
- Medications (past and current)
- Allergies

FAMILY HISTORY

- Illnesses in related family members (e.g., seizures, mental disorders, mental retardation, hyperactivity, drug and alcohol abuse, diabetes, cancer)
- Background of family members (occupation, education, social activities, religion)
- Family relationship (separation, divorce, deaths, contact with extended family, support system)

MENTAL STATUS ASSESSMENT

- General appearance
- Activity level
- Coordination/motor function
- Affect
- Speech
- Manner of relating
- Intellectual functions
- Thought processes and content
- Characteristics of child's play

---

can be completed by parents and teachers. A genogram can be used to document family composition, history, and relationships. (See Chapter 35 for an example of a genogram.) Numerous assessment tools are available and, with training, nurses can learn to use them effectively.

The observation/interaction part of a mental health assessment begins with a semistructured interview in which the child or adolescent is asked about life at home with parents and siblings and life at school with teachers and peers. Since the interview is not structured, children are free to describe their current problems, even giving information about their own developmental history. Play activities such as games, drawings, puppets, and free play are used for younger children who cannot respond to a direct approach. An important part of the first interview is observing the interactions among the child, the caregiver, and siblings (if available). Whenever possible, the child is observed in situations involving interactions with peers.

Mental Status Assessment

Mental status assessment in children is similar to that in adults except that the developmental level is considered. The developmental and mental status assessments have many areas in common, and for this reason any observation or interaction will provide data for both assessments.

This assessment provides information about the child's mental state at the time of the examination, which identifies problems with thinking, feeling, and behaving. The mental status assessment categories are general appearance, activity level, speech, coordination/motor function, affect, manner of relating, intellectual function, thought processes and content, and characteristics of play.

Developmental Assessment

The developmental assessment provides information about the child's current maturational level which, when compared with the child's chronological age, identifies developmental lags and deficits. One popular assessment tool that provides this comparison is the Denver II Developmental Screening Test for infants and children up to 6 years of age.

Abnormal findings in the developmental and mental status assessment are often related to stress, adjustment problems, or more serious disorders. Pediatricians no longer automatically say: "It's just a stage. The child will grow out of it." Although many children will outgrow a difficulty, nurses need to evaluate which behaviors indicate stress and minor regressions and which indicate more serious psychopathology. A child's stress behaviors and minor regressions can usually be handled by working with the parents. More serious psychopathology needs to be evaluated by the clinical nurse specialist in collaboration with workers in other mental health disciplines.

Suicide Risk

The number of suicidal children and adolescents not only increases each year but also increases throughout the teenage years, making it the third leading cause of death in adolescence (Centers for Disease Control and Prevention 1999). Because the nurse is often the first health care professional to have contact with the child or adolescent, the nurse needs to know how to assess suicidal ideation and risk. Pfeffer (1986) defines suicidal behavior in children as "any self-destructive behavior that has the intent to hurt oneself seriously or to cause death." Some children do make idle threats about killing themselves. However, any child or adolescent who expresses the wish to die needs to be carefully listened to in order to determine the cause of the distress and the risk of suicide. The areas to explore when assessing suicidal risk include

■ Suicidal thoughts, threats, or attempts
■ Circumstances and motivation at the time of suicidal thoughts or behaviors
■ Concepts about suicide and death, and experiences with the same
■ Depression and other moods/feelings (anger, guilt, rejection)

■ These areas are also applicable to assessing adolescents, but additional questions are asked about acting out behaviors and about listening to music or reading books with morbid themes.

Assessing lethality in a child's or young adolescent's suicide plan is complicated by a distorted concept of death, immature ego functions, and a lack of understanding of lethality. A child might think a few aspirins will cause death and the adult knows it will not, yet the child might be highly suicidal. Another child might believe that jumping off a bridge is not fatal and make threats when in fact he or she does not want to die. Early intervention is important, and parents need to understand that suicidal behavior must be evaluated by mental health professionals.

Cultural Influences

Psychiatric professionals recognize the importance of culture in evaluating psychiatric disorders (Canino and Spurlock 1994), especially when working with families. DSM-IV-TR identifies culture-bound syndromes of mental illness that are not diagnostic categories in Western medicine. Sensitivity to cultural influences in mental illness is a necessity in order to avoid stereotyping behavior and clouding assessment. However, overidentification with children from one's own cultural background causes a loss of objectivity (Canino and Spurlock 1994).

The nurse considers the influence of culture on the child's behavior, thoughts, and emotions. The lack of eye contact when relating to adults is characteristic of respect in African, Caribbean, and Vietnamese children. The American Indian child is taught to withhold the expression of feelings, especially anger, both verbally and nonverbally. The Japanese child learns to play using polite, social manners in interactions, whereas other cultures encourage aggressive retaliation when one is bullied by another.

In assessing speech, the characteristics and the content are considered. For example, the Navajo child's speech is slow and methodical, with pauses that could lead the nurse to believe the child has finished the sentence. The African American child is expected to be verbal, following the oral tradition in which there are multiparty conversations and children are encouraged to demonstrate their wit by outperforming peers. The Hawaiian child whose speech overlaps another's speech might be considered rude. Nonstandard English dialects make speech difficult for the outsider to assess and can contribute to stereotyping. A child's bilingual ability always needs evaluation because proficiency in interpersonal communication does not guarantee academic success. Whenever possible, a child should be interviewed in his or her native language to obtain a more accurate description of their problems.

In evaluating a child's cognition, it is important to know whether expressed beliefs are in keeping with his or her culture's belief system or are bizarre and indicative of disturbed thought processes. For example, the belief in witchcraft or in communicating with the spirits of the dead might not be pathological if the child is from a Caribbean culture. Folk medicine practices are also considered when evaluating the child. Cambodian refugees, who believe that illness is caused by a bad wind, will rub their child's skin with oil and a heated coin *(kos khyal)* in order to raise red welts through which the bad wind escapes (Frye and McGill 1993). In Western culture, these red welts would be mistaken for child abuse. (See Chapter 7 for folk beliefs.)

Pervasive Developmental Disorders

Pervasive developmental disorder (PDD) is characterized by severe and pervasive impairment in reciprocal social interaction and communication skills, usually accompanied by stereotypical behavior, interests, and activities (APA 2000). Mental retardation is often evident in these disorders. The latest diagnostic refinement in DSM-IV-TR identifies the four subtypes as autistic, Asperger's, Rett's, and childhood disintegrative disorders.

AUTISTIC DISORDER

Autistic disorder is usually observed before 3 years of age, and the prognosis is related to the child's overall intellectual level and the development of social and language skills (APA 2000).

Some children show improvement as they develop, but puberty can be a turning point toward either improvement or further deterioration. Cognitive function and social skills can decline or improve independently of each other. Autism is more common in siblings than in the general population. A small percentage of autistic children go on to develop seizure disorders, schizophrenia, or both. Few are ever able to live and work independently and about one third can achieve partial independence.

Autism is viewed as a behavioral syndrome resulting from abnormal brain function. Problems with left hemisphere functions (e.g., language, logic, reasoning) are evident, whereas music and visual-spatial activities can be enhanced, such as in savant syndrome.

Autism is first noticed by the mother or caretaker when the infant fails to be interested in others or to be socially responsive through eye contact and facial expressions. The autistic infant or child seems indifferent to, or has an aversion to, affection and physical contact. Later, the child may treat adults as interchangeable objects or may cling to one person. Odd responses to sensory input may be present, such as being oversensitive to or ignoring sounds. The development of intellectual skills is uneven, and impairments are noted in both verbal and nonverbal communication.

PRESENTING SYMPTOMS FOR AUTISM. As adapted from DSM-IV-TR:

1. *Impairment in communication and imaginative activity*

   - Language delay or total absence of language
   - Immature grammatical structure, pronoun reversal, inability to name objects
   - Stereotypical or repetitive use of language (echolalia, idiosyncratic words, inappropriate high-pitched squealing or giggling, repetitive phrases, unusual babbling or clicking, singsong speech quality)
   - Lack of spontaneous make-believe play or imaginative play
   - Failure to imitate

2. *Impairment in social interactions*

   - Lack of responsiveness to and interest in others
   - Lack of eye-to-eye contact and facial responses
   - Indifference to or aversion to affection and physical contact
   - Failure to cuddle or be comforted
   - Lack of seeking or sharing enjoyment, interest, or achievement with others
   - Failure to develop cooperative play or imaginative play with peers
   - Lack of friendships

3. *Markedly restricted, stereotypical patterns of behavior, interest, and activities*

   - Rigid adherence to routines and rituals with catastrophic reactions to minor changes in them or to changes made in the environment (e.g., moving furniture)
   - Stereotypical and repetitive motor mannerisms (hand or finger flapping, clapping, rocking, dipping, swaying, spinning, dancing around and walking on toes, head banging or hand biting)

- Preoccupation with certain repetitive activities (pouring water or sand, spinning wheels on toys, twirling string) that is abnormal in intensity or focus
- Abnormalities in behavior

- Problems with coordination and gait
- Severe psychomotor retardation
- Severe problems with expressive and receptive language
- Loss of interest in social interactions

ASPERGER'S DISORDER

Asperger's disorder differs from autistic disorder in that it appears to have a later onset and there is no significant delay in cognitive and language development (APA 2000). The cause is also unknown, although there appears to be a familial pattern. As in autism, restricted and repetitive patterns of behavior and idiosyncratic interests (e.g., fascination with remembering train schedules or dates) may develop. In the movie *Rain Man*, Dustin Hoffman portrayed a young man who would fall into this classification. The distinguishing characteristics of Asperger's disorder are as follows:

- Recognized later than autistic disorder
- No significant delays in cognitive and language development
- No significant delays in self-help skills
- Severe and sustained impairment in social interactions
- Development of restricted, repetitive patterns of behavior
- Interests and activities that resemble autistic disorder
- Possible presence of delayed motor milestones, with clumsiness noted in preschool
- Social interaction problems that become more noticeable when the child enters school
- Problems with empathy and modulating social relationships that may continue into adulthood

RETT'S DISORDER

Rett's disorder differs from autistic and Asperger's disorders in that it has been observed only in females, with the onset before 4 years of age (APA 2000). The exact cause is unknown, but the disorder has been associated with electroencephalographic abnormalities, seizure disorder, and severe or profound mental retardation. The distinguishing characteristics of Rett's disorder are

- Loss of acquired hand skills and the development of stereotypical hand movements (hand wringing)

CHILDHOOD DISINTEGRATIVE DISORDER

The rare childhood disintegrative disorder occurs in both sexes but is more common in males (APA 2000). The age of onset is between 2 and 10 years, with most cases occurring between 3 and 4 years of age. The onset can be abrupt or insidious and the cause is unknown, although it is thought to be related to an insult to the central nervous system. The distinguishing characteristics of childhood disintegrative disorder are

- Marked regression in multiple areas of function after at least 2 years of normal development
- Loss of previously acquired skills in at least two of the following areas: communication, social relationships, play, adaptive behavior, bowel/bladder control, motor skills
- Deficits in communication and social interactions (same as in autistic disorder)
- Stereotypical behaviors (same as in autistic disorder)
- Loss of skills reaching a plateau, which may be followed by limited improvement

Refer to Table 31–2 for comparisons and contrasts of these disorders.

Assessment Guidelines

ASSESSMENT GUIDELINES: PERVASIVE DEVELOPMENTAL DISORDERS

1. Assess for developmental spurts or lags, uneven development, or loss of previously acquired abilities. Use baby books and diaries, photographs, films or videotapes. (First-time mothers may not be aware of developmental lags and family members may need to be consulted.)
2. Assess the quality of the relationship between the child and parents or caregivers for evidence of bonding, anxiety, tension, and difficulty of fit between the parents' and child's temperament.
3. Be aware that children with behavioral and developmental problems are at risk for abuse.

TABLE 31–2 *Characteristics and Differential Diagnosis of the Pervasive Developmental Disorders*

CHARACTERISTICS	AUTISTIC DISORDER	CHILDHOOD DISINTEGRATIVE DISORDER	RETT'S DISORDER	ASPERGER'S DISORDER
Feature	Standard autism	Delayed onset but severe autism	Midchildhood autism	High-functioning autism
Intelligence	Severe MR to normal	Severe MR	Severe MR	Mild MR to normal
Age at recognition	0–3 years	>2 years	0.5–2.5 years	Usually >2 years
Communication skills	Usually limited	Poor	Poor	Limited to fair
Social skills	Very limited	Very limited	Varies with age	Limited
Loss of skills	Usually none	Marked	Marked	Usually none
Restricted interests	Variable	Not applicable	Not applicable	Marked
Seizure disorder	Uncommon	Frequent	Uncommon	Common
Family history of similar problems	Uncommon	No	No	Common
Gender ratio	M > F	M > F	F	M > F
Course in adulthood	Stable	Declining	Declining	Stable
Outcome	Poor	Very poor	Very poor	Fair to poor

MR, mental retardation.
Adapted from Volkmar, F. R., and Cohen, D. J. (1991). Nonautistic pervasive developmental disorders. In R. Michels et al. (Eds.), *Psychiatry*. Chapter 27.2. Philadelphia: J. B. Lippincott.

Nursing Diagnosis

The child with pervasive developmental disorders has severe impairments in social interactions and communication skills. Often these are accompanied by stereotypical behavior, interests, and activities. The severity of the impairment is demonstrated by the child's lack of responsiveness to or interest in others, lack of empathy or sharing with peers, and lack of cooperative or imaginative play with peers. Therefore, **Impaired social interactions** are almost always present. Language delay or absence of language and the unusual stereotypical or repetitive use of language are other areas for nursing assessment and intervention. **Impaired verbal communication** and **Delayed growth and development** (language delay) are useful nursing diagnoses. See Table 31–3 for a list of other potential nursing diagnoses.

Other behaviors not specifically addressed by NANDA categories include the following:

- Anger
- Bizarre behaviors
- Low frustration tolerance
- Abnormal, stereotypical body movements
- Clinging and dependent behaviors
- Poor impulse control
- Ritualistic behaviors

Children with PDD are treated in therapeutic nursery schools, day treatment programs, and special education classes in public schools, as their education/treatment is mandated under the Children with Disabilities Act. Treatment plans include working with parents, who are taught how to modify the child's behavior and to foster the development of skills when the child is home. Pharmacological agents such as haloperidol and fenfluramine have been used with some success.

Intervention

NURSING GOALS FOR INTERVENTIONS

Help the child with PDD reach his or her full potential by fostering developmental competencies and coping skills:

- Increase the child's interest in reciprocal interactions
- Foster the development of social skills
- Facilitate the expression of appropriate emotional responses, including the development of trust, empathy, shame, remorse, anger, pride, independence, joy, and enthusiasm
- Foster the development of reciprocal communication, especially language skills

TABLE 31–3 *Potential Nursing Diagnoses for Disorders of Childhood and Adolescence*

SIGNS AND SYMPTOMS	NURSING DIAGNOSIS
Lack of responsiveness or interest in others	Impaired social interaction
Lack of empathy and sharing	
Lack of cooperation or imaginative play with peers	
Disruptive, hostile behaviors leading to difficulty in making or keeping friends	
Language delay or absence, stereotyped or repetitive use of language	Impaired verbal communication
	Delayed growth and development
Head banging, face slapping, hand biting	Risk for injury
Catastrophic reactions, e.g., severe temper tantrums, rage reactions	Risk for other-directed violence
Impulsiveness, anger, and aggression	Risk for self-mutilation
Thoughts or verbalizations regarding self	
Frequent disregard for bodily needs	Self-care deficit
Inability to feed, bathe, dress, or toilet self at age-appropriate level	
Conflict with authority, refusal to comply with requests	Impaired adjustment
Not following age-appropriate social norms	Ineffective coping
Blaming others for problems or for causing his or her actions	Defensive coping
Fear of being separated from parent, e.g., going to school, party	Anxiety
Refusal to attend school	Fear
	Ineffective coping
Inability to concentrate, withdrawal, difficulty in functioning, feeling down, change in vegetative symptoms	Risk for suicide
Re-experiences of past trauma (dreams, illusions, flashbacks)	Fear
Fearful of objects, people, or situations	Anxiety (identify level)

- Provide for the development of psychomotor skills in play and activities of daily living (ADLs)
- Facilitate the development of cognitive skills (attention, memory, cause and effect, reality testing, decision making, and problem solving)
- Foster the development of self-concepts (identity, self-awareness, body image, and self-esteem)
- Foster the development of self-control, including impulse control, tolerance of frustration, and delay of gratification

Nursing interventions for **Impaired verbal communication** and **Risk for self-mutilation** are described in more detail on the Simon/Varcarolis website.

Attention-Deficit Hyperactivity and Disruptive Behavior Disorders

ATTENTION-DEFICIT HYPERACTIVITY DISORDER

Children with ADHD show an inappropriate degree of inattention, impulsiveness, and hyperactivity. ADHD occurs in various cultures and is difficult to diagnose before 4 years of age.

Children with ADHD are often dually diagnosed as having **oppositional defiant disorder** or **conduct disorder**. They also have a higher incidence of disorders involving mood, anxiety, learning, and communication. ADHD is often associated with Tourette's disorder; at least 25% of males with Tourette's disorder have ADHD (Popper and West 1999).

ADHD in the preschool child manifests itself as excessive gross motor activity that is less pronounced as the child matures. The disorder is most often picked up when the child has difficulty making the adjustment to elementary school and exhibits excessive fidgeting, restlessness, talkativeness, impulsivity, and difficulty sticking to and completing tasks. The symptoms worsen in situations requiring sustained attention. The attention problems and the hyperactivity contribute to a low frustration tolerance, temper outbursts, labile moods, poor school performance, rejection by peers, and low self-esteem (Barkley 1990). Some children with ADHD exhibit enuresis. Children with ADHD are three times more likely to have nocturnal enuresis and five times more likely to have daytime enuresis than children without ADHD (Robson et al. 1997).

PRESENTING SYMPTOMS FOR ADHD. As adapted from the DSM-IV-TR:

1. Inattention

   - Has difficulty paying attention in tasks or play
   - Does not seem to listen, follow through, or finish tasks
   - Does not pay attention to details and makes careless mistakes

■ Is easily distracted, loses things, and is forgetful in daily activities (symptoms worsen in situations requiring sustained attention)

2. Hyperactivity

■ Fidgets, is unable to sit still or stay seated in school or at other times
■ Runs and climbs excessively in inappropriate situations
■ Has difficulty playing in leisure activities quietly
■ Acts as if "driven by a motor," constantly "on the go"
■ Talks excessively

3. Impulsivity

■ Blurts out answer before question has been completed
■ Has difficulty waiting for own turn
■ Interrupts, intrudes in others' conversations and games

Oppositional Defiant Disorder

Oppositional defiant disorder is a recurrent pattern of negativistic, disobedient, hostile, defiant behavior toward authority figures without serious violations of the basic rights of others (APA 2000). Such children exhibit persistent stubbornness and argumentativeness, persistent testing of limits, an unwillingness to give in or negotiate, and a refusal to accept blame for misdeeds. This behavior is evident at home but may not be elsewhere. These children and adolescents do not see themselves as defiant; instead, they feel they are responding to unreasonable demands or situations.

This disorder is usually evident before 8 years of age and is more common in males (until puberty, when the rates are equal). According to DSM-IV-TR, a child with oppositional defiant disorder displays at least four of the following characteristics, which persist for 6 or more months:

■ Often loses temper
■ Often argues with adults
■ Often actively defies or refuses to comply
■ Deliberately annoys people
■ Blames others for his or her mistakes
■ Is easily annoyed by others
■ Is often angry and resentful
■ Is often spiteful or vindictive

Conduct Disorder

Conduct disorder is characterized by a persistent pattern of behavior in which the rights of others and age-appropriate societal norms or rules are violated (APA 2000). It is the most frequently diagnosed disorder, with rates for males being 6% to 16% and for females, 2% to 9%. Predisposing factors are ADHD, oppositional child behaviors, parental rejection, inconsistent parenting with harsh discipline, early institutional living, frequent shifting of parental figures, large family size, absence of father or alcoholic father, antisocial and drug-dependent family members, and association with a delinquent group.

Childhood-onset conduct disorder occurs prior to age 10 and mainly in males who are physically aggressive, have poor peer relationships and little concern for others, and lack feelings of guilt or remorse. These children frequently misperceive the intentions of others as being hostile and believe their aggressive responses are justified. Although they try to project a tough image, they have low self-esteem, low frustration tolerance, irritability, and temper outbursts. They are more likely to have their conduct disorder persist through adolescence and develop into antisocial personality disorder.

In **adolescent-onset conduct disorder,** individuals demonstrate less aggressive behaviors and more normal peer relationships. These youths tend to act out their misconduct with their peer group (e.g., early-onset sexual behavior, smoking, drinking, substance abuse, risk-taking behaviors). Males are apt to fight, steal, vandalize, and have school discipline problems, whereas girls lie, are truant, run away, abuse substances, and engage in prostitution. The male-to-female ratio is not as high as for the childhood-onset disorder.

Complications associated with conduct disorder are academic failures related to below-average reading/verbal skills and learning disabilities, school suspensions and dropouts, juvenile delinquency, and the need for the juvenile court system to assume responsibility for youths who cannot be managed by their parents. Psychiatric disorders that frequently coexist with conduct disorder are anxiety, depression, ADHD, and learning disabilities. The outcome for children with conduct disorder is poor and they account for a large percentage of inpatient admissions and institutional placements (Harnett 1989). Studies indicate that the antisocial behaviors persist into adulthood and often result in the diagnosis of antisocial personality disorder.

Conduct disorder is identified by four types of behavior from the DSM-IV-TR: (1) aggression toward people and animals; (2) destruction of property; (3) deceitfulness or theft; (4) serious violations of rules.

1. Aggression toward people and animals

■ Often bullies, threatens, and intimidates others
■ Often initiates physical fights

- Has used a weapon that could cause serious injury
- Has been physically cruel to others and/or animals
- Has stolen while confronting a victim
- Has forced someone into sexual activity

2. Destruction of property

- Has deliberately set fires intending to cause damage
- Has deliberately destroyed another's property

3. Deceitfulness or theft

- Has broken into a house, building, or car
- Often lies to obtain goods or favors
- Has stolen items of nontrivial value (shoplifting)

4. Serious violations of rules

- Often stays out at night before age 13 despite parental prohibition
- Has run away from home at least twice, or once for a lengthy time
- Has often been truant from school before age 13

Assessment Guidelines

ASSESSMENT GUIDELINES: ATTENTION-DEFICIT HYPERACTIVITY AND DISRUPTIVE BEHAVIOR DISORDERS

1. Assess the quality of the relationship between the child and parent/caregiver for evidence of bonding, anxiety, tension, and difficulty-of-fit between the parents' and the child's temperaments, which can contribute to the development of disruptive behaviors.
2. Assess the parent/caregiver's understanding of growth and development, parenting skills, and handling of problematic behaviors, because lack of knowledge contributes to the development of these problems.
3. Assess cognitive, psychosocial, and moral development for lags or deficits, because immature developmental competencies result in disruptive behaviors.

For Attention-Deficit Hyperactivity Disorder:
1. Observe the child for level of physical activity, attention span, talkativeness, and the ability to follow directions and control impulses. Medication is often needed to ameliorate these problems.
2. Assess difficulty in making friends and performing in school. Academic failures and poor peer relationships lead to low self-esteem, depression, and further acting out.
3. Assess for problems with enuresis and encopresis.

For Oppositional Defiant Disorder:
1. Identify issues that result in power struggles—when they begin and how they are handled.

2. Assess the severity of the defiant behavior and its impact on the child's life at home, at school, and with peers.

For Conduct Disorder:
1. Assess the seriousness of the disruptive behavior, when it started, and what has been done to manage it. Hospitalization or residential placement may be necessary in addition to medication.
2. Assess the child's levels of anxiety, aggression, anger, and hostility toward others, and the ability to control destructive impulses.
3. Assess the child's moral development for the ability to understand the impact of hurtful behavior on others, to empathize with others, and to feel remorse.

Nursing Diagnosis

Children and adolescents with attention-deficit hyperactivity disorder, oppositional defiant disorder, and conduct disorder have disruptive behaviors that are impulsive, angry/aggressive, and often dangerous. There is a **Risk for other-directed violence, Risk for suicide,** and a **Risk for injury.** These children and adolescents are often in conflict with parents and authority figures, refuse to comply with requests, do not follow age-appropriate social norms **(impaired adjustment),** and have inappropriate ways of getting needs met **(Ineffective coping).** Refer to Table 31–3 for other potential nursing diagnoses.

Other behaviors not specifically addressed by NANDA categories include the following:

- Attention seeking
- Intrusive behaviors
- Disregard for social norms or rules
- Lack of remorse
- Lying
- Promiscuity
- Poor school performance
- Dangerous risk taking
- Running away
- Substance abuse
- Stealing
- Truancy

Intervention

NURSING GOALS FOR INTERVENTIONS

Help the child or adolescent with attention-deficit hyperactivity-impulsivity, oppositional, or conduct disorders to reach his or her full potential by fostering developmental competencies and coping skills.

- Protect the child/adolescent from harm and provide for biological and psychosocial needs while acting as a parental surrogate and role model.

- Increase the child/adolescent's ability to trust, and use interpersonal skills to maintain satisfying relationships with adults and peers.
- Increase the child/adolescent's ability to control impulses, tolerate frustration, and modulate the expression of affect.
- Increase the child/adolescent's ability to develop and use cognitive skills (e.g., concentrate, remember, test reality, recognize cause and effect, and solve problems).
- Foster the child/adolescent's identification with positive role models so that positive attitudes and moral values can develop that enable the youth to experience feelings of empathy, remorse, shame, and pride.
- Foster the development of a realistic self-identity and self-esteem based on achievements and the formation of realistic goals.
- Provide support, education, and guidance for parents/caregivers.

The interventions for ADHD are behavior modification and pharmacological agents for the inattention and the hyperactive/impulsive behaviors, special education programs for the academic difficulties, and psychotherapy and play therapy for the emotional problems that develop as a result of the disorder. Methylphenidate (Ritalin) is the most widely used psychostimulant because of its safety and simplicity of use (Scahill and Lynch 1994). Concerta, a newer drug for ADHD, has an extended-release formula which allows once-daily dosing and so can help keep the existence of the condition private.

Interventions for treating oppositional defiant and conduct disorder focus on correcting the child's or adolescent's faulty personality (ego and superego) development, which involves developing more mature and adaptive coping mechanisms. This process is gradual and cannot be accomplished during short-term hospitalization or brief treatment. With conduct disorder, inpatient hospitalization is often needed for crisis intervention, evaluation, and treatment planning, as well as transfer to therapeutic foster care or long-term residential treatment. Youths with oppositional defiant disorder are generally treated on an outpatient basis, with much of the focus on parenting issues using individual, group, and family therapy.

To control the **aggressive behaviors** of these disorders, a wide variety of pharmacological agents have been tried, including antipsychotics, lithium carbonate, anticonvulsants, antidepressants, and beta-adrenergic blockers. Cognitive-behavioral therapy is used to change the pattern of misconduct by fostering the development of internal controls, both cognitive and emotional. Problem solving, conflict

resolution, empathy, and social interaction skills are important components of the treatment program.

Families are involved in therapy and are given support in parenting skills designed to help them provide nurturance and set consistent limits. They are the key players in carrying out the treatment plan, using behavior modification techniques at home, monitoring the medication and its effects, collaborating with the teacher to foster academic success, and setting up a home environment that promotes the achievement of normal developmental tasks. When families are abusive, drug dependent, or highly disorganized, the child may benefit from out-of-home placement.

NURSING INTERVENTIONS FOR WORKING WITH PARENTS/CAREGIVERS

- Assess parents/caregivers' knowledge of the disorder and the related behaviors and provide needed information.
- Explore the impact of the behaviors on family life.
- Assess the family/caregivers' support system.
- Discuss how to make home a safe environment.
- Discuss realistic behavioral goals and how to set them.
- Teach behavior modification techniques.
- Give parents/caregivers support as they learn to apply techniques.
- Provide educational information about medications.
- Refer parents/caregivers to a local chapter of an appropriate self-help group.
- Be a child/parent advocate with the educational system.

Nursing interventions for **Defensive coping** and **Risk for other-directed violence** are described in more detail on the Simon/Varcarolis website. Techniques for managing disruptive behaviors are listed in Box 31–3.

Anxiety Disorders

Not all anxiety is abnormal in childhood or adolescence, as a number of fears and worries are part of normal development. Anxiety becomes a problem when the child or adolescent fails to move beyond the fears associated with a certain developmental stage or when anxiety and fear interfere with normal functioning. There may be a genetic vulnerability to anxiety disorders, as they seem to run in families. Anxiety disorders can develop in response to physical or psychosocial stressors and trauma. Cognitive theorists propose that anxiety is the result of

Box 31–3 *Techniques for Managing Disruptive Behaviors*

- **Planned ignoring:** Evaluate surface behavior and intervene when the intensity is becoming too great.
- **Use of signals or gestures:** Use a word, a gesture, or eye contact to remind the child to use self-control.
- **Physical distance and touch control:** Move closer to the child for a calming effect, maybe put an arm around the child.
- **Increased involvement in the activity:** Redirect the child's attention to the activity and away from a distracting behavior by asking a question.
- **Additional affection:** Ignore the provocative content of the behavior and give the child emotional support for the current problem.
- **Use of humor:** Use well-timed kidding as a diversion to help the child save face and relieve feelings of guilt or fear.
- **Direct appeals:** Appeal to the child's developing self-control: "Please, not now."
- **Extra assistance:** Give early help to the child who "blows up" and is easily frustrated when trying to achieve a goal; do not overuse this technique.
- **Clarification as intervention:** Help the child understand the situation and his or her own motivation for the behavior.
- **Restructuring:** Change the activity in ways that will decrease the stimulation or the frustration; e.g., shorten a story or change to a physical activity.
- **Regrouping:** Use total or partial changes in the group's composition to reduce conflict and contagious behaviors.
- **Strategic removal:** Remove a child who is disrupting or acting dangerously, but consider whether this gives the child too much status or makes the child a scapegoat.
- **Physical restraint:** Use therapeutic holding to control, to give comfort, and to assure children that they are protected from their own impulses to act out.
- **Setting limits and giving permission:** Use sharp, clear statements about which behavior is not allowed and give permission for the behavior that is expected.
- **Promises and rewards:** Use very carefully and very infrequently to avoid situations in which the child bargains for a reward.
- **Threats and punishment:** Use very carefully; the child needs to internalize the frustration generated by the punishment and use it to control impulses rather than externalize the frustration in further acting out.

Data from Redl, F., and Wineman, D. (1957). *The aggressive child.* New York: Free Press. Adapted with the permission of The Free Press, a division of Simon & Schuster. Copyright © 1957 by The Free Press.

---

dysfunctional efforts to make sense of life's events. The physiological, behavioral, and cognitive characteristics of anxiety in children and adolescents are basically no different from those in adults. Anxiety disorders are the most common mental disorders of childhood and adolescence, affecting 13% of youth between the ages of 9 and 17 (NIMH 1999). Chapter 14 discusses the anxiety disorders that are also evident in children and adolescents. Separation anxiety and posttraumatic stress disorder are briefly discussed here as they relate to children and adolescents.

SEPARATION ANXIETY DISORDER

Children and adolescents with separation anxiety disorder become excessively anxious when separated from or anticipating a separation from their home or parental figures (APA 2000). Separation anxiety disorder may develop after a significant stress, such as the death of a relative or pet, an illness, a move or change in schools, or even a physical or sexual assault. The onset can be any time between preschool years and age 18. The prevalence of the disorder in children is estimated to be 4%, with a higher incidence of the disorder in females. The disorder is common in first-degree biological relatives, and the incidence may be related to having a mother with panic disorder. Although the remission rates are high, the disorder can persist and lead to panic disorder with agoraphobia. A **depressed mood** often accompanies the anxiety.

The DSM-IV-TR characteristics of separation anxiety disorder are

- Excessive distress when separated from or anticipating separation from home or parental figures
- Excessive worries about being lost or kidnapped or that parental figures will be harmed
- Fear of being home alone or in situations without other significant adults
- Refusal to sleep unless near a parental figure and refusal to sleep away from home

■ Refusal to attend school or other activities without a parental figure
■ Physical symptoms as a response to anxiety

POSTTRAUMATIC STRESS DISORDER

Posttraumatic stress disorder (PTSD) can occur at any age and has now been recognized in children. Rather than reliving the traumatic event as an adult might, younger children with PTSD tend to react with behaviors indicative of internalized anxiety. In older children and adolescents the anxiety is more often externalized.

Posttraumatic Stress Behaviors

Preschool Children. Internalizing behavior is common in the posttraumatic stress behaviors of preschool children, who exhibit the following responses (Amaya-Jackson and March 1993):

■ Agitated and disorganized behavior
■ Separation anxiety
■ Sleep difficulties (including falling or staying asleep, sleeping alone)
■ Nightmares/night terrors with unknown content, or changing to dreams of monsters
■ Reliving the trauma in repetitive play of the event
■ Increase in specific fears, especially those related to the trauma stimuli (storms, noise, a specific place)
■ Irritability, whining, angry outbursts, temper tantrums
■ Regression or loss of previously learned skills
■ Somatic complaints
■ Withdrawal from activities

School-Age Children. Externalizing behaviors are common in posttraumatic stress behaviors of school-age children, who exhibit the following responses:

■ Sleep difficulties, especially nightmares of monsters, rescuing others, or being threatened
■ Irritability and increased fighting with friends and siblings
■ Difficulty concentrating, with impaired academic performance
■ Repetitive playing out of the traumatic event
■ Feeling jumpy and hypervigilant and having an increased startle response
■ Belief that their lives will be short
■ Belief that they can foresee untoward events in the future ("omen formation")
■ Somatic complaints

Assessment Guidelines

ASSESSMENT GUIDELINES: ANXIETY DISORDERS

1. Assess the quality of the child–parent/caregiver relationship for evidence of anxiety, conflicts, or difficulty-of-fit between child and parent temperaments.
2. Assess for recent stressors and their severity, duration, and proximity to the child.
3. Assess the parent/caregiver's understanding of developmental norms, parenting skills, and handling of problematic behaviors (lack of knowledge contributes to increased anxiety).
4. Assess the developmental level and whether regression has occurred.
5. Assess for physical, behavioral, and cognitive symptoms of anxiety.

Separation Anxiety Disorder
1. Assess the child's previous and current ability to separate from parent/caregiver (the separation/individuation process may not be completed or the child may have regressed).

Posttraumatic Stress Disorder
1. Assess for personal exposure to an extreme traumatic stressor and evidence of internalized or externalized anxiety symptoms.

Nursing Diagnosis

As the name indicates, the anxiety disorders have as their chief characteristic disabling anxiety. The nursing diagnoses most applicable in all these disorders are **Anxiety** and **Ineffective coping. Delayed growth and development** can be used for a child with separation anxiety.

Refer to Table 31–3 for potential nursing diagnoses.

Intervention

NURSING GOALS FOR INTERVENTIONS

Help the child/adolescent reach his or her full potential by fostering developmental competencies and coping skills.

■ Protect the child from panic levels of anxiety by acting as a parental surrogate and providing for biological and psychosocial needs.
■ Accept regression, but give emotional support to help the child progress again.
■ Increase the child's self-esteem and feelings of competence in the ability to perform, achieve, or influence the future.
■ Help the child accept and work through traumatic events or losses.

Children and adolescents with anxiety disorders are most often treated on an outpatient basis with cognitive behavioral therapies in individual, group, or family modalities. Medications such as antihistamines, antianxiolytics, and antidepressants are also used; selective serotonin reuptake inhibitors have been proved to be most effective. Cognitive therapy focuses on the underlying fears and concerns, and behavior modification is used to reinforce self-control behaviors. Children who refuse to start primary school are introduced gradually into the school environment with a parent/caregiver present for support for part of the day. When adolescents develop school phobia, the goal is to return them to the classroom at the earliest possible date and to give parents support in setting limits on truancy. For further discussion of treatment of anxiety disorders, see Chapter 15.

Specific nursing interventions for **Anxiety** are described in more detail on the Simon/Varcarolis website.

Mood Disorders

It was once believed that children did not suffer from the same type of depression that adults did and that a child's sadness in reaction to an event or situation would be short-lived. Now, with increasing suicide rates in childhood and with suicide the third leading cause of death in adolescence (CDC 1999), depression is being treated with psychotherapy and medication rather than letting it run its course. The most frequently diagnosed mood disorders are **major depressive disorder, dysthymic disorder,** and **bipolar disorder.** (See Chapter 18 for depressive disorders.) Symptoms of depression in children and adolescents may be similar to symptoms in adults, with feelings of sadness, pessimism, hopelessness, and anhedonia and social withdrawal and thoughts of suicide. Children are more apt to have somatic complaints, be critical of themselves and others, and feel unloved. Adolescents are more apt to have psychomotor retardation and hypersomnia (APA 2000). Both children and adolescents often have irritability leading to aggressiveness. They are less likely than adults to have psychotic symptoms, and auditory hallucinations are more common than delusions. The acting out behaviors of children and adolescents, once considered symptoms of masked depression, can clearly be related to the presence of mood disorders. The signs of depression in both children and adolescents are listed in Table 31–4.

Factors associated with child and adolescent depression are physical and sexual abuse, neglect, homelessness, marital discord, death, divorce, separation of parents, separation from parents, learning disabilities, chronic illness, conflicts with family or peers, and rejection by family or peers. The complications of depression are school failure and dropping out, drug and alcohol abuse, sexual promiscuity, pregnancy, running away, illegal and antisocial behavior, and suicide.

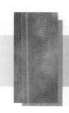

TABLE 31–4 *Signs of Depression in Children and Adolescents*

AREA OF CHANGE	BEHAVIOR
Mood/Affect	Apathy
	Anhedonia
	Anger
	Sadness or crying
	Irritability
	Guilt
	Decreased self-esteem
	Decreased spontaneity
	Monotone speech
Cognition	Apathy
	Boredom
	Decreased concentration
	Loss of interest in school
	Decreased school performance
	Decreased creativity
	Loss of interest in activities
	Preoccupation with illness
	Preoccupation with death
	Thoughts of dying
	Suicidal ideation
	Suicidal threats
Physical activity	Loss of energy
	Insomnia or hypersomnia
	Nightmares
	Appetite changes
	Weight loss or gain
	Physical complaints (aches in head, stomach, or legs)
Behavior and social function	Isolation (self-imposed or rejection by peers)
	Change in friends
	Loss of girlfriend or boyfriend
	Risk taking
	Drug or alcohol use
	Running away or truancy
	Misuse of sex
	Decrease in after-school activity and playtime
	Interest in morbid music and literature
	Suicidal gestures or attempts

Tourette's Disorder

Tourette's disorder involves motor and verbal tics that cause marked distress and significant impairment in social and occupational function (APA 2000). Tics may appear as early as 2 years of age, but the average age of onset for motor tics is 7 years. Motor tics usually involve the head but can also involve the torso or limbs, and they change in location, frequency, and severity over time. In one half of the cases the first symptom is a single tic, most often eye blinking. Other motor tics are tongue protrusion, touching, squatting, hopping, skipping, retracing steps, and twirling when walking. Vocal tics include words and sounds (barks, grunts, yelps, clicks, snorts, sniffs, coughs). Coprolalia (uttering obscenities) is present in less than 10% of cases. The disorder is usually permanent, but there can be periods of remission, and the symptoms often diminish during adolescence and sometimes disappear by early adulthood. There is a familial pattern in about 90% of cases. Vulnerability is transmitted in an autosomal-dominant pattern, with 70% of females and 99% of males who have inherited the gene developing the disorder. Nongenetic Tourette's disorder often coexists with PDD, a seizure disorder, obsessive-compulsive disorder, or ADHD (Popper and West 1999).

Symptoms associated with Tourette's disorder are obsessions, compulsions, hyperactivity, distractibility, and impulsivity. In addition, a child or adolescent with tics has low self-esteem as a result of feeling ashamed, self-conscious, and rejected by peers. The fear of having tic behavior in public situations causes the individual to limit activities severely. Central nervous system stimulants increase the severity of the tics, so children with coexisting ADHD must have their medications carefully monitored. The DSM-IV-TR characteristics for Tourette's disorder are

- Multiple motor and one or more vocal tics, which do not have to occur concurrently
- Tics occurring many times a day, nearly every day, for more than 1 year
- Tics causing marked distress or significant impairment in important areas of function (e.g., school, occupation)

Adjustment Disorder

Adjustment disorder is a residual category used for emotional responses to an identifiable stressor that do not meet the criteria for a DSM-IV-TR Axis I psychiatric disorder (APA 2000). It is a category commonly used for children and adolescents whose problems are not severe enough to require hospitalization, but who are showing decreased performance at school and temporary changes in social relationships. The disorder begins within 3 months of the stress and lasts no longer than 6 months after the stress has ceased. The subtypes are classified according to the presenting symptoms: adjustment disorder (1) with anxiety, (2) with mixed anxiety and depressed mood, (3) with disturbance of conduct, (4) with mixed disturbance of emotions and conduct, and (5) unspecified.

Feeding and Eating Disorders

Three feeding and eating disorders are pica, rumination disorder, and feeding and eating disorder of infancy or early childhood (APA 2000). Pica is the persistent eating of nonnutritive substances, although there is no aversion to eating food. Infants and toddlers may eat paint, plaster, string, or cloth. Older children may eat sand, pebbles, insects, or even animal droppings. This behavior is frequently associated with mental retardation. Rumination disorder is the repeated regurgitation and rechewing of food without apparent nausea, retching, or gastrointestinal problems. This disorder may occur with developmental delays between 3 and 12 months of age. It occurs later in mentally retarded children. In a feeding and eating disorder, the infant or child fails to eat adequate amounts of food, despite availability, and there is no medical condition or mental retardation. The individual fails to gain weight or has a significant weight loss, which then contributes to developmental delays. Chapter 17 addresses anorexia, bulimia, and compulsive eating.

Overall Interventions for Child and Adolescent Disease

The forms of treatment described in this section can be used in a variety of settings: inpatient, residential, outpatient, day treatment, and outreach programs. Many of the modalities involve the normal activities of a child's day, such as activities of daily living (ADLs), learning activities, multiple forms of play and recreational activities, and interactions with adults and peers.

FAMILY THERAPY

Children and adolescents are part of a family, and that family needs to be included in the treatment of the client. In the past, children who were treated in long-term facilities had limited contact with parents. This approach changed as family dynamics were viewed as causative factors in the child's disorder, and family therapy was developed as a treatment modality. Goren (1992) advocates involving parents in treatment decisions and in designing a plan that considers potential parental competencies and family organization. Scharer (1999) identified the process of nurse-parent relationship building on a child psychiatric unit and noted its importance in therapeutic outcomes. Thus, the family remains an integral part of the supportive and educative system for the child or adolescent. To ensure optimal treatment outcomes, it is vital to educate the family and involve family members in the treatment process.

In addition to therapy with a single family, multiple family therapy is being used (Bender 1992). This modality engages families as co-therapists for other families as they work through the problems of daily life. During the process, the families learn to (1) like and respect others, (2) accept shortcomings and capitalize on strengths, (3) develop insight and improve judgment, (4) use new information, and (5) develop lasting and satisfying relationships.

GROUP THERAPY

Group therapy for younger children takes the form of play; for grade-school children, it combines playing and talking about the activity. These groups help children learn social skills by taking turns and sharing with their peers. For adolescents, group therapy involves more talking, and focuses largely on peer relationships and specific problems (West and Evans 1992). The difficulty in using groups when working with children and adolescents lies in the contagious effect of disruptive behavior.

There is a wealth of information in the nursing literature about how to use group therapy with children and adolescents. For example, adolescent group therapy might use a popular TV show or soap opera as the basis for a group discussion. Groups have been used effectively to deal with specific issues in a child's life (e.g., bereavement and loss, physical and sexual abuse, substance abuse,

sexuality and dating, teenage pregnancy, chronic illnesses, depression, suicidal ideation). The mental health promotion and prevention activities, which nurses are now carrying out in school-based clinics, involve working with multiple groups (e.g., students, teachers, parents, community leaders). See Chapter 34.

MILIEU THERAPY

Milieu therapy remains the philosophical basis for structuring inpatient, residential, and day treatment programs. According to both the *Scope and Standards of Psychiatric and Mental Health Nursing Practice,* the ANA's combined adult and child standards of practice (2000), the nurse collaborates with other health care providers in structuring and maintaining a therapeutic environment, which facilitates the individual's growth and positive behavioral change.

1. Provide physical and psychological security
2. Promote growth and mastery of developmental tasks
3. Ameliorate psychiatric disorders

The physical milieu is designed to provide a safe, comfortable place to live, play, and learn, with areas for private time as well as group activity. There may be a gym, outdoor playground, swimming pool, garden, cooking and other recreational facilities, and even pets. No matter what physical facilities exist, the essential parts of a therapeutic milieu are the multidisciplinary team and the therapeutic activities. The daily schedule structures the activities (e.g., school, therapy sessions, group activities and outings, family or home visits). The multidisciplinary team shares a philosophy regarding how to provide physical and psychological security, promote personal growth, and work with problematic behaviors. The youth's behavior, emotions, and cognitive processes are the focus of the therapeutic interventions in the milieu. The therapeutic factors operating in the milieu's structure, activities, and interactions with staff are listed in Box 31-4.

BEHAVIOR THERAPY

Behavior modification is based on the principle that behavior that is rewarded is more likely to be repeated. Developmentally appropriate behaviors are normally rewarded with validation by a significant adult in the child's life, so modifying behavior in this manner is a standard parenting technique **(operant conditioning).** Behavior modification is easy to learn and does not require an understanding of the

BOX 31–4 *Therapeutic Factors in the Milieu*

- Holding environment, with roles, boundaries, and limits
- Reduction in stressors
- Situations for expression of feelings without fear of rejection or retaliation
- Available emotional support and comfort
- Assistance with reality testing and support for weak or missing ego functions
- Interventions in impulsive/aggressive and inappropriate behaviors
- Opportunities for learning and testing new adaptive behaviors and mastering developmental tasks
- Consistent, constructive feedback
- Reinforcement of positive behaviors and development of self-esteem
- Corrective emotional experiences
- Role models for making healthy identifications and positive attachments
- Opportunities to develop better peer relationships and be influenced by positive peer pressure
- Opportunities to be spontaneous and creative
- Experiences leading to identity formation

child's psychopathology. It is necessary only to identify the desired behavior and its reward and to apply the process systematically. To extinguish undesirable behavior, either the behavior is ignored or, if it is too disruptive, limits that have specified consequences are set.

Although there is an individualized treatment plan for each child or adolescent, most treatment settings use a behavior modification program to motivate and reward age-appropriate behaviors. One popular method is the **point and level system,** in which points are awarded for desired behaviors, and increasing levels of privileges can be earned. The point value for specific behaviors and the privileges for each level are spelled out on a large memo board. Each child's status and points acquired for the day are recorded. Older children and adolescents can be made responsible for keeping their own daily point sheet and for requesting points for their behaviors. Points are given for age-appropriate behaviors (e.g., dressing, attending school and activities on time and without disruptive behaviors, demonstrating social skills). Children who work on individual behavioral goals (e.g., seeking out staff for help in problem solving) are also rewarded with points. Points are collected and used to obtain a specific reward such as visiting the point store at the

end of the week to pick out a toy, or moving from one privilege level to the next.

The level system defines privileges, with the lowest level confining the child to the unit for all activities. Each level has increasing privileges (e.g., going off the unit with a staff member, later bedtime on weekends). At the highest level, the privilege might be to go off the unit unescorted.

Modifying Disruptive Behavior

Managing and modifying disruptive behaviors in group activities and in the therapeutic milieu are a real challenge for the nurse. If the disruptive behavior is not interrupted early, the contagion effect will derail the group activity and cause chaos. Intervention techniques for working with disruptive behaviors are rarely described in the nursing literature. Delaney (1992) advocates taking a proactive approach by increasing the structure of a group activity, using all available resources (e.g., increasing staff presence), and anticipating the contagious effects by means of "antiseptic bouncing" of a disruptive child from the activity. Refer back to Box 31–3 for a description of a series of classic intervention techniques developed by Redl and Wineman (1957) that modify disruptive behaviors and prevent the contagion effect.

REMOVAL AND RESTRAINT

Seclusion

Controversy over the use of seclusion in dealing with children continues, there being no clear evidence that it is therapeutic (Walsh and Randell 1995). Child and adolescent units may have a seclusion room, but its use is limited because youths who are out of control can become self-destructive. Seclusion is most frequently used for noncompliant behaviors that might have been managed in other ways before the behavior escalated. The persistent use of seclusion reflects the staff's lack of confidence in their ability to handle behaviors and their adherence to traditional practices (Goren and Curtis 1996). Seclusion may bring about superficial compliance, but it has little to do with real behavioral change (Goren 1991). The child or adolescent will always perceive seclusion as punishment, and the experience of being overpowered by adults is terrifying for one who has been abused.

Quiet Room

Instead of seclusion, a unit may have an unlocked **quiet room** for a child who needs to be removed from the situation for either self-control or control by the staff (Joshi et al. 1988). Other approaches include the **feelings room**, which is carpeted and supplied with soft objects that can be punched and thrown (Samenfeld 1991), and the **freedom room**, which contains a large ball for throwing and kicking (Herrmann 1982). The child is encouraged to express freely and work through feelings of anger, frustration, and sadness in private and with staff support. When a child has difficulty being in touch with or expressing feelings, staff can provide practice sessions and act as role models.

Time Out

Time out from the group or unit activity is another method for intervening in disruptive or inappropriate behaviors. Time-out procedures are designed so that staff can be consistent in their interventions. Time out may require going to a designated room or sitting on the periphery of an activity until the child gains self-control and reviews the episode with a staff member. The child's individual behavioral goals are considered in setting limits on behavior and using time-out periods.

Therapeutic Holding

At times a child's behavior is so destructive that physical restraint is needed. Although a mechanical restraint such as a helmet for head banging may be used, therapeutic holding is a long-established practice for the control of destructive behaviors (Miller et al. 1989). This intervention requires prompt, firm, nonretaliatory protective restraint that is gently and continuously personal in order to lead to a reduction in the child's distress and to greater relaxation, a return of self-control, and trust in the staff (Langley Porter Neuropsychiatric Institute 1965). One technique, the basket hold, involves one nurse holding the child from behind by the wrists, while the child's arms are crossed over the torso. The nurse can immobilize the child's legs if necessary by sitting and crossing one or both legs over the child's legs.

Throughout the episode, the nurse talks to the child in a reassuring manner, providing comfort and keeping the child's self-esteem intact (Klotz 1982). To make each restraint situation therapeutic, the nurse reviews the event with the child after restraint is released. This review of the event and a discussion of alternative ways of coping foster learning and self-control.

COGNITIVE-BEHAVIORAL THERAPY

The goal of this therapy is to change cognitive and behavioral processes, thereby reducing the frequency of maladaptive responses and replacing them with new cognitive and behavioral competencies. This therapy is carried out in individual or group sessions. An example of its use in group work is *Teaching Kids to Cope*, a 10-session psychoeducational program for adolescents that teaches youth how to cope with problems and stress through a series of cognitive and behavioral activities (e.g., cognitive rehearsal, social skills and assertiveness training, relaxation techniques) (Puskar et al. 1997).

PLAY THERAPY

Play is the work of childhood and the way a child learns to master impulses and adapt to the environment. Play is the language of childhood and the communication medium for assessing developmental and emotional status, determining diagnosis, and instituting therapeutic interventions. Melanie Klein (1955) and Anna Freud (1965) were the first to use play as a therapeutic tool in their psychoanalysis of children in the 1920s and 1930s. Axline (1969) identified the guiding principles of play therapy, and they are still used by mental health professionals:

- Accept the child as he or she is and follow the child's lead.
- Establish a warm, friendly relationship that helps the child express feelings completely.
- Recognize the child's feelings and reflect them back, so the child can gain insight into the behavior.
- Accept the child's ability to solve personal problems.
- Set limits only to provide reality and security.

There are many forms of play therapy that can be used individually or in groups. The term *play therapy* usually refers to a one-to-one session the therapist has with a child in a playroom. Most playrooms are equipped with art supplies, clay or playdough, dolls and doll houses, hand puppets, toy telephones, building blocks, and trucks and cars. The dolls, puppets, and doll house provide the child with opportunities to act out conflicts and situations involving the family, to work through feelings, and to develop more adaptive ways of coping. The following vignette shows how play therapy can help a child cope with a significant loss.

Vignette

- *Jennie, a 6-year-old, began having nightmares and refusing to go to school after her babysitter grandmother died. Her parents did not let her attend the funeral, thinking it would upset her. Jennie became fearful and preoccupied with the events surrounding the death. In play sessions, she repeatedly used dolls to act out her grandmother's hospitalization, death, and funeral. She then pretended to bury her grandmother in a small, coffin-like box. Her parents had told Jennie that Grandma had gone to heaven. Jennie demonstrated the concept by removing "Grandma" from the box and placing her high up on a bookshelf in the playroom, looking down on the rest of the doll family.*

DRAMATIC PLAY

Psychodrama, now more commonly referred to as theater, is a treatment modality that uses dramatic techniques to act out emotional problems, examine subjective experience, develop new perspectives, and try out new behaviors. This modality may be used with groups of verbal children and adolescents. If they are psychotic, reality-based role plays are substituted for fantasies.

Dramatic play, less formal than psychodrama, is used in many settings and with one child or several children. Hand puppets and puppet shows are a favorite way to act out problems and solutions. Uninhibited children and adolescents enjoy acting roles in dramas that they have created spontaneously or scripted. The dramas can be videotaped so that the nurse can review the experience and facilitate new learning with the group. A favorite type of dramatic play for children is dress-up, and a box of clothes is all that is needed. It is normally unstructured, and the staff observe the activity and intervene only if behavior becomes destructive.

Mutual storytelling is a psychodramatic technique developed by Gardner (1971) to help young children express themselves verbally. The child is asked to make up a story; it cannot be a known fairy tale, movie, or TV show. The story must have a beginning, a middle, and an ending. At the end of the story, the child is asked to state the lesson or the moral of the story. The nurse determines the psychodynamic meaning of the story and selects one or two of its important themes. Using the same characters and a similar setting, the nurse retells the story, providing a healthier resolution. The lesson of the story is also reformulated to help the child become consciously aware of the better resolution. If the child has trouble starting a story, the nurse can assist by beginning the story with "Once upon a time in a faraway land there lived a . . . " and then pointing to the child to continue. After the child has identified the main characters, the nurse may need to keep prompting the child with comments such as "and then . . . " until the story is completed. The story can be audio- or videotaped, which increases the child's motivation to participate and allows for a review to reinforce the learning.

THERAPEUTIC GAMES

Children enjoy games, so this treatment modality is ideal for children who have difficulty talking about their feelings and problems. Playing a game with the child facilitates the development of a therapeutic alliance and provides an opportunity for conversation. The game might be as simple as checkers, but therapeutic games are more effective in eliciting children's fears and fantasies. Gardner (1979) developed a series of therapeutic games for children, one of which, Board of Objects, can be used for children 4 to 8 years of age. The game pieces are small items (people, animals, various objects) that are placed on a checker board. The players roll dice on which one side of each die is colored red. If the red side lands face up, the player selects an object. To get a reward chip, the player must say something about the object; if the player tells a story about the object, he or she gets two reward chips. The child's statement or story can be used in a therapeutic interchange (e.g., to communicate empathy or make a statement suggesting a more adaptive way to cope with a difficult situation). In the end, the player with the most chips wins (usually the child).

A board game appropriate for latency and preadolescent children is Gardner's (1986) Talking, Feeling, and Doing Game. The player throws the dice and advances his or her playing piece along a pathway of different-colored squares. Depending on the color landed upon, the player draws a talking, feeling, or doing card, which gives instructions or asks a question. A reward chip is given when the player responds appropriately. For example, a feeling card might read, "All the girls in the class were invited to a birthday party except one. How did she feel?" If this game is played with more than one child, the nurse can elicit additional responses and engage the whole group in the therapeutic interchange. The nurse may stack the deck to make sure that cards relating to the child's problems will be selected.

BIBLIOTHERAPY

Bibliotherapy involves using children's literature to help the child express feelings in a supportive environment, gain insight into feelings and behavior, and learn new ways to cope with difficult situations. While children listen to a story, they unconsciously identify with the characters and experience a catharsis of feelings. The books selected by the nurse should reflect the situations or feelings the child is experiencing. It is important to assess not only the needs of the child but also the child's readiness for the particular topic and the child's level of understanding. A children's librarian has access to a large collection of stories and knows which books are written specifically to help children deal with particular subjects. Whenever possible, the nurse consults with the family to make sure the books do not violate the family's belief systems. A choice of several books is offered, and a book is never forced upon the child.

THERAPEUTIC DRAWING

Children love to draw and paint and will spontaneously express themselves in artwork. The drawings capture the thoughts, feelings, and tensions children may not be able to express verbally, are unaware of, or are denying. Children do not have to draw themselves. In drawing any human figure, children leave an imprint of the inner self, revealing personality traits, relationships with others, attitudes and values of the family and cultural group, behavioral characteristics, and perceived strengths or weaknesses (Klepsch and Logie 1982). Drawings are most reliable after children are able to create objective representations of what is seen (usually between 5 and 7 years of age). Drawings are less reliable when children have cognitive impairments. To use this modality, the nurse needs to be familiar with the drawing capabilities expected of children at particular developmental levels.

Therapeutic drawing may be used in play therapy with individuals or groups. The use of this modality involves observing children while they draw, asking questions about the pictures, and looking for messages in what has been drawn. Often children draw or are asked to draw human figures. The following characteristics of human figures are general indicators of children's emotions and are not necessarily indicative of psychopathology (Klepsch and Logie 1982):

- Size of figures very large (aggression, poor impulse control); very small (shyness, insecurity)
- Emphasis on and exaggeration of body parts: large heads (desire to be smarter), large mouths (speech problems), large arms (desire for strength and power)
- Omissions of body parts: hands (trauma, insecurity), arms (inadequacy), legs (lack of support), feet (insecure, helpless), mouth (difficulty relating to others)

- Facial expressions: mood and affect
- Integration of body parts: scattered or disorganized parts indicate cognitive or psychological problems or both

Drawing can be used in working with children and families. In the following vignette, the art therapist and the nurse used a family art session to identify family dynamics and begin interventions.

Vignette

- *Melvin, a highly intelligent 15-year-old with obsessive-compulsive behaviors and severe insecurity, lives with his parents and younger sister. In the art session, all family members are given paper on an easel and asked to draw themselves and the other members of the family. Melvin draws his parents and sister as being the same size and standing together shoulder to shoulder. He draws himself as a tiny figure in a box that appears to be suspended in space. When questioned, he reports feeling as though he were trapped in a falling elevator and disconnected from the family.*

  The family is surprised that he feels isolated (he was a normal size in their drawings). After completing a series of drawings and discussing them, the family is asked to draw a joint picture that requires them to work together. The picture they draw shows a smiling family standing by a house near a tree and a fence. The picture clearly demonstrates how the family does view Melvin as separate and different, for although he is standing beside the family, he is placed behind the fence. This observation is discussed, and as an intervention, the family is given the task of finding ways to make Melvin feel included.

PSYCHOPHARMACOLOGY

Rarely, if ever, is medication alone the treatment of choice. However, there are many indications for the use of medications. Medications that target specific symptoms can make a decided difference in a family's ability to cope and in their quality of life, and they can enhance the child's or adolescent's optimal potential for growth. Table 31-5 identifies some child and adolescent disorders and the medications used in the treatment of such disorders.

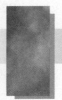

DISORDER OR SYMPTOM	TYPE OF DRUG	EXAMPLES AND COMMENTS
Pervasive developmental disorders	Antipsychotics, SSRIs	
Autistic disorder	Antipsychotics	Haloperidol (Haldol) can reduce irritability and labile affect
	Propranolol	Inderal reduces rage outbursts, aggression, and severe anxiety
	SSRIs	Clomipramine (Anafranil) may help treat anger and compulsive behavior
Attention-deficit hyperactivity disorder	Stimulants	Methylphenidate (Ritalin)
		Mixture of salts and L-amphetamine (Adderall)
		Methamphetamine
	Antidepressants	Nortriptyline (Aventyl)
		Bupropion (Wellbutrin)
		Fluoxetine (Prozac)
	Alpha-adrenergic agonists	Clonidine (Catapres) can be used for aggressiveness, impulsivity, and hyperactivity in ADHD clients
Conduct disorders	Antipsychotics	
	Stimulants	
	Antidepressants	
	Mood stabilizers	Carbamazepine (Tegretol)
	Alpha-adrenergic agonists	Clonidine (Catapres) may help with impulsive and disordered behaviors
Anxiety disorders		
Panic and school phobia	Antidepressants	
	MAOIs	
	SSRIs	
	TCAs	Imipramine (Tofranil) is commonly used
	Benzodiazepines	Alprazolam use is short-term
OCD	Antidepressants	
	SSRIs	Clomipramine (Anafranil)
	Atypical anxiolytics	Buspirone (BuSpar) is used as adjunct treatment of refractory OCD
Separation anxiety disorder	Antidepressants	
	TCAs	Imipramine (Tofranil)
		Protriptyline (Vivactil)
	SSRIs	Fluoxetine (Prozac)
Social phobia	Antidepressants	
	TCAs	Protriptyline (Vivactil)
	Antianxiolytics	Buspirone (BuSpar)
PTSD	Atypical antipsychotics	Risperidone (Risperdal) is being used to control the flashbacks and aggression in PTSD
Anxiety symptoms		
Insomnia	Antihistamines	Diphenhydramine (Benadryl)
Depressive symptoms		
Major depression and dysthymia	SSRIs	
	TCAs	
	Atypical antidepressants	Venlafaxine, Nefazodone
Major depression with		
Sleep disorders		Trazodone
Anxiety		Nefazodone
Bipolar depression		Bupropion
Psychotic symptoms	Antipsychotics	Chlorpromazine (Thorazine)
		Haloperidol (Haldol)
		Thioridazine (Mellaril)
		Trifluoperazine (Stelazine)

MAOI, monoamine oxidase inhibitor; OCD, obsessive-compulsive disorder; PTSD, posttraumatic stress disorder; SSRI, selective serotonin reuptake inhibitor; TCA, tricyclic antidepressant.

Data from Sylvester, C., and McKenna, K. (1997). Disorders in children: Autistic disorder, psychosis, attention deficit/hyperactivity disorder, anxiety disorders, and mood disorder. In D. L. Dunner (Ed.) *Current psychiatric therapy* (2nd ed.). Philadelphia: W.B. Saunders. (pp 446–452); and Schatzberg, A. F., Cole, J. O., and DeBattista, C. (1997). *Manual of Clinical Psychopharmacology* (3rd ed.). Washington, DC: American Psychiatric Press.

SUMMARY

Between 12% and 22% of children and adolescents are estimated to have emotional problems, and only a small percentage of these youths actually receive treatment. The mentally disturbed child or adolescent is one whose progressive personality development is interfered with or arrested by a variety of factors, resulting in impairments in the capacities expected for age and physical and cognitive endowment. Risk factors known to contribute to the development of mental and emotional problems in children and adolescents include genetic, biochemical (pre- and postnatal), temperament-based, psychosocial developmental, social/environmental, and cultural factors. However, not all at-risk children develop problems. The characteristics of a resilient child have been identified as follows: an adaptable temperament, the ability to form nurturing relationships with surrogate parental figures, the ability to distance the self from emotional chaos in parents and family, and good social intelligence and problem-solving skills.

The most commonly diagnosed child psychiatric disorders are ADHD, adjustment reactions, conduct and oppositional disorders, separation anxiety disorder, and mood disorder (depression). The PDDs are rarer.

Treatment of childhood and adolescent disorders requires a multimodal approach in almost all instances. Close work with schools, the availability of remediation services, and the incorporation of behavior modification techniques should be part of the intervention. Cognitive-behavioral therapies, social skills groups, family therapy, parent training in behavioral techniques, and individual therapy focused on esteem issues are therapies that have been found useful. Skills training may focus on a variety of areas, depending on the child's or adolescent's presenting symptoms. For example, some children need to learn basic ADLs; others have difficulty with impulse control and frustration tolerance, and those with anxiety disorders may benefit from anxiety reduction skills. Many children and adolescents benefit from training in a variety of social skills (problem solving, decision making, initiating and maintaining contacts with peers) that will help them to negotiate satisfying and productive relationships and friendships in the outside world. Many young people suffer from severe symptoms of depression, and although medication may be immediately useful, family and individual therapies should be made a pivotal part of the youngster's treatment.

Child and adolescent psychiatric nurses are increasingly becoming aware of the need to educate the family and involve the members in the treatment process. The family remains an integral part of the supportive and educative system for the child and adolescent.

Visit the **Evolve** website at
http://evolve.elsevier.com/Varcarolis
for a post-test on the content in this chapter.

Visit the **Evolve** website at
http://evolve.elsevier.com/Varcarolis
for additional self-study exercises.

Critical Thinking and Chapter Review

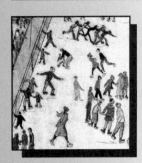

Critical Thinking

1. T. S. is 4 years old and he has been diagnosed with a pervasive developmental disorder (PPD)—autism.

   a. Describe the specific behavioral data you would find on assessment in terms of (1) communication, (2) social interactions, (3) behaviors and activities.
   b. Name at least six realistic goals that should be set for a child with PPD.
   c. Which interventions do you think are the most important for a child with PPD? Identify at least six.
   d. What kinds of support should the family receive?

2. N. T. is a 7-year-old girl who has been diagnosed with attention-deficit hyperactivity disorder (ADHD).

   a. N. is in the second grade. What clinical behaviors might she be exhibiting at home and in the classroom? Give behavioral examples for her (1) inattention, (2) hyperactivity, and (3) impulsivity.
   b. Identify at least six intervention strategies one might use for N. What medications might help her?
   c. Describe the concept of time out.

3. J. F. is an 8-year-old boy who has been diagnosed with conduct disorder.

   a. Explain to one of his classmates J.'s probable behaviors in terms of (1) aggression toward others, (2) destruction of property, (3) deceitfulness, or (4) violation of rules.
   b. What are the goals of interventions for J? What is the overall prognosis for children with this disorder?
   c. What are at least seven ways you could support J.'s parents? Where could you refer this family within your own community?

Chapter Review

Choose the most appropriate answer.

1. Which of the following should not be identified by the nurse as a risk factor associated with child psychiatric disorders?

   1. Resiliency
   2. Severe marital discord
   3. Low socioeconomic status
   4. Maternal psychiatric disorder

2. The nurse working in the emergency department usually assesses adult clients. In order to assess a child's suicide potential adequately, which additional topic must be explored in the assessment?

   1. Understandings about and experiences with suicide and death
   2. The presence of ideas about hurting self seriously or causing death

3. Circumstances at the time suicidal thoughts are experienced
4. Identification of feelings such as depression, anger, guilt, rejection

3. G. L., age 5, has been diagnosed with a pervasive developmental disorder based on loss of previously acquired abilities, deficits in communication, lack of responsiveness to and interest in others, and rigid adherence to routines and rituals. An applicable nursing diagnosis would be

1. Altered mobility
2. Impaired social interaction
3. Personal identity disturbance
4. Risk for self-directed violence

4. Which topic would be of the least relevance as a focus during the assessment of a 12-year-old with suspected attention-deficit hyperactivity disorder?

1. Impact of defiant behavior on the child's life at home and school
2. The child's level of physical activity and attention span
3. The child's ability to make friends and perform in school
4. Progress with toilet training and self-care habits

5. A method of modifying the disruptive behavior of a child that will be perceived by the child as punishment is

1. Therapeutic holding
2. Planned ignoring
3. Restructuring
4. Seclusion

NURSE, CLIENT, AND FAMILY RESOURCES

Books for Parents

Barkley, R. A. (1995). *Taking charge of ADHD: The complete authoritative guide for parents.* New York: Guilford Press.

Barkley, R. A., and Benton, C. M. (1998). *Your defiant child: 8 steps to better behavior.* New York: Guilford Press.

Burt, S., and Perlis, L. (1998). *Parents as mentors.* Rocklin, CA: Prima Publishing.

Gardner, R. A. (1997). *Understanding children.* Northvale, NJ: Jason Aronson.

Greenspan, S. I., and Salmon, J. (1995). *The challenging child: Understanding, raising and enjoying five different types of children.* Reading, PA: Perseus Books.

Maurice, C., Green, G., and Luce, S. (1996). *Behavioral interventions for your children with autism: A manual for parents and professionals.* Austin, TX: PRO-ED.

Powers, M. D. (Ed.) (1993). *A parent's guide to autism.* Rockville, MD: Woodbine House.

Schaefer, C. E. (1991). *Teach your child to behave.* New York: Viking Penguin.

References for Nurses

Berg, B. (1986). The changing family game. Cognitive-behavioral interventions for children of divorce. In C. E. Schaefer and S. E. Reid (Eds.), *Game play: Therapeutic use of childhood games.* New York: John Wiley.

Cittone, R. A., and Madonna, J. M. (1997). *Play therapy with sexually abused children.* New York: Jason Aronson.

Greenspan, S. I., and Wieder, S. (1998). *The child with special needs: Encouraging intellectual and emotional growth.* Reading, PA: Perseus Books.

Kaduson, H. (1997). Play therapy for children with attention-deficit hyperactivity disorder. In H. Kaduson, D. Cangelosi, and C. E. Schaefer (Eds.), *The playing cure: Individualized play therapy for specific childhood problems.* New York: Jason Aronson.

Kaduson, H., and Schaefer, C. E. (1997). *101 favorite play therapy techniques.* New York: Jason Aronson.

King, N. J., and Ollendick, T. H. (1997). Treatment of childhood phobias. *Journal of Child Psychology and Psychiatry,* 38:389–400.

Maurice, C., Green, G., and Luce, S. (1996). *Behavioral interventions for your children with autism: A manual for parents and professionals.* Austin, TX: PRO-ED.

Shelby, J. S. (1997) Rubble, disruption, and tears: Helping young survivors of natural disaster. In H. Kaduson, D. Cangelosi, and C. E. Schaefer (Eds.), *The playing cure: Individualized play therapy for specific childhood problems.* New York: Jason Aronson.

Tait, D., and Depta, T. (1997). Play group therapy for bereaved children. In N. B. Webb (Ed.), *Helping bereaved children.* New York: Guilford Press.

Internet Sites

Autism Society of America Home Page
http://www.autism-society.org

Autism Resources
http://www.autism-resources.com

Children and Adults with Attention-Deficit Hyperactivity Disorder
http://www.chadd.org

ADD Medical Treatment Center of Santa Clara Valley
http://www.addmtc.com

Oppositional Defiant Disorder
http://www.conductdisorders.com

Children and Anxiety
Anxiety-Panic Internet Resource
http://www.algy.com/anxiety/children.html

Adolescent Depression
Internet Mental Health
http://www.mentalhealth.com/mag1/p51-dp01.html

Mood Disorders in Children and Adolescents
Mental Health Info Source
http://www.mhsource.com/advocacy/narsad/childhood.html

American Academy of Child and Adolescent Psychiatry
http://www.aacap.org

Association of Child and Adolescent Psychiatric Nurses (ACAPN)
http://www.acapn.org

REFERENCES

Amaya-Jackson, L., and March, J. (1993). Post-traumatic stress disorders in children and adolescents. *Child and Adolescent Psychiatric Clinics of North America,* 2(4):639–654.

American Nurses' Association (2000). *Scope and standards of psychiatric and mental health nursing practice.* Washington, DC: ANA.

American Psychiatric Association (2000). *Diagnostic and statistical manual of mental disorders* (4th ed.) text revised. Washington, DC: American Psychiatric Association.

Anderson, J., and McGee, R. (1994). Comorbidity of depression in children and adolescents. In W. Reynolds and H. Johnson (Eds.), *Handbook of depression in children and adolescents* (pp 5081–601). New York: Plenum.

Anthony, J. E., and Cohler, B. J. (1987). *The invulnerable child.* New York: Guilford Press.

Axline, V. (1969). *Play therapy.* New York: Ballantine Books.

Barker, P. (1995). *Basic child psychiatry* (6th ed.). Cambridge, MA: Blackwell Science.

Barkley, R. (1990). *Attention deficit hyperactivity disorder: A handbook for diagnosis and treatment.* New York: Guilford Press.

Bender, P. A. (1992). Multiple family therapy for adolescents. *Journal of Child and Adolescent Psychiatric Nursing,* 5(1):27–31.

Canino, I. A., and Spurlock, J. (1994). *Culturally diverse children and adolescents: Assessment, diagnosis, and treatment.* New York: Guilford Press.

Carbray, J. A., and Rogers Pitula, C. (1991). Trends in adolescent psychiatric hospitalization. *Journal of Child and Adolescent Psychiatric Nursing,* 4(2):68–71.

Centers for Disease Control and Prevention. (1999). *Suicide deaths and rates per 100,000.* Online, http://www.cdc.gov/ncipc/data/us9794/suic.htm

Christ, A., Critchley, D., Larson, M., and Brown, M. (1965). The role of the nurse in child psychiatry. *Nursing Outlook,* 13(1):30–32.

Cook, E., et al. (1995). Association of attention-deficit disorder and the dopamine transporter gene. *American Journal of Human Genetics,* 56:993–998.

Dalton, S. T., and Howell, C. C. (1989). Autism: Psychobiological perspectives. *Journal of Child and Adolescent Psychiatric Nursing,* 2(3): 92–96.

Delaney, K. R. (1992). Nursing in child psychiatric milieus: Part I: What nurses do. *Journal of Child and Adolescent Psychiatric Nursing,* 5(1):10–14.

Delaney, K. (1999). Time-out: An overused and misused milieu intervention. *Journal of Child and Adolescent Psychiatric Nursing,* 12(2):53–60.

Freud, A. (1965). *Normality and pathology in childhood: Assessments of development.* New York: International Universities Press.

Frye, B. A., and McGill, D. (1993). Cambodian refugee adolescents: Cultural factors and mental health nursing. *Journal of Child and Adolescent Psychiatric Nursing,* 6(4):24–31.

Gardner, R. A. (1971). *Therapeutic communication with children: The mutual story-telling technique.* New York: Jason Aronson.

Gardner, R. A. (1979). Helping children cooperate in therapy. In J. D. Noshpitz and S. I. Harrison (Eds.), *Basic handbook of child psychiatry: Therapeutic interventions* (pp 414–432). New York: Basic Books.

Gardner, R. A. (1986). The talking, feeling and doing game. In C. E. Schaefer and S. E. Reid (Eds.), *Game play: Therapeutic use of childhood games* (pp 41–72). New York: John Wiley.

Garvey, M., Giedd, J., and Swedo, S. (1998). PANDAS: The search for environmental triggers of pediatric neuropsychiatric disorders: Lessons from rheumatic fever. *Journal of Child Neurology,* 13:413–423.

Goren, S. (1991). What are the considerations for the use of seclusion and restraint with children and adolescents? (letter to the editor). *Journal of Psychosocial Nursing and Mental Health Services,* 29(2):32–33.

Goren, S. (1992). Practicing in partnership with families in the inpatient setting. *Journal of Child and Adolescent Psychiatric Nursing,* 5(3):43–46.

Goren, S., and Curtis, W. (1996). Staff members' beliefs about seclusion and restraint in child psychiatric hospitals. *Journal of Child and Adolescent Psychiatric Nursing,* 9(4):7–14.

Gorzka, P. (1999). Homeless parents: Parenting education to prevent abusive behaviors. *Journal of Child and Adolescent Psychiatric Nursing,* 12(3):101–109.

Harnett, N. E. (1989) Conduct disorder in childhood and adolescence: An update. *Journal of Child and Adolescent Psychiatric Nursing,* 2(2):74–76.

Herrmann, C. (1982). The freedom room. In J. Schulman and M. Irwin (Eds.), *Psychiatric hospitalization of children* (pp 151–159). Springfield, IL: Charles C. Thomas.

Inder, T. (2000). Advances and application of psychopharmacology in pediatrics. Paper presented at Advancing Children's Health 2000: Pediatric Academic Societies (PAS) and the American Academy of Pediatrics (AAP) yearly joint meeting. www.medscape.com/medscape/cno/2000/PAS-AAP/PAS-AAP

Jenson, P. (1998). Developmental psycho-pathology courts developmental neurobiology: Current issues and future challenges. *Seminars in Clinical Neuropsychiatry,* 3:333–337.

Jemerin, J. M., and Phillips, I. (1988). Changes in inpatient child psychiatry: Consequences and recommendations. *Journal of the American Academy of Child and Adolescent Psychiatry,* 27:397–403.

Joshi, P., Capozzoli, J., and Coyle, J. (1988). Use of a quiet room on an inpatient unit. *Journal of the American Academy of Child and Adolescent Psychiatry,* 27:642–644.

Kelley, S. J. (1992). Child maltreatment, stressful life events, and behavior problems in school-aged children in residential treatment. *Journal of Child and Adolescent Psychiatric and Mental Health Nursing,* 5(2):5–13.

Kendall, J., and Peterson, G. (1996). A school-based mental health clinic for adolescent mothers. *Journal of Child and Adolescent Psychiatric Nursing,* 9(2):7–17.

Klein, M. (1955). The psychoanalytic play technique. *American Journal of Orthopsychiatry,* 25:223–237.

Klepsch, M., and Logie, L. (1982). *Children draw and tell.* New York: Brunner/Mazel.

Klotz, N. (producer/director, film). (1982). *The anger within.* Available from NAK 1 Productions, P.O. Box 39108, Washington, DC 20016.

Kovacs, M., et al. (1997). A controlled family history study of childhood-onset depressive disorder. *Archives of General Psychiatry,* 54:613–623.

Langley Porter Neuropsychiatric Institute. (1965). *Guidelines for child psychiatric unit.* San Francisco: Langley Porter Neuropsychiatric Institute.

Lewis, D. (1994). Etiology of aggressive conduct disorder. *Child and Adolescent Psychiatric Clinics of North America,* 3:303–320.

Lovrin, M. (1999). Parental murder and suicide: Posttraumatic stress disorder in children. *Journal of Child and Adolescent Psychiatric Nursing,* 12(3):110–117.

Mental health: A report of the Surgeon General. On-line, http://www.surgeongeneral.gov/library/mentalhealth/chapter3/sec 8.html

Middleton, A., and Fothier, P. (1970). The nurse in child psychiatry: An overview. *Nursing Outlook,* 18(5):52–56.

Miller, D., Walker, M., and Friedman, D. (1989). The use of a holding technique to control the violent behavior of seriously disturbed adolescents. *Hospital and Community Psychiatry,* 40:520–524.

National Institute of Mental Health. (1998). *Genetics and mental disorders: Report of the National Institute of Mental Health's genetic workgroup* (NIH Publication No. 98-4268). Rockville, MD: National Institute of Mental Health.

National Institute of Medical Health. (1999). Mental Health: A Report by the Surgeon General. Washington, DC: NIMH www.sg.gov/library/mentalhealth/home.html.

Ogbu, J. U. (1981). Origins of human competence: A cultural ecological perspective. *Child Development,* 52:413–429.

Pfeffer, C. R. (1986). *The suicidal child.* New York: Guilford Press.

Popper, C., and West, S. A. (1999). Disorders usually first diagnosed in infancy, childhood, or adolescence. In R. E. Hales, S. C. Yudofsky, and J. A. Talbott (Eds.), *The American Psychiatric Press textbook of psychiatry,* 3rd ed. Washington, DC: APA.

Puskar, K., Lamb, J., and Tusaie-Mumford, K. (1997). Teaching kids to cope A preventive mental health nursing strategy for adolescents. *Journal of Child and Adolescent Psychiatric Nursing,* 10(3):18–28.

Raphel, S. (1999). Eye on Washington: Access to health care for America's children. *Journal of Child and Adolescent Psychiatric Nursing,* 12(2):87–88.

Redl, F., and Wineman, D. (1957). *The aggressive child.* New York: Free Press.

Robson, W. L., et al. (1997). Enuresis in children with attention deficit hyperactivity disorder. *South Medical Journal,* 90:503–505.

Ross, C. (1989). *Multiple personality disorder: Diagnosis, clinical features and treatment.* New York: John Wiley.

Rutter, M. (1987). Psychosocial resilience and protective mechanisms. *American Journal of Orthopsychiatry,* 57:316–339.

St. John Seed, M. (1999). Identification and measurement of maladaptive behaviors in preschool children: Movement toward a preventive model of care. *Journal of Child and Adolescent Psychiatric Nursing,* 12(2):62–69.

Samerfeld, L. G. (1991). The feelings room. *Journal of Child and Adolescent Psychiatric Nursing,* 4(2):80–81.

Scahill, L., and Lynch, K. (1994). Pharmacology notes: The use of methylphenidate in attention deficit/hyperactivity disorder. *Journal of Child and Adolescent Psychiatric Nursing,* 7(4):44–47.

Shaffer, D., et al. (1996). The NIMH diagnostic interview schedule for children, version 2.3 (DISC 2.3): Description, acceptability, prevalence rates and performance in the MECA study. *Journal of the American Academy of Child and Adolescent Psychiatry,* 35:865–877.

Scharer, K. (1999). Nurse-parent relationship building in child psychiatric units. *Journal of Child and Adolescent Psychiatric Nursing,* 12(4):153–167.

Siantz, M. L. (1993). The stigma of mental illness on the children of color. *Journal of Child and Adolescent Psychiatric Nursing,* 6(4):10–17.

Smetana, J., and Kelly, M. (1989). Social cognition in maltreated children. In D. Chicetti and V. Carlson (Eds.), *Child maltreatment: Theory and research on causes and consequences of child abuse and neglect* (pp 620–666). New York: Cambridge University Press.

Spiegel, D., and Maldonado, E. (1999). Hypnosis. In R. E. Hales, S. C. Yudofsky, and J. A. Talbott (Eds.), *The American Psychiatric Press textbook of psychiatry,* 3rd ed. Washington, DC: APA.

Thomas, A., and Chess, S. (1977). *Temperament and development.* New York: Brunner/Mazel.

Walsh, E., and Randell, B. P. (1995). Seclusion and restraint: What we need to know. *Journal of Child and Adolescent Psychiatric Nursing,* 8(1):28–40.

West, P., and Evans, C. L. (1992). *Psychiatric and mental health nursing with children and adolescents.* Gaithersburg, MD: Aspen.

FORENSIC NURSING AND THE INCARCERATED INDIVIDUAL

Mental Illness in Jail

The number of mentally ill people in prisons and jails has increased over the past 30 years. With few long-term psychiatric facilities, many people who were previously cared for in state hospitals are now found in jails or prisons. The increase in numbers is also related to the lack of support for the severely and persistently mentally ill within the community. About one third of these individuals are part of a cycle of homelessness, mental hospitals, and jail. The incarceration results from lack of psychiatric facilities to manage a psychiatric emergency, so the individual ends up in jail instead of the hospital. These individuals may then be placed in solitary confinement as a result of their behavior—the symptoms then worsen as a result of the sensory deprivation, excessive use of force by guards, use of restraints as punishment, and lack of adequate medical care. (Fontaine and Fletcher 1999)

Lewine, Marsh, and Towner (1998) describe a typical scenario: a male paranoid schizophrenic does not take his medication and becomes psychotic, demonstrating hostile and threatening behavior. The family members of this individual may be desperate for immediate treatment and use the emergency system of police intervention rather than seeking support within the mental health system. In this scenario, the immediate treatment is necessary because the individual is a threat to others and the primary resource would be the law enforcement community rather than those within the mental health community.

Forensic units within psychiatric units help to reduce the numbers of mentally ill locked in jail cells for vagrancy, stealing, or other behaviors that were a result of their mental illness. Treatment was available for the individuals within the psychiatric units, and they were treated like patients rather than criminals. Some states have forensic psychiatric units or hospitals that are for individuals that are found "not guilty by reason of insanity." These individuals are too dangerous to be released but too ill to be within the confines of the state or federal prison system (Carson 2000).

Prior to deinstitutionalization prison inmates could be transferred to local mental health facilities for evaluation and treatment as the need arose, e.g., a person demonstrating a danger to himself or herself or others. Today such transfers are not feasible, and prisons must provide those services within the confines of the institution. Large state and federal prisons now employ nurses and other psychiatric staff to provide services for the mentally ill prisoners. Psychiatric care for prisoners can be problematic for those inmates who are not cooperative for they do not lose their civil rights. Unless they are a danger to themselves or others, they cannot be medicated without their express consent (Frish and Frish 1998).

Forensic nursing is a nursing specialty that is rapidly expanding its scope of practice. The practice of forensic nursing originated in Canada with nurses who served as medical examiners. Forensic nursing has expanded from concerns solely with death investigation to include the living survivors and perpetrators of violent crime. Correctional/institutional nurses work in secure settings providing treatment, rehabilitation, and health promotion to clients who have been charged with or convicted of crimes. Settings include jails, state and federal prisons, and halfway houses. Some nurses have created private practices in which they identify the health needs of people in custody and arrange for their care (Townsend 2000).

Nurses working in forensic units must have a conscious understanding of this specialty and examine their reasons for selecting this type of nursing. Those who are motivated by punishment should reconsider and opt for a different specialty (Evans 2000). Nurses should enhance their counseling skills, clarify their values, reduce defensiveness, become comfortable with their own sexuality, and demonstrate self-confidence in order to effectively work with the prison population (Evans 2000).

Laws

The legal system must demonstrate the concept of fairness. Psychiatric testimony is expected to assist the courts to understand how mental illness and other physical disorders affect the individual's ability to participate fairly in the legal process, always keeping in mind that the court has the final decision (Gutheil 1999). A legal system that treats the incompetent and mentally ill like everyone else may be seen to fail the test of fairness; therefore, the legal system must convince the court that mental illness might affect the defendant's ability to participate fairly in the legal process (Gutheil 1999).

The adversarial process of a trial is problematic for mentally ill individuals who need to be alert, be oriented, and able to understand the complexities of the situation they are facing while on trial. These components are essential for the test of whether the individual is competent to stand trial. The law rests on the moral assumption that certain mental states should qualify individuals for exoneration because they do not have the understanding or knowledge of what is right and wrong or understand the consequences of their actions (Table 32–1). Individuals who are psychotic, mentally retarded, or have some other condition that prevents them from knowing right from wrong may be remanded to a treatment facility rather than jail.

Finally, there is the requirement that the prosecutor prove intent. Is the individual able to form the intent necessary to make that person legally guilty of the crime (Gutheil 1999)? The issue with all of this is that these assumptions are also affected by the trial itself (see Table 32–1). The defendant must have both rational and factual understanding of the charges and the penalties associated with them. In addition, the defendant must have the ability to cooperate with the attorney who is providing the defense. The defendant does not have to admit to the crime, but he or she does have to know the meaning of the charges and the relative seriousness of the consequences. It is also important to remember that the determination of competence concerns the time of the criminal act, because it is recognized that the person's mental state may change in response to the stressors of the trial, incarceration, or treatment.

Kravitz and Kelly (1999) explored rehospitalization rates and criminal recidivism among offenders with mental illness and found the individuals remanded to outpatient treatment programs remained impaired, but were rehospitalized rather than reincarcerated. Rehospitalization is preferable to rearrest in the forensic population. Special forensic community programs are designed to reduce or eliminate the potential for criminal recidivism by accurately identifying and treating mental illness. Mentally disordered offenders are described as individuals who are charged with, but not necessarily convicted of, a crime and who demonstrate a mental disorder that affects how they are dealt with by the criminal justice system. These individuals often demonstrate violent behavior; therefore treatment of their psychopathology must include a reduction in their aggression and hostility (Kravitz and Kelly 1999).

Needs

The number of individuals with mental illness in prison is increasing. Yurkovich and Smyer (2000) reported that of the estimated 283,800 mentally ill individuals incarcerated in the United States, only 60% received treatment. They go on to point out that an additional 547,800 mentally ill offenders have been released into the community on probation. The severely and persistently mentally ill individuals are in the prison system at rates that are significantly greater than in the general population. Their research identified the need for health maintenance behaviors in order for these individuals to survive (Table 32–2). For more detailed discussion on the need for crisis intervention and rehabilitation of persons with severe mental illness (SMI), see Chapter 28.

Health professionals within the correctional facility have a responsibility to assist severely mentally ill individuals to understand their environment, identify role behaviors, and define maintenance of wellness within the confines of the prison. Health care providers have a responsibility to educate and advocate for the mentally ill prisoner in addition to providing care. Working with the mentally ill prisoner can identify how the prisoner lost control in the outside environment and determine methods for establishing a feedback network to prevent recurrence of such behaviors (Yurkovich and Smyer 2000).

Interventions

The health care provider within the prison system has limitations; health care within this system is a

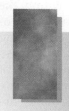

TABLE 32–1 *Description of Assumptions Made by Observers of Legal Proceedings and the Concepts Explaining the Misconceptions*

ASSUMPTION	REALITY
"He looks OK to me"	Defendants may sit quietly for many reasons during a trial. This is not an indication of innocence or guilt.
"I'm a bit of a psychologist myself"	Laypersons, though not formally trained, believe they have instinctive insight despite the evidence.
"If experts disagree, this is not valid"	Psychiatrists testify on both sides of the trial. This *mandatory* testimony may be viewed as a weakness when both sides agree on the basic point that the person is mentally ill.
"They are just trying to get him off"	Public may lose sight of the fact that psychiatrists must testify for both sides in the adversarial system; then the jury weighs the arguments.

Adapted from Gutheil, T.G. (1999) A confusion of tongues: Competence, insanity, psychiatry, and the law. *Psychiatric Services.* 50:767–773.

TABLE 32–2 *Comparison of Health Maintenance Behaviors in Incarcerated and Hospitalized Mentally Ill Individuals*

Variable	Behavior Incarcerated	Behavior Hospitalized
Relationships	Superficial	Established interpersonal
	Based on needs: protection, prolonged safety, reduction of boredom, access, or respect	Based on balance within family and friendships
Feelings	Controls through withdrawal or self-imposed solitude	Controls negative feelings and prevents anger—takes energy
	Controls fear and distrust	Attempts to balance mood
	Blocks thought about crime	
Functional behavior	Limited personal choices	Performs activities of daily living
		Participates in treatment program

Adapted from Yurkovich, E., and Smyer, T. (2000). Health maintenance behaviors of individuals with severe and persistent mental illness in a state prison. *Journal of Psychosocial Nursing*, 38(6):26–29.

privilege not a right (Yurkovich & Smyer 2000). Nurses must establish themselves as health care providers, not a part of the punishment process. Developing trust within the prison population is a powerful tool with great therapeutic promise. Health education is needed not only to control the mental illness of the prisoners but also to provide for their physical needs. It is important for these individuals to understand how poor physical health can have an impact on their mental health.

Nurses working with incarcerated individuals can also work as liaisons between the prison and community mental health systems to provide for a smoother transition from jail to the community. Continuity of care is essential to maintain the individual outside the structure of the prison system. Collaboration between mental health professionals and the prison system to meet the needs of offenders on probation encourages a close working relationship between the two systems, thus preventing misunderstanding of the goals of each system. There is an ongoing need for public safety that must be incorporated into the treatment program that is paramount in the minds of the probation officers. Mental health professionals focus on the treatment of the mental illness. Cooperation between the two agencies results in an understanding of the necessity of voluntary (or sometimes involuntary) hospitalization prior to other sanctions.

Swartz and Lurigio (1999) examined the prevalence of psychiatric disorders in male jail detainees and found there was also a need for treatment of substance abuse along with the presenting mental illness of the individual. Prisoners dependent on al-

cohol, marijuana, PCP, or other drugs are in need of an integrated program to treat their substance abuse in conjunction with their mental illness within the criminal justice system. Treatment programs that focus on dealing with addiction and not addressing the mental illness that may have led to it are less effective than ones that recognize the comorbidity of the disorders. Those individuals who are schizophrenic or bipolar or who demonstrate major depression are more difficult to treat, but these individuals have an increased risk for HIV infection and other poor outcomes if the comorbidity is not addressed (Swartz & Lurigo 1999). Currently there are only a few programs within the criminal justice system for chemically dependent prisoners with mental illnesses. Treatment programs that provide screening and intervention are in need of expansion within the forensic/mental health system.

Hartwell and Orr (1999) found that mentally ill individuals often experience extreme social isolation when returning to the community. These individuals are at great risk for returning to substance abuse which, in turn, can result in their becoming a danger not only to themselves but also to others in the community.

Roskes and Feldman (1999) identified the need for continued research in the effectiveness of community-based treatment programs. Research is needed into the effectiveness of the current jail diversion programs and to determine characteristics and service requirements of mentally ill offenders (Badger, 1999; Steadman, 1999). Further research is needed to determine the frequency that homelessness, deinstitutionalization, lack of community support, poor access to treatment, and public attitudes are factors in the incarceration of the mentally ill individual (Lamb and Weinberger 1998).

Deane and associates (1999) found that partnerships between mental health professionals and law enforcement are evolving through the development of special programs for responding to mentally ill individuals. Lamb, Weinberger, and Gross (1999) found that large numbers of severely mentally ill individuals fall under the jurisdiction of the criminal justice system. The treatment systems for these individuals differs from typical mental health programs because mentally ill offenders must comply with restrictions on their behavior and treatment that is often based first on protecting the public from harm rather than on alleviating symptoms.

SLEEP DISORDERS

Assessment

Sleep is a basic human need that appears to be a fundamental process, but for individuals who cannot sleep it becomes an extreme problem. The normal sleep cycle evolves throughout the life cycle and becomes decreased with increasing age (Vitiello 1999) (Table 32–3). Sleep disorders may result from clinical syndromes, biological factors, or environmental issues, but whatever the cause, the individual will have impaired functioning if the problems persist (Table 32–4). Sleep deprivation results in the attempt by the individual to alleviate the problem, sometimes by staying in bed longer, taking naps, or resorting to either pharmacological or herbal remedies in an effort to restore a normal sleep pattern.

Sleep disorders may range from simply annoying to persistent life-threatening problems. Those individuals with disorders such as undiagnosed sleep apnea may have problems that are potentially life

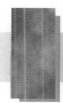

TABLE 32–4 *Specific Causes of Sleep Disorders*
Physical illness
Mental illness
Sleep apnea
Poor sleep habits
Unrealistic appraisal of sleep needs

Adapted from Vitiello, M.V. (1999). Effective treatments for age-related sleep disturbances. *Geriatrics,* 54(11):47–52.

threatening, yet they are focusing on the fact that they are not sleeping, not the underlying cause. Cardiovascular, endocrine, psychiatric, behavioral, and environmental problems all may manifest themselves with a sleep-related problem. Something as simple as a new environment with strange noises can have a significant impact on the sleep pattern of some individuals. If this is a frequent occurrence, it may then have an impact on the individual's health as she or he becomes more sleep deprived.

The DSM-IV-TR indicates that a sleep disorder—primary insomnia—must be of at least one month's duration, cause significant impairment of functioning, and may not be due to the effects of a substance, medical condition, or mental disorder. This disorder is manifested by difficulty falling asleep and intermittent wakefulness. This becomes a cyclical problem that may result in significant distress in the individual experiencing the problem. Lack of sleep may result in daytime sleepiness, irritability, and problems with attention and concentration. This disorder is typically seen in early to middle adulthood but may increase in occurrence as one ages.

When assessing an individual for a sleep disorder, a thorough history is necessary to determine daily routines, nightly rituals, diet, physical activity, stressors, and any other potential issues that might have an impact upon one's ability to go to sleep and stay asleep. The history should include information related to napping (daytime or evening), level of daily alertness (differing during day), total sleep time, impact of sleep on performing activities of daily living, total sleep time, snoring, restless, body movement or restlessness, and general emotional well-being. The history may suggest a sleep disorder, but a thorough physical and psychosocial assessment may indicate an underlying cause that should be evaluated. Underlying problems may include physical or mental illness, drug or alcohol use or abuse, sleep apnea, restless leg syndrome, or poor sleep habits (see Table 32–4). Referral to a sleep disorder center may

TABLE 32–3 *Normal Age-Related Changes in Sleep Patterns in the Elderly Individual*
Increased time in bed
Decreased total time sleeping
Reduction in REM sleep
Increased wakefulness during the night

Adapted from Vitiello, M.V. (1999). Effective treatments for age-related sleep disturbances. *Geriatrics,* 54(11):47–52.

assist with the diagnostic process (Vitiello 1999). See Table 32–3 for common sleep patterns in the elderly that may be interpreted as sleep problems.

Intervention

Traditional Pharmacologic Treatment

Over half of all patients who complain to their physicians about insomnia are treated with hypnotics. These medications are effective in treating transient insomnia, but when used over the long-term, patients run the risk of developing dependence on the drug itself. Hypnotics can worsen existing sleep disturbances when they induce drug dependency insomnia, for once the drug is discontinued, the individual then has a rebound insomnia and nightmares (Vitiello 1999).

When these individuals have undiagnosed sleep apnea, they run the risk of having an increase in the apnea. Hypnotics may cause daytime problems, which include impaired cognition, psychomotor retardation, and falling. Cautious use of hypnotics is recommended, especially in the elderly population. A sedative-hypnotic should only be prescribed for the shortest possible time at the lowest possible dose and then only intermittently.

Sleep apnea can also lead to excessive daytime sleepiness. This condition should be carefully evaluated at a sleep clinic to determine the extent of the apnea and necessary treatment. Sleep apnea is most frequently identified by the individual (or others) who complains of excessive snoring. When left untreated, sleep apnea can result in compromised cardiac function and increased mortality. This disorder is more common in men than women, and the incidence increases with age (Vitiello 1999).

Nontraditional Pharmacologic Treatment

The use of melatonin is becoming popular as a sleep therapy, especially in the older population. In studies of melatonin levels in the elderly population, the levels of melatonin have been shown to decrease as much as 50% during the night, thus the rationale for supplementation with melatonin (Ereshefsky 2000). The use of melatonin appears to be effective in assisting the elderly as well as those who work at night or have jet lag to sleep more effectively.

Careful evaluation of comorbid conditions is essential to ensure that the individual is not manifesting sleeplessness as a symptom of a much more serious condition. It is also important to educate the individual who is sleepless that poor sleep habits frequently are the underlying cause of the insomnia. Individuals who have irregular sleep-wake times, nap in the daytime or early evening, or consume caffeine or alcohol may demonstrate symptoms of insomnia that can be eradicated by reducing or eliminating the underlying cause (Neubauer 1999).

SEXUAL DISORDERS

The concept of what is normal in adult relationships and sexuality is related to values and religious beliefs, in addition to physical responses, and covers a wide spectrum of human behavior. Keeping in mind the range of normal, it is necessary when studying sexual disorders and dysfunction that abnormalities be considered those things that cause the client discomfort, pain, or interference with a healthy adult sexual response. It is necessary that a nurse be familiar with both the terms and the symptoms of sexual disorders. Without additional education, a nurse is limited in the type of therapeutic interactions that can be used to assist a client in making a significant change. It is appropriate that the basic-level nurse be able to identify alterations in normal sexuality and relationships in order to gain confidence about when to refer the client for additional assistance.

The Diagnostic and Statistical Manual of Mental Disorders, fourth edition, revised (DSM-IV-TR) (APA 2000) classifies sexual disorders in four categories: sexual dysfunction, gender identity disorders, paraphilias, and sexual disorder not otherwise specified (NOS).

Sexual Dysfunction

Sexual dysfunction includes sexual desire disorders, sexual arousal disorders, orgasmic disorders, sexual pain disorders, sexual dysfunction due to a general medical condition, and substance-related sexual dysfunction. General characteristics of a sexual dysfunction include a "disturbance in the processes that characterize the sexual response cycle or by pain associated with sexual intercourse" (APA 2000). When working with a person who has a sexual dysfunction, it is important to note that an individual's ethnic, cultural, religious, and social background play a significant role and may influence sexual desire, expectations, and attitudes about performance (APA 2000).

Orgasmic Disorders

Orgasmic disorder is a persistent or recurrent delay in, or absence of, orgasm after a normal sexual excitement phase. Orgasmic disorder in females is referred to as female orgasmic disorder and is the most commonly presented female problem. Some women are not interested in orgasm, but many are very interested in being able to enjoy sex fully.

Male orgasmic disorder entails persistent or recurrent delay in, or absence of, orgasm after a normal sexual excitement phase (DSM-IV-TR). Most commonly, it takes the form of inability to reach coital orgasm during intercourse, although manual or oral stimulation by a partner can bring the man to orgasm.

Premature ejaculation used to be the most commonly presented sexual difficulty of males, but the effective therapeutic techniques used for this problem have relegated it to second place, behind inhibited desire. There are many ways to define what is premature. Some have suggested that any ejaculation occurring before the partner is satisfied is premature. Others suggest that ejaculation occurring more than 50% of the time before the man wishes it is premature. DSM-IV-TR defines this disorder as "persistent or recurrent ejaculation with minimal sexual stimulation before, on, or shortly after penetration and before the person wishes it." The usual duration of coitus is between 4 and 7 minutes, so anything less than maintaining a 2-minute erection could be considered premature.

Sexual Pain Disorders

This disorder is found in both males and females and consists of genital pain associated with sexual intercourse. Symptoms range from mild discomfort to sharp pain and may be chronic in nature. Vaginismus is the persistent and recurrent involuntary contraction of the peritoneal muscles surrounding the outer third of the vagina when vaginal penetration with a penis, finger, tampon, or speculum is attempted. Some women may experience vaginismus in anticipation of vaginal penetration. A woman, however, may still experience desire and pleasure and be brought to orgasm if penetration is not attempted or anticipated. The disorder is found mostly in young women, especially if there is a history of sexual abuse or trauma, and in females with negative attitudes toward sex.

Biological Causes of Sexual Dysfunction

It is believed that there are biological causes of sexual dysfunction in less than 20% of presenting cases. Biological causes include general illness (e.g., influenza, colds, and fatigue) and those of more severe and persistent origin (e.g., diabetes, hepatitis, and multiple sclerosis). Hormonal disorders, in which

medications cause a decrease in androgen levels, such as hypopituitary problems and the feminizing effects of testicular tumors, may also cause sexual dysfunction. Alcohol and drug use (e.g., cocaine and heroin) decrease sexual drive. Hypertensive drugs and the phenothiazines (e.g., Prolixin, Trilafon, and Mellaril) affect sexual performance in some clients. Many of the SSRIs and other antidepressants may also cause sexual difficulties for some individuals.

Physical conditions that can cause pain during sex include arthritis, back pain, obesity, vaginal infection, and late stages of pregnancy. Age can be a factor in sexual dysfunction. Postmenopausal women may need additional vaginal lubrication, and older men may find they do not ejaculate as frequently as they did when they were younger. Also, if a partner is lost through death or divorce and the remaining partner has no sexual activity for a period of years, it may be difficult to regain sexual function. Age in itself does not cause dysfunction; many people report active and satisfactory sex lives well into their eighties and nineties.

Gender Identity Disorder

Gender, the physical fact of maleness or femaleness, is usually the first thing known about a person. Social groups prescribe different role models for males and females. Boys and girls are treated differently from birth, ranging from areas such as choice of toys and clothing to the amount of handling and cuddling each receives.

Children early in life become aware of the psychological and physiological differences between the sexes, and most are firmly committed to the societal expectations for their gender as early as 18 months of age. In rare cases in which gender was misassigned at birth owing to physical abnormality or in which accidental damage has been suffered, it is considered almost impossible to reassign a child to the opposite sex after 18 months of age. By then, the sense of gender identity, of being male or female, is too firmly ingrained to change.

For most people, the private sense they have of themselves as being male or female is congruent with their physical make-up. Most children enter adolescence aware that they are to be a man or a woman and, regardless of heterosexual or homosexual preferences, they are satisfied with their gender identity. Some people do not have this match between biological gender and psychological gender identity. These individuals have early and persistent feelings that they are trapped in a body with the wrong genitals. In reality, they believe they are and were always meant to be of the opposite sex (DSM-IV-TR).

Little is known about the origins of gender identity disorder, but childhood patterns seem to be fairly consistent. As early as 2 and 4 years of age some children may have cross-gender interests and activities. However, only a small percentage of children who display gender identity disorder characteristics will continue these characteristics into adolescence or adulthood. Typically, children who become transsexual relate better to the other sex. Boys prefer female friends and activities and cross-dress whenever possible. Girls imitate what they consider to be masculine behavior and refuse to be involved in activities usually assigned to females.

At puberty, the individual is greatly concerned and often self-conscious about the physical changes taking place; this is not true for most homosexuals or transvestites. About 75% of boys who had a childhood history of gender identity disorder report a homosexual or bisexual orientation. The remainder report a heterosexual orientation (DSM-IV-TR). The corresponding percentages for women are not known. People with gender identity disorder continue to prefer the opposite-sex behavioral style into adulthood; often, they come to desire sexual reassignment as they find partners whom they wish to live with or marry. These individuals never consider themselves to be homosexual. The biological female who falls in love with a woman believes herself actually to be a man who loves that woman. Thus, a desire for congruity in gender identity and physiology becomes important for many (Green and Blanchard 1995).

Adults with gender identity disorder seek various solutions when they suffer from gender dysphoria. Some people seek to have help in suppressing their cross-gender feelings, others want more information, and others come for surgery resulting in sex reassignment. When gender dysphoria is severe and intractable, sex reassignment may be the best solution (Green and Blanchard 1995). Hormone therapy is usually the first step (males taking estrogen and females taking androgen). Hormones help develop the bodily characteristics of the gender desired: for example, hips and breasts in the biological male, and body hair and lack of menstruation in the biological female. Most clinics in North America and Western Europe require their clients to live in the cross-gender role for 1 to 2 years before surgery (Green and Blanchard 1995). This includes going to work or attending school, to help the client determine if he or she can interact successfully with members of society in the cross-gender mode (Green and Blanchard 1995). Legal and social arrangements are made: name change on various documents, and new employment if it is necessary to leave a former job owing to discrimination. Relationship issues, such as what to tell parents, children, and former spouses need to be resolved. Only after it appears that a successful outcome is likely is the second step, surgery, performed.

Paraphilias

The essential features of paraphilias are recurrent and intense sexually arousing fantasies, sexual urges, or behaviors, generally involving inanimate objects, the suffering or humiliation of oneself or one's partner, or the use of children or other nonconsenting persons (APA 1994). Certainly history, culture, and experience play a role in what is considered paraphilia. Currently, the following are considered unusual enough to be called paraphilias: fetishism, pedophilia, exhibitionism, voyeurism, transvestitism, sexual sadism and masochism, and frotteurism. All paraphilias include (1) presence for at least 6 months and (2) the fantasies, sexual urges, or behaviors causing significant distress or impairment, in social, occupational, or other areas of functioning.

Fetishism is the presence of intense sexually arousing fantasies, sexual urges, or behaviors involving the use of inanimate objects (e.g., female undergarments). **Pedophilia** involves sexual activity with a prepubescent child (generally 13 years or younger). Because of the illegal nature of pedophilia, its incidence is unknown. A typical profile of a pedophile is that of a somewhat conservative, married male. When pedophilia involves family members, it is called incest.

Exhibitionism is the intentional display of the genitals in a public place. Sometimes the individual masturbates while exposing himself. Although illegal, it seems to be done more for shock value than as a preamble to sexual assault or rape. It has been suggested that this behavior is triggered by stress; the usual perpetrators are sedate, middle-class males. **Voyeurism** is the viewing of other people in intimate situations (e.g., naked, in the process of disrobing, or engaging in sexual activity). Voyeurs are also called "peeping Toms." Voyeurism is considered one of the paraphilias only when the "peeping" becomes compulsive and preferable to other sexual activity. The voyeur is almost always a heterosexual male who wishes no contact with those on whom he is spying. Often the man is described as shy, socially unskilled, and without close friends.

Transvestitism involves sexual satisfaction by means of dressing in the clothing of the opposite gender. This behavior is related to fetishism but often goes beyond the use of one particular object. Usually this behavior develops early in life. Unlike gender identity disorders, there are no sexual orientation issues, and transvestites do not desire a sex change. Usually heterosexual, many transvestites cross-dress only in specific sexual situations, and they often receive the cooperation and support of their partners.

Sexual sadism and **masochism (S/M)** are two related paraphilias involving the giving (sadism) and receiving (masochism) of psychological and/or physical pain or domination to achieve sexual gratification. Much of what may be labeled as S/M falls outside the definition as outlined by DSM. Masters and Johnson (1979) reported that S/M fantasies are frequent among both homosexuals and heterosexuals.

Frotteurism involves touching, rubbing against, or fondling an unfamiliar woman to achieve sexual satisfaction. This behavior usually occurs in busy public places where he can escape after touching his victim.

Many of the people involved in nonstandard sexual practices find no need for therapy because their sexual activities are carried out with a consenting adult partner and neither involve illegal actions nor are physically or emotionally harmful to either partner. If, however, the person is experiencing relationship difficulties, wishes to change the sexual behaviors, becomes involved in illegal activity, or is physically or emotionally harming others or being harmed, therapy is indicated.

The usual treatment design for working with paraphilias is cognitive and behavioral therapy. An attempt is made to help the person learn a new sexual response pattern that will eliminate the need for the activity that is causing the problem. Techniques range from positive reinforcement for appropriate object choices to aversion techniques, in which mild electric shocks may be used for inappropriate choices. Other treatment modalities include psychodynamic techniques designed to help the client understand the origin of the paraphilia. Psychotropic agents may also be used in those practices that are acutely or dangerously compulsive. No matter what the treatment employed (pharmacological, cognitive, behavioral, dynamic, or combinations of those), it is unlikely to be effective unless extended over a very long period (Meyer 1995).

SUMMARY

Adults requiring specialized interventions by the psychiatric nurse include individuals who have been a part of the legal system or others who have demonstrated sleep or sexual disorders. Specialized needs of patients require nurses to move beyond understanding the needs and care of the mentally ill individual and to expand their knowledge base into other areas. Nurses entering the specialty of forensic nursing are able to assist with needed treatment and rehabilitation while encouraging health promotion for individuals who have been charged with or convicted of crimes. It is essential that the nurse have effective communication, counseling, and assessment skills when working in an environment such as a jail, a state or federal prison, or a halfway house.

Nurses come into contact with individuals of varying backgrounds and belief systems. One's sexuality is very basic to the individual and how it is expressed will vary from individual to individual. Nurses can provide a warm and caring environment that makes individuals more comfortable when discussing issues related to their sexuality. It is important that the nurse is comfortable with sexual issues and has done some research to stay fully informed on information related to sexuality and other sexual issues.

Sleep disorders affect the individual's ability to function. The understanding of sleep disorders and their impact on health and wellness is a rapidly expanding area of research. Nurses must rely on their ability to effectively communicate when identifying the underlying issues or problems that may have an impact upon the individual's routines and the resultant lack or perceived lack of sleep. Knowledge of sleep disorders and interventions provide nurses with information that can help them effectively educate the individual with sleeping problems.

Visit the **Evolve** website at
http://evolve.elsevier.com/Varcarolis
for a post-test on the content in this chapter.

Visit the **Evolve** website at
http://evolve.elsevier.com/Varcarolis
for additional self-study exercises.

Critical Thinking and Chapter Review

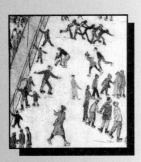

Critical Thinking

1. Discuss the components of the legal system that may result in problems for the mentally ill individual who has been charged with a criminal offense.
2. Your patient has complained that he never sleeps. You have observed that he often takes short frequent naps during the day and during this time he snores quite loudly. What questions would you ask to determine if this patient has a sleeping disorder?
3. As a nurse on an adolescent psychiatric nursing unit you often encounter teenagers who are misinformed about growth and development as well as about sexuality. Discuss information you might include in a series of teaching sessions that would help the adolescents have a greater understanding of the developmental changes they are going through.

Chapter Review

Choose the most appropriate answer.

1. Mr. O. has the psychiatric diagnosis of paranoid schizophrenia. He stopped taking his medication, became more delusional, began accosting people on the street and haranguing them. He was arrested and jailed. Once a medication regimen is reinstituted, a focus for intervention that the nurse in the jail should pursue is

   1. persuading Mr. O to be screened for HIV infection
   2. identifying the reason Mr. O stopped taking medication to prevent recurrence
   3. advocating for Mr. O's charges to be dropped so he can return to the community
   4. teaching Mr. O the importance of maintenance of physical health via regular physical examinations

2. Mrs. H, an elderly client, tells the nurse, "The only medication I take is melatonin." Based on this statement the nurse should ask questions designed to assess for

   1. sleep disorder
   2. depression
   3. paraphilia
   4. sexual dysfunction

3. Which of the following sleep patterns observed among elderly clients would be assessed by the nurse as a sleep disorder?

   1. reduction in REM sleep
   2. increased wakefulness at night
   3. taking several short naps daily
   4. loud snoring followed by periods of not breathing

4. Which sexual disorder is illegal?

1. fetishism
2. transvestism
3. pedophilia
4. gender dysphoria

5. Which responsibility would not be found in the job description of the psychiatric nurse working with mentally ill clients within a correctional facility?

1. providing direct care
2. planning health education
3. taking part in the punishment process
4. functioning as liaison between correctional facility and community mental health system

REFERENCES

American Psychiatric Association (2000). *Diagnostic and statistical manual of mental disorders* (4th ed, Text Revised) (DSM-IV-TR). Washington, DC: APA.

Badger, D., Vaughan, P., Woodward, M., and Williams, P. (1999). Planning to meet the needs of offenders with mental disorders in the United Kingdom. *Psychiatric Services*, 50(12):1624–1627.

Carson, V. B. (2000). *Mental health nursing—The nurse-patient journey* (2nd Ed). Philadelphia: W. B. Saunders.

Cauffield, J. S. (1999). Dietary supplements used in the treatment of depression, anxiety, and sleep disorders. *Primary Care Practice*, 3(3):290.

Deane, M. W., Steadman, H. J., Veysey, B. M., and Morrissey, J. P. (1999). Emerging partnerships between mental health and law enforcement. *Psychiatric Services*, 50(1):99–101.

Erikson, E. H. (1963). *Childhood and society.* New York: W. W. Norton.

Ereshefsky, T. G. (2000). Sleep disorders: Assisting patients to a good night's sleep *Journal of American Pharmacological Association*, 40(5 Suppl 1):S46–S47.

Evans, M. (2000). Re-visioning nurses' punitive attitudes within forensic psychiatric and correctional nursing: The significance of ethical sophistication. *Journal of Psychosocial Nursing*, 38(4):8–13.

Fontaine, K. L., and Fletcher, J. S. (1999). *Mental health nursing.* (4th Ed.). Menlo Park, CA: Addison-Wesley.

Freud, S. (1961). *The standard edition of the complete psychological works of Sigmund Freud*, translated and edited by James Strachey. London: Hogarth Press.

Frish, N. C. and Frish, L. E. (1998). *Psychiatric mental health nursing—Understanding the client as well as the condition.* New York: Delmar Publishers.

Green, R., and Blanchard, R. (1995). Gender identity disorder. In H. I. Kaplan and B. J. Sadock (Eds.), *Comprehensive textbook of psychiatry* (6th ed.), Vol I. Baltimore: Williams & Wilkins.

Gutheil, T. G. (1999). A confusion of tongues: Competence, insanity, psychiatry, and the law. *Psychiatric Services*, 50(6):767–773.

Hartwell, S. W. & Orr, K. (1999). The Massachusetts forensic transition program for mentally ill offenders re-entering the community. *Psychiatric Services*, 50(9):1220–1222.

Hoptman, M. J., Patalinjug, M. B., Wack, R. C., and Convit, A. (1999). Clinical prediction of assaultive behavior among male psychiatric patients at a maximum-security forensic facility. *Psychiatric Services*, 50(11):1461–1466.

Kravitz, H. M. and Kelly, J. (1999). An outpatient psychiatry program for offenders with mental disorders found not guilty by reason of insanity. *Psychiatric Services*, 50(12):1597–1605.

Lamb, H. R. and Weinberger. L. E. (1998). Persons with severe mental illness in jails and prisons: A review. *Psychiatric Services*, 49(4):483–492.

Lamb, H. R., Weinberger, L. E., and Gross, B. H. (1999). Community treatment of severely mentally ill offenders under the jurisdiction of the criminal justice system: A review. *Psychiatric Services*, 50(7):907–913.

Lewine, R., Marsh, K, and Towner, L. (1998). Incarceration as "therapy." *Psychiatric Services*, 49(8):1094–1095.

Meyer, J. K. (1995). Paraphilias. In H. I. Kaplan and B. J. Sadock (Eds.), *Comprehensive textbook of psychiatry* (6th ed.) Vol I. Baltimore: Williams & Wilkins.

McClanahan, S. F., McClelland, G. M., Abram, K. M., and Teplin, L. A. (1999). Pathways into prostitution among female jail detainees and their implications for mental health services. *Psychiatric Services*, 50(12):1606–1613.

Neubauer, D. N. (1999). Sleep problems in the elderly. *American Family Physician* 59(9):2551–2558.

Roberts, R. E., Kaplar, G. A., and Strawbridge, W. J. (2000). Sleep complaints and depression in an aging cohort: A prospective perspective. *American Journal of Psychiatry*, 157:81–88.

Roskes E. (1999). Offenders with mental disorders: A call to action. *Psychiatric Services*, 50(12):1596.

Roskes, E., and Feldman, R. (1999). A collaborative community-based treatment program for offenders with mental illness. *Psychiatric Services*, 50(12):1614–1619.

Steadman, H. J., Deane, M. W., Morrissey, J. P., Westcott, M. L., Salasin, S., and Shapiro, S. (1999). A SAMHSA research initiative assessing the effectiveness of jail diversion programs for mentally ill persons. *Psychiatric Services*, 50(12):1620–1623.

Swartz, J. A., and Lurigio, A. J. (1999). Psychiatric illness and comorbidity among adult male jail detainees in drug treatment. *Psychiatric Services*, 50(12):1628–1630.

Townsend, M. C. (2000). *Psychiatric mental health nursing—Concepts of care* (3rd Ed). Philadelphia: F. A. Davis Company.

Ventura, L. A., Cassel, C. A., Jacoby, J. E., and Huang, B. (1998). Case management and recidivism of mentally ill persons released from jail. *Psychiatric Services*, 49(10):1330–1337.

Vitiello, M. V. (1999) Effective treatments for age-related sleep disturbances. *Geriatrics*, 54(11):47–52.

Yurkovich, E., and Smyer, T. (2000). Health maintenance behaviors of individuals with severe and persistent mental illness in a state prison. *Journal of Psychosocial Nursing*, 38(6):20–31.

Outline

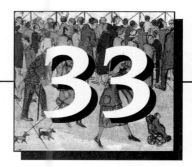

33

Psychosocial Needs of the Older Adult

Sally K. Holzapfel

Objectives

After studying this chapter, the reader will be able to

1. Assess personal knowledge on aging by taking quiz in Table 33–1, and discuss any misconceptions.

2. Compare the purpose, format, and desired outcomes among the following group treatments: remotivation, reminiscing, and psychotherapy.

3. Analyze how ageism affects your attitudes and willingness to care for the elderly.

4. Summarize problems with the use of physical and chemical restraints in the elderly, and cite most recent research findings.

5. Assess at least two elderly clients by using the Faces Scale with an elderly person.

6. Identify the problems associated with accurate pain assessment among elderly persons.

7. Discuss institutional requirements for the Patient Self-Determination Act (1990), and how it is applied in a facility the reader is familiar with.

8. Discuss differences between a living will, a directive to physician, and durable power of attorney for health care.

9. State end-of-life directives (comfort, hydration, resuscitation) and what should be expected of health care workers to help you meet clients' wishes.

10. Summarize the concept of a hospice program.

11. Identify some of the differences in assessment for depression and suicide in the elderly versus people 55 or under.

12. Discuss at least five unique assessment and treatment considerations for the addicted elderly individual.

THE OLDER POPULATION AND THE HEALTH CARE SYSTEM

The growing number of elderly people and their percentage in the general population of the United States have had a significant impact on the country's economy and its health and social services. By the year 2040, the United States will have more individuals over 65 than people under 20 years of age (Bureau of the Census 1995). Among the elderly, the fastest-growing age groups are the minorities, the poor, and those aged 85 and over. By the year 2030, the minority population will make up 25% (up from 13% in 1995) of all aged (Bureau of the Census 1995; Harper 1995).

As the population is living longer, chronic illness and disability have become major threats to the health of the elderly. Almost one third of all older persons consider their health only fair to poor. This is a significantly higher percentage than in persons under age 65, among whom only 10% hold this view (Harper 1995).

At least 80% of all individuals over age 65 have at least one chronic condition; many elderly people have more than one. The likelihood of developing one or more chronic illnesses increases notably with age: individuals 75 years of age and older are the most prone to chronic illnesses and functional disabilities. Chronic illness is responsible for more than 70% of all deaths. After age 85, there is a one-in-three chance of developing dementia, immobility, incontinence, or other age-related disabilities (Walsh 1992).

According to the Bureau of the Census (1995), today's life expectancy at birth is 72 years for men and 79 years for women, with an average of 76 years for both sexes. Upon reaching age 65, the elderly, on average, can expect to live 17 more years. The death rate for men at every age is higher than that for women. Elderly women outnumber elderly men in a ratio of 3:2. At age 85 and over, this ratio increases to 5:2.

As a general rule, women outlive men. Since husbands more often predecease their spouses, they have their wives' assistance and support when their health starts to fail. On the other hand, many older women do not have this support because of the earlier death of their husbands (Bureau of the Census 1995). Women's greater longevity has significant ramifications for society at large and for the health care profession in particular. Not only do women form the largest bloc among the elderly, they also utilize health care services more frequently than men do, and seek such services earlier, even for minor conditions (Sapp and Bliesmer 1995).

The elderly population can be categorized as 65–74 "young-old," 75–84 "middle-old," and 85 and above "old-old." Therefore, a distinction should be made between the needs of persons in the age group 85 and older (the "old-old") and the elderly who have not yet reached that age. There are noticeable differences between individuals in their sixties and people in their eighties. While the younger group is relatively healthy, the older group is much more vulnerable, frail, and at risk for visual problems, cognitive impairment, and falls. They also have more limited economic resources and community supports, and are more affected by the chronic diseases and disorders of aging (Ebersole and Hess 1994).

Elderly individuals with mental health problems are less likely than young adults to be accurately diagnosed or receive mental health treatment (Rabins et al. 2000). This is especially true for depression (Sahr 1999).

As it is, per capita health care expenses for the elderly are nearly four times higher than those for the rest of the population (Sapp and Bliesmer 1995). Questions of appropriate care and issues about health care delivery—in particular, managed care—need to be addressed. Since the aged population is expected to grow proportionally in the twenty-first century (as is managed care), nursing, to maintain its professional identity with its unique skills and expertise, will have to adjust to these developments and identify new strategies and approaches.

THE ROLE OF THE NURSE

Nurses have made a substantial contribution to the care and health promotion of the older adult. However, questions arise as to whether nurses in training are given enough information and sufficient exposure to the elderly during their nursing education. It is important for all nurses to develop an interest in the elderly and gain a better understanding of the older adult and the aging process. Adequate theory and principles are needed to provide safe and excellent care for the elderly. Any lack of specific information necessary for a student nurse to make sound decisions in regard to elderly clients is in part a result of the following:

- Negative faculty attitudes toward the elderly
- Lack of exposure to and lack of clinical emphasis on older persons
- Negative student attitudes toward the elderly because of information based on myths and stereotypes
- Unfamiliarity with gerontological information and resources

The negative view frequently held by nurses (as well as the general population) toward the elderly is part of the phenomenon of ageism. Studies have found that recruits to nursing hold ageist views, indicating significant implications for practice, education, and research (Lueckenotte 2000).

Ageism Among Health Care Workers

Ageism has been defined as a bias against older people because of their age; it is a system of destructive, erroneous beliefs. In essence, ageism reflects a dislike by the young of the old, depicting the disparaging effect of society's attitudes toward the elderly. This age prejudice is based on the notion that aging makes people increasingly unattractive, unintelligent, asexual, unemployable, and senile (Atchley 1994).

Ageism is not limited to the way the young may look at the old. It also includes older people's views, which tend to be critical about themselves and their peers. Indeed, the attitudes of the elderly toward their peers, particularly those with mental disabilities, are often more negative than the views held by the young (although this is not always the case). The threat of social contagion by association with the frail and infirm may simply be too strong to bear. Age proximity raises feelings of vulnerability (Ebersole and Hess 1990). This may explain why older persons often do not like to be referred to as "old." By seeing themselves as "young" rather than "old," they adjust better to their advancing years (Hogstel 1990).

Ageism differs from other forms of discrimination in that it cuts across gender, race, religion, and national origin. Old age does not award a desirable status or membership in a sought-after club; rather, it is a social category with negative connotations (Matthews 1979). According to Butler (1975):

> Ageism is manifested in a wide range of phenomena, both on individual and institutional levels—stereotypes and myths, outright disdain and dislike, or simply subtle avoidance of contact; discriminatory practices in housing, employment, and services of all kinds; epithets, cartoons, and jokes.

Butler (1993) is also concerned about the recent development of a new ageism that puts elderly in a no-win situation: the well-to-do elderly are envied for their economic progress, the middle class is blamed for making Social Security too costly, while the poor elderly are resented for being tax burdens.

The results of ageism can be observed throughout every level of society; even health care providers are not immune to its effects. Negative values can surface in a myriad of ways in the health care system. Financial and political support for programs for the elderly is difficult to obtain; their needs are addressed only after those of younger, albeit smaller, population groups. The Grey Panthers and American Association of Retired Persons (AARP) are, however, powerful lobbying groups that are fighting to change this trend.

Health care personnel do not always share medical information, recommendations, and opportunities with the elderly. A study of over 200 cardiac patients found that, compared with younger persons, those over age 60 receive considerably less information on available resources, practices to reduce the risk of future problems, and health management measures (USDHHS 1990). Another study showed that only about one half of all physicians believe that the older adult should receive maximal evaluation and treatment for an acute illness (USDHHS 1990). This reluctance to provide information and treatment also applies to mental health. The elderly are often not considered suitable to receive this care in the belief that providing such resources would be wasteful (Moak 1990).

Health care workers who deal on a daily basis with the confused, ill, and frail older adult may tend to develop a somewhat negative and biased view of the elderly. Their attitudes often reflect society's values, which are characterized by negativism and stereotyping. The rendering of medical care to older adults has been burdened with pessimism, defeatism, and professional aversion. Such thinking can be found among professionals as well as among ancillary personnel working in nursing homes and other institutional settings.

Other factors affecting the health care worker's approach are the clients' social conduct and level of functional independence. Nursing assistants, which as a group are likely to have the closest daily contact with the elderly, have expressed negative feelings about caring for extremely dependent clients. Independence in self-care and pleasing conduct by the client elicit more positive feelings on the part of the health care worker; conversely, socially unacceptable behaviors provoke unfavorable attitudes.

Positive attitudes toward the elderly and their care need to be instilled during basic nursing education and should be included in the curriculum. If the goal of nursing programs is to prepare the students to practice in the future, then preparing students to care for the older adult in a wide variety of settings is mandatory, for that *is* the future (Lueckenotte 2000).

To overcome existing misconceptions about older adults (the elderly) and to improve their care, educational programs are recommended and should provide (1) information about the aging process, (2) discussion of attitudes relating to the care of the elderly, (3) sensitization of participants to their clients' needs, and (4) exploration of the dynamics of nurse/staff and client interactions.

Such programs, designed to prepare nurses to function more effectively and be more receptive to working with the elderly, should help to increase the numbers of nurses wanting to work with the elderly. In addition, since the implementation of managed care makes employment opportunities in the acute care setting more limited, nurses will look for professional work in other areas. Table 33–1 presents a quiz on the facts and myths about aging.

Generalist vs. Gerontological Nursing Practice

Some elements of nursing practice remain the same between generalist nursing practice and gerontological nursing practice. For example:

■ Goals of nursing
■ Generic nursing process and methods
■ Professional practice roles:
    Standards of practice
    Code of ethics
    Accountability to clients

Yet there are differences requiring that the geriatric nurse have special expertise and interest. Nurses who care for the elderly need to have specific knowledge of aging and the interaction of health, aging, and illness, as well as knowledge and skill to modify and implement nursing methods.

The advanced practice nurses who work with the elderly experiencing mental health problems also need to know about normal aging and interactions between aging and illness, which are discussed in most medical-surgical nursing components of the nursing curriculum.

Unique Assessment Strategies

Nurses who work with the elderly benefit from specific knowledge about normal aging, drug interactions, and chronic disease. Those who work with

TABLE 33–1		***Facts and Myths About Aging***

T	F	1. Most adults past the age of 65 are demented.
T	F	2. The senses of vision, hearing, touch, taste, and smell all decline with age.
T	F	3. Muscular strength decreases with age.
T	F	4. Sexual interest declines with age.
T	F	5. For the older adult, regular sexual expressions are important to maintain sexual capacity and effective sexual performance.
T	F	6. At least 50% of restorative sleep is lost as a result of the aging process.
T	F	7. As a group, the elderly are major consumers of prescription drugs.
T	F	8. Older adults are not able to learn new tasks.
T	F	9. The elderly have a high incidence of depression.
T	F	10. As individuals age, they become more rigid in their thinking and set in their ways.
T	F	11. The aged are well off and no longer impoverished.
T	F	12. Many individuals experience difficulty when they retire.
T	F	13. The elderly are prone to become victims of crime.
T	F	14. Most elderly people are infirm and require help with daily activities.
T	F	15. Older individuals are more dependable and have fewer accidents than younger persons.
T	F	16. Most older adults are socially isolated and lonely.
T	F	17. Medicaid is a federally assisted program providing health care benefits to anyone over the age of 65.
T	F	18. The term *ageism* reflects society's positive views toward the elderly.
T	F	19. Widowers are more likely to remarry than widows.
T	F	20. Older widows appear to adjust better than younger ones.

Answers at end of chapter in Table 33–1A

elderly clients who have mental health problems also need to have special skills (e.g., interviewing, assessing, and knowing effective treatment modalities). Table 33–2 can be used as a guideline during the initial assessment. Because examination and interviews can produce anxiety in the elderly, and because the initial interview is often in unfamiliar surroundings, the guidelines are useful no matter what the setting or purpose of the interview.

There are a number of assessment tools that can be used with the elderly. Because effective coping, problem-solving, and adaptive behaviors are necessary for healthy social functioning, the degree of social dysfunction needs to be assessed. The Social

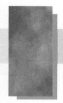

TABLE 33-2   Overall Guidelines for the Initial Assessment

APPROACH	PROCESS COMMENTS
1. Approach the client: note appearance, posture, spontaneous activity, grooming, hygiene, comfort, presence of others, facial expression, attentiveness, interest.	1. Cues gathered about musculoskeletal, neurological, genitourinary, gastrointestinal, cardiovascular, and pulmonary systems; cognitive and emotional function; senses; and social support.
2. Address the client by name. Introduce self: "My name is . . . I prefer to be called . . . What do you like to be called?	2. Hearing. Ability to respond to social situation and to cues about cognitive and affective function.
3. Offer to shake hands or grasp the client by the hand.	3. Neuromuscular function, strength, skin temperature, and texture.
4. Establish eye contact; ask about visual ability and use of glasses. Position self in full view of client. Adjust lighting.	4. Assess vision for brightness, but avoid glare.
5. Ask the client about any hearing difficulties and if the client can hear you clearly. Ask about the use of hearing aid, lip reading, better hearing in one ear than the other.	5. Cues about hearing and cognitive function.
"How are you feeling today?" If a clinic visit, "What brings you here today?" or "Is anything troubling you lately?" Probe specifically with open-ended questions, e.g., "Oh, you're hurting, tell me more about that." "What would you like help with today?" Note the issues identified and the order of concerns.	Self-assessment of health, symptoms assessment, cognitive and verbal function, communication skills, optimism, and emotional response. Cues about client's priorities, expectations, response to health, or social problems or concerns.
6. Summarize the interaction so far. "Mrs. J., we have approximately 45 minutes together to address your concerns. I think that will give us time to deal with the concerns you have voiced. I would like to proceed now by asking you a few more questions and then do the following examination procedures for these reasons."	6. Establish trust, contract for and set mutual expectations for the encounter, prioritize concerns, and validate inferences with the client.

From Matteson, M. A., and McConnell, E. S. (Eds.). (1988). *Gerontological nursing: Concepts and practice* (p. 80). Philadelphia: W. B. Saunders.

Dysfunction Rating Scale (Table 33-3) is widely used for this purpose. Depression and substance abuse among the elderly are both major health problems. Because depression and substance abuse affect each other, a special scale for detecting the presence of depression among the elderly has been devised (Box 33-1). Always ask about suicidal thoughts/suicidal intent, e.g., "Have you ever thought about killing yourself?" "Have you ever tried to in the past?"

Unique Intervention Strategies

Most older persons function quite well in their lives. The mental problems manifested by some are often treatable and responsive to treatment. Psychotherapeutic approaches need to be simplified and modified for older clients. Certain psychotherapeutic techniques are useful for the elderly client:

■ Using crisis intervention techniques (see Chapter 22)

■ Providing empathetic understanding
■ Encouraging ventilation of feelings
■ Reestablishing emotional equilibrium when anxiety is moderate to severe
■ Explaining alternative solutions
■ Assisting in the use of problem-solving approaches

Burnside (1988) offers specific guidelines for caring for older adults, urging nurses to pace themselves, not to move quickly or rush the client. She suggests that nurses "truly listen" and make the quality of their time important, not the quantity. Burnside's instructions for one-to-one relationships and interviews are found in Box 33-2.

Inpatient Settings

When clients are institutionalized, group therapy is an economical way to provide therapeutic intervention. Remotivation therapy, reminiscing therapy, and group psychotherapy are three modalities often

TABLE 33–3 *Social Dysfunction Rating Scale*

Directions: Score each of the items as follows:
1. Not present 2. Very Mild 3. Mild 4. Moderate 5. Severe 6. Very Severe

Self-esteem

1. _____ Low self-concept (feelings of inadequacy, not measuring up to self-ideal)
2. _____ Goallessness (lack of inner motivation and sense of future orientation)
3. _____ Lack of a satisfying philosophy or meaning of life (a conceptual framework for integrating past and present experiences)
4. _____ Self-health concern (preoccupation with physical health or somatic concerns)

Interpersonal System

5. _____ Emotional withdrawal (degree of deficiency in relating to others)
6. _____ Hostility (degree of aggression toward others)
7. _____ Manipulation (exploiting of environment or controlling at others' expense)
8. _____ Overdependency (degree of parasitic attachment to others)
9. _____ Anxiety (degree of feeling of uneasiness or impending doom)
10. _____ Suspiciousness (degree of distrust or paranoid ideation)

Performance System

11. _____ Lack of satisfying relationships with significant persons (spouse, children, kin, or significant persons serving in a family role)
12. _____ Lack of friends or social contacts
13. _____ Expressed need for more friends or social contacts
14. _____ Lack of work (remunerative or nonremunerative, productive work activities that normally give a sense of usefulness, status, or confidence)
15. _____ Lack of satisfaction from work
16. _____ Lack of leisure time activities
17. _____ Expressed need for more leisure, self-enhancing, and satisfying activities
18. _____ Lack of participation in community activities
19. _____ Lack of interest in community affairs and activities that influence others
20. _____ Financial insecurity
21. _____ Adaptive rigidity (lack of complex coping patterns to stress)

PATIENT: _____ RATER: _____ DATE: _____

From Linn, M.W., et al. (1969). A social dysfunction rating scale. *Journal of Psychiatric Research*, 6:299. Copyright 1969, with kind permission from Elsevier Science Ltd., The Boulevard, Langford Lane, Kidlington 0X5 1GB, United Kingdom.

led by nurses who have special training or education. Table 33–4 outlines the purpose, format, and desired outcomes for each type of group. Box 33–3 gives an example of a remotivation therapy session.

Community-Based Programs

The hazards of institutionalization are numerous. Increased mortality may be caused by an increased risk for nosocomial infections. Injuries may occur due to initial disorientation to a new setting. Residents may develop learned helplessness, losing interest in self-care activities. There also may be a decrease in opportunities for socialization. In contrast, community-based programs are an alternative whose purpose is to promote the elder's independent functioning and reduce the stress on the family system. Multipurpose Senior Centers fall within these groups. A broad range of services is provided: (1) health promotions and wellness programs; (2) health screening; (3) social, educational, and recreational activities; (4) meals; (5) information and referral services. For those in need of nursing care and custodial care services, adult day care would be an appropriate choice (Fultner and Raudonis 2000).

As a result of the negative view and rising costs of institutionalization, interest in day care programs has increased, in particular when rising costs of a nursing home cannot be afforded. Most individuals who use day care are physically frail or cognitively

BOX 33–1   *Geriatric Depression Scale (Short Form)*

■ Are you basically satisfied with your life? Yes/No
■ Have you dropped many of your activities and interests? Yes/No
■ Do you feel that your life is empty? Yes/No
■ Do you often get bored? Yes/No
■ Are you in good spirits most of the time? Yes/No
■ Are you afraid that something bad is going to happen to you? Yes/No
■ Do you feel happy most of the time? Yes/No
■ Do you often feel helpless? Yes/No
■ Do you prefer to stay at home, rather than go out and do new things? Yes/No

■ Do you feel you have more problems with memory than most? Yes/No
■ Do you think it is wonderful to be alive now? Yes/No
■ Do you feel pretty worthless the way you are now? Yes/No
■ Do you feel full of energy? Yes/No
■ Do you feel that your situation is hopeless? Yes/No
■ Do you think that most people are better off than you are? Yes/No

From Sheikh, J. I., Yesavage, J. A. (1986). Geriatric Depression Scale (GDS): Recent evidence and development of a shorter version. *Clinical Gerontology: A Guide to Assessment and Intervention* (165–173). New York: The Haworth Press.

BOX 33–2   *Helpful Interview Techniques With the Older Adult*

1. **Select a setting** that provides privacy for the interview.
2. Make certain that the **client is physically comfortable.**
3. Ask the client what name he or she prefers to be called and then use it often.
4. **Touch may be effective** in getting the client's attention.
5. **Assess the client's mental status,** e.g., look for any deficits in recent or remote memory and determine if any mental confusion exists. Be aware of *all* medications that the client is taking and their effects, any side effects, and possible drug interactions. A patient taking many medications can be confused.
6. **Ascertain the status of the client's sight and hearing faculties.** If the client has a hearing aid or glasses, or both, make certain they are being worn.
7. **Lighting in the interview setting is important,** as the older adult may need three times more light to see than the teenager. Do not allow sunlight or bright lights to shine directly into the client's face, as the older adult's eyes may be very sensitive to glare.
8. **Sit close to and speak directly to any clients who have hearing deficits.** Maintain direct eye contact with the client when sitting or standing not more than 5 feet away. When speaking, do *not* exaggerate lip movements; this action distorts the mouth and what is being said. Talk in a moderate voice

with a slower than normal rate of speech. Do *not* shout; this action accentuates the vowel sounds and obscures the consonants, which are already hard for the elderly person to hear.
9. **Observe the client for any signs of fatigue.** Gauge his or her attention span and keep the interview short if necessary.
10. **Pace the interview,** slowing it, if necessary, to match the client's needs. At the same time, allow the client enough time to think and respond to any questions, instructions, or discussions.
11. Try to include the client in all decisions.
12. Explain clearly to the client all the possible options from which to choose when making a decision. (Remember that choices may be more limited for the aged.)
13. When possible, **use reminiscing strategies to keep obtaining information.** Stimulate memory chains by attempting to recall patterns of association that will improve the client's recollection.
14. If the client verbalizes low self-esteem or negative views of aging, pick up on his or her strengths and point them out.
15. **Give instructions to the client slowly and clearly; print them in letters large enough to be read later, when the client's anxiety level may be lower.** If you are using handouts, make sure the type is large enough for the client to read.

Box continued on following page

BOX 33–2 *Helpful Interview Techniques With the Older Adult (Continued)*

16. **Make an appointment for the next meeting.** The client should understand what is expected both of the interviewer and of the client before the next meeting.

17. If possible, **include family members** in part of the interview for added input, clarification, support, and reinforcement.

18. **Be an advocate** for the elderly.

Adapted from Burnside, I. (1988). *Nursing and the aged: A self-care approach* (pp. 194–209). New York: McGraw-Hill.

TABLE 33–4 *Useful Group Modalities for Elderly Clients*

REMOTIVATION THERAPY	REMINISCING THERAPY (LIFE REVIEW)	PSYCHOTHERAPY
Purpose of Group		
■ Resocialize *regressed* and *apathetic* clients. ■ Reawaken interest in their environment.	■ Share memories of the past. ■ Increase self-esteem. ■ Increase socialization. ■ Increase awareness of the uniqueness of each participant.	■ Alleviate psychiatric symptoms. ■ Increase ability to interact with others in a group. ■ Increase self-esteem. ■ Increase ability to make decisions and function more independently.
Format		

■ Groups are made up of 10–15 clients.
■ Meetings are held once or twice a week.
■ Meetings are highly structured in a classroom-like setting.
■ Group uses props.
■ Each session discusses a particular topic.
■ See Box 33–3 for the five basic steps used in each session.
	■ Groups are made up of 6–8 people.
	■ Meetings are held once or twice weekly for 1 hour.
	■ Topics include holidays, major life events, birthdays, travel, and food.
		■ Group size is 6–12 members.
		■ Group members should share similar
		  a. Problems
		  b. Mental status.
		  c. Needs.
		  d. Sexual integration.
		■ Group meets at regularly scheduled times (number of times a week, duration of session) and place.

Desired Outcomes		

■ Increases participant's sense of reality.
■ Offers practice of health roles.
■ Realizes more objective self-image.
	■ Alleviates depression in institutionalized elderly.
	■ Through the process of reorganization and reintegration, provides avenue by which elderly can
	  a. Achieve a new sense of identity.
	  b. Achieve a positive self-concept.
		■ Decreases sense of isolation.
		■ Facilitates development of new roles and reestablishes former roles.
		■ Provides information for other group members.
		■ Provides group support for effecting changes and increasing self-esteem.

Data from Matteson, M.A., and McConnell, E. S. (Eds.). (1988). *Gerontological nursing: Concepts and practice.* Philadelphia: W. B. Saunders.

BOX 33–3 Example of Remotivation Session (Bodies of Water)

STEP 1: CLIMATE OF ACCEPTANCE

The leaders personally welcomed each participant as he or she arrived at the group session. After the leaders introduced themselves, each group member made a self-introduction. The leader used a calendar to orient the members to the date and time of the current remotivation session. The theme for session four was introduced by the leader as "bodies of water—rivers, lakes, and oceans." All group members had some familiarity with bodies of water because of their residence in Seattle.

STEP 2: CREATING A BRIDGE TO REALITY

The world globe was used as a visual aid to stimulate discussion on bodies of water. The leader asked questions, such as "How are bodies of water formed from glaciers?" Pictures of glaciers, rivers, and lakes were shown.

The leader read poems about tide pools, sea shells, and fishing written by anonymous grade school children. Discussion was stimulated by the leader asking, "What can we do at the ocean?" Visual aids and props were provided for direct sensory stimulation. Some examples of these aids and props included (1) different types of sea shells, (2) fishing tackle and bait, (3) suntan lotion, (4) sun hat, and (5) sunglasses.

A poem by an anonymous author about fishing was read to the group. This was followed by recorded music with lyrics about fishing experiences.

STEP 3: SHARING THE WORLD WE LIVE IN

Group discussion focused on jobs related to bodies of water. Topics the participants discussed in regard to self or others included crabbing, clamming, shrimping, and fishing. Visual aids were provided to stimulate further discussions of past-related experiences involving bodies of water. Pictures of river-rafting, canoeing, scuba diving, and sailing were shared.

STEP 4: AN APPRECIATION OF THE WORLD OF WORK

This time was used for the members to think about work in relation to others. More experiences in past-related work roles as well as hobbies and pastimes were discussed. The group then participated in singing a familiar old song, "Love Letters in the Sand," written in 1931 by J. Fred Coots and revived in 1957 when sung by Pat Boone.

STEP 5: CLIMATE OF APPRECIATION

The group members were thanked individually by the leaders for coming to the group and sharing their experiences. The next remotivation session theme and meeting date were announced prior to terminating the session.

GROUP RESPONSE TO SESSION FOUR

Most members of the group appeared to enjoy discussing their experiences in relation to bodies of water. Many members recalled fishing and boating experiences. Other members expressed interest in this topic by their nonverbal participation in touching and smelling some physical props and observation of visual aids. All but two participants touched the seashells and smelled the fish eggs. One lady in the group stood up and modeled the sun hat and glasses, while a man demonstrated how to reel in the line on a fishing pole. Several participants remarked on how beautiful the pictures of the glaciers were. All but a couple of group members sang to the recorded lyrics on fishing. One member stood up and danced to the music while many others clapped to her movements.

From Janssen, J. A., and Giberson, D. L. (1988). Remotivation therapy. *Journal of Gerontological Nursing*, 14(6):31.

---

impaired (Fultner and Raudonis 2000). There are three types of day care programs: (1) social day care, (2) adult day health or medical treatment model, and (3) maintenance model. In each, the elderly are taken care of during the day while staying in a home environment at night. The boundaries of these programs blend and overlap.

Social day care affords the participants the opportunity for recreation and social interaction. Nursing, medical, or rehabilitative care is usually not provided. This is the more common type of day care and is less expensive to operate. Generally, the clients are older adults who need socialization or continued physical activities, or individuals with mild dementia or physical frailty (Buckwalter et al. 1995; Nikolassy 1995).

The **adult day health** or medical treatment model goes beyond meeting recreational and social needs: it provides services such as medical interventions, psychiatric nursing, and rehabilitation for the high-risk elderly, and psychosocial interventions for the frail aged. Qualified personnel (nurses, pharmacists, physicians, physical therapists, occupational therapists, and social workers) are available, forming a broad base of support necessary for such care. This program, which requires physician referral, aims to prevent or slow down any mental, physical, or social deterioration and thus seeks to maximize the older adult's full potential regardless of disease or condition. If clients reach their full potential, they can be discharged from the program (Buckwalter et al. 1995).

The **maintenance day care** program assists clients at high risk for institutionalization. Placement is usually upon physician referral. An interdisciplinary team, including a psychiatrist, plans the care. The client mix includes frail persons with dementia and those with persistent and severe psychiatric disorders (e.g., schizophrenia, personality disorders) (Buckwalter and Piven 1995). The program's emphasis is on maintaining clients' functional abilities. Although the inevitable cognitive decline cannot be prevented in clients with dementia, the clients' quality of life is enhanced and psychosocial dysfunction may be decreased. The restlessness, anxiety, and agitation that frequently occur in the demented client are kept to a minimum with the aid of individualized treatment plans (Ebersole and Hess 1990). Discharge from this program is most often to an increased level of care such as found in an inpatient hospital or nursing home.

All three models are meant to provide a safe, supportive, and nonthreatening environment and play a vital function for older adults and their families. The programs permit the elderly to continue their present living arrangements and maintain their social ties to the community. This service relieves families of the burden of 24-hour daily care for their elderly dependents. If institutionalization becomes necessary, day care staff can work with elderly clients and their families to assess the present situation and make recommendations for placement.

ISSUES THAT AFFECT THE MENTAL HEALTH OF SOME ELDERLY

The issues chosen here for discussion are six of the most prevalent problems for some older adults:

1. Use of restraints
2. Pain management
3. Death and dying
4. AIDS
5. Suicide
6. Alcoholism

Elder abuse, another serious problem for many elderly people, is addressed in Chapter 25.

Use of Restraints

The use of restraints in the elderly is an issue of ethical, legal, and safety concern. Restraints can be both physical and chemical. Physical restraints are any manual method or mechanical device, material, or equipment that inhibits free movement. Chemical restraints are drugs given for the very specific purpose of inhibiting a specific behavior or movement.

Physical Restraints

According to a Health Care Financing Administration (HCFA) report on state and federal licensure surveys of nursing facilities in the United States in the 1980s, almost half of all nursing home residents are tied, at one time or another, to their beds or chairs (Stilwell 1991). In hospitals and nursing homes combined, every day more than 500,000 persons had some form of restraint (Evans and Strumpf 1989). Furthermore, once residents were restrained, there was a greater likelihood that they would continue to be restrained regularly for an indefinite period (Blakeslee et al. 1991).

Paradoxically, the use of physical restraints can increase the risk of serious falls (Meiner and Miceli 2000). A study by Arbesman and Wright (1999) concluded that the risk of falling was highest soon after a person was placed in mechanical restraints, since clients may become agitated and fight to get free. Another study by Neufield and colleagues (1999) found that serious injuries declined significantly when restraint orders were discontinued. The researchers concluded that restraint-free care is safe when a comprehensive assessment is done and alternatives to restraints are used.

There has always been the question of whether health care providers have the right to restrain another individual physically. Being physically restrained can be a humiliating and demoralizing experience. The elderly have responded to such action with anger, fear, anxiety, depression, and stress-related syndromes (Meiner and Miceli 2000).

Besides falls, physical restraints pose a risk of death through strangulation or asphyxiation (Blakeslee et al. 1991). Residents in restraint-free facilities have experienced fewer injuries from falls than have those in facilities using restraints. Although minor injuries such as bruises, abrasions, scratches, and cuts increased in a nonrestraint environment, moderate and serious injuries are substantially decreased (Neufield et al. 1999).

In addition to these most severe consequences, all

nurses are aware of the adverse effects of immobilization, which are compounded in the elderly:

■ Chronic constipation or impaction
■ Disrupted vestibular function
■ Reduced or impaired circulation
■ Incontinence of urine and feces
■ Abrasions and skin tears or pressure sores
■ Loss of bone mass
■ Reduced metabolic rate
■ Electrolyte losses
■ Muscle atrophy, decreased tone and strength, and contractures

Any confused behavior exhibited by restrained residents may become intensified through immobilization. Restraints also have a dehumanizing effect on both the caregiver and the resident. Their use is in conflict with the concept of human dignity and individual independence (Blakeslee et al. 1991).

To correct these injustices, the Omnibus Budget Reconciliation Act (OBRA) became a law in 1990. Nursing homes are now held accountable to a higher standard of care that focuses on the resident's "highest practicable, physical, mental, and psychosocial well-being," and are directed to support "individual needs and preferences" and to "promote maintenance or enhancement of the quality of life" (National Citizens' Coalition for Nursing Home Reform 1991). The OBRA mandates that each resident has the right to be free from unnecessary drugs and physical restraints and is provided treatment to reduce dependency on chemical and physical intervention (Hogstel 1990).

Since OBRA's implementation, rates of restraint usage have been steadily declining. While HCFA reported a decade ago a restraint rate of 22.5% nationally, more recent numbers show a reduction to less than 7% and in some facilities total elimination (Sullivan-Marx et al. 1999).

Restraints to ensure the physical safety of the resident and/or other residents may be imposed upon the written order of a physician that specifies the duration and the circumstances under which the restraints are to be used (National Citizens' Coalition for Nursing Home Reform 1991). The Food and Drug Administration (FDA) issued a safety alert in 1992 on the potential dangers of restraint devices. The agency mandated that all physical restraints be labeled with directions informing health care providers of the dangers of physical restraints and the specific usage (Myers 1994; Hogstel 1995). In addition, the FDA advised that patients or their representatives be informed of the contemplated action and its risks and benefits (Stolley 1995).

The federal government has set standards of care for every nursing home receiving Medicare or Medicaid funds. The HCFA has been charged with enforcing these standards through inspections or "surveys." The guidelines (National Citizens' Coalition for Nursing Home Reform 1991) direct HCFA surveyors to evaluate the use of physical restraint and determine whether

■ Less-restrictive measures were attempted.
■ Occupational or physical therapists were consulted.
■ The client and family received a complete explanation.
■ The device was used only for definite periods as an "enabler" to the resident or for brief periods to provide necessary life-saving treatment.
■ Use of restraints was detrimental to the resident's physical, mental, or psychosocial well-being.

Chemical Restraints

HCFA will investigate to determine whether

■ Residents are free from unnecessary drugs.
■ Residents are given antipsychotic drugs only to treat a specific condition.
■ Residents are given gradual dose reductions, drug holidays, and behavioral programming whenever possible, in lieu of medications.

The guidelines for antipsychotic drugs list certain circumstances for which they can be prescribed, e.g., cognitive impairment disorders including dementia, with associated psychotic or agitated features (National Citizens' Coalition for Nursing Home Reform 1991), defined by

■ Specific behaviors defined quantitatively and objectively that cause residents to present a danger to themselves or to others or actually hinder the staff in its ability to provide care.
■ Psychotic symptoms that cause the resident "frightful distress."

Nurses can avoid liability by knowledge of the law, adherence to the policies and procedures of the institution, and use of good nursing judgment. All nursing homes and hospitals should have written restraint procedures and policies available to all health care providers. If restraints are used, the nurse is responsible for the safety of the client during the time of their use. The client should be restrained only for a limited time and for a limited purpose. Restraints do not enhance resident care. Creative nursing skills and interventions are frequently more beneficial.

After the enactment of OBRA for long-term care institutions, the Joint Commission on the Accreditation of Healthcare Organizations (JCAHO) developed recommendations on the use of physical restraints in acute care facilities. Generally following OBRA's guidelines, JCAHO stipulates as a basis for physical restraints (Myers 1994):

■ A physician's order.
■ Time-limited application.
■ Documentation of alternative approaches.
■ Documentation of ongoing observation and assessment of the patient.
■ Documentation of care interventions (e.g., food, fluids, toileting, ADLs, and response to attempted release).

Pain and Older Adults

Pain is very common in this age group, affecting well-being and quality of life. Up to 85% of this population is thought to have problems that predispose them to pain, e.g., arthritis, peripheral vascular disease, diabetic neuropathy (Luggen 1998; 2000). Pain can be of chronic or acute origin. Even though the prevalence of pain in the older adult is not accurately known, it is thought to occur in as many as 70% of noninstitutionalized adults, a level that may also be found in acute care settings. It is estimated that about one half of patients having postoperative pain will not obtain adequate pain relief, and up to 80% of those with cancer will not receive sufficient analgesics (Luggen 1998). Pain management in the elderly frequently is not adequate and, in any event, is thought to be less effective than what is provided for other age groups (Celia 2000).

The elderly person's functioning and ability to perform activities of daily living such as walking, toileting, and bathing can be affected by pain, especially from musculoskeletal disease. Pain can also lead to increased stress, delayed healing, decreased mobility, and interference with sleep and appetite. Chronic pain can cause psychological and emotional distress, including depression, low self-esteem, social isolation, and feelings of hopelessness (Wynne et al. 2000).

Assessment and treatment of pain is one of the main tasks and responsibilities of the geriatric nurse (Bergh and Sjostrom 1999). It requires more than asking the client if there is any pain and should consist of a full pain assessment, i.e., pain pattern, duration, location, character, and any exacerbating factors or relieving factors, and the most likely cause of the pain. Once an initial pain assessment has been done, the elderly client should be monitored for any changes. Pain assessment instruments, which are discussed below, are helpful in this regard.

Barriers in Assessment

When assessing elderly clients, the health care provider should be aware of the physical/sensory changes that affect the elderly. Frequently, older adults tend to hinder the assessment process. They may perceive and report pain differently from younger adults because of physical and psychological changes associated with aging (Galloway and Turner 1999). Since pain for them is often considered normal and expected, they may belittle it or fail to mention it entirely unless carefully questioned. Unlike a younger adult, the elderly may refer to their pain with words such as discomfort, hurting, or aching. They are often reluctant to label a painful experience as pain (AGS 1998; Luggen 1998). Older adults may attribute a low ranking to the pain as compared with other health problems. Concerns about learning what the pain really signifies, exposure to additional costs, and fear of diagnostic tests or medications that may have side effects can make them reluctant to talk about their pain. They may be resigned to accept serious disease or imminent death as a natural consequence of aging or accept pain as retribution for past actions. Neither attitude encourages the client to talk about the pain (Miakowski 1999; AGS 1998). Changes in behavior may indicate pain and should be assessed, especially as they relate to clients who have difficulty communicating their needs (e.g., dementia).

In the aged, several chronic painful problems may occur together. Sorting out new pain from preexisting pain can be difficult. Sensory impairments, memory loss, dementia, and depression can exacerbate this. Any of these factors can add to the difficulty of obtaining an accurate pain assessment. An interview with close family members or friends is vital in such situations (Luggen 1998). A number of assessment tools may facilitate this process.

Assessment Tools

Many tools exist to assess pain. All of them require some sort of communication, e.g., pictorial, verbal, or graphic, between the client and health care provider. Because the elderly frequently may suffer from sensory deficits or cognitive impairments, simply worded questions and simple drawings, which can be easily understood, are most effective tools (Flaherty 2000). The **Visual Analog Scales (VAS)** (Jacox et al. 1994) and the **Faces Scale** (AGS 1998) are highly effective assessment instruments. Figure 33–1 shows the Faces Scale and three VAS variations, all having a horizontal line between two pain extremes and division with numbers or words. Clients are asked to choose a position on the line that

Visual Analogues Scales

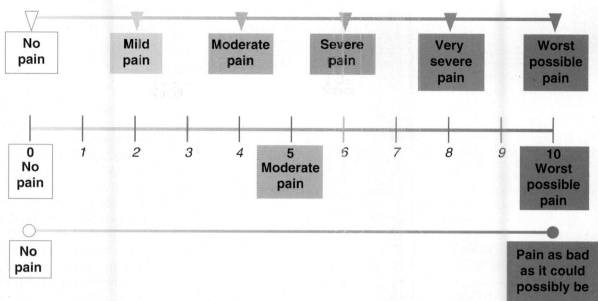

Figure 33–1 Visual analogue scales in the management of cancer pain. (From Clinical Practice Guideline No. 9. AHCPR Publication No. 94-0952. Rockville, MD: Agency for Health Care Policy and Research, Public Health Service, U.S. Department of Health and Human Services, March 1994; and Bieri D., Reeve K. A., Champion G. D. (1990). The Faces pain scale for the self-assessment of the severity of pain experienced by children: development, initial validation, and preliminary investigation for ratio scale properties. *Pain* 41(2):139–150.

indicates their level of pain. The Faces Scale shows facial expressions on a scale of 0 (a smile) to 6 (crying grimace). Respondents are asked to choose the face that depicts the pain they feel. Studies have shown that 86% of nursing home residents could complete either the VAS or Faces Scale (Flaherty 2000).

The Present Pain Intensity (PPI) Rating from the **McGill Pain Questionnaire (MPQ)** (Davis 1997; Chapman and Syrjala 1990) is another accepted tool on a scale of 0 to 5. Clients are asked to respond by selecting the word (which goes from no pain [0] to excruciating pain [5]) that they believe identifies the pain they feel. Wynne et al. (2000) found that the PPI of the McGill Pain Scale was the most useful instrument for nursing home residents who were either cognitively intact or impaired.

For the elderly who are unable to communicate or have a temporarily altered mental state, **Amy's Guide** (Galloway and Turner 1999) can be helpful. It lists in four groups (verbal, facial, behavioral, and physical expressions) several different types of behavior. The health care provider observes the clients and checks off the most pertinent descriptive factors in these groups, e.g., wincing with touch, grunting, closing their eyes, and not wanting to eat.

Since pain assessment is an ongoing process, regular communication among staff along with the development of comprehensive care plans is essential. Many health care workers refer to pain assessment as the fifth vital sign, and make it a routine

assessment among individuals who are likely to experience pain.

Pain Management

If pain is present, it should be addressed with pharmacological or nonpharmacological measures or both. Since the elderly may not always be able to express the level of pain adequately, they are often undertreated. Therefore, careful assessment of their pain and selection of effective interventions are essential.

Pharmacological pain management includes the use of prescriptive and nonprescriptive medications, frequently based on the recommendation of the health care provider. Included are the use of analgesics, opioid analgesics, and adjuvant medications. Some considerations in analgesic management in the elderly are given in Box 33–4.

Nonpharmacological management of pain includes a range of interventions and modalities. Physical treatment may consist of exercise, positioning, acupuncture, heat/cold, massage, and transcutaneous electrical nerve stimulation (TENS). Cognitive strategies may emphasize relaxation, distraction techniques, biofeedback, and hypnosis. Clients may also seek out alternative medicine approaches such as the use of homeopathy, naturopathy preparations, and spiritual healing. These techniques are often combined and all involve helping the patient deal with pain and gain some control over it. Education

Box 33–4   *Tips on Pharmacological Pain Management in the Elderly*

■ Remember that older adults often receive less pain medication than younger adults, resulting in inadequate pain relief. Compensate for this.

■ Safe administration of analgesics is complicated because of possible interactions with drugs used to treat multiple chronic disorders, nutritional alterations, and altered pharmacokinetics in the elderly.

■ The peak and length of action of analgesics are greater and longer in the elderly than in younger individuals. Start with 1/4 to 1/2 the adult dose and titrate up carefully.

■ Give oral analgesics around the clock. Administer on a p.r.n. basis later on as indicated by patient's pain status.

■ If acute confusion occurs, assess for other contributing factors before changing the medication or stopping analgesic use. Confusion in postoperative patients has been found to be associated with unrelieved pain rather than opiate use.

■ **Acetaminophen** is an effective analgesic in the elderly. Although there is an increased risk of end-stage renal disease with long-term use, it does not produce the gastrointestinal bleeding that is seen in the **NSAIDs.**

■ Analgesics and adjuvants, such as **anticholinergics** and **pentazocine,** may produce increased confusion in the elderly. The **NSAIDs** can have the same effect during their initial period of administration.

■ **Opiates** have a greater analgesic effect and longer duration of action. Avoid the use of **meperidine** whose active metabolite may stimulate the central nervous system (CNS), resulting in confusion, seizures, and mood alterations. If used, do not do so for more than 48 hours. Avoid intramuscular administration because of tissue irritation and poor absorption. **Morphine sulfate** is a safer choice than meperidine because its duration of action is longer, so a smaller overall dose is required.

■ Assess bowel function daily, as constipation can be a frequent side effect.

Data from Young, D. (1999). Acute pain management protocol. *Journal of Gerontological Nursing,* 25(6):10–21. © University of Iowa Gerontological Nursing Interventions Research Center Research Development and Dissemination Care.

the client be encouraged to be familiar with and practice the interventions to gain control so that they can work to their full potential (Seers 1999).

Nursing Implications

As individuals age, the body's ability to eliminate drugs via the kidney decreases. Nurses should be aware of this process, which can result in overdosing. Fear of narcotic overmedicating, which may lead to respiratory depression, can lead the nurse to give less pain medication to elderly individuals than may actually be needed for effective treatment (Celia 2000). Bergh and Sjostrom (1999) found that nurses tend to overestimate mild pain and underestimate severe pain. The latter may result in a situation in which the nurse believes that appropriate pain relief was administered although the pain was not adequately alleviated. It is a common misconception to assume that pain perception decreases with aging. No physiological changes in pain perception in the elderly have been demonstrated. In fact, older adults may feel pain even more keenly than do younger persons (Celia 2000). Careful and continuing assessments and an understanding of pain physiology are necessary for effective pain management in the elderly (Luggen 2000).

The Promotion of Comfort and Relief of Pain in Dying Patients (ANA 1991) states:

> Nurses should not hesitate to use full and effective doses of pain medication for the proper management of pain in the dying patient. The increasing titration of medication to achieve adequate symptom relief, even at the expense of life, thus hastening death, secondarily, is ethically justified.

Nurses must acquire increased knowledge regarding pain and its management and change outmoded practices when rendering treatment. Refer to Chapter 30 on care for the dying.

Death and Dying

In the early 1950s, the elderly approaching death found themselves not in a nursing home or hospital but at home, with death usually taking place in familiar surroundings. The individual could thus move through the dying process in the more intimate home setting.

As a more youth-oriented society, Americans tend to view death not as an immediate concern but rather as a remote prospect. By turning their sick over to the medical experts, Americans expect advanced technologies to answer all problems; thus, they insulate themselves from death (Ross 1981).

is an important component for both the client and caregivers and cannot be underestimated (AGS 1998). The key to successful pain management lies in the application of a variety of techniques that the client should learn and practice. It is important that

Polls have been conducted on themes of death and prolonging life. When members in a retirement community were asked to assess the extent of intervention they would like should they be dying, the majority desired only comfort care; they were not interested in the life-extending processes. It is interesting to note that a much greater percentage of older persons than younger ones said they would refuse intensive care or tube feeding. The elderly wanted to ensure that their wishes were followed by having a written document of such wishes accessible to their physicians (Snow and Atwood 1985).

Advances in Technology

Physicians and nurses often have a difficult time making decisions affecting the care of their dying clients. Frequently the lives of the dying persons are prolonged regardless of their mental capacity. Medical technology has frequently outpaced our ability to apply it judiciously (Pinch and Parsons 1992). The lives of those who would have died sooner are often prolonged regardless of their mental capacity.

On one hand the client's wishes (e.g., in a living will) should be respected. On the other hand for legal (malpractice charges) or ethical reasons, such requests may frequently be disregarded.

No specific cure exists for many of the severe and persistent diseases afflicting the elderly (e.g., senile dementia, stroke, osteoporosis, advanced cancer, rheumatic disease, arteriosclerosis). A definite aging population has evolved, which means that physicians, the elderly, and their families are facing more treatment decisions than ever before (Pinch and Parsons 1992).

Since the 1960s, the public's desire to have a voice in making decisions about its care has been increasing. This interest in client advocacy has been recognized with the passage of the Patient Self-Determination Act (PSDA) of 1990. Although the elderly are becoming better-educated consumers of health care, some are still reluctant to make health care decisions about the extent of medical interventions or to create a living will, instead, they prefer to rely informally on family members to make choices for them (Shawler et al. 1992). As a result of the passage of PSDA, the share of the population with some form of written directives has increased.

Patient Self-Determination Act (PSDA) of 1990

With the Patient Self-Determination Act becoming law, more health care providers have come into con-

tact with **advance directives.** The PSDA establishes guidelines regarding clients' requests regarding serious illness. It fosters clearer communication between the clients, their families, physicians, and health care workers. Health care institutions that receive federal funds are now required to provide, at the time of admission, written information to each client regarding his or her right to execute advance health care directives and to inquire if such directives have been made by the client. The client's admission records should state whether such directives exist. The ANA (1992) recommends that specific questions should be part of every nurse's admission assessment. See Box 33–5.

Such directives indicate preferences for the types of medical care or amount of treatment desired. The directives come into effect should physical or mental incapacitation prevent clients from making their health care decisions. These wishes can be communicated through one or more of the following instruments: (1) a living will, (2) a directive to physician, and (3) a durable power of attorney for health care. These documents must be in writing and witnessed; depending on state and institutional provisions, they may require notarization.

Living wills express clients' wishes about their future medical care. During times of crisis, living wills can influence the course of therapy. A competent client may alter a living will at any time. The question of whether an incompetent person can change a living will has to be addressed on a state-by-state basis.

Health care providers are obligated to abide by the advanced care directive unless their clients are told beforehand in writing that one or more of the provisions are against the institution's policy (within confinement of applicable state law) (Olson 1997).

Executing a living will may not always guarantee its application. American medicine is still largely ignoring end-of-life decisions. A study monitoring over 5000 critically ill individuals was conducted in five teaching hospitals in the United States and found that physicians often disregard or misunderstand their clients' requests. The result is that a significant number of individuals die against their wishes in intensive care units, isolated and in pain after days or weeks of futile treatment. Significant differences were found between what the clients desired and what they actually received. Less than half of all physicians knew when their clients did not want cardiopulmonary resuscitation (CPR). Even when there was knowledge, almost half of the do-not-resuscitate (DNR) orders were written only within two days of death in instances when they should have been written much earlier (SUPPORT Investigators 1995).

Box 33–5 *Nurses' Responsibilities and the Patient Self-Determination Act (1990)*

PART OF NURSING ADMISSION ASSESSMENT

Nurses should know the laws of the state in which (they) practice . . . and should be familiar with the strengths and limitations of the various forms of advance directive.

The ANA recommends that the following questions be part of the nursing admission assessment:

1. Do you have basic information about advance care directives, including living wills and durable power of attorney?
2. Do you wish to initiate an advance care directive?
3. If you have already prepared an advance care directive, can you provide it now?
4. Have you discussed your end-of-life choices with your family or designated surrogate and health care workers? (ANA 1992)

RESPONSIBILITIES OF HEALTH CARE WORKERS UNDER THE PATIENT SELF-DETERMINATION ACT OF 1990

Hospitals, skilled nursing facilities, home health agencies, hospice organizations, and health maintenance organizations serving Medicare and Medicaid clients must:

1. Maintain written policies and procedures for providing information to their clients for whom they provide care.
2. Give written material to clients concerning their rights under state law to make decisions about medical care, including the right to accept or refuse surgical or medical care and to formulate advance directives and provide written policies and procedures for the realization of these rights.
3. Document in clients' records whether they have advance directives.
4. Not discriminate in care or other ways against clients who have or have not prepared advance directives.
5. Make sure that policies are in place to ensure compliance with state laws governing advance directives.

Schlossberg, C., and Hart, M. A. (1992). Legal perspectives. In M. Burke and M. Walsh (Eds.), *Gerontologic nursing care of the frail elderly* (p. 469). St. Louis: Mosby—Year Book.

American Nurses Association (ANA) (1992). *Position statement on nursing and the patient self-determination act.* Washington, DC: The Association.

With a directive to physician, a physician is appointed by the individual to serve as proxy. This directive must be completed on a prescribed form. Many of the features parallel those of a living will (presence of terminal illness, verification by the physician, competency at time of signing).

The directive to physician can be particularly useful in cases in which a terminally ill individual with no family or close ties to others feels most comfortable with having the physician act as surrogate. The physician must agree in writing to be the client's agent and must also be one of the two physicians who made the original determination that the client is terminally ill (MacKay 1992). Like the living will, the directive to physician can be revoked orally at any time without regard to client competency.

The durable power of attorney for health care (DPAHC) differs from the two earlier instruments in that a person (other than a physician) is appointed to act as the client's agent and there is no waiting period for implementation. Furthermore, with the DPAHC, the client must not only be competent and of age when making the appointment but must also be competent to revoke the power. Designating a health care proxy is generally a simple step. Individuals do not have to be terminally ill or incompetent in order to allow the empowered individual to act on their behalf. No physician's certification is required.

The DPAHC provides the best option for most clients (MacKay 1992). Since relying only on a living will to make life or death decisions can be uncomfortable for the health care provider, the DPAHC individual can be called upon. On the other hand, some individuals may choose to supplement a DPAHC with a living will, keeping the latter in reserve in case of the possible need for clarification of their wishes.

Medical Futility

End-of-life decisions are a matter of concern not only for the client, family, or surrogate but also for the health care provider. Problems may arise when the clients (and more frequently the family or surrogate) express desires that life-prolonging actions be taken while, on the other hand, physicians recommend that treatment be withheld. The concept of medical futility is developing as an ethically acceptable rationale to withhold treatment. It has been defined thus (Futility: The Concept and Its Use 1993):

A treatment is considered medically futile when the treatment affords no benefit weighing the intrusiveness, burdens, and risks against the ultimate outcome.

In applying this concept to clinical practice, the health care provider will consider the beneficial effects of continued therapy or intervention. If treatment is highly unlikely to benefit certain clients, it may be deemed futile to continue.

Hospice Care

One alternative to dying in a hospital or nursing home setting is the hospice approach. In its original concept a hospice was a place of shelter and rest for pilgrims or strangers. Today this idea has broadened beyond the physical setting to recognize a program to meet the needs of the dying. The hospice approach to dying is covered more fully in Chapter 30.

The hospice philosophy is characterized by the acceptance of death as a natural conclusion to life, with clients rather than health care providers making the decisions how they want to live and die. Terminally ill clients can remain at home and receive supportive care. The focus is on keeping them comfortable, free of pain, as active as possible, and close to their families. They need not fear being subjected to prolonged medical care against their wishes.

Recently, some health care facilities have set aside hospice beds whose occupants are treated in accordance with the hospice philosophy. The hospice approach may constitute for many an acceptable equilibrium between clients' needs and wishes and the emotional and financial strain on their relatives.

Withholding Hydration

Contrary to earlier teaching, hydration is no longer advised when a terminally ill client facing imminent death is dehydrated. Although many nurses have been taught that dehydration causes suffering and that skilled care requires hydration, it is necessary to readjust this thinking (Zerwekh 1993). Research has shown that terminally ill clients in end-stage dehydration experience less discomfort than clients receiving medical hydration at that stage (Taylor 1995; Printz 1992). With respect to food, McCann and colleagues (1994) found that those terminally ill with cancer generally did not experience hunger, and those who did needed only small amounts of food for alleviation.

Hydration needlessly extends the dying process. Withholding artificial hydration and nutrition from an individual in an irreversible coma does not bring on a destructive state but rather permits an already existing fatal condition to take its natural course. When death is imminent, the moral responsibility to prolong life is outweighed by not unnecessarily burdening the dying process (Taylor 1995).

Nursing Role in the Decision-Making Process

In working with the client's family, the nurse should orient family members and significant others about the ethicolegal policies of the institution and assist them to understand the concepts of dying and death. The nurse should explain that the family need not feel morally obligated to provide for all possible medical care when it would only extend the suffering of a loved one. This is especially true when such extraordinary measures do not represent the person's values and beliefs.

Maintaining an open and continuing dialogue among client, family, nurse, and physician is of principal importance. The nurse should serve as an advocate for competent clients in their decision making and should be supportive of any surrogates appointed to act on the client's behalf.

In the absence of a living will or other directives, any indication that clients might have given in the past about their view toward death and dying should be given consideration with respect to medical care. Each health care institution should have a written policy on coding to serve as a guideline for physicians and nurses. For affected clients, there must be a physician's do-not-resuscitate order (DNR). **The nurse should never accept verbal "no-code" orders from physicians** (Alford 1986).

Each health care facility receiving federal funds must have written policies, procedures, and protocols in compliance with the Patient Self-Determination Act of 1990 (PSDA). Such guidelines result in more, not less, involvement and responsibilities for nurses. Nurses must prepare themselves for the legal, ethical, and moral issues involved when giving advance directive counseling. The new law does not specify who must talk with clients about treatment decisions, but in many facilities nurses are being asked to do this.

Although the nurses, especially in nursing homes, may discuss options with their clients, they may not assist clients to write advance directives as this could be considered a conflict of interest.

If an advance directive of a client is not being followed, the nurse should intervene on the client's behalf. If the problem cannot be resolved with the physician, the facility's protocol providing for notification of the appropriate supervision should be followed.

Nurses are often involved in decisions about whether to treat clients aggressively or allow them to die without the use of life-support equipment. All nurses should:

■ Know their state's nursing practice act and understand the state laws and the institution's policies concerning death and the termination of the life support systems.

■ Understand that it is the client's will, not health, that is all important.

Making decisions regarding the treatment of an incapacitated client is never easy. The existence of an advance directive can guide the health care providers in this process. Clear-cut answers will not always be found. However, a conscientious and informed health care provider, together with clear and established written policies and procedures of the institution, will facilitate the process of following the client's wishes.

AIDS *and the Elderly*

Not only does the acquired immunodeficiency syndrome (AIDS) affect young persons and intravenous drug users, but 10% of all AIDS cases are among people 50 years or older (Chiao et al. 1999).

Blood transfusions are a main cause for the spread of AIDS in the elderly. Consequently, the aged who received blood transfusions before 1985, and their spouses, are particularly at risk. The same applies to the elderly who participated in unprotected sex outside a monogamous relationship. Elderly individuals are less likely to use a condom during sexual intercourse or to participate in routine HIV testing (Chiao et al. 1999).

Older adults are frequently not considered targets for acquiring human immunodeficiency virus (HIV) infection through sexual activity. However, their sexual behavior should not be underestimated. Most have a high degree of interest in sexuality and continued sexual activity when a partner is available.

Older women may be at greater risk for getting the virus from an infected partner than are older men. Changes in vaginal tissue because of the aging process can lead to tears in the vaginal mucosa during intercourse, allowing the HIV virus to penetrate. In addition, since pregnancy is no longer a threat, use of condoms in this age group is uncommon. This puts the older woman at greater risk of exposure.

Because dementia caused by AIDS and Alzheimer's dementia (AD) can be easily confounded, a careful assessment and work-up are required. The health care provider must be aware that AIDS can occur in the elderly. Early symptoms of AIDS dementia that may mimic AD can be apathy, withdrawal, forgetfulness, and confusion.

Generally, health care providers have directed their educational efforts in HIV prevention toward an age group younger than that of the elderly. Society tends to ignore and discourage sex among older adults. Those who are sexually active may not feel comfortable discussing their sex lives with their health care providers. Because of this cultural denial, older adults are being excluded from HIV education (Wooten-Bielski 1999). Consequently, appropriate information may not be reaching the older adult. The nursing and medical community must realize that age does not preclude sexual activity and that a potential exposure of the older adult to AIDS exists. In the recognition that the elderly may fall victim to AIDS, educational programs should address prevention strategies for both the elderly and health care providers, as well as providing information on assessment and treatment of AIDS across the life span.

Suicide

Although suicide is often associated with the young, the suicide rates of the elderly in the United States are the highest of any age group. Suicide is now one of the top ten causes of death among the aged. While older adults account for 13% of the population, death by suicide accounts for 20% of all deaths of individuals 65 years of age or older (NIMH 1999). Refer to Chapter 23 on Suicide.

The elderly white male has the highest prevalence of suicide. One explanation for the high white male suicide rate may lie in changes of occupational status and measures of success in men at the time of retirement and thereafter. Such changes seem to affect white males, as a group, more than other elderly people, including women (Ebersole and Hess 1994). The Protestant white male living alone in his home is at highest risk. His appearance is likely to be neat and behavior calm. He is often taking either antianxiety or antipsychotic medication (Hogstel and Weeks 2000). With retirement, a man may lose status, influence, contact with fellow workers, and standing in the community. On the other hand, the older woman retains many of her earlier activities and roles. It remains to be seen whether women and other groups becoming more active in the work force will suffer the same effects as men upon retirement.

Other factors that can lead to suicide are feelings of hopelessness, uselessness, and despair. For older adults, suicide may be seen as a final gesture of control at a stage when independence is at risk or activities are limited. For this reason, the suicide attempts of the elderly are more likely to succeed. Unlike younger persons, whose suicidal gestures may be intended to draw attention to their problems, those of older adults do not signify a call for help but rather a desire to die (Atchley 1994; Stanley and Beare 1995). Persistent and terminal illness also contributes to increased suicide rates in the elderly.

Financial need can add to the high suicide rate. Federal reductions in programs such as Medicare, Medicaid, and food stamps, along with state-ordered cuts in medical care, cause many elderly Americans to worry about their future. An inverse relationship between economic conditions and suicide rate has been identified.

Even though the elderly's suicide rates are high, they are probably underreported. Suicide is often not listed on the death certificate, even if it may be suspected. The numbers also do not reflect those who passively or indirectly commit suicide by abusing alcohol, starving themselves, overdosing or mixing medications, stopping life-sustaining drugs, or simply giving up the will to live (Stanley and Beare 1995).

Assessing Suicide Risk in the Elderly

Among the high-risk suicide factors that should be included in the assessment in the elderly are (Hogstel and Weeks 2000):

- widowhood
- illnesses and intractable pain
- status change
- chronic pain
- chronic illness
- family history of suicide
- chronic sleep problems
- alcoholism
- losses
- depression

Losses may be personal in nature (death of a family member or close friend), economic (loss of earnings or job), or social (loss of prestige or position) (McIntosh 1985; Boxwell 1988). These changes and losses intensify the potential for suicide.

Multiple losses accompany the aging process. These losses increase stress at a time when the older adult may be the most vulnerable and least resistant to stress, thus precipitating a depressive state. Nevertheless, older adults are able to function despite their losses. Those who give in may do so because of hopelessness.

The technological advances that extend the lives of older adults sometimes bring a quality of life that is not acceptable to them. Some elderly people may decide that their lives are not worth living under such circumstances and opt for "rational" suicide. In these instances, they may have the tacit support of their children, who may resent the cost and problems involved in keeping their parents alive (Tolchin 1989). Placement in a nursing home can be another catalyst. The fear of this event was highest on a list

of reasons given in suicide notes in one study of the elderly (Loebel 1991).

The nurse must remain vigilant against the possible suicide tendencies of clients later in life. The significant increase in the sheer numbers of elderly people is expected to lead to a doubling in the number of suicides within the next 40 years. These rates are anticipated to swell as baby boomers grow older. Although life expectancy has increased, individuals continue to retire at about the same age. Fears about their livelihood, inflation, and possible collapse of pensions become crucial factors. Any cutbacks in medical care will cause anxiety about an increase in health care costs. All these factors are likely to contribute to an increase in the suicide rate.

In assessing suicide risk, the health care provider must examine previous suicidal behavior and understand that the elderly make fewer suicidal gestures than the population at large. They must realize that these older adults, as opposed to younger age groups, are less likely to communicate their intent to commit suicide. This has led many health care providers to the erroneous assumption that suicide is not an important issue among older adults (Hogstel and Weeks 2000).

In the elderly, suicide is most closely associated with untreated depression (Zerbe 1999). As the most frequent functional psychiatric disorder of later life, depression accounts for up to 70% of late-life suicides (Richardson et al. 1989). Research has shown that the majority of the elderly who commit suicide suffer from the most treatable kind of depression and yet do not receive needed mental health services (Buckwalter and Piven 1999). Early identification of and treatment for depression, therefore, are key measures for suicide prevention (Moody 1994).

Right to Suicide

One concern of nursing is the question of whether an elderly individual has the right to commit suicide. Accentuating the ethical and moral dilemma of suicide is the distinction that must be made between suicide and voluntary active euthanasia. Although society frowns on suicide in general, there seems to be a growing recognition that elderly persons with terminal illnesses should be able to control their own deaths. If an alert elderly client is confronted with an intractable, lingering, and painful illness, with no hope of relief except by committing suicide, is the intervention of the health care provider to prevent suicide justifiable? Several nursing scholars support the nursing perspective that affirms life by enhancing the individual's quality of life as opposed to assuring them of their right to die (Moore 1993).

Although suicide is discussed in Chapter 23, specific factors that concern the elderly are noted here, such as retirement-related difficulties, physical illness, economic problems, loneliness, social isolation, and ageism. Innovative methods to deal with these factors need to be developed for the elderly. Education of the public in general—and health care providers in particular—is necessary to raise the level of awareness of this geriatric problem.

Depression versus Dementia

Depression is often confused with dementia and not always recognized. This is important for nurses to keep in mind. A careful systematic assessment is therefore necessary to properly identify the illness. Unlike dementia, depression is treatable with medication and other interventions. In the elderly, symptoms of memory loss and other intellectual impairments, or asocial or agitated behavior, may be associated with dementia while actually caused by depression. See Chapter 21 for comparisons between dementia and depression.

In making an assessment, the nurse needs to be familiar with the symptoms of later-life depression (Osgood 1988; Zerbe 1999), which may include one or more of the following:

■ Changes in sleep patterns (insomnia)
■ Changes in eating patterns (loss of appetite)
■ Loss of interest or pleasure in usual activities (anhedonia)
■ Excessive fatigue (anergia)
■ Increased concern with bodily functions
■ Feeling depressed
■ Apprehension and anxiety without any reason
■ Low self-esteem (feeling insignificant or pessimistic)

A careful evaluation of the cause of the depression is also necessary. Depression can be caused by drugs (e.g., reserpine and other *Rauwolfia* derivatives, steroids, phenothiazines) as well as by metabolic and endocrine disorders (e.g., hepatitis and adrenal and thyroid insufficiency). Chronic health problems may also augment the depression and suicide potential. Thorough assessment for any medical or drug-induced side effects should be performed.

Antidepressants

In choosing a drug to treat depression in the elderly, primary emphasis should be placed on avoiding possible side effects rather than on efficacy. When starting therapy, low antidepressant dosages (usually half the routine recommended dose) are recommended, with subsequent slow and gradual increases if needed (**Start Low, Go Slow**).

Selective serotonin reuptake inhibitors (SSRIs) have become the first-line antidepressant for elderly individuals because of their more benign side effects profile and lack of toxicity when taken in overdose (Newhouse 1996). However, they are not problem free.

Fluoxetine and paroxetine can cause symptoms of central nervous system stimulation (e.g., increased awakenings, reduced time in rapid-eye-movement sleep, insomnia) (Lehne 1998). Age does not appear to affect the pharmacokinetics of sertraline. However, the metabolism of fluoxetine and paroxetine in the elderly is impaired, resulting in higher plasma levels (Young and Koda-Kimble 1995). This makes sertraline a good choice for an antidepressant among the SSRIs for the older population. Reboxetine, a noradrenaline reuptake inhibitor (selective NRI), has also been found to be effective and a well-tolerated antidepressant for both long- and short-term treatment of the elderly (Aguglia 2000)

Depressed elderly are at high risk for physical decline. Prevention and treatment of depression can be a practical intervention to reduce physical decline in later years (Penninx et al. 1998). Client and family education is an important component of successful management (Kelsey 1998).

Psychotherapy should also be considered. Groups are useful for the elderly because they can diminish social isolation and loneliness and help the members understand that they are not alone in their situation. Group members can learn creative ways to increase their mood as well as quality of life. Individual therapy is also useful. Cognitive-behavioral therapy, focus therapy, and psychodynamic therapy may all be helpful depending on the individual. A combination of some kind of therapy and medication usually has the best outcomes. Primary care providers must, therefore, acquire sensitive assessment skills for depression and suicidal risk and be knowledgeable about methods of intervention.

Alcoholism

The American Medical Association has termed alcohol abuse among the elderly a hidden epidemic. Alcohol abuse in the elderly is often difficult to identify. This is particularly true when an elder person is no longer in the familiar surroundings of work or when relatives, family members, friends, and employers are not available to notice changes in behavior and personality attributable to substance abuse. Health care providers may fail to assess the elderly for drinking problems because of the stereotype that older people are kindly grandparents (McCracken 1998). More than 10% of all older Americans in the community at large, and 20% of elders who are hospitalized, have serious problems with alcohol (Ebersole and Hess 1994; Ostrander 1992). Unfortunately, most (85%) receive no treatment (Parette et al. 1990). There are two major types of abusers: (1) the early-onset alcoholic or aging alcoholic and (2) the late-onset alcoholic or geriatric problem drinker. The aging alcoholic has generally had alcohol problems intermittently throughout life, with a regular alcohol-abuse pattern starting to evolve in late middle age or later. The geriatric problem drinker, on the other hand, has no history of alcohol-related problems but develops an alcohol-abuse pattern in response to the stresses of aging (Egbert 1993; Johnson 1989).

The stressful, or reactive, factors that precipitate late-onset alcohol abuse are often caused by environmental conditions that may include retirement, widowhood, and loneliness. These stressors in the older adult, who may have retired, may not drive, and may be isolated from family and friends, are often greater than the problems faced by the middle-aged adult, who has to manage a job or career and care for a family and household. Work and family responsibilities may help keep a potential alcoholic from drinking too much. Once these demands are gone and the structure of daily life is disrupted, there is little impetus to remain sober. Older adults who lose a spouse through death, divorce, or legal separation are at the highest risk of becoming late-in-life alcoholics (Kashka and Tweed 1995).

Alcohol and Aging

Excessive consumption of alcohol can create particular problems for the elderly. The older adult has an increased biological sensitivity to (a decreased tolerance for) the effects of alcohol. This diminished resistance, combined with age-related changes such as weakened manual dexterity, balance, and postural flexibility, can increase the likelihood of falls, burns, or other accidents.

Some drinkers, as they get older, note changes in their response to alcohol, such as headaches, reduced mental abilities with memory losses or lapses, and feelings of malaise rather than well-being. These problems start to occur at lower levels of consumption than was the case in earlier years. Older persons are likely to drink more frequently but in lesser quantities than younger individuals, who tend to drink larger amounts less often (Gomberg 1980). Thus, the possibility of alcohol abuse in cases of only moderate ingestion by the elderly is not often recognized by the alcoholic's friends or family.

With aging, the body becomes less resilient; healing from injury or infection is slower, and stress is more likely to cause a loss of physiological equilibrium. As the proportion of fatty tissues to lean body mass increases with age, the individual's metabolic rate usually slows down, increasing the amount of time it takes the body to eliminate drugs (Parette et al. 1990).

Alcohol and Medication

The interaction of drugs and alcohol in the elderly can have serious consequences. There is a decreased functioning of the liver enzymes that break down the alcohol, which on a short-term basis has the effect of prolonging the action of many medications, potentiating their effect. On the other hand, chronic ingestion of alcohol enhances the metabolism of many drugs by causing faster turnover of medication.

Older individuals can expect higher blood alcohol levels than younger persons for an equivalent intake of alcohol (Cavanaugh 1993). The effects of alcohol on the brain may be one reason that alcohol abuse sometimes mimics or exacerbates normal changes of aging, because even a moderate intake of alcohol can impair the cognition and coordination skills that are already decreased with age.

Extreme care is required when treating the older alcoholic with medication. Toxicity in the central nervous system from psychoactive drugs increases with aging. Ingestion of antidepressants or tranquilizers can be particularly harmful because their effect is further potentiated by alcohol. The toxicity of other drugs (e.g., acetaminophen) is enhanced by alcohol and by the decrease in age-related clearance (Egbert 1993).

Alcohol consumption produces a change in sleep patterns, particularly in older adults. Unlike younger persons, the elderly take longer to fall asleep and do not sleep as restfully. Although alcohol may decrease the time it takes to fall asleep, this benefit is offset by frequent awakenings during the night caused by alcohol.

Symptoms of Elder Dependence

Health practitioners working with the elderly need to be concerned with, and sensitive to, possible alcohol abuse among their older clients. Signs of alcohol abuse in younger individuals (e.g., alcohol-induced pancreatitis or liver disease, blackouts, major trauma) occur infrequently in older adults. Instead, the elder alcoholic displays vague geriatric syndromes of contusions, malnutrition, self-neglect, depression, and falls. Also present may be symptoms of diarrhea, urinary incontinence, a decrease in functional status, failure to thrive, and apparent dementia (Egbert 1993). Symptoms of poor coordination or visual changes may also mimic the normal aging process while actually being due to excessive drinking. Although confusion and disorientation in an older client are often associated with dementia or Alzheimer's disease, they could be caused by other factors, including alcohol abuse. Assessment of the conditions is necessary to differentiate the normal physiological changes of aging from those due to excessive drinking.

Treatment for the Elderly Alcoholic

Because many elderly people do not live in big families or have work-related contacts, they are less likely to be referred for treatment than are younger drinkers. Too often, by the time the elderly alcoholic comes to the notice of any treatment agencies, the client's support systems and resources are severely decreased or depleted. Declining social, physical, and psychological performances are frequently found in the elderly alcoholic, thus exacerbating the difficulties of loneliness, depression, monotony, accidents, social conflict, loss, and the physiological changes of aging (Burns 1988).

Ageism has deterred the development of treatment programs specially designed for the elderly. Beliefs about the elderly as being too isolated, too embedded in denial of their illness, and too old to function have been detrimental in encouraging health professionals to work with chemically dependent seniors (Lindblom et al. 1992). Another factor that may play a role is that older adults often try to hide alcohol dependence because they consider such abuse sinful or feel they can handle any problems themselves (Ebersole and Hess 1994).

Whenever there is a suspicion or indication that an older adult is abusing alcohol, the health care provider should conduct a screening test. Although commonly used screening tests for alcohol abuse have focused on younger individuals, there is now a screening test designed specifically for older patients. This test, MAST-G, which consists of 24 questions and is the geriatric version of the Michigan Alcohol Screening Test (MAST), gives the health care provider a more efficient instrument to assess the elderly (Alcoholism 1993).

Treatment plans for the elderly problem drinker should emphasize social therapies. Elderly alcoholics tend to be more passive than younger alcoholics and may benefit from interpersonal involvement with professional health care personnel. Old people respond easily to emotional and social support (Gulino and Kadin 1986). Family therapy should be encouraged. Group therapy made up of middle-aged and older alcoholics can also be effective.

The older alcoholic who does seek help may be confronted with serious gaps and inadequacies in the health care delivery system. Substance abuse counselors must therefore be in contact with other agencies providing services to the elderly so that their help can be coordinated. They should be cognizant of the financial and transportation abilities of their elderly clients.

The aging alcoholic is difficult to treat. On the other hand, the prognosis for the geriatric problem drinker—a person who had lived to this point without recourse to alcohol and whose drinking is caused by losses and stress—is excellent. This individual often responds very positively to an alcohol recovery program, especially if it is accompanied by environmental interventions (Salisbury 1999). It is important that health care providers recognize this recovery potential. Proper education and awareness of a positive outcome for the geriatric problem drinker could increase the availability of resources; if the prognosis is good, providers and agencies should be more willing to spend resources on treatment.

Considering the magnitude of the problems and the likelihood that the numbers of older abusers will continue to increase, efforts need to be intensified to identify the causes and to develop appropriate interventions for treating alcohol dependence among the elderly. If not, such dependence can overwhelm those charged with meeting the health and social service needs of older adults (Parette et al. 1990).

TABLE 33–1A	*Answers to Facts and Myths About Aging*

| 1. | **False.** | 90% of older adults possess a healthy mental ability, 5% exhibit symptoms of chronic mental dysfunction, and another 5% display signs of acute mental impairment (Ebersole and Hess 1994. |
| 2. | **True.** | All the senses decrease with aging. Many of the changes begin slowly when the individual is in his or her mid-forties and increase with aging. (1) Vision: Particularly affected are peripheral |

TABLE 33–1A *Answers to Facts and Myths About Aging (Continued)*

vision, visual acuity, adaptation to dark, and accommodation (presbyopia). (2) Hearing: Decreased ability to hear high-frequency sounds with later changes possibly involving middle- and low-frequency sounds (presbycusis); males tend to show hearing loss earlier than women. (3) Taste: The number of functioning taste buds is reduced, which particularly affects the ability to taste sweet and salty flavors. (4) Touch: Simultaneously occurring with age are the loss of receptors and an increased threshold for stimulation; pain and pressure are thus not as easily sensed. (5) Smell: A decline in the number of fibers in the olfactory nerve has been reported, leading to speculation that smell also undergoes age-related changes.

3.	True.	As one ages, muscle fibers atrophy and decrease in number, with fibrous tissue slowly displacing muscle tissue. Overall muscle mass, muscle strength, and muscle movements decrease. The arm and leg muscles, which become particularly flabby and weak, also show these changes. Exercise is important to minimize the loss of muscle tone and strength.
4.	False.	Sexual interest and activity continue to play a pivotal role in providing life satisfaction (Atchley 1994).
5.	True.	Masters and Johnson, in their work on human sexuality, found that regular sexual expressions in the older adult are important for maintained sexual capacity and effective sexual performance (Atchley 1994).
6.	True.	Changes in sleep patterns occur along the entire life span. Restorative sleep declines rapidly with aging and by age 50 is reduced by 50%. It takes the elderly more time to achieve restorative sleep than younger adults, and also with aging, sleep is less effective (Burke and Walsh 1992).
7.	True.	Making up 13% of the population, the elderly accounted for more than 25% of all prescription drugs sold. This is not surprising, since the incidence of chronic diseases among the elderly is high and prescription drugs are often used with chronic disease (Cadieux 1993; Census Bureau 65 Plus in the U.S. 1995).
8.	False.	All age groups can learn. Limited, of course, by any physical limitations, older adults can usually master anything others can do if allowed a little more time. Jobs involving manipulation of objects or symbols or requiring discrete and clear responses are particularly well performed by older people (Atchley 1994; Burggraf and Stanley 1989).
9.	True.	Clinical depressive disorders increase in both prevalence and intensity with age. They may be called the "common cold" of the elderly and are expected to further increase in the years ahead (Ebersole and Hess 1990).
10.	False.	The ability to change and adapt has little to do with one's age but more with one's character.
11.	False.	Although a small number of aged are very well off and many are moderately comfortable, a large segment remains poor. According to government statistics, 12% of older adults live in poverty (Burke and Walsh 1992).
12.	True.	One out of three retirees encounters difficulty adjusting to retirement. Adapting to a diminished income and no longer being in a job-related environment were two of the most frequently listed causes of difficulty (Atchley 1994).
13.	True.	Senior citizens make up 13% of the population but constitute about 30% of the victims of crime. Business and investment frauds rank high on the list of white-collar crimes perpetrated against the elderly. Aged widows are particularly vulnerable (Ebersole and Hess 1994).
14.	False.	Eighty percent of older adults are healthy enough to carry on their normal life styles; 15% have chronic health conditions interfering with their lives; about 5% are institutionalized (Ebersole and Hess 1990).
15.	True.	Older persons are more reliable workers; their accuracy, performance, and stability are better; and the number of accidents is lower except in situations requiring rapid reaction time (Palmore 1979).
16.	False.	Most elderly have relatives, friends, and organizations that are significant to them. About two thirds do not consider loneliness a problem (Ebersole and Hess 1990).
17.	False.	Medicaid is a federally assisted, state-administered program that provides health care benefits to low-income persons. Medicare, on the other hand, provides health insurance basically to individuals 65 and over.
18.	False.	The term *ageism* reflects the negative prejudicial views of older people that pervade our youth-oriented society.
19.	True.	Nearly twice as many widowers wed annually as widows in spite of the fact that older widows outnumber older widowers four times. In addition, half of those widowers who do remarry choose wives under 65 years of age (Atchley 1994).

Table continued on following page

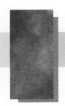

TABLE 33–1A   *Answers to Facts and Myths About Aging* (Continued)

20.   **True.**   Sociologists have found that, for the older widow, widowhood is viewed as ordinary with supports available from family, friends, and the community. The younger widow, however, is viewed differently; widowhood is not a normal occurrence. Young women are permitted to play the widow role for only a brief time and are considered to be single rather than widowed. Because they are in the minority, these women feel stigmatized by widowhood. The younger the widow, the more problems she encounters (Atchley 1994).

SUMMARY

There are a number of issues that older adults face as they age, and many myths exist that foster negative attitudes. Ageism is found in all levels of society and even among health care providers, thereby affecting the way we render care to our elderly clients.

Nurses who care for the elderly in various settings may function at various levels. All should be knowledgeable about the process of aging and be cognizant of the differences between normal and abnormal aging changes. Older adults face increasing problems of alcohol and suicide. The OBRA (Omnibus Budget Reconciliation Act) sets guidelines and a philosophy of care for clients to be free from unnecessary drugs and physical restraints.

Adequate pain assessment is important, with the nurse bearing in mind that the elderly tend to understate their pain. Sufficient pain medication should be administered. Nurses working with the mentally ill client should also know about psychotherapeutic approaches to the elderly. Nurses with special training and education may provide a variety of therapeutic modalities such as remotivation, reminiscing, or psychotherapy groups geared toward the special needs of this population.

When it comes to dying and death, older adults' wishes and those of their families are frequently ignored. The implementation of the PSDA (Patient Self-Determination Act) of 1990 can afford some clients autonomy and dignity in death.

Visit the **Evolve** website at
http://evolve.elsevier.com/Varcarolis
for a post-test on the content in this chapter.

Visit the **Evolve** website at
http://evolve.elsevier.com/Varcarolis
for additional self-study exercises.

Critical Thinking and Chapter Review

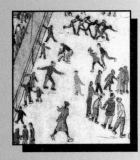

Critical Thinking

Mr. Morales, 72, is admitted to the ICU unit with alcohol withdrawal delirium.

■ He is combative and striking out with his hands, and the nurse on duty immediately restrains his hands.

1. Identify what legal and ethical problems existed with the nurse restraining Mr. Morales. What are the guidelines for physical restraints as presented in this chapter? What would be the best way to intervene with Mr. Morales during his acute withdrawal?

■ After treatment for withdrawal, he seems quiet, doesn't eat, sleeps very little during the night, and has many somatic complaints. He sighs a lot, and answers most questions with a "no" or "yeah" or not at all. He does admit to a suicide attempt three years ago after his wife died, and has stated that is when he started drinking. He has let his friends and activities drop and states he doesn't get much out of life anymore. For the most part he is hostile and suspicious of the health team, and prefers to be alone without visitors.

2. Assess Mr. Morales for depression and possible suicide using the Scale. How much can you complete using the Social Dysfunction Rating Scale provided in the chapter? What might be some interventions that would be appropriate for him once he leaves the hospital? (Is he a good candidate for alcohol treatment? Could his depression be compounded by his substance use? How could his depression be best treated? What kinds of social supports and referrals may be potentially helpful to Mr. Morales?)

■ Three years after discharge he is readmitted with lung cancer that has metastasized to almost every organ. He states that he wants to be comfortable but not to have his life prolonged. He knows he doesn't have much time to live, and the nurse talks to him about hospice. He is interested in hospice, and asks to see a priest.

3. When Mr. Morales is readmitted, you are his admitting nurse. How would you approach Mr. Morales (using the ANA's guidelines included)? What would be some of your other responsibilities in seeing that Mr. Morales got the best possible care for his situation? If the physician wanted to use radiation and chemotherapy, and you knew that Mr. Morales didn't want this, how would you proceed? What other ways could you help Mr. Morales? Identify other ways Mr. Morales could get spiritual support at this time.

4. Mr. Simon, age 85, lives with his family. He has advanced Alzheimer's disease and often has short-lived angry outbursts. Mr. Simon's family wants to keep him at home for as long as possible, but they are overwhelmed with his constant needs. Many well-meaning relatives have suggested that he be placed in a nursing home on a unit specifically designed for Alzheimer's clients.
Which of the following community placements might be best for Mr. Simon? Explain why.

A. Social day care
B. Adult day health (medical model)
C. Maintenance day care
D. Community mental health clinic

Chapter Review

Choose the most appropriate answer.

1. Which of the following is most essential to the provision of high-quality nursing assessment of elderly clients? The nurse's knowledge of

   1. normal aging
   2. drug interactions
   3. chronic diseases
   4. community supports

2. Mrs. W is an 82-year-old physically healthy widow who lives with her daughter and son-in-law, both of whom work during the day. Mrs. W states that she is lonely at home, since all her friends are elderly and unable to visit her. Mrs. W's daughter reports that her mother "isn't as sharp as she once was"

and mentions that she doesn't keep up with current news events and converses less during the evenings. The daughter asks if there are any programs that would be suitable for her mother. Assuming each is available, which should the nurse suggest?

1. Social day care center
2. Adult day health care center
3. Maintenance day care center
4. Skilled nursing facility

3. Knowledge the nurse needs when caring for an elderly client in restraint is

1. Restraint use appreciably enhances the overall safety of the client.
2. The nurse is responsible for client safety during the time the client is restrained.
3. Chemical restraint presents less potential for client harm than physical restraint.
4. Restraint may be used to prevent extubation if a nursing protocol exists.

4. Which understanding held by a nurse may prevent adequate intervention for an elderly client experiencing pain?

1. Pain perception decreases with aging.
2. Nonpharmacological interventions may provide control over pain.
3. Research has demonstrated that nurses tend to underestimate severe pain.
4. The nurse should assess verbal, facial, behavioral, and physical expressions of pain.

5. Which of the following is an action that is ethically unsuitable for a nurse?

1. Ignoring a DNR order for an elderly client in ICU
2. Implementing physician's orders to withhold artificial hydration from an elderly client in irreversible coma
3. Adhering to the choices made for an elderly client by the individual with DPAHC
4. Advocating for an elderly client in the terminal stage of cancer who wishes to discontinue chemotherapy

REFERENCES

Adelson, R., et al. (1982). Behavioral ratings of health professionals' interactions with the geriatric patient. *Gerontologist*, 22(3): 227.

AGS panel on chronic pain in older persons (1998). *Journal of American Geriatric Society*, 96:635–651.

Aguglia, E. (2000). Reboxetine in the maintenance therapy of depressive disorder in the elderly: A long-term open study. *International Journal of Geriatric Psychiatry*, 15(9):784–793.

Alcoholism (1993). New test designed to screen older patients. *Geriatrics*, 48(4):14.

Alford, D. (1986). *Managing ethical and legal dilemmas in the care of the elderly*. Presentation at Current Directions in Gerontological Nursing, Bethesda, MD.

American Nurses Association (ANA) (1991). *Position statement: The promotion of comfort and relief of pain in dying patients*. Washington, DC: The Association.

American Nurses Association (ANA) (1992). *Position statement on nursing and the patient self-determination act*. Washington, DC: The Association.

Arbesman, M. C., and Wright, C. (1999). Mechanical restraints, rehabilitation therapies, and staffing adequacy as risk factors for falls in an elderly hospitalized population. *Rehabilitation Nursing*, 24(3):122–128.

Atchley, R. (1994). *Social forces and aging*. Belmont, CA: Wadsworth.

Bergh, I., and Sjostrom, B. (1999). A comparative study of nurses' and elderly patients' ratings of pain and pain tolerance. *Journal of Gerontological Nursing*, 25(5):30.

Blakeslee, J. A., et al. (1991). Making the transition to restraint-free care. *Journal of Gerontological Nursing*, 17(2):4.

Blazer, D., et al. (1986). Suicide in late life: Review and commentary. *Journal of the American Geriatrics Society*, 34:519.

Boxwell, A. (1988). Geriatric suicide: The preventable death. *Nurse Practitioner*, 13(6):10.

Boyle, L. (1992). Legal implications of the Patient Self-Determination Act. *Nurse Practitioner Forum*, 3(1):12.

Brower, H. T. (1991). The alternatives to restraints. *Journal of Gerontological Nursing*, 17(2):18.

Buckwalter, K., et al. (1995). Community programs. In M. Hogstel (Ed.), *Geropsychiatric nursing*. St. Louis: Mosby–Year Book.

Buckwalter, K., and Piven, M. (1999). Depression. In J. Stone et al.

(Eds.), *Clinical gerontological nursing* Philadelphia: W.B. Saunders Company.

Bureau of the Census (1995). *Sixty-Five Plus in the United States.* Statistical brief. Washington, DC: U.S. Department of Commerce, Economics, and Statistics Administration.

Burggraf, V., and Stanley, M. (1989). *Nursing the elderly: A care plan approach.* Philadelphia: J. B. Lippincott.

Burke, M., and Walsh, M. (1992). *Gerontologic nursing care of the frail elderly.* St. Louis: Mosby–Year Book.

Burns, B. (1988). Treating recovering alcoholics. *Journal of Gerontological Nursing,* 14(4):18.

Burnside, I. (1988). *Nursing and the aged. A self-care approach.* New York: McGraw-Hill.

Butler, R. (1975). *Way survive? Being old in America.* New York: Harper & Row.

Butler, R., et al. (1991). *Aging and mental health.* New York: Macmillan.

Butler, R. (1993). Dispelling ageism: The cross-cutting intervention. *Generations,* 17(2):75.

Cadieux, R. (1993). Geriatric psychopharmacology. *Postgraduate Medicine,* 93(4):281.

Caserta, J. (1983). Public policy for long term care. *Geriatric Nursing,* 4(4):244.

Catina, J., et al. (1989). Older Americans and AIDS. Transmission, risks and primary prevention. *Gerontologist* 29(3):373.

Cavanaugh, J. (Ed.) (1993). *Health, adult development and aging.* Belmont, CA: Brooks Cole.

Celia, B. (2000). Age and gender differences in pain management. *Journal of Gerontological Nursing,* 26(5):7.

Centers for Disease Control (CDC) (1993). HIV/AIDS Surveillance Report. Atlanta, GA: 5(2):8.

Centers for Disease Control and Prevention (CDC) (1998). Prevent chronic diseases. Center for Disease Control and Prevention.

Chapman, C. and Syrjala, K. (1990). Measurement of pain. In J. Bonica (Ed.), *The management of pain.* Philadelphia Lea & Febiger, p. 580.

Chiao, E. Y., Ries, K. M., Sande, M. A. (1999). AIDS and the elderly. *Clinical Infectious Disease,* 28(4):740–745.

Curtis, J., et al. (1995). Use of the medical futility rationale in do-not-attempt-resuscitation orders. *Journal of American Medical Society,* 273(2):124.

Davis, G. (1997). Chronic pain management of older adults in residential settings. *Journal of Gerontological Nursing* 26(6) 16.

Devons, C. (1996). Suicide in the elderly: How to identify and treat patients at risk. *Geriatrics,* 51(3):67.

Donius, M., and Rader, J. (1994). Use of side-rails: Rethinking a standard practice. *Journal of Gerontological Nursing,* 20(11):23.

Ebersole, P., and Hess, P. (Eds.) (1990). *Toward healthy aging human needs and nursing response* (3rd ed.). St. Louis: Mosby–Year Book.

Ebersole, P., and Hess, P. (Eds.) (1994). *Toward healthy aging human needs and nursing response* (4th ed.). St. Louis: Mosby–Year Book.

Edwards, B. (1995). Physicians won't provide "futile" care. *American Journal of Nursing,* 95(9):56.

Egbert, A. (1993). The older alcoholic: Recognizing the subtle clinical clues. *Geriatrics,* 48(7):63.

Elliot, B., and Hybertson, D. (1982). What is it about the elderly that elicits a negative response? *Journal of Gerontological Nursing,* 8(10):568.

Evans, L., and Strumpf, N. (1989). Tying down the elderly: A review of the literature on physical restraints. *Journal of the American Geriatrics Society,* 37(1):65.

Flaherty, E. (2000). Assessing pain in older adults. *Journal of Gerontological Nursing,* 26(3):5.

Fultner, D., and Raudonis, B. (2000). Home care and hospice. In A. Lueckenotte (Ed.), *Gerontologic nursing* St. Louis: Mosby, p. 771.

Futility: The Concept and Its Use (1993). Northport Regional Medical Educational Center, National Center for Clinical Ethics. Northport, NY: Department of Veterans Affairs Medical Center.

Gadow, S. (1979). Advocacy nursing and new meanings of aging. *Nursing Clinics of North America,* 14:81.

Galloway, S., and Turner, L. (1999). Pain assessment in older adults who are cognitively impaired. *Journal of Gerontological Nursing,* 25(7):34.

Gambert, S. (1997). Alcohol abuse: medical effects of heavy drinking in later life. *Geriatrics,* 52(6):30.

Gobis, L. (1992). Recent developments in health care law relevant to health care providers. *Nurse Practitioner,* 17(3):77.

Goeber, B. (1996). Who decides if there is "triumph in the ultimate agony"? Constitutional theory and the emerging right to die with dignity William and Mary Law Review, Winter 37; 803.

Gomberg, E. (1980) Drinking and problem drinking among the elderly. Publication #1. *Alcohol, drugs, and aging: Usage and problems.* University of Michigan: Institute of Gerontology.

Gomez, G., et al. (1985). Beginning nursing students can change attitudes about the aged. *Journal of Gerontological Nursing,* 11(1):6.

Green, C. (1981). Fostering positive attitudes toward the elderly: A teaching strategy for attitude change. *Journal of Gerontological Nursing.* 7(3):169.

Gulino, C., and Kadin, M. (1986). Aging and reactive alcoholism. *Geriatric Nursing.* 7(3):148.

Harper, M. (1995). An overview of mental health. In M. Hogstel (Ed.), *Geropsychiatric nursing* (2nd ed.). St. Louis: Mosby–Year Book.

Hogstel, M. (1990). *Geriatric nursing.* St. Louis: C. V. Mosby.

Hogstel, M. (1995) *Geropsychiatric nursing* (2nd ed.). St. Louis: Mosby–Year Book.

Hogstel, M., and Weeks, S. (2000). Mental health. In A. Lueckenotte (Ed.), *Gerontologic nursing.* St. Louis: Mosby, p. 256.

Horne, A., and Blazer, D. (1992) The prevention of major depression in the elderly Clinics in Geriatric Medicine, 8(1):143.

Jacox, A., et al. (1994). Management of cancer pain. *Clinical Practice Guideline No. 9.* Agency for Health Care Policy and Research Publication and Human Services, Public Health Service, Agency for Health Care Policy and Research.

Janofsky, J. (1990). Assessing competency in the elderly. *Geriatrics,* 45(10):45.

Janssen, J. A., and Giberson, D. L. (1988). Remotivation therapy. *Journal of Gerontological Nursing,* 14(6):31.

Jenike, M. (Ed.) (1994). Ethical considerations in the care of the hopelessly ill patient. *Topics in Geriatrics,* 3(4):13.

Johnson, L. (1989). How to diagnose and treat chemical dependency in the elderly. *Journal of Gerontological Nursing,* 15(12):22.

Kashka, M. S., and Tweed, S. H. (1995). Substance related disorders. In M. Hogstel (Ed.), *Geropsychiatric nursing* (2nd ed.). St. Louis: Mosby–Year Book.

Kaufman, I. (1989). Life and death decisions. *New York Times,* October 6, 1989, p 21.

Kelsey, J. (1998). The use of antidepressants in long-term care and the geriatric patient: primary care issues. *Geriatrics* 53 (suppl 4): S12.

Kleiman, D. (1985). Uncertainty clouds of dying. *New York Times,* January 18:B1.

Lamy, P. P. (1988). Actions of alcohol and drugs in older people. *Generations,* 12(4):9

Lehne, R. (1998) *Pharmacology for nursing care* (3rd ed.). Philadelphia: W. B. Saunders.

Lekan-Rutledge, D. (1988). Functional assessment. In M. A. Matteson and E. S. McConnell (Eds.), *Gerontological nursing: Concepts and practice.* Philadelphia: W. B. Saunders.

Lueckenotte, A. (2000). Gerontologic assessment. In A. Lueckenotte (Ed.), *Gerontologic nursing.* St. Louis: Mosby.

Lindblom, L., et al. (1992). Chemical abuse: An intervention program for the elderly. *Journal of Gerontological Nursing,* 18(4):6.

Linn, M. W., et al. (1969). A social dysfunction rating scale. *Journal of Psychiatric Research,* 6:299.

Loebel, J. P. (1991) Precipitants to elder suicide. *Journal of the American Geriatric Society,* 39:407.

Luggen, A. (1998). Chronic pain in older adults a quality of life issue. *Journal of Gerontological Nursing,* 24(2):48.

Luggen, A. (2000). Pain. In A. Lueckenotte (Ed.), *Gerontologic nursing.* St. Louis: Mosby, p. 281.

MacKay, S. (1992). Durable power of attorney for health care. *Geriatric Nursing,* 13(2):99.

Marshall, J. (1978). Changes in aged white male suicide: 1948–1972. *Gerontologist,* 33:763.

Masters, R., and Marks F. (1990). The use of restraints. *Rehabilitation Nursing,* 15(1):22.

Matteson, M. A., and McConnell, E. S. (1988). *Gerontological nursing: Concepts and practice*. Philadelphia: W. B. Saunders.

Matteson, M. A., et al. (1997). *Gerontological nursing: Concepts and practice* (2nd ed.). Philadelphia: W. B. Saunders.

Matthews, S. (1979). *The social world of old women: Management of self-identity*. Sage Library of Social Research 78. Beverly Hills, CA: Sage Publications.

McCann, R., et al. (1994). Comfort care for terminally ill patients. *Journal of the American Medical Association, 272*(5):1263.

McCracken, A. (1998). Aging and alcohol. *Journal of Gerontological Nursing, 24*(4):37.

McIntosh, J. (1985). Suicide among the elderly: Levels and trends. *American Journal of Orthopsychiatry, 55*(2):287.

Meiner, S.E., and Miceli, D. G. (2000). Safety. In A. Lueckenotte (Ed.), *Gerontologic nursing*. St. Louis: Mosby.

Mezey, M., et al. (1994). Advance directives protocol: Nurses helping protect patients' rights. *Geriatric Nursing, 17*(5):204.

Miakowski, C. (1999). Pain and discomfort. In J. Stone (Ed.), *Clinical gerontological nursing*. Philadelphia: W.B. Saunders Company, p. 647.

Moak, G. (1990). Improving quality in psychogeriatric treatment. *Psychiatric Clinics of North America, 13*(1):99.

Moody, H. (1994). *Aging concepts and controversies*. Thousand Oaks, CA: Pine Forge Press.

Moore, C. V. (1992). Self-determined advance directives: New issues in primary care. *Nurse Practitioner Forum, 3*(1):10.

Moore, S. (1993). Rational suicide among older adults: A cause of concern? *Archives of Psychiatric Nursing, 8*(2):106–110.

Myers, R. (1994). Health legislation update. Restraint free environment for the elderly. *Ostomy Wound Management, 40*(19):12.

NANDA (1994). *Nursing diagnoses: Definitions and classification 1997–1998*. Philadelphia: NANDA.

National Citizens' Coalition for Nursing Home Reform (1991). *Nursing home reform law: The basics*. Washington, DC: National Citizens' Coalition for Nursing Home Reform.

National Institute of Mental Health (1999). Older adults: Depression and suicide facts. Washington, DC: NIMH. www.nimh.nih/gov/publicat/elderlydepsuicide.cfm pub#99-4593

Nelson, L. (1982). Questions of age. Doctors debate right to stop "heroic" effort to keep elderly alive. *Wall Street Journal*, September 7:20.

Neshkes, R., and Jarvik, L. (1986). Depression in the elderly: Current management concepts. *Geriatrics, 41*(9):51.

Neufield, R. R., et al. (1999). Restraint reduction reduces serious injuries among nursing home residents. *Journal of the American Geriatrics Society, 47*(10):1202.

Newhouse, P. A. (1996). Use of serotonin selective reuptake inhibitors in geriatric depression. *Journal of Clinical Psychiatry, 57*(5): 12–22.

Nikolassy, S. (1995). Nurses' role with the elderly in the community. In M. Stanley and P. Beare (Eds.), *Gerontological nursing*. Philadelphia: F. A. Davis.

Olson, M. (1997). *Healing the dying* (pp. 151–155). Albany, NY: Delmarr Publishers.

Osgood, N. (1988). Suicide in the elderly: Clues and prevention. Belle Mead, NJ: *Carrier Foundation Letter No. 133*, April 1988.

Ostrander, N. (1992). Alcoholism and aging—A rural community's response. *Aging Today*, February/March:19.

Palmore, E. (1979). Advantages of aging. *Gerontologist, 17*:220.

Parette, H., et al. (1990). Nursing attitudes toward geriatric alcoholism. *Journal of Gerontological Nursing, 16*(1):26.

Penninx, B. W. (1998). Depressive symptoms and physical decline in community-dwelling older persons. *Journal of American Medical Association, 279*:832–836.

Pfeiffer, E. (1978). Sexuality in the aging individual. In R. Solnick (Ed.), *Sexuality and aging*. Los Angeles, CA: University of Southern California Press.

Pinch, W. J., and Parsons, M. E. (1992). The patient self-determination act. *Nurse Practitioner Forum, 3*(1):16.

Preston, T. (1986). Ageism undermines relations with elderly. *Medical World News*, December 8:26.

Printz, L. A. (1992). Terminal dehydration, a compassionate treatment. *Archives of Internal Medicine, 152*:697.

Rabins, P. V., et al. (2000). Effectiveness of a nurse-based outreach program for identifying and treating psychiatric illness in the elderly. *Journal of American Medical Association, 283*(21):2802–2809.

Reynolds, C. (1994). Treatment of depression in later life. *American Journal of Medicine, 97*(Suppl. 6A):395.

Richardson, R., Lowenstein, S., and Weissberg, M. (1989). Coping with the suicidal elderly: A physician's guide. *Geriatrics, 44*(9):43.

Ronsman, K. (1987). Therapy for depression. *Journal of Gerontological Nursing, 13*(12):18.

Rosenthal, E. (1991). Filling the gap where a living will won't do. *New York Times*, January 17:B9.

Ross, H. (1981). Society/cultural views regarding death and dying. *Topics in Clinical Nursing, 3*(3):3.

Sabin, J. D. (1987). AIDS: The new "great imitator." *Journal of American Geriatric Society, 35*(5):467.

Sahr, N. (1999). Assessment and diagnosis of elderly depression. *Clinical Excellent Nurse Practice, 3*(3):158–164.

Salisbury, S. (1999). Alcoholism. In J. Stone (Ed.), *Clinical gerontological nursing* (p. 537). Philadelphia: W.B. Saunders Company.

Sapp, M., and Bliesmer, M. (1995). A health promotion/protection approach to meeting elders' health care needs through public policy and standards of care. In M. Stanley and P. Beare (Eds.), *Gerontological nursing*. Philadelphia: F. A. Davis.

Schlossberg, C., and Hart, M. A. (1992). Legal perspectives. In M. Burke and M. Walsh (Eds.), *Gerontologic nursing care of the frail elderly* (p. 469). St. Louis: Mosby–Year Book.

Schuerman, D. (1994). Clinical concerns. AIDS in the elderly. *Journal of Gerontological Nursing, 20*(7):11.

Seers, K. (1999). Pain and older people. In S. Redfern and F. Ross (Eds.), *Nursing older people*. London: Harcourt-Brace, 495–510.

Shawler, C., et al. (1992). Clinical considerations: Surrogate decision making for hospitalized elders. *Journal of Gerontological Nursing, 18*(6):5.

Smith, D. (1992). Advance directive editorial. *Journal of Enterostomal Therapy, 19*(4):109.

Snow, R., and Atwood, K. (1985). Probable death: Perspectives of the elderly. *Southern Medical Journal, 78*:851.

Stanley, M., and Beare, P. (1995). *Gerontological nursing*. Philadelphia: F. A. Davis.

Steingart, A. (1991). Day programs. In J. Sadovoy et al. (Eds.), *Comprehensive review of psychiatry*. Washington, DC: American Psychiatry Press.

Stilwell, E. M. (1991). Nurses' education related to the use of restraints. *Journal of Gerontological Nursing, 17*(2):23.

Stolley, J. (1995). Freeing your patients from restraints. *American Journal of Nursing, 95*(2):27.

Suicide Rate Among Elderly Rises, Study Says (1991). *New York Times*, September 19:A25.

Sullivan-Marx, E., et al. (1999). Restraint-free care. In J. Stone (Ed.), *Clinical gerontological nursing* (p. 573). Philadelphia: W.B. Saunders Company.

SUPPORT Investigators (1995). A controlled trial to improve care for seriously ill hospitalized patients. *Journal of American Medical Association, 27*(20):1591.

Taylor, M. (1995). Benefits of dehydration in terminally ill patients. *Geriatric Nursing, 16*(6):271.

Tolchin, M. (1989). When long life is too much: Suicide rises among elderly. *New York Times*, July 19:A15.

USDHSS (1990). United States Department of Health and Human Services National Institute on Aging: Special Report on Aging 1990. National Institute of Health. Public Health Service. Bethesda, MD: Government Printing Office.

Valanis, D., et al. (1987). Alcohol use among bereaved and non-bereaved older persons. *Journal of Gerontological Nursing, 13*(5): 26.

Virmani, L., et al. (1994). Relationship of advance directives to physician-patient communication. *Archives of Internal Medicine, 154*:909.

Wallace, R., et al. (1993). HIV infection in older patients: When to expect the unexpected. *Geriatrics 48*(6):61.

Wallis, C. (1986). To feed or not to feed? *Time*, March 31:60.

Walsh, M. (1992). The frail elderly population. In M. Burke and M. Walsh (Eds.), *Gerontologic nursing care of the frail elderly*. St. Louis: Mosby–Year Book.

Wooten-Bielski, K. (1999). HIV and AIDS in older adults. *Geriatric Nursing, 20*(5):268.

Wynne, C., et al. (2000). Comparison of pain assessment instruments. *Geriatric Nursing*, 21(1):20.

Young, L., and Koda-Kimble, M. (1995). *Applied therapeutics: The clinical use of drug*. Vancouver, WA: Applied Therapeutics.

Young, D. (1999). Acute pain management protocol. *Journal of Gerontological Nursing*, 25(6):10.

Zerbe, K. J. (1999). *Women's health in primary care*. Philadelphia: W.E. Saunders Company.

Zerwekh, J. (1993). Dehydration: A natural analgesic when death is imminent. *Critical Care Specialist*, 1(1):3.

Zung, W. K. (1965). A self-rating depression scale. *Archives of General Psychiatry* 12:63.

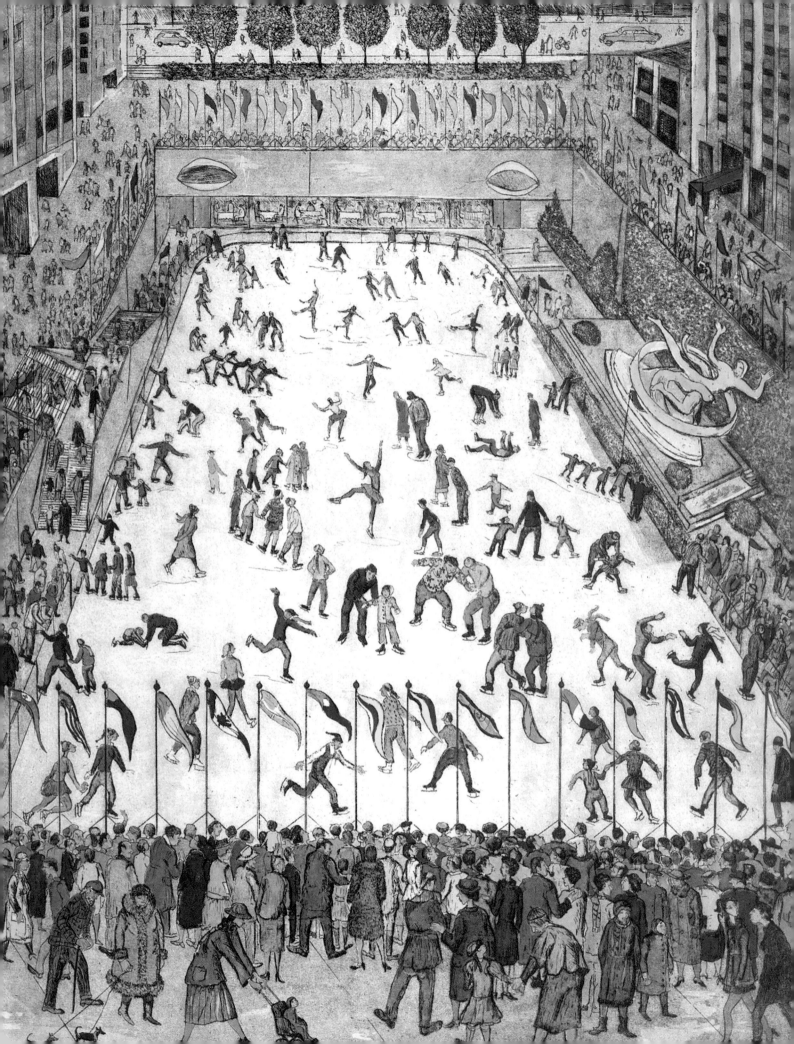

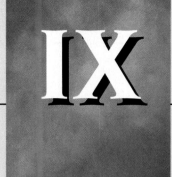
Other Intervention Modalities

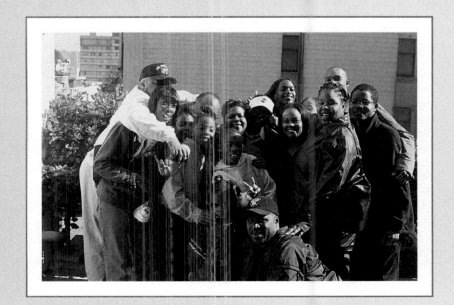

Do not protect yourself by a fence,
but rather by your friends.

CZECH PROVERB

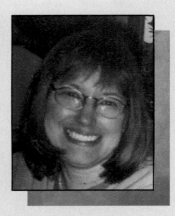

MARIKEN E. WOGSTAD-HANSEN

I am a clinical specialist in psychiatric nursing and a licensed psychologist in the State of Minnesota. While in my doctoral program, I was offered the opportunity to create a new role in a women's center where I had done my master's level internship. The center is a nonprofit agency developed as a small, grass-roots resource organization in the 1970s. It has since grown into a place where women can come for support and resource counseling, legal advice, chemical dependency treatment, and mental health services. The mental health clinic provides individual, group, and family psychotherapy as well as psychiatric services. As the first nurse to work at the clinic, I was hired initially to assist the psychiatrist in managing the medication clinic. This soon evolved into a collaborative practice in which I have been free to develop a unique, integrative role of nurse clinician and psychologist.

As a nurse, I am able to take a holistic approach to psychiatric care. This includes counseling on health promotion, including the role of nutrition, exercise, and various alternative modalities, as well as traditional psychotherapy and psychotropic medications. My colleagues come from a range of disciplines and approaches, including clinical social work, psychology, art therapy, music therapy, nursing, and psychiatry. The clinic offers a variety of therapy groups, including four dialectical behavioral therapy (DBT) groups, featuring a blend of Eastern meditative philosophies and Western cognitive behavior therapy (CBT), focusing on a team approach to assisting clients with borderline characteristics. Other groups offered are mixed issues, depression education and support, sexual abuse survivors, grieving, divorce, and sexuality. Childcare facilities are available while women receive services at the center. Transportation is provided for clients receiving chemical dependency treatment, and the center is located on a major bus line.

Part of my role is to function as a resource person to other staff members. The therapists refer clients for psychiatric evaluation and medication management, and I provide consultation and collaboration. I also have my own caseload of individual psychotherapy clients and co-lead a long-term psychotherapy group. In addition, I coordinate psychiatric services with primary clinics around the five-county metro area, as clients come from a variety of locations and insurance plans. There are no lab facilities on site, so women who need blood levels monitored are directed to use their primary care provider, and I coordinate services with them. The psychiatrist is on site four hours per week and is available for phone consultation. We meet weekly for forty-five minutes of face-to-face case management.

I see women from a wide spectrum of ages, socioeconomic, and ethnic backgrounds. Trauma is a common theme, and many of the women have post-traumatic stress syndrome (PTSD), depression, anxiety, dissociation, and psychotic symptoms. I try to provide an integrative approach, offering a variety of modalities and options. For example, several therapists at the clinic are trained in thought field therapy (TFT), a technique based on acupuncture meridians, in which the client is taught a series of tapping sequences which they can utilize on their own when needed, for symptoms such as anxiety, depression, or addictive cravings. The clinic also has a massage therapist available two days a week with reasonable rates. I may refer to local resources for alternative approaches such as acupuncture as well as counseling her on nutrition specific to mood disorders, or suggesting a combination of herbal preparations for depression and anxiety. My background in nursing has been a foundation for incorporating a collaborative, educational approach to psychiatric care.

Vignette

■ *One client, Sally, is a woman in her late 50s who is just now having memories of childhood sexual abuse by her father. She is working through many losses, including those of her husband, children, and her own childhood. For many years, she has been closed down emotionally, isolated, with few supports. Through encouragement in individual therapy, she reluctantly agreed to attend a day* treatment program. She gradually was able to participate in the groups there, and recently graduated. She is showing great courage in coming to terms with her past and how it has affected her life. She is also struggling with multiple health problems, including COPD, obesity with gastric stapling, and cataracts. I referred her for thought field therapy to use PRN to manage symptoms of PTSD, especially flashbacks, and anxiety, and distraction techniques. In addition, I communicate frequently with her primary care provider in the clinic to coordinate care and avoid drug-drug interactions while prescribing anti-depressants.

Vignette

■ Another client, Janet, came to me following an abusive relationship. She had almost constant panic attacks, depression, and flashbacks, as well as physical pain from the assaults on her body. She had had a bad reaction to side effects from antidepressant medication in the past, and was terrified to try traditional medication. I offered her a combination of cognitive-behavioral and meditation approaches in therapy, and gradually titrated her up to 1800 mg per day of St. John's wort. She also attended biofeedback sessions at a neurology clinic and learned relaxation techniques. After six months, she is no longer having panic attacks, attends a support group for abuse survivors, and is successfully supporting herself at a new, higher paying job.

The ability to combine skills from both nursing and psychology enables the application of an integrative, holistic approach to working with women in a setting specializing in their needs. This also illustrates the ways in which career development can take twists and turns in the life of one nurse.

Outline

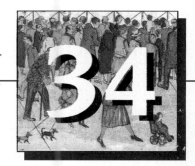

34

Therapeutic Groups

CATHERINE M. LALA

Key Terms and Concepts

The key terms and concepts listed here also appear in color where they are first defined or discussed in this chapter.

behavioral group therapy

cognitive-behavioral group therapy

feedback

flooding

insight

self-help groups

support groups

systematic desensitization

universality

Yalom's therapeutic factors

Objectives

After studying this chapter, the reader will be able to

1. Identify basic concepts used in group therapy.

2. Distinguish between Peplau's three phases of group development.

3. Describe the different roles group members may adopt within a group.

4. Discuss the approaches to group therapy for (a) therapeutic milieu groups, (b) time-limited-psychotherapy groups, (c) cognitive-behavioral therapy groups, (d) behavioral group therapy, and (e) self-help groups.

5. Use three facilitating techniques in a small group setting.

6. Act out an intervention for a group member who (a) monopolizes a group, (b) complains but rejects help, (c) is demoralizing, and (d) is silent.

7. Contrast and compare the guidelines for establishing an inpatient versus an outpatient therapy group.

GROUP CONCEPTS

Definition of Group

Thompson (1999) defines a group as "a number of people coming together, sharing some purpose, interest, or concern, and staying together long enough for the development of a network of relationships which includes them all. Recognition of this network brings the concept of group. Each member of the group is influenced by the emotional climate creating an interdependence."

Group work, by its very format, offers unique opportunities to experience and work through issues of intimacy, differentiation, and individuation. It is usually impossible for individuals to view themselves as existing alone and affecting no one after participating in a group therapy for a significant period. Individuals are brought together in groups and are expected to work at their relationships with others in the group. The easy escape response of changing relationships is highly discouraged in favor of resolving conflicts in the group setting (Rutan and Waller 1993).

Common Group Phenomena

Groups are based on different models and theoretical orientations. However, they have the following in common:

Group acceptance: Individuals feel that they are respected by, accepted by, and belong to the group.

Reality testing: Group members can monitor each person's reactions and behaviors, providing feedback in an open and nonthreatening manner.

Universality: Group members feel secure when they realize that they do not have unique problems and are not so different from other persons.

Ventilation: The expression of suppressed feelings, ideas, or events to other group members in the service of a better understanding of self.

Learning: Members gain insight into their problems by learning to examine or explore symptoms in themselves as well as in other group members. They gain knowledge about new areas, such as social skills and sexual behavior.

Altruism: Members give advice, support, and encouragement to one another. It involves **putting another's needs before one's own.**

Transference: The projection of feelings, thoughts, and wishes onto the group leader.

Interactions: Group therapy provides group members with the opportunity to assert themselves to improve communication.

Phases of Group Development

Three phases of group development are described by Peplau: (Belcher and Fish 1995): (1) orientation, (2) working, and (3) termination phase.

For group psychotherapy, there is also a pre-orientation phase in which the nurse leader assesses a potential member for therapy and begins the necessary therapeutic alliance that contains the member's anxiety. Clients need to feel safe in a group if they are expected to participate.

ORIENTATION. The leader's role is to set up an atmosphere of respect, confidentiality, and trust. The purpose of the group is stated, and members are helped to relax and feel comfortable. The group task is getting to know one another, to observe each other, and begin to take steps toward the working phase.

WORKING PHASE. The leader's role is to keep the group focused on the work of the group and to support individual members in accomplishing their goals. The nurse leader ties together common themes, encourages honest expression, and yet prevents any member from being verbally attacked. The members are actively involved in participating in working toward the group's goals.

TERMINATION. The group leader's task is to acknowledge the contributions of each member and the experience as a whole. Group members prepare for separation and help each other prepare for the future.

Roles of Group Members

Roles are dynamic and have an expected set of behaviors. Some roles, such as initiator and elaborator, promote growth in groups, while roles such as the blocker inhibit growth in groups. Nurse group leaders use their knowledge of roles to lead individual members to increase their personal growth. For example, a leader could help the opinion seeker develop his or her ability to be more assertive.

- **Opinion giver**—States beliefs or values.
- **Opinion seeker**—Asks for clarification of beliefs or values.
- **Information giver**—Offers facts or personal experience.
- **Information seeker**—Asks for facts pertinent to what is being discussed.
- **Initiator**—Proposes new ideas on how the goal can be reached or how the problem can be viewed.
- **Elaborator**—Expands on another person's idea and takes the idea and works out what would happen if it were adopted.

- **Coordinator**—Brings together ideas or suggestions.
- **Orientor**—Keeps the group focused on goals or questions the direction taken by the group.
- **Evaluator or Critic**—Examines possible group solutions against group standards and goals.
- **Clarifier**—Checks out what someone said by restating or testing.
- **Recorder**—Acts as the group's memory (e.g., takes notes).
- **Summarizer**—Pulls together related ideas, restates suggestions, and offers decisions or conclusions.

Terminology That Reflects the Group Process

The nurse learns to recognize a number of processes and phenomena when working with people in groups. Box 34–1 identifies terminology that is central to group work.

FACILITATING TECHNIQUES USED BY GROUP LEADERS

The following examples are scenarios for techniques adapted from Van Servellan (1984). Each nurse can build upon and develop a list that fits his or her own style. The basis for all communication is therapeutic communication skills, as described more fully in Chapter 11. Refer to Table 34–1.

THERAPEUTIC FACTORS COMMON TO ALL GROUPS

In the group, clients hear others share similar concerns, fantasies, and life experiences. The realization that they are not alone in their situation may offer considerable relief and a "welcome to the human race experience." The name of this concept is **universality.** Universality is one of the therapeutic factors of group therapy described by Yalom (1995) that can guide therapeutic interventions. Another therapeutic factor is **instilling hope.** Groups can instill hope in clients who are demoralized or pessimistic. Group members can gain hope from others with similar problems that have made positive changes in their lives through therapy. Other therapeutic factors include **developing social skills,**

interpersonal learning, expression of feelings (**catharsis**), and learning that each member can be useful to other members, which can in turn prevent morbid self-absorption and promote growth (**altruism**). People in groups may also learn to identify with healthier aspects of other group members or the leader and imitate behaviors that the clients wish to develop (**imitative behavior**) (Wolfe 1993).

BOX 34–1 *Terms Central to Group Work*

Group content—all that is said in the group
Group process—constant movement as members seek to reduce tensions that arise when people attempt to have their individual needs met while working to meet group goals; also includes all nonverbal behavior, such as yawning, facial expressions, and body posture
Confrontation—the process whereby problems or conflicts that have been covert are brought into the open
Covert content—the deeper, underlying meaning of messages or what is happening in the group
Dynamics—the ebb and flow of power and energy within a group
Feedback—letting group members know how they affect each other
Hidden agenda—individual, subgroup, or leader goals that are at cross-purposes to the group's goals
Cohesiveness—the bond between members of a group, measured by the group's willingness to work toward common goals; members' sense of identification with the group
Conflict—open disagreement among members; may be positive, indicating involvement with the task, or negative, indicating frustration with an impossible task or intergroup conflict
Closed group—membership is restricted; no new members are added when others leave
Open group—a group in which new members are added as others leave
Subgroup—an individual or a small group that is isolated within a larger group and functions separately; members of a subgroup may have more loyalty, similar goals, or perceived similarities to one another than they do to the larger group
Milieu therapy—therapy focused on positive environmental manipulation to effect positive change
Behavior modification—a treatment modality that focuses on modifying and changing specific observable dysfunctional patterns of behavior by means of stimulus and response conditioning.

TABLE 34–1   *Useful Communications Techniques*

COMMUNICATION TECHNIQUE	EXAMPLE	OUTCOME
Seeking Clarification	**Leader:** "Are you trying to tell us that you feel upset?" **Member:** (Jill) "Yes, I suppose I was."	Jill becomes aware of not being clear and learns to take responsibility for feelings.
Encouraging Description	**Leader:** "How did you feel when Mrs. X said that?" **Member:** "I was angry because it devalued the group and reminded me of my mother."	Member deals in greater depth with an experience.
Presenting Reality	**Leader:** "Would other group members feel Jill was unstable if they interviewed her for a job? You don't appear shaky to me." **Member:** Jill listens and considers other possibilities.	Member compares perception of self with others' perception of her.
Focusing	**Leader:** "Let's identify one problem you have and talk more about that." **Member:** Jill channels her thinking, and the group identifies specific topics they can resolve before the session ends.	Members increase their understanding of one problem before jumping to others. Other techniques include:
Reframing	**Leader:** "You have been so involved in your career, you chose not to get married until later on in life." **Member:** "That's true. I thought I was a loser for not being married yet."	Frames the situation in a positive, healthier manner that fits the facts of the situation.
Feedback	**Member:** "No one talks to me on the unit." **Leader:** "I notice that you go straight to your room after meals and avoid all other activities. Perhaps you give a message that you are not available." **Member:** "Maybe that is true. . . ."	Delivers a new perspective on the processing of information. The high degree of immediacy focuses on the sender of a message in a nonthreatening way.
Helping Clients gain Insight Into Their Behavior	**Member:** "I don't know why I am so shy. . . . I will never change." **Leader:** "Perhaps if you help the recreation therapist set up the Sunday movie snacks, you can feel more involved."	Member considers new behavior, and the member's experience of self is validated by the leader, providing a practical response that acknowledges her emotion and promotes increased responsibility for the outcome.

GROUP PROTOCOLS

A **protocol,** or description, of the actual nursing care involved in a group, includes:

- The clear, concise objectives of the group.
- The methods or means to evaluate the success of the group.
- The organization of such features as:
  Frequency and times of group meetings
  Qualifications of group leaders
  Descriptions of types of clients, their behaviors, and the diagnoses that are most suited to a type of group

An example of a standard group protocol format is provided in Box 34–2.

EXPECTED OUTCOMES

After a group experience, when members are presented with qualitative outcome criteria such as a questionnaire based on the therapeutic factors of groups (Yalom 1995), they tend to respond in these ways:

- "I do not feel alone."
- "I need this."
- "Why don't they have more groups like this?"
- "Extend the group from 1 hr to 2 hrs."
- "I'm more able to open up."
- "After being in this group, I am more capable of reaching out to others."
- "If I want to change a behavior or something about myself, I'll try it in group first."

It may be easier to achieve measurable outcomes with education and psychoeducation groups than with therapy groups. A nurse can define key quality indicators and can track those indicators over a period of time. For example, the key quality indicators for successful outcome (client education) in a medication education group could be any of the following: The clients will (1) ask questions about medication, (2) maintain compliance while hospitalized (or in the community), and (3) report side effects.

Outcome criteria can also be used by an outside evaluator (e.g., another trained staff member) to help evaluate the effectiveness of group. For example (Paleg and Jongsma 2000):

■ Therapist gives feedback to group members about their behavior.
■ Therapist facilitates interactions between group members.
■ Therapist checks for understanding of what is being said.

THE ROLE OF THE NURSE IN THERAPEUTIC GROUPS

Education and Preparation

Psychiatric mental health nurses can be involved in therapy groups as well as other groups. Psychiatric

mental health nurses who conduct group psychotherapy need specific education and experience. The American Nurses' Association (2000) sets the standard for graduate study (master's degree or higher) for psychiatric advanced practice nurses, which includes the necessary theory, supervision, and clinical practice.

Training obtained through college courses, workshops, and ongoing clinical supervision is essential. Psychiatric advanced practice nurses can serve as role models and mentors for nurses who wish to learn about various types of groups. Group therapy always has a theoretical base; this base is one that the leader believes in, is educated in, and believes to be appropriate for the outcome criteria of the group.

Nurse group therapists need to have individual or peer-group supervision. In supervision, the nurse reviews the process of therapy and his or her own biases and intuitions with a more experienced therapist or peers. Group work provides a rich learning environment. All psychotherapeutic work with clients—whether it is individual, couple, family, child, group, or any other type—requires interpersonal learning with a senior clinician who is trained in that particular therapy (Critchley and Maurin 1985). In supervision, a relationship exists between the supervisor and the nurse supervised that helps the supervised nurse become a better therapist.

Many master's-prepared nurses pursue additional training, certification, or credentials in group psychotherapy. On the bachelor and associate degree levels, nurses with an understanding of group therapy and process may be actively involved in leading therapeutic groups such as milieu groups and psychoeducational groups.

The major groups discussed here are:

■ Psychoeducational groups
■ Therapeutic milieu groups
■ Time-limited therapy groups
■ Cognitive-behavioral groups
■ Spirituality groups
■ Behavioral groups
■ Self-help groups

Psychoeducational Groups

Medication Groups

Psychiatric nurses are the ideal professionals to teach in a medication education group for long-term self-management care. Sharing a concrete and objective here-and-now subject such as medication information in a group setting can also facilitate discussion. Clients often listen to the experience of others who have taken medication, and have an opportunity to ask questions without the fear that they will

Box 34–2   *Standard Group Protocol*

1. Name of the group
2. Identify group leader(s).
3. Identify the purpose and goals of the group.
4. Identify the conceptual/theoretical framework for the group.
5. State objectives of the group.
6. Group format/group structure

   ■ Where to meet, when, how long each session; duration of group (if known)
   ■ Roles and responsibility of group members/of group leaders

7. Measurement of outcomes, evaluation methods, tools, frequency of evaluations
8. Clarify method of documenting group process and individual client progress.

go against the prescriber's recommendations. Medication groups are designed to teach clients about their medications, answer their questions, and prepare them for discharge. Clients are encouraged to know which medications they are taking before they come to group. Resources provided by a leader might include pencils, an overhead projector, transparencies, and handouts. To promote medication compliance, one transparency (or handout) could ask:

■ What medicines are you taking now?
■ What is the main action of these medications?
■ What are the side effects of these medications?

Prior to inviting a client to a group, the ability of a potential group member to concentrate and tolerate a group needs to be evaluated. It is helpful to keep a group focused on one class of medication, such as mood stabilizers for persons diagnosed with bipolar disorder. The nurse provides medication education so the client will be knowledgeable about the following (Ramos 1996):

■ Name of medication
■ Reasons for taking the medication
■ Exact dose of the medication
■ Appropriate time to take medication
■ Common side effects
■ A wish to change the medication regimen will first be discussed with a health care provider prior to any changes
■ Favorite ways to remember to take the medication on time
■ The importance of informing other health care providers of medication treatment, in order to avoid adverse medication interactions
■ What foods and over-the-counter medications to avoid
■ Approximately how long medication will be needed

Clients can be given a drug information sheet before they leave and are encouraged to review the material several times. Clients are encouraged to participate in treatment by being informed, and communication with the prescriber of the medication is stressed. Box 34–3 gives a protocol for setting up a medication group. For clients who have reading or cognitive difficulties, it is helpful to underscore the main advantages and possible side effects of their medication in one-on-one sessions. Table 34–2 is an example of a medication group questionnaire that the nurse leader can use as a guide to understanding a client's teaching needs. Clients who have used particular medicines can be helpful to others who are weighing the risks and benefits of starting a

Box 34–3 *Example of Medication Education Group*

DESCRIPTION OF GROUP

A group for all clients, regardless of level of concentration, that prepares clients for self-management of medication on discharge.

CRITERIA FOR PATIENT SELECTION

Open to all clients, except those who are displaying the following behaviors: suicidal, homicidal, potential for assault.

MEDIA

Overhead transparencies, films, patient medication education sheets.

PURPOSE

1. To educate clients on the primary function of their medications.
2. To provide information on side effects (that benefits can outweigh risks).
3. To describe a mechanism to negotiate relationships with health care workers.
4. To enhance a sense of self-control over treatment.

PROCEDURE

1. Orientation and introduction to the group.
2. Brief description of major symptoms in a diagnosis.
3. Overview of antipsychotics or antidepressants.
4. Use of Albany Medical Center patient medication education sheets.
5. Specific open-question period.

BEHAVIORAL OBJECTIVES

At the end of the 45-minute session, patients will be able to

1. State one symptom they have that is treated by their medication.
2. Be able to ask at least one question about their medicine.
3. Identify one mechanism that helps with compliance with medicine.

THEORETICAL JUSTIFICATION

Even people who think they are compliant only take 80% of doses. Counseling and therapy are always adjuncts to drug therapy.

Ott, C. A. [2000]. *Pediatric psychopharmacology*. Wheaton, MD: American Healthcare Institute.

TABLE 34–2 *Medication Group Evaluation*

CRITERIA	STRONGLY AGREE	SOMEWHAT AGREE	AGREE	DISAGREE	STRONGLY DISAGREE
1. I know the names of the medications I am taking.					
2. I know what symptoms the medications can help me with.					
3. I know the common side effects of my medication(s).					
4. I feel comfortable talking to my prescriber if I am having problems with my medications.					
5. It is important to take my medication at the same time every day.					

medication. Clients often need to attend more than one medication group to clarify questions and reinforce knowledge.

Sexuality Groups

Acquired immunodeficiency syndrome (AIDS) remains one of the most serious public health issues in the United States and throughout the world. Psychiatric diagnoses associated with AIDS include organic mental disorders, adjustment disorder with depressed or anxious mood, panic disorder, major depression, psychoactive substance abuse, and sleep disorders. Clients who, as a result of the manic phase of bipolar disorder or the abuse of substances, have used poor judgment in sexual liaisons are at high risk for AIDS and other sexually transmitted diseases. Topics for discussion include:

■ AIDS
■ Modes of transmission and treatment of sexually transmitted diseases
■ Education on how to use a condom and other forms of safer sex
■ Sexuality and the use of psychotropic drugs
■ The effect of antidepressants on sexuality

Nutrition groups and women's and men's health groups are other examples of psychoeducational groups.

Therapeutic Milieu Groups

Therapeutic milieu groups aim to help increase clients' self-esteem, decrease social isolation, encourage appropriate social behaviors, and educate clients in basic living skills. These groups are often led by occupational or recreational therapists, although nurses frequently co-lead them. Examples of therapeutic milieu groups are recreational groups, physical activity groups, creative arts groups, self-care groups, and story-telling groups (Table 34–3).

Recreational Groups

Recreational groups focus on engaging in teamwork, learning how to spend leisure time, and increasing self-esteem by completing a project. Nostalgia groups encourage clients to talk about earlier years and about the good things in life. Exercise groups let clients experience physical and psychological release through physical exercise and games.

Physical Activity Groups

In many treatment programs for the mentally ill, exercise programs are typically prescribed by the recreational, occupational, or activity therapist. However, in any psychiatric treatment setting, a group of clients exists for which standard exercise tests and prescriptions are not effective and in some cases are actually contraindicated. In these cases, nurses are in the best position to offer guidance and prescriptions (Dexter 1992).

The nurse should discuss an exercise prescription with the client's psychiatrist and define with clients the kind of exercise they like best. Depending on the frequency, intensity, and duration of exercise, medical laboratory tests may be recommended, along with a full history and physical examination by an internist for medical clearance.

TABLE 34–3 *Therapeutic Milieu Groups*

MILIEU GROUPS	TARGET POPULATION	GOALS	FREQUENCY AND DURATION
Activity groups (hospital) **Recreational:** Current events, nostalgia, exercise, horticulture, pets, crafts **Self-care:** Reality, cooking, grooming, discharge group, community meeting **Creative arts:** Art, dance/movement, poetry, psychodrama, music, bibliotherapy **Self-awareness:** Feelings (men's groups, women's group) **Education:** Stress reduction, skills training, medication groups, assertiveness training, ways to increase self-esteem **Physical activity**	The psychiatric client in the hospital or in a day treatment program.	*Overall goal:* Increase in self-esteem: 1. Help clients manage time. 2. Increase cooperation. 3. Teach specific knowledge, skills, or both, related to patient's illness, treatment, or interpersonal communication (psychoeducational).	*Meets:* Once per week or more, often depending on the program.

Creative Arts Groups

The goal of creative arts therapy is for clients to get in touch with feelings and emotions through books, poems, music, and dance. Dance therapy, art therapy, and music therapy are helpful to clients who are demonstrating withdrawn behaviors and are not amenable to "talk" therapy. Specially trained therapists lead these groups with withdrawn clients.

Social Skills Groups

Examples of social skills groups include cooking groups, activities of daily living or grooming groups, and client government groups. These types of groups educate clients and provide an opportunity for staff members to assess a client's ability to function in areas such as planning, budgeting, and other basic skills needed for living.

Time-Limited Therapy Groups

Kanas, et al. (1989) describes an example of a time-limited psychotherapy group for persons diagnosed with schizophrenia. All persons in the group demonstrate the symptoms of auditory hallucinations and social isolation. After eliciting information from each member by encouraging them to share their experiences, the nurse therapist inquires about their coping strategies. For example: "How do you handle the voices that you hear?"

The goal of the group is to diminish clients' feelings of isolation and find ways of coping with psychotic symptoms. The group is co-led, is closed, includes 6 to 10 individuals, is 45 to 60 minutes long, and is limited to 10 to 12 sessions. This type of group is for an outpatient setting, or it can be adjusted to fit an inpatient setting with rapid turnover.

Cognitive-Behavioral Groups

Cognitive and behavioral therapies differ from traditional psychotherapy in that they are both usually short-term, problem-oriented, and deal with the here-and-now. Cognitive behaviorists see in the group model an opportunity for clients to rethink old cognitive schemas (world views) and to question some of their prior cognitive distortions (Alonso 1999). Cognitive behaviorists find that the social influences that occur in groups can have a pivotal role in altering maladaptive response by the use of modeling and reinforcement of new behaviors (Alonso 1999).

There are specific formats for dealing with the client's negative thoughts, distortions, and attitudes. Cognitive-behavioral group therapy can be useful in a wide range of client problems. Some areas where cognitive-behavioral groups have been found to be effective are: with HIV-infected persons (Mulder et al. 1994), the depressed elderly (Rolke et

Nurse's Role: Assessment and selection to exclude clients who may be at risk of harm from an active approach.

Nurse's Role: Establish an explicit verbal agreement regarding circumscribed goals.

Nurse's Role: Focus on goals.

Nurse's Role: Encourages members to stick to the topic.

Nurse's Role: Establishes an expectation that ideas will be actively applied to outside circumstances.

Nurse's Role: Expects and encourages clients to assume responsibility for initiating therapy tasks.
Nurses Role: Encourages the mobilization of outside resources that can reinforce positive change.

Example: Exclude clients who are having active command hallucinations of self-harm. A group at this time may be too overwhelming.
Example: Weeks 1–2: Coping with auditory hallucinations. Weeks 3–4: dealing with family's reactions to illness.
Example: Use Peplau's technique of dealing with hallucinations. For example: "Tell those so-called voices you hear to go away when you are with other people" (O'Toole and Weldt 1989).
Example: Structure provides a means of organization and teaching an interpersonal skill (being attentive to others in discussion).
Example: At the end of the group, the nurse reminds clients to practice, for example, asking a peer to go to a museum exhibit to avoid social isolation.
Example: Chooses an active member to be a co-leader.

Example: Encourages obtaining medication information from pharmacists, and how to speak to prescribers about medication.

---

al. 2000), and with persons who have a chronically depressed mood and pessimistic view of the world (Ravindran et al. 1999). For example:

Spiritual Groups

There is a growing awareness of the need to incorporate spiritual concerns and the spiritual process in healing, both mentally and physically. In recent years, the predominantly Judeo-Christian societies of the West have adopted some of the beliefs of Eastern religions, such as Hinduism, Buddhism, and Taoism. One example is the idea of karma (the law of cause and effect, sometimes loosely interpreted as "what goes around comes around"). There has also been increasing interest in, and respect for, the sometimes spiritually based healing practices of other cultures, including those indigenous to the United States (e.g., American Indian medicine). A spiritual assessment tool (Burkhardt 1989) can be used in a group. Questions are grouped into catego-

POPULATION	GOAL	INTERVENTION
HIV-infected	Reframe a sense of hopelessness	Identify distortions of emotional reasoning, challenge those distortions, and reframe problem areas in healthier, more hopeful ways, using existing facts about the person's situation.
Depressed elderly	Provide high level of structure appropriate for persons whose mental and cognitive functions are changing (e.g., memory loss).	Change black and white thinking (all or nothing), e.g., "My spouse died, so I am nothing now." **Reframe to:** "My spouse died and this is a great loss. We shared so many activities together. Even though I won't be able to be with my spouse, eventually I can find people to share activities, provide companionship, and value my friendship."
Chronically depressed and negative persons (dysthymia)	Change tendency to magnify (catastrophize) events	**Reframe:** "My husband and I got into a terrible argument, therefore he will divorce me." **Change to:** "We had a terrible argument. However, we can use this as an opportunity to look at the issues and make changes once we both calm down. We have had arguments before and lived through them."

ries. For example, the following questions relate to the person's ability to connect with others interpersonally. To assess inner strength, ask

- What brings you joy and peace in your life?
- What are your personal strengths?
- What life goals have you set for yourself?
- How aware were you of your body before you became sick?
- How has your illness influenced your faith?
- Does faith play a role in regaining your health?

Behavioral Group Therapy

Behavioral group therapy can help members of a group eliminate certain undesirable behaviors, such as phobias. The Diagnostic and Statistical Manual (DSM)–IV-TR defines a phobia as a marked and persistent fear that is excessive or unreasonable, cued by the presence or anticipation of a specific object or situation (APA 2000). Persons with phobias recognize that the fear is excessive, unless they are children. A compulsion, on the other hand, is a repetitive behavior, such as excessive hand washing, that takes up a significant part of the day, that the person feels driven to perform.

A professional who is trained in behavioral therapy leads this type of group, either as an adjunct to medication or for patients who have not responded to medication. The group is generally homogeneous (e.g., clients have the same phobias or compulsions). Behavioral therapy seeks to bring about change by altering the client's environment or the client's response to the environment.

The principles of behavioral therapy are guided by the tenets of behavioral theory. According to behavioral theorists,

1. The frequency of a specific behavior is influenced by a negative stimulus, a positive stimulus, or both;
2. Events are associated when they occur together, and
3. Through teaching and role modeling, new behaviors can be learned.

During behavioral group therapy, basic behavioral techniques such as systematic desensitization and other anxiety-reducing regimens (e.g., flooding), are used.

Systematic desensitization involves having a client gradually approach the feared object or situation while the client is in a state of relaxation. Flooding is the process of saturating the client with the anxiety-producing experience without allowing the client to escape. This method causes the client to experience the anxiety, and usually within 5 to 20 minutes, the anxiety decreases. During behavioral group therapy, clients discuss each person's problems, such as phobias, and how they interfere with the client's quality of life. Each week, at the end of the session, the therapist gives clients individual homework assignments designed to help them overcome their undesirable behaviors. Clients are expected to complete their assignments and to report their results the following week. The homework begins with small, easy steps and progressively becomes more difficult.

An example of desensitization in a group in which all members have a fear of elevators would start with the leader talking group members through an imagined elevator ride. Next, the leader would walk the members to the elevator, and the next step would be the members getting into the elevator. A subsequent step would be having the door close and immediately reopen, and then allowing clients to get out. Eventually, they would ride the elevator up one floor, then up several floors.

During these short, progressive steps, the group members would be encouraged to use stress-reduction techniques such as deep breathing and visualization throughout the experience. Group support and encouragement are important aspects of behavioral group therapy. Table 34–4 identifies those who would best benefit, the goal, and the group leader's activity.

Self-Help Groups

Self-help groups or support groups are based on the premise that people who have experienced a particular problem are able to help others who have the same problem. Nurses may serve as resource people for their clients and need to be aware of the wide array of self-help groups available. Self-help groups are designed to serve people who have a common problem. One of their most important functions is to demonstrate to individuals that they are not alone in having a particular problem. Thus, these groups provide members with support, and their members help each other by telling their stories and providing alternative ways to view and to resolve problems.

A prototype for many self-help groups is the 12-step program developed by Alcoholics Anonymous (AA). For further description of the 12 steps, refer to Chapter 27. The first step is admitting to having a problem (e.g., substance abuse, overeating, internet addictions, gambling). Integral to the program is the acknowledgement of a power higher than one's self. The first meeting is an open or general meeting at which several members tell their stories. As new members gain confidence and make a commitment

TABLE 34–4 *Behavioral Group Therapy*

TARGET POPULATION	GOALS	GROUP LEADER ACTIVITIES	FREQUENCY AND DURATION
People with specific symptoms they want to modify, e.g., Phobias Sexual problems Passivity Smoking Overeating	*Overall goal:* Relief of a specific symptom or change in a specific behavior.	1. Works to create new defenses. 2. Uses an active and directive approach. 3. Uses techniques of behavior modification.	*Meets:* 1–3 times per week. *For:* 6–12 sessions or more.

to healing, they are encouraged to work through the 12 steps of the program with the help of a sponsor. The sponsor is an experienced member of AA who volunteers to be available for support whenever the sponsored individual needs special help (i.e., is tempted to drink alcohol).

Not all self-help groups use the 12-step method, but all support groups are organized around one particular problem or crisis that has been experienced by all members of that group. A nurse may be included as a group member and may be asked to speak as a resource person, but unless the nurse has personally overcome the problem that the group members have, the nurse would not be asked to lead the group.

Strategies used by group leaders include promotion of dialogue, self-disclosure, and encouragement among members (Kane et al. 1990). Concepts used in groups include psychoeducation, self-disclosure, and mutual support. These groups can also prevent physical, emotional, or social health problems; improve an individual's or a family's quality of life; and provide education necessary to further develop the member's potential.

Vignette

■ Bob and Jill, a married couple, are having difficulty conceiving a child. Their infertility is affecting their marriage, and they are depressed and angry. They begin to attend a RESOLVE group, in which everyone is having the same difficulty. Through the group process, they explore their options for having children or living childfree. Bob and Jill realize they are not alone, and through the group they gain insight that helps them deal with their anger and depression.

Examples of groups initiated by nurses include a support group for parents who have a child with a terminal illness or whose child has died, and a support group for persons with anorexia (Staples, et al.

1990). Other self-help groups include Weight Watchers, Parents Without Partners, and National Alliance for the Mentally Ill. Some support groups have formed for those who are not in the mainstream population (e.g., Fat Women Unite, Coming Out). Characteristics of these groups include peer support, group teaching, counseling, and use of shared experiences. Refer to Table 34–5 for supportive and self-help groups.

CHALLENGING CLIENT BEHAVIORS

Leading a group is anxiety-provoking for most group leaders, especially in the beginning. Many defensive behaviors used by some clients interfere with their attaining satisfaction in their lives. At the same time, these behaviors can be disruptive to a group process and disturbing to the leader. The client who monopolizes the group, the client who complains but continues to reject help, the demoralizing client, and the silent client often challenge a group leader.

Person Who Monopolizes the Group

This person's compulsive speech is an attempt to deal with anxiety. As the client sees group tension grow, the client's level of anxiety rises and the client's tendency to speak increases even more. Therefore, no one else gets a chance to be heard, and other group members eventually lose interest and begin to withdraw.

Vignette

■ Holly is the most talkative member of the group until the nurse intervenes. Initially, Holly talks at length about her early experiences relating to the deaths of both her mother *and her father and to having to live with her grandparents. The other members of the group become bored with the same old story, and they drift off. They have heard these stories many times, not only in group therapy but also during other activities.*

INTERVENTION. The leader asks group members why they have permitted the monopolizer to go on and on. This serves to validate the other members' feelings of anger. After the group members become angry, they may see how they, too, are responsible for allowing themselves to be victimized. Some members may be angry with the therapist for pointing out their passivity, but they may subsequently realize that they are responsible adults with the right to say what they feel. They may then discuss their fears of being assertive or of hurting the feelings of the monopolizer. Placing responsibility on the group members also takes the therapist out of the authoritative position.

Group members may need help disclosing their own feelings and responses. The therapist encourages statements such as, "When you speak this way, I feel. . . ." The therapist helps by saying that feel-ings are not right or wrong but simply exist. People feel less defensive with "I feel" statements than they do with "you are" statements. They help members feel like part of the group, not alienated from it.

Person Who Complains But Continues to Reject Help (yes . . . but)

The client who complains but continues to reject help continually brings environmental or somatic problems to the group and often describes them in a manner that makes the problems seem insurmountable; in fact, the client appears to take pride in the insolubility of his or her problems. The client seems entirely self-centered. The group's attempts to help the person are continually rejected. The person who uses these tactics usually has highly conflicting feelings about his or her own dependency. Any notice from the therapist temporarily increases the client's self-esteem; on the other hand, the client has a pervasive mistrust toward all authority figures. Most clients who complain but continue to reject help have been subjected to severe deprivation early in their lives. For example, they may have been emotionally and physically abused.

TABLE 34–5 *Supportive Self-Help Group Therapy*

TARGET POPULATION	GOALS	GROUP LEADER ACTIVITIES	FREQUENCY AND DURATION
People who have experienced a common tragedy, crisis, illness, or self-destructive behavior, e.g.: **Support groups** Bereavement: For those who have experienced the loss of a loved one Rape: For those who have been raped Cancer: For those families and patients coping with the ramifications of cancer and its treatment RESOLVE: For couples experiencing infertility **Self-help groups** Alcoholics Anonymous (AA)—the prototype Gamblers Anonymous (GA) Overeaters Anonymous (OA) Narcotics Anonymous (NA) Co-Dependents Anonymous Adult Children of Alcoholics (ACOA)	*Overall goal:* Provision of support and encouragement of positive coping behaviors: Decrease feelings of isolation Provide mutual support Provide psychoeducation and health education Reduce stress Help people cease self-destructive behaviors or come to terms with an overwhelming event or situation	May or may not have a specific leader Strengthens existing defenses Is actively involved in the group process Provides information to educate and give direction	*Meets:* Once or more per week *For:* Indefinite period of time, ongoing and open membership

Vignette

■ *Michelle is always complaining about how horrible her relationship with her boyfriend is, and she manages to get the entire group worked up over this. Members tell her to leave him, not to spend all her time with him, and not to spend all her money on him, but each week she reports a new escapade or crisis. In every session, the group members become concerned and offer encouragement, advice, and solutions. Each time, the group becomes angry at her lack of change, and she is frustrated by her own inability to change. She asserts that the group is not helpful.*

INTERVENTION. The therapist agrees with the content of the client's pessimism and maintains a detached affect. If the client stays in the group long enough and the group develops a sense of cohesion, the therapist helps this individual recognize the pattern of his or her relationships. The therapist encourages the client to look at his or her "yes . . . but" behavior.

Person Who Demoralizes Others

Some people who are extremely self-centered, lack empathy or concern for other members of the group, are highly depressive, are angry, and refuse to take any personal responsibility can challenge the group leader and negatively affect the group process.

Vignette

■ *Becky came to the support group on the inpatient psychiatric unit. She was very angry, stating, 'I don't know why I come to these groups anyway! They don't help." Becky was to be discharged the next day to a 28-day alcohol rehabilitation program. She had a previously scheduled dental appointment before the rehabilitation intake interview, and she was being strongly encouraged by her therapist to reschedule the appointment. The therapist feared she was at high risk for drinking again, since Becky stated that she constantly had the urge to drink. When a group member, who was an addictions therapist, confronted Becky about not being flexible and prioritizing her need for alcohol treatment, she exploded. "I thought this group was for support. This is outrageous!" Group members were obviously uncomfortable with her anger.*

Clients who are severely narcissistic may have difficulty in group therapy for the following reasons:

■ They are defensive, exhibiting a grandiose sense of self-importance. This creates a resistance to treatment because they experience a wounding reaction to any comment perceived as criticism.
■ They may be initially charming, then demanding.
■ They may devalue the therapist and then feel elated.
■ They may monopolize the group.

INTERVENTION. The group therapist needs to listen to the content that is being avoided. Listening requires the participant-observer to stay therapeutically objective. Only then can the therapist be empathetic (Liebenberg 1990). In being empathetic, however, the therapist must be aware that a narcissistic client may fear excessive warmth because it stimulates a great deal of anxieties or fears. Underneath, these clients may be extremely vulnerable, and devaluing or demoralizing others keeps them at a distance and maintains their precarious sense of "safety." Therapists need to empathize with the client in a matter-of-fact manner, e.g., "You seem angry that the group wants to support you in sobriety over your dental needs."

Silent Person

Clients who are silent in group may be observing intently until they decide the group is safe for them or believe they are not as competent as other, more assertive group members. Often, these clients can offer valuable insights about others' behavior, but they may avoid speaking in order to avoid conflict.
    INTERVENTION. The leader needs to exhibit patience but also encourage each member as offering something worthwhile to the group. This encouragement is offered in a supportive manner. The leader makes an observation without putting the client on the defensive. For example, the leader says, "What do you think, Jill?" instead of, "Do you want to say anything about Linda's problem, Jill?"

ESTABLISHING AN INPATIENT OR OUTPATIENT PSYCHOTHERAPY GROUP

General Guidelines

Nurse therapists interview each prospective group member before the actual group begins. The nurse provides an introduction to group therapy, establishes ground rules, provides a time frame, and helps socialize clients into being members of the group. A brief synopsis of some of the topics to be discussed in the group, for example, problems in interpersonal relationships, disturbing feelings, how to manage one's mental health problems if employed. Discussing confidentiality now and in the first group helps ensure a feeling of safety. The nurse therapist also decides whether this will be an open or closed group. The beginning level nurse may find conducting a closed group more manageable than an open group. A closed group has a fixed number of members. An open group is one where new members replace others who have left.

A group experience is often anxiety-provoking for many members at first. Many people have never been in any type of group treatment. They do not understand how their behavior affects others, so the group is an ideal opportunity to receive honest feedback that can be gently reframed by the group leader, if needed. There is an opportunity for truthfulness, so essential for human growth. It is important that this truth not be wounding in order for people to return to the group without feeling attacked.

The ideal number of clients in a psychotherapy group ranges from 7 to 10. Having more than 10 members is not recommended, because the group will subdivide, which is counterproductive. Too large a group can also create more opportunities for acting out, as opposed to working through issues.

Members should vary in age, gender, race, and psychodynamics. The presence of both men and women helps members work through personal issues with persons of both genders. People have different personalities and coping styles, which helps members "try on" another member's way of dealing with an issue.

Clients who should not be included in psychotherapy groups include those who are acutely psychotic, those with antisocial personality disorder, those experiencing drug or alcohol withdrawal, those who are actively using drugs or alcohol, and those who are violent.

However, persons diagnosed with schizophrenia can greatly benefit from some modes of group therapy. Persons diagnosed with antisocial personality disorder should not be included in groups, because they are often disruptive to a psychotherapy group and are unable to relate in a way that is helpful to themselves or to others (Lego 1996). Certain special groups may benefit people with antisocial traits. Other groups are effective for persons with schizophrenia and people with addictions. Groups specific to these populations are discussed in Chapter 20 and Chapter 27.

Group therapy may take place in an inpatient or an outpatient setting. Table 34–6 contrasts and compares the differences between inpatient and outpatient group therapy.

Inpatient Groups

One popular method of structuring an inpatient therapy group is by focusing on the here and now (Yalom 1995). The group therapist should

1. **Begin with a brief orientation for new clients.** Clients enter the hospital for different reasons, and everyone can benefit from examining how he or she relates to other people. Group members and the therapist or therapists provide feedback. Members have important and painful problems other than interpersonal ones, but given the brief

TABLE 34–6 *Differences Between Outpatient and Inpatient Groups*

OUTPATIENT GROUPS	INPATIENT GROUPS
The group has a stable composition.	The group is rarely the same for more than 1 or 2 meetings.
Clients are carefully selected and prepared.	Clients are admitted to the group with little prior selection or preparation.
The group is homogenous regarding ego function.	The group has a heterogenous level of ego functioning.
Motivated, self-referred clients make up the group; therapy is growth-oriented.	Clients are ambivalent, often therapy is compulsory; therapy is relief oriented.
Treatment proceeds as long as required: 1–2 years.	Treatment is limited to the hospital period: 1–3 weeks, with rapid patient turnover.
The boundary of the group is well maintained, with few external influences.	Whatever happens on the unit affects the group.
Group cohesion develops normally, given sufficient time in treatment.	There is no time for cohesion to develop spontaneously; group development is aborted at an early stage.
The leader allows the process to unfold; there is ample time to set up group norms.	The group leader structures time and is not passive.
No extragroup contact is encouraged.	Clients eat, sleep, and live together outside of the group; extragroup contact is endorsed.

Adapted from Leszcz, M. (1986). Inpatient groups. In A. J. Frances and R. E. Hales (Eds.), *Psychiatric update* (Vol. 5). Washington, DC: American Psychiatric Press. Reprinted with permission. Copyright 1986 American Psychiatric Association.

duration of most inpatient hospitalizations, these problems may need to be addressed in individual therapy.

2. **Provide spatial boundaries.** No table is used. The group meets in the same place each time. The nurse leader and members sit in a circle so everyone can see each other.

3. **Start and end the session on time.** Encourage clients and other therapists not to interfere with group time. One to one-and-a-half hours is usually sufficient. Obtain administrative support.

4. **Encourage clients to stay, but do not lock the door.** If a client attempts to leave, ask him or her what is happening. Try to connect the behavior to a feeling. For example, a client who stated the day before that she isolates herself when she is feeling depressed would need encouragement to stay. If the client still leaves, follow up with the client after the group therapy session and find out more about the client's thoughts and feelings.

5. **Be directive and decisive.** For example, if a manic person monopolizes the group, suggest that the client stop talking and try listening to others.

6. **Maintain group safety.** If a client threatens to act out physically (e.g., by striking somebody), tell the client, "You may talk about your anger, but you cannot act on it in this group." Get help if the client becomes increasingly threatening, and escort the client from the room. Follow up after the group session, and do not allow the client to come back until the reason for the threatening behavior has been explored with the client's primary therapist.

An example of a basic protocol for an inpatient group could be

■ Orientation or preparation (3 to 5 minutes).
■ Agenda "go round": Each member offers a personal agenda for the meeting (20 to 30 minutes).
■ Agenda "fitting": The therapist fits the agendas together by finding commonalities in the group.
■ Review.

In many inpatient settings, the group leader is often not the client's primary therapist. Information is obtained from the client, the primary therapist, and the chart. The nurse should keep in mind that the client's ease in communicating in the group setting is often based heavily on his or her feelings of comfort with the group leader.

The nurse should encourage clients to discuss individual group issues with their therapists. If the client brings up any issues in group therapy that affect his or her safety, such as suicide, the nurse must discuss this with the client's therapist, the treatment team, or both. This situation is set up as part of the ground rules, and everyone knows this from the beginning.

Outpatient Groups

Nurses often run outpatient psychotherapy groups in clinics, in community health units, and in private practice. Outpatient groups are a cost-effective treatment, in that several clients are seen together over a period of time. At times, more experienced group clients can share leadership with the group leader. The group leader promotes independent thoughts and feelings, promoting a sense of individuality. In outpatient psychiatric groups, prospective members are seen at least once individually before they are admitted to a group.

In contrast to pre-group preparation that occurs in an inpatient group, in an outpatient group, the client is often not prepared for what happens in group therapy or who will be there. Only a general statement is made (e.g., "The group is a place to discuss feelings, problems, or reactions.") (Lego 1996). Setting general goals (e.g., wanting closer relationships, improving work life, relieving painful symptoms) is useful. It may be unrealistic to set goals that are too specific. Goal setting that is too specific is antithetical to the natural process of developing ongoing intimate relationships. Clients often have specific, conscious goals that for a time are unobtainable because of unconscious factors. For instance, a woman may state that she wants to find a man and get married but may consistently choose to go out with men who are unsuitable (e.g., married men, men not interested in making a commitment).

SUMMARY

Nurses have many opportunities for professional, creative, and thoughtful work in groups. The beginning group therapist is encouraged to use modalities initially that concentrate on education (e.g., medication groups, sexuality) on the inpatient psychiatric unit in order to become familiar with group dynamics, roles, and psychiatric diagnoses. Staff nurses in a hospital unit or in a community health center may run milieu groups, such as recreational, social skills, creative arts, storytelling, physical activity, and educational groups.

Advanced nurse practitioners are encouraged to seek ongoing clinical supervision. Leading groups such as behavioral, cognitive, psychoanalytic, and family therapy requires specialized training and education. Beginning group therapists can benefit from observing such groups.

When working with groups, the nurse identifies the theoretical base that is the most comfortable for the nurse. To prepare clients adequately for therapy in an inpatient psychotherapy group, the advanced-practice nurse needs to assess clients, provide a cognitive structure, and tell them what to expect. The focus is on the here-and-now and on relationships. The nurse psychotherapist is always active, analyzing both the group process and the content and continually striving to link the universal aspects of clients' common issues. The group becomes a microcosm of the inpatient unit, and the therapy group may be the first group with which a client feels a sense of belonging.

Outpatient groups that provide ongoing therapy may be less structured and tend to have the same members over an extended period of time, particularly those outpatient groups that are insight-oriented psychotherapy groups. Cognitive/behaviorally oriented groups are often more goal directed, and clients may stay only until they meet their goal. The nurse therapist in an outpatient group may see the client for individual therapy as well. This therapist usually provides less structure and does less preparation than the inpatient therapist and generally has more time to see the group develop through the three phases of group development.

Visit the **Evolve** website at
http://evolve.elsevier.com/Varcarolis
for a post-test on the content in this chapter.
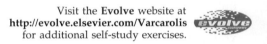

Visit the **Evolve** website at
http://evolve.elsevier.com/Varcarolis
for additional self-study exercises.

Critical Thinking and Chapter Review

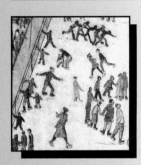

Critical Thinking

1. Construct a formula for a medication teaching group that would cover information useful for your client or clients.
2. If possible, co-lead this group with a staff member or a fellow student with instructor guidelines.
3. Identify which milieu groups are offered in your clinical setting and ask to either co-lead or participate in at least two, with your instructor's guidance.
4. Using the nursing process, assess your unit and prioritize the groups that need to be developed. Discuss your findings with the team/nurse manager and propose one group, utilizing the standard group protocol Box 34–2.
5. Ms. Rodriguez is a 22-year-old Puerto Rican–born medical student admitted to the psychiatric unit after a nearly lethal overdose of Tylenol. She is at risk of failing school. She has complained of a loss of interest in her studies, decreased concentration, irritability, social isolation, and forgetfulness. In the group, she rolls her eyes, and has a smirk on her face when another member of the group asks for help with a problem.

   A. What is your evaluation of Ms. Rodriguez's situation?
   B. What might Ms. Rodriguez's nonverbal behavior mean?
   C. How could you get Ms. Rodriguez to notice her nonverbal behavior?
   D. What approaches would you use to involve her in the group?
   E. What criteria could you use to evaluate the effectiveness of your intervention?

Chapter Review

1. The nurse leader of the behavioral health inpatient unit wishes to assign a BSN-prepared staff nurse who has just completed orientation to co-lead a unit group. Which type of group should the nurse leader choose?

   1. Family therapy
   2. Cognitive therapy
   3. Dual diagnosis group
   4. Medication education group

2. The nurse who plans to begin working with a new group of clients on the inpatient unit needs one additional client to complete the group. Of the clients listed below, the best choice would be

   1. Mr. F., who is diagnosed as having an antisocial personality.
   2. Miss G., who is newly admitted for alcohol detoxification.
   3. Mrs. H., who has strong paranoid delusions and a high potential for violence.
   4. Ms. J., who was hospitalized following a suicide attempt.

3. In which self-help group would a nurse expect to observe the use of a 12-step method?

   1. Weight Watchers
   2. Alcoholics Anonymous
   3. Parents Without Partners
   4. National Alliance for the Mentally Ill

4. A student nurse asks the co-assigned staff nurse, "I've been assigned to observe in a time-limited therapy group focusing on problems in interpersonal relationships. What can you tell me about the role of the group therapist?" The best explanation would be, the therapist focuses on

   1. Creating harmony within the group.
   2. Offering facts and personal experience.
   3. Examining possible group solutions in light of group goals.
   4. Stimulating group interaction and group analysis of the interaction.

5. Which factors can the nurse conducting a therapeutic group rely upon to promote client growth and behavioral change?

   1. Acting out and flooding
   2. Resistance and subgrouping
   3. Universality and imitative behavior
   4. Creating defenses and altering the environment

NURSE, CLIENT, AND FAMILY RESOURCES

Ormont, L. (2000). Where is group treatment going in the 21st century? GROUP, 24:185–92.

Ormont, L. R. (1999b). Progressive emotional communication: Criteria for a well-functioning group. *Group Analysis*, 32(1):139–150.

Van Sevellen, G., et al. (1991). Nursing-led group modalities in a psychiatric inpatient setting: A program evaluation. *Archives of Psychiatric Nursing*, 5(3):128.

Internet Resources

Alzheimer's Association
http://www.alz.org

American Institute for Cognitive Therapy
e-mail: AICT@aol.com

American Psychiatric Association
http://www.psych.org

Anxiety Disorders Association of America
http://www.ndma.org

Grief and Bereavement
http://www.bereavement.org/index.html

International Association of Group Psychotherapy
http://www.psych.mcgill.ca/labs/iagp

National Alliance for the Mentally Ill
http://www.nami.org.

National Institute of Mental Health
http://www.nimh.nih.gov

REFERENCES

Alonso, A. (1999). Group psychotherapy, combined individual and group therapy. In H. I. Kaplan and B. J. Sadock (Eds.), *Comprehensive textbook of psychiatry*, 7th ed. Philadelphia: Lippincott Williams & Wilkins.

American Psychiatric Association (2000). *Diagnostic and statistical manual of mental disorders* (4th ed, revised.). Washington, DC: Author.

Befler, P.L., et al. (1995). Cognitive behavioral group psychotherapy, for agoraphobia and panic disorder. *International Journal of Group Psychotherapy*, 45(2):185–206.

Belcher, J., and Fish, L. (1995). Hildegard E. Peplau. In George, J. (ed.) *Nursing theories: The base for professional nursing practice* (4th ed.) (pp. 49–66) Norwalk, Ct.: Appleton and Lange.

Burkhardt, M. (1989). Spirituality: An analysis of the concept. *Holistic Nursing Practice*, 3(3):69.

Ciarmiello, S. (1992). Medication Group Questionnaire. Unpublished material. Albany Medical Center, Albany, NY.

Critchley, D., and Maurin, J. (1985). *The clinical specialist in psychiatric mental health nursing* (pp. 178–198). New York: John Wiley & Sons.

Dexter, N. (1992). Physical exercise as a nursing intervention. Unpublished paper. Stormant-Vail Regional Medical Center, Topeka, Kan.

Dobson, K., and Craig, K. (1996). *Advances in cognitive behavioral therapy*. London: Sage Publishing.

Ellis, A., and Harper, R. (1975). *A new guide to rational living*. North Hollywood, Calif: Wilshire.

Hamilton, J., et al. (1993). Quality assessment and improvement in group psychotherapy. *American Journal of Psychiatry* 150(2): 316, 320.

Kanas, N., Deri, J., Kitter, T., and Fein, G. (1989). Short-term outpatient therapy groups for schizophrenics. *International Journal of Group Psychotherapy* 31:517–520.

Kane, C. F., DiMarino, E., and Jiminez, M. (1990). A comparison of short-term psychoeducational supports for relatives coping with chronic schizophrenia. *Archives of Psychiatric Nursing*, 4(6): 343.

Kaplan, H. I., and Sadock, B. J. (1998). *Synopsis of psychiatry* (8th ed.). Baltimore: Williams & Wilkins.

Kuipers, J., et al. (1988). Designing a psychiatric medication program. *Journal of Rehabilitation Research and Development*. 54(3): 55.

Lego, S. (ed.) (1996). *Psychiatric nursing—A comprehensive reference* (2nd ed.). Philadelphia: Lippincott-Raven.

Leszcz, M. (1986). Inpatient groups. In A. J. Frances and R. E. Aoles (Eds.), *Psychiatry update* (p. 729). Washington, DC: American Psychiatric Press.

Leszcz, M. (1989). Group psychotherapy of the characterologically difficult patient. *International Journal of Group Psychotherapy*, 39(3):311.

Levin, J. (1991). When the patient abuses alcohol. In H. Jackson (Ed.), *Using self-psychology in psychotherapy* (pp. 203–221). Northvale, NJ: Jason Aronson.

Liebenberg, B. (1990). The difficult patient in group. Group psychotherapy with borderline and narcissistic disorders. In B. E. Roth, W. N. Stone, and H. O. Kibel (Eds.), *The unwanted and unwanting patient*. Madison, Conn: International Universities Press. (pp. 311–322).

Mackenzie, K. R. (1993). Time-limited group theory and technique. In A. Alonso and H. Swiller (Eds.), *Group therapy in clinical practice* (pp. 423–444). Washington, DC: American Psychiatric Press.

Morgan, A. J., and Moreno, J. W. (1973). *The practice of mental health nursing: A community approach*. Philadelphia: J. B. Lippincott.

Mulder, C. L., et al. (1994). Cognitive behavioral and experiential group psychotherapy for HIV-infected men: Comparative studies. *Psychosomatic Medicine*, 56(5):423–431.

Naegle, M. (Ed.) (1993). *Substance abuse education in nursing* (Vol. III, press publication no. 15-2464). New York: National League for Nursing.

O'Toole, A. W., and Weldt, S. (Eds.) (1989). *Interpersonal theory in nursing practice: Selected works of Hildegard E. Peplau*. New York: Springer.

Ott, C. A. (2000). *Pediatric psychopharmacology*. Wheaton, Md: American Healthcare Institute.

Paleg, K., and Jongsma, A. E. Jr. (2000). *The group therapy treatment planner*. New York: John Wiley & Sons.

Peplau, H. E. (1991). *Interpersonal relations in nursing—A conceptual frame of reference for psychodynamic nursing*. New York: Springer.

Ramos, F. (1996). Teaching self-medication in psychiatric nursing. In S. Lego, (Ed.), *Psychiatric nursing—A comprehensive reference* (2nd ed.). Philadelphia: Lippincott-Raven.

Ravindran, A. V., et al. (1999). Treatment of primary dysthymia with group cognitive therapy and pharmacotherapy. *The American Journal of Psychiatry*, 156(10):1608–1617.

Rokke, P. D., Tomhave, J. A., and Zefjko, J. (2000). Self-management therapy and educational group therapy for depressed elders. *Cognitive Therapy and Research*, Feb. 24:99–119.

Rutan, J. S., and Waller, S. (1993). *Psychodynamic group psychotherapy* (2nd ed.). New York: Guilford Press.

Salvendy, J. T. (1999). Ethnocultural considerations in group psychotherapy. *International Journal of Group Psychotherapy*, 49(4): 429–464.

Staples, N., and Schwartz, M. (1990). Anorexia nervosa support group: Providing transitional support. *Journal of Psychosocial Nursing*, 28(2):6.

Thompson, S. (1999). *The group context*. London: Jessica Kingsley Publishers.

Tuckman, B. (1965). Developmental sequence in small groups. *Psychological Bulletin*, 63.

Van Servellen, G., et al. (1992). Methodological concerns in evaluating psychiatric nursing care modalities and a proposed standard group protocol format for nurse-led groups. *Archives of Psychiatric Nursing*, 6(2):117–124.

Van Servellan, G. M. (1984). *Group and family therapy*. St. Louis: Mosby

Wenckus, E. (1994). Storytelling: Using an ancient art to work with groups. *Journal of Psychosocial Nursing*, 32:7, 30–32.

Yalom, I. D. (1995). *The theory and practice of group psychotherapy* (4th ed.). New York: Basic Books.

Wolfe, M. (1993). Group modalities in the care of clients with drug and alcohol problems. In M. A. Naegle (Ed.), *Substance abuse education in nursing* (Vol. III, pp. 6–7). New York: National League for Nursing Press.

Outline

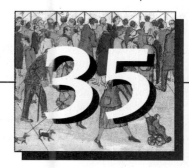

Chapter 35

Family Therapy

ELIZABETH M. VARCAROLIS

Key Terms and Concepts

The key terms and concepts listed here also appear in color where they are defined or first discussed in this chapter.

boundaries

clear boundaries

cognitive behavioral family therapy

diffused or enmeshed boundaries

double bind theory

family systems theory

family triangle

flexibility

genogram

insight family therapy

multigenerational issues

nuclear family

psychoeducational family therapy

rigid or disengaged boundaries

sociocultural context

Objectives

After studying this chapter, the reader will be able to

1. Discuss the characteristics of a healthy family using clinical examples.

2. Differentiate between functional and dysfunctional family patterns of behavior as they relate to the five family functions.

3. Compare and contrast the insight-oriented models of family therapy with behavioral family therapy.

4. Identify five family theorists and their contributions to the family therapy movement.

5. Analyze the meaning and value of the family's sociocultural context when assessing and planning intervention strategies.

6. Construct a genogram by use of a three-generation approach.

7. Formulate seven outcome criteria that a counselor and family might develop together.

8. Identify some strategies for family intervention.

9. Distinguish between the nursing intervention strategies of a basic level nurse and a certified nurse specialist regarding counseling/psychotherapy and psychobiological issues.

10. Explain the importance of the nurse's role in psychoeducational family therapy.

Family therapy is a psychotherapeutic approach that focuses on altering interactions between a couple, within a nuclear family or extended family, or between a family and other interpersonal systems, with the goal of alleviating problems initially presented by individual family members, family subsystems, the family as a whole, or other referral sources (Wynne 1988, p 9).

Family therapy is essentially about changing relationships through changing the interactions among the people who make up the family or marital unit. Kadis and McClendon (1999) point out that the principles and techniques used in family therapy are the same for those used by consultants (corporate and family business), attorneys (arbitration among groups), and social scientists (understanding cultural groups). All evaluate the complex web of relationships, patterns of transactions that repeat themselves, and the unspoken rules that drive these transactions.

Families today are composed of numerous configurations of reciprocal arrangements in which people have commitments to each other, which is vastly different from the traditional view of the traditional nuclear family. Fewer than 15% of American children living today grow up in traditional two-parent nuclear families (Kadis and McClendon 1999).

> [M]ore than three-fifths of married women with dependent children are in the labor force, as well as a majority of mothers with infants, while there are more than twice as many single-mother families as married, home-maker-mom families (Stacey 1996, p 6).

What is a family? A family is a married couple with children. A family is two people of the same sex committed to each other and living together. A family is a married couple without children. A family is a remarriage in which a parent, stepparent, children, and or stepchildren all live together. A family is a single adult with an adopted child. A family can be tri-generational where grandparent(s), parent(s), and child(ren) all live together as a cohesive unit. This is not an exhaustive list; pets are family members also.

The family is the primary system to which a person belongs, and in most cases, it is the most powerful system to which a person may ever belong. Birth, puberty, marriage, and death are all considered to be family experiences. The family can be the source of love or hate, pride or shame, security or insecurity. Although individual family members

have roles and functions, the overriding value in families lies in the relationships among family members. It is these family relationships that provide the primary context of human development. "Family" comprises the entire emotional system of at least three, and frequently four, generations. In their discussion of the changing family life cycle, Carter and McGoldrick (1989) emphasized the intergenerational connectedness of the family as being one of our greatest human resources.

As pointed out, most people no longer live in families that conform to the prevailing cultural ideal of the 1950s, and the definition of family has become more complicated over the past two decades.

THEORETICAL PREMISES

Family Functions

Healthy families provide individuals with the tools that guide how they will function in intimate relationships, in the workplace, within their culture, and in society generally. These tools are acquired through the activities that are associated with family life. These activities can be divided into five functions: (1) management, (2) boundary, (3) communication, (4) emotional-supportive, and (5) socialization (Roberts 1983). Although family counselors may use various assessment strategies, these five areas are always included. Figure 35–1 presents an assessment tool developed by Roberts that the family counselor can use to evaluate five areas of functions. The following sections explain these functions more fully.

Management Function

Every day in every family, decisions are made regarding issues of power, rule making, and provision of financial support. Other management issues include future planning and goods allocation (who gets what within the family). In healthy families, it is usually the adults in the family who agree as to how these functions are to be performed. In families with a single parent, these management functions may sometimes become overwhelming, and single parents can benefit from discussions with other adults. In more chaotic families, an inappropriate member, such as a teenager or a grandparent, may be the one who makes these decisions. Although children learn decision-making skills as they mature and increasingly make decisions and choices about their own lives, they should not have to take on this responsibility for the family of origin.

The editor would like to thank Jeannemarie G. Baker for her contributions to this chapter in the third edition of *Foundations of Psychiatric Mental Health Nursing*.

FAMILY FUNCTION CHECKLIST

Client Family _____ Date of Assessment _____

FAMILY FUNCTIONS	OBSERVED BEHAVIOR	ASSESSED NEED LEVEL (I–IV)	SUGGESTED NURSING RESPONSES
I. *Management function* 　A. Use of power for all family members 　B. Rule making clear, accepted 　C. Fiscal support adequate 　D. Successful negotiations with extrafamilial systems 　E. Future planning present II. *Boundary function* 　A. Clear individual boundaries 　B. Clear generational boundaries 　C. Clear family boundaries III. *Communication function* 　A. Straight messages 　B. No manipulation 　C. Expression of positive and negative feelings safely IV. *Emotional-supportive function* 　A. Mutual positive regard 　B. Deals with conflict 　C. Uses resources for all family members 　D. Allows growth for all family members V. *Socialization function* 　A. Children growing and developing in a healthy pattern 　B. Mutual negotiation of roles by age and ability 　C. Parents feeling good about parenting 　D. Spouses happy with each other's role behavior			

Figure 35–1 Family Function Checklist. From Roberts, F. B. (1983). An interaction model for family assessment. In I. W. Clements and F. B. Roberts (Eds.), *Family health: a theoretical approach to nursing care* (p. 202). New York: John Wiley. Copyright © 1983 John Wiley & Sons. Reprinted by permission of John Wiley & Sons, Inc.

Boundary Function

Boundaries maintain a distinction between individuals in the family. Boundaries may be clear, diffuse, rigid, or inconsistent. Clear boundaries are well understood by all members of the family; they help to define the roles of members within the family and allow for differences among members. To a great extent, a person's emotional, social, and physical functioning is related to his or her level of role differentiation within the family and the amount of anxiety within the family system (Cooley 1995).

Diffused or enmeshed boundaries refer to a blending together of the roles, thoughts, and feelings of the individuals so that clear distinctions among family members fail to emerge. The members of a family that operates with diffused, rigid, or inconsistent boundaries are more prone to psychological or psychosomatic symptoms. A common phenomenon within families with diffuse boundaries is that individuals expect other members of the family to

know what they are thinking ("Why did you take that? You know I wanted it.") and to believe they know what other family members are thinking ("I know exactly why you did that").

Rigid or disengaged boundaries are those in which the rules and roles are adhered to no matter what; thus, rigid boundaries prevent family members from trying out new roles or, in some cases, from taking on more mature functions as time goes on. In families in which rigid boundaries predominate, isolation may be marked. The family is often cut off from the community and outside influences, and even from each other.

Vignette

■ Lucy M. is a single parent with two preschool-aged children. The family is living on public assistance. Lucy is a teenage mother who is working toward a general equivalency degree and who also works "under the table" part *time as a seamstress. Her mother, Maria, watches the children for Lucy, and discipline is a hot issue between Lucy and Maria.*

If the boundary functioning of this family were clear, Lucy and Maria would have worked out an arrangement in which Maria would be in charge of disciplining the children when Lucy is away and when both Lucy and Maria are present, Lucy would make the decisions without interference from Maria. The children would be made aware of these arrangements and would clearly understand who is in charge and when. They would know that Lucy and Maria have different operating styles, to which they would learn to adjust. If the boundary functioning of this family were blurred, Lucy and Maria would likely be interfering with each other's mode of discipline, which undoubtedly would lead to tension between them as their anxiety levels increase, and angry outbursts around many issues would eventually ensue. The children, in turn, would become confused as to where their loyalties lie and would probably engage in manipulative behaviors because of the unclear boundaries. If the boundary functioning of this family were rigid, Lucy and Maria would likely have great difficulty agreeing on issues of discipline if their perceptions of rules and roles differed. The children would probably be triangled into a double bind position between a warring mother and daughter in which no correct response exists. All family members would likely become stuck in this established, rigid pattern with no available alternatives.

Communication Function

Communication patterns are extremely important in family life. Healthy communication patterns include clear and comprehensible messages (e.g., "I would like to go now," or "I don't like it when you interrupt what I'm saying"). Healthy communication within the family encourages members to ask for what they want and to express their feelings appropriately. Feelings of affection and conflict are both openly expressed. Family members are able to ask for what they want and get the attention they need without resorting to manipulation to get their needs met. When communication among family members is not clear, it cannot be used as a means to solve problems or to resolve conflict; therefore, the cardinal rule for effective and functional communication in families is "Be clear and direct in saying what you want and need."

As simple as this may seem, it is one of the hardest skills to activate in a family system. To be direct,

individuals must first have a sense that the self is respected and loved; this sense entitles them to take a stand and to set boundaries with others. The consequences for being clear and direct may be unpleasant in a family system in which boundaries are enmeshed and confusion is the norm. To attempt to change a family pattern is to pit oneself against the status quo. Saying what one wants and needs is especially difficult when one believes that family members should already know—especially if the family member is a spouse, a parent, or a close sibling. In fact, most family members cannot read each other's minds, although emotionally undifferentiated members may think that this is possible. The following is a spousal situation that shows how easily communication can be misunderstood when clear and direct messages are not sent.

Vignette

■ *Mary would like to spend more time with her husband John on the weekends; however, John always seems to be busy with projects around the house or talking with friends on the telephone. Mary feels that he does not notice her, or maybe is not interested in her, so she spends a lot of time working out or playing tennis. John figures that Mary is doing what she wants to do, and that it makes her happy, so he contents himself by finding things to do alone. The net result is that Mary and John spend little time together.*

Mary finally confronts John clearly and directly about his "disinterest" in her, saying what she wants and needs, that is, it is her desire to spend more time together on the weekends. John replies that he had no idea she felt that way. He had thought she enjoyed the way things were. Actually, he, too, would like to have more time together. What a learning experience for them both!

Box 35–1 identifies some unhealthy communication patterns.

Emotional-Supportive Function

All families encounter conflicts, and no family is 100% "functional." However, in a healthy family, feelings of affection are generally uppermost, and anger and conflict do not dominate the family's pattern of interaction. Healthy families are concerned with each other's needs, and most of the family members' emotional and physical needs are met most of the time. When people's emotional needs are met, they feel support from those around them and are free to grow and explore new roles and facets of their personalities. A family that is domi-

Box 35–1   *Examples of Dysfunctional Communication*

MANIPULATING

Instead of asking directly for what one wants, family members manipulate others into getting what they want. For example, a child starts a fight with a sibling in order to get attention. Another example is a family member's making requests with strings attached, so that the other person has a difficult time refusing the request, "If you do this for me, then I won't tell Daddy that you are getting poor grades in school."

DISTRACTING

In order to avoid functional problem solving and resolve conflicts within the family, family members introduce irrelevant details into problematic issues.

GENERALIZING

When dealing with problematic family issues, members use global statements, like "always" and "never," instead of dealing with specific problems and areas of conflict. Family members may say "Harry is always angry" instead of "Harry, what is upsetting you?"

BLAMING

Family members blame others for failures, errors, or negative consequences of an action in order to keep the focus away from themselves. This is a response to fear of being blamed by others.

PLACATING

Family members "pretend" to be inadequate but well meaning in order to keep peace in the family at any price. "Don't yell at the children, dear, I put the shoes on the stairs."

---

nated by conflict and anger alienates its members, leaving them isolated and fearful. This is not an atmosphere in which personality growth can take place, so this family would not be considered functional.

Socialization Function

It is within families that each member learns socialization skills. People learn how to interact, negotiate, and plan; they adopt coping skills. This is most evident in the socialization of children. Children learn how to function effectively within their family, and then they apply those skills in society. Parents are socialized into their family role by the demands of each child throughout the developmental stages of their children. The role of the parents changes again when the children mature and leave home, and the partners may renegotiate the pattern of their lives together. As time goes on, the parents may need their adult children's help if they become less able to care for their needs. Each phase brings new demands and requires new approaches to deal with changes as people become socialized into new roles. Families have difficulty negotiating role change, and changes often increase the stress within families for a time. In response to the family's developmental life cycle, healthy families use flexibility to adapt to new roles.

Family Life Cycle

The life cycle of the individual takes place within the family life cycle, which is the primary context of human development. The family is a system that moves through time, and family stress is often the greatest at transition points from one stage to another of the family developmental process. Symptoms are most likely to appear when an interruption or a dislocation occurs in the unfolding family life cycle; this interruption or dislocation could be a serious illness, a death, or a divorce. At these times, therapeutic efforts often need to be directed toward helping family members reorganize so that they can then proceed developmentally. Unlike all other organizations, families incorporate new members only by birth, adoption, or marriage, and members can leave only by death. If no way can be found to function within the system, the pressures of family membership with no available exit can, in the extreme, lead to mental illness or suicide. The development of symptoms should be viewed not only as a response to an interruption or a dislocation in the family life cycle but also as a solution to a stressful situation. This model takes a traditional family approach and would need to be modified for less traditional family consultations.

Six main stages exist in the changing family life cycle: (1) launching the single young adult, (2) joining families through couple formation, (3) becoming parents—families with young children, (4) families with adolescents, (5) launching children and moving on, and (6) families in later life, as identified in the middle-class North American family. Four stages are identified for the divorce and post-divorce family life cycle, and two phases for the remarried life cycle (Table 35–1).

TABLE 35–1   *Family Life-Cycle Stages and Tasks for Three Types of Family Life Cycles*

STAGE	TASK
I. Middle-class North American Family Life Cycle	
1. Launching the single youth adult	a. Differentiating self in relation to family of origin b. Developing intimate peer relationships c. Establishing self in relation to work and financial independence
2. Marriage: the joining of families	a. Establishing couple identity b. Realigning relationships with extended families to include spouse c. Making decisions about parenthood
3. Families with young children	a. Adjusting marital system to make space for child b. Joining in child-rearing, financial, and household tasks c. Realigning relationships with extended families to include parenting and grandparenting roles
4. Families with adolescents	a. Shifting parent-child relationships to permit adolescents to move into or out of system b. Refocusing on midlife marital and career issues c. Beginning to shift toward joint caring for older generation
5. Launching children and moving on	a. Renegotiating marital system as a dyad b. Developing adult-to-adult relationships between grown children and their parents c. Dealing with disabilities and death of grandparents
6. Families in later life	a. Maintaining own and/or couple functioning and interest in the face of physiological decline: exploration of new familial and social role options b. Making room in the system for the wisdom and experience of the seniors c. Dealing with loss of spouse, siblings, and other peers and preparation for death
II. Divorce and Postdivorce Family Life Cycle	
1. Deciding to divorce	a. Accepting one's own part in the failure of the marriage
2. Planning the breakup of the system	a. Working cooperatively on problems of custody, visitation, and finances b. Dealing with extended family about the divorce
3. Separation	a. Mourning loss of nuclear family b. Restructuring marital and parent-child relationships and finances; adapting to living apart c. Realigning relationships with extended family; staying connected with spouse's extended family
4. Divorce	a. Retrieving hopes, dreams, and expectations from the marriage
Postdivorce: single-parent (custodial)	a. Making flexible visitation arrangements with ex-spouse and his or her family b. Rebuilding own financial resources c. Rebuilding own social network
Postdivorce: single-parent (noncustodial)	a. Finding ways to continue effective parenting relationships with children b. Maintaining financial responsibilities to ex-spouse and children c. Rebuilding own social network
III. Remarried Family Life Cycle	
1. Entering new relationship; conceptualizing and planning the new marriage and family	a. Recommitting to marriage and to forming a family b. Developing openness and avoiding pseudomutuality in the new relationship c. Planning financial and coparental relationships with ex-spouse d. Planning to help children deal with fears, loyalty conflicts, and membership in two systems e. Realigning relationships with extended family to include new spouse and children f. Planning maintenance of connections for children with extended family of ex-spouse(s)
2. Remarriage and reconstruction of family	a. Restructuring family boundaries to allow for inclusion of new spouse-stepparent b. Realigning relationships and financial arrangements throughout subsystems to permit interweaving of several systems c. Making room for relationships of all children with custodial and noncustodial parents and grandparents d. Sharing memories and histories to enhance stepfamily integration

From Friedman, M. (1992). *Family nursing: Theory and practice* (3rd ed.) (pp. 82–105). Norwalk, CT: Appleton & Lange.

THEORIES, THEORISTS, AND APPROACHES TO FAMILY THERAPY

There are many different approaches to family therapy. Treatment possibilities have become too numerous to count (Kadis and McClendon 1999). Many therapists today use an integrative approach.

The basic framework of family therapy took root in the 1960s and 1970s during societal upheaval. In clinical settings, therapists were beginning to notice the effects of the social milieu on their clients. The therapeutic community was established as a treatment modality at this time, and group therapy and psychodrama were developed. All of these changes were rooted in observations of the client and viewing treatment in terms of social systems. An **interactive** (interpersonal) rather than an **indwelling** (intrapsychic) model of mental illness was becoming more widely accepted. These influences paved the way for an interest in the family system as it related to psychiatric disorders.

One of the original shapers of family theory and therapy was Haley (1980), who was associated with the Mental Research Institute in Palo Alto, California, where the double bind theory was developed. The **double bind theory** describes a situation in which two conflicting messages are given simultaneously on two levels, verbal and nonverbal. Since the messages conflict, people find themselves in a double bind, in which no acceptable response exists. For example, a recently divorced and lonely mother says to her teenaged daughter, "Go on out, have fun with your friends. I'll be just fine." However, the nonverbal message is that the mother will be left alone and lonely. The nonverbal message is made clear by the mother's dejected face, slumped posture, and sad tone of voice. The daughter is now in a no-win situation. If she goes out with her friends, she will feel guilty for leaving her mother alone. If she stays home with her mother, she will miss out on the friendships and activities that are important for teenage development.

Virginia Satir (1972, 1983), a leading theorist of the same era, moved the focus from the patient's symptom to the patient's position and relationships within the family. The Milan Group, especially Palazolli, Cecchia, and Prata, established the use of paradox (i.e., "Don't Change") as a way to work with families. Probably more than anyone, Minuchin (1974), a structural therapist, established the legitimacy of family therapy within psychiatry. Bowen (1985) was a leading proponent of the family systems model; he underplayed problem resolution, focusing instead on the long-term differentiation process of individual family members.

The terms **strategic** and **structural** are used to identify a framework from which specific therapists operate. A **strategic model of family therapy** assumes that by changing any single element in the family system, change can be brought about in the entire system. Briefly, the aim of strategic therapy is to change the patterns, the rules, and the meaning of family interactions. For example, in the Gomez family, whom you will read about shortly, a pattern of communicating, partly cultural, exists that excludes any discussion with the children. All decisions, whether or not they involve the children, are made without consulting the children. Consequently, the children in this family often feel powerless, and the 12-year-old has begun to engage in destructive behavior at school, which has precipitated a visit to a family therapist. A family therapist who uses the strategic model might work with the family to change their rigid pattern of communicating, allowing the children to be present when important decisions are being made. The children could comment and offer suggestions about how issues could be resolved. This could result in a resolution of the 12-year-old's negative behavior by giving him a sense of control over aspects of his life and a more positive outlet for being heard and recognized. This intervention would result in a systemic change in the way the Gomez family communicates.

The **structural model of family therapy** is based on a normative concept of a healthy family, emphasizing the boundaries between family subsystems and the establishment and maintenance of a clear hierarchy based on parental competence. A therapist using the structural model with the Gomez family, rather than focusing on changing a specific pattern, would highlight the importance of boundaries between the parental and sibling subsystems (children). At the same time, the therapist would emphasize the importance of flexibility in the family system that would allow for the changes inherent to normal growth and development.

The aims of family systems theory are to decrease emotional reactivity and to encourage differentiation among individual family members (i.e., increase each member's "sense of self"). In family therapy, no one model exists; all the shapers of family theory have made substantial contributions to the field of family therapy. In addition, all techniques are not applicable to all problems, and the experienced clinician must be discerning.

According to outcome research, there are two basic forms of marital family therapy (MFT). These two approaches are organized through a combination of theory and commonality of approach (Snyder 1991). They are:

1. Insight-oriented marital and family therapy, and
2. Behavioral marital and family therapy.

All of the theoretical schools or approaches fall into these two categories. Table 35–2 identifies some of the basic therapies under each group, identifies basic concepts and approaches, and lists the major theorists.

Kadis and McClendon (1999) state that insight alone does not result in major changes, and behavioral change by itself may not be long lasting, either. What is needed is a mix that factors in the family's immediate situation, helping them develop insight on how their behaviors impact on other family members, and the development of new skills, behaviors, and guidelines for relationships.

Basic Concepts in Family Therapy

Many concepts are widely used in working with families. The concepts of the identified patient, the family triangle, and the nuclear family emotional system are discussed here. Table 35–3 identifies other concepts relevant to family work.

The Family as a System

All families can be viewed as unique systems. All have their own structure, rules, and history of how it handles life problems and crisis. Focusing on family patterns and interaction is basic to MFT. The

---

TABLE 35–2 *Insight-Oriented and Behavioral Therapy*

TYPE OF THERAPY	CONCEPTS	MAJOR THEORISTS
Insight-Oriented Family Therapy		
Psychodynamic	Problems arise from ■ Developmental arrest ■ Current interactions ■ Projections ■ Current stresses Improvement through insight into problematic relationships originating in the past	Nathan Ackerman James Framo Ivan Boszormenyi-Nagy
Family of Origin Therapy	Family is an emotional relationship system ■ Goal is to foster differentiation and decrease emotional reactivity ■ Concept of **triangulation** ■ Emphasize the family of origin	Murray Bowen
Experimental/Existential	Goal of therapy is to encourage the growth of family ■ Symptoms express family pain ■ The family is responsible for its own solutions ■ The therapist uses nurturing and identifies dysfunctional communication patterns	
Behavioral Family Therapy		
Structural	Focus on organizational patterns, boundaries, systems and subsystems, and use of scapegoating ■ Restructures dysfunctional triangles ■ Clarifies boundaries ■ Looks at enmeshment and disengagement (excessive distance) issues	Salvador Minuchin
Strategic	Goal to change repetitive and maladaptive interaction patterns ■ Identifies inequality of power, life cycle perspectives, and use of **double bind** messages ■ Uses paradox ■ Prescribes rituals	Jay Haley Chloe Madanes Milan Group (Palazzoli, Cecchia, Prata)
Cognitive/Behavioral	Based on learning theory; focus on changing cognition and behavior ■ Problem solving and solutions focus on present situations ■ Skills training	

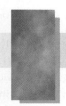

TABLE 35–3 *Central Concepts of Family*

Boundaries	**Clear boundaries** are those that maintain distinctions between individuals within the family and between the family and the outside world. Clear boundaries allow for balanced flow of energy between members. **Roles of children and parent or parents are clearly defined. Diffuse or rigid boundaries** are more often seen in families with problematic functioning. **Enmeshed versus disengaged,** and degree of flexibility and individuation: enmeshed boundaries are the result of the fusion or blending together of individuals so that the distinct person fails to emerge.
Triangulation	When two-person relationships tend to be stressful and unstable, the tendency is to draw in a third person to stabilize the system by forming a coalition in which the two join the third.
Scapegoating	A form of displacement whereby a family member (usually the least powerful) is blamed for another's or other family members' distress. The purpose is to keep the focus off the painful issues and the problems of the blamers. **In a family, the blamers are often the parents, and the scapegoat a child.**
Double bind	A positive command (often verbal) followed by a negative command (often nonverbal), leaving the recipient confused, trapped, and immobilized since there is no way to act.
Hierarchy	The function of power and its structures in families, differentiating parental and sibling roles and generational boundaries.
Family life cycle	The family's developmental process over time; refers to the family's past course, its present tasks, and its future course.
Differentiation	Developing a strong identity and sense of self while at the same time maintaining an emotional connectedness with one's family of origin.
Sociocultural context	The framework for viewing the family in terms of the influence of gender, race, ethnicity, religion, economic class, and sexual orientation.
Multigenerational emotional transition process	The continuation and persistence from generation to generation of certain emotional interactive family patterns, e.g., reenactment of fairly predictable and almost ritual-like patterns; repetition of themes or toxic issues; and repetition of reciprocal patterns, e.g., overfunctioner and underfunctioner.

focus is NOT on an individual, as it is in traditional therapy, but rather on the family group's interpersonal process. "The task of the therapist is to describe the sequence of interactions in such a way that appropriate intervention can result in possible change" (Kadis and McClendon 1999, p. 1315).

The Identified Patient

The identified patient is the individual in the family whom everyone regards as "the problem." This problem family member generally bears most of the family system's anxiety. When a family comes for treatment, the presenting problem must be addressed before the underlying systematic problem is dealt with. The family member who is the identified patient is not always the one who initially seeks help from inpatient or outpatient services.

Nurses generally tend to be more aware of the biophysical aspects of an individual than of the interpersonal aspects. Understandably, nurses also tend to subscribe to the medical model of cause-and-effect thinking. However, when a client is assessed

in the context of family, the nurse clinician must think in a less linear way (cause and effect) and more in terms of a circular causality. In circular causality, the presenting problem is viewed from many different perspectives. For example, the nurse considers a particular family's stressors and strengths in light of the family's current life cycle stage, its sociocultural context and multigenerational issues, and the family's impact on the presenting problem. Thus, there is more than one perspective to be considered when looking at the identified patient from a family system's perspective. The focus is on the family system's anxiety.

Vignette

■ *Eight-year-old Tommy, who is hyperactive and disruptive at school and at home, is brought to the community mental health clinic to be evaluated for attention-deficit hyperactivity disorder. The nurse clinician performs an assessment and finds that a great deal of turmoil exists within the family. The family is composed of a heterosexual couple (married and the parents of the three children) and a grandmother. Tommy's father has just lost his job, and his grandmother was recently diagnosed with bladder cancer. Tommy's mother is planning to file for separation because of constant, unresolved arguments with her husband. The nurse clinician who views this family from a position of circular causality would not focus solely on Tommy but would view Tommy's symptoms as a function of many difficult losses and transitions that are stressing the entire family's coping mechanisms.*

The nurse identifies the multiple stressors in this family, believing that Tommy's symptoms of hyperactivity and acting out are related to the severe stresses in the family system. Once the issues within the family are addressed and plans are made to deal with these issues, perhaps Tommy's symptoms will subside. She refers the couple to a family therapist. In the meantime, she encourages the couple to focus more on their own issues and less on Tommy's behavior. An appointment is made to go to the clinic in 1 month, where Tommy will be reevaluated.

Family Triangles

Bowen (1985) described a relationship process in families that can be seen as a system of interlocking triangles. In relationships between two people, the major tension lies in the struggle between closeness and independence. When the tension in a close twosome builds, a third person (child, friend, parent) is brought in to help lower the tension. The **family triangle** (Figure 35–2) then becomes the basic building block of interpersonal relationships. All triangles contain a close side, a distant side, and a side in which conflict or tension exists between two people (Andrus 1996). The intensity of the triangling process varies among families and within the same family over time; this is because triangles are related to lack of emotional stability. **Differentiation** refers to the ability of the individual to establish a unique identity and still remain emotionally connected to the family of origin. The lower the level of differentiation in a family, the higher the tension, and the more important the role of triangling is to the lowering of tension and the preservation of emotional stability. As the family becomes stressed, for whatever reasons, the anxiety in the system gets triggered, and the triangles become more active.

A common problem that occurs in families is the setting up of a triangle among two parents and a child, in which one parent is overinvolved with the child and the other plays a more peripheral role. In this situation, the child eventually becomes the means by which the parents communicate with each other about issues they cannot deal with directly. In other words, spousal conflicts may be brought into the parental arena, where they clearly do not belong.

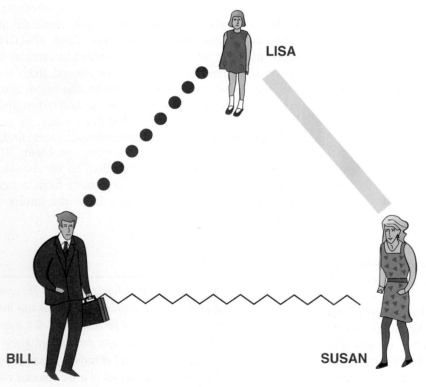

LISA

BILL   SUSAN

Key:
Distance   ● ● ● ● ● ● ●
Over-involvement ▬▬▬▬
Conflict   ∿∿∿∿

Figure 35–2 Example of a family triangle.

Vignette

- Six-year-old Lisa is having trouble making friends. Her mother, Susan, has been feeling anxious and helpless as she tries to find ways to engage Lisa with other youngsters. Susan develops an overprotectiveness with Lisa that further inhibits Lisa from venturing out to make friends. Susan feels that her husband Bill is uncaring and disinterested because he thinks that she should be more relaxed about Lisa's social life, letting things develop naturally. Bill's job requires that he travel most of the week, so he is not involved with Susan's daily experiences and struggles with Lisa.

  In the spousal arena, Susan and Bill have been avoiding intimacy for almost a year. Susan is angry with Bill for spending so much time with his parents, which further casts him in a peripheral role in their nuclear family, and Bill is angry with Susan, sensing her rejection of him.

  Both parents are feeling isolated and alienated and are consequently angry at each other. Neither Bill nor Susan addresses this issue directly. Instead, they play out their anger in the parental arena as they battle over how to handle Lisa's social isolation.

When working with families, nurse clinicians need to avoid becoming triangled into the family's system. The nurse's personal work on his or her own differentiation process is an important way to maintain emotional stability in the face of a chaotic family situation, where the nurse's own issues may be playing out. Holding the family members accountable for themselves—making clear that the responsibility for change is theirs and not that of the nurse clinician—is a way of remaining clear of their triangles. For example, the nurse clinician could become triangled into a family system in any number of ways: perhaps the nurse recently experienced the loss of a member, or maybe the nurse belongs to an enmeshed family system, in which the children are regularly drawn into spousal arguments; or perhaps stubbornness is an unresolved issue for the nurse. Any of these possibilities could allow the nurse to become triangled into a family system, making good therapeutic intervention difficult, if not impossible. The likelihood is great that nurse clinicians will become triangled into others' family systems to engage in their own family battles. Nurse clinicians need to make regular concerted efforts to self-reflect (self-assessment) and to understand their own personal family issues through therapy or supervision. Regular supervision is always recommended when nurse clinicians work with individuals, couples, or families. Supervision can be conducted with peer professionals, in groups, or privately with a more experi-

enced clinician. One indication that a nurse clinician is being triangled in is that his or her level of anxiety is greater than the situation warrants.

The Nuclear Family Emotional System

The term nuclear family refers to a parent or parents and the children under the parents' care. Bowen (1985) developed the concept of a nuclear family emotional system, which is defined as the flow of emotional processes within the nuclear family. In this concept, symptoms are viewed as belonging to the nuclear family emotional system rather than to any one individual. Within the system, a distinction is made between conventional medical (psychiatric) diagnosis and family diagnosis; rather than viewing a symptom as reflecting a disease that is confined to a client, Bowen identified an emotional process that transcends the boundaries of a client and encompasses the family relationship system. The earlier example of 8-year-old Tommy, who was believed by his family and others to have attention-deficit hyperactivity disorder, is one in which Tommy's symptoms could be viewed as reflecting the family's conflicts and changes.

Many different models, theories, and therapies have been developed to enable people to be considered within a family context. Some therapists are committed to just one theory and interpret family activity exclusively through its concepts. Far more therapists are eclectic in their approach, combining concepts from different theories in their treatment of families. Nurses can draw from many theories as they develop a general understanding of the concepts related to families. Refer to Table 35–3 for a summary of these and other concepts central to family life.

APPLICATION OF THE NURSING PROCESS

ASSESSMENT

Assessment is typically intermixed with treatment, rather than a distinct phase (Legow 1998). Assessment should have multiple foci, including:

- The family system
- Its sub-systems
- The individuals

Essential information regarding sociocultural issues, past medical and mental illness, family interactions and communication styles, and areas of stress within the family need to be obtained.

Carter and McGoldrick (1989) developed a model for marital and family assessment that includes three important areas of consideration:

1. Stage of the family life cycle
2. Multigenerational issues
3. Sociocultural context

Sociocultural Context

The family must be viewed not as an isolated unit but in a sociocultural context, in which the issues of gender, race, ethnicity, class, sexual orientation, and religion are equally considered. Each of these contextual issues affects the family's specific values, norms, traditions, roles, and rules. For example, in the family with adolescents, the way the family relates to the terminally ill family member may be decidedly different in a first-generation Italian-American Catholic family than in an Asian family or in an African American Baptist family. Therefore, the nurse clinician needs to ask the question, How do this family's cultural and religious beliefs affect the patient's presenting problem, and what impact do they have on the family's available options?

In regard to gender, for example, the position of women in United States society needs to be understood in terms of job opportunity, earning power, and status, which for most women are secondary to those of men. Gender and culture must be viewed together since the relative status of males and females differs according to culture. In particular, people from Asian and Latin cultures living in the United States have difficulty understanding American gender roles. In the context of race and ethnicity, it is extremely important that nurses be aware of and understand the mores, practices, and beliefs of the many different cultures that currently make up America's fabric (refer back to Chapter 5). This sensitivity prepares the nurse clinician to make effective interventions for families in times of crisis or psychiatric emergency. Since our American society does not outwardly make class distinctions (as do the British, for example), viewing the family in the context of class may not come easily and indeed may be downright uncomfortable; in fact, class is often considered by most therapists to be the "last taboo." Yet, although it is unspoken, most Americans do have a definite sense of the class to which they belong. It is most often defined in terms of money, education, and taste, and only with gentle questioning do these defining issues come to the fore.

Sexual orientation is another part of the context that often gets overlooked. When gathering family information, the nurse must ask questions regarding sexual orientation (e.g., in terms of long-term relationships). Finally, the context of religion figures prominently in a large percentage of the population, and within this context are many issues regarding why a person becomes ill and how that person should be treated. When the family is viewed in a sociocultural context, religion and spiritual values are important issues for consideration.

Multigenerational Issues

The influence of family is not restricted to the members of a household. Family is composed of the entire emotional system of at least three, and frequently four, generations; this means that family has multigenerational issues. Through this intergenerational system, various patterns (e.g., geographical distance, suicide, divorce, addiction, affairs, grief, triangles, and loss) are passed down through the generations. The messages and legacies of the multigenerational family relate in some way to the client's presenting problem. For example, in a family with adolescents in which the grandmother is terminally ill with cancer, if a pattern of addiction is already established in the family, the impending loss of an important family figure may exacerbate an incipient addiction in one of the family members. An astute nurse may express concern to the family regarding this possibility, perhaps preventing the development of a serious problem. This family may also have a preferred pattern of dealing with grief by using denial and by not allowing the outward expression of painful feelings. If this is the case, the nurse guides the family into learning about other, more acceptable and healthier ways of dealing with grief, because unexpressed feelings of grief may lead to further symptomatic behaviors in other family members. One way to identify multigenerational issues is through constructing a genogram.

CONSTRUCTING A GENOGRAM

The genogram is an efficient format that provides a clinical summary of information and relationships across at least three generations. It is an invaluable family assessment tool that incorporates the three important areas of consideration in the evaluation of a family:

1. Stage of the family life cycle
2. Multigenerational issues
3. Sociocultural context

The genogram provides a graphic display of complex patterns, as well as a source of hypotheses that indicate how the presenting problem connects to the family context and the evolution of the family over time (McGoldrick and Gerson 1985). Patterns of illness, shifts in relationships, and changes in structure are easily noted by use of the genogram. The physical, social, and emotional functioning of family members is interdependent; therefore, change in one part of the family system results in changes in other parts. This concept of *homeostasis* is a pivotal one in family systems thinking. The family system constantly pushes toward stability (i.e., maintaining the status quo) in the continuing face of change. This move toward stability is compelling, and for families with a rigid style of operating, maintaining stability can become very problematic because of inflexibility and limited alternatives for adjusting to the inevitable changes that are part of every family life cycle. The genogram reflects the family system's adaptation to its total context at a given moment.

Bowen (1985) provided much of the conceptual framework for the analysis of genogram patterns. He proposed that the family is organized according to generation, age, sex, roles, functions, and interests, and that where each individual fits into the family structure influences the family functioning, the relational patterns, and the type of family formed in the next generation. He further contended that sex and birth order shape sibling relationships and characteristics. Also, some issues tend to be played out from generation to generation through persisting interactive emotional patterns. A major concept is that of triangling, which was discussed earlier. As mentioned earlier, triangling occurs when a two-person relationship tends to be unstable and under stress. The tendency of those in the relationship is to draw in a third person to stabilize the system by forming a coalition by which the two join in relation to the third.

In creating a genogram, the nurse clinician is able to map the family structure and record family information. This information should include demographics such as location, occupation, and educational level. Functional information regarding medical, emotional, and behavioral status is also recorded. Finally, critical events must be noted (e.g., important transitions, moves, job changes, separations, illnesses, and deaths). Figure 35–3 provides an example of a genogram derived from the data from the following vignette of the Schneider family.

Vignette

■ Hank and Catherine Schneider are both college educated, and each suffers from intermittent depression. Hank is an only child whose father died of a heart attack at age 55, Hank's present age. Hank's mother committed suicide at age 35. This is a toxic subject in Hank's family of origin. In Catherine's family of origin, she is the eldest, born after three miscarriages. Much pressure and expectation were placed on Catherine. Catherine's brother Mike was born 4 years after Catherine. Their mother died during Mike's birth. Mike never finished high school, has a serious alcohol addiction, and has had three marriages that ended in divorce. One can speculate about the level of guilt Mike may feel regarding the loss of his mother.

Hank and Catherine have two children, Bill and Mary. Bill, the identified patient, is 35 years old, has a college degree, and has not been able to hold down a job. He also has an addiction to alcohol. In 1989, Bill made a suicide attempt. In November 1995, Bill experienced a psychotic episode for which he was hospitalized and was diagnosed as having schizophrenia. His younger sister, Mary, has a college degree and works as a nurse. She married Bruce in 1989, the year that Bill attempted suicide. Mary and Bruce have two young children, 4 and 2 years old.

Self-Assessment

Nurses must be well trained when working with families in a counseling situation because the potential for multiple transferences and triangulations is high. Therefore, a nurse educated at the advanced practice level or a certified clinical specialist with special training in family work is usually best qualified to conduct family therapy. However, all nurses interact with families, whether in hospital acute care settings or in community-based settings. Most nurses come from a family, and since no family is perfect, all nurses are subject to forming triangles when anxious, to becoming defensive when personal family anxieties are aroused, or to experiencing role blurring or loosening of self-boundaries when sensitive personal issues and conflicts are triggered.

Often, when working with families, nurses are most helpful when they are able to draw back and recognize when a personal issue is increasing anxiety levels. When the nurse believes that he or she is getting drawn into the family dynamics rather than maintaining an objective stance, discussing these issues with a professional peer or supervisor is extremely important in order to maintain effectiveness. The nurse should identify a time when he or she reacted intensely (positively or negatively) to either a client or a client's situation. How was this issue dealt with later in conference? Common issues with which health care workers may intensely identify are alcohol or drug use, family abuse, codependency issues, rescue fantasies, and lifestyles. These and many other issues that evoke strong feelings need to be addressed before the nurse is able to see the client and the client's situation and needs clearly. Self-assessment is a crucial component of effective nursing care not only in psychiatric nursing but also in other nursing specialties.

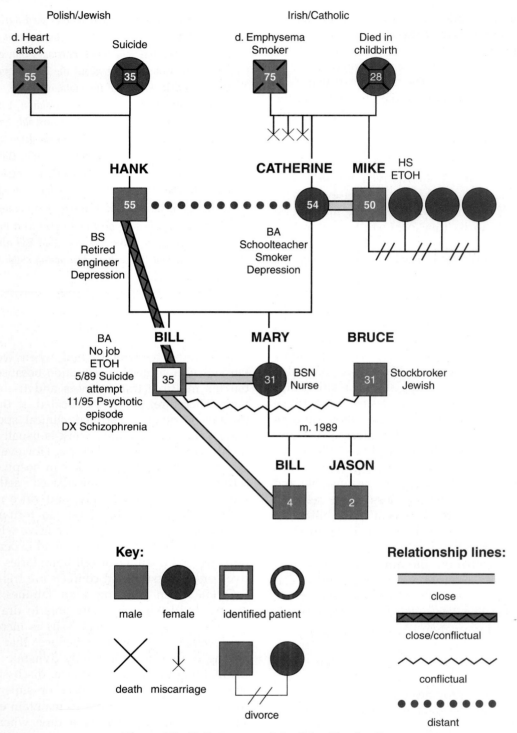

Figure 35–3 Genogram of the Schneider family.

Other Assessment Strategies

Other tools are available to help the practitioner assess how the family functions as a unit and identify individual member's perceptions of how the family communicates; how they deal with emotional issues, such as anger, conflict, and affection; how they work together as a unit to plan and solve problems; how

they make the important decisions for the family; and how they function generally. A focused interview, one in which the nurse can ask these questions directly, or an assessment device can be used to obtain this information.

A careful family assessment can be a vital part of the treatment if the family has as one of its members a person with a severe mental illness. Finkelman (2000) emphasizes the need to form a partnership with the family to reintegrate the ill person into the family and home.

NURSING DIAGNOSIS

Families have many needs at different times in their development. Family life often involves new members, deaths, mental and physical illness, economic reverberations, developmental crises, and unanticipated changes or decline. Severe dysfunctional patterns (e.g., marked relational conflict, sexual misconduct, abuse, violence, and suicide) exist within many families that cause physical or mental anguish to the members.

Numerous nursing diagnoses are useful in working with families. Box 35–2 identifies some useful family nursing diagnoses. DSM-IV-TR (APA 2000) has also identified areas that can be used to target medical or psychiatric attention. These areas come under the heading "other conditions that may be a focus of clinical attention." These DSM-IV-TR categories are listed below:

Relational Problems	Relational problems related to a mental disorder or a generic medical condition, sibling relational problem or problems
Problems related to abuse or neglect	Includes physical and sexual abuse and neglect of a child, and physical or sexual abuse of an adult
Bereavement	Bereavement may cause considerable impairment and complications
	Identity problems
	Religious or spiritual problems
	Age-related decline
	Acculturation problems

OUTCOME CRITERIA

Although different theories are held and a wide variety of methods are used by different therapists, the goals of family therapy are basically the same. These goals (Steinglass 1995) are to

■ Reduce dysfunctional behavior of individual family members.
■ Resolve or reduce intrafamily relationship conflicts.
■ Mobilize family resources and encourage adaptive family problem-solving behaviors.
■ Improve family communication skills.
■ Heighten awareness and sensitivity to other family members' emotional needs and help family members meet their needs.
■ Strengthen the family's ability to cope with major life stressors and traumatic events, including chronic physical or psychiatric illness.
■ Improve integration of the family system into the societal system, e.g., school, medical facilities, workplace, and especially the extended family.

Family psychoeducational treatment is often done by nurses. Goals a nurse can use for psychoeducational teaching with a family include:

■ Learning to accept the illness of a family member.
■ Learning to deal effectively with an ill member's symptoms, such as hallucinations, delusions, poor hygiene, physical limitations, paranoia, and aggression.
■ Understanding what medications can and cannot do and when the family should seek medical advice.
■ Assistance in locating community resources.
■ Reducing family anxiety and restoring or gaining a sense of control and balance in family life.

BOX 35–2   *Possible Nursing Diagnoses for Family Interventions*

Impaired parenting	Impaired adjustment
Sexual dysfunctioning	Ineffective denial
Interrupted family processes	Ineffective family therapeutic regimen management
Dysfunctional family processes: alcohol	Deficient knowledge
Caregiver role strain	Impaired verbal communication
Risk for caregiver role strain	Defensive coping
Spiritual distress	

PLANNING

Determine the kinds of immediate and long-term needs of the family. For example, is the family in crisis, e.g., is one of the members homicidal, suicidal, abusive, or being abused? Do protective services need to be called? Is hospitalization necessary to protect a suicidal or self-mutilating member?

Is there a crisis at one of the family's developmental stages? What are the family coping mechanisms at this time, what kinds of new skills can family members use to help them at this time in order to help facilitate resolution of normal life-cycle crises? Do family members need to be taught conflict management skills, problem-solving skills, parenting skills, limit-setting skills?

Is there a need for psychoeducational family interventions? Nurses are learning to be adept at helping family members learn about the physical illness of an afflicted family member (e.g., severe mental illness, dementia), understand what medications can do (as well as effects, etc.), and identify support groups and community resources to help the family cope with crisis and improve the quality of life for all of its members. How extensive is the family's knowledge deficit?

Where should a family be referred for optimal outcomes? Is there a problem with substance abuse, depression, and unrealistic expectations of members, anger, or conduct disorder?

A careful analysis of a sound assessment helps the nurse and other members of the health care team to identify the most appropriate family interventions for troubled families.

INTERVENTION

Outcome research has shown that family therapy works best in the following situations (Kadis and McClendon 1999):

■ The child is the patient and the disorder is one of conduct (Prince and Jacobson 1995, Pinsoff and Wynn 1998)
■ The wife in the couple is depressive
■ A substance-abusing person enters treatment and then is maintained after treatment
■ A schizophrenic individual is the client and family therapy is used to reduce relapse rates.

Communication Guidelines

The roles of the psychiatric mental health nurse and the advanced practice clinical specialist or practitioner vary in the ways in which the nurse clinician works with families in both the hospital and the community settings. Differences exist in counseling and psychobiological interventions. The basic-level nurse clinician may provide counseling by use of a problem-solving approach for a problem that represents an immediate family difficulty related to health or well-being. The advanced practice nurse, a certified clinical specialist who has postgraduate training in family therapy, may conduct private family therapy sessions. As to psychobiological interventions, the advanced practice certified specialists may have prescriptive authority (in accordance with their state nurse practice act and their qualifications).

The roles of the entry-level nurse and the staff nurse, although different in scope from that of the psychiatric mental health nurse and the clinical specialist, are equally important, especially in promoting and monitoring a family's mental health. Developing and practicing good listening skills and regarding family members in a positive, nonjudgmental way are critically important skills for all levels of nurses wherever one practices.

An important function of entry-level and staff nurses is to assess cues from various family members that indicate the degree and the amount of stress the family system is experiencing. These critical observations need to be readily reported so that appropriate interventions may be made in a timely manner. Some indicators of stress in a family system are

■ an inability by the family or a family member to process and act on certain recommended treatment directives
■ various somatic complaints among family members
■ a high degree of anxiety
■ depression
■ problems in school
■ drug use

Promoting and monitoring a family's mental health can occur in virtually any setting and often requires making the most of an opportune moment. It does not have to be a formal meeting. Sometimes, an informal conversation (**therapeutic encounter**) can have the greatest effect. A few general guidelines help the nurse clinician be nonjudgmental in the information presented, as well as in tone of voice and questions asked. For example, the question "Don't you think you should at least try to comply with your medical regimen?" would probably cause the patient to tune the nurse out, while the invitation "Tell me what this medical regimen of yours is like" could open the door to understanding and problem solving in a collaborative rather than a hierarchical way.

1. The nonblaming manner promotes open and flexible communication among all professionals and family members in the caregiving system. If other family members are involved in the conversation, be it on the hospital unit or in a family therapy session, the nurse should get each member's view of how the individual member's medical regimen affects the way the family functions and what the individual members consider a possible solution to the problem.

2. A second guideline for the nurse clinician is to impart information that is clear and understandable to all family members and to allow them to choose and decide what to do with the information. This is both a respectful and an empowering way to work with families, which indicates to them that they are the ones who are accountable and responsible for how they choose to use the information.

3. Third, it is imperative that the perspective of each family member is elicited and heard. Often, some family members hear another member's view for the first time in this democratic forum, and many times, they are surprised ("I didn't know you felt that way"). The more family input there is, the more options usually exist for alternative ways of managing problematic situations. This approach defines the family as the central psychosocial unit of care. The following vignette provides an example of maintaining neutrality and of hearing from all members.

Vignette

■ *Ms. Conway, the head nurse on the adolescent psychiatric unit, was concerned about all the negative comments the staff members were making regarding the fact that none of Chip's family had been in to visit him for over a week. In fact, she was concerned that Chip was picking up the staff's feelings as well. After many attempts, Ms. Conway finally reached Chip's mother by telephone and began to assess the situation. She discovered that Chip's mom is divorced and is working double shifts to meet the family's expenses. There is a 2-year-old at home and a set of twins in the fourth grade.*

Chip's mom was planning to visit on the weekend, but the babysitter called to say she was sick. Once Ms. Conway was able to see the situation from another perspective, that this was a family with young children that was struggling to make ends meet, she called a staff meeting to address the situation.

Further interventions in this situation would be to process (problem solve) with Chip and his mother concerning what is realistic for each of them regarding visiting. Perhaps an extended family member or a friend can visit when the mother cannot. Longer-range planning for supervision for Chip when he is discharged should also be discussed as family supports are identified and assessed.

Unfortunately, the negative comments about family members by staff occur all too often. This can present a difficult situation for the student, who is entering the "culture" of the unit as an outsider and who realizes the negative effects that this behavior has on family members. An intervention is in order; however, it would be appropriate for the student to first seek supervision from the instructor, so that the most effective approach can be planned out beforehand. One useful technique is for the student to ask questions of the head nurse and staff in such a way that alternative ways to view the family in a broader perspective are embedded in the questions. An example of this might be "Has anyone had a chance to contact Chip's mom to see if there are any problems?" or "I wonder what it's like for Chip's mom to have her son in a psychiatric unit?"

Family Interventions

Family therapy is viewed by professionals as appropriate for most situations, although there are some contraindications: (Kadis and McClendon 1999)

■ When the therapeutic environment is not safe and someone will be harmed by information, uncontrolled anxiety, or hostility
■ When there is a lack of willingness to be honest
■ When there is an unwillingness to maintain confidentiality

However, in most other situations, family therapy is useful, especially when it is combined with psychopharmacology in the treatment of families who have a member with a mental illness, such as bipolar disorder, depression, and schizophrenia. However, not all families can afford the money or the time for traditional family therapy. Therefore, many families greatly benefit from psychoeducational family therapy and from self-help groups. The first part of this section introduces the student to (1) traditional family therapy intervention strategies, (2) psychoeducational groups, and (3) self-help groups that may benefit families and family members.

TRADITIONAL FAMILY THERAPY

Family therapists use a wide variety of theoretical philosophies and techniques to bring about change in dysfunctional patterns of behavior and interaction. Some therapists may focus on the here and now, while others may rely more heavily on the family's history and reports of what happened between sessions. As stated earlier, most family therapists use an eclectic approach, drawing on a variety of techniques that are designed to fit the particular personality and strengths of the family (Steinglass 1995).

Multiple-family group therapy is often used with families who have a hospitalized family member in an inpatient setting. These groups can help family members identify and gain insight into their own problems as they are reflected in the problems of other families. Several families meet in one group with one or more therapists, usually once a week until their ill family member is discharged; these groups often continue for a specific period of time after the client is discharged.

PSYCHOEDUCATIONAL FAMILY THERAPY

Psychoeducational groups have proved immensely effective, especially as a family treatment modality combined with other modalities (e.g., psychopharmacology). One of the most successful areas of psychoeducational family training is schizophrenia. Some studies have shown that psychoeducational family therapy reduces the long-term need for rehospitalization by as much as 50% to 80% (Steinglass 1995). Gamble and Midence (1994) emphasize that families are extremely valuable and positive resources for clients. Family work promotes and supports families in coping with a family member with a severe mental illness.

The primary goal of psychoeducational family therapy is the sharing of mental health care information. Family education groups help family members better understand their member's illness, prodromal symptoms (symptoms that may appear before a full relapse), medications needed to help reduce the symptoms, and more. The modes of psychoeducational family meetings or multiple family meetings allow feelings to be shared and strategies for dealing with these feelings to be developed. Painful issues of anger or loss, feelings of stigmatization or sadness, and feelings of helplessness can be shared and put in a perspective that the family and individual members can deal with more satisfactorily. Psychoeducational family groups are extremely useful for people with all kinds of mental as well as medical disorders.

Psychoeducational groups have also proved helpful in parent management training such as working with a child with conduct disorder.

SELF-HELP GROUPS

Self-help groups can be divided into two types. One type is for groups of people who have a personal problem or social deprivation. The second is for families with a member who has a specific problem or condition. Self-help groups acknowledge the needs of family members. Some groups may focus on families with healthy members, while others offer assistance to families whose members may be experiencing a health disorder or crisis. Most health professionals are aware that for any developmental event, life crisis, or health disorder, a comparable mutual-aid group exists. These health professionals are in the best position to help their clients and their families find additional support and information. For many people, self-help groups can be healing.

Case Management

Although the nursing profession has always interacted with families to some degree in the process of meeting a client's needs, our current knowledge of family systems dictates that the family be the primary focus when the management of the individual client is planned. The family's culture, ethnicity, socioeconomic status, and stage of family life cycle, as well as its unique patterns and beliefs about illness, all affect an individual's progress and response to case management. The family is the most powerful group to which an individual may ever belong, and it is vital that the nurse not discount or ignore the importance of the family's influence on its members when planning care.

To a great extent, case management entails teaching, giving appropriate referrals, and offering emotional support.

Vignette

■ *David Gardiner, age 21, is leaving the hospital after having experienced his first psychotic episode while taking his final examinations before graduation from college. David is being discharged back to his family, which consists of his mother and father; his maternal grandfather, who has been recently bedridden; and a younger brother Todd, who is 17 years of age. David's diagnosis is paranoid schizophrenia. The nurse takes a psychoeducational approach with the family.*

Issues and needs are addressed by the nurse during family meetings while David is still hospitalized and later in follow-up family therapy after discharge. Initial interventions involve imparting information about David's mental illness through reading materials and discussion. The nurse also gives the family information and telephone numbers of psychosocial support groups and affiliation with a local chapter of the National Alliance for the Mentally Ill (NAMI).

The nurse maintains ongoing assessment of the family's strengths and weaknesses, including family supports as well as community support. She identifies some of the areas that may need to be addressed during the next few meetings.

Some of these issues include reorganizing family roles to accommodate a family member with a newly diagnosed, severe and persistent mental illness; managing their bedridden grandfather; attending to Todd's probable fears that he, too, may have this illness; dealing with potential parental guilt feelings from a genetic point of view; planning how to mobilize should David experience another psychotic episode; managing medication and emphasizing the importance of compliance; dealing with concerns about David's future and formulating realistic expectations; coping with feelings of loss for what was, and what was hoped for; and, finally, maintaining the integrity and functioning of the spousal subsystem.

The nurse discusses these and other issues with the family and identifies where and how these issues can best be addressed. For example, the visiting nurse was called in to evaluate the grandfather's situation and need for support in the home, and a multiple family psychoeducation group was formed to continue the family's understanding of David's illness, to learn ways to cope with common problems that may arise, and to provide a place for the family to share their feelings of loss and grief.

Psychopharmacology Issues

The nurse is often the first to explain to the family the purpose for a prescribed medication as well as the desired effects and possible side effects and adverse reactions. The following situation took place at the time of discharge.

Vignette

■ Susan Harris, a 45-year-old account executive and mother of three teenagers, had been referred by her physician to the mental health center for acute depression. The psychia-

trist there had prescribed an antidepressant. Routinely, new clients are seen by the nurse clinician for a review of medications as a part of the health teaching. Unfortunately, the nurse clinician was engaged with another client in crisis at the time and missed meeting with Susan and her husband.

One week later, Susan made an appointment with the clinical specialist for symptoms of insomnia and lack of sexual desire, which was a concern for both Susan and her husband. She feared that she was getting worse and "going crazy." During the appointment, the nurse clinician reviewed the side effects and adverse reactions of antidepressants with Mrs. Harris. She informed Mrs. Harris that the medication she was taking might take 3 weeks or longer to take effect. She also explained that common side effects of the group of medications she was taking (selective serotonin reuptake inhibitors [SSRIs]) were sleeplessness and lowered sexual drive. They discussed ways to combat these side effects (see Chapter 18). The nurse urged Susan to continue taking the medication; however, if the side effects were to continue, the medication could be changed. Susan was due to visit the clinic 2 weeks later for follow-up. The nurse urged Susan to discuss the side effects of the medication with her husband and encouraged him to come with her to the clinic at her next appointment.

Certainly, the more information the family has at its disposal, the less anxiety will distort their observations and decision making after discharge. Because of untoward circumstances in this case, the nurse clinician on the unit did not review Susan's medication with her before she was discharged. The clinical specialist needs to closely monitor Susan to determine whether her symptoms represent an exacerbation of her depression or a reaction to the antidepressant medication. If Susan is having a reaction to the medication, the nurse may consult with a physician and try another medication.

Visit the **Evolve** website at
http://evolve.elsevier.com/Varcarolis
for more Case Studies.

CASE STUDY 35–1	*Ortega Family*

The Ortega family has just arrived on the locked unit of a large city psychiatric hospital. Maria Ortega is an 18-year-old female college student and the eldest of four siblings. She is admitted through the emergency department after having slashed her wrists and losing a lot of blood. Her parents and extended family members are talking loudly, crying hysterically, and pacing about the waiting area. Having finished the usual admitting procedures, the nurse clinician now turns her attention to the family members.

ASSESSMENT

The tendency for some families in a time of crisis is to overreact and be unable to focus on the problem at hand. This may happen in families in which the boundaries are blurred and unclear, and individuation of family members is not well defined. The primary initial goal was to calm down the family system. Chairs were provided for everyone, and the nurse clinician proceeded to talk in a soft, slow, emphatic manner, answering any questions that the family had. Once the nurse clinician joined with the family in this way, she then began to construct a genogram as she asked the family for information. During this process, the nurse clinician discovered that the youngest child in the Ortega family, Tony, age 4, has an autistic disorder. Maria was Tony's primary caretaker before she left for college. The family was stressed both financially and emotionally because of the "loss" of Maria before the present emergency.

NURSING DIAGNOSIS

Maria's suicide attempt seems to be related to her depression and feelings of hopelessness. These feelings appear to originate from what is taking place in the family system. The nursing diagnosis was: **Ineffective role performance related to loss of financial and caregiving support.**

OUTCOME CRITERIA

Maria would most likely be in the hospital overnight. A family meeting session was to begin on the unit that day, and follow-up sessions would take place at the community mental health center after discharge. **Outcome criteria** included helping the family stabilize and meet their needs, allowing Maria to leave home and become an independent young adult. **Short-term goals** centered around helping the family identify alternative ways to deal with Tony's care and the management of Maria's tuition.

CASE STUDY 35–1	*Ortega Family (Continued)*

INTERVENTION

Once Maria is discharged, the family decides to continue with family therapy sessions in a community mental health clinic, where they meet weekly with a certified specialist. Here, the work that was begun during hospitalization is continued, and the family, which is no longer in a crisis situation, is able to work toward making changes that will prevent a similar situation from occurring. If the clinical specialist is licensed for prescriptive privileges, she would take over the management of Maria's antidepressant medication prescribed by the hospital psychiatrist. Otherwise, she would report her observations and progress to the medicating psychiatrist when necessary.

The family is eventually able to work together and find ways to expand their financial resources. With information they obtain from the nurse, they are able to contact two community resources that increase their understanding of how to work with Tony as well as ways to divide up the responsibility for Tony's care so the family does not seem so overwhelmed.

EVALUATION

Shortly after discharge, Maria stops taking the antidepressant. She states the problem is no longer overwhelming and that once her anxiety and feelings of helplessness subsided, so did her suicidal thoughts.

The process of rebalancing the family system after such a disruption will take time. However, timely interventions by the nurse clinician can make a tremendous difference in providing the family with direction and with the belief that they are indeed capable of adapting to these untoward changes in the family's life cycle.

SUMMARY

The aim of family therapy is to decrease emotional reactivity among family members and to encourage differentiation among individual family members. The primary characteristics that are essential to healthy family functioning are flexibility and clear boundaries. The stages in the changing family life cycle of a traditional family, a divorced family, and a remarried family have been introduced. There are many approaches to family therapy that are based on theoretical concepts; those approaches that include helping a family gain insight and helping a family make behavioral changes are most successful.

The genogram is an efficient clinical summary and format for information and relationships across at least three generations. The family's culture, ethnicity, socioeconomic status, and life cycle stage, as well as its unique patterns and beliefs about illness, all affect the individual patient's progress and response to case management.

The impact of the family and the family's effect on the health and progress of the ill family member is invaluable. It is imperative that the nurse clinician assess the identified patient in the context of the family. Using a multicontextual framework, the nurse clinician observes the stage of the family life cycle, the multigenerational issues, and the family's sociocultural status. The nurse clinician must continually be sensitive to the many different perspectives of individual family members in terms of how they view the problem and what their ideas are regarding negotiating within the family system to accommodate to the changes required. Nurses with basic training are frequently called upon to conduct psychoeducation with families. Nurses with specialized training and who are certified use a variety of theoretical approaches in family therapy.

Visit the **Evolve** website at
http://evolve.elsevier.com/Varcarolis
for a post-test on the content in this chapter.

Visit the **Evolve** website at
http://evolve.elsevier.com/Varcarolis
for additional self-study exercises.

Critical Thinking and Chapter Review

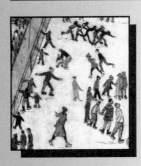

Critical Thinking

1. Use a family from your clinical experience. Evaluate this family's functional/dysfunctional status using the five family functions described in the text, i.e., management, boundary, communication, emotional-supportive, and socialization functions.
2. Using the same family from above, create a genogram that identifies their stage in the family life cycle and describe the sociocultural context of this family.
3. Create your own personal genogram, including at least three generations. Be sure to include
   A. Location, occupation, and educational level
   B. Critical events, such as births, marriages, moves, job changes, separations, divorce, illnesses, death
   C. Relationship patterns, such as cut-offs, distancing, over-involvement, and conflict
4. A family has just found out that their young son is going to die. The parents have been fighting and blaming each other for ignoring the child's ongoing symptoms of leg pain, which was eventually diagnosed as advanced cancer. There are two other siblings in the family. How would you as the primary nurse apply family concepts to help this family? What would be your outcome criterion?

Chapter Review

Choose the most appropriate answer.

1. When assessed within the context of the family system, the nurse determines that the identified patient is

   1. the family member the others say is the problem
   2. the individual member of the family who first seeks help
   3. the person who is triangled in to help lower tension between spouses
   4. the person who makes the rules about who participates in a particular family function.

2. When a nurse assesses a family system as being healthy, the two primary characteristics found to be present are

   1. generalizing and placating
   2. flexibility and clear boundaries
   3. diffusion and enmeshment
   4. socialization and management

3. A realistic goal for improved communication in a family engaged in family therapy could be stated as "Communication among family members will be

1. clear and direct."
2. altruistic and supportive."
3. distant and guarded."
4. emotional and conflictual."

4. A function of the entry-level staff nurse in promoting a family's mental health is to

   1. conduct family therapy sessions
   2. identify each member's unmet needs and devise plans for meeting these needs
   3. assess cues that indicate the amount of stress the family is experiencing
   4. give assignments designed to change defensive coping styles and limit denial

5. Jim, a 20-year-old college student, has been hospitalized for treatment of bipolar disorder. His discharge plan is to live with his parents and 17-year-old sister until stabilized. His return to college is planned for the following semester. The nurse believes rehospitalization can be avoided if Jim and his family understand his illness and his medication. The type of family therapy that will produce these outcomes is

   1. crisis intervention
   2. traditional family therapy
   3. psychoeducational family therapy
   4. a self-help group for families with mentally ill members

REFERENCES

American Psychiatric Association (2000). *Diagnostic and statistical manual of mental disorders DSM-IV-TR* (4th ed.). Washington, DC: American Psychiatric Association.

Andrus, K. (1996). Family therapy. In V. B. Carson and E. N. Arnold (Eds.), *Mental health nursing: The nurse-patient journey*. Philadelphia: W. B. Saunders.

Bowen, M. (1985). *Family therapy in clinical practice*. New Jersey: Jason Aronson.

Carter, B., and McGoldrick, M. (Eds.) (1989). *The changing family life cycle: A framework for family therapy* (2nd ed.). Boston: Allyn & Bacon.

Clements, I. (1983). Stress adaptation. In I. W. Clements and F. B. Roberts (Eds.), *Family health: A theoretical approach to nursing care* (pp. 133–144). New York: John Wiley.

Cooley, M. (1995). A family perspective in community health nursing. In C. M. Smith and F. A. Mauer (Eds.), *Community nursing: Theory and practice* (pp. 205–220). Philadelphia: W. B. Saunders.

Finkleman, A. W. (2000). Psychiatric patients and families Moving from catastrophic event to long-term coping. *Home Care Providers*, 5(4):142–147.

Gamble, C., and Midence, K. (1994). Schizophrenic family work: Mental health nurses delivering an innovative service. *Journal of Psychosocial Nursing and Mental Health Services*, 32(10):13–16.

Haley, J. (1980). *Leaving home*. New York: McGraw-Hill.

Kadis, L. B., and McClendon, R. (1999). Marital and family therapy. In R. E. Hales, S. C. Yadofsky, and J. A. Talbot (Eds.). *The American Psychiatric Press textbook of psychiatry* (3rd ed.). Washington, DC: The American Psychiatric Press.

Lebow, J. L. (1998). Conducting couple and family therapy. In G. P. Koochen, J. C. Norcross, and S. S. Hill (Eds.). *Psychologists' desk reference*. New York: Oxford University Press.

McGoldrick, M., and Gerson, R. (1985). *Genograms in family assessment*. New York: W. W. Norton.

Minuchin, S. (1974). *Families and family therapy*. Cambridge, MA: Harvard University Press.

Pinsoff, W., and Wynne, L. (1995). The efficacy of marital and family therapy: Overview and conclusions. *Journal of Marital and Family Therapy*, 21:585–616.

Prince, S., and Jacobson, N. (1995). A review and evaluation of marital and family therapy for affective disorders. *Journal of Marital and Family Therapy*, 21:377–402.

Roberts, F. B. (1983). An interaction model for family assessment. In I. W. Clements and F. B. Roberts (Eds.), *Family health: A theoretical approach to nursing care* (pp. 189–204). New York: John Wiley.

Rolland, J. (1994). *Families, illness, and disability: An integrative treatment approach*. New York: Basic Books.

Satir, V. (1972). *Peoplemaking*. Palo Alto, CA: Science and Behavior Books.

Satir, V. (1983). *Conjoint family therapy*. Palo Alto: Science and Behavior Books.

Steinglass, P. L. (1995). Family therapy. In H. I. Kaplan and B. J. Sadock (Eds.), *Comprehensive textbook of psychiatry VI* (Vol. 1, pp. 1838–1846). Baltimore: Williams & Wilkins.

Wynne, L. C. (1988). *The state of the art in family therapy research: Controversies and recommendations*. New York: Family Process Press.

Outline

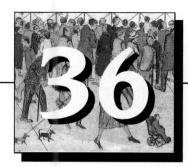

36

Alternative and Complementary Therapies and Practices

GLORIA KUHLMAN

Key Terms and Concepts

The key terms and concepts listed here also appear in color where they are defined or first discussed in this chapter.

acupressure

acupuncture

alternative medicine

complementary therapy

herbal therapies

homeopathy

Objectives

After studying this chapter, the reader will be able to

1. Explore philosophies behind various complementary and alternative therapies, including acupressure or acupuncture, aromatherapy, chiropractic medicine, herbal medicine, homeopathy, and massage.

2. Discuss the techniques used in the various complementary therapies and the nurse's role.

3. Discuss how the public can be misled through quackery and fraud related to the use of alternative and complementary therapies.

4. Identify research projects that are exploring the efficacy of alternative and complementary therapies.

5. Explore information resources available through literature and online sources.

OVERVIEW OF ALTERNATIVE AND COMPLEMENTARY MEDICINE

Complementary and alternative medicine (CAM) is a broad domain of healing resources that encompasses all health systems, modalities, and practices and their accompanying theories and beliefs, other than those intrinsic to the politically dominant health system of a particular society or culture in a given historical period. CAM includes all such practices and ideas self-defined by their users as preventing or treating illness or promoting health and well-being. Boundaries within CAM and between the CAM domain and that of the dominant system are not always sharp or fixed. (Zollman and Vickers 1999)

This chapter explores issues and raises questions related to the increasing number of Americans who are turning to complementary therapy and alternative medicine (CAM) to help manage or sometimes prevent the onset of chronic illness, increase longevity, improve cognitive function, or increase their feeling of well-being (Ness, Sherman, and Pan 1999). These individuals often learn about these resources from the media or friends. CAM therapies are now in demand by health consumers and are available to the general public through every known means of communication including the internet, a primary source of information for some people in this information age. Caution is advised, since information from the internet may not be reliable.

The dominant health care system of biomedicine in the United States is frequently based on scientific research. Alternative and complementary treatments are based on cultural or historical beliefs but do not always have scientific underpinnings. The dominant system of biomedicine, commonly called allopathy, may utilize traditional psychotropic medications that may have limited efficacy and often-significant side effects. The newer generations of psychotropic medications are increasingly beneficial for the treatment of mental illness but are not always available to those who need them (Lake 2000).

Clinicians recognize the connection between mind and body and their interaction, especially in the mental health field. This connection is understood in all areas of medicine when symptoms are exaggerated by stress. Conventional medicine often treats the disease, while CAM focuses on healing the whole person.

Alternative and Complementary Medicine Defined

The National Institutes of Health (NIH) established an Office of Alternative Medicine (OAM) in 1992. Complementary and alternative medicine (CAM) covers a broad range of healing philosophies. Most often it is defined as those treatments and health care practices that are not taught widely in medical schools, not generally used in hospitals, and usually not reimbursed by insurance companies (NCCAM). These therapies may be termed "holistic," that is, therapies that incorporate the entire person—biological, psychological, social, and spiritual. It is important to recognize, however, that holistic practitioners do thorough assessments with the client's active participation and then determine the best approach, which may be CAM or may in fact be conventional medical care (Eliopoulos 1999). The philosophy of complementary and alternative medicine often espouses the prevention of health problems rather than the treatment of symptoms once health problems arise. Therapies may be used alone (referred to as alternative), with other alternative therapies, or in tandem with conventional treatments (referred to as complementary) (NCCAM). These therapeutic modalities incorporate therapies consistent with Western medicine, in some cases, and in other cases, healing processes that have originated in other areas of the world are used. Some complementary and alternative medicine practices are becoming incorporated into mainstream medical practice, but others are still considered outside the realm of accepted medical care.

Consumers and Health Care

Consumers of traditional health care practices are requesting information about complementary and alternative medical treatments from their health care practitioners. The knowledgeable consumer, relying on readily available medical information through public libraries, popular bookstores, and databases on the internet, are questioning the traditional practice of biomedicine. People who already use alternative or complementary health services have created a need for health care providers to become informed about the current literature related to those treatments. Herbal remedies, for example, may be used to treat psychiatric symptoms but may also produce a change in mood, thinking, or behavior as a side effect as do psychotropic medications. Herbal remedies can also interact with other psychiatric medications that the individual is taking (Wong and Boon

1998). There are an increasing number of people who use medicinal herbs or seek the advice of their health care provider regarding their use. More than one third of Americans use herbs for health purposes, yet clients often lack accurate information about the safety and efficacy of herbal remedies (O'Hara, Kiefer, Farrell, and Kemper 1998). The University of Washington Health Services Center through the Robert Wood Johnson Clinical Scholars Program undertook a project to review data on 12 of the most commonly used herbs in the United States and provide practical information on the judicious use of the medicinal herbs studied (O'Hara et al. 1998).

Many practitioners are expanding their understanding of CAM practices by utilizing literature available from professional associations, educational organizations, and research institutions that provide information on complementary and alternative medical practices. Since many of these organizations have developed internet websites, the consumer may now access information once available only to professionals. All professionals and consumers must be aware that the health information disseminated by a particular organization presenting a therapy may be less than objective, therefore everyone should research a desired therapy by consulting and reviewing several sources. An up-to-date resource that may be utilized is the institutes and centers supported by the National Institutes of Health.

Categories of Alternative and Complementary Therapies

Complementary alternative health care and medical practices may be grouped into five major domains according to the NCCAM (Table 36–1). These domains include (1) alternative medical systems, (2) mind-body interventions, (3) biologically based treatments, (4) manipulative and body-based methods, and (5) energy therapies. Alternative medical systems are often traditional systems of medicine that are practiced in cultures throughout the world. Traditional oriental medicine falls within this category and emphasizes the proper balance or disturbances of chi or vital energy, in health and disease. The techniques that are incorporated into this category include acupuncture, herbal medicine, and oriental massage. **Homeopathy** and naturopathy are also examples of alternative medical systems. **Homeopaths** use small doses of specially prepared plant extracts and minerals to stimulate the body's defense mechanism and healing processes in order to treat illness. **Naturopathy** emphasizes health restoration rather

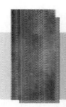

TABLE 36–1 *Complementary and Alternative Therapies Grouped by Health Care Domain*
■ Alternative medical systems Traditional oriental medicine Acupuncture Herbal medicine Oriental massage Homeopathy Naturopathy ■ Mind-body interventions Hypnosis Dance, music, art therapy ■ Biologically based treatments Herbal therapy Dietary therapy Orthomolecular therapy Individual biologic therapies ■ Manipulative and body-based methods Chiropractic Massage therapy ■ Energy therapies Bioelectromagnetic therapy Reiki Therapeutic touch

than disease treatment and uses diet and clinical nutrition, homeopathy, acupuncture, herbal medicine, hydrotherapy, spinal and soft-tissue manipulation, physical therapies involving electric currents, ultrasound, and light therapy, and therapeutic counseling.

Mind-body interventions employ techniques designed to facilitate the mind's capacity to affect bodily function and symptoms. Many of these interventions, such as cognitive-behavioral approaches and patient education, are considered mainstream, but hypnosis, dance, music, and art therapy, as well as prayer are categorized as complementary and alternative. Biologically based therapies may overlap with conventional medicine's use of dietary supplements. These therapies include herbal, special dietary, orthomolecular, and individual biological therapies.

Manipulative and body-based methods are based on manipulation or movement of the body. Chiropractors focus on the relationship between structure and function, and how that relationship affects the preservation and restoration of health by using manipulative therapy as a treatment tool. Massage therapists manipulate the soft tissues to normalize these tissues. Energy therapies focus on energy fields originating within the body and those from

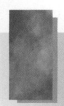

TABLE 36–2 *Grouping of Treatments by Classification: Alternative Medicine or Complementary Therapy*

■ Alternative medicine
  Diet and nutrition
■ Complementary therapy
  Acupressure and acupuncture
  Aromatherapy
  Chiropractic medicine
  Herbal medicine
  Homeopathy
  Therapeutic touch

other sources. An example of these therapies is Reiki, which is based on the belief that by channeling spiritual energy through the practitioner the spirit is healed and, in turn, it heals the physical body.

Cost of Alternative Therapies

The use of alternative therapies is also spreading from another influence. The increasing pressure to control health care spending in most countries has resulted in a need for the development of alternative less expensive means for treatment of mental illnesses. In order to identify cost-effective care, we must also have reliable information about the treatment methods that are being utilized. With the increased use of herbal remedies, some of which have become commonly used, it is imperative that data be available to identify the efficacy of those treatments being employed.

The remainder of the chapter reviews some common alternative and complementary therapies that have direct relationships with the practice of mental health (Table 36–2). There are many indications for these therapies in the treatment of other types of nonpsychiatric disorders. The National Center for Complementary and Alternative Medicine (NCCAM) and the National Institutes of Health (NIH) web sites provide information on other treatments and reviews of other complementary and alternative therapies. Literature in medical and nursing journals provide information related to the use of complementary and alternative therapies for a variety of physiological disorders.

ALTERNATIVE MEDICINE

Diet and Nutrition

Dietary supplements, once regulated like foods, are now sold without the premarketing safety evaluations required of new food ingredients. This changed with the Dietary and Supplemental Health and Education Act of 1994 (DSHEA). Prior to this Act, dietary supplements were nutrients such as vitamins and protein; now other substances (essential nutrients, plus herbs, botanicals, enzymes, and hormones) once considered in this category of supplements. The FDA no longer has the power to regulate supplements of vitamins, minerals, herbs, amino acids, and other compounds (Yen 1999). Dietary supplements can be labeled with certain health claims if they meet published FDA requirements and contain a disclaimer saying that the supplement has not been evaluated by the FDA and is not intended to diagnose, treat, cure, or prevent any disease.

Nutritional therapies have been used for a variety of disorders, most commonly addictions. The majority of the information available is anecdotal and often related to treatments of addictions. The American Dietetic Association (ADA) has issued a position statement that nutritional supplements are able to improve the effectiveness of the treatment of chemical dependency. Culliton, Boucher, and Bullock (1999) reviewed multiple treatment modalities, including nutritional supplements to reduce alcohol and cocaine intake. However, there are still few research trials that have been undertaken to demonstrate scientific efficacy. The use of specific vitamin and mineral supplements appears to result in significantly reduced alcohol intake. The nutritional programs, if standardized through research programs, may result in having a significant impact on the treatment of addictions.

Druss and associates (1998), examining data from a National Health and Nutrition Examination Survey, found that individuals who experienced major depression were twice as likely to be taking nonprescription dietary supplements as were individuals without depression. The researchers suggest that individuals may seek self-medication for depressive symptoms rather than seeking traditional means of treatment.

Of additional concern to health care providers is the fact that many of the nutritional supplements may have problematic interactions with medications. There are known interactions with vitamins, but other supplements are not as easily recognized. As the use of nutritional supplements increases, especially in megadoses, there is a need to assess the interactions between nutritional supplements and medications. Food and drug interactions should be available to consumers, and individuals who take dietary supplements should be encouraged to discuss their intake of all supplements with their health care practitioner (Miller 1999).

COMPLEMENTARY THERAPY

Acupressure and Acupuncture

Acupuncture and other forms of Asian therapies, such as acupressure, have become increasingly part of the complementary and alternative health care in the last two decades in the United States. Information is available in professional and popular literature related to the use of acupuncture for a variety of health care needs (Beal 2000). Acupuncture, a therapy used in traditional Chinese medicine, consists of the placement of needles into the skin at certain points to modulate the flow of energy called *chi*, which flows through the body along specific pathways called meridians.

Most people use acupuncture for pain relief (headache, back pain, osteoarthritis, neck pain, or organic pain), but this therapy also has been used to treat substance abuse and other emotional disorders (Lorenzi 1999; Ackerman 1999; Freeman and Lawlis 2001). Puncturing the skin is the most common method of application, but practitioners may use heat, pressure, friction, or suction (Freeman and Lawless 2001). Acupuncture is an intervention with few side effects when used for drug detoxification but has not been reviewed through traditional research methods. Because of the nature of acupuncture, it is difficult to perform research that meets the traditional trials of Western medicine, although NIDA and NIMH have conducted studies.

Research studies in 1987 and 1989 by Bullock (1989) found acupuncture was effective in the treatment of severe alcoholism. Patients in the treatment group reported less desire for alcohol, had fewer drinking episodes, and fewer admissions to detoxification centers than those patients receiving acupuncture to nonspecific treatment points. At six months post treatment, patients in the control group had twice the number of drinking episodes and expressed a stronger need for alcohol.

While the treatment of addiction is a multidimensional problem, the expectation that only one treatment modality would resolve this is probably unreasonable. The National Institutes of Health in a Consensus Statement in 1997 identified the treatment of addiction through acupuncture as an acceptable adjunct treatment that could be included in a comprehensive management program (NIH 1997).

The NCCAM fact sheet of Acupuncture Information and Resources identifies anxiety, depression, insomnia, and other conditions appropriate for acupuncture therapy. These are among 40 conditions identified by the World Health Organization (WHO) for which acupuncture can be used. The researchers at the NCCAM are conducting randomized clinical trials for these and other conditions to identify the efficacy of the treatment. Researchers in Minnesota and New Jersey are also conducting clinical trials in the treatment of emotional disorders, among other conditions. It is important to remember that acupuncture should be administered by a physician or a practitioner certified by NCCAM.

Reiki

Reiki is a practice reconnecting individuals to their innate power of self-healing through the gentle laying on of hands by the practitioner (Neild-Anderson and Ameling 2000). It is a healing therapy that provides comfort and healing through gentle touch. There is no attempt to manipulate the recipient's body or energy fields. The most frequently documented use of Reiki is for the relief of pain or relaxation in palliative care. Practitioners of Reiki report a reduction of stress as well as spiritual and emotional well-being along with a sense of deep relaxation. There are also reports of improved communication between caregivers and recipients as their emotional distress is diminished.

Aromatherapy

Aromatherapy, the use of essential oils for inhalation, works to activate the body's healing energy to balance mind, body, and spirit. Essential oils have been used to enhance the quality of life through reducing stress, regulating emotions, relief of anxiety, and reduction of insomnia (Lorenzi 1999). The National Association for Holistic Aromatherapy web site provides information on the use of essential oils from plant materials. They indicate that aromatherapy works through the stimulation of the olfactory nerve when the essential oils are inhaled. This stimulation sends messages to the limbic area, the seat of memory, learning, and emotion. Psychological changes may bring comfort, warmth, and security, often due to the association of the aroma with pleasant events. Positive responses may occur even when there are no specific memories associated; these events are what therapists use to determine the therapeutic benefits of the treatment.

Aromatherapy may also be experienced through application of the essential oils (diluted in a carrier base) to the skin. The topical use of the oils provides a sense of well-being. The use of the oils may not only relieve the muscle tension that was the original focus but also provide a sense of relaxation through the reduction of mental and emotional tension.

Chiropractic Medicine

Chiropractic care is the most widely used complementary and alternative therapy. Contemporary chiropractic care most frequently involves relief of musculoskeletal pain. Chiropractic medicine is based on the theory that energy flows from the brain to all parts of the body through the spinal cord and spinal nerves. Manipulation of the spinal column, called adjustment, puts the vertebrae back in their normal positions. Individuals seek chiropractic treatment for a variety of illnesses ranging from headaches, pain, allergies, asthma, and other disorders (NCCAM). The use of manipulation for headache has often focused on the treatment of migraine, tension, or cervicogenic headache pain. In randomized clinical trials of the treatment of tension headaches, both groups experienced relief of pain, but there were fewer side effects from the manipulation than from the use of medication (Freeman and Lawlis 2001).

Herbal Medicine

A growing number of Americans are using herbal products for preventive and therapeutic purposes (Cohen, Rousseau, and Robinson 2000). Manufacturers are not required to submit proof of safety or efficacy to the FDA. Providers must provide close scrutiny of herbal therapies used by their patients. Food products now are being sold with herbs—the drug-like action of herbs is important to disease treatment, but addition to foods may result in untoward reactions, especially when individuals do not realize the supplement is in the food they are consuming (Yen 1999).

With the vast availability of lay literature on herbal remedies and the ready availability of the products in health food and other stores, individuals are seeking less conventional therapies for their health problems. Information on the safe and effective use of the products is necessary. Currently, there is a lack of standardization and regulation of herbal products. There is a need for further standardization and information on the use of herbs (Youngkin and Israel 1996). The compounds are truly psychoactive substances and are neither benign nor without potential for drug-drug interactions as consumers often believe, since the substance is "nat-

TABLE 36–3 *Commonly Accepted Uses for Selected Herbal Remedies*

USE	HERBAL REMEDY
Sedative	St. John's wort, valerian
Memory loss	Gingko biloba
Tranquilizing	Black cohosh, kava kava

ural" rather than a "synthetic chemical" (McEnany 1999).

Alternative therapies are widely used by consumers. A number of herbs and supplements have recognizable effects on mood, memory, and insomnia (Table 36–3). Hypericum perforatum (St. John's wort) is used for mild to moderate depression, and gingko biloba for dementia. Research is now being conducted on the use of vitamins, amino acids, and fatty acids to determine their effects on mood and other mental phenomena. (Fugh-Berman and Cott 1999). People who seek conventional therapy commonly use herbs and related products. All physicians and health care providers should determine if the client's symptom is from the "remedy" that was not prescribed. (Winslow and Kroll 1998)

St. John's wort has been used for centuries to treat mental disorders and pain. In the past decade it has become the second most common herbal remedy in Germany and the United States. It is estimated that 17% of Americans have taken products containing St. John's wort (Beaubrun and Gray 2000). Herbalists in ancient times wrote about the efficacy of it as a sedative, antimalarial agent, and a balm for burns and wounds (NCCAM). People are turning to St. John's wort because side effects from traditional antidepressants are unpleasant (dry mouth, nausea, headache, diarrhea, or impaired sexual function). St. John's wort is far less costly, has fewer side effects (dry mouth, dizziness, gastrointestinal symptoms, photosensitivity, and fatigue), and does not require a prescription (NCCAM).

St. John's wort has been studied by a number of research teams over the last few years. Lantz, Buchalter, and Giambanco (1999) reported five cases of serotonin syndrome in older persons when combining St. John's wort and other antidepressants. Crupp (1999) reports that St. John's wort may have monoamine oxidase-inhibiting (MAOI) effects or may cause increased levels of serotonin, dopamine, and norepinephrine. Singer (1999) showed that St. John's wort inhibits serotonin reuptake by elevating extracellular sodium. The FDA published a warning in the Journal of the American Medical Association in April 2000, indicating that St. John's wort may interact with medications for HIV infection and immunosuppressants (JAMA 2000).

St. John's wort is thought to be useful in the treatment of mild to moderate depression. A study of St. John's wort on major depression found no significant change between placebo and St. John's wort (N = 200) (Shelton et al. 2001). Further studies looking at the effects of St. John's wort vs. SSRIs on mild to moderate major depression will aid in clarifying its efficacy. It reduces depression but causes photosensitivity. It is important to understand that the different preparations at the natural food store may vary in strength, quality, and potency of active ingredients, so individuals taking the compound may have varied responses (McEnany 1999). Ness, Sherman, and Pan (1999) report that regulated preparations of St. John's wort are reasonably safe. Side effects include dry mouth, dizziness, fatigue, constipation, nausea, and photosensitivity. The combination of St. John's wort with SSRIs has resulted in serotonergic syndrome (tremors, hypertonicity, autonomic dysfunction, hyperthermia, and even death). Therefore, the combination is contraindicated (Ness, Sherman, and Pan 1999; Beaubrun and Gray 2000).

Gingko biloba has been used for the treatment of cerebral insufficiency, but this is broadly defined and ranges from memory loss to emotional instability (Ness, Sherman, and Pan 1999). A recent clinical trial of mild to severely demented individuals demonstrated cognitive improvement after 4 to 6 weeks in individuals with mild cognitive impairment. Gingko is well tolerated, with rare, nonspecific side effects of gastrointestinal distress, headache, and allergic skin reactions. Gingko improves cognitive function, but it interacts with anticoagulants and antiplatelet agents and may cause spontaneous bleeding. Gingko should be used with caution by patients who consume alcohol or who have other risk factors for hemorrhagic stroke (Beaubrun and Gray 2000).

There are other herbs that are available as over-the-counter remedies at health food and other stores. These herbal remedies have been used over time, but most of them have not been extensively tested to determine their efficacy. Because these are dietary supplements (often found next to vitamins on store shelves), there is no FDA approval or standardization.

Black cohosh is an extract from a root that has been identified to have a calming effect. It is toxic in high doses and should be avoided if there is a history of hypertension or heart conditions. Kava kava, used in the Pacific Islands for thousands of years, has significant analgesic and anesthetic properties. It is considered a potential option in the treatment of anxiety but should not be combined with other tranquilizing agents, especially benzodiazepines (McEnany 2000, Beaubrun and Gray 2000). Kava kava also may potentiate the effects of alcohol and other sedative-hypnotic agents (Beaubrun and Gray 2000).

Valerian is a root that when made into a tea has sedative, tranquilizing, and sleep-inducing effects (McEnany 2000). Valerian can also be made into a variety of extracts and tinctures, which may also contain other ingredients (Beaubrun and Gray 2000). It is generally recognized as safe for the treatment of insomnia when taken at the recommended dosages. Side effects at recommended doses include headache and upset stomach. At higher than recommended dosages, side effects include blurred vision and severe headaches (NCCAM). The major drug interactions are with other sedative-hypnotic agents, and the sedative effect of valerian may potentiate the effects of other central nervous system depressants (Beaubrun and Gray 2000).

Herbal teas have long been used for their sedative-hypnotic effect. Common ingredients in these teas, besides valerian, consist of hops, lemon balm, chamomile, and passion flower. The most studied of these is chamomile, a tea widely used as a folk remedy. Chamomile extract has been found to bind with gamma-aminobutyric acid (GABA) receptors, but far less is known of the effectiveness of the other herbs (Beaubrun and Gray 2000).

Homeopathy

Homeopathy is based on the concept that like items cure like items (Law of Similars). Small doses of diluted preparations that mimic an illness are used to heal the body or help the body heal itself. Patients receiving homeopathic care frequently feel worse before they get better because homeopathic medicines often stimulate, rather than suppress, symptoms (Stehlin 1996). The first law is that healing occurs from inside (mental, to emotional, to physical). The treatments are designed to heal both the physical injury and the mental insult (Lorenzi 1999).

The substances given to stimulate healing are homeopathic remedies. Homeopathic remedies are dilutions of natural substances from plants, minerals, and animals. Dilutions are prescribed that match the patient's illness-symptom profile. Homeopathic treatments are individualized, and each individual, even with the same diagnosis, is given different medicines because the symptoms are different (Freeman and Lawlis 2001). Homeopathy has been indicated in treatment of short-term, acute illnesses, migraine pain, allergies, chronic fatigue, otitis media, immune dysfunction, digestive disorders, and colic.

It is contraindicated as a treatment for advanced diseases, cancer, sexually transmitted diseases, irreparable damage (heart valves), or brain damage because of stroke (Freeman and Lawlis 2001).

The use of homeopathic remedies has been studied in the treatment of depression, anxiety, social phobia, and panic disorder (Spencer and Jacobs 1999). The patients in the trials were self-selected or referred after a poor response to other therapies. In each of the individuals there was some response, but the numbers were small and each individual's treatment was different, so there can be no generalizability in the results. Spencer and Jacobs (1999) reported an additional study that did have a double-blind format. The post-test comparisons were nonsignificant. It is difficult to develop such a study protocol when each individual's treatment is different.

QUACKERY AND FRAUD

Consumers waste billions of dollars on unproved, fraudulently marketed, and sometimes useless health care products and treatments. To make matters worse, some of the treatments can in fact cause harm. Plants and herbs are natural and unprocessed, but that does not mean they can not be harmful or abused. Herbs and other food supplements do not have to undergo the same safety review that over-the-counter and prescription medications must clear. There are some typical phrases or marketing techniques that the National Center for Complementary and Alternative Medicine website provides:

■ The product is advertised as a quick and effective cure-all for a wide range of ailments.
■ The promoters use words like scientific breakthrough, miraculous cure, exclusive product, secret ingredient, or ancient remedy.
■ The text is written using impressive terminology to disguise lack of good science.
■ The promoter claims the government, the medical profession, or research scientists have conspired to suppress the product.
■ The advertisement includes undocumented case histories claiming amazing results.
■ The product is advertised as available from only one source, and payment is required in advance.
■ The promoter promises a "no-risk money-back guarantee."

Phrases such as these should set off warning signals to the nurse that further investigation is necessary from resources such as the NCCAM.

RESEARCH

More complementary medical research exists than is commonly recognized—the *Cochrane Library* lists over 4000 randomized trials—but the field is still poorly researched compared with conventional medicine. There are several reasons for this, some of which also apply to conventional disciplines like occupational and speech therapy. However, complementary practitioners are increasingly aware of the value of research, and many complementary training courses now include research skills. Conventional sources of funding, such as the NHS research and development program and major cancer charities, have become more open to complementary researchers (Zollman and Vickens, 1999, p. 693).

The National Institutes of Health Office of Alternative Medicine (OAM) was established in 1992 and has been mandated to facilitate evaluation of alternative treatments, serve as an information clearinghouse, and support research training in therapies not usually incorporated in health professional's educational programs. The OAM does not advocate specific treatment modalities; instead it supports fair and scientific evaluation of the therapies. The OAM was elevated in October of 1998 to a Center and renamed the National Center for Complementary and Alternative Medicine (NCCAM). In response to these mandates, health insurance companies have begun to include coverage for certain modalities. Additionally, almost two thirds of medical schools have integrated alternative/complementary approaches into their course of study (Hayes and Alexander 2000).

INFORMATION RESOURCES

The National Institutes of Health (NIH) National Center for Complementary and Alternative Medicine (NCCAM) conducts and supports basic and applied research and training. The Center disseminates information on complementary and alternative medicine to practitioners and the public through the NCCAM Clearinghouse. The NCCAM with a congressional mandate to "establish a clearinghouse to exchange information with the public about alternative medicine" developed that resource in the fall of 1996. The NCCAM provides fact sheets, information packages, and publications to increase the public's understanding of complementary and alternative medicine and research supported by the NIH. This is not a referral agency; the agency conducts and facilitates biomedical research. Consumers and practitioners are able to access information from the clearinghouse through its website (*http://nccam.nih.gov*) or request information through addressing the clearinghouse:

NCCAM Clearinghouse
P.O. Box 8218
Silver Spring, MD 20907-8218
Toll-Free: 1-888-564-6226
TTY/TDY: 1-888-644-6226
FAX: 301-495-4957

The NCCAM online database contains bibliographic records that describe CAM research that has been published over the last 35 years. Searches of various diseases or conditions, alternative medicine techniques, and literature are available. The National Library of Medicine MEDLINE may be used to search for a particular condition. The NCCAM makes available a fact sheet entitled "Alternative Medicine Research Using MEDLINE" through their clearinghouse.

The NCCAM Clearinghouse also provides literature on "Considering Complementary and Alternative Therapies," which provides information related to questions a consumer might ask when choosing an alternative health care practitioner. Medical regulatory and licensing agencies in each state also serve as a clearinghouse for information.

SUMMARY

Alternative complementary therapies are in greater demand as consumers seek a broader range of therapies other than those offered by traditional medicine. With the availability of information on the internet, consumers are more likely to have researched their symptoms or condition and identified potential alternative or complementary treatments. Unfortunately, not all sites are reliable or present information in a nonbiased or factual manner. Nurses are in a position of providing resources to clients and other individuals seeking assistance. Therefore, the nurse must also review the latest information on alternative and complementary treatments and check on accuracy and reliability. The National Center for Complementary and Alternative Medicine (NCCAM) provides up-to-date information for health care practitioners and consumers. Sites such as these will help all individuals select those therapies that have a high safety record and have been proven to be effective.

Visit the **Evolve** website at
http://evolve.elsevier.com/Varcarolis
for a post-test on the content in this chapter.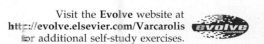

Visit the **Evolve** website at
http://evolve.elsevier.com/Varcarolis
for additional self-study exercises.

Critical Thinking and Chapter Review

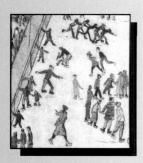

Critical Thinking

1. As a nurse you may have patients who use alternative therapies in conjunction with the therapies prescribed by the health care provider. In doing an assessment, identify those communication techniques that would be most effective in determining the extent to which a patient is following the therapeutic regimen. How would you determine whether patients were using alternative health care treatments in addition to prescribed treatments?
2. Discuss how herbal products sold in the United States can vary in quality. How does a patient identify the efficacy of the herb. What can a patient do to guarantee the quality and dosage of an herbal product.
3. Utilizing the internet, determine how the NCCAM provides information for the consumer and professionals.

Chapter Review

Choose the most appropriate answer.

1. Kim, 24, has had several hospitalizations for treatment of schizophrenia. She presently takes psychotropic medication. She tells the nurse, "I'm going to stop taking my medication. It makes me feel awful. I'm thinking of searching the internet to find an alternative herbal remedy that will be a holistic treatment." The best response for the nurse would be

    1. "Information on the internet isn't always objective and reliable."
    2. "You shouldn't do that! Herbals can be harmful to your general health."
    3. "Tell me what you mean when you say the medicine makes you feel awful."
    4. "Your medication treats your disease. Since nothing else is wrong with you, no other treatment is necessary."

2. A client tells the nurse, "I've been reading about Asian medicine. I think my alcoholism may be related to chi imbalance. I am going to seek alternative treatment." The nurse can expect the client to turn to

    1. chiropractic care
    2. acupuncture
    3. aromatherapy
    4. reiki

3. A client tells the nurse, "I've been using St. John's wort to try to get back on track." The nurse should pursue assessment related to the client's experiencing symptoms of

    1. depression
    2. diminished cognitive abilities
    3. altered reality perception
    4. sensory perceptual disturbances

4. The nurse who wishes to access accurate information on complementary and alternative medicine should contact

    1. AMA
    2. NLN
    3. NAMI
    4. NCCAM Clearinghouse

5. Mrs. Nash, 72, has had two small strokes. Her physician has prescribed Coumadin daily. Mrs. Nash tells the nurse that she is considering taking gingko biloba to help her with her failing memory. Which information should the nurse give?

    1. Gingko biloba seems to have a positive effect on memory.
    2. Coumadin and gingko biloba taken together may cause spontaneous bleeding.
    3. Gingko biloba may cause sedation and increased danger of falls.
    4. There is no medical reason not to try the herbal preparation.

NURSE, CLIENT, AND FAMILY RESOURCES

Books

Micozzi, M.S. (Ed.). (2001). *Fundamentals of Complementary and Alternative Medicine*. London: Churchill Livingstone.

Fontaine, K.L. (2001). *Healing Practices: Alternative Therapies for Nursing*. Upper Saddle River, N.J.: Prentice Hall.

Journal Articles

McEnany, G. (2000). Herbal psychotrophics, Part 3: Focus on kava, valerian, and melatonin. *Journal of the American Psychiatric Nurses Association*, 6(4):126–130.

Zahourek, R. (2000). Alternative, complementary, or integrative approaches to treating depression. *Journal of the American Psychiatric Association* 6(3):77–86.

Internet Sites

British Medical Journal—ABC of Complementary Medicine–What is Alternative Medicine?
http://www.bmj.com/cgi/content/full/319/7211/693

Complementary and Alternative Medicine Research—Stanford University
http://scrdp.stanford.edu/camps.html

NIH National Center for Complementary and Alternative Medicine
http://nccam.nih.gov

REFERENCES

Ackerman, J.M. (1999). Acupuncture in psychiatry. *Psychiatric Services*, 50:117.

Acupuncture, NIH Consensus Statement, 1997, November 3–5. 15(5):1–34.

Ashcroft, D.M. (1999). Herbal remedies: Issues in licensing and economic evaluation. *Pharmacoeconomics*, 16(4):321–328.

Beal, M.W. (2000). Acupuncture and oriental bodywork: Traditional and biomedical concepts in holistic care: History and basic concepts. *Holistic Nursing Practice*, 14(3):69–78.

Beaubrun, G., and Gray, G.E. (2000). A review of herbal medicines for psychiatric disorders. *Psychiatric Services*, 51(9):1130–1134.

Bullock, M.L. (1989) Controlled trial of acupuncture for severe recidivist alcoholism. *Lancet*, 1:1435–1439.

Cohen, S.M., Rousseau, M.E., and Robinson, E.H. (2000). Therapeutic use of selected herbs. *Holistic Nursing Practice*, 14(3):59–68.

Culliton, P.D., Boucher, T.A., and Bullock, M.L. (1999). Complementary/alternative therapies in the treatment of alcohol and other addictions. In J.W. Spencer and J.J. Jacobs (Eds.), *Complementary/alternative medicine*. St. Louis: Mosby.

Crupp, M.J. (1999). Herbal remedies: Adverse effects and drug interactions. *American Family Physician*. 59(5):1239–1245.

Druss, B.G., Rohrbaugh, R., Kosten, T., Hoff, R., and Rosenheck, R.A. (1998). Use of alternative medicine in major depression. *Psychiatric Services*, 49(11):1397.

Eliopoulos, C. (1999). Using complementary and alternative therapies wisely. *Geriatric Nursing*, 20(3):139–143.

Freeman, L.W., and Lawlis, G.F. (2001). *Mosby's complementary and alternative medicine: A research-based approach*. St. Louis: Mosby.

Fugh-Berman, A., and Cott, J.M. (1999). Dietary supplements and natural products as psychotherapeutic agents. *Psychosomatic Medicine*, 61(5):712–728.

Glisson, J., Crawford, R., and Street, S. (1999). The clinical applications of ginko biloba, St. John's wort, saw palmetto, and soy. *Nurse Practitioner*, 24(6):28, 31, 35–36.

Hagemaster, J. (2000). Use of therapeutic touch in treatment of drug addictions. *Holistic Nursing Practice*, 14(3):14–20.

Hayes, K.M., and Alexander, I.M. (2000). Alternative therapies and nurse practitioners: Knowledge, professional experience, and personal use. *Holistic Nursing Practice*, 14(3):49–58.

Henney, J.E. (2000). Risk of drug interactions with St. John's wort. *JAMA*, 283(3):1679

Lake, J. (2000). Psychotropic medications from natural products: A review of promising research and recommendations. *Alternative Therapeutic Health Medicine*, 6(3):36, 39–45, 47–52.

Lantz, M.S., Buchalter, E., and Giambanco, V. (1999). St. John's wort and antidepressant drug interactions in the elderly. *Journal of Geriatric Psychiatry and Neurology*, 12(1):7–10.

Lorenzi, E. (1999). Complementary/Alternative therapies: So many choices. *Geriatric Nursing*, 20:125–133.

McEnany, G. (1999). Herbal psychotropics. Part 1: Focus on St. John's wort and SAMe. *Journal of the American Psychiatric Nurses Association*, 5(6):192–196.

McEnany, G. (2000). Herbal psychotropics. Part 3: Focus on kava, valerian, and melatonin. *Journal of the American Psychiatric Nurses Association*, 6(4):126–130.

National Association for Holistic Aromatherapy information sheet. http://www.naha.org/at.html.

NCCAM Clearinghouse—St. John's wort fact sheet. http://nccam.nih.gov/nccam/fcp/factsheet/stjohnswort.

Neild-Anderson, J., and Ameling, A. (2000). The empowering nature of Reiki as a complementary therapy. *Holistic Nursing Practice*, 14(3):21–29.

Ness, J., Sherman, F.T., and Pan, C.X. (1999). Alternative medicine: What the data say about common herbal therapies. *Geriatrics*, 54(10):33–43.

O'Hara, M., Kiefer, D., Farrell, K., and Kemper, K. (1998). A review of 12 commonly used medicinal herbs. *Archives of Family Medicine*, 7(6):523–536.

Shelton, R.C., Keller, M.B., Gelenberg, A., Dunner, D.L., et al. (2001). Effectiveness of St. John's wort in major depression: A randomized controlled trial. *JAMA*, 285(15):1978–1986.

Singer, A., Wonnemann, M., and Muller, W.E. (1999). Hyperforin, a major constituent of St. John's wort, inhibits serotonin uptake by elevating free intracellular sodium. *Journal of Pharmacology and Experimental Therapeutics*, 290:1363–1368.

Spencer, J.W., and Jacobs, J.J. (1999). Complementary/Alternative medicine—An evidence-based approach. St. Louis: Mosby.

Stehlin, I. (1996). Homeopathy: Real medicine or empty promises? FDA Home Page. www.fda.gov/fdac/features/096_home.

Straneva, J.A. (2000) Therapeutic touch coming of age. *Holistic Nursing Practice*, 14(3):1–13.

Winslow, L.C., and Kroll, D.J. (1998). Herbs as medicines. *Archives of Internal Medicine*, 158(20):2192–2199.

Wong, A.H., and Boon, H.S. (1998). Herbal remedies in psychiatric practice. *Archives of General Psychiatry*, 55(11):1033–1044.

Yen, P.K. (1999). The Supplement Dilemma. *Geriatric Nursing*, 20(3):167–168.

Youngkin, E.Q., and Israel, D.S. (1996). A review and critique of common herbal alternative therapies. *Nurse Practitioner*, 21(10): 39, 43–46, 49–52.

Zollman, C., and Vickers, A. (1999). ABC of complementary medicine: What is complementary medicine? *British Medical Journal*, 319(10):693–696.

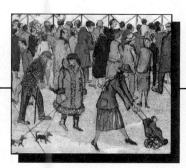

Appendix A: DSM-IV-TR Classification

DISORDERS USUALLY FIRST DIAGNOSED IN INFANCY, CHILDHOOD, OR ADOLESCENCE (39)

Mental Retardation (41)

Note: These are coded on Axis II.

F70.9 Mild Mental Retardation (43)
F71.9 Moderate Mental Retardation (43)
F72.9 Severe Mental Retardation (43)
F73.9 Profound Mental Retardation (44)
F79.9 Mental Retardation, Severity Unspecified (44)

Learning Disorders (49)

F81.0 Reading Disorder (51)
F81.2 Mathematics Disorder (53)
F81.8 Disorder of Written Expression (54)
F81.9 Learning Disorder NOS (56)

Motor Skills Disorder (56)

F82 Developmental Coordination Disorder (56)

Communication Disorders (58)

F80.1 Expressive Language Disorder (58)
F80.2 Mixed Receptive-Expressive Language Disorder (62)
F80.0 Phonological Disorder (65)
F98.5 Stuttering (67)
F80.9 Communication Disorder NOS (69)

Pervasive Developmental Disorders (69)

F84.0 Autistic Disorder (70)
F84.2 Rett's Disorder (76)
F84.3 Childhood Disintegrative Disorder (77)
F84.5 Asperger's Disorder (80)
F84.9 Pervasive Developmental Disorder NOS (84)

Attention-Deficit and Disruptive Behavior Disorders (85)

___.__ Attention-Deficit/Hyperactivity Disorder (85)
F90.0 Combined Type
F98.8 Predominantly Inattentive Type
F90.0 Predominantly Hyperactive-Impulsive Type

F90.9 Attention-Deficit/Hyperactivity Disorder NOS (93)
F91.8 Conduct Disorder (93)
Specify type: Childhood-Onset Type/Adolescent-Onset Type
F91.3 Oppositional Defiant Disorder (100)
F91.9 Disruptive Behavior Disorder NOS (103)

Feeding and Eating Disorders of Infancy or Early Childhood (103)

F98.3 Pica (103)
F98.2 Rumination Disorder (105)
F98.2 Feeding Disorder of Infancy or Early Childhood (107)

Tic Disorders (108)

F95.2 Tourette's Disorder (111)
F95.1 Chronic Motor or Vocal Tic Disorder (114)
F95.0 Transient Tic Disorder (115)
Specify if: Single Episode/Recurrent
F95.9 Tic Disorder NOS (116)

Elimination Disorders (116)

___.__ Encopresis (116)
R15 With Constipation and Overflow Incontinence (also code K59.0 constipation on Axis III)
F98.1 Without Constipation and Overflow Incontinence
F98.0 Enuresis (Not Due to a General Medical Condition) (118)
Specify type: Nocturnal Only/Diurnal Only/Nocturnal and Diurnal

Other Disorders of Infancy, Childhood, or Adolescence (121)

F93.0 Separation Anxiety Disorder (121)
Specify if: Early Onset
F94.0 Selective Mutism (125)
F94.x Reactive Attachment Disorder of Infancy or Early Childhood (127)
.1 Inhibited Type
.2 Disinhibited Type
F98.4 Stereotypic Movement Disorder (131)
Specify if: With Self-Injurious Behavior
F98.9 Disorder of Infancy, Childhood, or Adolescence NOS (134)

Numbers in parentheses indicate page numbers in DSM-IV-TR where disorders can be found.

DELIRIUM, DEMENTIA, AND AMNESTIC AND OTHER COGNITIVE DISORDERS (135)

Delirium (136)

F05.0   Delirium Due to . . . *[Indicate the General Medical Condition] (code F05.1 if superimposed on Dementia)* (141)

___._   Substance Intoxication Delirium *(refer to Substance-Related Disorders for substance-specific codes)* (143)

___._   Substance Withdrawal Delirium *(refer to Substance-Related Disorders for substance-specific codes)* (143)

___._   Delirium Due to Multiple Etiologies *(code each of the specific etiologies)* (146)

F05.9   Delirium NOS (147)

Dementia (147)

F00.xx   Dementia of the Alzheimer's Type, With Early Onset *(also code G30.0 Alzheimer's Disease, With Early Onset, on Axis III)* (154)
.00   Uncomplicated
.01   With Delusions
.03   With Depressed Mood
    Specify if: With Behavioral Disturbance

F00.xx   Dementia of the Alzheimer's Type, With Late Onset *(also code G30.1 Alzheimer's Disease, With Late Onset, on Axis III)* (154)
.10   Uncomplicated
.11   With Delusions
.13   With Depressed Mood
    Specify if: With Behavioral Disturbance

F01.xx   Vascular Dementia (158)
.80   Uncomplicated
.81   With Delusions
.83   With Depressed Mood
    Specify if: With Behavioral Disturbance

F02.4   Dementia Due to HIV Disease *(also code B22.0 HIV disease resulting in encephalopathy on Axis III)* (163)

F02.8   Dementia Due to Head Trauma *(also code S06.9 Intracranial injury on Axis III)* (164)

F02.3   Dementia Due to Parkinson's Disease *(also code G20 Parkinson's disease on Axis III)* (164)

F02.2   Dementia Due to Huntington's Disease *(also code G10 Huntington's disease on Axis III)* (165)

F02.0   Dementia Due to Pick's Disease *(also code G31.0 Pick's disease on Axis III)* (165)

F02.1   Dementia Due to Creutzfeldt-Jakob Disease *(also code A81.0 Creutzfeldt-Jakob disease on Axis III)* (166)

F02.8   Dementia Due to. . . *[Indicate the General Medical Condition not listed above] (also code the general medical condition on Axis III)* (167)

___._   Substance-Induced Persisting Dementia *(refer to Substance-Related Disorders for substance-specific codes)* (168)

F02.8   Dementia Due to Multiple Etiologies *(instead code F00.2 for mixed Alzheimer's and Vascular Dementia)* (170)

F03   Dementia NOS (171)

Amnestic Disorders (172)

F04   Amnestic Disorder Due to . . . *[Indicate the General Medical Condition]* (175)
    Specify if: Transient/Chronic

___._   Substance-Induced Persisting Amnestic Disorder *(refer to Substance-Related Disorders for substance-specific codes)* (177)

R41.3   Amnestic Disorder NOS (179)

Other Cognitive Disorders (179)

F06.9   Cognitive Disorder NOS (179)

MENTAL DISORDERS DUE TO A GENERAL MEDICAL CONDITION NOT ELSEWHERE CLASSIFIED (181)

F06.1   Catatonic Disorder Due to . . . *[Indicate the General Medical Condition]* (185)

F07.0   Personality Change Due to . . . *[Indicate the General Medical Condition]* (187)
    Specify type: Labile Type/Disinhibited Type/Aggressive Type/Apathetic Type/Paranoid Type/Other Type/Combined Type/Unspecified Type

F09   Mental Disorder NOS Due to . . . *[Indicate the General Medical Condition]* (190)

SUBSTANCE-RELATED DISORDERS (191)

The following specifiers may be applied to Substance Dependence:
[a] With Physiological Dependence/Without Physiological Dependence
[b] Early Full Remission/Early Partial Remission/Sustained Full Remission/Sustained Partial Remission
[c] In a Controlled Environment
[d] On Agonist Therapy

The following specifiers apply to Substance-Induced Disorders as noted:
[I]With Onset During Intoxication/[W]With Onset During Withdrawal

Alcohol-Related Disorders (212)

Alcohol Use Disorders (213)

F10.2x   Alcohol Dependence[a] (213)
F10.1   Alcohol Abuse (214)

Alcohol-Induced Disorders (214)

F10.00   Alcohol Intoxication (214)
F10.3   Alcohol Withdrawal (215)
    Specify if: With Perceptual Disturbances
F10.03   Alcohol Intoxication Delirium (143)
F10.4   Alcohol Withdrawal Delirium (143)
F10.73   Alcohol-Induced Persisting Dementia (168)
F10.6   Alcohol-Induced Persisting Amnestic Disorder (177)
F10.xx   Alcohol-Induced Psychotic Disorder (338)
.51   With Delusions[I,W]
.52   With Hallucinations[I,W]
F10.8   Alcohol-Induced Mood Disorder[I,W] (405)
F10.8   Alcohol-Induced Anxiety Disorder[I,W] (479)
F10.8   Alcohol-Induced Sexual Dysfunction[I] (562)
F10.8   Alcohol-Induced Sleep Disorder[I,W] (655)
F10.9   Alcohol-Related Disorder NOS (223)

Amphetamine (or Amphetamine-Like)-Related Disorders (223)

Amphetamine Use Disorders (224)

F15.2x Amphetamine Dependence[a] (224)
F15.1 Amphetamine Abuse (225)

Amphetamine-Induced Disorders (226)

F15.00 Amphetamine Intoxication (226)
F15.04 Amphetamine Intoxication, With Perceptual Disturbances (226)
F15.3 Amphetamine Withdrawal (227)
F15.03 Amphetamine Intoxication Delirium (143)
F15.xx Amphetamine-Induced Psychotic Disorder (338)
  .51   With Delusions[I]
  .52   With Hallucinations[I]
F15.8 Amphetamine-Induced Mood Disorder[I,W] (405)
F15.8 Amphetamine-Induced Anxiety Disorder[I] (479)
F15.8 Amphetamine-Induced Sexual Dysfunction[I] (562)
F15.8 Amphetamine-Induced Sleep Disorder[I,W] (655)
F15.9 Amphetamine-Related Disorder NOS (231)

Caffeine-Related Disorders (231)

Caffeine-Induced Disorders (232)

F15.00 Caffeine Intoxication (232)
F15.8 Caffeine-Induced Anxiety Disorder[I] (479)
F15.8 Caffeine-Induced Sleep Disorder[I] (655)
F15.9 Caffeine-Related Disorder NOS (234)

Cannabis-Related Disorders (234)

Cannabis Use Disorders (236)

F12.2x Cannabis Dependence[a] (236)
F12.1 Cannabis Abuse (236)

Cannabis-Induced Disorders (237)

F12.00 Cannabis Intoxication (237)
F12.04 Cannabis Intoxication, With Perceptual Disturbances (237)
F12.03 Cannabis Intoxication Delirium (143)
F12.xx Cannabis-Induced Psychotic Disorder (338)
  .51   With Delusions[I]
  .52   With Hallucinations[I]
F12.8 Cannabis-Induced Anxiety Disorder[I] (479)
F12.9 Cannabis-Related Disorder NOS (241)

Cocaine-Related Disorders (241)

Cocaine Use Disorders (242)

F14.2x Cocaine Dependence[a] (242)
F14.1 Cocaine Abuse (243)

Cocaine-Induced Disorders (244)

F14.00 Cocaine Intoxication (244)
F14.04 Cocaine Intoxication, With Perceptual Disturbances (244)
F14.3 Cocaine Withdrawal (245)
F14.03 Cocaine Intoxication Delirium (143)
F14.xx Cocaine-Induced Psychotic Disorder (338)
  .51   With Delusions[I]
  .52   With Hallucinations[I]
F14.8 Cocaine-Induced Mood Disorder[I,W] (405)
F14.8 Cocaine-Induced Anxiety Disorder[I,W] (479)
F14.8 Cocaine-Induced Sexual Dysfunction[I] (562)
F14.8 Cocaine-Induced Sleep Disorder[I,W] (655)
F14.9 Cocaine-Related Disorder NOS (250)

Hallucinogen-Related Disorders (250)

Hallucinogen Use Disorders (251)

F16.2x Hallucinogen Dependence[a] (251)
F16.1 Hallucinogen Abuse (252)

Hallucinogen-Induced Disorders (252)

F16.00 Hallucinogen Intoxication (252)
F16.70 Hallucinogen Persisting Perception Disorder (Flashbacks) (253)
F16.03 Hallucinogen Intoxication Delirium (143)
F16.xx Hallucinogen-Induced Psychotic Disorder (338)
  .51   With Delusions[I]
  .52   With Hallucinations[I]
F16.8 Hallucinogen-Induced Mood Disorder[I] (405)
F16.8 Hallucinogen-Induced Anxiety Disorder[I] (479)
F16.9 Hallucinogen-Related Disorder NOS (256)

Inhalant-Related Disorders (257)

Inhalant Use Disorders (258)

F18.2x Inhalant Dependence[a] (258)
F18.1 Inhalant Abuse (259)

Inhalant-Induced Disorders (259)

F18.00 Inhalant Intoxication (259)
F18.03 Inhalant Intoxication Delirium (143)
F18.73 Inhalant-Induced Persisting Dementia (168)
F18.xx Inhalant-Induced Psychotic Disorder (338)
  .51   With Delusions[I]
  .52   With Hallucinations[I]
F18.8 Inhalant-Induced Mood Disorder[I] (405)
F18.8 Inhalant-Induced Anxiety Disorder[I] (479)
F18.9 Inhalant-Related Disorder NOS (263)

Nicotine-Related Disorders (264)

Nicotine Use Disorder (264)

F17.2x Nicotine Dependence[a] (264)

Nicotine-Induced Disorder (265)

F17.3 Nicotine Withdrawal (265)
F17.9 Nicotine-Related Disorder NOS (269)

Opioid-Related Disorders (269)

Opioid Use Disorders (270)

F11.2x Opioid Dependence[a] (270)
F11.1 Opioid Abuse (271)

Opioid-Induced Disorders (271)

F11.00 Opioid Intoxication (271)
F11.04 Opioid Intoxication, With Perceptual Disturbances (272)
F11.3 Opioid Withdrawal (272)
F11.03 Opioid Intoxication Delirium (143)
F11.xx Opioid-Induced Psychotic Disorder (338)
  .51   With Delusions[I]
  .52   With Hallucinations[I]
F11.8 Opioid-Induced Mood Disorder[I] (405)
F11.8 Opioid-Induced Sexual Dysfunction[I] (562)
F11.8 Opioid-Induced Sleep Disorder[I,W] (655)
F11.9 Opioid-Related Disorder NOS (277)

Phencyclidine (or Phencyclidine-Like)-Related Disorders (278)

Phencyclidine Use Disorders (279)

F19.2x Phencyclidine Dependence[a] (279)
F19.1 Phencyclidine Abuse (279)

Phencyclidine-Induced Disorders (280)

F19.00   Phencyclidine Intoxication (280)
F19.04   Phencyclidine Intoxication, With Perceptual Disturbances (280)
F19.03   Phencyclidine Intoxication Delirium (143)
F19.xx   Phencyclidine-Induced Psychotic Disorder (338)
    .51   With Delusions[I]
    .52   With Hallucinations[I]
F19.8   Phencyclidine-Induced Mood Disorder[I] (405)
F19.8   Phencyclidine-Induced Anxiety Disorder[I] (479)
F19.9   Phencyclidine-Related Disorder NOS (283)

Sedative-, Hypnotic-, or Anxiolytic-Related Disorders (284)

Sedative, Hypnotic, or Anxiolytic Use Disorders (285)

F13.2x   Sedative, Hypnotic, or Anxiolytic Dependence[a] (285)
F13.1   Sedative, Hypnotic, or Anxiolytic Abuse (286)

Sedative-, Hypnotic-, or Anxiolytic-Induced Disorders (286)

F13.00   Sedative, Hypnotic, or Anxiolytic Intoxication (286)
F13.3   Sedative, Hypnotic, or Anxiolytic Withdrawal (287)
    Specify if: With Perceptual Disturbances
F13.03   Sedative, Hypnotic, or Anxiolytic Intoxication Delirium (143)
F13.4   Sedative, Hypnotic, or Anxiolytic Withdrawal Delirium (143)
F13.73   Sedative-, Hypnotic-, or Anxiolytic-Induced Persisting Dementia (168)
F13.6   Sedative-, Hypnotic-, or Anxiolytic-Induced Persisting Amnestic Disorder (177)
F13.xx   Sedative-, Hypnotic-, or Anxiolytic-Induced Psychotic Disorder (338)
    .51   With Delusions[I,W]
    .52   With Hallucinations[I,W]
F13.8   Sedative-, Hypnotic-, or Anxiolytic-Induced Mood Disorder[I,W] (405)
F13.8   Sedative-, Hypnotic-, or Anxiolytic-Induced Anxiety Disorder[W] (479)
F13.8   Sedative-, Hypnotic-, or Anxiolytic-Induced Sexual Dysfunction[I] (562)
F13.8   Sedative-, Hypnotic-, or Anxiolytic-Induced Sleep Disorder[I,W] (655)
F13.9   Sedative-, Hypnotic-, or Anxiolytic-Related Disorder NOS (293)

Polysubstance-Related Disorder (293)

F19.2x   Polysubstance Dependence[a] (293)

Other (or Unknown) Substance-Related Disorders (294)

Other (or Unknown) Substance Use Disorders (294)

F19.2x   Other (or Unknown) Substance Dependence[a] (192)
F19.1   Other (or Unknown) Substance Abuse (198)

Other (or Unknown) Substance-Induced Disorders (295)

F19.00   Other (or Unknown) Substance Intoxication (199)
F19.04   Other (or Unknown) Substance Intoxication, With Perceptual Disturbances (199)
F19.3   Other (or Unknown) Substance Withdrawal (201)
    Specify if: With Perceptual Disturbances
F19.03   Other (or Unknown) Substance-Induced Delirium (*code F19.4 if onset during withdrawal*) (143)

F19.73   Other (or Unknown) Substance-Induced Persisting Dementia (168)
F19.6   Other (or Unknown) Substance-Induced Persisting Amnestic Disorder (177)
F19.xx   Other (or Unknown) Substance-Induced Psychotic Disorder (338)
    .51   With Delusions[I,W]
    .52   With Hallucinations[I,W]
F19.8   Other (or Unknown) Substance-Induced Mood Disorder[I,W] (405)
F19.8   Other (or Unknown) Substance-Induced Anxiety Disorder[I,W] (479)
F19.8   Other (or Unknown) Substance-Induced Sexual Dysfunction[I] (562)
F19.8   Other (or Unknown) Substance-Induced Sleep Disorder[I,W] (655)
F19.9   Other (or Unknown) Substance-Related Disorder NOS (295)

SCHIZOPHRENIA AND OTHER PSYCHOTIC DISORDERS (297)

F20.xx   Schizophrenia (298)
    .0x   Paranoid Type (313)
    .1x   Disorganized Type (314)
    .2x   Catatonic Type (315)
    .3x   Undifferentiated Type (316)
    .5x   Residual Type (316)
Code course of Schizophrenia in fifth character.
    2 = Episodic With Interepisode Residual Symptoms (*specify if:* With Prominent Negative Symptoms)
    3 = Episodic With No Interepisode Residual Symptoms
    0 = Continuous (*specify if:* With Prominent Negative Symptoms)
    4 = Single Episode In Partial Remission (*specify if:* With Prominent Negative Symptoms)
    5 = Single Episode In Full Remission
    8 = Other or Unspecified Pattern
    9 = Less than 1 year since onset of initial active-phase symptoms
F20.8   Schizophreniform Disorder (317)
    Specify if: Without Good Prognostic Features/With Good Prognostic Features
F25.x   Schizoaffective Disorder (319)
    .0   Bipolar Type
    .1   Depressive Type
F22.0   Delusional Disorder (323)
    Specify type: Erotomanic Type/Grandiose Type/ Jealous Type/Persecutory Type/Somatic Type/ Mixed Type/Unspecified Type
F23.xx   Brief Psychotic Disorder (329)
    .81   With Marked Stressor(s)
    .80   Without Marked Stressor(s)
    Specify if: With Postpartum Onset
F24   Shared Psychotic Disorder (332)
F06.x   Psychotic Disorder Due to . . . [*Indicate the General Medical Condition*] (334)
    .2   With Delusions
    .0   With Hallucinations
___.___   Substance-Induced Psychotic Disorder (*refer to

Substance-Related Disorders for substance-specific codes) (338)

Specify if: With Onset During Intoxication/With Onset During Withdrawal

F29   Psychotic Disorder NOS (343)

MOOD DISORDERS (345)

Depressive Disorders (369)

F32.x   Major Depressive Disorder, Single Episode (369)
F33.x   Major Depressive Disorder, Recurrent (369)

Code current state of Major Depressive Episode in fourth character:

0 = Mild
1 = Moderate
2 = Severe Without Psychotic Features
3 = Severe With Psychotic Features
   Specify: Mood-Congruent Psychotic Features/Mood-Incongruent Psychotic Features
4 = In Partial Remission
4 = In Full Remission
9 = Unspecified

F34.1   Dysthymic Disorder (376)
   Specify if: Early Onset/Late Onset
   Specify: With Atypical Features

F32.9   Depressive Disorder NOS (381)

Bipolar Disorders (382)

F30.x   Bipolar I Disorder, Single Manic Episode (382)
   Specify if: Mixed

Code current state of Manic Episode in fourth character:

1 = Mild, Moderate, or Severe Without Psychotic Features
2 = Severe With Psychotic Features
8 = In Partial or Full Remission

F31.0   Bipolar I Disorder, Most Recent Episode Hypomanic (382)
F31.x   Bipolar I Disorder, Most Recent Episode Manic (382)

Code current state of Manic Episode in fourth character:

1 = Mild, Moderate, or Severe Without Psychotic Features
2 = Severe With Psychotic Features
7 = In Partial or Full Remission

F31.6   Bipolar I Disorder, Most Recent Episode Mixed (382)
F31.x   Bipolar I Disorder, Most Recent Episode Depressed (382)

Code current state of Major Depressive Episode in fourth character:

3 = Mild or Moderate
4 = Severe Without Psychotic Features
5 = Severe With Psychotic Features
7 = In Partial or Full Remission

F31.9   Bipolar I Disorder, Most Recent Episode Unspecified (382)
F31.8   Bipolar II Disorder (392)
   Specify (current or most recent episode): Hypomanic/Depressed
F34.0   Cyclothymic Disorder (398)
F31.9   Bipolar Disorder NOS (400)

F06.xx   Mood Disorder Due to . . . *[Indicate the General Medical Condition]* (401)
   .32   With Depressive Features
   .32   With Major Depressive–Like Episode
   .30   With Manic Features
   .33   With Mixed Features
____.__   Substance-Induced Mood Disorder *(refer to Substance-Related Disorders for substance-specific codes)* (405)
   Specify type: With Depressive Features/With Manic Features/With Mixed Features
   Specify if: With Onset During Intoxication/With Onset During Withdrawal
F39   Mood Disorder NOS (410)

ANXIETY DISORDERS (429)

F41.0   Panic Disorder Without Agoraphobia (433)
F40.01   Panic Disorder With Agoraphobia (433)
F40.00   Agoraphobia Without History of Panic Disorder (441)
F40.2   Specific Phobia (443)
   Specify type: Animal Type/Natural Environment Type/Blood-Injection-Injury Type/Situational Type/Other Type
F40.1   Social Phobia (450)
   Specify if: Generalized
F42.8   Obsessive-Compulsive Disorder (456)
   Specify if: With Poor Insight
F43.1   Posttraumatic Stress Disorder (463)
   Specify if: Acute/Chronic
   Specify if: With Delayed Onset
F43.0   Acute Stress Disorder (469)
F41.1   Generalized Anxiety Disorder (472)
F06.4   Anxiety Disorder Due to . . . *[Indicate the General Medical Condition]* (476)
   Specify if: With Generalized Anxiety/With Panic Attacks/With Obsessive-Compulsive Symptoms
____.__   Substance-Induced Anxiety Disorder *(refer to Substance-Related Disorders for substance-specific codes)* (479)
   Specify if: With Generalized Anxiety/With Panic Attacks/With Obsessive-Compulsive Symptoms/With Phobic Symptoms
   Specify if: With Onset During Intoxication/With Onset During Withdrawal
F41.9   Anxiety Disorder NOS (484)

SOMATOFORM DISORDERS (485)

F45.0   Somatization Disorder (486)
F45.1   Undifferentiated Somatoform Disorder (490)
F44.x   Conversion Disorder (492)
   .4   With Motor Symptom or Deficit
   .5   With Seizures or Convulsions
   .6   With Sensory Symptom or Deficit
   .7   With Mixed Presentation
F45.4   Pain Disorder (498)

Specify type: Associated With Psychological Factors/Associated With Both Psychological Factors and a General Medical Condition
Specify if: Acute/Chronic

F45.2 Hypochondriasis (504)
Specify if: With Poor Insight

F45.2 Body Dysmorphic Disorder (507)

F45.9 Somatoform Disorder NOS (511)

FACTITIOUS DISORDERS (513)

F68.1 Factitious Disorder (513)
Specify type: With Predominantly Psychological Signs and Symptoms/With Predominantly Physical Signs and Symptoms/With Combined Psychological and Physical Signs and Symptoms

F68.1 Factitious Disorder NOS (517)

DISSOCIATIVE DISORDERS (519)

F44.0 Dissociative Amnesia (520)

F44.1 Dissociative Fugue (523)

F44.81 Dissociative Identity Disorder (526)

F48.1 Depersonalization Disorder (530)

F44.9 Dissociative Disorder NOS (532)

SEXUAL AND GENDER IDENTITY DISORDERS (535)

Sexual Dysfunctions (535)

The following specifiers apply to all primary Sexual Dysfunctions:

Lifelong Type/Acquired Type/Generalized Type/Situational Type/Due to Psychological Factors/Due to Combined Factors

Sexual Desire Disorders (539)

F52.0 Hypoactive Sexual Desire Disorder (539)

F52.10 Sexual Aversion Disorder (541)

Sexual Arousal Disorders (543)

F52.2 Female Sexual Arousal Disorder (543)

F52.2 Male Erectile Disorder (545)

Orgasmic Disorders (547)

F52.3 Female Orgasmic Disorder (547)

F52.3 Male Orgasmic Disorder (550)

F52.4 Premature Ejaculation (552)

Sexual Pain Disorders (554)

F52.6 Dyspareunia (Not Due to a General Medical Condition) (554)

F52.5 Vaginismus (Not Due to a General Medical Condition) (556)

Sexual Dysfunction Due to a General Medical Condition (558)

N94.8 Female Hypoactive Sexual Desire Disorder Due to . . . *[Indicate the General Medical Condition]* (558)

N50.8 Male Hypoactive Sexual Desire Disorder Due to . . . *[Indicate the General Medical Condition]* (558)

N48.4 Male Erectile Disorder Due to . . . *[Indicate the General Medical Condition]* (558)

N94.1 Female Dyspareunia Due to . . . *[Indicate the General Medical Condition]* (558)

N50.8 Male Dyspareunia Due to . . . *[Indicate the General Medical Condition]* (558)

N94.8 Other Female Sexual Dysfunction Due to . . . *[Indicate the General Medical Condition]* (558)

N50.8 Other Male Sexual Dysfunction Due to . . . *[Indicate the General Medical Condition]* (558)

___.___ Substance-Induced Sexual Dysfunction (*refer to Substance-Related Disorders for substance-specific codes*) (562)
Specify if: With Impaired Desire/With Impaired Arousal/With Impaired Orgasm/With Sexual Pain
Specify if: With Onset During Intoxication

F52.9 Sexual Dysfunction NOS (565)

Paraphilias (566)

F65.2 Exhibitionism (569)

F65.0 Fetishism (569)

F65.8 Frotteurism (570)

F65.4 Pedophilia (571)
Specify if: Sexually Attracted to Males/Sexually Attracted to Females/Sexually Attracted to Both
Specify if: Limited to Incest
Specify type: Exclusive Type/Nonexclusive Type

F65.5 Sexual Masochism (572)

F65.5 Sexual Sadism (573)

F65.1 Transvestic Fetishism (574)
Specify if: With Gender Dysphoria

F65.3 Voyeurism (575)

F65.9 Paraphilia NOS (576)

Gender Identity Disorders (576)

F64.x Gender Identity Disorder (576)
.2   in Children
.0   in Adolescents or Adults
Specify if: Sexually Attracted to Males/Sexually Attracted to Females/Sexually Attracted to Both/Sexually Attracted to Neither

F64.9 Gender Identity Disorder NOS (582)

F52.9 Sexual Disorder NOS (582)

EATING DISORDERS (583)

F50.0 Anorexia Nervosa (583)
Specify type: Restricting Type; Binge-Eating/Purging Type

F50.2 Bulimia Nervosa (589)
Specify type: Purging Type/Nonpurging Type

F50.9 Eating Disorder NOS (594)

SLEEP DISORDERS (597)

Primary Sleep Disorders (598)

Dyssomnias (598)

F51.0 Primary Insomnia (599)

F51.1 Primary Hypersomnia (604)
Specify if: Recurrent

G47.4 Narcolepsy (609)

G47.3 Breathing-Related Sleep Disorder (615)

F51.2 Circadian Rhythm Sleep Disorder (622)
Specify type: Delayed Sleep Phase Type/Jet Lag Type/Shift Work Type/Unspecified Type

F51.9 Dyssomnia NOS (629)

Parasomnias (630)

F51.5 Nightmare Disorder (631)
F51.4 Sleep Terror Disorder (634)
F51.3 Sleepwalking Disorder (639)
F51.8 Parasomnia NOS (644)

Sleep Disorders Related to Another Mental Disorder (645)

F51.0 Insomnia Related to . . . [Indicate the Axis I or Axis II Disorder] (645)
F51.1 Hypersomnia Related to . . . [Indicate the Axis I or Axis II Disorder] (645)

Other Sleep Disorders (651)

G47.x Sleep Disorder Due to . . . [Indicate the General Medical Condition] (651)
.0 Insomnia Type
.1 Hypersomnia Type
.8 Parasomnia Type
.8 Mixed Type
___.__ Substance-Induced Sleep Disorder (*refer to Substance-Related Disorders for substance-specific codes*) (655)
Specify type: Insomnia Type/Hypersomnia Type/Parasomnia Type/Mixed Type
Specify if: With Onset During Intoxication/With Onset During Withdrawal

IMPULSE-CONTROL DISORDERS NOT ELSEWHERE CLASSIFIED (663)

F63.8 Intermittent Explosive Disorder (663)
F63.2 Kleptomania (667)
F63.1 Pyromania (669)
F63.0 Pathological Gambling (671)
F63.3 Trichotillomania (674)
F63.9 Impulse-Control Disorder NOS (677)

ADJUSTMENT DISORDERS (679)

F43.xx Adjustment Disorder (679)
.20 With Depressed Mood
.28 With Anxiety
.22 With Mixed Anxiety and Depressed Mood
.24 With Disturbance of Conduct
.25 With Mixed Disturbance of Emotions and Conduct
.9 Unspecified
Specify if: Acute/Chronic

PERSONALITY DISORDERS (685)

Note: *These are coded on Axis II.*
F60.0 Paranoid Personality Disorder (690)
F60.1 Schizoid Personality Disorder (694)
F21 Schizotypal Personality Disorder (697)

F60.2 Antisocial Personality Disorder (701)
F60.31 Borderline Personality Disorder (706)
F60.4 Histrionic Personality Disorder (711)
F60.8 Narcissistic Personality Disorder (714)
F60.6 Avoidant Personality Disorder (718)
F60.7 Dependent Personality Disorder (721)
F60.5 Obsessive-Compulsive Personality Disorder (725)
F60.9 Personality Disorder NOS (729)

OTHER CONDITIONS THAT MAY BE A FOCUS OF CLINICAL ATTENTION (731)

Psychological Factors Affecting Medical Condition (731)

F54 . . . [Specified Psychological Factor] Affecting . . . [Indicate the General Medical Condition] Choose name based on nature of factors (731):
Mental Disorder Affecting Medical Condition
Psychological Symptoms Affecting Medical Condition
Personality Traits or Coping Style Affecting Medical Condition
Maladaptive Health Behaviors Affecting Medical Condition
Stress-Related Physiological Response Affecting Medical Condition
Other or Unspecified Psychological Factors Affecting Medical Condition

Medication-Induced Movement Disorders (734)

G21.0 Neuroleptic-Induced Parkinsonism (735)
G21.0 Neuroleptic Malignant Syndrome (735)
G24.0 Neuroleptic-Induced Acute Dystonia (735)
G21.1 Neuroleptic-Induced Acute Akathisia (735)
G24.0 Neuroleptic-Induced Tardive Dyskinesia (736)
G25.1 Medication-Induced Postural Tremor (736)
G25.9 Medication-Induced Movement Disorder NOS (736)

Other Medication-Induced Disorder (736)

T88.7 Adverse Effects of Medication NOS (736)

Relational Problems (736)

Z63.7 Relational Problem Related to a Mental Disorder or General Medical Condition (737)
Z63.8 Parent-Child Relational Problem (*code Z63.1 if focus of attention is on child*) (737)
Z63.0 Partner Relational Problem (737)
F93.3 Sibling Relational Problem (737)
Z63.9 Relational Problem NOS (737)

Problems Related to Abuse or Neglect (738)

T74.1 Physical Abuse of Child (738)
T74.2 Sexual Abuse of Child (738)
T74.0 Neglect of Child (738)
T74.1 Physical Abuse of Adult (738)
T74.2 Sexual Abuse of Adult (738)

Additional Conditions That May Be A Focus of Clinical Attention (739)

Z91.1 Noncompliance With Treatment (739)
Z76.5 Malingering (739)

Z72.8   Adult Antisocial Behavior (740)
Z72.8   Child or Adolescent Antisocial Behavior (740)
R41.8   Borderline Intellectual Functioning (740)
R41.8   Age-Related Cognitive Decline (740)
Z63.4   Bereavement (740)
Z55.8   Academic Problem (741)
Z56.7   Occupational Problem (741)
F93.8   Identity Problem (741)
Z71.8   Religious or Spiritual Problem (741)
Z60.3   Acculturation Problem (741)
Z60.0   Phase of Life Problem (742)

ADDITIONAL CODES (743)

F99   Unspecified Mental Disorder (nonpsychotic) (743)
Z03.2   No Diagnosis or Condition on Axis I (743)
R69   Diagnosis or Condition Deferred on Axis I (743)
Z03.2   No Diagnosis on Axis II (743)
R46.8   Diagnosis Deferred on Axis II (743)

Appendix B: Some Contributions to Psychiatric and Mental Health Nursing

Pre-1860

Nursing care for the young, ill, and helpless historically has existed as long as the human race. Care was given by family members, relatives, servants, neighbors, members of religious orders or humanitarian societies, or by convalescing patients or prisoners.

1860

Florence Nightingale. Established Nightingale School at St. Thomas Hospital in London after Crimean War and worked with untrained women caring for soldiers. *Founder of modern day nursing.*

1860–1880

Emphasized maintaining healthful environment, personal hygiene, cleanliness, and healthful living habits, such as adequate nutrition, exercise, and sleep so that nature could heal. Emphasized kindness toward patients along with custodial care.

Linda Richards. *First graduate nurse and first psychiatric nurse in the United States.* After study under Miss Nightingale, organized nursing services and educational programs in Boston City Hospital and in several state mental hospitals in Illinois.

Dorothea Dix. *Worked to reform psychiatric care in mental hospitals* and to correct overcrowding and the insufficient number of physicians and attendants.

1882

First school to prepare nurses to care for acutely and chronically mentally ill opened at McLean Hospital, Waverly, Massachusetts, through collaboration of Linda Richards and Dr. Edward Cowles.

1890–1930

Nurses recognized by some administrative psychiatrists in state and private hospitals for their preparation. Nurses relieved of menial housekeeping chores to engage in physical custodial care of patients. Role primarily to assist physician or carry out procedures for physical care. Few psychological nursing skills. Psychologically concerned with maintaining kind, tolerant attitude and humane treatment.

1920

Harriet Bailey. *First nurse educator to write a psychiatric nursing text, Nursing Mental Disease,* 1920. She wrote of the importance of a nurse's knowing mental illness and of teaching mental health nursing, and she worked for student experiences in psychiatry. She argued for more holistic care of patients.

1937

The incorporation of psychiatric nursing was recommended by the National League for Nursing for inclusion in basic nursing curriculum.

1946

National Mental Health Act passed, authorizing establishment of National Institute of Mental Health, with funds and programs to train professional psychiatric personnel, conduct psychiatric research, and aid in development of mental health programs at the state level. Provided impetus for psychiatric nursing as a specialty.

1950–1960

Nurse's role included physical care and medications and maintenance of therapeutic milieu. Less emphasis on physical restraints.

Ruth Matheney and Mary Topalis. Emphasized importance of milieu therapy and the nurse's using this intervention.

1952

Hildegard E. Peplau. *Formulated first systematic theoretical framework in psychiatric nursing; presented in Interpersonal Relations in Nursing,* 1952. Emphasized that nursing is an interpersonal process and that psychological techniques and theoretical concepts are essential to nursing practice. Emphasized steps in nurse-patient relationship:

1. Nurse helps patient examine situational factors through observation of behavior.
2. Nurse helps patient describe and analyze behavior.
3. Nurse formulates with patient connections between feelings and behavior.
4. Nurse encourages patient to improve interpersonal competence through testing new behavior.
5. Nurse validates with patient when new behavior is integrated into personality structure. Psychoanalytical, interpersonal, and communication theories used by nurses.

1953

The Therapeutic Community, by Maxwell Jones in Great Britain, laid basis for movement in United States toward therapeutic milieu and nurse's role in this therapy.

1956

National Conference on Graduate Education in Psychiatric Nursing introduced concept of psychiatric clinical nurse specialist. Theoreticians begin to differentiate functions based on master's level of preparation in nursing.

1957

June Mellow. *Introduced second theoretical approach to psychiatric nursing, called Nursing Therapy,* using psychoanalytical theory in one-to-one approach with schizophrenic patient. *Emphasized providing corrective emotional experience rather than investigating pathological processes or interpersonal developmental processes in order to facilitate integration of overwhelmed ego.*

1958

American Nurses' Association established Conference Group on Psychiatric Nursing.

1959

Accredited schools of nursing had to have own psychiatric nursing curriculum and instructor, per National League for Nursing. Could no longer buy services of hospitals to supply education.

1960–1970

Hildegard E. Peplau, Gertrude Ujhely, Joyce Travelbee, Shirley Burd, Loretta Bermosk, Joyce Hays, Catherine Norris, Gertrude Stokes, Anne Hargreaves, Dorothy Gregg, and Sheila Rouslin. Nursing leaders emphasized importance of self-awareness and use of self, nurse-patient relationships therapy, therapeutic communication, and psychosocial aspects of general nursing. Peplau formulated the manifestations of anxiety and steps in anxiety intervention, now used by all health care professions. All of these nursing leaders developed various psychological concepts into operational definitions for use in nursing.

1960

Ida Orlando. *Initiated term nursing process and began to delineate its components.* Presented general theoretical framework for all nurse-patient relationships, with focus on client ascertaining meaning of behavior and explaining help needed. Wrote the classic book *The Dynamic Nurse-Patient Relationship,* 1961.

Comprehensive Community Mental Health Act passed, 1960; provided impetus for nurses moving from hospital to community setting.

1961

Anne Burgess and Donna Aguilera. *Engaged in crisis work and short term therapy* as well as in long-term therapy. *Applied crisis theory to psychiatric nursing.*

Hildegard E. Peplau. Promoted *primary role of nurse as psychotherapist or counselor* rather than as mother surrogate, socializer, or manager.

1960–1965

Sheila Rouslin and Suzanne Lego. Opened private practices in psychotherapy.

1967

American Nurses' Association presented Position Paper on Psychiatric Nursing, endorsing role of clinical specialist as therapist in individual, group, family, and milieu therapies.

American Nurses' Association, Division in Psychiatric and Mental Health Nursing Practice, published first *Statement on Psychiatric and Mental Health Nursing Practice.*

1970–1980

Sheila Rouslin. *Certification of clinical specialists in psychiatric nursing begun* by Division of Psychiatric Mental Health Nursing, New Jersey State Nurses' Association, *because of her leadership.* Later, certification developed by American Nurses' Association.

Shirley Smoyak. *Client defined as individual, group, family, or community;* nurse defined as family therapist. Expanding role of psychiatric nurse.

Gwen Marram and Irene Burnside. *Group and family psychotherapy by graduate-prepared nurses* emphasized by nursing leaders.

Carolyn Clark. *Systems framework was used increasingly* by psychiatric nurses.

Change agent, health maintenance, and research roles emphasized in latter half of decade.

Bonnie Bullough. *Legal and ethical aspects of psychiatric care emphasized.*

Madeleine Leininger. *Care of whole person reemphasized.* Introduced implications of cultural diversity for mental health services and psychiatric treatment.

Hector Gonzales, Doris Mosley and Paulette D'Angi. Practice as autonomous member of team and in independent or private practice increased in latter half of decade. Work with citizens, consumer groups, and consumer organizations increased toward end of decade.

1976

American Nurses' Association Division of Psychiatric and Mental Health Nursing Practice published revised *Statement on Psychiatric and Mental Health Nursing Practice.*

1978

President's Commission Report of 1978 concluded that effects of de-institutionalization and discharge of patients to community facilities have not worked as expected because of lack of financial, social, medical, and nursing resources and lack of coordination of services.

1980s

Anne Burgess. *Formulated theory of victimology,* based on extensive studies of adult and child victims of rape and abuse, child victims of neglect, and family violence of incest and battering. Described rape trauma syndrome, silent rape trauma, and compounded reactions to rape.

Lee Ann Hoff. *Expanded crisis theory to be used in nursing practice. Contributed to theory of suicidology.* Described battering syndrome after research on battered women and battered elderly.

1982

American Nurses' Association Executive Committee and Standards Committee, Division of Psychiatric and Mental Health Nursing Practice, published *Standards of Psychiatric and Mental Health Nursing Practice.*

1987

Maxine E. Loomis, Anita O'Toole, Marie Scott Brown, Patricia Pothier, Patricia West, and Holly S. Wilson. Began the development of a classification system for Psychiatric and Mental Health Nursing, first published in *Archives of Psychiatric Nursing,* 1(1):16–24, 1987, a new journal.

1990

Suzanne Lego. *Opened the first psychoanalytic training program for nurses* at Columbia School of Nursing.

1994

Carolyn V. Billings, Jean Blackburn, Mickie Ceimone, Carol Dashiff, Kathleen Scharer, Anita O'Toole, and Carole A. Shea. Composed a Task Force to:
- Revise: *A statement on psychiatric-mental health clinical nursing practice* updating the scope and functions for nurses certified at the basic level and those certified at the advanced practice level.
- Revise: *Standards of psychiatric-mental health clinical nursing practice* describing professional nursing activities that are demonstrated by the nurse through the nursing process for both the Basic Level Certified Psychiatric Nurse and the Advanced Practice Psychiatric Nurse, and *Standards of professional performance.*

2000

Grace Sills, Karen A. Ballard, Carolyn V. Billings and others. *Revision of the Scope and Standards of Psychiatric Mental Health Nursing Clinical Practice.*

Adapted from Murray R.B. (1991). The nursing process and emotional care. In Murray RB, Huelskoetter MMW (Eds.). Psychiatric Mental Health Nursing—Giving Emotional Care (3rd ed) (pp 94–97). Norwalk, CT: Appleton & Lange.

Appendix C:　NANDA-Approved Nursing Diagnoses

Activity intolerance
Activity intolerance, Risk for
Adjustment, Impaired
Airway clearance, Ineffective
Allergy response, Latex
Allergy response, Risk for latex
Anxiety
Anxiety, Death
Aspiration, Risk for
Attachment, Risk for impaired parent/ infant/child
Autonomic dysreflexia
Autonomic dysreflexia, Risk for
Body image, Disturbed
Body temperature, Risk for imbalanced
Bowel incontinence
Breastfeeding, Effective
Breastfeeding, Ineffective
Breastfeeding, Interrupted
Breathing pattern, Ineffective

Cardiac output, Decreased
Caregiver role strain
Caregiver role strain, Risk for
Comfort, Impaired
Communication, Impaired verbal
Conflict, Decisional
Conflict, Parental role
Confusion, Acute
Confusion, Chronic
Constipation
Constipation, Perceived
Constipation, Risk for
Coping, Ineffective
Coping, Ineffective community
Coping, Readiness for enhanced community
Coping, Defensive
Coping, Compromised family
Coping, Disabled family
Coping, Readiness for enhanced family

Denial, Ineffective
Dentition, Impaired
Development, Risk for delayed
Diarrhea
Disuse syndrome, Risk for
Diversional activity, Deficient
Energy field, Disturbed
Environmental interpretation syndrome, Impaired
Failure to thrive, Adult
Falls, Risk for
Family processes: alcoholism, Dysfunctional
Family processes, Interrupted
Fatigue
Fear
Fluid volume, Deficient
Fluid volume, Excess
Fluid volume, Risk for deficient
Fluid volume, Risk for imbalanced

Diagnoses in italics are the ones most recently added to the list. Copyright © 2001 by the North American Nursing Diagnosis Association.

Gas exchange, Impaired
Grieving
Grieving, Anticipatory
Grieving, Dysfunctional
Growth and development, Delayed
Growth, Risk for disproportionate
Health maintenance, Ineffective
Health-seeking behaviors
Home maintenance, Impaired
Hopelessness
Hyperthermia
Hypothermia
Identity, Disturbed personal
Incontinence, Functional urinary
Incontinence, Reflex urinary
Incontinence, Stress urinary
Incontinence, Total urinary
Incontinence, Urge urinary
Incontinence, Risk for urge urinary
Infant behavior, Disorganized
Infant behavior, Risk for disorganized
Infant behavior, Readiness for enhanced organized
Infant feeding pattern, Ineffective
Infection, Risk for
Injury, Risk for
Injury, Risk for perioperative-positioning
Intracranial, adaptive capacity, Decreased
Knowledge, Deficient
Loneliness, Risk for
Memory, Impaired
Mobility, Impaired bed
Mobility, Impaired physical
Mobility, Impaired wheelchair
Nausea
Neglect, Unilateral
Noncompliance

Nutrition: less than body requirements, Imbalanced
Nutrition: more than body requirements, Imbalanced
Nutrition: more than body requirements, Risk for imbalanced
Oral mucous membrane, Impaired
Pain, Acute
Pain, Chronic
Parenting, Impaired
Parenting, Risk for impaired
Peripheral neurovascular dysfunction, Risk for
Poisoning, Risk for
Post-trauma syndrome
Post-trauma syndrome, Risk for
Powerlessness
Powerlessness, Risk for
Protection, Ineffective
Rape-trauma syndrome
Rape-trauma syndrome, compound reaction
Rape-trauma syndrome, silent reaction
Relocation stress syndrome
Relocation stress syndrome, Risk for
Role performance, Ineffective
Self-care deficit, Bathing/hygiene
Self-care deficit
Self-care deficit, Feeding
Self-care deficit, Toileting
Self-esteem, Chronic low
Self-esteem, Situational low
Self-esteem, Risk for situational low
Self-mutilation
Self-mutilation, Risk for
Sensory perception, Disturbed
Sexual dysfunction
Sexuality patterns, Ineffective

Skin integrity, Impaired
Skin integrity, Risk for impaired
Sleep deprivation
Sleep pattern, Disturbed
Social interaction, Impaired
Social isolation
Sorrow, Chronic
Spiritual distress
Spiritual distress, Risk for
Spiritual well-being, Readiness for enhanced
Suffocation, Risk for
Suicide, Risk for
Surgical recovery, Delayed
Swallowing, Impaired
Therapeutic regimen management, Effective
Therapeutic regimen management, Ineffective
Therapeutic regimen management, Ineffective community
Therapeutic regimen management, Ineffective family
Thermoregulation, Ineffective
Thought processes, Disturbed
Tissue integrity, Impaired
Tissue perfusion, Ineffective
Transfer ability, Impaired
Trauma, Risk for
Urinary elimination, Impaired
Urinary retention
Ventilation, Impaired spontaneous
Ventilatory weaning response, Dysfunctional
Violence, Risk for other-directed
Violence, Risk for self-directed
Walking, Impaired
Wandering

Appendix D: Drug Information

Visit the Evolve website at http://evolve.elsevier.com/Varcarolis for the complete version of Appendix D.

Appendix E: Answers to Chapter Review Questions

CHAPTER 1

1. 3
2. 4
3. 3
4. 2
5. 4

CHAPTER 2

1. 4
2. 1
3. 1
4. 3
5. 1

CHAPTER 3

1. 1
2. 3
3. 1
4. 2
5. 3

CHAPTER 4

1. 3
2. 2
3. 4
4. 4
5. 1

CHAPTER 5

1. 1
2. 4
3. 3
4. 3
5. 4

CHAPTER 6

1. 2
2. 1
3. 2
4. 2
5. 1

CHAPTER 7

1. 3
2. 3
3. 4
4. 2
5. 3

CHAPTER 8

1. 4
2. 1
3. 1
4. 1
5. 3

CHAPTER 9

1. 2
2. 1
3. 2
4. 1
5. 1

CHAPTER 10

1. 1
2. 3
3. 4
4. 3
5. 4

CHAPTER 11

1. 1
2. 3
3. 1
4. 2
5. 1

CHAPTER 12

1. 1
2. 2
3. 1
4. 3
5. 3

CHAPTER 13

1. 3
2. 3
3. 3
4. 1
5. 2

CHAPTER 14

1. 1
2. 3
3. 4
4. 4
5. 2

CHAPTER 15

1. 2
2. 3
3. 4
4. 2
5. 2

CHAPTER 16

1. 4
2. 2
3. 4
4. 2
5. 1

CHAPTER 17

1. 1
2. 3
3. 2
4. 1
5. 1

CHAPTER 18

1. 2
2. 4
3. 1
4. 3
5. 2

CHAPTER 19

1. 1
2. 2
3. 1
4. 2
5. 2

CHAPTER 20

1. 4
2. 4
3. 1
4. 1
5. 3

CHAPTER 21

1. 1
2. 4
3. 1
4. 1
5. 1

CHAPTER 22

1. 1
2. 3
3. 1
4. 1
5. 1

CHAPTER 23

1. 4
2. 2
3. 4
4. 4
5. 1

CHAPTER 24

1. 3
2. 1
3. 1
4. 4
5. 2

CHAPTER 25

1. 1
2. 4
3. 2
4. 1
5. 4

CHAPTER 26

1. 1
2. 4
3. 2
4. 2
5. 4

CHAPTER 27

1. 3
2. 1
3. 4
4. 1
5. 1

CHAPTER 28

1. 2
2. 1
3. 3
4. 1
5. 4

CHAPTER 29

1. 2
2. 3
3. 2
4. 4
5. 3

CHAPTER 30

1. 1
2. 2
3. 4
4. 1
5. 1

CHAPTER 31

1. 1
2. 1
3. 2
4. 4
5. 4

CHAPTER 32

1. 2
2. 1
3. 4
4. 3
5. 3

CHAPTER 33

1. 1
2. 1
3. 2
4. 1
5. 1

CHAPTER 34

1. 4
2. 4
3. 2
4. 4
5. 3

CHAPTER 35

1. 1
2. 2
3. 1
4. 3
5. 3

CHAPTER 36

1. 3
2. 2
3. 1
4. 4
5. 2

GUIDELINES FOR CHAPTER 8 CRITICAL THINKING QUESTIONS

1. ■ Yes, even if Beth denies taking the medications, Joe should discuss the problem with the supervisor.
   ■ The supervisor and agency will report after investigating.
   ■ If Beth has admitted it, Joe should identify Beth.
   ■ Yes, most state boards do mandate reporting, although often the agency will accept this responsibility (not suspicions, but admitted facts).
   ■ No. This is a legal duty to intervene.
2. ■ Legally practice? The nurse's license allows her to practice in an ICU, *but* it is unreasonable to expect a psychiatric nurse to understand all of the equipment. It would probably be found to be negligent to place a psychiatric nurse in an ICU.
   ■ Yes
   ■ Yes, as far as medical-surgical expectations. If unfamiliar with current practice, the RN should seek

continuing education proper to working with patients in a specialty area. To avoid insubordination charges, the nurse must clarify the expectations and areas of care to which he or she will be assigned when hired.
   ■ Harm to patient, negligence, liability if patient injured, misrepresentation.
   ■ Insubordination; charges of abandonment.
   ■ Clarify expectations with employer when being hired (in writing).
   ■ Request the assistance of another professional (nurse, supervisor, doctor) during nurse B's absence.
   ■ Both the hospital and nurse A will likely be named as defendants. The hospital breached its duty to provide competent care providers, especially if they knew of nurse A's limited scope of practice abilities.
3. ■ Yes, but the nasal packs in this case call for a higher standard of care, e.g., more frequent checks. The question will revolve around what behavior was/is

reasonable and prudent to protect the client (Negligence Standard).

- No. Nasal packing increases the need to check more often.
- No. The doctor does not avoid any responsibility, but nurses are licensed professionals and as such are expected to exercise their own sound judgment when a client's safety is jeopardized.
- No, the order for the restraint was inappropriate.
- (a) The client is in a private room (isolated, where there is less opportunity for observation), and (b) this client could go into delirium tremens, which is a contraindication for restraints. The client could have had seizures with nasal packs in place.
- No. Closer observation was warranted. The statute identified a standard found acceptable by the state, but more frequent checks (every 15 to 30 minutes) are generally recommended. Federal regulations would overrule less restrictive state regulations.
- No restraints. Check the client more frequently. Don't place the client in an isolated private room. Question the doctor on the order to restrain and refuse to place the client in an unsafe position.

(Don't confront the doctor, but rather share your concerns in a professional manner.)

4. ■ No, the nurse has a legal duty to notify the boy's therapist, who, in turn, should warn the boy's mother.
- Ethical principles cannot be valued over a human life that is threatened. The client will be in greater trouble if the nurse does not intervene and allows the boy to harm his mother. Preventing this legal and human dilemma is more ethical toward the client than maintaining confidentiality. Preventing a crime is in the client's best interest (beneficence); justice could not allow harm to an innocent victim; our society cannot allow total autonomy or we'd have no law and order.
- The "special relationship" is recognized by the law as with the therapist, whom the nurse must notify, who in turn should warn the mother.
- Would need to warn in either case.
- No difference when discussing legal duty to warn and ethics.
- Talk to the supervisor to have discharge reconsidered and to decide who should warn the mother.

Glossary

Abstract thinking The ability to conceptualize ideas (e.g., finding meaning in proverbs).

Abuse An act of misuse, deceit, or exploitation; wrong or improper use or action toward another, resulting in injury, damage, maltreatment, or corruption.

Accommodation The ability to change one's way of thinking in order to introduce new ideas, objects, or experiences.

Acrophobia Fear of high places.

Acting out behaviors Behaviors that originate on an unconscious level to reduce anxiety and tension. Anxiety is displaced from one situation to another in the form of observable behavioral responses (e.g., anger, crying, or violence).

Activities of daily living For a person with a chronic mental illness, this term refers to the skills necessary to live independently as an adult.

Acute anxiety Anxiety that is precipitated by an imminent loss or a change that threatens an individual's sense of security.

Addiction Addiction incorporates the concepts of loss of control with respect to use of a drug (e.g., alcohol), taking the drug despite related problems, and a tendency to relapse. *Addiction* is an older term that has been replaced by the term *drug dependence.*

Adult Children of Alcoholics (ACOA) A support group for adult children of alcoholics, who often experience similar difficulties and problems in their adult lives as a result of having an alcoholic parent or parents.

Adventitious crises Crises that are not part of everyday life; they are unplanned and accidental. They include natural disasters, national disasters, and crimes of violence such as rapes or muggings.

Affect An objective manifestation of an experience or emotion accompanying an idea or feeling. The observations one would make on assessment. For example, a client may be said to have a flat affect, meaning that there is an absence or a near absence of facial expression. Some people, however, use the term loosely to mean a feeling, emotion, or mood.

Ageism A system of destructive, erroneous beliefs about the elderly; defined as a bias against older people based solely on their age.

Aggression Any verbal or nonverbal (actual or attempted, conscious or unconscious) forceful means to harm or abuse another person or object.

Agnosia Loss of the ability to recognize familiar objects. For example, a person may be unable to identify familiar sounds, such as the ringing of a doorbell (auditory agnosia), or familiar objects, such as a toothbrush or keys (visual agnosia).

Agoraphobia The most serious and the most common phobia for which people seek treatment. It is fear and avoidance of being alone or being in open spaces from which escape might be difficult. At its most severe, a person with agoraphobia may not be able to leave his or her own home.

Agraphia Loss of a previous ability to write, resulting from brain injury or brain disease.

Akathisia Regular rhythmic movements, usually of the lower limbs; constant pacing may also be seen; often noticed in people taking antipsychotic medication.

Akinesia Absence or diminution of voluntary motion. Akinesia is usually accompanied by a parallel reduction in mental activity.

Al-a-Teen A nationwide network for children over 10 years of age who have alcoholic parents.

Al-Anon A support group for spouses and friends of alcoholics.

Alcohol withdrawal delirium An organic mental disorder that occurs 40 to 48 hours after cessation or reduction of long-term heavy alcohol intake and that is considered a medical emergency; often referred to by the older term *delirium tremens* (DTs).

Alcoholic hallucinations Auditory hallucinations reported to occur approximately 48 hours after heavy drinking by alcohol-dependent clients.

Alcoholics Anonymous (AA) A self-help group of recovering alcoholics that provides support and encouragement to those involved in continuing recovery.

Alcoholism The end stage of the continuum that includes addiction to and dependence on the drug alcohol.

Alliance for the Mentally Ill A national support group for families of the mentally ill, with many local and state affiliates; provides educational programs and political action.

Alzheimer's disease A primary cognitive impairment disorder characterized by progressive deterioration of cognitive functioning, with the end result that a person may not recognize once-familiar people, places, and things. The ability to walk and talk is absent in the final stages.

Ambivalence The holding, at the same time, of two opposing emotions, attitudes, ideas, or wishes toward the same person, situation, or object.

Amnesia Loss of memory for events within a specific period of time; may be temporary or permanent.

Anergia Lack of energy; passivity.

Anger An emotional response to the perception of frustration of desires or threat to one's needs.

Anhedonia The inability to experience pleasure.

Anorexia A medical term that signifies a loss of appetite. A person with anorexia nervosa, however, may not have any loss of appetite and often is preoccupied with food and eating. A person with this condition may suppress the desire for food in order to control his or her eating.

Antabuse (disulfiram) A drug given to alcoholics that produces nausea, vomiting, dizziness, flushing, and tachycardia if alcohol is consumed.

Anticholinergic side effects Side effects caused by the use of some medications, e.g., neuroleptics and tricyclics. Symptoms include dry mouth, constipation, urinary retention, blurred vision, and dry mucous membranes.

Anticipatory grief Grief that occurs before an actual loss. During this time, painful feelings may be partially resolved.

Antidepressants Drugs predominantly used to elevate mood in people who are depressed.

Antimanic drugs Drugs used in the treatment of a manic state to lower an elevated and unstable mood and to reduce irritability and aggressiveness.

Antipsychotic drugs (neuroleptics, major tranquilizers) Drugs that have the ability to decrease psychotic, paranoid, and disorganized thinking and positively alter bizarre behaviors; they are thought to reduce the effects of the neutrotransmitter dopamine by blocking the dopamine receptors.

Antisocial (sociopathic, psychopathic) These terms are often used interchangeably to refer to a syndrome in which a person lacks the capacity to relate to others. These people do not experience discomfort in inflicting or observing pain in others, and they constantly manipulate others for personal gain. Common behaviors seen in people with this disorder include crimes against society, aggressiveness, inability to feel remorse, untruthfulness and insincerity, unreliability, and failure to follow any life plan.

Anxiety A state of feeling apprehension, uneasiness, uncertainty, or dread resulting from a real or perceived threat whose actual source is unknown or unrecognized.

Anxiolytics (antianxiety drugs, minor tranquilizers) Drugs prescribed usually on a short-term basis to reduce anxiety.

Apathy A state of indifference.

Aphasia Difficulty in the formulation of words; loss of language ability. In extreme cases, a person may be limited to a few words, may babble, or may become mute.

Apraxia Loss of purposeful motor movements. For example, a person may be unable to shave, to dress, or to do other once-familiar and purposeful tasks.

Assault An intentional act that is designed to make the victim fearful and that produces reasonable apprehension of harm.

Assertiveness Asking for what one wants or acting to get what one wants in a way that respects the rights and feelings of other people.

Assertiveness training Communications skills that help people ask directly in appropriate (nondemanding, nonthreatening, and nondemeaning) ways for what they want.

Assimilation The ability to incorporate new ideas, objects, and experiences into the framework of one's thoughts.

Associative looseness Disturbance of thinking in which ideas shift from one subject to another in an oblique or unrelated manner. When this condition is severe, speech may be incoherent.

Attention-deficit hyperactivity disorder A behavioral disorder usually manifested before the age of 7 that includes over-activity, chronic inattention, and difficulty dealing with multiple stimuli.

Autistic thinking Thoughts, ideas, or desires derived from internal, private stimuli or perceptions that often are incongruent with reality.

Automatic obedience The performance of all simple commands in a robot-like fashion; may be present in catatonia.

Aversion therapy A behavioral technique that uses negative reinforcement or "conditioning" to alter or eliminate an unwanted or negative behavior.

Avolition Lack of motivation.

Axon The part of the neuron that conveys electrical impulses away from the cell body.

Basal ganglia Pockets of integrating gray matter deep within the cerebrum that are involved in the regulation of movement, emotions, and basic drives.

Battering Refers to physical assaults, such as hitting, kicking, biting, throwing, and burning.

Battery The harmful or offensive touching of another's person.

Behavioral modification A treatment modality that focuses on modifying and changing specific observable dysfunctional patterns of behavior by means of stimulus-and-response conditioning. Examples of behavioral therapy techniques include operant conditioning, token economy, systematic desensitization, aversion therapy, and flooding.

Binge-purge cycle An episodic, uncontrolled, rapid ingestion of large quantities of food over a short period of time, often followed by "purging" (vomiting); a characteristic seen in people with bulimia nervosa.

Biofeedback A technique for gaining conscious control over unconscious body functions, such as blood pressure and heartbeat, to achieve relaxation or the relief of stress-related physical symptoms; involves the use of self-monitoring equipment.

Bipolar disorders Mood disorders that include one or more manic episodes and usually one or more depressive episodes.

Bisexuality Sexual attraction toward both males and females, which may be acted on by engaging in both heterosexual and homosexual activities.

Blocking A sudden obstruction or interruption in the spontaneous flow of thinking or speaking that is perceived as an absence or deprivation of thought.

Blurred or diffused boundaries Refers to a blending together of roles, thoughts, and feelings of an individual so that clear distinctions among family members (or others) fail to emerge.

Body image One's internalized sense of self.

Borderline personality disorder Disorder characterized by impulsive and unpredictable behavior and marked shifts in mood. Instability is seen predominantly in the areas of behavior, mood, relationships to others, and images of self.

Boundaries Those functions that maintain a clear distinction among individuals within a family or group and with the outside world. Boundaries may be clear, diffuse, rigid, or inconsistent.

Bulimia An eating disorder characterized by the excessive and uncontrollable intake of large amounts of food (binges), alternating with purging activities such as self-induced vomiting; use of cathartics, diuretics, or both; and self-starvation. These alternating behaviors characterize the eating disorder *bulimia nervosa.*

Case management Duties of a health care worker (e.g., a nurse) that involve assuming responsibility for a client or group of clients—arranging assessments of need, formulating a comprehensive plan of care, arranging for delivery of services to address individual client needs, and assessing and monitoring the services delivered.

Catatonia A state of psychologically induced immobilization at times interrupted by episodes of extreme agitation.

Catecholamines A group of biogenic amines derived from phenylalanine and containing the catechol nucleus. Certain of these amines, such as *epinephrine, norepinephrine,* and *dopamine,* are neurotransmitters and exert an important influence on peripheral and central nervous system activity.

Cathexis A psychoanalytical term used to describe the emotional attachment or bond to an idea, an object, or most commonly, a person.

Character The sum of a person's relatively fixed personality traits and habitual modes of response.

Chemical restraints Drugs given for the specific purpose of inhibiting a specific behavior or movement.

Child abuse—neglect This abuse can be *physical* (e.g., failure to provide medical care), *developmental* (e.g., failure to provide emotional nurturing and cognitive stimulation), *educational* (failure to provide educational opportunities to the child according to the state's education laws), or a combination.

Child abuse—physical battering Physical assaults such as hitting, kicking, biting, throwing, and burning.

Child abuse—physical endangerment The reckless behaviors toward a child that could lead to the child's serious physical injury, such as leaving a young child alone or placing a child in a hazardous environment.

Child abuse—sexual Sexual abuse of children can take many forms. Essentially it is those acts designated to stimulate the child sexually or to use a child for sexual stimulation, either of the perpetrator or of another person.

Chronic anxiety Anxiety that a person has lived with for a long period of time. Chronic anxiety may take the form of chronic fatigue, insomnia, discomfort in daily activities, or discomfort in personal relationships.

Chronic illness The process of progressive deterioration, with a resulting increase in functional impairment, symptoms, and disability over time.

Chronic pain Pain that a client has had for more than 6 months.

Circadian rhythm A 24-hour biological rhythm that influences specific regulatory functions such as the sleep-wake cycle, body temperature, and hormonal and neurotransmitter secretions. The 24-hour biological rhythm is controlled by a "pacemaker" in the brain that sends messages to various systems in the body such as those mentioned above.

Circumstantial speech A pattern of speech characterized by indirectness and delay before the person gets to the point or answers a question; the person gets caught up in countless details and explanations.

Clang association The meaningless rhyming of words, often in a forceful manner.

Clinical (or critical) pathway A written plan or "map" that identifies predetermined times that specific nursing and medical interventions (e.g., diagnostic studies, treatments, activities, medications, teaching, client outcomes, discharge teaching) will be implemented (e.g., day 1 or day 2 for hospital settings, or week 1 or month 2 for community-based settings).

Co-dependent Coping behaviors that prevent individuals from taking care of their own needs and have as their core a preoccupation with the thoughts and feelings of another or others. It usually refers to the dependence of one person on another person who is addicted in one form or another.

Co-therapist A therapist who shares responsibility for therapeutic work, usually work done with groups or with families.

Cognition The act, process, or result of knowing, learning, or understanding.

Cognitive impairment syndromes/disorders A term that refers to disturbances in orientation, memory, intellect, judgment, and affect due to physiological changes in the brain. Delirium and dementia are examples of two cognitive impairment syndromes. An older term is *chronic mental disorders*

Cognitive rehearsal A technique of having a client imagine each successive step in the sequence leading to the completion of a task, identifying potential "roadblocks" (cognitive, behavioral, or environmental) and planning strategies to deal with them before they produce an unwanted failure experience.

Cognitive therapy A treatment method (particularly useful for depressive disorders) that emphasizes the rearrangement of a person's maladaptive processes of thinking, perceptions, and attitudes.

Community nursing centers (CNCs) Nurse-managed centers that provide direct access to professional nurses who offer holistic, client-centered health services for reimbursement.

Compensation Making up for deficits in one area by excelling in another area in order to raise or maintain self-esteem.

Compulsions Repetitive, seemingly purposeless behaviors performed according to certain rules known to the client in order to temporarily reduce escalating anxiety.

Concrete thinking Thinking characterized by immediate experience rather than abstraction. There is an overemphasis or specific detail as opposed to general and abstract thinking.

Confabulation Filling in a memory gap with a detailed fantasy believed by the teller. The purpose is to maintain self-esteem. This is seen in organic conditions, such as Korsakoff's psychosis.

Confidentiality The ethical responsibility of a health care professional that prohibits the disclosure of privileged information without the patient's informed consent.

Conscious All experiences that are within a person's awareness.

Consensual validation The reality-checking of thoughts, feelings, and actions with others. If a child grows up in an environment in which the chance to validate thoughts, feelings, and behaviors is decreased, the child's ability to perceive reality is greatly impaired.

Conversion The unconscious transfer of anxiety to a physical symptom that has no organic cause.

Coping mechanisms Ways of adjusting to environmental stress without altering one's goals or purposes; they include both conscious and unconscious mechanisms.

Countertransference The tendency of the nurse (therapist, social worker) to displace onto the client feelings that are a response to people in the counselor's past. Strong positive or strong negative reactions to a client may indicate possible countertransferential reactions.

Crisis A temporary state of disequilibrium (high anxiety) in which a person's usual coping mechanisms or problem-solving methods fail. Crisis can result in personality growth or personality disorganization.

Crisis intervention A brief, active, and collaborative therapy that uses an individual's personal coping abilities and resources within the family, health care setting, or community.

Culture The total life style of a people, the social legacy the individual acquires from his or her group, or the environment that is the creation of humankind.

Cyclothymia A chronic mood disturbance (of at least 2 years' duration) involving both hypomanic and dysthymic mood swings. Delusions are never present, and these mood swings usually do not warrant hospitalization or grossly impair a person's social, occupational, or interpersonal functioning.

Decode Interpret the meaning of autistic communications, such as in looseness of associations.

Defense mechanisms (DMs) Unconscious intrapsychic processes used to ward off anxiety by preventing conscious awareness of threatening feelings. They can be used in a healthy and a not-so-healthy manner. Examples of defense mechanisms include repression, projection, sublimation, denial, and regression.

Delayed grief A dysfunctional reaction to grief in which a person may not experience the pain of loss; however, that pain is modified by chronic depression, intense preoccupation with body functioning (hypochondriasis), phobic reactions, or acute insomnia.

Delirium An acute, usually reversible brain syndrome with multiple causes (APA 1987).

Delirium tremens (DTs) An older term now replaced by *alcohol withdrawal delirium.*

Delusion A false belief held to be true even with evidence to the contrary (e.g., the false belief that one is being singled out for harm by others).

Dementia An insidious, chronic, often irreversible brain syndrome (APA 1987).

Dendrite The part of the neuron that conveys electrical impulses toward the cell body.

Denial Escaping of unpleasant realities by ignoring their existence.

Depersonalization A phenomenon whereby a person experiences a sense of unreality or self-estrangement. For example, one may feel that one's extremities have changed, that one is seeing oneself from a distance, or that one is in a dream.

Depressive mood syndrome This term can be defined as "a depressed mood or loss of interest, of at least two weeks' duration, accompanied by several associated symptoms, such as weight loss and difficulty concentrating" (APA 1987).

Derealization The false perception by a person that his or her environment has changed. For example, everything seems bigger or smaller, or familiar objects have become strange and unfamiliar.

Desensitization The reduction of intense reactions to a stimulus (e.g., phobia) by repeated exposure to the stimulus in a weaker or milder form.

Detachment An interpersonal and intrapersonal dissociation from affective expression. Therefore, individuals appear cold, aloof, and distant. This behavior is thought to be learned and is viewed as defensive.

Diagnostic and Statistical Manual of Mental Disorders **(DSM-IV)** Classification of mental disorders that includes descriptions of diagnostic categories. DSM-IV is the most widely accepted system of classifying abnormal behaviors used in the United States today.

Diffused boundaries See *Blurred or diffused boundaries.*

Disorientation Confusion and impaired ability to identify time, place, and person.

Displacement Transfer of emotions associated with a particular person, object, or situation to another person, object, or situation that is nonthreatening.

Dissociation Technique of putting threatening thoughts or feelings out of conscious awareness before they are able to trigger overwhelming and intolerable anxiety; similar to Freud's defense mechanisms of repression.

Dissociative disorders Disorders that involve sudden temporary disturbances or loss of one's normal ability to integrate identity or motor behavior. Psychogenic amnesia and fugue are two examples.

Distractibility Inability to maintain attention; shifting from one area or topic to another with minimal provocation.

Double-bind message A message that contains two contradictory messages given by the same person at the same time, to which the receiver is expected to respond. Constant double-bind situations result in feelings of helplessness, fear, and anxiety in the receiver of the message.

Drug abuse The maladaptive and consistent use of a drug despite social, occupational, psychological, or physical problems exacerbated by the drug; or recurrent use in situations that are physically hazardous, such as driving while intoxicated (APA 1994).

Drug dependence Impaired control of drug use despite adverse consequences, the development of a tolerance to the drug, and the occurrence of withdrawal symptoms when drug intake is reduced or stopped.

Drug interaction The effects of two or more drugs taken simultaneously, producing an alteration in the usual effects of either drug taken alone. The interacting drugs may have a potentiating or an additive effect, and serious side effects may result.

Dual diagnosis A high prevalence for other psychiatric disorders in identified addicts (Talbott et al. 1988). A person with a dual diagnosis is chronically dependent on a drug or alcohol and also has another psychiatric disorder such as a depressive or personality disorder.

Dyskinesia Involuntary muscular activity, such as tic, spasm, or myoclonus.

Dyspareunia Persistent genital pain in either a male or a female before, during, or after sex.

Dysthymia A depression that is mild to moderate in degree and is characterized by a chronic depressive syndrome that is usually present for many years. The depressive mood disturbance is hard to distinguish from the person's usual pattern of functioning, and the person has minimal social or occupational impairment.

Dystonia Muscle spasms of the face, head, neck, and back; usually an acute side effect of neuroleptic (antipsychotic) medication.

Echolalia Mimicking or imitating the speech of another person.

Echopraxia Mimicking or imitating the movements of another person.

Ego One of three psychological processes that make up the Freudian system of personality (id, ego, and superego). The ego is one's "sense of self" and provides such functions as problem solving, mobilization of defense mechanisms, reality testing, and the capability of functioning independently. The ego is said to be the mediator between one's primitive drives (the id) and internalized parental and social prohibitions (the superego).

Ego boundaries A person's perception of the boundaries between him- or herself and the external environment.

Ego-alien/Ego-dystonic Synonymous terms used to describe symptoms that are unacceptable to the person who has them and not compatible with the person's view of him- or herself (e.g., fear of cats).

Ego-syntonic Symptoms that include behaviors or beliefs that do not seem to bother the person or that seem right to the person. For example, a very paranoid person who wrongly believes that the government is out to get him or her truly believes this thought, and it is consistent with the way this person experiences life.

Egocentric Self-centered.

Electroconvulsive therapy (ECT) An effective treatment for depression that consists of inducing a grand mal seizure by passing an electrical current through electrodes that are applied to the temples. The administration of a muscle relaxant minimizes seizure activity, preventing damage to long bones and cervical vertebrae.

Elopement Escape.

Emotional abuse Essentially, emotional abuse is depriving a child of a nurturing atmosphere in which the child can thrive, learn, and develop. This takes many forms (e.g., terrorizing, demeaning, consistently belittling, withholding warmth).

Empathy The ability of one person to get inside another's world and see things from the other person's perspective and to communicate this understanding to the other person.

Enabling Helping a chemically dependent individual avoid experiencing the consequences of his or her drinking or drug use. It is one component of a person in a co-dependency role.

Endorphins A naturally produced chemical (peptide) with morphine-like action. It is usually found in the brain and associated with the reduction of pain and with feelings of well-being.

Enmeshed boundaries See *Blurred or diffused boundaries.*

Enuresis Nocturnal and daytime involuntary discharge of urine.

Epinephrine (adrenaline) A catecholamine secreted by the adrenal gland and by fibers of the sympathetic nervous system. It is responsible for many of the physical manifestations of fear and anxiety.

Ethics The discipline concerned with standards of values, behaviors, or beliefs adhered to by individuals or groups.

Eustress A positive emotion that demonstrates a person's confidence in the ability to master given demands or tasks with success.

Euthymia A normal mood state.

Extrapyramidal side effects A variety of signs and symptoms that are often side effects of the use of certain psychotropic drugs, particularly the phenothiazines. Three reversible side effects include acute dystonia, akathisia, and pseudoparkinsonism. A fourth, tardive dyskinesia, is most serious and is not reversible.

Family system Those individuals who make up the family unit and contribute to the functional state of the family as a unit.

Family therapy A treatment modality that focuses on the relationships within the family system.

Family triangle A dysfunctional phenomenon in which a third person is brought into a family system to help relieve anxiety or stress between two family members. Triangles are dysfunctional because the lowering of anxiety comes from *diversion* from the conflict rather than from *resolution* of the conflict between the two members.

Fantasy A retreat from reality and an attempt to solve problems in a private world. The difference between a healthy person and a schizophrenic, for example, is that a schizophrenic may not know where fantasy leaves off and reality begins.

Fear A reaction to a specific danger.

Feedback Communication of one person's impressions of and reactions to another person's actions or verbalizations.

Fellatio Oral sexual contact with the penis.

Fetish An object or part of the body to which sexual significance or meaning is attached.

Fight-or-flight response (sympathetic response) The body's physiological response to fear or rage that triggers the sympathetic branch of the autonomic nervous system as well as the endocrine system. This response is useful in emergencies; however, a sustained response can result in pathophysiological changes such as high blood pressure, ulcers, and cardiac problems.

Flight of ideas A continuous flow of speech in which the person jumps rapidly from one topic to another. Sometimes the listener can keep up with the changes; at other times, it is necessary to listen for themes in the incessant talking. Themes often include grandiose and fantasized estimation of personal sexual prowess, business ability, artistic talents, and so on.

Formication Tactile hallucination or illusion involving insects crawling on the body or under the skin.

Frustration Curtailment of personal goals, satisfaction, or security by conditions of external reality or by internal controls.

Fugue An altered state of consciousness involving both memory loss (as does psychogenic amnesia) and traveling away from home or from one's usual work locale. Therefore, fugue involves flight as well as forgetfulness (psychogenic fugue).

General adaptation syndrome (GAS) The body's organized response to stress, as demonstrated by Hans Selye. It progresses through three stages: (1) the stage of alarm, (2) the stage of resistance, and (3) the stage of exhaustion.

Genogram A systematic diagram of the three-generational relationships within a family system.

Grandiosity Exaggerated belief in or claims about one's importance or identity.

Grief The subjective feelings and affect that are precipitated by a loss.

Group Two or more individuals who have a relationship with one another, are interdependent, and may share some norms.

Group dynamics The interactions and interrelations among members of a therapy group and between members and the therapist. The effective use of group dynamics is essential in group treatment.

Group process Interaction continually taking place among members of a group.

Group therapy Psychotherapy based on the examination of group interaction with a view toward understanding and eventually changing the ways in which clients interact with others.

Hallucination A sense perception (seeing, hearing, tasting, smelling, or touching) for which no external stimulus exists (e.g., hearing voices when none are present).

Health Maintenance Organization (HMO) An organization that contracts with a group or individuals to offer designated health care services to plan members for a fixed, prepaid premium (an example of a managed care program).

Histrionics A dramatic presentation of oneself with pervasive and excessive emotionality in order to seek attention, love, and admiration.

Homelessness—chronic The final stage in a lifelong series of crises and missed opportunities. It is the culmination of a gradual disengagement from supportive relationships and institutions.

Homosexuality Sexual attraction to or preference for persons of the same sex.

Hopelessness The belief by a person that no one can help him or her; extreme pessimism about the future.

Hospice philosophy A philosophy characterized by the acceptance of death as a natural conclusion to life, with clients rather than health care providers making the decisions how they want to live and die.

Hostility Anger that is destructive in nature and purpose.

Hotline A telephone crisis counseling service often used in crisis intervention centers to provide immediate contact between a person in crisis and a counselor.

Hypermetamorphosis The need to touch everything in sight.

Hyperorality The need to taste everything, chew everything, and put everything in one's mouth.

Hypersomnia Increased time spent in sleep, possibly to escape from painful feelings; however, the increased sleep is not experienced as restful or refreshing.

Hypochondriasis Excessive preoccupation with one's physical health, without the presence of any organic pathology.

Hypomania An elevated mood with symptoms less severe than those of mania. A person in hypomania does not experience impairment in reality testing, nor do the symptoms markedly impair the person's social, occupational, or interpersonal functioning.

Hysterical personality disorder A disorder characterized by dramatic, emotionally intense, unstable behavior.

Id One of three psychological processes that make up the Freudian system of personality (id, ego, and superego). The id is the source of all primitive drives and instincts and is thought of as the reservoir of all psychic energy.

Ideas of reference False impressions that outside events have special meaning for oneself.

Identification Unconsciously taking on the thoughts, mannerisms, or behaviors of a person or group, in order to decrease anxiety.

Identity The sense of one's self based on experience, memories, perceptions, and emotions.

Illusion An error in the perception of a sensory stimulus. For example, a person may mistake polka dots on a pillow for hairy spiders.

Impotence The inability to achieve or maintain a penile erection of sufficient quality to engage in successful sexual intercourse.

Impulsiveness An action that is abrupt, unplanned, and directed toward immediate gratification.

Incest A sexual relationship between persons related biologically.

Insight Understanding and awareness of the reasons for and meanings behind one's motives and behavior.

Insomnia Inability to fall asleep or to stay asleep, early morning awakening, or both.

Intellectualization The use of thinking and talking to avoid emotions and closeness.

Intimacy Emotional closeness.

Intoxication Excessive use of a drug or alcohol that leads to maladaptive behavior.

Intrapsychic Within the self.

Introjection Process by which a person incorporates or takes into his or her own personality qualities or values of another person or group with whom or with which intense emotional ties exist.

Intuition Emotional knowing without thinking or talking.

Isolation Separation of thoughts, ideas, or actions from their emotional aspects.

Judgment The ability to make logical, rational decisions.

La belle indifference The affect or attitude of unconcern about a symptom that is used when the symptom is unconsciously used to lower anxiety. The lack of concern is thought to be a sign that the primary gain has been achieved.

Labile Having rapidly shifting emotions; unstable.

Lesbian A female homosexual.

Libido Sexual drive.

Limbic system The part of the brain that is related to emotions and referred to by some as the "emotional brain." It is associated with fear and anxiety; anger and aggression; love, joy, and hope; and sexuality and social behavior.

Limit setting The reasonable and rational setting of parameters for client behavior that provide control and safety.

Lithium carbonate This agent is known as an antimanic

drug because it can stabilize the manic phase of a bipolar disorder. When effective, it can modify future manic episodes and protect against future depressive episodes.

Living will An expression by a person, while competent, that states the individual's preference that life-sustaining treatment be withheld or withdrawn if he or she becomes terminally ill and no longer able to make health care decisions.

Looseness of association A state in which thinking is haphazard, illogical, and confused, and connections in thought are interrupted; it is seen mostly in schizophrenic disorders.

Magical thinking The belief that thinking something can make it happen; it is seen in children and psychotic clients.

Malingering A conscious effort to deceive others, often for financial gain, by pretending physical symptoms.

Managed care A term that refers to an organized system that integrates the issues of cost management and health care. Health maintenance organizations (HMOs), preferred provider organizations (PPOs), and managed care options from government and private indemnity health insurance plans are the basic types of managed care organizations.

Mania An unstable elevated mood in which delusions, poor judgment, and other signs of impaired reality testing are evident. During a manic episode, clients have marked impairment in their social, occupational, and interpersonal functioning.

Manipulation Purposeful behavior directed at getting needs met. According to Chitty and Maynard (1986), manipulation is maladaptive when (1) it is the primary method used for getting needs met, (2) the needs. goals, and feelings of others are disregarded, and (3) others are treated as objects in order to fulfill the needs of the manipulator.

Masochism Unconscious or conscious gratification obtained when a person experiences mental or physical pain; often used to refer to deviant sexual behaviors.

Maturational crisis Normal state in growth and development in which specific maturational tasks must be learned while old coping mechanisms are no longer acceptable.

Mental status exam A formal assessment of cognitive functions such as intelligence, thought processes, and capacity for insight.

Milieu The physical and social environment in which an individual lives.

Milieu therapy Therapy focused on positive environmental manipulation (both physical and social) in order to effect positive change.

Mnemonic disturbance Loss of memory.

Modeling A technique in which desired behaviors are demonstrated. The client learns to imitate these behaviors in appropriate situations.

Mood A "pervasive and sustained emotion that, in the extreme, markedly colors the person's perception of the world" (APA 2000).

Mood syndrome An alteration in mood along with associated symptoms that occur for a minimal period.

Mourning The processes (grief work) by which grief is resolved.

Multiple personality disorder A severe dissociative disorder in which one or more distinct subpersonalities exist within an individual, each of which may be dominant at different times Each subpersonality is a complex unit with its own memories, behavioral patterns, and social relationships, which may be very different from those of the primary personality.

Narcissism (narcism) Self-involvement with lack of empathy for others; the narcissistic person is very self-centered and self-important; it is normal in children but pathological when experienced in adults to the same degree.

Narcissistic personality disorder A disorder characterized by a pervasive pattern of grandiosity, need for admiration, and lack of empathy for others.

Negativism Opposition or resistance, either covert or overt, to outside suggestions or advice.

Negligence The act, or failure to act, that breaches the duty of due care and results in or is responsible for a person's injuries.

Neologisms Words a person makes up that have meaning only for that person; often part of a delusional system.

Neuroleptic malignant syndrome A rare and sometimes fatal reaction to high-potency neuroleptic drugs. Symptoms include muscle rigidity, fever, and elevated white blood cell count. It is thought to result from dopamine blockage on the basal ganglia and hypothalamus.

Neurons Specialized cells in the central nervous system. Each neuron has a cell body, an axon, and a dendrite.

Neurotransmitter A chemical substance that functions as a neural messenger. Neurotransmitters are released from the axon terminal of the presynaptic neuron when stimulated by an electrical impulse.

Nihilism A delusion that the self or part of the self does not exist.

No-suicide contract A contract made between a nurse or counselor and client, outlined in clear and simple language, in which the client states that he or she will *not* attempt self-harm and in which specific alternatives are given for the person instead.

Nonverbal communication Communication without words, such as body language, facial expressions, or gestures.

Nursing The diagnosis and treatment of human responses to actual or potential health problems.

Obesity A weight gain of at least 20% over the acceptable standard or ideal weight.

Obsession An idea, impulse, or emotion that a person cannot put out of his or her consciousness; it can be mild or severe.

Organic mental disorders Specific brain syndromes in which an etiology is known; for example, alcohol withdrawal delirium and Alzheimer's disease (APA 1987).

Orientation The ability to relate the self correctly to time, place, and person.

Overt anxiety Anxiety in which the attendant physical, physiological, and cognitive symptoms are evident and may be assessed.

Panic Sudden, overwhelming anxiety of such intensity that it produces disorganization of the personality, loss of rational thought, and inability to communicate, along with specific physiological changes.

Paranoia Any intense and strongly defended irrational

suspicion. These ideas cannot be corrected by experiences and cannot be modified by facts or reality.

Passive-aggressive behavior Indirect expression of anger. Behavior may seem passive but is motivated by unconscious anger, often triggering anger and frustration in others. Examples of passive-aggressive behavior include lateness, forgetting, "mistakes," and obtuseness.

Peer review Review of clinical practice with peers, supervisors, or consultants.

Perception Mental processes by which intellectual, sensory, and emotional data are organized logically or meaningfully.

Perseveration The involuntary repetition of the same thought, phrase, or motor response (e.g., brushing teeth, walking); it is associated with brain damage.

Personality Deeply ingrained personal patterns of behavior, traits, and thoughts that evolve, both consciously and unconsciously, as a person's style and way of adapting to the environment.

Phobia An intense irrational fear of an object, situation, or place. The fear persists even though the object of the fear is harmless and the person is aware of the irrationality.

Physical restraints Any manual method or mechanical device, material, or equipment that inhibits free movement.

Play therapy An intervention that allows a child to symbolically express feelings such as aggression, self-doubt, anxiety, and sadness through the medium of play.

Pleasure principle A tendency to seek immediate gratification of impulses and tension reduction; the id operates according to the pleasure principle.

Polydrug abuse The pathologic use of more than one drug.

Polypharmacy The taking of more than one drug at any given time.

Postvention Therapeutic interventions with the significant others of an individual who has committed suicide.

Poverty of speech Speech that is brief and uncommunicative.

Pressure of speech Forceful energy heard in a manic individual's frantic, jumbled speech as he or she struggles to keep pace with racing thoughts.

Primary anxiety Anxiety that is due to intrapersonal or intrapsychic causes, such as a phobia.

Primary depression A depressive mood episode that *is not* due to a known organic factor and *is not* part of another psychotic disorder, such as schizophrenia (APA 1987).

Primary gain The anxiety relief resulting from the use of defense mechanisms or symptom formation, such as somatizing (e.g., getting a headache instead of feeling angry).

Primary process A primitive and unconscious psychological activity in which the id attempts to reduce tension through formation of an image or by hallucinating the object that would satisfy its need.

Projection The unconscious attributing of one's own intolerable wishes, emotional feelings, or motivation to another person.

Projective identification A primitive form of projection used to externalize aggressive feelings. Once projection

has occurred, fear of the person who is the object of the projection is coupled with a desire to control the person.

Prolonged grief A dysfunctional reaction to grief in which the bereaved remains intensely preoccupied with the memories of the decreased many years after the person has died.

Psychiatric liaison nurse A master's prepared nurse with a background in psychiatric and medical-surgical nursing. The liaison nurse functions as a nursing consultant in the management of psychosocial concerns and as a clinician in helping the client deal more effectively with physical and emotional problems.

Psychiatry The science of treating disorders of the psyche. It is the medical specialty that is derived from the study, diagnosis, treatment, and prevention of mental disorders.

Psychoeducational therapy A strategy of teaching clients and their families about disorders, treatments, coping techniques, and resources. It helps empower clients and families by having them become more involved and prepares them to participate in their own care once they have the knowledge.

Psychogenic Physical conditions affected by psychological factors.

Psychogenic amnesia The loss of memory for an event or period of time that contains overwhelming anxiety and pain. The loss of memory is related to psychological stress.

Psychomotor agitation The constant involvement in some tension-relieving activity, such as constantly pacing, biting one's nails, smoking, or tapping one's fingers on a tabletop.

Psychomotor retardation Extremely slow and difficult movements that in the extreme can entail complete inactivity and incontinence.

Psychosexual development Emotional and sexual growth from birth to adulthood.

Psychosis An extreme response to psychological or physical stressors that affects a person's affective, psychomotor, and physical behavior. Evidence of impairment in reality testing is evident by hallucinations or delusions.

Psychosocial rehabilitation The development of the skills necessary for people with chronic mental illness to live independently.

Psychosomatic An older term describing the interaction of the mind (psyche) and the body (soma). The term was used in reference to certain diseases thought to be caused by psychological factors. Referred to in DSM-I.

Psychotherapy A treatment modality based on the development of a trusting relationship between client and therapist for the purpose of exploring and modifying the client's behavior in a satisfying direction.

Psychotropic Affecting the mind.

Psychotropic drugs Drugs that have an effect on psychic function, behavior, or experience.

Racism A belief that inherent differences between races determine one's achievement and that one's own race is superior.

Rape See *Sexual assault/rape.*

Rape-trauma syndrome This syndrome comprises the acute phase and the long-term reorganization process that occurs after an actual or attempted sexual assault. Each phase has separate symptoms.

Rationalization Justifying illogical or unreasonable ideas, actions, or feelings by developing acceptable explanations that satisfy the teller as well as the listener.

Reaction-formation (overcompensation) The process of keeping unacceptable feelings or behaviors out of awareness by developing the opposite emotion or behavior.

Reality principle The gradual development of the ability to delay immediate gratification and modify desires in accordance with the demands of society and external reality.

Receptors Protein molecules located in the cell membrane of neurons, muscles, and blood vessels. Receptors receive chemical stimulation that causes a chemical reaction resulting in either stimulation or inhibition of activity of the neuron, muscle, or blood cell.

Reframing A technique of changing the viewpoint of a situation and replacing it with another viewpoint that fits the facts equally well but changes the entire meaning.

Regression In the face of overwhelming anxiety, the ego returns to an earlier, more comforting (although less mature) way of behaving.

Relapse The process of becoming dysfunctional in sobriety that ends in a return to chemical use.

Relaxation response The opposite of the fight-or-flight response. This response is synonymous with the functioning of the parasympathetic branch of the nervous system. The relaxation response has a stabilizing effect on the nervous system.

Repression The exclusion of unpleasant or unwanted experiences, emotions, or ideas from conscious awareness; thought of as the first line of psychological defense.

Respite care Temporary supervision and care of a client who lives with his or her family. The purpose of respite care is to provide the family with some relief from the demands of the client's needs for continuous care.

Restraints See *Physical restraints* and *Chemical restraints*.

Reuptake The process of neurotransmitters' returning to the presynaptic cell after communication with receptor cells.

Rigid or disengaged boundaries Those boundaries in which the "rules and roles" are adhered to no matter what the situation. Rigid boundaries prevent family members from trying out new roles or taking on more mature functions.

Rituals Repetitive actions that a person must do over and over until he or she is exhausted or anxiety is decreased; they are often done to lessen the anxiety triggered by an obsession.

Role playing A technique used in individual, group, or family therapy in which the therapist or a group member acts out the behavior of another member in order to increase the other person's ability to see a situation from another point of view. It is also a useful tool that therapists, teachers, and others use to help people practice skills in a safe environment before they try them in real-life situations, such as practicing asking for a raise, discussing a crucial topic with a person in authority, or saying no to someone without getting defensive or angry.

Sadism Sexual pleasure and erotic gratification obtained by inflicting pain, abuse, or humiliation on another.

Scapegoat A member of a group or family who becomes the target of aggression from others but who may not be the actual cause of hostility or frustration in them.

Schizoaffective disorder A disorder that includes a mixture of schizophrenic and affective symptoms (i.e., alterations in mood as well as disturbances in thought); it is thought by some to be a severe form of bipolar disorder.

Schizoid personality disorder A personality disorder in which there is a serious defect in interpersonal relationships. Other characteristics include lack of warmth, aloofness, and indifference to the feelings of others.

Schizophrenia A severe disturbance of thought or association, characterized by impaired reality testing, hallucinations, delusions, and limited socialization.

Seasonal affective disorder (SAD) A recently studied syndrome that appears to affect mostly women. It is characterized by hypersomnia, fatigue, weight gain, irritability, and interpersonal difficulties during the winter months. It has been successfully managed with daily treatments of 2 to 3 hours of bright light.

Seclusion The last step in a process to maximize safety to a client and others whereby a client is placed alone in a specially designed room for protection and close observation.

Secondary anxiety Anxiety that is due to physiological abnormalities such as certain medical disorders (e.g., neurological, endocrine, or circulatory) or is secondary to a pervasive psychiatric disorder such as depression.

Secondary dementia A result of some other pathological process, such as a metabolic, nutritional, or neurological process. AIDS-related dementia is an example.

Secondary depression A depressive mood syndrome that is caused by a physical illness or another psychiatric disorder or is part of an organic mental disorder; essentially, it is depression secondary to other causes.

Secondary gain Those advantages a person realizes from whatever symptoms or relief behaviors he or she employs. These advantages include increased attention from others, getting out of expected responsibilities, financial gain, and the ability to manipulate others in the environment.

Secondary process A process consistent with the reality principle: that is, realistic thinking.

Selective inattention Characterized by not noticing an almost infinite series of more-or-less meaningful details of one's own living that might cause anxiety. A concept articulated by H. S. Sullivan.

Selective serotonin reuptake inhibitors (SSRIs) First-line antidepressants that block the reuptake of serotonin, permitting serotonin to act for an extended period at the synaptic binding sites in the brain.

Self-concept A person's image of the self.

Self-esteem Feelings individuals have about their own worth and value.

Self-help group An organization of people who share similar problems who meet to receive peer support and encouragement and work together using their strengths to gain control over their lives.

Self-mutilation The act of self-induced pain or injury without the intent to kill oneself.

Sexual assault/rape Forced and violent vaginal or anal penetration against the victim's will and without the victim's consent. Legal definitions vary from state to state.

Situational crises Crises arising from external sources, as opposed to internal sources; most people have them to some extent during the course of their lives (e.g., with the death of a loved one, marriage, divorce, or a change in health status).

Social phobias These include phobias of an interpersonal nature, such as fear of public speaking, fear of eating in front of others, or fear of writing or performing in public.

Social skills training Training that utilizes the principles of guidance, demonstration, practice, and feedback to enhance a client's skills in community living. Training focuses on skills such as introducing oneself, starting and ending a conversation, asking for assistance, and other simple yet essential social interactions; it is often helpful in combating the negative symptoms of schizophrenia.

Somatic therapy Treatment that involves manipulations of the body, such as the use of medications or electroconvulsive therapy.

Somatization The expression of psychological stress through physical symptoms.

Somatizing Experiencing an emotional conflict as a physical symptom.

Specific phobias These are very common in the general population; essentially, a specific phobia is fear and avoidance of a single object, situation, or activity.

Spirituality The devotion or receptiveness to religious/moral values.

Splitting A primitive defense in which persons see themselves or others as all good or all bad, failing to integrate the positive and negative qualities of the self and others into a cohesive whole.

Spouse abuse The intentional act or perceived intention of physically injuring one's spouse. It is an act of mental cruelty.

Stereotype The assumption that all people in a similar cultural, racial, or ethnic group think and act alike.

Stereotyped behaviors Motor patterns that originally had meaning to the person (e.g., sweeping the floor or washing windows) but have become mechanical and lack purpose.

Stress The body's arousal response to any demand, change, or perceived threat.

Stupor A state in which a person is dazed and awareness of reality in his or her environment appears deadened. For example, a person may sit motionless for long periods of time and in extreme cases may appear to be in a coma.

Subconscious Often called the preconscious; includes experiences, thoughts, feelings, and desires that might not be in immediate awareness but can be recalled to consciousness. The subconscious mind helps repress unpleasant thoughts or feelings.

Subintentioned suicide Term used by Schneidman to describe self-destructive behaviors people employ that could hasten their own death, such as compulsive use of drugs, hyperobesity, and medical noncompliance (Schneidman 1963).

Sublimation The unconscious process of substituting constructive and socially acceptable activities for strong impulses that are not acceptable in their original form, such as strong aggressive or sexual drives.

Suicidal ideation Thoughts a person has regarding killing him- or herself.

Suicide The ultimate act of self-destruction in which a person purposefully ends his or her own life.

Suicide attempt Any willful, self-inflicted, life-threatening attempt that has not led to death.

Suicide gesture A suicide attempt that is planned to be discovered and is made for the purpose of influencing or manipulating others.

Sundown syndrome Increasing destabilization of cognitive abilities (e.g. confusion, lability of mood) during the late afternoon, early evening, or night. Seen in people with cognitive disorders.

Superego One of three psychological processes that make up the Freudian system of personality (id, ego, and superego). The superego is the internal representative of the values, ideals, and moral standards of society. The superego is said to be the moral arm of the personality.

Support groups Groups that help people during stressful periods using a variety of modalities in order to overcome overwhelming situations or unwanted behaviors.

Suppression The conscious putting off of awareness of disturbing situations or feelings; the only defense mechanism that operates on a conscious level.

Symbolization The process by which one object or idea comes to represent another. For example, the nurse's keys on a locked unit may represent power and autonomy, or a fancy house may represent prestige and power.

Synapse The gap between the membrane of one neuron and the membrane of another neuron. The synapse is the point at which the transmission of nerve impulses occurs.

Synesthesia A phenomenon experienced by people on hallucinogenic drugs; described as hearing colors or seeing sounds.

Tangentiality An association disturbance in which the speaker goes off the topic. When it happens frequently and the speaker does not return to the topic, interpersonal communication is destroyed.

Tarasoff **decision** A California court decision that imposes a duty on the therapist to warn the appropriate person or persons when the therapist becomes aware that a client may present a risk of harm to a specific person or persons.

Tardive dyskinesia A serious and irreversible result of the use of phenothiazine-like drugs. It consists of involuntary tonic muscular spasms typically involving the tongue, fingers, toes, neck, trunk, or pelvis.

Therapeutic encounter A brief, informal meeting between nurse and client in which the relationship is useful and important for the client.

Therapeutic nurse-client relationship A therapeutic relationship requiring that the nurse maximize his or her communication skills, understanding of human behaviors, and personal strengths in order to enhance personal growth in the client. This relationship applies to *all* clinical settings, not just those on a psychiatric unit.

Time out Removing or disengaging a child from a situation so that the child might regain self-control.

Token economy A behavioral approach to eliciting desired behaviors involving the application of the principles and procedures of operant conditioning; it is usually used in the management of a social setting such as a ward, classroom, or halfway house. Targeted behaviors are awarded "tokens" that can be exchanged for desired goods or privileges.

Tolerance A need for higher and higher doses of a drug in order to achieve intoxication or the desired effect.

Torts Civil wrongs for which money damages are collected by the injured party (plaintiff) from the wrongdoer (defendant).

Transference The experiencing of thoughts and feelings toward a person (often the therapist) that belong to a significant person in one's past. Transference is a valuable tool used by therapists in psychoanalytical psychotherapy.

Transsexuals People who have an early and persistent feeling that they are trapped in a body with the wrong genitals. They believe they are, and were always meant to be, of the opposite sex.

Triangle See *Family triangle.*

Unconscious Repressed memories, feelings, thoughts, or wishes that are not available to the conscious mind. Usually, these unconscious memories, feelings, thoughts, or wishes harbor intense anxiety and can greatly affect an individual's behavior.

Undoing An act or behavior unconsciously motivated to make up for or negate a previous act or behavior (e.g., bringing the boss a present after talking about him or her unfavorably to co-workers).

Validate See *Consensual validation.*

Values clarification A process of self-discovery whereby a person can explore and determine his or her personal values and identify what priority these values hold in personal decision making. The result of this process can increase awareness about why the person behaves in certain ways.

Vegetative signs of depression During a depressive episode, these represent a significant change from normal functioning of those activities necessary to support physical life and growth, such as eating, sleeping, elimination, and sex.

Waxy flexibility Having one's arms or legs placed in a certain position and holding that same position for hours.

Withdrawal symptoms The negative physiological and psychological reactions that occur when a drug taken for a long period of time is reduced or no longer taken.

Word salad A mixture of phrases meaningless to the listener and to the speaker as well.

Index

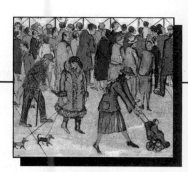

Note: Page numbers followed by the letter b refer to boxed material, and those followed by f and t refer to figures and tables, respectively.